# Clinical Laboratory Science
*The Basics and Routine Techniques*

FOURTH EDITION

**FOURTH EDITION**

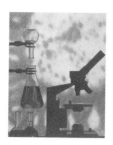

# Clinical
# Laboratory Science
## THE BASICS AND ROUTINE
## TECHNIQUES

*Jean Jorgenson Linné*, B.S., M.T.(A.S.C.P.)

Assistant Professor,
Department of Laboratory Medicine and Pathology,
University of Minnesota Medical School,
Minneapolis, Minnesota

*Karen Munson Ringsrud*, B.S., M.T.(A.S.C.P.)

Assistant Professor,
Department of Laboratory Medicine and Pathology,
University of Minnesota Medical School,
Minneapolis, Minnesota

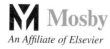 Mosby
*An Affiliate of Elsevier*

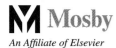
*An Affiliate of Elsevier*

*Editor:* Janet Russell
*Developmental Editor:* Sarahlynn Lester
*Project Managers:* Mark Spann, Patricia Tannian
*Production Editor:* Steve Hetager
*Book Design Manager:* Judi Lang
*Interior Designer:* Jeanne Wolfgeher
*Cover Designer:* Jeanne Wolfgeher

Permissions may be sought directly from Elsevier's Health Sciences Rights Department in Philadelphia, USA: phone: (+)215-238-7869, fax: (+)215-238-2239, email: healthpermissions@elsevier.com. You may also complete your request on-line via the Elsevier Science homepage (http://www.elsevier.com), by selecting 'Customer Support' and then 'Obtaining Permissions'.

Printed in the United States of America.

Mosby, Inc.
11830 Westline Industrial Drive
St. Louis, Missouri 64146

**ISBN 1-55664-505-8**

04 05 06 07 08 / 9 8 7 6

# Reviewers

**Mary Breci-Swendrzynski, M.A., B.S.M.T.**
Program Director,
Medical Laboratory Technology,
Midlands Technical College,
Columbia, South Carolina

**Margaret L. Charette, M.Ed.,**
**M.T.(A.S.C.P.)S.C.**
Program Director, MLT-AD,
MaineGeneral Medical Center,
Augusta, Maine

**Judith A. Cowan, B.S., R.N., C.M.A.**
Medical Assisting Program,
Kirkwood Community College,
Cedar Rapids, Iowa

**Patrick Debold**
Concord Career Colleges,
Kansas City, Missouri

**Patricia Etnyre-Zacher, Ed.D.,**
**C.L.S.(N.C.A.), M.T.(A.S.C.P.)**
Associate Professor,
Program in Clinical Laboratory Sciences,
School of Allied Health Professions,
Northern Illinois University,
Dekalb, Illinois

**Jeanne M. Isabel, M.S.Ed., C.L.Sp.H.,**
**M.T.(A.S.C.P.)**
Assistant Professor,
Program in Clinical Laboratory Sciences,
School of Allied Health Professions,
Northern Illinois University,
Dekalb, Illinois

**Beverly J. Philpott, B.Sc., C.M.A.**
Assistant Professor,
Medical Assisting Program,
Kirkwood Community College,
Cedar Rapids, Iowa

**George D. Smith, M.T.(A.S.C.P.)**
Consultant,
Anderson Continuing Education,
Sacramento, California

*To David, David, and Jonathan*
*Peter and Erik*

# Preface

Close to thirty years have passed since the publication of the first edition of this textbook, and in these years much has changed in the practice of clinical laboratory science. It is interesting to note, however, that although technology has produced drastic changes in how clinical laboratory tests are done, many of the techniques and procedures used today continue to be based on fundamentals that have been in place for many years. The clinical laboratory will continue in this evolution, with procedures changing for carrying out the tests, while the basic theory is left intact. Because introductory information is necessary for anyone engaged in performing laboratory tests, a thorough understanding of basic concepts and general background material continues to be an essential first step in the practice of clinical laboratory science, regardless of the technology or specific procedural steps required in a given laboratory setting.

This fourth edition has been completely rewritten in light of the need both to retain the necessary basic information that is essential for understanding the routine procedures done in typical clinical laboratories of various sizes and locations and to include new information of importance. The primary aim of this book remains unchanged: it is a source of general background information for performing the many basic and routine clinical laboratory tests, presented in an understandable manner—information often difficult to find in any other single textbook. Understandably, because we have chosen to include laboratory assays that we consider to be routine and basic, certain other assays are not included. It is our hope that the decisions we have made about what to include have resulted in a book that is pertinent to the work being done today in clinical laboratories without attempting to be exhaustive. We have tried to retain the writing style, organization, and level of presentation used in previous editions so that the material can be used by students and laboratorians of many levels, as it has been in past editions.

New pedagogy, including learning objectives, review questions (and answers), and, where applicable, case studies, has been added to this edition. A new chapter, "Examination of Extravascular Fluids and Miscellaneous Specimens," with information about tests on extravascular body fluids and feces, taken from separate chapters in previous editions, and miscellaneous CLIA '88–waived or provider-performed microscopy (PPM) tests is also included.

To satisfy a demand for a more limited version of this textbook—one containing only Part I, "Fundamentals of the Clinical Laboratory," and therefore a version that does not include the divisions of the clinical laboratory, such as hematology, chemistry, and urinalysis—a separate textbook has been prepared by Mosby, entitled *Clinical Laboratory Science: The Basics*.

Most of the photographs in Chapter 14 were taken by Karen Ringsrud. A few are very old slides used in teaching at the University of Minnesota, for which the photographer is unknown. In addition, Figures 14-66 and 14-126 were photographed by Dr. G. Mary Bradley, University of Minnesota, retired; Figures 14-70 and 14-80 were photographed by Helen Louise Yates, UMHC, retired; and Figures 14-10, 14-40, 14-63, 14-100, 14-101, 14-106, 14-107, 14-112, and 14-114 were photographed by Dr. Patrick C.J. Ward, School of Medicine, University of Minnesota, Duluth. We thank them for the use of these photomicrographs. In addition, we thank Mosby for permission to use many illustrations from our book *Urinalysis and Body Fluids: A ColorText and Atlas*. We also thank our colleagues and friends at the University of Minnesota who have given us both technical and moral support in this endeavor. We appreciate the support of the Department of Laboratory Medicine and Pathology at the University of Minnesota, Leo T. Furcht, M.D., Professor and Head.

We once again acknowledge the unconditional support of our families during the process of completing these textbook revisions—no project of this magnitude can be undertaken without this support. We are thankful to our husbands, David Linné and Peter Ringsrud, and to our children, who have, in these almost thirty years, gone from infants to adults.

**Jean Jorgenson Linné**

**Karen Munson Ringsrud**

# Brief Contents

# Detailed Contents

# Clinical Laboratory Science
*The Basics and Routine Techniques*

FOURTH EDITION

# PART I

# Fundamentals of the Clinical Laboratory

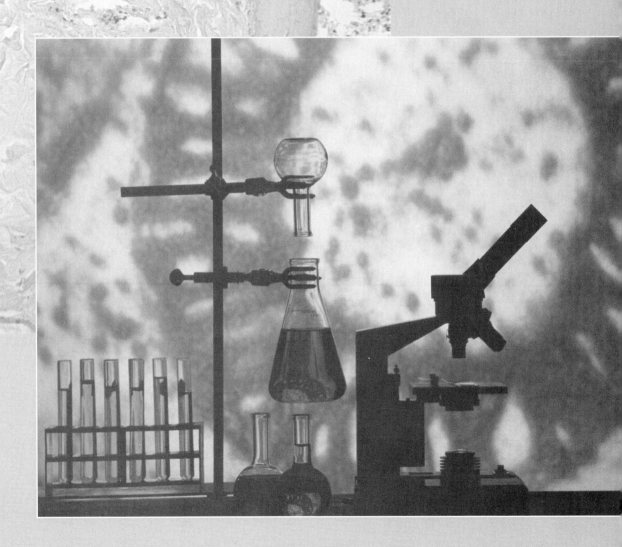

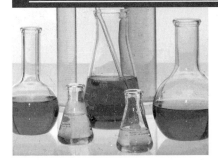

# Introduction to Clinical Laboratory Science

## Learning Objectives

*From study of this chapter, the reader will be able to:*

➤ Understand the organization of a clinical laboratory and its various parts, purposes, and personnel.

➤ Compare and contrast the uses of various sites for laboratory testing—central laboratory, point of care, physician office laboratory, reference laboratory.

➤ Appreciate the importance of federal, state, and institutional regulations concerning the quality and reliability of work being done—become familiar with the terms OSHA, CLIA '88, HCFA, JCAHO, NCCLS, and CAP.

➤ Understand the CLIA '88 regulations in particular and the concept of classification of laboratory testing by complexity of the test—waived, moderately complex, highly complex, and provider-performed microscopy.

➤ Understand the purpose of participation in CLIA '88–mandated proficiency testing programs and how they relate to quality assurance.

# INTRODUCTION TO THE CLINICAL LABORATORY

The goal of medical practice is to resolve the problems presented to the physician by the patient. This includes establishing or ruling out a diagnosis, deciding on a management plan for the particular diagnosis and patient, giving the patient the prognosis for the presenting problem, and monitoring any follow-up therapy needed. Included in the process a physician uses is an interview with the patient and an organized analysis of the patient's presenting problem. This process includes the taking of a complete history, a physical examination, and the ordering of appropriate laboratory or other diagnostic tests. The findings are sorted and expanded where necessary, to make a diagnosis, formulate a prognosis, and decide on a course of management. Abnormal laboratory findings constitute only one aspect of the patient's problems, and any action taken because of these findings should be predicated on how this action will affect the patient as a whole. The ultimate goals of medical practice should be relief of patient suffering and prolonging the general well-being of the patient.

## Laboratory Medicine or Clinical Pathology

**Laboratory medicine** or **clinical pathology** is the medical discipline by which clinical laboratory science and technology are applied to the care of patients. Several different disciplines make up this practice—chemistry, hematology, microbiology, urinalysis, immunology, and blood banking, to name the more traditional ones. Each will be described in more detail in later chapters of this book. Many changes are taking place in the clinical laboratory, and these are already affecting the types of tests being offered. A possible system for the organization of a clinical laboratory is seen in Fig. 1-1. In addition to the traditional areas already mentioned, the disciplines of cytogenetics, toxicology (often a part of the chemistry laboratory), and other specialized divisions are present in the larger laboratories. Molecular pathology diagnostics and the use of polymerase chain reaction (PCR), DNA probes, and other genetic testing are evident in many laboratories.

Another change is to move from tests being done in a centralized laboratory setting to point-of-care testing (POCT). Alternative testing sites, such as at the bedside of the patient, in the operating rooms or recovery areas, or even in the home of the patient, should be a part of any discussion of the clinical laboratory and its organization. Automation has already changed the way in which testing is done, and more changes are likely to come. The diversity available in the clinical laboratory is necessary to provide the clinicians seeing patients with the best, most appropriate information for the total care of their patients.

## Utilization of the Clinical Laboratory

The appropriate utilization of the clinical laboratory is of the utmost importance in the practice of laboratory medicine. It is important that the laboratory serve to educate the physician and other health care providers so that the information available through the results reported for the various tests ordered can be utilized in an appropriate manner. When tests are being ordered, the clinical laboratory should assume a role of leadership and education in assisting the physician to understand the most useful pattern of ordering, for example, to serve the best interest of the patient, the clinical decision-making process for the physician, and the costs involved. Continuing education is always a part of any laboratory's program for ensuring high-quality service as well as for maintaining the morale of the laboratory staff.

Hundreds of different laboratory tests are readily available in the larger laboratories, but it is often the case that only a percentage of these tests are routinely ordered. Only 50 to 60 tests of the hundreds available account for 70% of the results generated by a modern hospital clinical laboratory.[5] The implication of these data is that common diseases are investigated

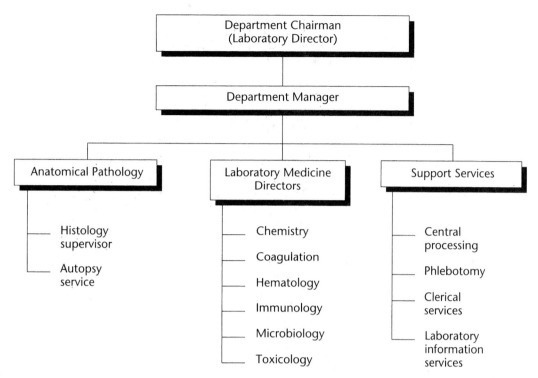

**FIG 1-1.** Organization of a clinical laboratory. (From Kaplan LA, Pesce A: *Clinical Chemistry: Theory, Analysis, and Correlation,* ed 3. St Louis, Mosby, 1996, p 49.)

by using common laboratory tests. When the results of these common tests are utilized appropriately in the context of the patient's clinical case, physical examination findings, and the medical history, clinical decision making will be improved. It is unusual that the results from a single laboratory assay will make a diagnosis. Certain additional laboratory tests may be needed to take decision making to the next step. Generally a small number of appropriately chosen laboratory tests may be sufficient to confirm, or rule out, one or more of the possibilities in a differential diagnosis.

## Future Directions for Laboratory Medicine

Biotechnology is a fast-growing discipline of the diagnostic laboratory. Molecular biology or the discipline of **molecular diagnostics** utilizes this technology. Molecular pathology applies the

principles of basic molecular biology to the study of human diseases. New approaches to human disease assessment are being developed by clinical laboratories because of the new information about the molecular basis of disease processes in general. The use of traditional laboratory analyses gives results based on a description of events currently going on in the patient—blood cell counts, infectious processes, blood glucose concentration. Molecular biology introduces a predictive component: findings from these tests can be used to anticipate events that may occur in the future, when patients may be at risk for a particular disease or condition. This predictive component reinforces, more than ever, the importance of how laboratory test results are utilized and emphasizes ethical considerations and the need for use of genetic counseling. Genetic counseling has gained an important status in the utilization of the laboratory results obtained from molecular biologic tests. Nucleic acids form the chemical basis for transmission of genetic information, and genetic information is sustained as sequences of nucleic acids. Chromosomes contain DNA as a primary component, and genetic traits can be transmitted through DNA.

## Patient Specimens

Clinical laboratorians work with many types of specimens. Blood and urine specimens are probably the ones most often tested, but tests are also ordered on body tissues and other body fluids, such as synovial, cerebrospinal, peritoneal, and pericardial fluids. Since the purpose of the clinical laboratory is to provide information regarding the assay results for the specimens analyzed, it is most important that the specimens be properly collected in the first place. In the testing process, analytes or constituents are measured by using only very small amounts of the specimens collected, but in interpreting the results, it is assumed that the results obtained do represent what the actual concentrations of the analytes are in the patient. It is only by use of the various quality assurance systems discussed later in this book that the reliability of results can be ensured. No matter how carefully a laboratory assay has been carried out, valid laboratory results can be reported only when preanalytical quality control has also been ascertained. Special patient preparation considerations for some specimen collections, along with proper transportation to and handling in the laboratory prior to the actual analytical assay, are very important. Appropriate **quality assurance programs** must be in place in the laboratory to make certain that each patient specimen is given the very best analysis possible and that the results reported will benefit the patient in the best possible way.

## REGULATION OF THE CLINICAL LABORATORY

In current laboratory settings, many governmental regulations, along with regulations and recommendations from professional, state, and federal accreditation agencies and commissions of various types, govern the activities of the laboratory, all of which must be explicitly understood and followed. Many of these groups are working toward similar goals, two primary ones being (1) ensuring that the quality of work being done in the laboratory is such that reliable results are reported to the physician who is treating the patient and (2) assuring the laboratory workers that the workplace provided to them is safe and healthful. Adhering to the regulatory mandates must constantly be balanced with also making certain that the testing of specimens and the results reporting are being done in a cost-effective manner. The regulations and standards are designed specifically to protect the people working in the laboratory, other health care personnel, the patients being treated in the health care facility, and society as a whole. **Federal regulations** exist to meet these objectives. Certain regulatory mandates have been issued externally, such as the **Clinical Laboratory Improvement Amendments of 1988 (CLIA '88)**, others are internal, and some are combinations of both.[2-4] Many of the factors governing the standards and their resulting regulations are associated with laboratory-acquired infections or accidents involving hazards in the workplace. These are discussed in Chapter 2.

A laboratory that wishes to receive payment for its services from Medicare or Medicaid must be licensed under the **Public Health Service Act**. To be licensed, the laboratory must meet the conditions for participation in those programs. The **Health Care Financing Administration (HCFA)** has the administrative responsibility for both the Medicare and CLIA '88 programs. Facilities accredited by approved private accreditation agencies, such as the College of American Pathologists, must also follow the regulations for licensure under CLIA '88. States with equivalent CLIA '88 regulations are reviewed individually as to possible waiver for CLIA '88 licensure.

The Health Care Financing Administration, under the U.S. **Department of Health and Human Services (HHS),** has also established regulations to implement CLIA '88. Any facility performing quantitative, qualitative, or screening test procedures or examinations on materials derived from the human body is regulated by CLIA '88. This includes hospital laboratories of all sizes; physician office laboratories; nursing home facilities; clinics; industrial laboratories; city, state, and county laboratories; pharmacies, fitness centers, health fairs; and independent laboratories.

The leaders and managers of the clinical laboratory must be certain that all legal operating regulations have been met and that all persons working in the laboratory setting are fully aware of the importance of compliance with these regulations. Those in leadership positions in a clinical laboratory must be well grounded in their expertise in medical, scientific, and technical areas in addition to fully understanding the regulatory matters. All laboratory personnel must be aware of these regulatory considerations, but it is up to the management to make certain that this information is communicated to everyone who needs to know.

## Quality Assurance Requirements

Quality assurance programs are now also a requirement in the federal government's implementation of CLIA '88. The standards mandated are for all laboratories, with the intent that the medical community's ability to provide good-quality patient care will be greatly enhanced. Included in the CLIA '88 provisions are requirements for quality control and quality assurance, for the use of proficiency testing, and for certain levels of personnel to perform and supervise the work in the laboratory (see also Chapter 8).

## External Regulations

Much of how the work of the clinical laboratory is carried out is delineated by federal regulations or other external regulations. The Clinical Laboratory Improvement Amendments of 1988 govern most of the activities of a particular laboratory.[2] The goals of these amendments are to ensure that the laboratory results reported are of high quality regardless of where the testing is done—small laboratory, physician's office, large reference laboratory, or something in between. CLIA '88 regulations include aspects of proficiency testing programs, management of patient testing, quality assurance programs, the use of quality control systems, personnel requirements, inspections and site visits, and consultations. Several federal agencies govern practices in the clinical laboratory. These regulatory agencies or organizations are primarily concerned with setting standards, conducting inspections, and imposing sanctions, when necessary. External standards have been set to ensure that all laboratories provide the best, most reliable information to the physician and the patient. It was to this end, primarily, that CLIA '88 was enacted.

In addition to the CLIA '88 regulations, other state and federal regulations are in place to regulate chemical waste disposal, use of hazardous chemicals, and issues of laboratory safety for the personnel working there; safety issues include the handling of biohazardous materials and the application of standard precautions (see Chapter 2).

Based on the complexity of tests performed by a laboratory, a tiered grouping has been devised, with varying degrees of regulation for each level. The law contains a provision to exempt certain laboratories from standards for personnel and from quality control programs, proficiency testing, or quality assurance programs. These laboratories are defined as those that perform only simple, routine tests, which, as determined by HHS, have an insignificant risk of an erroneous result. These laboratories receive a "certificate of waiver." Another category based on complexity of testing is provider-performed microscopies (PPM); generally it is the physician himself or herself who is performing the testing in the office setting. The PPM category is also exempt from some of the CLIA requirements. The moderate-complexity and high-complexity levels are more regulated, with some minimal personnel standards required, as well as proficiency testing and quality assurance programs. The level to which the laboratory is assigned depends on the complexity of the tests performed. The criteria for classification include risk of harm to the patient, likelihood of erroneous results, type of testing method used, degree of independent judgment and interpretation needed, and availability of the particular test in question for home use. A panel of experts will periodically review the test complexity criteria for the categories and make suggestions for any changes needed.

External standards have been set to ensure quality of results reported—quality assurance, as imposed by CLIA '88 and administered by the Health Care Financing Administration. A clinical laboratory must be certified by HCFA, by a private certifying agency, or by a state regulatory agency that has been given approval by HCFA. Once certified, the laboratory is scheduled for regular inspections to determine that there has been compliance with the federal regulations, including CLIA '88. Two certifying agencies, the **College of American Pathologists (CAP)** and the **Joint Commission on Accreditation of Healthcare Organizations (JCAHO)**, have been given *deemed status* to act on the federal government's behalf. From an external source, guidelines and standards have also been set to govern safe work practices in the clinical laboratory (see also Chapter 2). Through labor laws and environmental regulations, assurance has been given to laboratory workers that they are in a safe atmosphere and that every precaution has been taken to maintain that safe atmosphere. The **Occupational Safety and Health Administration (OSHA)** has been involved in setting these practices into motion, and it is through OSHA that the mandates have come to be a part of the daily life of the laboratory workplace. Other external controls include standards mandated by public health laws and reporting requirements via the **Centers for Disease Control and Prevention (CDC)** and via certification and licensure requirements issued by the **Food and Drug Administration (FDA)**. State regulations are imposed by Medicaid agencies, state environmental laws, and state public health laws and licensure laws. Local regulations include those determined by building codes and fire prevention codes.

Independent agencies also have influence over practices in the clinical laboratory through accreditation policies or other responsibilities. These include groups such as the College of American Pathologists, the Joint Commission on Accreditation of Healthcare Organizations, and other specific proficiency-testing programs.

## Internal Regulations

Local, internal programs must be in place to carry out the external mandates. Internal regulation also comes from the need to ensure quality performance and reporting of results for the many laboratory tests being done—a process of quality assurance. It is the responsibility of the clinical laboratory, to both patient and physician, to ensure that the results reported from that laboratory are reliable and also to provide the physician with an estimate of what constitutes the reference range or "normal" for an analyte being measured. Internal monitoring programs are concerned with **total quality management (TQM), quality assurance (QA),** or **continuous quality improvement (CQI),** each of which is designed to monitor and improve the quality of services provided by the laboratory.

## CLIA '88: Federal Regulation of the Clinical Laboratory

Regulation of clinical laboratories in general began at about the same time as the Medicare law in 1965. Since then, the federal government has been moving closer to regulation of all types of clinical laboratories, beginning with larger hospital and reference laboratories engaging in interstate commerce, and including physician office laboratories (POLs) with the implementation of CLIA '88. Until 1988, regulation applied only to hospitals and independent laboratories under the Clinical Laboratory Improvement Act of 1967 (CLIA '67). This act provided for licensing of laboratories that accepted specimens for testing from across state lines (interstate commerce). In addition, Medicare law provided for inspection and accreditation of laboratories (hospital and independent) that performed tests on and were billed for reimbursement of Medicare patients. These two laws generally did not apply to smaller laboratories such as physician office laboratories.

On October 31, 1988, Congress passed the Clinical Laboratory Improvement Amendments of 1988 in response to a series of newspaper articles about poor Pap smear testing in the Washington, D.C., area. According to federal law, under CLIA '88, a laboratory is now defined as " . . . a facility for the biological, microbiological, serological, chemical, immunohematological, hematological, biophysical, cytological, pathological, or other examination of materials derived from the human body for the purpose of providing information for the diagnosis, prevention, or treatment of any disease or impairment of, or the assessment of the health of human beings."[2] As a result of CLIA '88, any facility that performs testing on material derived from humans for the purpose of diagnosis, assessment, or treatment is subject to federal regulation. Proposed regulations implementing CLIA '88 were published on May 21, 1990. These were met with more than 60,000 comments and protests. On February 28, 1992, the Secretary of Health and Human Services published the final rules implementing CLIA '88.[2] These regulations replaced the Medicare, Medicaid, and CLIA '67 standards and apply to almost all laboratory testing of human specimens. The regulations set standards for laboratory personnel, quality assurance and quality control, and proficiency testing, which are based on test complexity and risk factors. In addition, the regulations establish application procedures and fees for CLIA certification, plus enforcement procedures and sanctions if laboratories fail to meet standards. The regulations were generally effective (implemented) on September 1, 1992, although some parts of the regulations were effective at a later date and modifications are ongoing.[3,4]

### CLIA Categories Based on Complexity of the Tests Done by the Laboratory

CLIA regulations divide laboratories into groups based on the "complexity" of the tests being performed: **waived, moderately complex**, and **highly complex test** categories. Included in the moderately complex category are two subcategories: (1) **provider-performed microscopies (PPM),** specific microscopies (wet mounts) usually performed by a physician or provider for his or her own patients, and (2) **accurate and precise technology (APT),** or "easy," automated quantitative tests or easy qualitative tests such as agglutination patterns or color change end points. Most laboratory tests are classified as moderately complex. Tests are categorized by the federal government on the basis of the analyte tested and the method or instrumentation used to perform the test. For example, reagent strip or tablet urine tests are categorized as waived tests when results are read visually, but as moderately complex when results are read by instrumentation. The microscopic analysis of the urine sediment is categorized as a moderately complex test, unless performed by a physician or provider, in which case it falls under the PPM category.

**Waived Tests.** As currently defined, waived laboratory tests or procedures are those cleared by the Food and Drug Administration (FDA) for home use, which employ methodologies that are so simple that the likelihood of erroneous results is negligible and which pose no reasonable risk of harm to the patient if a test is performed incorrectly.

*Procedures in the Waived Test Category.* Waived tests listed in the April 1995 Federal Register regulations (with revisions in February 1996) are: dipstick or tablet reagent urinalysis (nonautomated) for bilirubin, glucose, hemoglobin, ketone, leukocytes, nitrite, pH, protein, specific gravity, and urobilinogen; fecal occult blood;

ovulation tests—visual color comparison tests for human luteinizing hormone; urine pregnancy tests—visual color comparison tests; erythrocyte sedimentation rate—nonautomated; hemoglobin—copper sulfate, nonautomated (an extremely outdated testing methodology); blood glucose by glucose monitoring devices cleared by the FDA specifically for use at home; spun microhematocrit; hemoglobin by single analyte instruments with self-contained or component features to perform specimen-reagent interaction, providing direct measurement and readout; blood cholesterol test by cholesterol monitoring device approved by the FDA for use at home; and Cholestech L*D*X System for total cholesterol, HDL cholesterol, triglycerides, and glucose.[3] As technology changes, this list may be expanded.

**Provider-Performed Microscopy.** To meet the criteria for being in this category, procedures must follow these specifications: the examination must be personally performed by the practitioner (defined as a physician, a midlevel practitioner under the supervision of a physician, or a dentist), the procedure must be categorized as moderately complex, the primary instrument for performing the test is the microscope (limited to brightfield or phase-contrast microscopy), the specimen is labile, control materials are not available, and there is limited specimen handling.

*Procedures in the PPM Category.* As currently defined, all direct wet mount preparations for the presence or absence of bacteria, fungi, parasites, and human cellular elements in vaginal, cervical, or skin preparations, all potassium hydroxide (KOH) preparations, pinworm examinations, fern tests, postcoital direct, qualitative examinations of vaginal or cervical mucus, urine sediment examinations, nasal smears for granulocytes (eosinophils), fecal leukocyte examinations, and qualitative semen analysis (limited to the presence or absence of sperm and detection of motility) are included in the PPM category.

## Other Regulatory or Accreditation Agencies and Organizations

In addition to CLIA '88 regulations, other agencies and private organizations that regulate or provide accreditation to clinical laboratories include the following:

> Occupational Safety and Health Administration (OSHA)
> Environmental Protection Agency (EPA)
> Food and Drug Administration (FDA)
> State agencies (such as state departments of health)
> College of American Pathologists (CAP).
> Commission on Office Laboratory Accreditation (COLA)
> Joint Commission on Accreditation of Healthcare Organizations (JCAHO)
> National Committee for Clinical Laboratory Standards (NCCLS)
> Americans with Disabilities Act (ADA)

### Commission on Office Laboratory Accreditation

As of December 29, 1993, the HCFA approved the accreditation program developed by the **Commission on Office Laboratory Accreditation (COLA)** for the physician office laboratory. This means that COLA accreditation requirements are recognized by HCFA as being equivalent to those established by CLIA. The COLA accreditation established a peer-review option in place of the CLIA regulatory requirements. COLA-accredited laboratories are surveyed every two years to see that they meet requirements developed by their peers in family practice, internal medicine, or pathology.

### National Committee for Clinical Laboratory Standards

The **National Committee for Clinical Laboratory Standards (NCCLS)** is a nonprofit, educational organization created for the development, promotion, and use of national and international laboratory standards. It was founded in

1968 and accredited by the American National Standards Institute. It employs voluntary consensus standards that are intended to maintain the performance of the clinical laboratory at the high level necessary for quality patient care. Participants include individual laboratories, laboratory professional associations, industries, and agencies of the federal and state governments. NCCLS guidelines and standards are cited throughout this text when applicable. NCCLS recommendations, guidelines, and standards follow the CLIA '88 mandates and therefore serve to inform and assist the laboratory in following the federal regulations.

### Americans with Disabilities Act

The **Americans with Disabilities Act (ADA)** of 1990 (signed into law in 1992) prohibits employment discrimination against qualified persons who have disabilities, in both the public and the private sectors. Under this Act, specific plans must be developed for any known disabled person working in the laboratory to make certain that he or she is working in a safe atmosphere.

## QUALITY ASSURANCE UNDER CLIA REGULATIONS

According to CLIA '88 regulations, quality assurance (QA) activities in the laboratory must be documented and be an active part of the ongoing organization of the laboratory. It is essential that all persons working in the clinical laboratory be totally committed to the concepts of the quality assurance process as it is defined by their institution. The dedication of sufficient planning time to the topic of quality assurance and the implementation of the program in the total laboratory operation are critical. All persons working in the clinical laboratory must be willing to work together to make the quality of service to the patient their top priority. It is not a system meant to penalize the laboratory staff but a means of giving self-confidence to the persons performing tests. Because the total laboratory staff must be involved in carrying out any

quality assurance process, it is important to develop a comprehensive program to include all levels of laboratorians. See also Chapter 8.

### Continuous Quality Improvement

The ongoing process of making certain that the correct laboratory result is reported for the right patient in a timely manner and cost is known as Continuous Quality Improvement, or CQI. This is a process of assuring the clinician ordering a test that the testing process has been done in the best possible way to provide the most useful information in diagnosing or managing the particular patient in question.

### Proficiency Testing

According to CLIA '88, a laboratory must establish and follow written quality control procedures for monitoring and evaluating the quality of the analytical testing process of each method, to ensure the accuracy and reliability of patient test results and reports. **Proficiency testing (PT)** is a means by which quality control between laboratories is maintained. Provisions of CLIA '88 require enrollment in an external proficiency testing program for laboratories performing moderately complex or highly complex tests. Only the waived tests under CLIA '88 are exempt from proficiency testing regulations. The PT program being used must be approved by CLIA. Proficiency testing programs are available through the CAP, the Centers for Disease Control and Prevention, and the health departments in some states.

Laboratories enrolled in a particular PT program test samples for specific analytes and send the results to be tabulated by the program managers. Results of the assays are graded for each participating laboratory according to designated evaluation limits, and the results are compared with those of other laboratories participating in the same PT program.

If a laboratory performs only waived tests, it is not required to participate in a proficiency testing program. However, it must apply for and be given a certificate of waiver from the

United States Department of Health and Human Services. If a laboratory performs moderate- or high-complexity tests for which no proficiency testing is available, it must have a system for verifying the accuracy and reliability of its test results at least twice a year.

## LABORATORY DEPARTMENTS OR DIVISIONS

The organization of a particular clinical laboratory will depend on factors of size, numbers of tests done, and the facilities available. Larger laboratories tend to be departmentalized; there is a separate area designated for each of the various divisions. There is a trend currently to have a more open design, in which personnel can work in any of several areas or divisions. Aspects of cross-training are important considerations in the open model. There is more chance for cooperation and interfacing when the open model is used. As consultation and cooperation are encouraged in health care in general, this trend would appear to be supported by use of the open model for the clinical laboratory. With either the more traditional divisions by separate areas or the open model, there are still several distinct departments or divisions to the organization of the clinical laboratory. Some of these are hematology, coagulation, urinalysis, blood bank (immunohematology), chemistry, immunology/serology, and microbiology. Each will be addressed in separate sections of this book.

### Hematology

Hematology is the study of blood. The formed elements of the blood, or blood cells, include erythrocytes (red blood cells, RBC), leukocytes (white blood cells, WBC), and thrombocytes (platelets). The routine hematology screening test for abnormalities in the blood is the complete blood count, or CBC. This test includes several parts; the following are included in most CBCs: RBC count, WBC count, platelet count, hemoglobin concentration, hematocrit, and a percentage differential of the white blood cells present. The results of the CBC are useful in diagnosing anemias, in which there are too few red blood cells or too little hemoglobin, in leukemias, in which there are too many white blood cells, and in infectious processes of several etiologies, in which changes in white cells are noted. These tests are done in most hematology laboratories by use of an automated instrument. Many of these automated cell counters also provide automated white cell differential analyses, separating the types of white cells present by size, maturity, and nuclear and cytoplasmic characteristics. Cell counts for other body fluids, such as cerebrospinal fluid or synovial fluid, are also performed in some hematology laboratories. There is also a microscopy component to work done in the hematology laboratory, as microscopic assessment of a stained blood film is done as part of some CBCs, especially when automated instrumentation is not readily available or when a more complete morphologic examination is necessary.

Other tests done in hematology laboratories are reticulocyte counts and erythrocyte sedimentation rate measurements. Examination of bone marrow is done in special hematology divisions where trained hematopathologists and technologists are present to examine the slides. The process of obtaining the bone marrow from the patient is done by a trained physician.

### Coagulation

Work done in the coagulation laboratory assesses bleeding and clotting problems. In some laboratories, hematology and coagulation tests are part of the same laboratory department. The two most commonly performed tests in the coagulation laboratory are prothrombin time (PT) and activated partial thromboplastin time (aPTT). These tests can be used to identify potential bleeding disorders and to monitor anticoagulant therapy. Patients who have had a heart attack or stroke, both due to formation of blood clots, are given medications that anticoagulate their blood or slow the clotting process and must be monitored because too large a dose of these drugs can lead to bleeding problems.

## Urinalysis

In this laboratory division, the routine urine screening tests are done. The routine urinalysis was one of the earliest laboratory tests performed, historically, and it still serves to give valuable information regarding the detection of disease related to the kidney and urinary tract. By evaluating the results of the three component parts of the urinalysis—observation of the physical characteristics of the urine specimen itself, such as color, clarity, and specific gravity; screening for chemical constituents such as pH, glucose, ketone bodies, protein, blood, bilirubin, urobilinogen, nitrites, and leukocyte esterase; and microscopic examination of the urinary sediment—metabolic diseases such as diabetes mellitus, kidney diseases, or infectious diseases of the urinary bladder or kidney can be diagnosed and monitored.

## Clinical Chemistry

The clinical chemistry laboratory performs quantitative analytic procedures on a variety of body fluids, but primarily on serum or plasma that has been processed from whole blood collected from the patient. Tests are also done on urine or, less frequently, on body fluids such as cerebrospinal fluid. Several hundred analytes can be tested in the chemistry laboratory, but a few tests are used much more often in the aid of diagnosis of disease. Probably the most common chemistry tests done are for blood glucose, cholesterol, electrolytes, and serum proteins. Blood glucose tests are used to diagnose and monitor diabetes mellitus. Cholesterol is a test that is part of a battery of tests to monitor the lipid status of the patient. Electrolytes affect many of the metabolic processes in the body; among these processes are maintenance of osmotic pressure and water distribution in various body compartments, maintenance of pH, regulation of the functioning of heart and other muscles, and oxidation-reduction processes. Elevated protein levels can indicate disease states of several types. Serum enzyme tests are done to identify damage to or disease of specific organs, such as heart muscle damage or liver cell damage. Tests to monitor drug therapy and drug levels, toxicology, are also performed in chemistry laboratories. Most routine chemistry testing is done by automated methods, using computerized instruments that are very sophisticated and fast and that provide reliable results. Persons working in chemistry laboratories will be using automated analytic equipment, and having a good working knowledge of the various types of methodologies and instrumentation used is essential.

## Blood Bank (Immunohematology)

When blood is donated for transfusion purposes, it must undergo a rigorous protocol of testing to make certain that it is safe for transfusion. Proper sample identification is particularly crucial in blood banking procedures, as a mislabeled specimen could result in a severe transfusion reaction or even death for the recipient. Most of the testing done in the blood bank laboratory is based on antigen-antibody reactions. In the specific tests performed in the blood bank laboratory, the antigens are specific proteins that are attached to the red and white blood cells. The nature of these antigens determines the blood group assigned, whether it is group A, B, O, or AB: group A red cells have antigen A, group B have antigen B, group AB have both antigens A and B, and group O have neither antigen A nor antigen B. Rh typing is also done, with blood being classified as Rh positive or Rh negative. Donated blood is also screened for any unusual antibodies present and for the presence of infectious antibodies such as hepatitis virus or human immunodeficiency virus. The donor blood must be matched to that of the prospective recipient to ensure that the recipient will not suffer any ill effects from the transfusion as a result of incompatible antibodies. When a blood transfusion is ordered, it is extremely important that only properly matched blood is transfused.

Blood banks are also engaged in the practice of transfusion medicine using components of blood or blood products. A patient does not usually need the whole unit of blood, only a particular part of it, such as the red blood cells, platelets, or specific clotting factors. By use of blood component therapy, one unit of donated blood can help several different patients who have different needs. The blood bank laboratorian will separate the donated unit into its components and store them for transfusion at a later time.

## Immunology/Serology

The normal immune system functions to protect the body from foreign microorganisms that may invade it. When foreign material—that is, something that the body does not already have as part of itself—enters the body, the immune system works to eliminate the foreign material. This foreign material can be bacteria, viruses, fungi, or parasites, for example. The body's defensive action is carried out by its white blood cells—lymphocytes, monocytes, and other cells—by which the invading organism is eliminated or controlled. As in the blood bank laboratory, many of the immunology/serology laboratory's procedures are based on antigen-antibody reactions. When foreign material (antigen) is introduced into the body, the body reacts by means of its immune system to make antibodies to the foreign antigen. The antibodies formed can be measured in the laboratory.

In the evaluation of certain infectious diseases, the detection of antibodies in the serum of the patient is an important step in making and confirming a diagnosis and in the management of the illness. The use of serologic testing is based on the rise and fall of specific antibody titers in response to the disease process. In many instances serologic testing is done retrospectively, as the disease must progress to a certain point before the antibody titers will rise—often it takes several days or weeks for the antibody titer to rise after the first symptoms appear. In general, serologic testing is most useful for in-

fectious organisms that are difficult to culture, cause chronic conditions, or have prolonged incubation periods.

In addition to its use in the diagnosis of infectious disease, the immunology laboratory can identify normal and abnormal levels of immune cells and serum components. Immune cellular function can also be determined.

## Microbiology

In the microbiology laboratory, microorganisms that cause disease are identified; these are known as pathogens. Generally, the common bacteria, viruses, fungi, and parasites are identified in a typical clinical laboratory. Specimens sent to the microbiology laboratory for culture include swabs from the throat or wounds, sputum, vaginal excretions, urine, and blood. It is important that the microbiology laboratorian be able to differentiate the normal flora—those organisms which are part of the normal constituents of the host—from the pathogenic flora. Various differential testing is done, from the inoculation and incubation of the classic culture plate to observe an organism's growth characteristics, to the use of Gram staining techniques to separate gram-positive from gram-negative organisms. Once a pathogen is suspected, more testing is done to confirm its identity. Rapid testing methods have been developed to identify routine pathogens. For example, immunologic tests have been devised using monoclonal antibodies to identify the streptococcal organism causing pharyngitis or "strep" throat.

Another task for the microbiology laboratory is to identify the appropriate antibiotic to use for treatment of the offending pathogen. The pathogen is tested by using a panel of antibiotics of various types and dosages to determine the susceptibility of the organism to the various antibiotics. By doing this, the most effective antibiotic along with its correct dosage can be used to treat the specific patient's pathogenic organism in the most cost-effective and beneficial way.

# PERSONNEL IN THE CLINICAL LABORATORY

Physicians generally do not perform the needed laboratory tests themselves but rely on trained laboratory personnel to do this for them. Clinical laboratorians, persons working in clinical laboratories, are an important component of the medical team. This clinical laboratory team generally is made up of the medical director, or pathologist, medical technologists/clinical laboratory scientists, laboratory assistants, phlebotomists, and specialists in the various laboratory disciplines, such as chemists, microbiologists, and hematologists. The categories of laboratory personnel and their titles vary from facility to facility. Generally the more highly trained persons will do the more complex work and administrative tasks, leaving the routine work to others. Many clinical laboratories are highly automated, and the job duties will reflect this. In some laboratories personnel are cross-trained to work in all disciplines; in others there may be specialists in certain areas such as clinical chemistry or microbiology. The size and work load of the laboratory may determine the organization of the work load for the personnel.

## CLIA Requirements for Personnel

The personnel section of the CLIA regulations defines the responsibilities of persons working in each of the testing sites where tests of moderate or high complexity are done, along with the educational requirements and training and experience needed. Minimum education and experience needed by testing personnel to perform the specific laboratory tests on human specimens are also regulated by CLIA '88. These job requirements are listed in the CLIA '88 final regulations, along with their amendments published from 1992 to 1995.[2-4] There are no CLIA regulations for testing personnel who work at sites performing only the waived tests or the PPMs. For laboratories where only tests of moderate complexity are performed, the minimum requirement for testing personnel is a high school diploma or equivalent, as long as there is

documented evidence of an amount of training sufficient to ensure that the laboratorian has the skills necessary to collect, identify, and process the specimen, and to perform the laboratory analysis itself. For tests of the highly complex category, the personnel requirements are more stringent. Anyone who is eligible to perform highly complex tests can also perform moderate-complexity testing. The Occupational Safety and Health Administration requires that training in handling chemical hazards, as well as training in handling infectious materials (standard precautions), be included for all new testing personnel. The laboratory director is ultimately responsible for all personnel working in the laboratory.

## Pathologist

Most clinical laboratories are operated under the direction of a **pathologist**. The clinical laboratory can be divided into two main sections: clinical pathology and anatomic pathology. Many pathologists have training in both anatomic and clinical pathology. The anatomic pathologist is a licensed physician trained, usually for an additional four to five years after graduating from medical school, to examine (grossly and microscopically) all of the surgically removed specimens from patients, which include frozen sections, tissue samples, and autopsy specimens. Examination of Pap smears and other cytologic and histologic examinations are also generally done by an anatomic pathologist.

A clinical pathologist is also a licensed physician, with additional training in clinical pathology or laboratory medicine. As described earlier, laboratory medicine is the medical discipline by which clinical laboratory science and technology are applied to the care of the patient. Under the direction of the clinical pathologist, many common laboratory tests are performed on blood and urine, including assays such as blood cell counts and white cell differentials, urinalysis, common chemistry tests for blood sugar and cholesterol, microbiologic cultures of throat swabs and urine, coagulation studies such as prothrombin time tests, and immunoassays of various types—tests described in later sections of this book. With training and advanced education in the use of various laboratory assays of the patient's blood, urine, tissue, or other body fluids or excretions, and with the effective utilization of these findings to present an informative result report to the patient's attending clinician, the clinical pathologist fulfills his or her role in the practice of laboratory medicine. The interpretation of laboratory findings in a timely and useable fashion is very important. Consultation with clinicians along the course of this process is also important; any and all information gained concerning the patient's case is actually the result of collaborative activity between the laboratory and the attending physician.

The pathologist will perform only certain of the services, such as examination of the surgical specimens, which is done primarily by the anatomic pathologist. Other work, such as the routine tests for blood cell counts and urinalysis, will be performed by trained laboratory personnel with various levels of education and experience, under the pathologist's responsibility and supervision.

## Other Laboratory Personnel

Depending on the size of the laboratory and the numbers and kinds of laboratory tests performed, various levels of trained personnel are needed. CLIA '88 regulations set the standards for personnel, including their levels of education and training. Generally, the level of training or education of the laboratorian will be taken into consideration in the roles assigned in the laboratory and the kinds of laboratory analyses performed. In addition to the categories described below, various specialist categories are available to laboratorians; specific extra training and education will earn certification in areas such as blood banking or chemistry, for example. Other specialized training includes that for cytotechnologists, histotechnologists, and phlebotomists.

## Laboratory Supervisor/Manager/Chief Technologist

Typically, a laboratory has a supervisor or manager who is responsible for the technical aspects of management of the laboratory. This person is most often a clinical laboratory scientist (also known as a medical technologist) with additional experience and skills in administration. In very large laboratories, a chief technologist may be in place to supervise the technical aspects of the facility (matters dealing with assay of analytes), including quality control programs and maintenance of the laboratory instruments. In addition, a business manager may be hired specifically to handle administrative details. The supervisor or administrative manager may also be the chief technologist in the case of smaller laboratories. Section-supervising technologists are in place as needed, depending on the size and work load of the laboratory. A major concern of administrative technologists, no matter what the job titles are called, is making certain that all federal, state, and local regulatory mandates are being followed by the laboratory. Persons in leadership and management positions in the clinical laboratory must be certain that all legal operating conditions have been met and that they are balanced with the performance of work in a cost-effective manner.

It is important that the people serving in a supervisory position be able to communicate in a clear, concise manner, both to the persons working in their laboratory settings and to the physicians and other health care workers who utilize the services of the laboratory.

## Clinical Laboratory Scientist

**Medical technologists (MT)**, now also known as **clinical laboratory scientists (CLS)**, usually have earned a bachelor of science degree in medical technology or clinical laboratory science. Responsibilities vary; among other things, they may perform laboratory assays, supervise other laboratorians, or teach. Some are engaged in research. An important aspect of the training for a clinical laboratory scientist is to understand the science behind the tests being performed so that problems can be recognized when they occur and solutions undertaken. Troubleshooting is a constant consideration in the clinical laboratory. Because of his or her in-depth knowledge of technical aspects, principles of methodology, and instrumentation used for the various laboratory assays being done, the clinical laboratory scientist is able to correlate and interpret the data. Once educational requirements have been met at an accredited institution, certification for this level of laboratorian is offered through examination by the **Board of Registry of the American Society of Clinical Pathologists (ASCP)** and the **National Certification Agency for Medical Laboratory Personnel (NCA)**, an independent nonprofit certification agency.

### Medical Laboratory Technician, Clinical Laboratory Technician, Clinical Laboratory Assistant

These laboratorians generally have some limitations in what work they can do in the laboratory and have different titles according to where they trained and in which health care facility they are employed—**medical laboratory technician (MLT), clinical laboratory assistant (CLA), clinical laboratory technician (CLT)**. These titles (and possibly others) indicate laboratorians with similarities. These laboratory personnel generally have a lesser amount of formal education or training than the clinical laboratory scientist. They usually possess some formal training; some have completed associate degrees, while others have a certificate of completion from a technical school or other vocational program. Much of the general, routine laboratory testing is done by these persons. Their work is usually done under the supervision of a clinical laboratory scientist or a pathologist. The CLT, MLT, or CLA collects, processes, and tests specimens (mostly blood and urine specimens) for the many routine, high-volume, repetitive tests

done in a clinical laboratory. He or she is trained to seek help when a problem arises. Certification for CLT or MLT is offered through examination by ASCP and NCA.

## SITES OF TESTING

### Central Laboratory Testing vs. Point-of-Care Testing (Decentralization of Laboratory Testing)

The traditional setting for performance of diagnostic laboratory testing has been a centralized location in a health care facility (hospital) where specimens from patients are sent to be tested. The **centralized laboratory** setting remains in many institutions, but the advent of near-testing, bedside testing, or **point-of-care testing (POCT)** has changed the organization of many laboratories. In the POCT concept of testing, the laboratory testing actually comes to the bedside of the patient. Any changes to implement the use of POCT should show a significant improvement in outcome for the patient and should also show a total financial benefit to the patient and the institution and not just a reduction in the costs of equipment and supplies.

### Point-of-Care Testing

Decentralization of testing away from the traditional laboratory setting can greatly increase the interaction of laboratory personnel with patients and with other members of the health care team. POCT is an example of an interdisciplinary activity that crosses many boundaries in the health care facility. POCT is not always performed by laboratorians, however. Other health care personnel, such as nurses, respiratory therapists, anesthesiologists, operating room technologists, and physician assistants, often are the ones doing the testing. However, the CLIA '88 regulations associated with clinical laboratory testing must also be followed for POCT, even if nonlaboratorians are actually performing the tests. These CLIA regulations are considered "site neutral," meaning that all laboratory testing must meet the same standards for quality of work done, personnel, proficiency testing, quality control, and so on, regardless of where the tests are performed—in a central laboratory or at the bedside of the patient. Test complexity is also considered for POCT, and the categories described earlier in this chapter, under Regulation of the Clinical Laboratory (waived tests, tests of moderate complexity, tests of high complexity, and provider-performed microscopies) also apply in regulations for POCT. If these tests are performed in a facility that is JCAHO or CAP accredited, they are regulated in essentially the same way as tests done in a centralized laboratory.

Qualifications for POCT personnel are also set by federal, state, and local regulations.[1,2] The level of training varies with the analytical system being employed and with the background of the individual involved—this can range from a requirement for a high school diploma with no experience to a bachelor of science degree with two years of experience. The director of the laboratory is responsible for setting additional requirements, as long as the federal CLIA '88 regulations are also being followed.

With the immediate reporting of results being available and with the patient's case management depending on the result, it is essential that POCT devices have built-in quality control and quality assurance systems to prevent erroneous data from being reported to the physician. POCT has been found to provide cost-effective improvement of medical care. In a hospital setting, POCT provides immediate assessment and management of the critically ill patient—this is its most significant use for this setting. Tests commonly included in POCT are ones based on criteria of immediate medical need; these include blood gases, electrolytes ($Na^+$, $K^+$, $Ca^{++}$), prothrombin time (PT), partial thromboplastin time (PTT) or activated clotting time (ACT), hematocrit or hemoglobin, and glucose. POCT attempts to meet the demands of intensive care units, operating rooms, and emergency departments for the faster reporting of test results.

Other possible benefits of POCT are improved therapeutic turnaround times, less trauma and more convenience for the patient (when blood is collected and analyzed at the bedside), decreased preanalytical errors (errors formerly due to specimen collection, transportation, and handling by the laboratory), decreased manpower (the use of cross-training, whereby nurses can perform the laboratory analysis, eliminating a laboratorian for this step), more collaboration of clinicians with the laboratory, and shorter intensive care unit stays. Certain tests, such as the fecal screen for blood and the routine chemical screening of urine by reagent strips, can often be done more easily on the nursing unit, as long as the tests are properly performed and controlled using quality assurance protocol.

POCT in outpatient settings provides the ability to obtain test results during the patient's visit to the clinic or the physician's office, enabling diagnosis and subsequent case management in a more timely manner.

When central laboratory testing is compared with POCT, consideration must be given to which site of testing will provide the most appropriate testing mechanism. Centralized laboratories can provide "stat" testing capabilities, which can report results in a very timely manner. Sometimes laboratories will develop a laboratory satellite that is set up to function at the point of need—a laboratory located near or in the operating room, for example, or a laboratory that is portable and can be transported on a cart to the point of need.

## Reference Laboratories

When a laboratory performs only routine tests, specimens for the more complex tests ordered by the physician must be sent to a **reference laboratory** for analysis. It is often more cost-effective for a laboratory to actually perform only certain common, repetitive tests and to send out the others for another laboratory to perform. These reference laboratories can then perform the more complex tests for many customers, giving good turnaround times—this is their service to their customers. It is important to select a reference laboratory where the mechanisms for specimen transport and results reporting are managed well. The turnaround time is important, and it often is a function of how well the specimens are handled by the reference laboratory. There must be a good means of communication between the reference laboratory and its customers. The reference laboratory should be managed by professionals who recognize the importance of providing quality results, and information about the utilization of the results when needed, to the patient's clinician. Messengers or couriers are engaged to transport or drive specimens within a fixed, reasonable geographic area. The various commercial delivery systems are used for transport out of the area.

## Physician Office Laboratories

A **physician office laboratory (POL)** is a laboratory where the tests performed are limited to those done for the physician's own patients coming to the practice, group, or clinic. Because of the concern that some of these laboratories were lacking in quality of work done, the CLIA '88 regulations included POLs also. Prior to CLIA '88, the POLs were largely unregulated. Most POLs perform only the waived tests or provider-performed microscopy, as set by the CLIA. For a description of the tests included in the waived test category and for those in the PPM category, see CLIA Categories Based on Complexity of the Tests Done by the Laboratory, earlier in this chapter. Tests most commonly performed in POLs are reagent strip urinalysis, blood glucose, occult fecal blood, rapid strep A in throats, hemoglobin, urine pregnancy, cholesterol, and hematocrit.

The convenience to the patient of having laboratory testing done in the physician's office is a driving force for a physician to include a laboratory in his or her office or clinic. Manufacturers of laboratory instruments have accommodated the clinic or office setting with a modern generation of instruments that require less technical skill on the part of the person using them. The improved turnaround times for test results and patient convenience must be balanced, however, with cost-effectiveness and the potential for the physician to be exposed to problems that may be outside the realm of his or her expertise or training. Laboratorians, including pathologists, must be available to act as consultants when the need arises.

A physician office laboratory must submit an application to the Department of Health and Human Services or its designee. On this application form, details about the number of tests done, the methodologies used for each measurement, and the qualifications of each of the testing personnel employed to perform the tests are included. Certificates are issued for up to two years, and any changes in tests done or methodologies used, personnel hired, and so forth, must be submitted to HHS within 30 days of the change. This application may also be made through an accreditation agency whose requirements are deemed by HHS to be equal to or more stringent than the HHS requirements. Accreditation requirements from the Commission on Office Laboratory Accreditation have been recognized by the HCFA as being equivalent to the CLIA requirements. See Regulation of the Clinical Laboratory, earlier in this chapter.

When a POL performs only waived tests or PPM tests, there are no CLIA personnel requirements. The physician is responsible for the work done in the POL. When moderately or highly complex testing is done in a POL, the more stringent CLIA personnel requirements must be followed for the testing personnel; these POLs must also adhere to a program of quality assurance, including programs of proficiency testing.

## MEDICAL-LEGAL ISSUES

### Informed Consent

For laboratories, an important responsibility is that of obtaining informed consent from the patient. **Informed consent** means that the patient is aware of, understands, and agrees to the nature of the testing to be done and what will be done with the results reported. Generally, when a patient enters a hospital, there is an implied consent to the many routine procedures that will be performed while he or she is there. Venipuncture is one of the routine tests that carries this implied consent. The patient must sign specific consent forms for more complex procedures, such as bone marrow aspiration, lumbar puncture for collection of cerebrospinal fluid, or fine-needle biopsies, and for nonurgent transfusion of blood or its components. The patient should be given sufficient information about the reasons why the informed consent is needed and must be given the opportunity to ask questions. In the event the patient is incapable of signing the consent form, a guardian should be obtained—for example, when the patient is a minor, legally not competent, physically unable to write, or hearing impaired, or does not speak English. Health care institutions have policies in place for handling these situations.

## Confidentiality

Any results obtained for specimens from patients must be kept strictly confidential. Any information about the patient, including the types of measurements being done, must also be kept in confidence. Only authorized persons should have access to the information about a patient, and any release of this information to non–health care persons, such as insurance personnel, lawyers, or friends of the patient, can be done only when authorized by the patient. It is important to speak about a particular patient's situation only in the confines of the laboratory setting and not in any public place, such as elevators or hospital coffee shops.

## Chain of Custody

Laboratory test results that could potentially be used in a court of law—at a trial or judicial hearing—must be handled in a specific manner. For evidence to be admissible, each step of the analysis, beginning with the moment the specimen is collected and transported to the laboratory, to the analysis itself and the reporting of the results, must be documented—a process known as maintaining the **chain of custody.** The links between specimen collection and presentation in court must establish certainty that the material or specimen tested had not been altered in any way that would change its usefulness as admissible evidence. Any specimen that has potential evidentiary value should be labeled, sealed, and placed in a locked refrigerator or other suitable secure storage areas. Specimens that provide alcohol levels, specimens collected from rape victims, specimens for paternity testing, and specimens submitted from the medical examiner's cases are the usual types requiring the "chain of custody" documentation. See also Chapter 3.

## REFERENCES

1. Ancillary (Bedside) Testing in Acute and Chronic Care Facilities, Approved Guideline. Villanova, Pa, National Committee for Clinical Laboratory Standards, 1994, NCCLS Document C30-A.
2. Department of Health and Human Services, Health Care Financing Administration: Clinical Laboratory Improvement Amendments of 1988. *Federal Register*, February 28, 1992. CLIA '88; Final Rule. 42 CFR. Subpart K, 493.1201.
3. Department of Health and Human Services, Health Care Financing Administration: Clinical Laboratory Improvement Amendments of 1988. *Federal Register*, April 24, 1995, vol 60, no 78. Final rules with comment period.
4. Department of Health and Human Services, Health Care Financing Administration: Clinical Laboratory Improvement Amendments of 1988. *Federal Register,* September 15, 1995, vol 60, no 179. Proposed rules.
5. Tietz NW (ed): *Applied Laboratory Medicine.* Philadelphia, W.B. Saunders Co., 1992, p 1.

## BIBLIOGRAPHY

Clerc JM.: *An Introduction to Clinical Laboratory Science.* St Louis, Mosby, 1992.

Henry JB (ed.): *Clinical Diagnosis and Management by Laboratory Methods*, ed 19. Philadelphia, WB Saunders Co., 1996.

Kaplan LA, Pesce AJ: *Clinical Chemistry: Theory, Analysis, and Correlation*, ed 3. St Louis, Mosby, 1996.

Laboratory Design, Proposed Guideline. Villanova, Pa, National Committee for Clinical Laboratory Standards, 1994, NCCLS Document GP18-P.

NCCLS: *Clinical Laboratory Technical Procedure Manuals: Approved Guideline*, ed 3. 1996. Villanova, Pa, National Committee for Clinical Laboratory Standards, 1996, NCCLS Document GP2-A3.

NCCLS: *CLIA-NCCLS Index (A Collection of Documents)*. Villanova, Pa, National Committee for Clinical Laboratory Standards, NCCLS Document X2-R.

NCCLS: *CLIA Specialty Collection (A Collection of Documents)*. Villanova, Pa, National Committee for Clinical Laboratory Standards, NCCLS Document SC11.

NCCLS: *Continuous Quality Improvement: Essential Management Approaches and their Use in Proficiency Testing: Proposed Guideline*. Villanova, Pa, National Committee for Clinical Laboratory Standards, 1997, NCCLS Document GP22-P.

NCCLS: *Point-of-Care Testing (A Collection of Guidelines)*. Villanova, Pa, National Committee for Clinical Laboratory Standards, NCCLS Document SC17-L.

NCCLS: *Training Verification for Laboratory Personnel: Approved Guideline*. Villanova, Pa, National Committee for Clinical Laboratory Standards, 1995, NCCLS Document GP21-A.

*Physician Office Laboratory Policy and Procedure Manual*. Northfield, Ill, College of American Pathologists, 1993.

*Physician Office Laboratory Series*. Commonwealth of Pennsylvania, Department of Health, Bureau of Laboratories, 1988.

## STUDY QUESTIONS

1. **Which of the following acts, agencies, or organizations was created to make certain that the quality of work done in the laboratory is reliable?**

   A. Healthcare Finance Administration (HCFA)
   B. Occupational Safety and Health Administration (OSHA)
   C. Clinical Laboratory Improvement Amendments of 1988 (CLIA '88)
   D. Centers for Disease Control and Prevention (CDC)

2. **Match each of the following agencies or organizations (1 to 5) with the best description of its purpose pertaining to the clinical laboratory (A to E):**

   1. Healthcare Financing Administration (HCFA)
   2. Joint Commission on Accreditation of Healthcare Organizations (JCAHO)
   3. College of American Pathologists (CAP)
   4. Commission on Office Laboratory Accreditation (COLA)
   5. National Committee for Clinical Laboratory Standards (NCCLS)

   _____ A. Sets accreditation requirements for physician office laboratories (POLs).

   _____ B. Administers both the CLIA '88 and Medicare programs.

   _____ C. HCFA has given it *deemed status* to act on the government's behalf to certify clinical laboratories.

   _____ D. A nonprofit, educational group that establishes consensus standards for maintaining a high-quality laboratory organization.

   _____ E. Accredits health care facilities and sets standards for quality assurance programs in those facilities.

3. **Name the categories of laboratory tests based on the complexity of the test performed, as established by CLIA '88.**

4. Laboratories performing which of the following types of tests must be enrolled in a CLIA-approved Proficiency Testing Program? (More than one of the answers may be correct.)

A. Waived
B. Moderately complex
C. Highly complex
D. Provider-performed microscopies

5. Match the following terms (1 to 4) with the descriptive statements (A to D) that follow:

1. Proficiency testing (PT)
2. Quality assurance (QA)
3. Provider-performed microscopies (PPM)
4. Point-of-care testing (POCT)

_____ A. A continuing process of evaluating and monitoring all aspects of the laboratory to ensure accuracy of test results.

_____ B. Specific microscopies (wet mounts) performed by a physician for his or her own patients.

_____ C. A means by which quality control between laboratories is maintained.

_____ D. A process of performing the laboratory testing at the bedside of the patient; a means of decentralizing some of the laboratory testing.

# CHAPTER 2

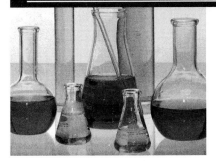

# Safety in the Clinical Laboratory

## Learning Objectives

*From study of this chapter, the reader will be able to:*

➤ Know the general safety regulations governing the clinical laboratory, including components of the OSHA-mandated plans for chemical hygiene and for occupational exposure to blood-borne pathogens, the importance of the safety manual, and general emergency procedures.

➤ Know the basic aspects of infection control policies, including how and when to use personal protective equipment or devices (gowns, gloves, goggles), and the reasons for using standard precautions.

➤ Know the importance of a safety program in the laboratory.

➤ Know how to take the necessary precautions to avoid exposure to the many potentially hazardous situations in the clinical laboratory, including biohazards and chemical, fire, and electrical hazards, along with dangers in using certain supplies and equipment (broken glassware, for example)—the successful implementation of the "right to know" rule.

➤ Know the pre-exposure and post-exposure prophylactic measures for handling potential occupational transmission of certain pathogens, namely hepatitis B and human immunodefiency viruses (HBV and HIV).

➤ Know how to properly decontaminate a work area when a hazardous spill has occurred and, in general, how to keep the workplace clean.

➤ Know how to properly segregate and dispose of the various types of waste products generated in the clinical laboratory, including the use of sharps containers for needles and lancets.

➤ Know the basic steps of first aid.

# IMPORTANCE OF LABORATORY SAFETY

The importance of safety and correct first-aid procedures cannot be overemphasized to anyone working in the clinical laboratory. Students as well as laboratory personnel should be constantly reminded of safety precautions. Many accidents do not just happen—they are caused by carelessness or lack of proper communication. For this reason, the practice of safety should be uppermost in the mind of anyone working in a clinical laboratory.

Most laboratory accidents are preventable by the exercise of good technique and by the use of common sense. There are many potential hazards in the laboratory, but most can be controlled by taking simple precautions. In every medical institution, the administration supplies the laboratory with safety devices for equipment and personal use, but it is up to the individual to make use of them. Safety is personal, and its practice must be a matter of individual desire and commitment. Real appreciation for safety requires a built-in concern for the other person, for an unsafe act may harm the bystander without harming the person who performs the act.

# SAFETY MANUAL

Each laboratory should have a **safety manual** readily available that covers all safety practices and precautions. The safety manual should be updated frequently with additional or new information as it becomes available and should also include regulations covering the proper use of laboratory equipment and the handling of all hazardous or infectious materials. Anything that poses a potential safety hazard for persons in the laboratory should be described in the safety manual. All persons in the laboratory setting should be familiar with the location and the contents of this manual.

# EMERGENCY PRECAUTIONS

A posted **plan for evacuation** of the laboratory in the event of an emergency must be readily available. Routes for exiting the room and the building must be made known to all persons working in that setting, as well as the locations of the various safety devices—fire extinguishers, emergency showers, eye washers, fire blankets, and other equipment such as respirators or goggles. Implementation of periodic unannounced safety drills may motivate the laboratory personnel to become familiar with current safety practices.

# SAFETY STANDARDS AND GOVERNING AGENCIES

Safety standards for clinical laboratories are initiated, governed, and reviewed by several agencies or committees. These include the U.S. Department of Labor's **Occupational Safety and Health Administration (OSHA);** the **National Committee for Clinical Laboratory Standards (NCCLS),** a nonprofit educational organization providing a forum for development, promotion, and use of national and international standards; the Centers for Disease Control and Prevention (CDC), a part of the U.S. Department of Health and Human Services' Public Health Service; and the College of American Pathologists (CAP).[5,6,9,12]

To ensure that workers have safe and healthful working conditions, the United States government created a system of safeguards and regulations under the **Occupational Safety and Health Act of 1970.**[7] This system touches almost every person working in the United states today. It is especially relevant to discuss the meaning of the act in terms of safety in the clinical laboratory, where there are special problems with respect to potential safety hazards. Diseases or accidents associated with preventable causes cannot be tolerated.

The Occupational Safety and Health Act regulations apply to all businesses with one or more employees and are administered by the U.S. Department of Labor through OSHA. The programs deal with many aspects of safety and health protection, including compliance arrangements, inspection procedures, penalties for noncompliance, complaint procedures, duties and responsibilities for administration and operation of the system, and how the many standards are set. Responsibility for compliance is placed on both the administration of the institution and the employee.

The **OSHA standards**, where appropriate, include provisions for warning labels or other appropriate forms of warning to alert all workers to potential hazards, suitable protective equipment, exposure control procedures, and implementation of training and education programs—all for the primary purpose of ensuring safe and healthful working conditions for every American worker.

A person who understands the potential hazards in a clinical laboratory and knows the basic safety precautions can prevent accidents. The Occupational Safety and Health Act requires a **safety program** in every clinical laboratory. Identification of potential hazards is an important part of any such program. Although many hazards are commonly found throughout the clinical laboratory, the specific type of hazard may be slightly different in the various departments. Two programs have been mandated by OSHA to ensure the safety of persons working in a clinical laboratory. One covers occupational exposure to chemical hazards; the other covers occupational exposure to blood-borne pathogens.[5,6] Both of these programs will be discussed in subsequent sections of this chapter.

## LABORATORY HAZARDS

### Biological Hazards and Infection Control

Because many hazards of the clinical laboratory are unique, a special term, **biohazard**, was devised. This word is posted throughout the laboratory to denote infectious materials or agents that present a risk or even a potential risk to the health of humans or animals in the laboratory. The potential risk can be either through direct infection or through the environment. Infection can occur during the process of specimen collection, or from handling, transporting, or testing the specimen. Biological infections are frequently caused by accidental aspiration of infectious material, accidental inoculation with con-

taminated needles or syringes, animal bites, sprays from syringes, aerosols from the uncapping of specimen tubes, or centrifuge accidents. Some other sources of laboratory infections are cuts or scratches from contaminated glassware, cuts from instruments used during animal surgery or autopsy, and spilling or spattering of pathogenic samples on the work desks or floors. Persons working in laboratories on animal research or other research involving biologically hazardous materials are also susceptible to the problems of biohazards. The symbol shown in Fig. 2-1 is used to denote the presence of biohazards.

One precaution that can be taken is to see that all containers are properly labeled. Labeling may be the simplest and the single important step in the proper handling of any hazardous substance. A label for a container should include a date and the contents of the container. When the contents of one container are transferred to another container, this information should also be transferred to the new container.

Laboratories must make every effort to implement a **program for infection control**. This can start with prevention of contamination when specimens are collected and when they

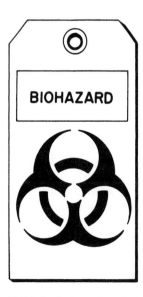

**FIG 2-1.** Biohazard symbol.

are delivered to the laboratory. A large percentage of the specimens sent to a laboratory contain blood, and their safe collection and transportation must take top priority in any discussion of safety in the laboratory (see also Chapter 3).

## Infection Control Programs

Since the clinical laboratory performs assays on various biological specimens from patients, one of the most important OSHA regulations covers exposure to biological hazards. Protection from **blood-borne pathogens** is of major importance. The OSHA-mandated program, Occupational Exposure to Bloodborne Pathogens, must be in place, and has been a law since March 1992.[4] Clinical specimens received from patients pose a potential hazard to laboratory personnel because of infectious agents they may contain. In addition, the CDC recommends safety precautions concerning the handling of all patient specimens. These are known as standard precautions (formerly known as universal precautions or universal blood and body fluid precautions). They are published by the Centers for Disease Control and Prevention as a guideline for hospital infection control practices and also published in *Morbidity and Mortality Weekly Report* (MMWR), which is a series of recommendations from the CDC to protect health care workers and others from infection by blood-borne pathogens.[2,10]

Recommendations from OSHA include an infection control plan, engineering and work practice controls, personal protective clothing and equipment, sufficient education and training, signs and labels, provision of hepatitis B virus (HBV) vaccination, and medical follow-up after exposure incidents. The CDC provides recommendations for chemoprophylaxis after occupational exposure to HIV.[1] The NCCLS has also issued guidelines for the laboratory worker in regard to protection from blood-borne diseases spread via contact with patient specimens.[9]

Together, these agencies are working to lessen the risk of exposure of health care workers to blood-borne pathogens. An infectious disease program must be in place in any health care facility to ensure the safety of the people working there. The U.S. Department of Labor (under OSHA) has developed standards of practice for health care institutions. The CDC has issued guidelines for implementation of these standards. The College of American Pathologists offers a voluntary accreditation program for clinical laboratories. The requirements include safe work practices, which, in turn, include biosafety measures.

## Standard Precautions

The term **standard precautions,** refers to a system of infectious disease controls that assumes that every direct contact with body fluids is infectious. These controls include personal protective devices, good work practices, and the proper implementation of engineering controls. They require that every employee who has direct contact with patients and with their body fluids be protected as though such body fluids contained an infectious pathogen such as **hepatitis B virus (HBV)** or **human immunodeficiency virus (HIV)**. Since not all patients carrying blood-borne pathogens are identified prior to the handling of their specimens, all persons who handle patient specimens or who come in contact with patients in a health care setting should exercise certain consistent precautions on a routine basis. These standard precautions recognize the infectious potential of any patient specimen. The CDC recommendations also recognize that although all patients are potentially infectious, not all types of specimens pose the same degree of risk for health care personnel.

Blood and certain body fluids pose the greatest risk for those persons whose activities involve contact with them. Body fluids included in this classification are semen and vaginal secretions, tissues, cerebrospinal fluid, synovial fluid, peritoneal fluid, and amniotic fluid. For the purposes of prudent laboratory practice, however, adherence to standard precautions for the handling of all biological patient specimens is recommended. Through the use of these precautions, both the prevention of cross-transmission of infectious disease to patients and the protection of laboratory personnel from infected patients will be addressed. In most health care institutions, all patient specimens and body substances encountered during patient care are regarded as infectious and are handled by using the standard precautions policy.

The essence of any standard precautions policy is the avoidance of direct contact with patient specimens in general. When contact with any patient specimen is anticipated, health care workers should use the appropriate barrier precautions to prevent cross-transmission and exposure of their own skin and mucous membranes.

### Protection from Specimen-Borne Pathogens

Precautions against exposure to possible specimen-borne infection focus mainly on HBV, HIV, and human T cell lymphotropic viruses (HTLV). Focus on HBV and HIV transmission is emphasized, owing to the severity of illnesses due to hepatitis B and acquired immunodeficiency syndrome (AIDS)—risks to health care workers that have grave consequences.[12] There are other viruses of concern to laboratory workers; **hepatitis C virus (HCV)**, formerly known as hepatitis non-A non-B virus, is one example. It is believed, however, that the standard precautions recommended for HBV and HIV are sufficient for most pathogens in general.

**Virus Transmission.** The major infectious pathogens, HBV and HIV, may be transmitted in the laboratory directly by three main routes:

1. Percutaneous: parenteral inoculation of blood, plasma, serum, or body fluids, which can occur by accidental needle sticks, scalpel cuts, and so forth, and by transfusion of infected blood or blood products
2. Nonintact skin: transfer of infected blood, plasma, serum, or body fluids in the absence of overt punctures of the skin, through the contamination of preexisting minute cuts, scratches, abrasions, burns,

weeping or exudative skin lesions, and so forth
3. Mucous membranes: contamination of mucosal surfaces with infected blood, plasma, serum, or body fluids, as may occur with mouth pipetting, splashes, spattering, or other means of oral or nasal mucosal or conjunctival contact

HBV and HIV can be transmitted indirectly from such common inanimate surfaces as telephones, test tubes, laboratory instruments, and work surfaces that have been contaminated with infected blood or certain body fluids to areas of broken skin or mucous membranes by hand contact. HIV has been isolated from blood, semen, vaginal secretions, saliva, tears, breast milk, cerebrospinal fluid, amniotic fluid, and urine. However, only blood, semen, vaginal secretions, and breast milk have been implicated in the transmission of HIV. Hepatitis B is of special concern in laboratories of hospitals where organ transplants are done, where large volumes of blood and blood products are used. Personnel most heavily exposed to these large amounts of blood, such as blood from renal transplant patients—for example, through accidental inoculation, ingestion of blood, or inhalation of blood aerosols during laboratory work on these samples—are at the greatest risk of infection.

Hepatitis B and C viruses cause the most frequent laboratory-associated infections. As a precautionary measure against potential exposure to HBV, a licensed inactivated vaccine (HB) is recommended. The CDC's Advisory Committee on Immunization Practices (ACIP) recommends the use of this vaccine as a precautionary step for persons who are at a substantially greater risk for HBV infection—clinical laboratorians, phlebotomists, and pathologists.[8]

**Hepatitis B Virus Exposure.** After skin or mucosal exposure to blood that is known to contain or might contain hepatitis B antigen, the ACIP recommends **immunoprophylaxis**, depending on several factors. If the worker has not been vaccinated against HBV, a single dose of hepatitis B immune globulin should be given as soon as possible, within 24 hours if practical, along with doses of HB vaccine at a later date. The specific protocol for these measures will rest with the institution's infection control division. Post-vaccination testing for the development of antibody to surface HB antigen (anti-HBsAg) for persons at occupational risk who may have had needle-stick exposures necessitating post-exposure prophylaxis should be done to ensure that the vaccination has been successful.

**Hepatitis C Virus Exposure.** After exposure to blood of a patient infected or suspected of being infected with HCV, immune globulin should be given as soon as possible. No vaccine is currently available.

**Human Immunodeficiency Virus Exposure.** Transmission of HIV is believed to result from intimate contact with blood and body fluids from an infected person. Casual contact with infected persons has not been documented as a mode of transmission. If there has been occupational exposure to a potentially HIV-infected specimen or patient, the antibody status of the patient or specimen source should be determined, if it is not already known. If the source is a patient, voluntary consent should be obtained, if possible, for testing for HIV antibodies as soon as possible. High-risk exposure prophylaxis includes the use of a combination of antiretroviral agents to prevent seroconversion. **Post-exposure prophylaxis (PEP)** guidelines from the CDC are based on the determined risks of transmission (stratified as highest, increased, and no risk). Highest risk has been determined to exist when there has been occupational exposure both to a large volume of blood (as with a deep percutaneous injury or cut with a large-diameter hollow needle previously used in the source patient's vein or artery) and to blood containing a high titer of HIV (known as a high viral load), to fluids containing visible blood, or to specific other potentially infectious fluids or tissue, including semen, vaginal secretions, and cerebrospinal, peritoneal, pleural, pericardial, and amniotic fluids.[9]

An enzyme immunoassay (EIA) screening test is used to detect antibodies to HIV. Before any HIV result is considered positive, the result is confirmed by Western blot (WB) analysis. A negative antibody test for HIV does not confirm the absence of virus. There is a window period after infection with HIV during which detectable antibody is not present. In these cases, detection of antigen is important; a polymerase chain reaction (PCR) assay for HIV DNA can be used for this purpose and a p24 antigen test is used for screening blood donors for HIV antigen.

If the source patient is seronegative, the exposed worker should be screened for antibody again at 3 and 6 months. If the source patient is at high risk for HIV infection, more extensive follow-up of both the worker and the source patient may be needed.

If the source patient or specimen is HIV positive (HIV antibodies, Western blot, HIV antigen, or HIV DNA by PCR), the blood of the exposed worker should be tested for HIV antibodies within 48 hours, if possible. Exposed workers who are initially seronegative for the HIV antibody should be tested again 6 weeks after exposure. If this test is negative, the worker should be tested again at 12 weeks and 6 months after exposure. Most reported seroconversions have occurred between 6 and 12 weeks after exposure. Post-exposure prophylaxis should be started immediately and according to policies set by the institution's infection control program. A policy of "hit hard, hit early" should generally be in place.

During the early follow-up period after exposure (especially the first 6 to 12 weeks), the worker should follow the recommendations of the CDC regarding the transmission of AIDS, including[1]:

1. Refrain from donating blood or plasma.
2. Inform potential sex partners of the exposure.

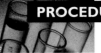

## PROCEDURE 2-1

### Hand Washing

1. Wet both hands and wrists with warm water only; do not use very hot or very cold water.

2. Apply soap from a dispenser to the palms first (about one teaspoonful).

3. Lather well and wash hands and wrists, fingernails, and between the fingers. Do this for a minimum of 10 seconds.

4. Rinse well with warm water and dry completely.

5. If the sink being used is not equipped with foot- or knee-operated controls, turn off the hand faucets with a paper towel to avoid recontamination of clean hands.

---

3. Avoid pregnancy.

4. Inform health care providers of their potential exposure, so that necessary precautions can be taken by them.

5. Do not share razors, toothbrushes, or other items that could become contaminated with blood.

6. Clean and disinfect surfaces on which blood or body fluids have spilled.

The exposed worker should be advised of and alerted to the risks of infection and evaluated medically for any history, signs, or symptoms consistent with HIV infection. Serologic testing for HIV antibodies should be made available to all health care workers who are concerned that they may have been infected with HIV.

**Tuberculosis Control.** For **tuberculosis control,** OSHA also now requires the use of certain types of masks and respirators for persons occupationally exposed to patients with suspected or confirmed cases of pulmonary tuberculosis.

### Safe Work Practices

To eliminate the risk of transmitting infectious pathogens, those working with blood specimens in the laboratory must take several precautions. Washing the hands frequently is one of the most important ways of preventing contamination. At least one sink in the laboratory should be equipped with a foot pedal for operating the faucets, and it should also have a foot pedal dispenser with a detergent solution for the hands.

**Hand Washing.** Hand washing is the most important means of interrupting transmission of infectious pathogens. Immediately after any accidental skin contact with blood, body fluids, or tissues, hands or other skin areas must be thoroughly washed. If the contact occurs through breaks in gloves, the gloves must be removed immediately and the hands thoroughly washed according to established procedure for the laboratory. It is also good practice to wash the hands any time there is visible contamination with blood or any body fluid, after completion of laboratory work and before leaving the laboratory, after removing gloves, and before any activities that involve contact with mucous membranes, eyes, or breaks in the skin.

*Hand Washing Procedure* (Procedure 2-1). Washing with soap and water is recommended, although any standard detergent product acceptable to the personnel may be used. Except in a unique situation, the use of hand towelettes and cleansing foams is not recommended, because they do not provide the necessary dilution and detergent action with the proper rinsing action to follow. No additional benefit has been established for washing with antiseptic soaps or solutions. Any product that disrupts the integrity of the skin should be avoided. Moisturizing hand creams or lotions may reduce skin irritation caused by the frequent hand washing that is so necessary.

**Food and Drink Restrictions.** Since the safety of the laboratory personnel is the reason for such scrutiny in the handling of specimens and other items, previously discussed, it is only prudent that there be no eating, drinking, smoking, or application of cosmetics in the laboratory. Hands may be contaminated with infectious organisms, which can easily be spread to the mouth during the above-mentioned activities.

### Personal Protective Equipment

**Personal protective equipment**, including that for eyes, face, head, and extremities, protective clothing, respiratory devices, and protective shields and barriers, are to be provided to laboratory personnel whenever necessary by reason of the potential hazards of processes or environment. This equipment not only should be provided but also should be maintained in a sanitary and reliable condition. OSHA requires that institutions provide their personnel with personal protective equipment.[5]

### Barrier Precautions

As discussed previously, precautions for exposure to possible specimen-borne infection focus mainly on HBV and HIV. With the emergence of multidrug-resistant strains of the bacteria causing pulmonary tuberculosis, OSHA now also requires the use of special types of masks or respirators when there will be exposure to patients with known or suspected pulmonary tuberculosis. **Protective devices** and **barrier precautions** will prevent transmission of most infectious disease if compliance is strictly maintained.

In the laboratory, the skin (especially when scratches, abrasions, dermatitis conditions, or lesions are present) and the mucous membranes of the eye, mouth, nose, and possibly the respiratory tract can be considered potential pathways for entry of infectious pathogens. Puncture with needles, sharp instruments, broken glass, or other sharp objects must be avoided. The handling and discarding of these objects must be done carefully and in a consistent manner. Constant vigilance and care must be exercised in the handling of infected cell-culture liquid or other virus-containing materials. Barrier precautions are implemented to prevent exposure to infectious pathogens.

**Gloves.** Protective gloves must be worn by all persons who engage in procedures that involve direct contact of skin with biological specimens. The implementation of standard precautionary practices is recommended for handling clinical specimens, body fluids, and tissues from humans or from infected or inoculated laboratory animals.

Gloves must be manufactured from the appropriate material, usually intact latex, of the appropriate quality for the procedures required, and of the appropriate size for each health care worker. Gloves should be thrown away and not washed and used again. Since barrier protection is the ultimate goal, gloves must be discarded if they are peeling, cracking, or discolored (indications of deterioration), or if they have tears or punctures. Proper discarding of used gloves is necessary.

Gloves are worn during phlebotomies and during the processing of body fluid and blood specimens in the laboratory. After the gloves are removed and discarded, the hands must be washed immediately.

**Gowns.** All laboratory workers should wear a long-sleeved laboratory coat or gown with a closed front. Gowns and coats worn in the laboratory should be removed when the worker leaves. If personnel desire to wear a laboratory coat out of the laboratory, it is recommended that they have coats of different colors—one color to be worn in the laboratory (considered to be contaminated) and a different color to be worn outside the laboratory (considered to be noncontaminated).

When splashes to the skin or clothing are likely to occur, a special protective gown, apron, or laboratory coat must be worn. This protective clothing should be manufactured of fluid-proof or fluid-resistant material and should protect all areas of exposed skin.

**Masks and Eye Protectors.** When contamination of mucosal membranes (mouth, eyes, or nose) is likely to occur, the use of masks and protective eye wear or face shields is required. Such contamination can occur with body fluid splashes or aerosolization. Protective eye wear should be worn for transferring blood from a collection syringe into the specimen container, for example. Potential splashes can also occur when chemicals are being used. Certain laboratory reagents are known to be especially caustic to the mucosa. Broken glassware projectiles and vapors from some chemicals can also cause serious eye injuries. The eyes should always be protected with goggles when glassware is being cleaned with analytic cleaners and when laboratory reagents are being prepared from strong acids or bases or any other hazardous material.

**Respirators or Masks for Tuberculosis Control.** A person must be exposed to the tuberculosis bacterium to be infected. This occurs through close contact over a period of time, when contaminated droplet nuclei from an infected person's respiratory tract enter another person's respiratory tract. A common-sense way to control transmission of these contaminated droplets is to cover the mouth during coughing and to use tissues. In addition, certain specialized types of masks or respirators are now OSHA-mandated for use by persons who are occupationally exposed to patients with suspected or confirmed cases of pulmonary tuberculosis. A "Special Respiratory Precautions" sign should identify rooms where there are patients fitting this criterion. Health care personnel caring for these patients must be fitted with and trained to use the proper respirator.

### Protection From Aerosols

Biohazards are generally treated with great respect in the clinical laboratory. The adverse effects of pathogenic substances on the body are well documented. The presence of pathogenic organisms is not limited to the culture plates in the microbiology laboratory. Airborne infectious particles, or **aerosols**, can be found in all areas of the laboratory where human specimens are used.

**Biosafety Cabinets.** Biosafety cabinets are protective workplace devices used to control the presence of infectious agents in the air. Microbiology laboratories selectively utilize biological safety cabinets for performing procedures that generate infectious aerosols. Several common procedures in the processing of specimens for culture—grinding, mincing, vortexing, centrifuging, and preparation of direct smears—are known to produce aerosol droplets. Air containing the infectious agent is sterilized by heat or ultraviolet light or, most commonly, by passage through a high-efficiency particulate air (HEPA) filter. Biosafety cabinets not only remove air contaminants through a local exhaust system but provide an added measure of safety by confining the aerosol contaminant within an enclosed area, thereby isolating it from the worker.

**Specimen Processing Protection.** Specimens should be transported to the laboratory in plastic leak-proof bags. Protective gloves should always be worn for handling biological specimens of any kind.

Substances can become airborne when the stopper (cap) is popped off a blood-collecting container, a serum sample is poured from one tube to another, or a serum tube is centrifuged. When the cap is being removed from a specimen tube or a blood collection tube, the top should be covered with a disposable gauze pad or a special protective pad. Gauze pads with an impermeable plastic coating on one side can reduce contamination of gloves. The tube should be held away from the body and the cap gently twisted to remove it. Snapping off the cap or top can cause some of the contents to aerosolize. When not in place on the tube, the cap should still be kept in the gauze and not placed directly on the work surface or counter top.

Specially constructed plastic splash shields are used in many laboratories for the processing of blood specimens. The tube caps are removed behind or under the shield, which acts as a barrier between the person and the specimen tube. This is designed to prevent aerosols from entering the nose, eyes, or mouth. Laboratory safety boxes are commercially available and can be used for unstoppering tubes or doing other procedures that might cause spattering. Splash shields and safety boxes should be periodically decontaminated.

When specimens are being centrifuged, the tube caps should always be kept on the tubes. Centrifuge covers must be used and left on until the centrifuge stops. The centrifuge should be allowed to stop by itself and not be manually stopped by the worker.

Another step that should be taken to lessen the hazard from aerosols is to exercise caution in handling pipettes and other equipment used to transfer human specimens, especially pathogenic materials. These materials should be discarded properly and carefully.

## Other Hazards

The fact that clinical laboratories present many potential hazards simply because of the nature of the work done there cannot be overemphasized. In addition to biological hazards, open flames, electrical equipment, glassware, chemicals of varying reactivity, flammable solvents, and toxic fumes are but a few of the other hazards present in the clinical laboratory.

### Flammable Substances

One serious hazard in laboratory work is the potential for fire and explosion when flammable solvents such as ether and acetone are used. These materials should always be stored in spe-

---

**BOX 2-1**

**Seven Rules for Biosafety in the Laboratory**

1. Never mouth-pipette.
2. Treat infectious fluids carefully to avoid spills and to minimize aerosolization.
3. Restrict use of needles and syringes to procedures in which there is no alternative; use needles, lancets, and other "sharps" carefully to avoid self-inoculation; dispose of sharps in leak- and puncture-resistant containers.
4. Use protective laboratory coats and gloves.
5. Wash hands frequently: after all laboratory activities, after removing gloves, and immediately after contact with infectious materials.
6. Decontaminate work surfaces before and after use; wipe up any spills immediately.
7. Never eat, drink, store food, or smoke in the laboratory.

---

cial safety containers in an appropriate storage cabinet. Even with proper storage of these materials, there is always some release of flammable vapors in a working laboratory. A good ventilation system for the room and vent sites for the storage area will help to eliminate some of the potential hazard. When flammable materials are being used, proper precautions must be taken; for instance, flammable liquids should be poured from one container to another slowly, they should never be used when there is an open flame in the room, and they should be kept in closed containers when they are not being used.

### Chemical Hazards

Other sources of injury in the laboratory are poisonous, volatile, caustic, or corrosive reagents, such as strong acids or bases. Chemicals and reagents can present different types of hazards. Some are dangerous when inhaled (sulfuric acid), some are corrosive to the skin (phenol), some are caustic (acetic acid), some are volatile (many solvents), and some combine these hazards. Acids and bases should be stored separately in well-ventilated storage units. When not in use, all chemicals and reagents should be returned to their storage units. Bottles of particularly volatile substances should not be left open for extended periods.

OSHA is also involved in setting standards directed at minimizing occupational **exposures to hazardous chemicals** in laboratories. The OSHA hazard communication standard (the **employee "right-to-know" rule**) is designed to ensure that laboratory workers are fully aware of the hazards associated with chemicals in their workplaces.[6] This OSHA-mandated program became law in January 1991. The occupational exposure to chemical hazards law necessitates the development of comprehensive plans at each work site to implement safety measures throughout the laboratory insofar as the use of laboratory chemicals is concerned. A **chemical hygiene plan** for each laboratory must outline the specific work practices and procedures that are necessary to protect workers from any health hazards associated with hazardous chemicals. Information and training regarding hazardous chemicals must be provided to all workers in the laboratory setting. The individual states have also enacted "right-to-know" laws to ensure that available information is disseminated at the local level.

Information about signs and symptoms associated with exposure to hazardous chemicals used in the laboratory must be communicated to all. Reference materials for this information are included in the **material safety data sheets (MSDS)** provided by all chemical manufacturers and suppliers. This information concerns hazards, safe handling, storage, and disposal of hazardous chemicals used in the laboratory.

**Material Safety Data Sheets.** Information is provided by chemical manufacturers and suppliers about each chemical. This information is to accompany the shipment of all chemicals and should be available for anyone to review. Each laboratory must have on file all MSDSs for the hazardous chemicals used in that laboratory. Use of MSDSs is a common way that potential product hazard information is made available, and OSHA requires their provision by all chemical manufacturers. The health care facility, in turn, is required to provide this information to its workers in the laboratory.

Each MSDS contains basic information about the specific chemical or product. Trade name, chemical name and synonyms, chemical family, manufacturer's name and address, emergency telephone number for further information about the chemical, hazardous ingredients, physical data, fire and explosion data, and health hazard and protection information are included for each chemical.

**Protection.** When any potentially hazardous solution or chemical is being used, protective equipment for the eyes, face, head, and extremities, as well as protective clothing or barriers, should be used. Volatile or fuming solutions should be used under a fume hood. In case of accidental contact with a hazardous solution or a contaminated substance, quick action is essential. The laboratory should have a safety shower where quick, all-over decontamination can take place immediately. Another safety device that is essential in all laboratories is a face or eye washer that streams aerated water directly onto the face and eyes to prevent burns and loss of eyesight. Any action of this sort must be undertaken immediately, so these safety devices must be present in the laboratory area.

Measures to limit exposure to hazardous chemicals must be implemented. Appropriate work practices, emergency procedures, and personal protective equipment are to be employed by all. Many of the measures taken are also those needed for protection from biologica hazards, as discussed previously (see under Personal Protective Equipment). These measures include the use of gloves, keeping the work area clean and uncluttered, the proper and complete labeling of all chemicals, and the use of proper eye protection, fume hood, respiratory equipment, and any other emergency or protective equipment as necessary.

Chemical waste must be deposited in appropriately labeled receptacles for eventual disposal.

**Specific Hazardous Chemicals.** Some specific chemicals that must be handled with care, and some potential hazards in their use, are as follows:

- *Sulfuric acid:* at a concentration above 65% may cause blindness; may produce burns on the skin; if taken orally may cause severe burns, depending on the concentration.
- *Nitric acid:* gives off yellow fumes that are extremely toxic and damaging to tissues; overexposure to vapor can cause death, loss of eyesight, extreme irritation, smarting, itching, and yellow discoloration of the skin; if taken orally can cause extreme burns, may perforate the stomach wall, or cause death.
- *Acetic acid:* severely caustic; continuous exposure to vapor can lead to chronic bronchitis.
- *Hydrochloric acid:* inhalation of vapors should be avoided; any acid on the skin should be washed away immediately to prevent a burn.
- *Sodium hydroxide:* extremely hazardous in contact with the skin, eyes, or mucous membranes (mouth), causing caustic burns; dangerous even at very low concentrations; any contact necessitates immediate care.
- *Phenol (a disinfectant):* can cause caustic burns or contact dermatitis even in dilute solutions; wash off skin with water or alcohol.
- *Carbon tetrachloride:* damaging to the liver even at an exposure level where there is no discernible odor.
- *Trichloroacetic acid:* very severely caustic; respiratory tract irritant.
- *Ethers:* cause depression of central nervous system.

**Select Carcinogens.** These are substances regulated by OSHA as carcinogens. **Carcinogens** are any substances that cause the development of cancerous growths in living tissue; they are considered hazardous to people working with them in laboratories. When possible, substances that are potentially carcinogenic have been replaced by ones that are less hazardous. If necessary, with the proper safeguards in place, potentially carcinogenic substances can be used in the laboratory. Lists of potential carcinogens used in a particular laboratory must be available to all who work there. These lists can be long.

**Hazard Warning.** A **hazard identification system** was developed by the National Fire Protection Association.[4] This system provides at a glance, in words, symbols, and pictures, information on the potential health, flammability, and chemical reactivity hazards of materials used in the laboratory. This information is provided on the labels of all containers of hazardous chemicals.

The hazard identification system consists of four small, diamond-shaped symbols grouped into a larger diamond shape (Fig. 2-2). The top diamond is red and indicates a flammability hazard. The diamond on the right is yellow and indicates a reactivity-stability hazard. These materials are capable of explosion or violent chemical reactions. The diamond on the left is blue and indicates a possible health hazard. The diamond on the bottom is white and provides special hazard information. It can provide information about radioactivity, special biohazards, and other dangerous elements. The system also indicates the severity of the hazard by using numerical designations from 4 to 0, with 4 being extremely hazardous and 0 being no hazard.

### Electrical Hazards

Shocks from electrical apparatus in the clinical laboratory are a common source of injury if one is not aware of the potential hazard. This may be one of the most serious hazards in the laboratory.

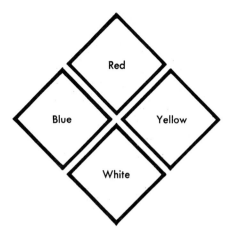

**FIG 2-2.** Identification system of the National Fire Protection Association. (From Kaplan LA, Pesce AJ: *Clinical Chemistry: Theory, Analysis, and Correlation,* ed 3. St Louis, Mosby, 1996.)

The important thing to understand with respect to danger to the human body is the effect of an electrical current. Current flows when there is a difference in potential between two points, and this knowledge is used in determining the approach to safety in the use of electrical equipment. Grounding of all electrical equipment is essential. If there is no path to ground, such a path might be established through the human in contact with the apparatus, resulting in serious injury. Attempts to repair or inspect a disabled electrical device should be left to someone who is trained to do this work.

## Hazards With Glassware

The use of many kinds of glassware is basic to work in the clinical laboratory. Caution must be used to prevent unnecessary or accidental breakage. Some types of glassware can be repaired, but most glassware used today is discarded when it is broken. Any broken or cracked glassware should be discarded in a special container for broken glass, and not thrown into the regular waste container. Common sense should be used in storing glassware, with heavy pieces being placed on the lower shelves and tall pieces being placed behind smaller pieces. Shelves should be placed at reasonable heights; glassware should not be stored out of reach. Broken or cracked glassware is the cause of many lacerations, and care should be taken to avoid this laboratory hazard.

## Fire Hazards

Various types of fire-extinguishing agents must be available and their use must be understood. Fire in clothing should be smothered with a fire blanket or heavy toweling, or the flame should be beaten out; it should not be flooded with water. Everyone in the laboratory should know the correct use of the fire alarm and the procedure to follow in the event of a fire (see under Emergency Precautions).

## Pipetting Safeguards: Automatic Pipetting Devices

It is a generally accepted rule that all pipetting must be done by mechanical means, either mechanical suction or aspirator bulbs. This procedure guards against burning the mouth with caustic reagents and against contamination by pathogenic organisms in samples. All specimens of human origin that are used in the laboratory (blood, urine, spinal fluid, stools, and so on) should be considered potentially infectious. To eliminate the use of aspirator bulbs and to provide increased pipetting accuracy, a form of automatic pipetting device is frequently used. Such devices offer fast, accurate ways of dispensing repetitive volumes. They can be set to deliver volumes in different ranges, depending on the device used. In general, a syringe reservoir is filled with the reagent to be measured, the volume to be delivered is determined by setting the dispenser dial, and the dispensing button is depressed to deliver the amount selected. The syringe mechanisms are usually autoclavable, and the pipette tips are disposable. Another device, a bottle top dispenser, can be used to deliver repetitive aliquots of reagents. Such a device is designed as a bottle-mounted system that can dispense repetitive selected volumes in an easy, precise manner. It is usually trouble free and requires a minimum of maintenance.

# DECONTAMINATION

It is important to keep the laboratory workplace in a clean and sanitary condition. Cleaning and **decontamination** of the working surfaces after contact with blood or other potentially infectious materials are of prime importance. Most disinfectants are less active in the presence of high concentrations of protein. Because blood and other body fluids contain high concentrations of protein, these specimens, if spilled, should first be absorbed as completely as possible with disposable towels or gauze pads prior to disinfection. After absorption of the liquid, all contaminated materials (paper towels, etc.) should be discarded as **biohazard waste**. After absorption, the spill site should be cleaned with an aqueous detergent solution, and then disinfected with a high-level hospital **disinfectant** such as a dilution of **household bleach**.

## Use of Bleach

Sodium hypochlorite, liquid household bleach, is often used as an intermediate-level disinfectant. Dilutions of bleach—a 0.5% solution made from a 5% solution (one part 5% sodium hypochlorite and nine parts water)—should be made up fresh weekly to prevent the loss of germicidal action during prolonged storage.

To clean up the laboratory work area, a strong bleach solution can be used for any spills of biological materials. Desk tops can be cleaned daily with a dilute solution of bleach. Any contaminated laboratory ware that must be reused cannot be cleaned with bleach, because it corrodes stainless steel containers and coagulates proteins. A strong detergent solution such as 3% phenolic detergent can be used before autoclaving. Contaminated pipettes should be placed in long horizontal covered trays that are deep enough to minimize the chance of spilling when they are transported to the autoclave.

## Autoclaves

Material that is to be autoclaved should be loosely packed so the steam can circulate freely around it. Autoclaving depends on humidity, temperature, and time. Under pressure, steam becomes hotter than boiling water and kills bacteria much more quickly. Autoclaves must be used with caution.

Autoclaves should be monitored regularly for their performance in adequately sterilizing the materials to be decontaminated. This monitoring procedure should be part of the ongoing quality assurance program for the laboratory.

# LABORATORY WASTE DISPOSAL

OSHA standards provide for the implementation of a **waste disposal program**.[11] Receptacles used for the disposal of medical wastes should be manufactured from leak-proof materials and be maintained in a sanitary condition. The purpose of waste disposal control is to confine or isolate any possible hazardous material from all workers—laboratory personnel as well as custodial and housekeeping personnel. The NCCLS has also published guidelines on management of clinical laboratory waste.[3]

## Infectious Waste

OSHA has defined **infectious waste** as blood and blood products, contaminated sharps, pathologic wastes, and microbiological wastes. Infectious waste is to be packaged for disposal in color-coded containers and should be labeled as such with the universal symbol for biohazards. Final disposal is by incineration or autoclaving.

## Containers for Waste

Containers must be easily accessible to personnel needing them and must be located in the laboratory areas where they are commonly used. They should be constructed in such a manner that their contents will not be spilled if the container is tipped over accidentally.

## Sharps Containers

After use, disposable syringes and needles, scalpel blades, and other sharp items should be placed in puncture-resistant **sharps containers** for disposal. The most widespread control measure required by OSHA and NCCLS is the use of puncture-resistant sharps containers.[5,9] The primary purpose of using these containers is to eliminate the need for anyone to transport needles and other sharps while looking for a place to discard them. Sharps containers are to be located in the patient areas as well as being conveniently placed in the laboratory. Use of the special sharps container permits quick disposal of a needle without recapping. This supports the recommendation against recapping, bending, breaking, or otherwise manipulating any sharp needle or lancet device by hand. Most needlestick accidents have occurred during recapping of a needle after a phlebotomy. If a needle must be recapped, it should be done in a one-handed fashion with one hand held behind the back. Injuries also can occur to housekeeping personnel when contaminated sharps are left on a bed, concealed in linen, or disposed of improperly in a waste receptacle. Most accidental disposal-related exposures can be eliminated by the use of sharps containers.

## Biohazard Containers

Body fluid specimens, including blood, must be placed in well-constructed **biohazard containers** with secure lids to prevent leakage during transport and for future disposal. Contaminated specimens and other materials used in laboratory tests should be decontaminated before reprocessing for disposal or should be placed in special impervious bags for disposal in accordance with established waste removal policies. If outside contamination of the bag is likely, a second bag should be used.

Hazardous specimens and potentially hazardous substances should be tagged and identified as such. The tag should read "biohazard," or the biological hazard symbol should be used. All persons working in the laboratory area must be informed about the meaning of the tags and about what precautions should be taken for each.

Contaminated equipment must be placed in a designated area for storage, washing, decontamination, or disposal. With the increased use of disposable protective clothing, gloves, and so forth, the volume of waste for discard will be on the increase.

## Biohazard Bags

Plastic bags are appropriate for disposal of most infectious waste materials, but rigid, impermeable containers should be used for disposal of sharps and broken glassware. Plastic bags with the biohazard symbols and lettering prominently visible can be used in secondary metal or plastic containers. These containers can be decontaminated or disposed of on a regular basis or immediately when visibly contaminated. These biohazard containers should be used for all blood, body fluids, tissues, and other disposable materials contaminated with infectious agents and should be handled with gloves.

## Final Decontamination of Waste Materials

Final decontamination of materials in bags or containers is done by either incineration or autoclaving, either off or on site.

Disposal of medical waste should be done by licensed organizations that will ensure that no environmental contamination or anything aesthetically displeasing occurs. Congress has passed various acts and regulations regarding the proper handling of medical waste to assist the Environmental Protection Agency (EPA) to carry out this process in the most prudent fashion.

## BASIC FIRST AID PROCEDURES

Since there are so many potential hazards in a clinical laboratory, it is easy to understand why a knowledge of **basic first aid** should be an

## BOX 2-2

General Rules for Safety in the Clinical Laboratory

1. Know where the fire extinguishers are located, the different types for specific types of fires, and how to use them properly.
2. Pipette all solutions by using mechanical suction or an aspirator bulb. Never use mouth suction.
3. Handle all flammable solvents and fuming reagents under a fume hood. Store in a well-ventilated cabinet.
4. Use an explosion-proof refrigerator to store ether. Never use ether near an open flame. It is highly flammable.
5. Do not use any flammable substance near an open flame.
6. Wear gloves when handling infectious substances or toxic substances such as bromine or cyanide.
7. Mercury is poisonous. Contact supervisor; institution-specific protocol for cleanup of mercury is necessary.
8. If glass tubing is to be cut, hold the tubing with a towel to prevent cuts of the hands. This precaution also applies to putting a piece of glass tubing through a rubber stopper.
9. Use extreme caution when handling laboratory glassware. Broken glass is probably the greatest source of injury in the laboratory. Immediately discard cracked or broken glassware in a separate container, not with other waste.
10. If strong acids or bases are spilled, wipe them up immediately, using copious amounts of water and great care. Keep sodium bicarbonate on hand to assist in neutralizing acid spillage.
11. Plainly label all laboratory bottles, specimens, and other materials. When a reagent bottle is no longer being used, store it away in its proper place.
12. Put away safely or cover any equipment that is not being used.
13. Replace covers, tops, or corks on all reagent bottles as soon as they are no longer being used. Never use a reagent from a bottle that is not properly labeled.
14. If water is spilled on the floor, wipe it up immediately. Serious injuries can result from falls caused by slipping on a wet floor.
15. Never taste any chemical. Smell chemicals only when necessary and then only by fanning the vapor of the chemical toward the nose.
16. When handling blades or needles, use extreme caution to avoid cuts and infections. Dispose of all blades and needles in sharps containers.
17. Always pour acid into water for dilution. Never pour water into acid. Pour strong acids or bases slowly down the side of the receiving vessel to prevent splashing.
18. Use standard precautions when obtaining any specimen from a patient. Handle blood, serum, plasma, cerebrospinal fluid, urine, or any other patient specimen carefully, as if it were infectious. Severe infections and illnesses can result from handling specimens carelessly.
19. Wear gloves when handling any biological specimen.
20. Wash hands frequently while working in the laboratory, especially after handling patient specimens or reagents. Always wash hands before leaving the laboratory.

## BOX 2-2

General Rules for Safety in the Clinical Laboratory—*cont'd*

21. Wear safety goggles when preparing reagents with strong chemicals. Some states (e.g., Minnesota) have enacted laws that require students, teachers, and visitors in educational institutions who are participating in or observing activities in eye-protection areas (areas where work is performed that is potentially hazardous to the eyes) to wear devices to protect their eyes.

22. In case of severe fire or burns, know where the safety shower is located and how to operate it.

23. Know the location of a fire blanket, which is used to smother flames in case of fire.

24. Most hospitals and teaching institutions have some type of warning signal and a procedure to follow in the event of a fire. This procedure should be understood thoroughly by anyone working in such an institution, whether as a student or as an employee. These institutions also have disaster plans, with which every worker must be thoroughly familiar.

25. When using burners and other heating devices, keep them far enough away from the working area that there is no possibility that anything will catch on fire.

26. Never lean over an open flame. Extinguish flames when not in use.

27. Learn the procedure used in the laboratory for discarding hazardous substances such as strong acids and bases.

28. Never pour volatile liquids or hazardous waste chemicals down a sink drain. Disposal of waste chemicals must be handled according to chemical hygiene protocol established by the facility.

29. To free a frozen glass stopper, run hot water over it, tap it lightly with a towel wrapped around it, or grasp it with a rubber glove or tourniquet.

30. Wear gloves when cleaning glassware, in case there is broken glass in the sink or soaking bucket.

31. Handle all hot objects with tongs, not hands. Extremely hot objects are to be handled with asbestos gloves.

32. If contaminated materials such as human specimens or bacterial agents are spilled on the work area, discard the contaminated material properly and wipe off the work area with bleach solution or other laboratory disinfectant.

33. Primary specimen (blood, primarily) collection tubes should be centrifuged with the caps left on them or by using sealed centrifuge cups for specimens without caps.

34. Cover all centrifuges to avoid flying broken glass and aerosols. Do not open centrifuges before they have stopped. Do not stop the centrifuge head by hand.

35. Be familiar with the OSHA rules and regulations, and be ready for an inspection by OSHA.

integral part of any educational program in clinical laboratory medicine. The first emphasis should be on removal of the accident victim from further injury; the next involves definitive action or first aid to the victim. By definition, first aid is "the immediate care given to a person who has been injured or suddenly taken ill." Any person who attempts to perform first aid before professional treatment by a physician can

be arranged should remember that such assistance is only a stopgap—an emergency treatment to be followed until the physician arrives. Stop bleeding, prevent shock, and then treat the wound—in that order.

A rule to remember in dealing with emergencies in the laboratory is to keep calm. This is not always easy to do, but it is very important to the well-being of the victim. Keep crowds of people

---

**PROCEDURE 2-2**

*First Aid for Skin Puncture or Mucosal Contamination*

1. For skin puncture or surface skin contamination, wash skin site with soap and water while encouraging bleeding. If appropriate, bandage the site. Report incident to supervisor.

2. For contaminated mucosal or conjunctival sites, wash with large amounts of water for an extended period of time. Report incident to supervisor.

---

away, and give the victim plenty of fresh air. Because so many of the possible injuries are of an extreme nature and because in the event of such an injury immediate care is most critical, application of the proper first-aid procedures must be thoroughly understood by every person in the medical laboratory. A few of the more common emergencies and the appropriate first-aid procedures are listed below. These should be learned by every student or person working in the laboratory.

1. *Alkali or acid burns on the skin or in the mouth:* Rinse thoroughly with large amounts of running tap water. If the burns are serious, consult a physician.

2. *Alkali or acid burns in the eye:* Wash out thoroughly with running water for a minimum of 15 minutes. Help the victim by holding the eyelid open so that the water can make contact with the eye. An eye fountain is recommended for this purpose, but any running water will suffice. Use of an eyecup is discouraged. A physician should be notified immediately, while the eye is being washed.

3. *Heat burns:* Apply cold running water (or ice in water) to relieve the pain and to stop further tissue damage. Use a wet dressing of 2 tablespoons of sodium bicarbonate in 1 quart of warm water. Bandage securely but not tightly. In the case of a third-degree burn (the skin is burned off), do not use ointments or grease, and consult a physician immediately.

4. *Minor cuts:* Wash carefully and thoroughly with soap and water. Remove all foreign material, such as glass, that projects from the wound, but do not gouge for embedded material. Removal is best accomplished by careful washing. Apply a clean bandage if necessary (see Procedure 2-2).

5. *Serious cuts:* Direct pressure should be applied to the cut area to control the bleeding, using the hand over a clean compress covering the wound. Call for a physician immediately.

In cases of serious laboratory accidents, such as burns, medical assistance should be summoned while first aid is being administered. For general accidents, competent medical help should be sought as soon as possible after the first-aid treatment has been completed. In cases of chemical burns, especially when the eyes are involved, speed in treatment is most essential. Remember that first aid is useful not only in your working environment, but at home and in your community. It deserves your earnest attention and study.

## REFERENCES

1. CDC update: provisional public health service recommendations for chemoprophylaxis after occupational exposure to HIV. *MMWR* 1996; 45:468-472.
2. Centers for Disease Control and Prevention (CDC): Hospital Infection Control Practices Advisory Committee (HICPAC), *Guidelines for Isolation Precautions in Hospitals*, 1996.

3. *Clinical Laboratory Waste Management: Approved Guideline.* Villanova, Pa, National Committee for Clinical Laboratory Standards, 1993, NCCLS document GP5-A.

4. National Fire Protection Association: *Hazardous Chemical Data.* Boston, National Fire Protection Association, 1975, no 49.

5. Occupational Safety and Health Administration (Department of Labor): Occupational exposure to bloodborne pathogens: final rule. *Federal Register* 29 CFR part 1910.1030(235), 64003-64182, Dec 6, 1991.

6. Occupational Safety and Health Administration (Department of Labor): Occupational exposure to hazardous chemicals in laboratories: final rule. *Federal Register* 29 CFR part 1910.1450, 55(21), 3327-3335, Jan 31, 1990.

7. Occupational safety and health standards. *Federal Register* 1978; 43(Oct 24, Nov 17).

8. Protection against viral hepatitis: recommendations of the Immunization Practices Advisory Committee. *MMWR* 1990; 39:1-23.

9. *Protection of Laboratory Workers from Infectious Disease Transmitted by Blood, Body Fluids, and Tissue: Tentative Guideline*, ed 2. Villanova, Pa, National Committee for Clinical Laboratory Standards, 1991, NCCLS document M29-T2.

10. Recommendations for prevention of HIV transmission in health-care setting. *MMWR* 1987; 36(suppl):3s.

11. Standards for the tracking and management of medical waste: interim final rule and request for comments. *Federal Register* 1989; 40(March 24): 12326.

12. Update: universal precautions for prevention of transmission of human immunodeficiency virus, hepatitis B virus, and other bloodborne pathogens in health-care settings. *MMWR* 1988; 37:377.

## BIBLIOGRAPHY

*Clinical Laboratory Safety: Approved Guideline.* Villanova, Pa, National Committee for Clinical Laboratory Standards, 1996, GP17-A.

Henry JB (ed): *Clinical Diagnosis and Management by Laboratory Methods*, ed 19. Philadelphia, WB Saunders Co, 1996.

Kaplan LA, Pesce AJ: *Clinical Chemistry: Theory, Analysis, and Correlation*, ed. 3, St Louis, Mosby, 1996.

## STUDY QUESTIONS

1. Which of the following acts, agencies, or organizations is primarily responsible for safeguards and regulations to ensure a safe and healthful workplace?

   A. Healthcare Finance Administration (HCFA)
   B. Occupational Safety and Health Administration (OSHA)
   C. Clinical Laboratory Improvement Act, 1988 '(CLIA '88)
   D. Centers for Disease Control and Prevention (CDC)

2. The OSHA hazard communication standard, the "right to know rule," is designed for what purpose?

3. To comply with various federal safety regulations, each laboratory must have which of the following? (More than one of the answers may be correct.)

   A. A chemical hygiene plan
   B. A safety manual
   C. Biohazard labels in place
   D. An infection control plan

4. What is the essence of any standard precautions policy?

5. If it is likely that an employee has been exposed to blood or any other potentially HBV-infected material, to what preventive measure is the employee entitled free of charge?

6. What is the single most important procedure that can be performed to prevent the transmission of most infectious agents?

7. If a chemical spill occurs, what is one important source of information about the potential hazards resulting from exposure to that chemical? Explain how this source is used.

8. What is the main purpose of any waste disposal program in place in the laboratory?

# CHAPTER 3

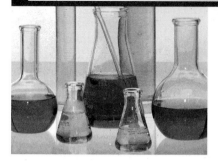

# Collecting and Processing Laboratory Specimens

## Learning Objectives

*From study of this chapter, the reader will be able to:*

➢ Appreciate the skills needed to interact with patients in the collection of specimens and the importance of the Patient's Bill of Rights.

➢ Understand the use of standard precautions and transmission-based precautions policies.

➢ Know the proper collection technique for venous blood.

➢ Know the proper collection technique for capillary or peripheral blood.

➢ Identify common anticoagulants and additives used to preserve blood specimens.

➢ Know the preferred urine specimen for a routine urinalysis, storage requirements for it, and the difference between the various types of urine collection—clean-catch, midstream, quantitative, and timed.

➢ Explain collection procedures for other body fluid specimens—cerebrospinal, pleural, synovial, and so forth.

➢ Collect a throat swab for culture.

➢ Collect feces for occult blood ("hidden" blood) tests and other tests.

➢ Know the importance of general specimen collection requirements prior to analysis—transport, processing, and storage.

**General Specimen Requirements**
    Quality Assurance Considerations
    Patient Identification
    Labels
**Use of Standard Precautions and Transmission-Based Precautions**
**Isolation Techniques**
    Protective Isolation
**Types of Specimens Collected**
    Blood: General Collection Information
        Circulation of Blood
        The Phlebotomist
        Approaching the Patient
        Types of Collection Procedures
        Capillary or Peripheral Blood
            Collection by Skin Puncture
        Venous Blood Collection by
            Venipuncture
        Additives and Anticoagulants
        Laboratory Processing of Blood
            Specimens
        Appearance of Processed
            Specimens
        Storage of Processed Specimens
    Urine: General Collection Information
        Types of Urine Collection
        Containers for Urine Collection
        Preservation of Urine Specimens
        Collecting Urine Specimens
    Body Cavity Fluids (Extravascular)
        Cerebrospinal Fluid
        Synovial Fluid
        Pericardial, Pleural, and Peritoneal
            Fluids
    Swabs for Culture
        Throat Culture Collection
    Feces
    Other Specimens
**Chain-of-Custody Specimen
    Information**
**Specimen Transportation**
    Shipping Specimens to Reference
        Laboratories

# GENERAL SPECIMEN REQUIREMENTS

The laboratory test can be no better than the specimen on which it is performed. If the specimen is improperly collected, not stored correctly, or mishandled in some way, the most quantitatively perfect determination is of no use because the results are invalid and cannot be used by the physician in diagnosis or treatment.

All samples sent to the laboratory must be processed according to certain established policies. Each division of the laboratory has unique requirements for specimens used in that division, but several general considerations apply to all specimens. Special requirements for the collection, preservation, and processing of laboratory specimens are discussed where appropriate in subsequent chapters.

## Quality Assurance Considerations

The term **quality assurance** is used to describe management of the treatment of the whole patient. As it applies to the clinical laboratory, quality assurance requires establishing policies that maintain and control, as much as possible, the many processes that involve the patient and any laboratory results for that patient. It includes properly preparing the patient for any specimens to be collected, collecting valid samples, correctly performing the laboratory analyses needed, validating the test results, correctly recording and reporting the test results, and getting those results into the patient's record. Another very important aspect of quality assurance is the policy regarding how records describing quality assurance practices and quality control measures used for laboratory analyses are documented, maintained, and made available, if needed, for review.

The purpose of a quality assurance policy is to make certain that over a long period of time, the laboratory provides reliable data that accurately reflect the status of the patient. Since physicians use laboratory test data to make diagnoses and to determine courses of therapy, it is essential that the results be reliable. As stated previously, the accuracy of a test result begins with the quality of the specimen received by the laboratory. The quality of a specimen depends on how it was collected, transported, and processed. The person collecting any patient specimen has the responsibility of ensuring that the collection is done in the best manner possible. By following established policy and with training and experience, specimens can be collected that will yield valid results, thus ensuring high-quality patient care.

## Patient Identification

Initial identification of the patient is extremely important. It is essential that a specimen from a particular patient be collected in the appropriate container and labeled for that patient. The patient's name, unique identification number and room number or clinic, and date and time of collection are commonly found on the label. All specimens sent to the laboratory must be properly labeled. For some tests, labels must include the time of collection of the specimen and the type of specimen. A properly completed request form should accompany all specimens sent to the laboratory.

## Labels

Quality assurance policies are implemented in the clinical laboratory to protect the patient from any adverse consequences of errors resulting from an improperly handled specimen—beginning with the collection of that specimen. Laboratory quality assurance and accreditation require that specimens be properly labeled at the time of collection.

An unlabeled container or one labeled improperly should not be accepted by the laboratory. Specimens are considered improperly labeled when there is incomplete or no patient identification on the tube or container holding the specimen. Many specimen containers are transported in leak-proof plastic bags. It is not acceptable that only the plastic bags be labeled—the container actually holding the specimen must also be labeled. If the identification is illegible, the specimen is also unacceptable. In laboratories where computers are used, labels are computer generated, which assists in making certain that the proper identification information is included for each patient. Bar-coded labels facilitate this process. A specimen is unacceptable if the specimen container identification does not match exactly the identification on the request form for that specimen. Each laboratory has a specific protocol for the handling of mislabeled or "unacceptable" specimens.

All specimen containers must be labeled by the person doing the collection, to ensure that the specimen is actually collected from the patient whose identification is on the label.

## USE OF STANDARD PRECAUTIONS AND TRANSMISSION-BASED PRECAUTIONS

With the use of **standard precautions (formerly known as universal precautions)** the need for the isolation category called "blood and body fluid isolation" (formerly referred to as "strict isolation") has been for the most part eliminated. The Centers for Disease Control and Prevention (CDC) recommends several disease-specific precautionary policies for patients known to be or suspected of being infected with certain pathogens.[6] With strict adherence to standard precautions, all sources of specimens (patients) are considered potentially pathogenic or infectious; that is, all specimens are treated in the same way. The use of proper personal protective equipment and barriers to prevent transmission of infectious agents is discussed in Chapter 2.

For known airborne pathogens (such as tuberculosis) or other highly communicable diseases that are spread by airborne or contact routes, specific additional **transmission-based precautions** should be taken for specimen collection. Respirators designed to control transmission of tuberculosis should be worn to enter the patient's room. CDC transmission-based precautions apply for patients (1) with known specific infection or suspected to be infected with specific microorganisms spread by airborne, droplet, or contact routes of transmission and (2) during the incubation period of certain easily transmitted diseases. The individual health care facility will initiate its specific precautions policies. Always follow the procedure of the hospital or patient care unit regarding transmission-based precautionary policies.

Contact precautions must be used for patients with volumes of drainage, skin infections, lice, scabies, cytomegalovirus infections, etc., when direct care is being given.

### Protective Isolation

**Protective isolation** is used to protect the patient from infectious agents. For example, a burn patient is very susceptible to infection, so anyone entering the room of a burn patient must use protective isolation procedures. When specimens are collected from patients with leukemia or severe burns, or those who are immunosuppressed in preparation for receiving organ or bone marrow transplants, body radiation therapy, or plastic surgery, who must be protected from exposure to pathogens and other bacteria, a sterile gown, cap, gloves, and mask should be worn. Shoe coverings may also be required. With patients needing these extra measures, protective isolation techniques should be used for their sake, as well as the usual standard precautions being used for the sake of the health care worker.

## TYPES OF SPECIMENS COLLECTED

Several different kinds of specimens are analyzed routinely in the clinical laboratory, but the specimen most often tested is blood. It is true that blood represents a large percentage of the specimens sent to the laboratory, but urine specimens are also sent in great numbers. Specific requirements for specimen collections are discussed throughout this book under the various laboratory divisions.

Many pathologic conditions may be associated with fluids that accumulate in the variou cavities of the body. Laboratory examination c body cavity fluid may yield useful information regarding its formation and constituents. The physician can also be alerted to the type of disease process present by the information obtained from the laboratory analysis of a patient's various body cavity fluids—presence of infection, inflammation, tumor, etc. Some of the body cavity fluids examined in the laboratory are pleural, pericardial, peritoneal, synovial, amniotic, and cerebrospinal.

Fecal specimens and other miscellaneous specimens such as throat cultures and swabs from wound abscesses are also sent to the laboratory for analysis.

## Blood: General Collection Information

Blood represents a large percentage of the specimens assayed in the clinical laboratory. Blood specimens are collected by several different types of health care personnel, depending on the facility. In some institutions, this work is done by the clinical laboratory scientists, medical technologists, or certified medical laboratory technicians. In other institutions, there are specially trained individuals who do the blood collecting. The person who practices this specialty is called a phlebotomist.

### Circulation of Blood

Blood, although a liquid, can also be called a tissue. It circulates throughout the body, acting as a transportation system. As it circulates through the system of blood vessels (the vascular system), oxygen is transported from the lungs to the tissues of the body, products of digestion are absorbed in the intestine and carried to the various body tissues, and substances produced in various organs are transferred to other tissues for use. Cellular elements of the blood may also be transported to fight infection or aid in the coagulation of the blood. At the same time, waste products from the body tissues are picked up by the blood, and these end products of metabolism are then excreted through the skin, kidneys, and lungs.

The heart is the pump that forces the blood, under pressure, out through the arteries to all parts of the body. If an artery is cut, blood spurts out in small bursts each time the heart contracts. Near organs and muscles, the arteries branch out into smaller and smaller blood vessels called arterioles. Still smaller branches from the arterioles are called capillaries. In the tiny capillaries, the blood cells give up the oxygen they have been carrying and exchange it for the waste product from the body tissues, carbon dioxide. The capillary blood carrying carbon dioxide flows into larger vessels called venules, and then into still larger vessels called veins. The veins carry the blood back to the heart. As the blood flows through the capillaries, it gradually loses pressure. In the veins it has still less pressure. Therefore, if a vein is cut, the blood oozes out; it does not spurt out. After the veins have carried the blood back to the heart, the blood is pumped into the alveoli, or air sacs of the lung. In the alveoli the carbon dioxide is removed from the red blood cells, which take up oxygen in its place. The blood then returns to the heart to be pumped out to the body once again through the arteries. It is important to understand the basics of the blood circulation so that the proper sites for blood collection are used.

The chemical compound in the red blood cells that actually picks up the oxygen and exchanges it for carbon dioxide is hemoglobin. When hemoglobin is saturated with oxygen, it is bright red. When oxygen is replaced by carbon dioxide, the hemoglobin becomes darker red. When blood from an artery is compared with blood from a vein, the arterial blood is a visibly brighter red because of the nature of the hemoglobin compound.

### The Phlebotomist

A professional **phlebotomist** has specific training in the technical skills of drawing blood. The phlebotomist is an important connection between the patient and the clinical laboratory. In addition to being skilled in obtaining blood by venipuncture, he or she is also trained to do capillary blood collections and perform special skin punctures, such as collecting specimens from infants in neonatal care units. Drawing specimens from indwelling lines is another collection specialty for those engaged in collecting blood.

Related areas of specimen transportation, handling, and processing must also be fully understood by the phlebotomist and by anyone who collects blood specimens. It is important therefore, to understand the proper means for collecting, preserving, and processing blood samples.

### Approaching the Patient

Because it is relatively easy to obtain a blood sample, numerous studies are done on blood in diseased and normal states. Much valuable information is readily available at relatively low cost and with little discomfort to the patient. Certain routine blood studies are part of new hospital admissions. Many of these studies are carried out in the hematology and chemistry departments (see Chapters 11 and 12). Blood is also cultured in the microbiology department.

Anyone who plans to assume a duty or occupation in which contact with patients is required must consider several factors. These persons are providing a service to the patient. Adequate performance of this service involves not only technical knowledge but also sincere and concerned interest in people. This is a quality that, unfortunately, cannot be taught readily. It is a quality that a person must learn as a part of being engaged in a professional endeavor. Those in the medical laboratory field must be not only academically capable but also psychologically and socially responsible.

**Patient's Bill of Rights.** When blood specimens are collected, it is important that the rights of patients be kept in mind at all times. Being cognizant of these rights is consistent with good patient care. Phlebotomy involves direct patient contact, and it is essential that all people engaged in this aspect of laboratory work remember to serve the patient well.

Many hospitals have adopted a **patient's bill of rights** as declared by the Joint Commission on Accreditation of Healthcare Organizations (JCAHO). In some states, laws have been passed making patients' rights mandatory (California and Minnesota have these laws). Such a law could become the basis of litigation if a patient feels that his or her rights have been violated. Box 3-1 is a summary of basic patient rights as endorsed by the JCAHO.

**Patient Considerations.** A patient in the hospital experiences several emotions, including anxiety and fear. The patient, separated from familiar surroundings, is also probably not feeling well, is concerned about his or her physical condition, and may be afraid of what is going to happen next. For these and other reasons, the patient's mental state is probably at its worst during hospitalization. It is extremely important that the patient be shown kindness and understanding. The collection of blood specimens is one area in which laboratory personnel have an opportunity to meet patients. It is essential, therefore, that those doing the blood collecting try to understand what the patient is feeling—to imagine what it would be like to be the patient—and act accordingly. Talking to the patient in a comfortable, friendly, pleasant, yet honest way is important.

When approaching a patient for the first time, there are certain procedures to remember. First, make certain that the patient on whom the test is being done is actually the right patient. Checking the identification number of the patient is essential. Check the wrist tag of the hospitalized patient to make certain that he or she is the right patient. For outpatients and for hospitalized patients, ask the patient's name—this is also a good way to start conversation. A mix-up in labeling tubes or drawing blood from the wrong patient can be disastrous. Always label the tubes of blood at the bedside of the patient or at the drawing site, as well as any slides, microcollection/capillary tubes, or other materials used for taking specimens. Proper and immediate labeling is essential.

Patient's Bill of Rights

The patient has a right to:

1. Impartial access to treatment or accommodations that are available or medically indicated, regardless of race, creed, sex, national origin, or sources of payment for care.

2. Respectful, considerate care and treatment.

3. Confidentiality of all communications and other records and data which pertain to the care received by the patient.

4. Expect that any discussion or consultation involving the patient's case will be conducted discreetly and respectfully and that persons not directly involved in the case will not be present without the permission of the patient or guardian.

5. Expect reasonable personal safety in accord with the hospital practices and environment.

6. Know the identity and professional status of individuals providing service and to know which physician or other practitioner is primarily responsible for his or her care.

7. Obtain from the practitioner complete and current information about diagnosis, treatment, and any known prognosis, in terms which can reasonably be understood by the patient.

8. Reasonable and informed participation in decisions involving his or her health care. The patient shall be informed if the hospital proposes to engage in or perform human experimentation or other research or educational projects affecting his or her care or treatment. The patient has the right to refuse participation in such activity.

9. Consult a specialist at the patient's own request and expense.

10. Refuse treatment to the extent permitted by law.

11. Request and receive an itemized and detailed explanation of the total bill for services rendered in the hospital regardless of the source of payment.

12. Be informed of the hospital rules and regulations.

**Pediatric Patients.** When working with a pediatric patient, one must first gain the patient's confidence. This may be the first time a child has had blood drawn. If this first experience is a bad one, it will be remembered and feared for years to come. It is therefore important to take some extra time to gain the child's confidence before going ahead with the collection procedure. Get acquainted with the child by using a book or a toy, for example. Keep your equipment tray as inconspicuous as possible. Be frank with the child. Sometimes it may be possible to tell a story about what you are doing. It is important in working with pediatric patients to bolster their morale as much as possible. Ask for help in restraining a very small or uncooperative child.

Older children may be more responsive when permitted to "help," by holding the gauze, for example. Working with a child often involves working with the parents also. This is best accomplished by allowing the parents to know, by the professional attitude assumed, that the laboratorian or phlebotomist is kind but very definitely in charge of the situation. This attitude, which is so basic for laboratory personnel, can be developed only with practice.

In the nursery, each hospital will have its own rules, but a few general precautions apply. After working with an infant in a crib, the crib sides must be returned to the position in which they were found when the collection process was begun. If an infant is in an incubator, the portholes should be closed as much as possible. When oxygen is in use, do not forget to close the openings when the collection process is completed. Dispose of all waste materials properly.

**Adult Patients.** Adult patients must be told briefly what is expected of them and what the test involves. With adults as well as with children, complete honesty is important. It is unwise to say that a finger puncture will not hurt, when it really will. However, if possible, avoid dwelling on that aspect of the collection process.

The patient should be greeted in a friendly and tactful manner; without becoming overly familiar, a conversation can be started in a quiet, pleasant, and calm manner. The patient should be told about the purpose of the blood collection. Any personal information the patient relates is being told in confidence. Religious beliefs of the patient should be respected, laboratory reports kept confidential, and any personal information about the patient also kept in confidence. Information about other patients or physicians is always kept in confidence. If the same patient is seen frequently, it is possible to become familiar with his or her interests, hobbies, or family and to use these as topics of conversation. Many patients in the hospital are lonely and need a friend. Occasionally, especially with the extremely ill patient, he or she will not wish to talk at all; in this case, respect these wishes. It is important to be honest, but to attempt to boost the patient's morale as much as possible.

Even if the patient is disagreeable (and many are), the laboratorian should remain pleasant. A smile can often work miracles. It is important to be firm when the patient is unpleasant, to remain cheerful, and to express confidence in the work to be done. Young children who do not understand words seem pacified by the sound of a confident voice. Talking pleasantly to every patient is essential.

In a hospital setting, before leaving the patient's room, the area should be checked to see that everything is in place in the laboratory tray and that the room has been left as it was found. The tray holding the blood collection supplies and equipment should always be kept out of reach of the patient. This is especially important in working with children, but it applies to all patients.

### Types of Collection Procedures

Any discussion concerning blood specimens must include collection procedures for blood—this applies to all areas of the clinical laboratory. There are two general sources of blood for clinical laboratory tests: peripheral, or capillary, blood and venous blood. The National Committee for Clinical Laboratory Standards (NCCLS) has set standards for the collection of both **capillary blood (skin puncture)** and **venous blood (venipuncture)**.[8,9] For small quantities of blood for some hematologic or microchemical determinations, capillary blood is suitable; it is obtained from the capillary bed by puncture of the skin (see Capillary or Peripheral Blood Collection by Skin Puncture, below). The tip of the finger is the site most commonly punctured. For larger quantities of blood, a puncture is made directly into a vein (phlebotomy), using a sterile syringe and needle collection system or evacuated tube and needle collection system (see Venous Blood Collection by Venipuncture later in this chapter). A vein in the upper forearm (or antecubital fossa) area is most often chosen for venipuncture, as these veins are easily palpable and fairly well fixed.

**Gloves.** Before any contact with the patient is made, the phlebotomist must put on protective gloves to implement the necessary barrier protection required by the standard precautions policy.

### Capillary or Peripheral Blood Collection by Skin Puncture

For the small quantities of blood required for most hematologic procedures and for microchemical techniques requiring serum or plasma, an adequate blood sample may be obtained from the capillary bed by puncture of the skin—a capillary puncture or skin puncture. The NCCLS has set standards for the collection of capillary blood by skin puncture.[8] (See Procedures 3-1 and 3-2.) From certain patients, such as babies, burned patients,

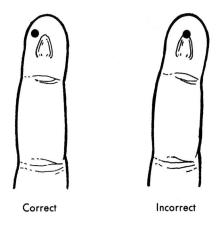

Correct              Incorrect

**FIG 3-1.** Sites for finger puncture. (From Powers LW: *Diagnostic Hematology.* St Louis, Mosby, 1989, p 433.)

very sick patients, or amputees, it may be necessary or desirable to obtain only a very small amount of blood. This can be accomplished quite easily by means of capillary puncture. This blood is collected into suitable capillary tubes, pipettes, or microcontainers or used directly to prepare blood films.

Capillary blood is often used for point-of-care tests (POCT)—bedside testing for glucose using one of several available reading devices and the accompanying reagent strips being a common one. This same procedure is done at home by countless diabetics on their own blood to ascertain the level of blood glucose for maintenance of good glucose control.

In adults and older children, the tip of the finger is punctured (Fig. 3-1) (see Procedure 3-1). In infants, the plantar surface of the heel or the large toe is punctured (Fig. 3-2) (see also

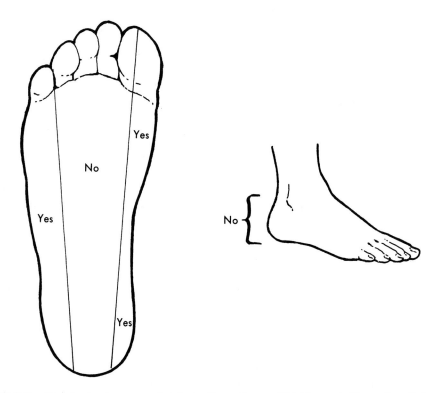

**FIG 3-2.** Sites for heel puncture in infants. (From Powers LW: *Diagnostic Hematology.* St Louis, Mosby, 1989, p 435.)

## PROCEDURE 3-1

### Finger Puncture

1. Assemble the necessary equipment: lancet device, alcohol pad, dry gauze, slides, and capillary tubes or other supplies necessary to receive the blood.

2. Be sure that the patient is seated comfortably.

3. Wash hands and put on gloves.

4. Choose an area for the puncture that is free from calluses, edema, or cyanosis. Warm the puncture site if it is cold by immersing it in warm water or by rubbing it.

5. Clean the skin of the puncture site on the third or fourth finger vigorously with a pad soaked in an alcohol solution. This will remove dirt and epithelial debris, increase the circulation, and leave the area relatively sterile. Allow the area to air-dry.

6. Grasp the finger firmly, and make a quick, firm puncture about 2 to 3 mm deep with a sterile disposable lancet or automated lancet device (see Fig. 3-4). This puncture should be made at right angles to the fingerprint striations on the patient's finger, midway between the edge and midpoint of the fingertip (see Fig. 3-1). The puncture should not be made too far down on the finger and should not be too close to the fingernail. A deep puncture hurts no more than a superficial one, and it gives a much more satisfactory flow of blood.

7. Discard the lancet in the sharps disposal container. Used lancets should never be left lying on the work area. They should be discarded immediately after use and should not be touched again.

8. Wipe away the first drop of blood, using a clean piece of dry gauze or tissue. This drop is contaminated with tissue fluid, which will interfere with some laboratory results. The succeeding drops are used for tests.

9. If a good puncture has been made, the blood will flow freely. If it does not, use gentle pressure to make the blood form a round drop. Excessive squeezing will cause dilution of the blood with tissue fluid.

10. Collect the specimens by holding a capillary tube to the blood drop or by touching the drop to a glass slide. Rapid collection is necessary to prevent coagulation, especially when several tests are to be done with blood from the same puncture site.

11. When the blood samples have been collected, have the patient hold a sterile, dry piece of gauze or cotton over the puncture site until the bleeding has stopped.

12. Remove gloves and wash hands.

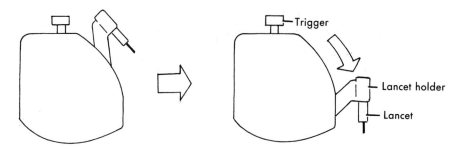

**FIG 3-3.** Automated lancet, spring-driven and trigger-activated (Autolet, Owen Munford Inc., Marietta, Ga). (From Powers LW: *Diagnostic Hematology.* St Louis, Mosby, 1989, p 430.)

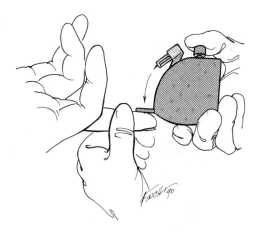

**FIG 3-4.** Finger puncture technique using automated lancet device (Autolet).

Procedure 3-2). In general, the ear lobe should be avoided for puncture because there is a slower flow of blood there and the concentrations of cells and hemoglobin will be greater. Blood obtained by skin puncture of these types is generally called capillary blood, but it is closer to arteriolar blood in its composition.

The results of tests from venous and capillary (fingertip) blood compare well if the capillary blood is free flowing. To ensure free flow of capillary blood, the finger must be warm.

Various types of disposable lancets or blades are used for skin puncture. Nondisposable lancets are not used, because of the risk of transmission of infectious pathogens. Lancets with safety gauges for depth of puncture are the best ones to use.

**Precautions to Note When Obtaining Capillary Blood.** If the patient's fingers are cold, slight rubbing may help to warm them. The finger or heel must not be squeezed excessively, because tissue fluid may dilute the blood sample or cause the blood to clot faster than it normally would. The first drop of blood is usually removed because it contains tissue fluid, alcohol, or perspiration, which will dilute the blood. Immediately after surgery, patients with low blood pressure and those in surgical shock may require more than one puncture. Only one sterile lancet is used at a time. The tip of the lancet should not touch anything until it punctures the skin of the patient. Contaminated lancets are discarded properly and new ones used. After the puncture is made, the lancet is discarded immediately. Hand washing before and after each new patient is encountered, along with wearing gloves, is essential.

**Skin Puncture Devices** A variety of automatic, **spring-activated skin puncturing devices** are commercially available. The NCCLS has set guidelines for skin puncture devices.[4] Clean, rapid incisions can be made of a consistent depth with the use of one of these devices. Devices such as the Autolet* have a

*Owen Munford Inc, Marietta, Ga.

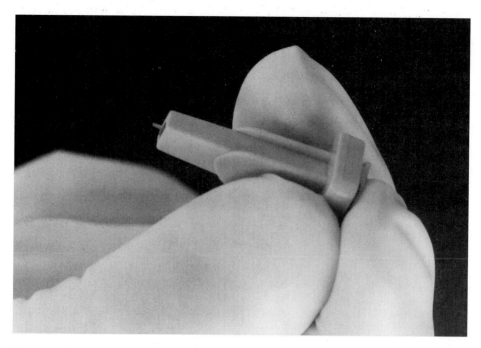

**FIG 3-5.** Microtainer Safety Flow Lancet. (Courtesy Becton Dickinson & Co, Becton Dickinson VACUTAINER Systems, Franklin Lakes, NJ.)

lancet held in place by a cocking lever (Figs. 3-3 and 3-4). When released, the blade penetrates the skin to a depth of 2 to 3 mm, depending on the choice of platform used. The platform regulates the depth of the puncture. Disposable lancets/blades and platforms or guards are used with these devices. The device itself can be cleaned with a bleach or disinfectant solution. It is important that all used lancets and platforms be discarded in a container for sharps. Transmission of blood-borne infections must be prevented (see under Standard Precautions in Chapter 2).

Individual spring-activated lancet devices are also available, in which case the entire device is disposable. One such lancet system, the Microtainer Safety Flow Lancet,* is a sterile, self-

contained spring-activated triggering device, containing a lancet housed in a protective plastic coating. These lancets are available in varying puncture depths (Fig. 3-5). To prevent accidental punctures once the device has been triggered, the lancet retracts into its protective covering once it has been used. Similar devices are available in a form used for neonatal heel punctures.

**Procedure for Heel Puncture** (Procedure 3-2). For infants under 3 months of age, the heel is the most commonly used site for obtaining a blood sample. Any wound-inflicting device can result in serious injury when excessive pressure and skin indentation accidentally allow the wound depth to reach the heel bone.

The foot must be held securely in place for the puncture (Fig. 3-6). The lateral or medial plantar surface of the foot should be used for the skin puncture (see Fig. 3-2). The site and depth of the

*Becton Dickinson VACUTAINER Systems, Becton Dickinson & Co, Franklin Lakes, NJ.

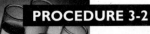

## PROCEDURE 3-2

### Heel Puncture

1. Wash hands and put on gloves.

2. Clean the puncture site with an alcohol sponge. Let it thoroughly dry.

3. Hold foot firmly to avoid sudden movement. Warm foot if needed.

4. Select lancet device with the appropriate depth for the size of the infant.

5. Perform the puncture on the most medial or most lateral portion of the plantar surface (see Figs. 3-2 and 3-5).

6. Puncture no deeper than 2.4 mm.

7. Do not perform punctures on the posterior curvature of the heel.

8. Do not puncture through previous sites, which may be infected.

9. Fill collection containers as needed.

10. When finished, elevate heel and place a piece of dry gauze on the puncture site. Keep pressure on the site until bleeding has stopped.

11. Discard used supplies in the appropriate waste containers. Notify nursing personnel that the procedure is complete.

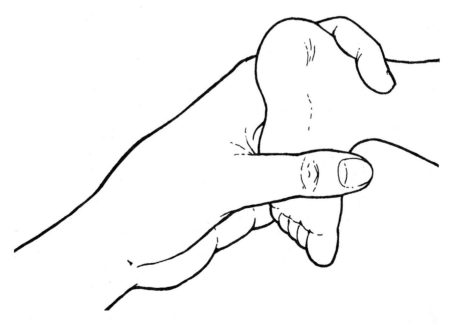

**FIG 3-6.** Holding an infant's heel for capillary puncture. (From Powers LW: *Diagnostic Hematology.* St Louis, Mosby, 1989, p 436.)

puncture are of critical importance. The depth should not exceed 2.4 mm. The central portion and posterior curvature of the heel are not used, because the bone lies too close to the surface. Puncture of the heel bone (calcaneus) can result in osteochondritis or osteomyelitis. The NCCLS has established recommendations for heel punctures in neonates[8] (see Procedure 3-2).

A semiautomatic device for performing heel punctures, called tenderfoot,* makes an incision that is 1 mm deep and 2.5 mm wide, allowing free-flowing collection of up to 3 mL of blood (Fig. 3-7). A tenderfoot device with a depth of puncture specifically designed for premature infants is also available. The blade of the device automatically retracts following the skin incision, ensuring that neither the blood collector nor the infant is accidentally punctured. When compared with other puncturing devices, tenderfoot causes less hemolysis of the sample, requires fewer punctures to obtain the desired sample, and produces less physical trauma to the heel of the infant. It is a sterile, completely disposable device, reducing the possibility of introducing infection in the infant. The depth and width of the incision are controlled, thus eliminating the possibility of calcaneal puncture and osteomyelitis. The amount of sample collected and the free-flowing nature of the blood following the puncture make squeezing the foot unnecessary. The device reduces the number of heel punctures needed. The detailed procedure for using this device accompanies the product.

**Blood Spot Collection for Neonatal Screening Programs.** Most states have passed laws requiring that newborn infants be screened for certain diseases that can result in serious abnormalities, including mental retardation, if they are not diagnosed and treated early. These diseases include phenylketonuria (PKU), galactosemia, hypothyroidism, and hemoglobinopathies. The

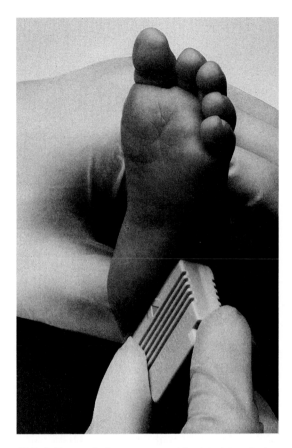

**FIG 3-7.** tenderfoot automated heel incision device for infant blood sampling. (Courtesy International Technidyne Corp, Edison, NJ.)

NCCLS has set standards for filter paper collection, or **blood spot collection**, of blood for these screening programs.[2] Blood should be collected 1 to 3 days after birth, before the infant is discharged from the hospital—at least 24 hours after birth and after ingestion of food for a valid PKU test. There is an increased chance of missing a positive test result when an infant is tested for PKU before 24 hours of age. When infants are discharged early, however, many physicians prefer to take a sample early rather than risk no sample at all.

In most **neonatal screening programs**, the specimen is collected onto filter paper and then sent to the approved testing laboratory for

---

*International Technidyne Corp, Edison, NJ.

analysis. Special collection cards with a filter paper portion are supplied by the testing laboratory—these are kept in the hospital nursery or central laboratory. There is an information section on these cards, and all requested information must be provided—it is to be treated as any other request form. The filter paper section of the card contains circles designed to identify the portion of the paper onto which the specimen should be placed, where the filter paper will properly absorb the amount of blood necessary for the test.

Collection is usually done by heel puncture, following the accepted procedure for the institution. When a drop of blood is present, the circle on the filter paper is touched against the drop until the circle is completely filled. A large enough drop should be formed so that the process of filling the circle can be done in only one step. The filter paper is allowed to air dry and then is transported to the testing laboratory in a plastic transport bag or other acceptable container. The procedure established by the testing laboratory should be followed for the collection step.

**Capillary Blood for Testing at the Bedside (Point-of-Care Testing).** Capillary blood samples for glucose testing and for other assays are used frequently in many health care facilities for **bedside testing, or point-of-care testing (POCT)**. Quantitative determinations for glucose are made available within 1 or 2 minutes, depending on the system employed. The NCCLS has set guidelines for these tests, as they are performed in acute care and long-term care facilities.[1] (POCT is also discussed in Chapter 1, under Sites of Testing.)

POCT for glucose is also performed at home by many outpatient diabetics, using their own blood and one of several glucose measuring devices. It is important for patients with diabetes, especially those with insulin-dependent diabetes mellitus, to monitor their own blood glucose levels several times a day and to be able to adjust their dosage of insulin accordingly to maintain good glucose control.

For the inpatient diabetes patient, POCT is also a valuable tool for management of the disease. The blood glucose level is often quite unstable in these patients, a situation that may necessitate frequent adjustments of insulin dosage. The POCT tests give results that are immediate, so dosages can be adjusted more quickly. Ordering and collecting venous blood specimens for glucose tests done by a central laboratory with the necessary frequency and rapidity of reporting required are often impractical, thereby making the POCT tests much more useful. Good quality-control programs must be used to ascertain the reliability of the POCT results, however. Whole blood samples should be collected by puncture from the heel (for infants only), finger, or flushed heparinized line, using policies for standard precautions to protect against the transmission of blood-borne pathogens. Arterial or other venous blood should not be used, unless the directions from the manufacturer of the POCT device being used specify the appropriateness of these alternative blood specimens. The POCT instrument should be calibrated and the test performed according to the manufacturer's directions. Results should be recorded permanently in the patient's medical record in a manner that distinguishes between bedside test results and central laboratory test results.

It is critical to understand the limitations of each POCT detection system so that reliable results are obtained. The specific limitations described by each manufacturer must be considered. The use of a quality assurance program is mandatory to ensure reliable performance of these procedures. The use of POCT—bedside testing or self-testing for glucose—is intended for management of diabetes patients and not for initial diagnosis. It is not used to replace the standard laboratory tests for glucose, but only as a supplement.

Several commercial instruments are available, and with each product a meter provides quantitative determination of glucose present when used with a reagent strip that is designed to accompany the meter. A drop of capillary blood is touched to the reagent strip pad and, according to the specific procedure, read in the meter. The instrument provides an accurate and standardized reading when used according to the manufacturer's directions. The reagent strips must be handled with care and used within their proper shelf life. The strips are specific only for glucose. The meters are packaged in convenient carrying cases and are small enough to be placed in a pocket or briefcase.

**Capillary Blood for Slides.** A finger or heel puncture is made and, after the first drop is wiped away, the glass slide is touched to the second drop formed. The slide is placed on a flat surface and a spreader slide used to prepare the smear (see Chapter 12). The slide is allowed to air dry, is properly labeled, and then is transported to the laboratory for examination.

**Capillary Blood Specimen Containers.** Once the skin has been punctured and the blood

is flowing, the capillary sample can be collected into a variety of containers. For general purposes, glass tubes with or without heparin can be used and the blood allowed to flow into the tube by capillary action. For example, a heparinized capillary tube is used to collect blood for performing the microhematocrit test in the hematology laboratory.

Another capillary sampling device is called the Unopette* (Fig. 3-8). It consists of a disposable capillary pipette that measures a fixed volume and a reservoir of diluent appropriate to the test being performed. This pipette and diluent system can be used with either capillary or venous blood, and the general system has been adapted for several chemical and hematologic determinations. Unopettes are described further in Chapter 12 in their use for measuring hemoglobin and for doing manual white cell and platelet counts.

Microcontainers are available to contain small volumes of blood. They consist of a small plastic

*Becton, Dickinson & Co, Franklin Lakes, NJ.

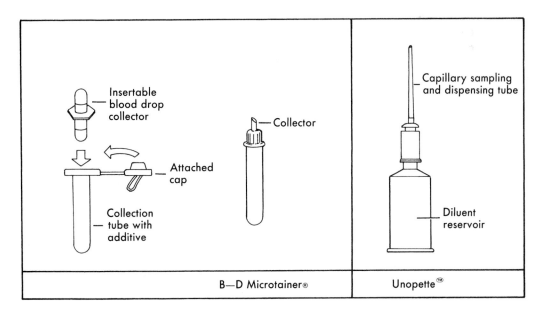

B—D Microtainer®                 Unopette™

**FIG 3-8.** Types of microcontainer tubes and collecting devices. (From Powers LW: *Diagnostic Hematology*. St Louis, Mosby, 1989, p 431.)

tube with a blood drop collector as part of the lid (see Fig. 3-8). One such commercially available system is the Microtainer.* This allows the specimen to be collected by capillary action and results in a relatively large amount of specimen in a single container. When the collection is finished, the container can be properly capped and processed by centrifugation, if serum is to be obtained. These microcontainers are available with various additives, including serum separator gels.

### Venous Blood Collection by Venipuncture

The veins that are generally used for venipuncture are those in the forearm, wrist, or ankle. The first choice for a venipuncture site is a vein in the forearm. Veins in this region are larger and fuller than those in the wrist, hand, or ankle. The wrist, hand, or ankle veins are used only if the forearm site is not available. Venipuncture must be performed with great care and technical skill. The NCCLS has set standards for the collection of venous blood.[9] The veins of the patient are the

---

*Becton, Dickinson & Co, Franklin Lakes, NJ.

main source of blood for testing, and the entry point for medications, intravenous solutions, and blood transfusions. A patient has only a limited number of accessible veins, and it is important that everything possible be done to preserve their good condition and availability. Part of this responsibility lies with the person doing the blood drawing.

Blood may be obtained directly from a vein (phlebotomy) by using a sterile **syringe and needle** or **evacuated tube and needle collection system** (Fig. 3-9). The use of the evacuated (vacuum) tube system allows the blood to pass directly from the vein into the collection tube. Veins in the forearm are most commonly used when this system is used. The three main veins in the forearm are the cephalic, median cubital, and median basilic (Fig. 3-10). The **median cubital vein** is usually chosen for venipuncture. The median basilic might roll or move, and the skin over the cephalic might be tougher to penetrate. Other sites may be used when necessary.

The phlebotomy may be done and blood collected by either the syringe method or the evac-

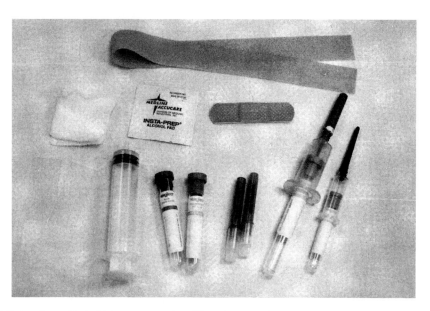

**FIG 3-9.**  Assembled phlebotomy supplies. (From Powers LW: *Diagnostic Hematology.* St Louis, Mosby, 1989, p 423.)

uated (vacuum) tube method (see Procedure 3-3). An infusion or butterfly set can be used in combination with the evacuated tube method (see Procedure 3-4) (see Fig. 3-11). In the syringe method, a needle is attached to a syringe and inserted into the vein. The plunger of the syringe is drawn back, which creates suction, drawing the blood into the syringe. In the evacuated tube method, one end of a two-way needle is partially attached by means of a holder device to the rubber stopper of a specially prepared vacuum tube. The other end of the two-way needle is inserted into the vein. Once that end is in the vein, the end of the needle in the rubber stopper is pushed through the stopper to make a direct connection to the vacuum tube (Fig. 3-12). The vacuum tube creates suction, which draws the

blood into the tube. One commercially available vacuum tube system is called Vacutainer.* The NCCLS has published standards for the use of evacuated tubes for blood specimen collection.[5]

When doing a venipuncture, the phlebotomist should remain in a standing position, which gives the greatest freedom of movement. The patient should assume a comfortable position. A bed patient should remain lying down, and an **ambulatory patient** should be seated comfortably with the arm in an inclined position. The seated patient should put an arm on a table or other firm support and extend it for the phlebotomist.

**Blood Collection Variables.** The majority of clinical laboratory determinations are done on whole blood, plasma, or serum. Many of these analyses are done in the hematology or chemistry laboratories, but many other areas of the laboratory also require venous blood for testing.

Most venous blood specimens are drawn from fasting patients. Most fasting blood is drawn in the morning before breakfast. This means that the food from the previous meals has been completely digested and absorbed and any excess has been stored. Food intake, medication, activity, and time of day can all influence the laboratory results for blood specimens. Some of these facts are rarely taken into account by the persons interpreting the laboratory results. The fasting state is one fact that is carefully noted, however, especially for glucose, triglyceride, and phosphorus determinations. Through numerous studies it has been found that the average meal has no significant effect on the concentration of most blood constituents, with certain exceptions. Blood collected directly after a meal is described as a **postprandial specimen.** Food intake significantly affects blood glucose and triglycerides, giving a falsely high result, and phosphorus, giving a falsely low result. Because it is the most efficient time of day to draw spec-

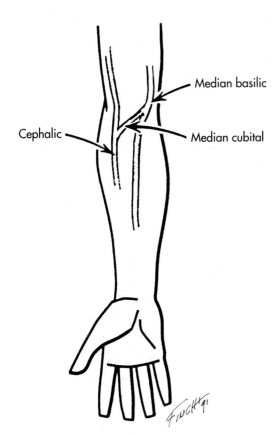

**FIG 3-10.** Major veins of the arms.

*Becton Dickinson VACUTAINER Systems, Becton Dickinson & Co, Franklin Lakes, NJ.

## PROCEDURE 3-3

### Venipuncture Using the Evacuated Tube System[3,9]

1. Wash hands and put on gloves to comply with policies for standard precautions for blood collection.

2. Identify and reassure the patient. Ask the patient to state his or her full name. Always check the wrist identification to confirm the identity of the patient. This is especially important when blood specimens are being drawn from unconscious or mentally impaired patients.

3. Assemble necessary equipment and supplies (Fig. 3-9).
   a. Thread the short end of the double-pointed needle (called the hub of the needle) into the plastic holder and tighten securely, using the needle sheath as a wrench (see Fig. 3-12).
   b. Assemble sterile evacuated blood collection tubes as needed for the tests desired, ascertaining the proper order for collection. Before using, tap all tubes that contain additives to make certain all the additive is dislodged from the stopper.
   c. Place the vacuum tube in the holder and push the stopper of the blood collection tube into the shorter shielded needle (within the holder) up to the recessed guideline on the needle holder. The needle will thus be embedded in the stopper without puncturing it and losing vacuum in the tube (see Fig. 3-12, *A*). Do not push the tube beyond the guideline, as a premature loss of vacuum may result. Because of this potential problem, some phlebotomists prefer not to attach the tube at this stage.
   d. Remove the needle shield, and inspect the tip of the longer needle visually to see if it is free of hooks at the end of the point and the opening is clear. Leave the needle covered loosely until the actual venipuncture can be performed. Do not contaminate it.

4. Position the patient. For ambulatory patients: a chair with side supports is used to prevent accidental falling. The patient should be seated comfortably in the chair, with the arm extended to form a straight line from the shoulder to the wrist and inclined in a downward position. The arm should rest across a narrow table or on a slanting armrest, which can be part of the chair. The arm and elbow should be supported firmly, and the arm should not be bent at the elbow. Add more support if needed.

   For patients in bed: make certain they are in a comfortable supine position. If additional support is needed, a pillow may be placed under the arm on which the venipuncture is to be done. The patient should extend the arm to form a straight line from the shoulder to the wrist.

5. Close the patient's hand (unnecessary if veins are prominent).

6. Select the vein site to be used. If possible, the site is selected without the tourniquet. However, on many patients the tourniquet is used at this point (Procedure 3-5). Observe both arms. Select the median cubital vein that appears fullest. These veins are usually easily palpable, fairly well anchored in place, and bruise less. If necessary, use the cephalic vein, in preference to the basilic vein. The cephalic vein does not roll and bruise as easily as the basilic, although the blood usually flows more slowly. Palpate and trace the vein several times with the tip of the index finger. Feel the "bounce" of a full vein. A vein feels much like an elastic tube and gives under pressure. Even if you can see the vein, palpate until you can be certain of its location and direction.

## PROCEDURE 3-3

### Venipuncture Using the Evacuated Tube System—cont'd

Unlike veins, arteries pulsate and have a thick wall. Thrombosed veins feel cordlike and roll. Muscle tendons are usually apparent.

Blood can be forced into the vein by gently massaging the arm from wrist to elbow. Several sharp taps at the vein site with the index and second fingers may cause the vein to dilate. Application of heat to the site may have the same result. Lowering the arm over the chair will allow the veins to fill to capacity. If a vein is not readily apparent, use a tourniquet temporarily. Do not leave the tourniquet in place for more than one or two minutes for this examination process.

The best location to perform the venipuncture is at the bend of the elbow, but if these sites are not usable, the flexor surfaces of the forearm, the wrist area above the thumb, the volar area of the wrist, or the back of the hand can be used. Use of the foot or ankle is rarely necessary.

Collection of blood from a site on which the tourniquet has been used for more than 2 minutes can result in inaccurate laboratory analyses. A tourniquet prevents blood from flowing freely, and the balance of fluid and blood elements may be disrupted.

Do not use areas of obvious hematomas, where blood has been collected before, as some laboratory results may be erroneous. If no other veins are available, collect below (distal to) the hematoma.

Do not collect blood from scarred areas or from an arm where intravenous fluids are being given. Use the other arm. Special procedures must be followed if blood is collected from an arm where an intravenous solution is being administered.

Only experienced phlebotomists should draw blood specimens from intravascular devices—cannula, fistula, vascular graft, or heparin-locked catheter.

7. Apply the tourniquet so that it can be easily released (Fig. 3-13 and Procedure 3-5). The tourniquet increases venous filling with blood and makes the veins more prominent and easier to enter. Do not leave the tourniquet on for longer than 1 minute, if possible; apply just before venipuncture is to be performed. Never apply a tourniquet above an intravenous site, a fistula, a shunt, a cannula, or a heparin-locked catheter. Avoid pinching the skin. The tourniquet should remain "flat" around the patient's arm.

8. Clean the skin at the venipuncture site. Usually the vein site is cleaned with an isopropyl alcohol solution or medicated alcohol on a gauze pad, using a circular motion starting from the actual site of entry and working toward the periphery. This is done to prevent any chemical or microbiologic contamination of either patient or specimen. Allow the area to air-dry in order to prevent hemolysis of the blood sample and alcohol seepage into the puncture. For blood culture collection, a triple application of povidone-iodine solution is required.

   If the area is touched before the puncture, it should be recleaned.

9. Place the selected collection tubes and needle assembly within easy reach.

10. Grasp the patient's arm and anchor the vein. The patient's arm should be grasped firmly, with the palm of the hand under the elbow. The patient's arm should be fully extended. Use the

*Continued*

## PROCEDURE 3-3

*Venipuncture Using the Evacuated Tube System—cont'd*

thumb, placed 1 or 2 in. below the puncture site, to anchor the vein by drawing the skin taut. Ask the patient to open and close the hand.

11. Perform the venipuncture:
    a. Keep the patient's arm in a downward position and maintain the tube below the site throughout the procedure to prevent backflow from the tube into the patient's vein.
    b. Turn the needle so that the bevel side is up.
    c. Line up the needle with the vein.
    d. Puncture the vein. The puncture of the skin and vein should be done in two steps, if possible, the skin first and then the vein, at approximately a 15- to 30 degree angle and in a direct line with the vein. A sensation of resistance will be felt, followed by ease of penetration as the vein is entered.
    e. As soon as the needle is positioned sufficiently in the vein, insert the vacuum tube into the needle holder as far as it will go so that blood can flow into the vacuum tube (see Fig. 3-12, *B*). Do this by grasping the flange of the needle holder from the top, between the index and third fingers, and triggering the tube forward by pushing with the thumb until the hub end of the needle punctures the stopper. This will activate the vacuum action to draw the blood into the collection tube.
    f. Allow the tube to fill until the vacuum is exhausted and blood flow ceases, in order to ensure the correct ratio of anticoagulant to blood. The tube normally will not be filled completely. As the blood flow ceases, remove the tube from the needle holder, being careful not to change the position of the needle in the vein. If multiple samples are to be drawn, remove the tube as soon as the blood flow stops and insert the next tube into the holder. The shut-off device on the hub of the needle covers the point at which the tube is removed and stops the blood from flowing until the next tube is inserted. Adhere to the proper order for the draw: first, sterile tubes for culture, then nonadditive tubes, tubes for coagulation studies, and finally the tubes with additives.
    g. As the tube containing an additive is removed, mix immediately by gently inverting the tube five to ten times. To avoid hemolysis, do not shake or mix vigorously.
    h. To collect multiple samples, carefully insert the next tube into the holder, taking care not to change the position of the needle in the vein. Collect as many tubes as needed, using the same technique.

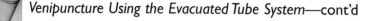

## PROCEDURE 3-3

*Venipuncture Using the Evacuated Tube System—cont'd*

12. Open the patient's hand. Ask the patient to open his or her hand; this reduces the amount of venous pressure.

13. Release the tourniquet (preferably at 1 minute). Remove the tourniquet as soon as blood flow is established in the last tube to be drawn. If the tourniquet has been left on too long before blood is acquired, some test results are altered owing to stasis of cells and movement of fluid out of the vein into the tissue. The arm will become cyanotic. **The tourniquet must always be released before the needle is removed from the vein.**

14. Position a dry gauze pad. Lightly place a gauze pad over (covering) the venipuncture site.

15. Quickly, but gently, remove the needle. Then apply pressure on the gauze pad. Hold the dry gauze pad over the needle and puncture site. Quickly remove the needle while keeping the bevel in an upward position, exercising care not to scratch the patient's arm. Apply mild pressure to the site as soon as the needle is withdrawn. Continue to apply pressure on the gauze pad until bleeding is stopped. Special attention should be given to patients with prolonged bleeding.

16. Bandage the arm, if needed. If the patient continues to bleed, apply a pressure bandage over the venipuncture site. Tell the patient to leave the bandage on for 15 to 30 minutes. It is recommended that adhesive bandages not be placed on small children; they may remove, chew, or swallow them.

17. Dispose of the puncturing unit. Avoid puncturing your own skin. **NEVER attempt to reshield the needle.** Special sharps biohazard disposal systems are available, which allow for direct disposal of the needle. Dispose of all waste supplies immediately in the proper disposal containers.

18. Label tubes. Be sure to properly label all tubes with the patient's name, identification number, date of collection, and other necessary patient information, and mix the tubes adequately with their additive or anticoagulant. In the clinical laboratory, blood tube labels must exactly match the patient data on the test request forms.

19. Remove gloves and wash hands.

20. Leave the patient only after all signs of bleeding have stopped.

## PROCEDURE 3-4

### Venipuncture Using an Infusion Set and the Evacuated Tube System

1. Attach the tube holder and adapter to the end of the infusion/butterfly needle tubing (Fig. 3-15).

2. Hold the butterfly needle with the bevel up, at approximately 15 to 30 degrees to the patient's skin and in a direct line with the vein to be entered.

3. Apply tourniquet (Fig. 3-13 and Procedure 3-5).

4. Anchor the vein.

5. Insert the needle into the vein with one smooth aggressive motion. Some blood will appear in the tubing if the vein has been entered.

6. When using the evacuated tube system, as soon as the needle enters the vein, insert the collection tube into the holder as far as it will go.

7. If multiple tubes are needed, remove the tube as the blood flow stops and insert the next tube into the holder.

8. When the last tube has filled, remove the tourniquet and then the needle and tubing, positioning a dry gauze over the needle and puncture site Apply mild pressure to the site as soon as the needle is withdrawn.

9. Apply pressure on the venipuncture site until bleeding has stopped.

10. Bandage the arm, if needed. If the patient continues to bleed, apply a pressure bandage over the venipuncture site. Tell the patient to leave the bandage on for 15 to 30 minutes. It is recommended that adhesive bandages not be placed on small children; they may remove, chew, or swallow them.

11. Dispose of the puncturing unit. Avoid puncturing your own skin. Special sharps biohazard disposal systems are available, which allow for direct disposal of the infusion system. Dispose of all waste supplies immediately in tthe proper disposal containers.

12. Label tubes. Be sure to properly label all tubes with the patient's name, identification number, date of collection, and other necessary patient information, and mix the tubes adequately with their additives or anticoagulants. In the clinical laboratory, blood tube labels must exactly match the patient data on the test request forms.

13. Remove gloves and wash hands.

14. Leave the patient only after all signs of bleeding have stopped.

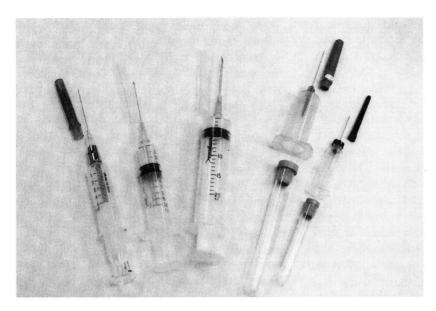

**FIG 3-11.** Phlebotomy equipment: syringe, needles, and evacuation system. *Left to right:* Syringe with Luer-Lok needle, disposable plastic syringes and needles, VACUTAINER evacuation systems. (From Powers LW: *Diagnostic Hematology.* St Louis, Mosby, 1989, p 418.)

imens for the laboratory, most of the blood collecting is done early in the morning, and for this reason most of the patients are in the **fasting state** (having had no food or liquid other than water for 8 to 12 hours). Fasting specimens, however, are not necessary for most laboratory determinations. Blood should not be collected while intravenous solutions are being administered, if possible.

Other controllable biological variations in blood include posture (whether the patient is lying in bed or standing up), immobilization (resulting from prolonged bed rest, for example), exercise, circadian/diurnal variations (cyclical variations throughout the day), recent food ingestion (caffeine effect, for example), smoking (nicotine effect), alcohol ingestion, and administration of drugs. The concentrations of certain plasma constituents are affected by some of these factors, and for some laboratory tests it is important to take into consideration the time of day, posture of the patient, dietary intake, and so forth, prior to collection of the blood specimen. Standardization of collection policies can

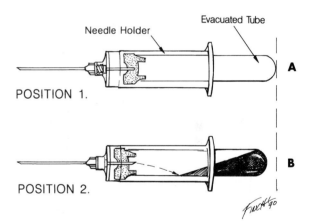

**FIG 3-12.** Standard double-ended blood collecting needle with holder using vacuum tube system. **A,** Preparation for venipuncture. **B,** Collection of specimen.

minimize the effect of these variables on test values, but in most health care facilities, this is difficult to do. Specimen requirements for the various tests to be done should always be kept in mind by the person collecting the blood.

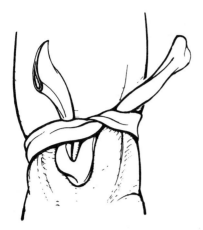

**FIG 3-13.** Application of a tourniquet.

**Application of the Tourniquet.** The use of a **tourniquet** is desirable to enlarge the veins, so that they become more prominent. A strip of flat tubing (about 1 in. wide) can serve as a tourniquet. It is applied around the arm just above the bend in the elbow and should be just tight enough to obstruct the venous blood flow (Fig. 3-13). The patient should also be instructed to close his or her hand to make the veins more prominent and easier to enter. The proper way to apply an elastic tubing tourniquet is described in Procedure 3-5.

**General Venipuncture Considerations.** The most prominent vein is usually chosen for venipuncture. If the veins are difficult to find, have the patient open and close the hand a few times; this will build up more pressure. Veins may be made more prominent by use of a tourniquet, by allowing the arm to hang down for 2 to 3 minutes, by massaging the vein toward the trunk of the body, or by sharply tapping the site of the puncture with the index and second fingers. If a tourniquet has been used to locate the vein site, release the tourniquet for a few minutes and then reapply to perform the venipuncture. The tourniquet should not be in place for more than one minute—or two at the maximum. Veins may be hardened or rubbery in elderly persons or in persons who have had re-

peated venipuncture. Rolling veins may be held in place by putting the thumb and index finger on the vein so that 2 to 5 cm of vein lies between them. As soon as the vein is entered, the thumb and finger are removed.

The veins can be felt by touching or palpating with the index finger. They reveal themselves as elastic tubes under the surface of the skin. By pressing up and down on the vein gently several times, the path of the vein can be felt.

Once the site for venipuncture has been chosen and the vein observed or palpated, the area is cleaned with an antiseptic solution. One suitable antiseptic is a solution of medicated alcohol (or isopropyl alcohol). The area of puncture is cleansed thoroughly with the antiseptic. After application of the antiseptic, the area must not be touched until after the actual puncture is made.

To insert the needle properly into the vein, the skin and vein are first fixed in place by grasping the patient's arm with the other hand and pulling the skin taut. This can be accomplished by placing the thumb about 1 or 2 in. below the puncture site (Fig. 3-14). The bevel of the needle should be facing up, and the needle should be positioned in the same direction as the vein. The syringe or evacuated tube assembly should be held so that the needle makes a 15- to 30-degree angle with the patient's arm. The tip of the needle is then placed on the vein and pushed deliberately forward. (See also Procedure 3-3.) A sensation of resistance is felt, followed by ease of penetration as the vein is entered. When the vein has been punctured and a suitable amount of blood collected into the tube or syringe, the patient releases the clenched hand, the tourniquet is released, a dry gauze is placed over the puncture site, and the needle is withdrawn. After the needle has been removed, pressure may be applied on the puncture site, using dry gauze, until bleeding has stopped. Special attention must be given to patients with prolonged bleeding times.

If difficulty is experienced in entering the vein (no blood appears in the tube or syringe) and especially if a **hematoma** (collection of

## PROCEDURE 3-5

### Application of a Tourniquet

1. Place the tourniquet under the patient's arm, just above the bend in the elbow (see Fig. 3-11).

2. Grasping the ends of the tourniquet, pull up so that tension is applied to the tourniquet. This tension must be maintained throughout the procedure.

3. With the proper tension, cross the end of the tourniquet and tuck a loop in the tourniquet from the top down, leaving the ends up and away from the venipuncture site. Do not tie a bow or a knot. The loop must be made in such a way that the tourniquet can easily be released by pulling on a free end of the tourniquet when it is to be removed (see Fig. 3-11). Avoid pinching the skin, if possible. The tourniquet should remain flat around the patient's arm.

4. Do not leave the tourniquet on for long periods of time because this will cause stoppage of the circulation (stasis). Prolonged stasis results in gross alterations in the blood constituents. Leave the tourniquet in place for no longer than one minute, if possible.

blood under the skin) starts to form, release the tourniquet and promptly withdraw the needle; then apply pressure to the wound. It is best to select an alternative site for repeated venipunctures on the same patient.

It is most important that the tourniquet be released before the needle is removed from the skin. If this is not done, excessive bleeding will occur. If the venipuncture is poorly done (if there is trauma to the tissues), a hematoma may result. This should be avoided, if at all possible.

The evacuated tube system is an ideal means of collecting multiple samples with ease. The NCCLS has published standards for the use of evacuated tubes for blood specimen collection.[5] A multiple-sample needle is used (see Fig. 3-12 and Procedure 3-3). After blood has filled the first tube, the tube is removed from the needle holder, leaving the needle anchored in the vein, and a second tube is inserted into the tube holder. Blood will fill the second tube just as it did the first. Each tube must be thoroughly and immediately mixed with any additive or anticoagulant in the tube by inverting the tube gently 5 to 10 times to ensure proper mixing of the additive and blood. The multiple-sample needle has a special adaptation that prevents blood

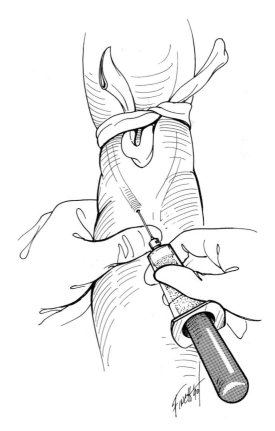

**FIG 3-14.** Venipuncture technique using evacuated tube system.

from leaking out during the exchange of tubes. Some vacuum tube collection systems can be purchased with an added guard closure, which helps to shield the laboratorian against exposure to blood specimens. All tubes must be immediately labeled according to the labeling protocol established for the facility.

If blood must be drawn from a patient who has intravenous equipment attached to one arm, the blood sample should be drawn from a vein in the other arm. If neither arm is free, an ankle vein is the site of choice for the venipuncture.

In weak or elderly patients, the venous pressure may be so low that the pressure of the needle or the negative pressure of the vacuum tube may collapse the vein. In these cases it may be advisable to use a syringe, for then the negative pressure can be controlled.

If the patient's clothing is too tight above the venipuncture site, it will slow down the flow of blood and may cause a hematoma. If the tourniquet is too tight, it will cause the arterial flow to stop. The radial pulse should be felt with the tourniquet in place correctly. A tight tourniquet can cause cyanosis, and it pinches the skin, causing unnecessary discomfort to the patient. It may also cause the vein to disappear before the puncture is made. When this happens, the vein has collapsed, and the tourniquet should be released for a few minutes and the procedure repeated.

The placement of the needle—the angle of entry and the entry itself—is important (Fig. 3-14). The angle of entry of the needle with the skin should be 15 to 30 degrees. If the skin and the vein are penetrated at one time, the needle may go straight through the vein. It is best to make the penetration in two steps: the skin first and then the vein. The bevel of the needle must always be covered by skin before the vacuum tube is fully engaged; otherwise the vacuum in the tube is lost. If there is a poor flow of blood, the needle may be half into the vein or the bevel may be partly occluded. To correct this problem, gently turn the needle, push in, or press down to keep the vein wall off the bevel. The needle bevel must be in the lumen of the vein and the needle itself in line with the vein in order to have a good flow of blood.

**Hemolysis**, when destruction of red cells has occurred, causes erroneous results in some chemistry measurements using serum. Hemolytic serum will appear pink. For a summary of general considerations for venipunctures using the evacuated tube system, see Box 3-2.

**Venipuncture Using Syringe and Needle.** A syringe and needle are often used to collect blood from patients with difficult veins. With the use of the same preparation procedures as for the vacuum tube system, the syringe and needle system is assembled and the vein entered. When making preparations for doing the venipuncture, remove the syringe from its protective wrapper and the needle from the sterile package and assemble them, allowing the covering to remain over the needle when not in use. Attach the needle so that the bevel faces in the same direction as the graduation marks on the syringe. Check to make sure the needle is sharp, the syringe moves smoothly, and there is no air left in the syringe.

Blood will enter the syringe spontaneously if a clean entry into the vein has been made. In persons with low venous pressure, the plunger of the syringe is withdrawn slightly to make certain that the needle has entered the vein. Withdraw the blood by using the left hand to pull back the plunger while steadying the syringe with the right hand (do not push in the plunger, as air will be injected into the patient's vein).

When sufficient blood has been withdrawn, release the tourniquet and remove the needle and syringe from the vein. Place a dry gauze pad over the site of the venipuncture, and maintain gentle pressure for a few minutes. Do not leave the patient until the bleeding stops.

Remove the needle from the syringe, and gently expel the blood into a collection tube (place used collection supplies into the proper disposal container immediately). Avoid foaming or rupture of the cells by using gentle pressure

**BOX 3-2**

General Considerations for Venipunctures Using the Evacuated Tube System

1. If a tube begins to fill and then stops, change the position of the needle, first in a forward direction, then slightly backward, or rotate the needle half a turn. Loosen the tourniquet. The bevel of the needle may not be fully in the lumen of the vein.

2. If a tube is not filling with blood but the needle is in the vein, try another vacuum tube; sometimes the vacuum tubes are defective and the vacuum has been lost.

3. Do not probe with the needle. It is painful for the patient.

4. If another venipuncture attempt is necessary, try the other arm in the cubital fossa, or another puncture in the same arm in a site below the first puncture.

5. Never attempt a venipuncture more than twice. Request that another phlebotomist or a physician draw the specimen.

6. Sometimes a capillary puncture may be used in place of the venipuncture.

7. Clothing may be too tight above the site of the venipuncture. This can slow the flow of blood and may cause a hematoma.

8. If the tourniquet is too tight (the radial pulse should be felt at all times), arterial flow of blood will stop and this may cause the vein to disappear before the puncture is done. A tight tourniquet may cause pinching of skin (an unnecessary discomfort), cyanosis, fluid shifts, and possible erroneous laboratory results.

9. Needle placement and angle of entry are important. The angle of the needle with the skin should be about 30 degrees. If the angle is greater than 30 degrees, the needle can pass straight through the vein. If skin and vein are penetrated at one time, blood may spurt from the puncture hole. The needle bevel should be well covered by skin before the vacuum tube is fully attached, or the vacuum will be lost. With small veins, the bevel may be rotated down to help increase blood flow.

10. If the vein disappears at puncture (some veins collapse when touched), the tourniquet pressure may be tightened slightly.

11. If the vacuum collapses the vein (the size and softness of veins vary), tighten the tourniquet, press the needle down gently, or rotate it so that the vein wall is not occluding the bevel.

12. Undue bleeding and hematoma formation can be prevented if the puncture is made only in the uppermost wall of the vein and by making certain that it is fully penetrated; by removing the tourniquet before removing the needle; by immediately applying pressure to the venipuncture site after removing the needle; by applying pressure on the gauze pad over the venipuncture site for several minutes until bleeding stops; or by covering the site with an adhesive dressing, except with small children. If bleeding appears to be excessive, a roll of gauze under an adhesive bandage may be effective. Patients with bleeding must be observed again at 5 minutes.

13. To prevent hemolysis in the blood specimen, avoid drawing blood from an area where there is a hematoma and, in general, do not mix blood in nonadditive tubes (except for serum separator tubes, which must be tipped two or three times to activate the clotting process). Allow blood to clot at room temperature for 30 minutes before centrifuging for serum separation. Mix anticoagulated specimens thoroughly but by gentle inversion five to ten times.

on the plunger of the syringe. Stopper the tube, and gently invert it 5 to 10 times to mix blood with additive, if one is used.

If an evacuated collection tube is used to hold the blood, push the needle through the stopper and allow the blood to collect in the tube by using the vacuum in the tube.

A syringe and needle or an **infusion set (Butterfly)** is often used for coagulation studies, for babies and small children with small veins, for very obese patients whose veins are hard to find, for patients receiving intravenous chemotherapy for cancer (whose veins have become scarred), for patients who have frequent venipunctures (leukemia patients), and for veins other than those in the antecubital fossa.

**Venipuncture Using the Infusion Set (Butterfly Needle).** The infusion set, or Butterfly Needle* is generally used for drawing a blood specimen from a patient with small, fragile, "rolly" veins or for drawing from veins in the wrist area, back of the hand, ankle, foot, or scalp. This system has generally replaced the syringe method of blood collection in many institutions. A 25-gauge needle is recommended for the smallest and most fragile veins. A syringe collection system, rather than an evacuated tube method, is recommended when the 25-gauge infusion set is used. The infusion set is often used for drawing blood specimens from pediatric patients (see Procedure 3-4).

An infusion set is used with an additional collection method—either by attaching it to a sterile syringe and manually filling the syringe or by attaching it to an adapter, which is in turn attached to an evacuated tube holder (Fig. 3-15). The specimen is eventually transferred to or collected directly into an evacuated tube.

**Obtaining Blood From Existing Intravascular Devices or Indwelling Lines.** When vascular access is needed over an extended period of time, for administration of therapeutic

*Becton Dickinson & Co, Franklin Lakes, NJ.

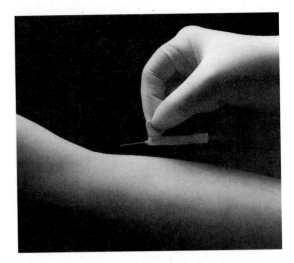

**FIG 3-15.** Butterfly Needle (infusion set). (Courtesy Becton Dickinson & Co, Becton Dickinson VACU-TAINER Systems, Franklin Lakes, NJ.)

blood products or for infusion of fluids, medications, or parenteral nutrition solutions, without the necessity for multiple venipunctures, **vascular access devices (VAD)** are used. These devices are also called **indwelling lines** or **intravascular devices.** It is also possible, with skill and experience, to collect a venous or arterial blood sample from these devices. Because infection and septicemia are serious consequences, especially in immunosuppressed patients, adherence to a strict asepsis control protocol for collection from intravascular devices is required. Each health care facility has its own policy and procedure for dealing with these devices, and this must be followed to prevent complications from infection due to improper use of the devices. For this reason, a special training program for phlebotomists drawing blood from intravascular devices is necessary.

An intravascular device consists of a silicone catheter and a self-sealing silicone septum encased in a metal or plastic port and may have other types of access ports. It is surgically implanted with the use of local or general anesthesia. The catheter is tunneled through the subcutaneous tissue to a major blood vessel, and the portal is secured to the fascia under the skin. The device is accessed by needle puncture through the skin into the port or through a diaphragm. For venous ports, catheters are placed in a vein. Several different intravascular devices are used.

The decision to use an intravascular device for obtaining a blood specimen is made by the attending physician.

**Obtaining Blood With Heparin Locks.** A **heparin-lock system** consists of an indwelling winged Butterfly Needle and can be used in a vein for 36- to 48-hour periods to administer medication intravenously or as a source for venous blood samples. This device is used to "save" veins for patients and to lessen trauma to the veins. Repeated venipunctures can be painful to patients and can, after time, result in scarring of the vein lining, which makes the vein unusable.

The Butterfly system is carefully placed in the vein and must be maintained by careful adherence to infection control procedures, since the needle is a foreign body being placed directly into the patient's vein. These procedures include the use of antibiotic ointments and careful monitoring for signs of inflammation.

A dilute heparin solution is used in the line to keep the blood in it from clotting. This heparin flush is injected through the tubing, and a plug at the end of the butterfly line holds the solution in place. Before any blood is used for analysis, a waste specimen of 2 to 3 mL must be withdrawn and discarded to free the specimen of the heparin solution. There must be a special period of training and education before a phlebotomist draws specimens from a heparin lock.

**Blood Collection for Culture.** To ensure that the blood collected for culture is free from contamination (from the patient, the phlebotomist, or other personnel), extra precautions are taken for cleaning the skin and the collection tube prior to the actual collection. The skin is cleaned three times with a povidone-iodine solution or a chlorhexidine gluconate preparation. By use of a scrub applicator, the povidone-iodine solution must be applied to the puncture site in a concentric outward-moving circle, beginning at the site. This step is repeated three times. After the triple cleaning, the povidone-iodine may be removed with an alcohol pad if the color of the solution makes it difficult to locate the vein. If for any reason the vein must be touched prior to the actual venipuncture, the phlebotomist's gloved finger must be triple-cleaned with povidone-iodine. Perform the venipuncture using a sterile syringe and needle, or collect directly into culture bottles using an evacuated (vacuum) system.

Each culture bottle top must be cleaned with an alcohol pad prior to injection of the required amount of blood sample into the bottle. Culture bottles are labeled and brought to the laboratory.

### Additives and Anticoagulants

Blood is a combination of formed elements (red cells, white cells, and platelets) in a liquid portion called plasma. In vivo (in the body) the blood is in a liquid form, but in vitro (outside the body) it will clot in a few minutes. Blood that is freshly drawn into a glass tube appears as a translucent, dark red fluid. In a matter of minutes it will start to clot, or coagulate, forming a semisolid jelly-like mass. If left undisturbed in the tube, this mass will begin to shrink, or retract, in about 1 hour. Complete retraction normally takes place within 24 hours. When coagulation occurs, a pale yellow fluid called serum separates from the clot and appears in the upper portion of the tube. During the process of coagulation, certain factors present in the original blood sample are depleted or used up (see also Chapter 13). Fibrinogen is one important substance found in the circulating blood (in the plasma portion) that is necessary for coagulation to occur. Fibrinogen is converted to fibrin when clotting occurs, and the fibrin lends structure to the clot in the form of fine threads in which the red cells (erythrocytes) and the white cells (leukocytes) are embedded. To assist in obtaining serum, collection tubes with a separator gel additive in them are commonly used

(Fig. 3-16). Serum is used extensively for chemical, serologic, and other laboratory testing, and can be obtained from the tube of clotted blood by centrifuging.

If coagulation is prevented by the addition of an **anticoagulant**, the formed elements of the

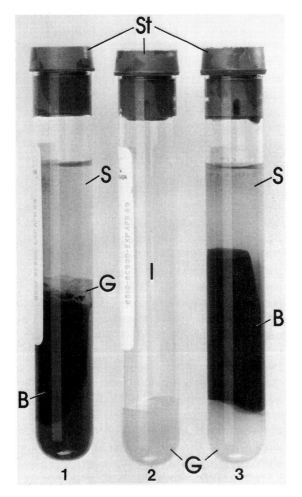

**FIG 3-16.** VACUTAINER phlebotomy tubes containing barrier gel (red-gray tops). *1*, Tube filled with blood and centrifuged. *2*, Unfilled tube. *3*, Tube filled with blood and not centrifuged. Note positions of gel before *(3)* and after centrifugation *(1)*. *B*, Clotted blood; *St*, red-gray stoppers; *G*, barrier gel; *S*, serum. (From Kaplan LA, Pesce AJ: *Clinical Chemistry: Theory, Analysis, and Correlation*, ed 2. St Louis, Mosby, 1989, p 43.)

blood— red cells, white cells, and platelets—can be separated from the plasma. If the anticoagulated blood is centrifuged, it separates into three main layers: the red cells, the buffy coat (consisting of white cells and platelets), and the plasma. Hematologic studies are done primarily on whole anticoagulated venous blood or on fresh capillary blood. It is important that everyone involved in collecting blood specimens thoroughly understand the reason for using anticoagulants. Use of the appropriate **additive** is essential, and to do this the type of determination to be done by the laboratory must be indicated on the request form.

Several anticoagulant additives are available for various purposes in the clinical laboratory. Some of the more commonly used anticoagulants are:

1. *Sodium fluoride:* This is a dry additive, a weak anticoagulant, used primarily for blood glucose specimens, since it is also an enzyme poison (preventing glycolysis, or destruction of glucose). More information on the use of this anticoagulant may be found under Glucose and Glucose Metabolism in Chapter 11.

2. *Oxalates:* These dry additives are available as sodium, potassium, ammonium, or lithium oxalates. The oxalate in the anticoagulant forms an insoluble complex with the calcium in the blood, inhibiting the clotting mechanism. When calcium ions are combined with oxalate and are therefore not available to participate in clotting, the blood does not clot.

3. *Ammonium and potassium oxalate:* Also called balanced oxalate, or double oxalate, this combination is a dry additive. It is used for some hematology work. It is not used in chemistry, as a rule, because the presence of ammonium in the anticoagulant interferes with some of the chemistry determinations. Use of this anticoagulant has been replaced in most laboratories by the use of EDTA.

4. *EDTA (ethylenediaminetetraacetic acid):* EDTA is used as a disodium or dipotassium salt. It prevents coagulation by chelating (binding) calcium in the plasma. It is available as a dry (potassium or sodium EDTA) or liquid (potassium EDTA) additive and is used primarily in the hematology laboratory. It is the anticoagulant of choice for blood to be used in cell counts, hematocrit, hemoglobin, and cell differentials on stained blood films, to name but a few tests, because it preserves the morphologic structure of the blood cell elements.

5. *Sodium citrate:* This additive is widely used for coagulation procedures, including prothrombin times and partial thromboplastin tests. It prevents coagulation by inactivating calcium ions. The citrate helps to prevent the rapid deterioration of labile coagulation factors such as factor V and factor VII.

6. *Heparin:* This additive is theoretically the best anticoagulant, because it is a normal constituent of blood and introduces no foreign contaminants to the blood specimen. Heparin is available as sodium, lithium, and ammonium salts. It prevents coagulation for approximately 24 hours by neutralizing thrombin, thus preventing the formation of fibrin from fibrinogen. Only a small amount of heparin is needed, so that simply coating the insides of tubes or syringes is often enough to give a good anticoagulant effect.

**Color Coding for Vacuum Tubes.** Stopper color codes for additives have been generally accepted by manufacturers of vacuum (evacuated) tubes for blood collection and also for microcontainer systems. Table 3-1 explains the color coding system for vacuum tube stoppers.

**Order for Drawing Blood Into Collection Tubes.** To avoid any possible cross-contamination of additives between tubes, it is recommended that blood collection tubes be drawn in a specific order. Each health care facility implements its own specific policy governing the order in which tubes for laboratory analyses are drawn. Policies on coagulation studies and blood cultures, for example, vary from place to place. In general, however, it is important to draw any sterile blood culture specimens first, then specimens that require no additives (plain

## TABLE 3-1

Color Coding for Vacuum Tubes

| Stopper Color | Use | Additive |
| --- | --- | --- |
| Gray | Plasma or whole blood; glycolysis inhibition | Potassium oxalate and sodium fluoride |
| Yellow, pale | Sterile interior of tube; cultures | Sodium polyanetholesulfonate (SPS) |
| Yellow, bright | Blood bank | Acid citrate dextrose (ACD) |
| Green | Plasma or whole blood chemistries; viable lymphocytes or neutrophils | Lithium, ammonium, or sodium heparin |
| Red | Serum Chemistries; serology; blood bank | No additive |
| Red and black | Serum chemistries | Inert serum separator gel |
| Light blue | Plasma or whole blood; coagulation assays | Sodium citrate |
| Dark blue | Tests for trace elements | Sodium heparin |
| Lavender | Plasma or whole blood; hematology, drug analyses | Sodium or potassium EDTA (dried), Potassium EDTA (liquid) |

tubes), followed by tubes needed for coagulation studies (usually sodium citrate or heparin), if they are drawn at the same time. Last, tubes with the various other additives are drawn, with gel separator tubes first, then EDTA, then oxalates and fluorides. It is possible that there can be additive contamination from tube to tube, especially if the blood drawing is slow and difficult. If, for example, the EDTA tube is collected prior to the heparin tube for electrolyte analysis, the potassium salt of EDTA may falsely elevate the potassium determination.

**Adverse Effects of Additives.** The additives chosen for specific determinations must be such that they do not alter the blood components and do not affect the laboratory tests to be done. The following are some adverse effects of using an improper additive or using the wrong amount of additive.

1. The additive may contain a substance that is the same, or reacts in the same way, as the substance being measured. An example would be the use of sodium oxalate as the anticoagulant for a sodium determination.

2. The additive may remove the constituent to be measured. An example would be the use of an oxalate anticoagulant for a calcium determination; oxalate removes calcium from the blood by forming an insoluble salt, calcium oxalate.

3. The additive may affect enzyme reactions. An example would be the use of sodium fluoride as an anticoagulant in an enzyme determination. Fluoride destroys many enzymes.

4. The additive may alter cellular constituents. An example would be the use of oxalate in cell morphology studies in hematology. Oxalate distorts the cell morphology; red cells become crenated, vacuoles appear in the granulocytes, and bizarre forms of lymphocytes and monocytes appear rapidly when oxalate is used as the anticoagulant. Another example is

the use of heparin as an anticoagulant for blood to be used in the preparation of blood films that will be stained with Wright's stain. Unless the films are stained within 2 hours, heparin gives a blue background with Wright's stain.

5. If too little additive is used, partial clotting will occur. This interferes with cell counts.

6. If too much liquid anticoagulant is used, it dilutes the blood sample and thus interferes with certain quantitative measurements.

### Laboratory Processing of Blood Specimens

Blood specimens must be properly handled after collection. The NCCLS has published standards for handling blood specimens after collection by venipuncture.[10] As discussed previously, if no anticoagulant is used, the blood will clot and serum is obtained. After being placed in a plain tube with no additives, the blood is allowed to clot. The serum is then removed from the clot by centrifugation. To prevent excessive handling of biological fluids, many laboratory instrumentation systems can now use the serum directly from the centrifuged tube, without another separation step and without removing the stopper. In the past, the serum was removed and placed in a clean, dry storage tube or vial prior to analysis.

**Serum Separator Devices.** To assist in the processing of clotted whole blood to obtain the serum, special **serum separator collection tubes** are available. An evacuated glass tube serves as the single system for both collection and processing of the blood. Serum separator tubes are of two major types, those used during centrifugation and those used after centrifugation.

The tubes used during centrifugation may be either integrated gel tube systems or devices inserted into the collection tube just before centrifugation. The integrated gel tubes contain a special silicone gel layer, which, because of its viscosity and density, moves to form a barrier between cells and serum during centrifugation (see Fig. 3-14). Blood is forced into the gel layer during centrifugation, causing a temporary change in viscosity. The gel starts out at the bottom of the collection tube. Blood is added to the tube and the clot allowed to form for a minimum of 30 minutes. After clot formation, the tubes are centrifuged. The gel rises and lodges between the packed red cells and the top layer of serum. The gel hardens and forms an inert barrier. These tubes do not have to be unstoppered before centrifugation, thus eliminating aerosol production and possible evaporation. The serum separator tubes also give a higher yield of serum as well as a shorter processing time because only a single centrifugation step is needed.

**Processing Blood for Serum.** Serum can be used in the chemistry laboratory for tests for sodium, potassium, calcium, phosphorus, acid and alkaline phosphatase, cholesterol, uric acid, and liver function, to mention but a few. Serum is also used for serology testing.

It is important to remove the plasma or serum from the remaining blood cells, or clot, as soon as possible. Since biological specimens are being handled, the need for certain safety precautions is stressed. The standard precautions policy should be used, since all blood specimens should be considered infectious (see Chapter 2). Blood specimens should be handled with protective gloves. The outsides of the tubes may be bloody, and initial laboratory handling of all specimens necessitates direct contact with the tubes. When stoppers must be removed from the tubes, they must be removed carefully and not popped off, as this could cause infection by inhalation or by contact of the infectious aerosol with mucous membranes. Stoppers should be twisted gently while being covered with protective gauze to minimize the risk from aerosol. This processing step can be done with the use of a protective plastic shield so that no direct splashes can take place. To separate the serum and plasma from the remaining blood cells, the tube must be centrifuged. It is generally best to test specimens as quickly as possible. If the specimen must be stored prior to analysis, remove

the serum/plasma from the clot/red cells to prevent alterations from taking place in the sample to be tested. It is especially important to remove the plasma quickly from the cell layer when potassium oxalate has been used as the anticoagulant, because the salt (potassium oxalate) shrinks the red blood cells and the intracellular water diffuses into the plasma (fluid inside the red cell leaves the cell and thus causes shrinkage). Centrifuge covers should always be in place during centrifugation to protect the worker from the specimens, and the centrifuge should be placed as far from laboratory personnel as possible. If the centrifuged serum or plasma must be removed into a separate tube or vial, the safest procedure for this step is pipetting instead of pouring. Pipette the serum or plasma by using mechanical suction and a disposable pipette; use a protective plastic shield so that no direct splashes can take place. All serum and plasma tubes, as well as the original blood tubes, should be discarded properly in biohazard containers when they are no longer needed for the determination.

### Appearance of Processed Specimens

Persons working with specimens in the laboratory must be able to recognize the appearance of normal as opposed to abnormal plasma or serum. Normally, serum or plasma is straw colored, but various shades of yellow are also normally seen. Abnormal-appearing serum and plasma can be clinical indications of serious disorders. Also, the use of such abnormal specimens can interfere with some determinations, especially chemistry tests.

**Hemolysis.** Hemolysis in specimens is perhaps the most common cause of the abnormal appearances to be considered. A specimen that is hemolyzed appears red, usually clear red, because the red blood cells have been lysed and the hemoglobin has been released into the liquid portion of the blood. Often the cause of hemolysis in specimens is the technique used for venipuncture. A poor venipuncture, with excessive trauma to the blood vessel, can result in a hemolyzed specimen. Collecting the blood in dirty tubes or tubes that are not entirely dry can also result in hemolysis. In these cases, carefully repeating the venipuncture and using clean, dry equipment will produce a normal-appearing specimen that can be used for chemical determinations. Hemolysis of blood can also be caused by freezing, prolonged exposure to warmth, unnecessarily forceful spraying of blood from the needle of a syringe when the blood is transferred to a specimen tube, or allowing the serum or plasma to remain too long on the cells before testing or removal to another tube. **Hemolyzed serum** or plasma is unsuitable for several chemistry determinations because substances usually present within cells can be released into the serum or plasma. If serum is left on the cells for a prolonged period, potassium will move out of the red cells and into the serum, resulting in falsely elevated levels of serum potassium. The procedure to be done should always be checked first to see if abnormal-appearing specimens can be used.

**Jaundice. Jaundiced serum** or plasma is another specimen with an abnormal appearance. When serum or plasma takes on a brownish-yellow color, there has most likely been an increase in bile pigments, namely bilirubin. Excessive intravascular destruction of red blood cells, obstruction of the bile duct, or impairment of the liver leads to an accumulation of bile pigments in the blood, and the skin becomes yellow. When this occurs, the skin of the patient is said to be jaundiced. The serum or plasma can also be jaundiced, or yellow. Those performing clinical laboratory determinations should note any abnormal appearance of serum or plasma and record it on the report form. Another term for jaundiced is icteric. Jaundiced serum or plasma is seen in patients with hepatitis. Once again, it is important to be observant in all areas of laboratory work—to notice things such as the appearance of a jaundiced specimen can assist the physician in making a diagnosis.

**Lipemia.** When the blood, serum, or plasma takes on a milky appearance, the specimen is said to be lipemic. The presence of lipids, or fats, in the serum causes this abnormal lipemic appearance. A blood specimen drawn from a patient soon after a meal may often appear lipemic. Use of a **lipemic serum** specimen, does not, for the most part, interfere with chemical determinations, except for triglyceride tests (see also Lipids-Fat in Chapter 11).

### Storage of Processed Specimens

The processing of individual serum or plasma tubes will depend on the analysis to be done and the time that will elapse before analysis. Serum or plasma may be kept at room temperature, refrigerated, frozen, or protected from light, depending on the circumstances and the determination to be done. Some specimens must be analyzed immediately after they reach the laboratory, such as specimens for blood gas and pH analyses. Blood specimens for hematology studies can be stored in the refrigerator for 2 hours before being used in testing. After storage, anticoagulated blood, serum, or plasma must be thoroughly mixed after it has reached room temperature.

Plasma and serum often can be frozen and preserved satisfactorily until a determination can be done. Whole blood cannot be frozen, because red blood cells rupture on freezing. Freezing preserves most chemical constituents in serum and plasma and provides a method of sample preservation for the laboratory. In general, refrigerating specimens retards alterations of many constituents. With all biological specimens, however, preservation should be the exception rather than the rule. A laboratory determination is best done on a fresh specimen.

## Urine: General Collection Information

The urine specimen has been referred to as a liquid tissue biopsy of the urinary tract that is painlessly and easily obtained. Urine yields a great amount of valuable information quickly and economically, but, as for all other human specimens used in the laboratory, the specimen must be carefully collected, preserved, and processed prior to analysis in order for the results reported to be regarded as reliable. A routine urine analysis (urinalysis) is included with many hospital admissions and visits to physicians' offices or clinics.

### Types of Urine Collection

The composition of urine in random samples collected at different times during the day is likely to vary considerably, because the work of the kidney is so variable. The NCCLS recommends that a specimen for routine urinalysis be from a well-mixed, **first morning specimen** (eight-hour concentrated), that it be uncentrifuged, and that it be tested at room temperature.[7] It is not practical to collect an entire day's specimen (24-hour specimen), as it would take too long for any results to be ready for the physician; also, as urine stands, many of the more important constituents found in it disappear or are altered. A 24-hour specimen, or other **timed urine collection,** is required only when it is necessary to know the entire day's volume of urine output, or for quantitative tests in which the exact amount of urine must be known so that the exact amount of substance present may be reported. The NCCLS describes several types of urine collection.[11] Some of these are random, first morning, timed, midstream, clean-catch, catheterized, and suprapubic.

Urine testing should be done within two hours of collection. If this is not possible, the specimen should be stored at 4°C as soon as possible after collection. Specimens can be stored under refrigeration for 6 to 8 hours with no gross alterations in constituents (see Chapter 14).

Since a 24-hour collection is not necessary for a routine urinalysis, any random specimen that is passed during the day may be used. A **voided midstream urine specimen** is suitable for most routine urine tests. As discussed above, the first urine voided in the morning is usually recommended. This is true primarily because the first morning urine specimen is the most concentrated one passed during the day. It is more concentrated because less fluid (or water) is excreted during the night, while the same amount of solid or dissolved substance must be excreted for the kidney to perform its function of maintaining the composition of the extracellular fluid. To test for the presence of urine sugar, the best specimen to use is one voided 2 to 3 hours after a meal. This is the one exception to the recommended use of the first morning specimen.

### Containers for Urine Collection

It is of prime importance that the containers used to collect the urine specimen be clean and dry. Containers should not be reused. Several types of containers are suitable for this purpose. The NCCLS has made several recommendations regarding urine collection containers.[7] Disposable, inert, plastic containers with sealable or screw-top lids and plastic bags or jars are most often used. These are available in several sizes and are preferred for routine screening urinalysis. Containers for routine urine tests should have a capacity of 50 to 100 mL with a round opening at least 2 in. in diameter and should have screw caps. Sterile containers with lids for collecting urine for microbiologic studies (cultures) are available. There are also special pediatric urine-collecting bags made of clear polyethylene. If a 24-hour pediatric specimen is required, a special tube can be attached to the bag, which is in turn connected to a collection bottle.

Large plastic containers with wide mouths and screw caps are used to collect timed specimens (24-hour collections) from adults, usually with added preservatives. The collection bottles should be refrigerated between voidings. Any bedpans that are used to collect voided urine must be scrupulously clean and free of cleaning agents or bleach. Any collection containers used must be labeled with complete patient identification. Labels must remain fixed to the container under refrigeration and must be on the container, not on the lid.

### Preservation of Urine Specimens

If a fresh specimen of urine is left at room temperature for a period of time, the urine rapidly undergoes changes. It is for this reason that a good routine urinalysis should include the use of a fresh specimen. Decomposition of urine begins within 30 minutes after collection. Specimens left at room temperature will soon begin to decompose, mainly owing to the action of bacteria in the urine. Urea-splitting bacteria produce ammonia, which on combination with hydrogen ions forms ammonium. This causes an increase in urine pH. The increase in pH will result in decomposition of casts and certain cells, if they are present in the urine. The various laboratory tests to be performed on a specimen of urine should be done within 30 minutes after collection, if possible; no longer than 1 or 2 hours should elapse before the tests are done, unless the urine is preserved in some way.

If it is impossible to examine the urine specimen when it is fresh or if a timed urine collection (2-, 12-, or 24-hour) is required, the urine must be preserved. Various methods of preserving urine are available, most of which inhibit the growth of bacteria, thus preventing many of the alterations from occurring.

The best method of preservation is immediate refrigeration during (for timed collection) and after collection. The specimen may be kept 6 to 8 hours under refrigeration, with no chemical preservative added, with no gross alterations. Several chemical preservatives are available as additives for routine urine specimens. Most of them interfere in some way with the testing procedures, however, and it is best if no chemical preservative is added.

Toluene is one chemical preservative that can be used. It is a liquid that is lighter than urine or water. It has its preservation effect by preventing the growth of bacteria by excluding contact of urine with air. A thin layer of toluene is added, just enough to cover the surface of the urine. The toluene should be skimmed off or the urine pipetted from beneath it when the urine is examined. Toluene (toluol) is the best all-around preservative, because it does not interfere with the various tests done in the routine urinalysis. Other common preservatives for urine specimens are formaldehyde (formalin), thymol, and boric acid. Thymol, a crystalline substance, works to prevent the growth of bacteria. However, thymol may interfere with tests for urine protein and bilirubin. Formalin, a liquid preservative, acts by fixing the formed elements in the urinary sediment, including bacteria. It may, however, interfere with the reduction tests for urine sugar and may form a precipitate with urea that interferes with the microscopic examination of the sediment. Preservative tablets that produce formaldehyde are commercially available. The tablets are more convenient to use than the liquid formalin and do not interfere with the usual chemical and microscopic examination.

Various disposable collecting systems are available commercially for collecting, storing, transporting, and testing urine specimens. New systems are continually being introduced to the market.

In general, it should be remembered that a fresh urine specimen is best for urinalysis tests. It is usually easy to collect and will give the most satisfactory results.

### Collecting Urine Specimens

As stated previously, the specimen for urinalysis should be collected in a clean, dry container, and the specimen should be fresh. For routine screening, a freshly voided, random, preferably midstream (freely flowing) urine specimen is usually suitable. For most routine urinalysis, including protein content and urinary sediment constituents, the concentrated first morning specimen is the most satisfactory one to use.

Occasionally it may be necessary to obtain a catheterized urine specimen, but this procedure is not encouraged because of the risk of patient infection. These urine specimens are obtained by introducing a catheter into the bladder, through the urethra, for the withdrawal of urine. This procedure should be avoided whenever possible, as there is always a risk of introducing bacteria into an otherwise sterile bladder—this could initiate a urinary tract infection. Catheterized specimens may be necessary in female patients

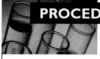

## PROCEDURE 3-6

### Clean-Catch, Midstream Urine Specimen For Culture (Patient Collection Instructions)[11]

1. Wash your hands thoroughly with soap and water.

2. Open the lid of the urine container provided. Be careful not to touch the inside.

3. Cleanse your genital area using the following procedure:

   *Man*

   a. If you are uncircumcised, draw back the foreskin before cleansing.

   b. Clean the tip of your penis using a sterile cleansing towelette, beginning at the tip and moving toward the base. Repeat the cleansing process using a second towelette.

   *Woman*

   a. Squat over the toilet, and use the fingers of one hand to separate and hold open the folds of the skin in your genital area.

   b. Clean the urinary opening and surrounding area with a sterile cleansing towelette, moving from front to back. Repeat the cleansing process using a second towelette.

4. Discard the towelettes in a trash receptacle (not in the toilet).

5. Begin urinating into the toilet bowl. After the urine has flowed for several seconds into the toilet, catch the midportion of the urine flow in the collection container. When sufficient urine has been collected (approximately one-half full), continue urinating into the toilet.

6. **Tightly** screw the cap on the specimen container.

7. Wash your hands thoroughly with soap and water.

8. Promptly give the specimen container to the nurse or laboratory personnel or leave in the place specified.

9. Ensure that the specimen label contains your proper identification.

---

when contamination by vaginal contents may alter the examination (especially during menstruation). Catheterization may also be necessary for obtaining urine specimens for bacteriologic examination when a sterile sample is needed. Under many conditions, however, a freely flowing voided specimen is satisfactory for bacteriologic cultures. Urine obtained by means of catheterization should be handled very carefully in the laboratory. Remember that catheterization is an invasive procedure for the patient and does involve some degree of risk.

When both a bacteriologic culture and a routine urinalysis are needed on the same specimen, the culture should always be done first and then the routine tests, so as not to contaminate the culture. See Procedure 3-6 for collection of specimens suitable for culture.

Since on most days many urine specimens are sent to the laboratory, it is especially important that each container be properly labeled when it is collected from the patient. Each specimen must be accompanied by a request form.

When a 24-hour urine specimen is sent to the laboratory, it must be ascertained first that the specimen has been properly collected. A preservative must have been added at the beginning of the collection time, and the correct collection time must have been used (24 hours total time, for example). In the laboratory, the total volume of specimen is measured and recorded, the urine is thoroughly mixed, and an aliquot is withdrawn for analysis.

**Collection of Timed Urine Specimens.** The patient is carefully instructed about details of the collection process, if the collection will be done on an outpatient basis. The bladder is emptied at the starting time (8 A.M., for example), and this time is noted on the collection container. This urine is discarded and not put into the container. All subsequent voidings are collected and put into the container, up to and including that at 8 A.M. the following day. This urine specimen will complete the 24-hour collection. For timed collections of other than 24 hours, the sample collection principle applies. The first urine voided at the beginning of the collection is always discarded. These timed collection specimens are preserved by refrigeration between collections, with the appropriate chemical preservative being added to the container prior to the beginning of the collection process.

The total volume of the timed collection sample is measured and recorded, and the sample well mixed, before a measured aliquot is withdrawn for analysis.

**Collection of Urine for Culture.** A clean, voided midstream urine specimen (often referred to as a "clean catch") is desirable for culture (see Procedure 3-6). It is important that the glans penis in the male and the urethral orifice in the female be thoroughly cleaned with a mild antiseptic solution by means of sterile gauze or cotton balls. The patient should be instructed to urinate forcibly, and to allow the initial stream of urine to pass into the toilet or bedpan. Throughout the urination process for the female, the labia should be separated so that no contamination results. The midstream specimen should be collected in a sterile container, and no portion of the perineum (female) should come in contact with the collection container. After the specimen has been collected, the rest of the urine is passed into the toilet or bedpan.

## Body Cavity Fluids (Extravascular)

When fluids normally found in small amounts in various cavities or spaces in the body—**body cavity fluids**—increase in amount and mechanically inhibit the action of certain key organs such as the heart or lungs, or when such a fluid is needed for diagnostic purposes, the fluid is aspirated. The procedure is done under sterile conditions by a physician. Fluids aspirated from the chest, abdomen, joints, cysts, or abscesses are often brought to the laboratory for various types of tests. The origin of the fluid and the tests to be done should be noted on the container and the request form, along with the usual label information required (patient name, hospital number, and so on.). Many different tests can be ordered on body cavity fluids, including chemistry determinations, cultures, cell counts and differentials, and examination for tumor cells.

The various types of extravascular fluids, or body cavity fluids, are examined in various departments of the clinical laboratory, depending on what test is to be done and what type of fluid is to be examined. Cell counts are done on most body fluid specimens. For this reason, in many institutions without a central specimen processing area, body cavity fluid specimens are brought first to the hematology laboratory, and are either examined there or sent on to a specific department for further analyses. Specific body fluids and their analysis will be discussed later in this book (see Chapter 15).

Most normal body cavity fluids are pale and straw colored. As the cell count and any abnormal debris and constituents increase, the fluid becomes more turbid.

Since cell counts are done on many body cavity fluid specimens, the specimen must be a fresh one. If it is not fresh, cell disintegration will occur. No cell counts may be done on a clotted specimen; anticoagulants must be used to prevent coagulation of the specimen when a cell count is needed. Specific gravity tests, when done, must also be done on a clot-free specimen. Tests for mucin and protein, however, can be done on clotted specimens. When a glucose determination is ordered, the specimen must be immediately preserved with sodium fluoride to prevent glycolysis. Generally, a blood glucose test is done simultaneously for comparison purposes. Body cavity fluid specimens to be cultured should be sent to the microbiology laboratory. Specimens to be tested for a chemical constituent should be sent to the chemistry laboratory as soon as possible. Sometimes only one specimen is sent to the laboratory, and several tests are required; except for culture, cell counts should always be done before other tests. For cell counts, the anticoagulant of choice is heparin or liquid EDTA. For examination for tumor cells, the fluid may be collected in EDTA or heparin. If the fluid is collected without any anticoagulant, clotting may be observed. The presence of clotting indicates a substantial inflammatory reaction. Sometimes so much fluid is aspirated that it must be collected in a gallon container instead of the usual tube. It is important to remember that the suitable anticoagulant must be placed in this large container just as in the tube. Many laboratory tests cannot be done on a clotted specimen of body fluid. With the standard precautions policy, all body cavity fluids should be considered contaminated, and all equipment must be decontaminated or discarded after being used.

### Cerebrospinal Fluid

**Cerebrospinal fluid (CSF)** is the most frequently tested body cavity fluid other than blood or urine. It fills the ventricles of the brain, the central canal of the spinal cord, and the subarachnoid spaces of the brain and spinal cord; it is formed in the ventricles. It has many of the same characteristics as plasma, since most of its components are derived from the blood plasma. The only known function of the cerebrospinal fluid is mechanical—providing protection for the brain and spinal cord. Examination of the cerebrospinal fluid is important in the diagnosis of neurologic disorders, inflammatory diseases, and hemorrhage in the meninges.

The cerebrospinal fluid, or spinal fluid, is obtained by puncturing one of the spaces between the lumbar vertebrae with a needle. It is collected by lumbar puncture into the L3-4 lumbar

interspace to avoid damaging the spinal cord. This procedure is done by a physician. The spinal fluid is usually collected into three or four sterile containers (numbered according to the order of collection), each containing between 1 and 3 mL of fluid. It is essential that the containers be properly labeled and handled with extreme care, as the procedure of collection cannot be easily repeated. There is a certain risk to the patient in this procedure, and for this reason the specimen is extremely precious and must be treated with the utmost care. Cerebrospinal fluid is considered infectious, and standard precautions must be used in connection with the specimen. A 5% phenol, concentrated bleach solution, alcohol solution, or other disinfectant solution can be used for decontamination of equipment that is not disposable. Specific decontamination protocol varies according to the laboratory facility. There is always the danger of spreading infectious pathogens if cerebrospinal fluid is not handled properly. Cell counts on a spinal fluid specimen must be done as soon as possible after the spinal tap has been completed, since the cells present will disintegrate within a short time. Tests for glucose in spinal fluid must also be performed immediately to prevent glycolysis. The use of sodium fluoride will slow down the glycolytic process. A blood specimen for a glucose assay should accompany a request for spinal fluid glucose for comparison purposes. For the chemical tests ordered, the specimen should be sent to the chemistry laboratory.

Normal cerebrospinal fluid appears clear and colorless. If the fluid is grossly bloody or blood tinged, the patient may have a serious brain or spinal injury. Sometimes, however, a drop of blood gets into the sample from the puncture needle. It is important for this reason to observe the collected tubes and to note the order in which they are collected. If blood has gotten into the tube from a **traumatic tap** (blood from the needle, skin, or muscle), the tubes will progressively clear. That is, the first tube collected will have more blood in it, and the succeeding tubes will have less. This is one reason why it is important to observe all the tubes collected, not just one. If all the tubes are bloody to the same degree, a hemorrhage in the brain or spinal cord is more likely. If the spinal fluid in the tubes appears cloudy, there is good reason to suspect an infection in the central nervous system. Most conditions for which spinal fluid testing is requested are very serious and require immediate diagnosis and treatment. This is why the laboratory tests are so important and why speed is essential.

### Synovial Fluid

**Synovial fluid** is the fluid that is contained in the joint spaces. Normal synovial fluid resembles uncooked egg white; it is straw colored and viscous, and does not clot. Examination of this fluid from the joints provides information about joint diseases such as infections, gout, and rheumatoid arthritis.

Synovial fluid differs from other body cavity fluids because of the importance of finding crystals in the specimen and because it is normally very viscous. Ideally the specimen should be collected into three tubes: a sterile tube for culture; a tube with either sodium heparin or liquid EDTA anticoagulant, preferably heparin, for cell counts, crystal identification, and prepared smears; and a plain tube without additive anticoagulant (and not in a serum separator gel tube) to observe for gross appearance, crystal analysis, and fibrinogen clots and for chemistry or immunologic tests. Sodium heparin or liquid EDTA is the additive of choice because other anticoagulants are likely to have undissolved crystals present when the amount of specimen aspirated is small. Normal joints have very little synovial fluid. The additive crystals can cause confusion when the specimen is being examined for the presence of crystals. To test for clot formation, the fluid must be collected in a plain tube without anticoagulant.

### Pericardial, Pleural, and Peritoneal Fluids

The fluids of the pericardial, pleural, and peritoneal cavities are called **serous fluids**. They normally are formed continuously in the body cavities and are reabsorbed, leaving only very small volumes. The normal appearance of these fluids is pale and straw colored. The fluid becomes more turbid as the cell count rises, an indication of inflammation. Increases in the amounts of these body cavity fluids formed are seen in inflammation and when the serum protein level falls. Serous fluids are aspirated because they are mechanically inhibiting the function of the associated organs or for diagnostic purposes. These aspirations are done by the physician. The specimen is collected into various containers, depending on the laboratory testing to be done. An EDTA tube is used for cell counts and smear evaluation, sterile tubes for cultures, and oxalate or fluoride tubes for protein, glucose, or other chemistry tests. If a large volume of fluid is aspirated, it is collected in a gallon jar with an appropriate additive to prevent clotting. If the fluid clots, it is useless for many analyses.

### Swabs for Culture

Swabs with samples of specimens from wounds, abscesses, throats, and so forth are brought to the laboratory in a sterile transport tube for culture. These swabs are potentially from infectious areas and should be treated very carefully in the laboratory. Again, the container with the swab in it must be properly labeled and the culture done immediately (see Chapter 16). Most bacteria will die if stored on a dry swab, so if the culture cannot be done immediately, a transport medium should be used—some means to keep the swab moist and cool. Most organisms can live for many hours if stored properly. Immediate culture is still best, however. Proper technique for disposal of contaminated material must be used.

### Throat Culture Collection

Throat swab specimens are used for detection of group A $\beta$-hemolytic streptococci causing pharyngitis (see Procedure 3-7). The specimen collected can be used for the classic culture on sheep blood media or for one of the rapid direct tests utilizing extraction of the cell wall polysaccharide antigen and its recognition by antibody. These rapid tests have gained popularity, especially in physicians' offices, because results are available within minutes instead of hours (see Chapter 16).

## PROCEDURE 3-7

### *Throat Culture*

1. Ask the patient to open his or her mouth.

2. Using a sterile tongue blade to hold the tongue down, and a sterile swab to collect the specimen, take the specimen directly from the back of the throat, being careful not to touch the teeth, cheeks, gums, or tongue when inserting or removing the swab (Fig. 3-17).

3. The tonsillar fauces and rear pharyngeal wall should be swabbed, not just gently touched, in order to remove organisms adhering to the membranes. White patches of exudate in the tonsillar area are especially productive for isolating the streptococcal organisms.

4. The swab containing the specimen can be placed in a special container with transport media. Commercial collection sets containing both swabs and transport media are available. Streptococci survive on dry swabs for up to 2 to 3 hours and on swabs in transport (holding) media at 4° C for 24 to 48 hours.

5. The specimen container must be labeled with the necessary patient identification.

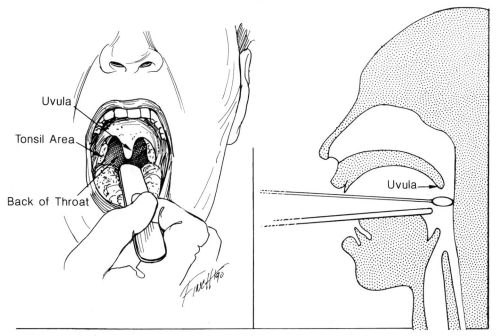

Uvula

Tonsil Area

Back of Throat

Uvula

A. DEPRESS TONGUE FIRMLY          B. COLLECT THROAT CULTURE

**FIG 3-17.** Obtaining a throat culture.

## Feces

Feces, or stool specimens, should be collected in a clean plastic container. The specimen should be collected and covered without being contaminated with urine. The amount collected depends on the test to be done. Most testing is done on a random specimen. The container should be labeled properly, including the time of collection (for a timed specimen) and the laboratory tests desired.

Small amounts of fecal material are frequently analyzed for the presence of occult, or hidden, blood. Occult blood is recognized as a most important sign of the presence of a bleeding ulcer or malignant disease in the gastrointestinal tract. The specimen is applied to commercially prepared filter paper slides that have been impregnated with reagent. These slides are then sent to the laboratory for analysis. Outpatients are often asked to recover small amounts of their own feces that have been excreted into the toilet and apply them directly to the slides, which have been supplied by the physician. These slides are then mailed back to the physician or laboratory for testing.

Feces from infants are usually recovered from the child's diaper for trypsin activity screening tests to detect cystic fibrosis. In adults, for certain metabolic balance studies and for measurement of fecal nitrogen and fat, 3-day (72-hour) fecal collections are needed.

## Other Specimens

Other types of specimens, such as gallstones, kidney stones, sputum, seminal fluid, or tissue samples, may be sent to the laboratory for analysis. Each requires special collection and processing considerations.

## CHAIN-OF-CUSTODY SPECIMEN INFORMATION

When specimens are involved in possible medicolegal situations, certain specimen handling policies are required. Medicolegal, or forensic, implications require that any data pertaining to the specimen in question be arrived at in such a way that they will be recognized by a court of law. Processing steps for such specimens, including the initial collection, transportation, storage, and analytic testing, must be documented by careful record keeping. Documentation ensures that there has been no tampering with the specimen by any interested parties, that the specimen has been collected from the appropriate person, and that the results reported are accurate. Each step of the collection, handling, processing, testing, and reporting processes must be documented—this is called the chain of custody.

**Chain-of-custody documentation** must be signed by every person who has handled the specimens involved in the case in question. The actual process may vary in different health care facilities, but the general purpose of this process is to make certain that any data obtained by the clinical laboratory will be admissible in a court of law and that all steps have been taken to ensure the integrity of the information produced.

## SPECIMEN TRANSPORTATION

Once the specimen has been collected and properly labeled, it must be transported to the laboratory for processing and analysis. In many institutions the specimen container is placed in a leak-proof plastic bag as a further protective measure to prevent pathogen transmission—the implementation of the standard precautions policy and the use of barriers. The request form must be placed on the outside of this bag. Many of these transport bags have a special pouch provided on the outside of the bag, into which the request form is placed.

Since some laboratory analyses require special handling of the specimens to be tested, beginning with the transporting of the specimen to the laboratory, specific requirements for specimens should be noted for each particular test to be done. For example, some tests require that the specimen be protected from light to prevent changes in the constituent to be measured. These specimens should be covered as soon as

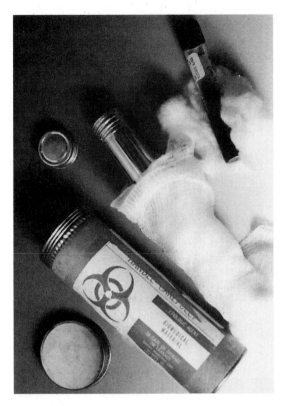

**FIG 3-18.** Proper containers for shipping biological specimens. (From Baron EJ, Finegold SM: *Bailey and Scott's Diagnostic Microbiology,* ed 8. St Louis, Mosby, 1990, p 15.)

possible with a light-protective foil wrap and then transported to the laboratory for processing and testing. Some tests must be done on the specimen as soon after collection as possible. For other tests, the specimen can be processed and stored until testing is done at a later time. It is always the best rule to transport the specimen to the laboratory as quickly as possible, however, using the transport system implemented by the health care institution.

## Shipping Specimens to Reference Laboratories

Sometimes it is necessary to ship a specimen to another laboratory, a large reference laboratory, for example, for testing. Tests infre-

quently performed, or those needing specialized technology, are sometimes more cost-effective if they are done in a central or reference laboratory setting where these special tests are performed. Such testing has become increasingly popular with the advent of the CLIA '88 regulations.

Since biological specimens are potentially infectious, care must be taken to ship them safely, according to the requirements established by the receiving laboratory. Leak-proof and crush-proof primary containers and mailing containers should be used (Fig. 3-18).

All specimen containers to be shipped must be labeled with the necessary patient identification information, and the mailing package must include the properly completed request form for the tests to be done.

## REFERENCES

1. *Ancillary (Bedside) Blood Glucose Testing in Acute and Chronic Care Facilities: Approved Guideline.* Villanova, Pa, National Committee for Clinical Laboratory Standards, 1994, NCCLS document C30-A.
2. *Blood Collection on Filter Paper for Neonatal Screening Programs: Approved Standard,* ed 3. Villanova, Pa, National Committee for Clinical Laboratory Standards, 1997, NCCLS document LA4-A3.
3. College of American Pathologists: *So You're Going to Collect a Blood Specimen: An Introduction to Phlebotomy,* ed 7. Northfield, Ill., College of American Pathologists, 1996.
4. *Devices for Collection of Skin Puncture Blood Specimens: Approved Guideline,* ed 2. Villanova, Pa, National Committee for Clinical Laboratory Standards, 1990, NCCLS document H14-A2.
5. *Evacuated Tubes for Blood Specimen Collection: Approved Standard,* ed 4. Villanova, Pa, National Committee for Clinical Laboratory Standards, 1996, NCCLS Document H1-A4.
6. *Guideline for Isolation Procedures Hospitals.* Hospital Infection Control Practices Advisory Committee (HICPAC), Centers for Disease Control and Prevention (CDC), 1996.

7. *Physician's Office Laboratory Guidelines: Tentative Guideline*, ed 3. Villanova, Pa, National Committee for Clinical Laboratory Standards, 1995, NCCLS document POL1/2-T3.

8. *Procedures for the Collection of Diagnostic Blood Specimens by Skin Puncture: Approved Standard*, ed 3. Villanova, Pa, National Committee for Clinical Laboratory Standards, 1991, NCCLS document H4-A3.

9. *Procedures for the Collection of Diagnostic Blood Specimens by Venipuncture: Approved* Standard, ed 4. Villanova, Pa, National Committee for Clinical Laboratory Standards, 1998, NCCLS document H3-A4.

10. *Procedures for the Handling of Blood Specimens by Venipuncture: Approved Standard*, ed 3. Villanova, Pa, National Committee for Clinical Laboratory Standards, 1990, NCCLS document H18-A.

11. *Routine Urinalysis and Collection, Transportation, and Preservation of Urine Specimens: Approved Guideline*. Villanova, Pa, National Committee for Clinical Laboratory Standards, 1995, NCCLS document GP16-A.

## BIBLIOGRAPHY

Burtis CA, Ashwood ER (eds): *Tietz Fundamentals of Clinical Chemistry*, ed 4. Philadelphia, WB Saunders Co, 1996.

Garza D, Becan-McBride K: *Phlebotomy Handbook*, ed 3. Norwalk, Conn, Appleton & Lange, 1993.

Henry JB (ed): *Clinical Diagnosis and Management by Laboratory Methods*, ed 19. Philadelphia, WB Saunders Co, 1996.

NCCLS: *Procedures for the Handling and Transport of Diagnostic Specimens and Etiologic Agents: Approved Standard*, ed 3. Villanova, Pa, National Committee for Clinical Laboratory Standards, 1994, NCCLS Document H5-A3.

Protection of Laboratory Workers From Infectious Disease Transmitted by Blood, Body Fluids and Tissue: Tentative Standard, ed 2. Villanova, Pa, *National Committee for Clinical Laboratory Standards*, 1991, NCCLS document M29-T2.

Slockbower JM, Blumenfeld TA: *Collection and Handling of Laboratory Specimens*. Philadelphia, JB Lippincott Co, 1983.

## STUDY QUESTIONS

1. **An evacuated blood collection tube with a lavender-colored top is used for almost all tests relating to:**

   A. Clinical chemistry
   B. Microbiologic cultures
   C. Coagulation studies
   D. Hematology

2. **A red-topped or red-and-black-topped blood collection tube is used for:**

   A. Plasma for coagulation tests
   B. Serum for chemistry tests
   C. Anticoagulated blood for hematologic tests
   D. Whole blood for glucose tests

3. **Fasting blood is necessary for some chemistry tests because certain values increase substantially after eating. Which of the following assays does *not* require a fasting blood specimen?**

   A. Glucose
   B. Cholesterol
   C. Triglyceride
   D. Phosphorus

4. **Blood specimens are not acceptable for laboratory testing when which of the following is noted?**

   A. There is no patient name or identification number on the label.
   B. The label on the request form and the label on the collection container do not match.
   C. The wrong collection tube has been used (i.e., anticoagulant additive instead of tube for serum).
   D. All of the above

5. **If serum is allowed to remain on the clot for a prolonged period, which of the following effects will be noted?**

   A. Elevated level of serum potassium
   B. Decreased level of serum potassium
   C. Elevated level of glucose
   D. Decreased level of glucose

6. Match each of the following abnormal serum appearances (1 to 3) with the likely cause for the color change (A to C).

   1. Red-pink
   2. Yellow
   3. Milky white
   _____ A. Elevated bilirubin (jaundice; icteric serum)
   _____ B. Lysis of red blood cells (hemolyzed serum)
   _____ C. Presence of lipids or fat (lipemic serum)

7. What is the preferred method for preserving a urine specimen if it cannot be tested within 2 hours of being voided?

8. What does the NCCLS recommend as a preferred specimen for routine urinalysis?

9. What instructions are necessary to convey to a patient about how a 24-hour urine collection should be done?

10. What would be the appearance of the cerebrospinal fluid in the series of tubes collected if there had been a traumatic tap?

# CHAPTER 4

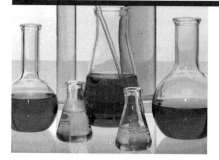

# Systems of Measurement and General Laboratory Equipment

## Learning Objectives

*From study of this chapter, the reader will be able to:*

➤ Understand the metric units of measurement for weight, length, volume, and temperature, how the metric system is used in the laboratory, and the conversion of English units to metric units.

➤ Convert temperatures from degrees Celsius to degrees Fahrenheit and vice versa.

➤ Know how normal and molar solutions are prepared.

➤ Know how to prepare solutions and reagents of specific composition, about the various forms and grades of water used in the laboratory and how each is prepared, about the various grades of chemicals used in the laboratory, including their levels of quality and the purposes for which they are intended, and how to properly label a container used to store a laboratory reagent or solution.

➤ Describe the various types of and uses for laboratory volumetric glassware (pipettes, flasks, burets), the techniques for their use, and the various types of glass used to manufacture them.

➤ Describe and interpret how laboratory volumetric glassware is calibrated and how the calibration markings are indicated on the glassware.

➤ Solve a titration problem—that is, solve for *x* normality when the volume and normality of one solution is known and only the volume of the second solution is known.

➤ Know how to properly clean laboratory glassware and plastic ware.

➤ Describe the operation of and uses for laboratory balances—analytical, torsion, triple beam.

➤ Describe types and uses of laboratory centrifuges.

# INTRODUCTION TO GENERAL LABORATORY MEASUREMENTS AND EQUIPMENT USED

If the results of laboratory analyses are to be useful to the physician in diagnosing and treating patients, the tests must be performed as accurately as possible. Many factors constitute the final laboratory result for a single determination. The use of high-quality analytic methods and instrumentation is of prime importance, but other basic principles and procedures also play a role.

In order to unify physical measurements worldwide, the International System of Units (SI units) has been adopted. Many of these units also relate to the metric system. A coherent system of measurement units is vital to precise clinical laboratory analyses. The pertinent SI units of measure are discussed in this chapter, as well as the use of metric measurements in the laboratory.

A general discussion of laboratory glassware and plastic ware, including types used for measuring volume, is included. The importance of knowing the correct use of these various pieces of glassware must be thoroughly appreciated. The four basic pieces of volumetric glassware—volumetric flasks, graduated measuring cylinders, burets, and pipettes—are specialized, with each having its own particular use in the laboratory.

The accuracy of laboratory analyses depends to a great extent on the accuracy of the reagents used. Traditional preparation of reagents makes use of balances and volumetric measuring devices such as pipettes and volumetric flasks—examples of fundamental laboratory apparatus. When reagents and standard solutions are being prepared, it is imperative that only the purest water supply be used in the procedure. For this reason, the various types of water are discussed. The careful preparation of reagents and standard solutions, along with the necessary knowledge about the chemicals used for these preparations, is basic to any analytic procedure in the clinical laboratory and therefore is discussed in this chapter.

Many and varied pieces of laboratory equipment are used in performing clinical determinations, and knowledge of the proper use and handling of this equipment is an important part of any laboratory work. Measurement of mass, using balances, and measurement of volume, using pipettes and burets, are important basic analytic procedures in the clinical laboratory. Centrifuges are also used in various ways in the laboratory. The use of photometry, and spectrophotometers in particular, is covered in Chapter 6. Autoclaves and incubators are discussed in Chapters 2 and 16.

# SYSTEMS OF MEASUREMENT

The ability to measure accurately is the keystone of the scientific method, and anyone engaged in performing clinical laboratory analyses must have a working knowledge of measurement systems and units of measurement. It is also necessary to understand how to convert units of one system to units of another system. Systems of measurement included here are the English, metric, and SI systems.

## Metric System

Traditionally, measurements in the clinical laboratory have been made in metric units. The **metric system** is based on a decimal system, a system of divisions and multiples of tens. It has not been widely used in the United States, except in the scientific community. The meter (m) is the standard metric unit for measurement of length, the gram (g) is the unit of mass, and the liter (L) is the unit of volume. Multiples or divisions of these reference units constitute the various other metric units.

## International System (SI System)

Another system of measurement, the **International System of Units** (from le Système International d'Unités, or **SI**) has been adopted by the worldwide scientific community as a coherent, standardized system, based on seven base units. There are also derived units and supplemental units, in addition to the base units. The SI base units describe seven fundamental, but independent, physical quantities. The derived units are calculated mathematically from two or more base units.

The SI system was established in 1960 by international agreement and is now the standard international language of measurement. The **International Bureau of Weights and Measures** is responsible for maintaining the standards on which the SI system of measurement is based.

The term *metric system* generally refers to the SI system and, for informational purposes, metric terms that remain in common usage are described where needed. Since the English system is common in everyday use, English system equivalents are also given in the discussion of units.

The National Committee for Clinical Laboratory Standards (NCCLS) recommends that an extensive educational effort be put forth to implement the SI system in clinical laboratories in the United States.[6] Any changes in units used to report laboratory findings should be done with great care, to avoid misunderstanding and confusion in interpretation of laboratory results.

### Base Units of the SI System

In the SI system the base units of measurement are the metre (meter), kilogram, second, mole, ampere, kelvin, and candela. These seven base units and their accepted abbreviations are listed in Table 4-1.

All units in the SI system can be qualified by standard prefixes that serve to convert values to more convenient forms, depending on the size of the object being measured. These prefixes are listed in Table 4-2.

Various rules should be kept in mind when one is combining these prefixes with their basic units and using the SI system; some of these rules follow. An *s* should not be added to form the plural of the abbreviation for a unit or for a prefix with a unit. For example, 25 millimeters should be abbreviated as 25 mm, not 25 mms. Do not use periods after abbreviations (use mm,

## TABLE 4-1

Base Units of the SI System

| Measurement | Unit Name | Abbreviation |
|---|---|---|
| Length | Metre* | m |
| Mass | Kilogram | kg |
| Time | Second | s |
| Amount of substance | Mole | mol |
| Electric current | Ampere | A |
| Temperature | Kelvin† | K |
| Luminous intensity | Candela | cd |

*The spelling *meter* is more commonly used in the United States and is used in this book.

†Although the basic unit of temperature is the kelvin, the degree Celsius is regarded as an acceptable unit, since kelvins may be impractical in many instances. Celsius is more commonly used in the clinical laboratory.

## TABLE 4-2

Prefixes of the SI System

| Prefix Name | Symbol | Factor | Decimal |
|---|---|---|---|
| Tera | T | $10^{12}$ | 1 000 000 000 000 |
| Giga | G | $10^9$ | 1 000 000 000 |
| Mega | M | $10^6$ | 1 000 000 |
| Kilo | k | $10^3$ | 1 000 |
| Hecto | h | $10^2$ | 100 |
| Deka | da | $10^1$ | 10 |
| Deci | d | $10^{-1}$ | 0.1 |
| Centi | c | $10^{-2}$ | 0.01 |
| Milli | m | $10^{-3}$ | 0.001 |
| Micro | μ | $10^{-6}$ | 0.000 001 |
| Nano | n | $10^{-9}$ | 0.000 000 001 |
| Pico | p | $10^{-12}$ | 0.000 000 000 001 |
| Femto | f | $10^{-15}$ | 0.000 000 000 000 001 |
| Atto | a | $10^{-18}$ | 0.000 000 000 000 000 001 |

not mm.). Do not use compound prefixes; instead, use the closest accepted prefix. For example, $24 \times 10^{-9}$ gram (g) should be expressed as 24 nanograms (24 ng) rather than 24 millimicrograms (25 mμg). In the SI system, commas are not used as spacers in recording large numbers, since they are used in place of decimal points in some countries. Instead, groups of three digits are separated by spaces. When recording temperature on the Kelvin scale, omit the degree sign. Therefore, 295 kelvins should be recorded as 295 K, not 295° K. However, the symbol for degree Celsius is ° C, and 22 degrees Celsius should be recorded as 22° C. Multiples and submultiples should be used in steps of $10^3$ or $10^{-3}$. Only one solidus or slash (/) is used when indicating *per* or a denominator: thus meters per second squared ($m/s^2$), not meters per second per second (m/s/s), and millimoles per liter-hour (mmol/L • hour), not millimoles per liter per hour (mmol/L/hour). Finally, although the preferred SI spellings are *metre* and *litre*, the spellings *meter* and *liter* remain in common usage in the United States and are used in this book.

The base units of measurement that are used most often in the clinical laboratory are those for length, mass, and volume.

**Length.** The standard unit for the measurement of length or distance is the **meter (m)**. The meter is standardized as 1,650,763.73 wavelengths of a certain orange light in the spectrum of krypton 86. One meter equals 39.37 inches (in.), slightly more than a yard in the English system. There are 2.54 centimeters (cm) in 1 in.

Further common divisions and multiples of the meter, using the system of prefixes previously discussed, follow. One tenth of a meter is a decimeter (dm), one hundredth of a meter is a centimeter (cm), and one thousandth of a meter is a millimeter (mm). One thousand meters equals 1 kilometer (km). The following examples show equivalent measurements of length:

$$25 \text{ mm} = 0.025 \text{ m}$$
$$10 \text{ cm} = 100 \text{ mm}$$
$$1 \text{ m} = 100 \text{ cm}$$
$$0.1 \text{ m} = 100 \text{ mm}$$

Other units of length that were in common usage in the metric system but are no longer recommended in the SI system are the angstrom and the micron. The angstrom (Å) is equal to $10^{-10}$ m or $10^{-1}$ nanometer (nm). This unit is permitted but not encouraged. The micron ($\mu$), which is equal to $10^{-6}$ m, has been replaced by the micrometer ($\mu$m).

**Mass (and Weight).** Mass denotes the quantity of matter, while weight takes into account the force of gravity and should not be used in the same sense as mass. However, they are commonly used interchangeably and may be so used in this book. The standard unit for the measurement of mass in the SI system is the **kilogram (kg).** This is the basis for all other mass measurements in the system. The standard kilogram is the mass of a block of platinum-iridium kept at the International Bureau of Weights and Measures. One kilogram weighs approximately 2.2 pounds (lb) in the English system. Conversely, 1 lb equals approximately 0.5 kg.

The kilogram is divided into thousandths, called grams (g). One thousand grams equals 1 kg. The gram is used much more often than the kilogram in the clinical laboratory. The gram is divided into thousandths, called milligrams (mg). Grams and milligrams are units commonly used in weighing substances in the clinical laboratory. One millionth of a gram, a microgram ($\mu$g), may also be encountered. Some examples of weight measurement equivalents follow:

$$10 \text{ mg} = 0.01 \text{ g}$$
$$0.055 \text{ g} = 55 \text{ mg}$$
$$25 \text{ g} = 25,000 \text{ mg}$$
$$1.5 \text{ kg} = 1,500 \text{ g}$$

Units that were once used to describe mass and that may still be encountered are the gamma and parts per million. The term gamma ($\gamma$) should not be used; instead, use microgram ($\mu$g). The term parts per million (ppm) should be replaced by micrograms per gram ($\mu$g/g).

**Volume.** In the clinical laboratory the standard unit of volume is the **liter (L).** It was not included in the list of base units of the SI system because the liter is a derived unit. The standard unit of volume in the SI system is the cubic meter ($m^3$). However, this unit is quite large, and the cubic decimeter ($dm^3$) is a more convenient size for use in the clinical laboratory. Thus in 1964 the Conférence Générale des Poids et Mésures (CGPM) accepted the litre (liter) as a special name for the cubic decimeter. Previously, the standard liter was the volume occupied by 1 kg of pure water at 4° C (the temperature at which a volume of water weighs the most) and at normal atmospheric pressure. On this basis, 1 L equals 1,000.027 cubic centimeters ($cm^3$), and the units milliliters and cubic centimeters were used interchangeably, although there is a slight difference between them. One liter is slightly more than 1 quart (qt) in the English system (1 L = 1.06 qt).

The liter is divided into thousandths, called milliliters (mL); millionths, called microliters ($\mu$L); and billionths, called nanoliters (nL). Some examples of volume equivalents are:

$$500 \text{ mL} = 0.5 \text{ L}$$
$$0.25 \text{ L} = 250 \text{ mL}$$
$$2 \text{ L} = 2,000 \text{ mL}$$
$$500 \text{ }\mu\text{L} = 0.5 \text{ mL}$$

Since the liter is derived from the meter (1 L = 1 $dm^3$), it follows that 1 $cm^3$ is equal to 1 mL and that 1 millimeter cubed ($mm^3$) is equal to 1 $\mu$L. The former abbreviation for cubic centimeter (cc) has been replaced by $cm^3$. Although this is a common means of expressing volume in the clinical laboratory, milliliter (mL) is preferred.

**Amount of Substance.** The standard unit of measurement for the amount of a (chemical) substance in the SI system is the mole (mol). The mole is defined as the quantity of a chemical equal to that present in 0.0120 kg of pure carbon 12. A mole of a chemical substance is the relative atomic or molecular mass unit of that substance. Formerly, the terms atomic and molecular weight were used to describe the mole. These are further defined and discussed below.

**Temperature.** Three scales are commonly used to measure temperature, namely, the Kelvin, Celsius, and Fahrenheit scales. The **Celsius scale** is sometimes referred to as the centigrade scale, which is an outdated term.

The basic unit of temperature in the SI system is the kelvin (K). However, as mentioned previously, the degree Celsius is regarded as an acceptable unit, since the kelvin may be impractical in many instances. The Celsius scale is the one used most often in the clinical laboratory. The Kelvin and Celsius scales are closely related, and conversion between them is simple since the units (degrees) are equal in magnitude. The difference between the Kelvin and Celsius scales is the zero point. The zero point on the Kelvin scale is the theoretical temperature of no further heat loss, which is absolute zero. The zero point on the Celsius scale is the freezing point of pure water. Remember, however, that the magnitude of the degree is equal in the two scales. Therefore, since water freezes at 273 kelvins (273 K), it follows that 0 degrees Celsius (0° C) equals 273 kelvins (273 K) and that 0 Kelvin (0 K) equals minus 273 degrees Celsius (–273° C). Thus, to convert from kelvins to degrees Celsius, add 273; to convert from degrees Celsius to kelvins, subtract 273.

$$K = {}^\circ C + 273$$
$$^\circ C = K - 273$$

Since the Celsius scale was devised so that 100° C is the boiling point of pure water, the boiling point on the Kelvin scale is 373 K.

Converting from Celsius to Fahrenheit is not as simple, since the degrees are not equal in magnitude on these two scales. The Fahrenheit scale was originally devised with the zero point at the lowest temperature attainable from a mixture of table salt and ice, while the body temperature of a small animal was used to set 100° F. Thus, on the Fahrenheit scale the freezing point of pure water is 32°, while the temperature at which pure water boils is 212°. It is rare that readings on one of these scales must be converted to the other, as almost without exception readings taken and used in the clinical laboratory will be on the Celsius scale.

Examples of comparative readings of the three scales with common reference points are given in Table 4-3.

It is possible, however, to convert from one scale to the other. The basic conversion formulas are:

1. $1^\circ C = \frac{9}{5}{}^\circ F$
   $1^\circ F = \frac{5}{9}{}^\circ C$
2. To convert Fahrenheit to Celsius:
   *Method A:* Add 40, multiply by $\frac{5}{9}$, and subtract 40 from the result.
   *Method B:*  $^\circ C = \frac{5}{9}({}^\circ F - 32)$

---

**TABLE 4-3**

Common Reference Points on the Three Temperature Scales

|  | Kelvin | Degrees Celsius | Degrees Fahrenheit |
|---|---|---|---|
| Boiling point of water | 373 | 100 | 212 |
| Body temperature | 310 | 37 | 98.6 |
| Room temperature | 293 | 20 | 68 |
| Freezing point of water | 273 | 0 | 32 |
| Absolute zero (coldest possible temperature) | 0 | –273 | –459 |

3. To convert Celsius to Fahrenheit:
    *Method A:* Add 40, multiply by ⅝, and subtract 40 from the result.
    *Method B:* $\degree F = \frac{9}{5}\degree C + 32$

### Non-SI Units

Several non-SI units are relevant to clinical laboratory analyses, such as minutes (min), hours (hr), and days (d). These units of time have such historic use in everyday life that it is unlikely that new SI units derived from the second (the base unit for time in the SI system) will be implemented. Another non-SI unit is the liter (L). This has already been discussed with the base SI units of volume. Pressure is expressed in millimeters of mercury (mm Hg) and enzyme activity in international units (IU) (1 IU is defined as the amount of enzyme that will catalyze the transformation of 1 mol/sec of substrate in an assay system).

### Reporting Results in SI Units

In order to give a meaningful laboratory result, it is important to always report both the numbers and the units by which the result is measured. The unit expresses or defines the dimension of the measured substance—concentration, mass, or volume—and it is an important part of any laboratory result.

Laboratory results can be reported as a mass concentration unit—mass/liter (as g/dL)—or as a molar unit (moles/L). Commonly, laboratories in the United States have been using the mass per liter system in results reporting. Worldwide, moles per liter units are used. Implementation, or conversion, to SI units (moles/L) would mean that some previously reported units will change. With SI units, whenever the molecular weight of the measured analyte is known, its concentration is to be expressed in moles per liter (mol/L) or a subunit, rather than in mass per liter. If the molecular weight is not known, as in specific proteins, mixtures of proteins, or other complex molecules, the concentration should be expressed in mass per liter.

Conversion to the molar (mol/L) unit from a mass concentration unit (g/dL) first involves multiplication by 10 for volume conversion and then division by the molecular weight of the substance. If any conversion is made, no greater precision should be given than was present in the original measurement.

## LABORATORY GLASSWARE AND PLASTIC WARE

The general laboratory supplies, or laboratory ware, described in this chapter are those used for storage, measurement, and containment. Laboratory glassware and plastic ware, as well as automatic pipetting and diluting devices, are included. Most laboratory glassware and other laboratory ware can be divided into two main categories according to the use to which they are put: containers and receivers and volumetric ware. Examples of containers and receivers are beakers, test tubes, Erlenmeyer flasks, and reagent bottles. Examples of volumetric ware are pipettes, automatic and manual; volumetric flasks; graduated cylinders; and burets.

### Glassware

Clinical laboratories still use glassware for the greater part of the analytic work done, even with the advent of plastic ware. Glassware is used in all departments of the laboratory, and special types of glass apparatus have been devised for special uses. These special types of glassware are discussed where applicable. The chemistry department probably has the greatest variety and amount of glassware. Certain types of glass can be attacked by reagents to such an extent that the determinations done in them are not valid. It is therefore important to use the correct type of glass for the determinations being done.

### Types of Glass

Clinical laboratory glassware can be divided into several types: glass with high thermal resistance, high-silica glass, glass with a high resistance to alkali, low-actinic glass, and standard flint glass.

**Thermal-Resistant (Borosilicate) Glass.** High-thermal-resistant glass is usually a borosilicate glass with a low alkali content. This type of glassware is resistant to heat, corrosion, and thermal shock and should be used whenever heating or sterilization by heat is employed. Borosilicate glass, known by the commercial name of Pyrex* or Kimax,[†] is used widely in the laboratory because of its high qualities of resistance. Laboratory apparatus such as beakers, flasks, and pipettes are usually made from borosilicate glass. Other brands of glassware are made from lower-grade borosilicate glass and may be used when a high-quality borosilicate glass is not necessary. If the various pieces of glassware found in the laboratory are examined, it will be seen that one or more of these brand names will be found on many different kinds of glassware. It is essential to choose glassware that has a reliable composition and that will be resistant to laboratory chemicals and conditions. In borosilicate glassware, mechanical strength and thermal and chemical resistance are well balanced.

**Alumina-Silica Glass.** Alumina-silica glass has a high silica content, which makes it comparable to fused quartz in its heat resistance, chemical stability, and electrical characteristics. It is strengthened chemically rather than thermally. Corex* brand is made from alumina-silica. This type of glassware is used for high-precision analytic work, is radiation resistant, and can also be used for optical reflectors and mirrors. It is not used for the general type of glassware found in the laboratory.

**Alkali-Resistant Glass.** Glass with high resistance to alkali was developed particularly for use with strong alkaline solutions. It is boron-free. It is often referred to as soft glass, as its thermal resistance is much less than that of borosilicate glass, and it must be heated and cooled very carefully. Its use should be limited to times when solutions of, or digestions with, strong alkalis are made.

**Low-Actinic Glass.** Low-actinic glassware contains materials that usually impart an amber or red color to the glass and reduce the amount of light transmitted through to the substance in the glassware. It is used for substances that are particularly sensitive to light, such as bilirubin or vitamin A.

**Standard Flint Glass.** Standard flint glass, or soda-lime glass, is composed of a mixture of the oxides of silicon, calcium, and sodium. It is the most inexpensive glass and is readily made into a variety of types of glassware. This type of glass is much less resistant to high temperatures and sudden changes in temperature, and its resistance to chemical attack is only fair. Glassware made from soda-lime glass can release alkali into solutions and can therefore cause considerable errors in certain laboratory determinations. For example, manual pipettes made from soda-lime glass may release alkali into the pipetted liquid.

**Disposable Glassware.** The widespread use of relatively inexpensive disposable glassware has greatly reduced the need to clean glassware. Disposable glassware is made to be used and discarded, and no cleaning is necessary either before or after use, in most cases. Disposable glass and plastic are used to manufacture test tubes of all sizes, pipettes, slides, Petri dishes for microbiology, and specimen containers, to mention but a few.

### Containers and Receivers

This category of glassware includes many of the most frequently used and most common pieces of glassware in the laboratory. Containers and

---

*Corning Glass Works, Corning, NY.
[†]Kimble Glass Co, Vineland, NJ.

receivers must be made of good-quality glass. They are not calibrated to hold a particular or exact volume, but rather are available for various volumes, depending on the use desired. Beakers, Erlenmeyer flasks, test tubes, and reagent bottles are made in many different sizes (Fig. 4-1). This glassware, like the volumetric glassware, has certain information indicated directly on the vessel. The volume and the brand name, or trademark, are two pieces of information found on items such as beakers and test tubes. Containers and receivers are not as expensive as volumetric glassware, because the process of exact volume calibration is not necessary.

**Beakers.** Beakers are wide, straight-sided cylindrical vessels and are available in many sizes and in several forms. The most common form used in the clinical laboratory is known as the Griffin low form. Beakers should be made of glass that is resistant to the many chemicals used in them and also resistant to heat. Beakers are used along with flasks for general mixing and for reagent preparation.

**Erlenmeyer Flasks.** Erlenmeyer flasks are used commonly in the laboratory for preparing reagents and for titration procedures. They, too, come in various sizes and must be made from a resistant form of glass.

**Test Tubes.** Test tubes come in many sizes, depending on the use for which they are intended. Test tubes without lips are the most satisfactory, because there is less chance of chipping and eventual breakage. Disposable test tubes are used for most laboratory purposes.

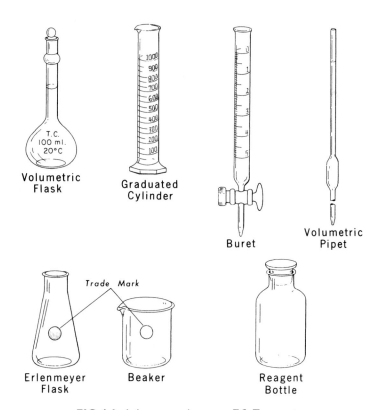

**FIG 4-1.** Laboratory glassware. *T.C.*, To contain.

Since chemical reactions occur in test tubes used in the chemistry laboratory, test tubes intended for such use should be made of borosilicate glass, which is resistant to thermal shock.

**Reagent Bottles.** All reagents should be stored in reagent bottles of some type. These can be made of glass or some other material; some of the more commonly purchased ones now are made of plastic. Reagent bottles come in various sizes; the size used should meet the needs of the particular situation.

**Photometry Cuvettes.** The special tubes used for photometry are called cuvettes or absorption cells. They may be round, square, or rectangular and may be made of glass, silica (quartz), or plastic. For most routine purposes in the clinical laboratory, a round cuvette made of good-quality glass is used. The amount of light transmitted by the cuvette varies significantly with the material used to make it. In order for cuvettes to be used interchangeably, they must be of uniform inside diameters so that the absorbance of a solution will be within a specified tolerance when measured in different cuvettes. To ensure this uniformity, only calibrated cuvettes must be used or plain tubes that have been optically matched (see also Chapter 6).

### Volumetric Glassware

**Volumetric glassware** must go through a rigorous process of volume **calibration** to ensure the accuracy of the measurements required for laboratory determinations. In very precise work it is never safe to assume that the volume contained or delivered by any piece of equipment is exactly that indicated on the equipment. The calibration process is lengthy and time consuming; therefore the cost of volumetric glassware is relatively high compared with the cost of noncalibrated glassware (beakers, test tubes, and so on).

**Volumetric Flasks.** Volumetric flasks are flasks with a round bulb at the bottom. This ta-

pers to a long neck, on which the calibration mark is found. The specifications set up by the National Bureau of Standards apply to all volumetric glassware and therefore to volumetric flasks (see Fig. 4-1).[4] Volumetric flasks are calibrated to contain a specific amount or volume of liquid, and therefore the letters TC are inscribed somewhere on the neck of the flask. There are many different sizes of volumetric flasks, for the different volumes of liquid that are used. The following are some of the sizes in which volumetric flasks can be purchased: 10, 25, 50, 100, and 500 mL, and 1 and 2 L.

Volumetric flasks have been calibrated individually to contain the specified volume at a specified temperature. They are not calibrated to deliver this volume. For each size of volumetric flask, there are certain allowable limits within which its volume must lie. These limits are called the tolerance of the flask. All volumetric glassware has a specific tolerance, the capacity tolerance, which is dependent on the size of the glassware. For example, if a 100-mL volumetric flask has a tolerance of $\pm0.08$ mL, conditions are controlled during the calibration of a 100-mL volumetric flask to guarantee these limits. A tolerance of $\pm0.08$ mL indicates that the allowable limits for the volume of a 100-mL volumetric flask are from 99.92 to 100.08 mL. A tolerance of $\pm0.05$ mL for a 50-mL volumetric flask indicates allowable limits of 49.95 to 50.05 mL for the volume of the flask. Volumetric flasks are used in the preparation of specific volumes of reagents or laboratory solutions. They should be used with reagents or solutions at room temperature. Solutions diluted in volumetric flasks should be repeatedly mixed during the dilution so that the contents are homogeneous before they are made up to volume. In this way, errors due to the expansion or contraction of liquids during mixing are made negligible. An important factor in the use of any volumetric apparatus is an accurate reading of the meniscus level. For more information on reading a meniscus, see under Pipetting Technique Using Manual Pipettes later in this chapter.

**Graduated Measuring Cylinders.** A graduated measuring cylinder is a long straight-sided cylindrical piece of glassware with calibrated markings on it. Graduated cylinders are used to measure volumes of liquids when a high degree of accuracy is not essential. They can be made from plastic or polyethylene as well as from glass (see Fig. 4-1). Graduated cylinders come in various sizes according to the volumes they measure: 10, 25, 50, 100, 500, and 1000 mL. A 100-mL graduated cylinder can measure 100 mL or a fraction thereof, depending on the calibration, or graduation, marks on it. Most graduated cylinders are calibrated to deliver. This will be indicated directly on the glassware by the inscription TD. The letters TD can be found on many kinds of volumetric glassware, especially on the numerous kinds of pipettes used in the laboratory (see under Pipettes).

Graduated cylinders can be used to measure a specified volume of a liquid, such as water, in the preparation of laboratory reagents. The calibration marks on the cylinder indicate its capacity at different points. If 450 mL of water is to be measured, the most satisfactory cylinder to use would be one with a capacity of 500 mL. Graduated cylinders are not calibrated as accurately as volumetric flasks. Therefore, the capacity tolerance for graduated cylinders allows a greater variation in volume. The capacity tolerance is greater for the larger graduated cylinders. A 100-mL graduated cylinder (TD) has a tolerance of ±0.40 mL, meaning that the allowable limits are 99.60 to 100.40 mL.

**Pipettes.** Pipettes are another type of volumetric glassware used extensively in the laboratory. Many types of pipettes are available. It is important, however, to use only pipettes manufactured by reputable companies. Care and discretion should be used in selecting pipettes for clinical laboratory use, since their accuracy is one of the determining factors in the accuracy of the procedures carried out. A pipette is a cylindrical glass tube used in measuring fluids. Pipettes are calibrated to deliver, or transfer, a specified volume from one vessel to another (see Fig. 4-1). Manual and automatic pipettes are available.

Each manual pipette has at least one calibration or graduation mark on it, as does all volumetric glassware. A pipette is filled by using mechanical suction or an aspirator bulb. Mouth suction is never used. Strong acids, bases, solvents, or human specimens are much too potent or contaminated to risk pipetting them by mouth. Caustic liquids and some solvents are very dangerous; some destroy tissue immediately on contact. Some solvents have harmful vapors (see Chapter 2).

For most general laboratory use, there are two main types of manual pipettes: the **volumetric (or transfer) pipette** and the **graduated (or measuring) pipette**. They are classified according to whether they contain or deliver a specified amount; thus they may be called **to-contain pipettes** or **to-deliver pipettes**. A to-contain pipette is identified by the inscribed letters TC and a to-deliver one by the letters TD. The TD pipette is filled properly and allowed to drain completely into a receiving vessel. Portions of nonviscous samples, such as filtrates, serum, and standard solutions, are accurately measured by allowing the volumetric pipette to drain while it is held in the vertical position and by using only the force of gravity (see under Pipetting Technique Using Manual Pipettes). For most volumetric glassware the temperature of calibration is usually 20° C, and this is inscribed on the pipette (see under Calibration of Volumetric Glassware).

The opening (orifice) at the delivery tip of the pipette is of a certain size to give a specified length of time for drainage when the pipette is held vertically. A pipette must be held vertically to ensure proper drainage. It will not drain as fast when held at a 45-degree angle. The actual procedure is discussed further under Measurement of Volume: Pipetting and Titration.

The use of diluting pipettes is discussed in Chapter 12.

*Volumetric Pipettes.* A pipette that has been calibrated to deliver a fixed volume of liquid by drainage is known as a volumetric pipette, or transfer pipette. These pipettes consist of a cylindrical bulb joined at both ends to narrow glass tubing. A **calibration mark** is etched around the upper suction tube, and the lower delivery tube is drawn out to a fine tip. Some important considerations concerning volumetric pipettes are that the calibration mark should not be too close to the top of the suction tube, the bulb should merge gradually into the lower delivery tube, and the delivery tip should have a gradual taper. To reduce drainage errors, the orifice should be of such a size that the flow out of the pipette is not too rapid. These pipettes should be made from a good-quality glass, such as Kimax or Pyrex (Fig. 4-2).

Volumetric pipettes are suitable for all accurate measurements of volumes of 1 mL or more. They are calibrated to deliver the amount inscribed on them. This volume is measured from the calibration mark to the tip. A 5-mL volumetric pipette will deliver a single measured volume of 5 mL, and a 2-mL volumetric pipette will deliver 2 mL. The **tolerance** of volumetric pipettes increases with the capacity of the pipette. A 10-mL volumetric pipette will have a greater tolerance than a 2-mL one. The tolerance of a 5-mL volumetric pipette is ±0.01 mL. When volumes of liquids are to be delivered with great accuracy, a volumetric pipette is used. Volumetric pipettes are used to measure standard solutions, unknown blood and plasma filtrates, serum, plasma, urine, cerebrospinal fluid, and some reagents.

Measurements with volumetric pipettes are done individually, and the volumes can be only whole milliliters, as determined by the pipette selected (e.g., 1, 2, 5, and 10 mL). To transfer 1 mL of a standard solution into a test tube volumetrically, a 1-mL volumetric pipette is used. To transfer 5 mL of the same solution, a 5-mL volumetric pipette is used. After a volumetric pipette drains, a drop remains inside the delivery tip. The specific volume the pipette is calibrated to deliver is dependent on the fact that the drop is left in the tip of the pipette. Information inscribed on the pipette includes the temperature of calibration (usually 20° C), capacity, manufacturer, and use (TD). The technique involved in using volumetric pipettes correctly is very important, and a certain amount of skill is required (see under Pipetting Technique Using Manual Pipettes).

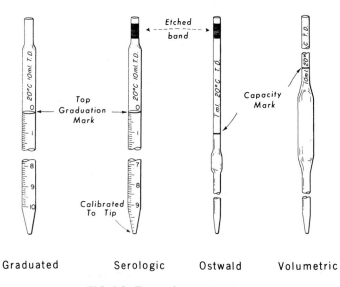

**FIG 4-2.** Types of manual pipettes.

**Graduated Pipettes.** Another way to deliver a particular amount of liquid is to deliver the amount of liquid contained between two calibration marks on a cylindrical tube, or pipette. Such a pipette is called a graduated pipette, or measuring pipette. It has several graduation, or calibration, marks (see Fig. 4-2). Many measurements in the laboratory do not require the precision of the volumetric pipette. Graduated pipettes are used when great accuracy is not required. This does not mean that these pipettes may be used with less care than the volumetric pipettes. Graduated pipettes are used primarily in measuring reagents, but they are not calibrated with sufficient tolerance to use in measuring standard or control solutions, unknown specimens, or filtrates.

A graduated pipette is a straight piece of glass tubing with a tapered end and graduation marks on the stem separating it into parts. Depending on the size used, graduated pipettes can be used to measure parts of a milliliter or many milliliters. These pipettes come in various sizes or capacities, including 0.1, 0.2, 1.0, 2.0, 5.0, 10, and 25 mL. If 4 mL of deionized water is to be measured into a test tube, a 5-mL graduated pipette would be the best choice. Since graduated pipettes require draining between two marks, they introduce one more source of error, compared with the volumetric pipettes, which have only one calibration mark. This makes measurements with the graduated pipette less precise. Because of this relatively poor precision, the graduated pipette is used when speed is more important than precision. It is used for measurements of reagents and is generally not considered accurate enough for measuring samples and standard solutions.

Two types of graduated pipettes are calibrated for delivery (see Fig. 4-2). One (called a Mohr pipette) is calibrated between two marks on the stem, and the other (a serologic pipette) has graduation marks down to the delivery tip. The serologic pipette has a larger orifice and therefore drains faster than the Mohr pipette (see under Serologic Pipettes).

The volume of the space between the last calibration mark and the delivery tip is not known in the Mohr pipette. In Mohr graduated pipettes, this space cannot be used for measuring fluids. Graduated pipettes are calibrated in much the same manner as volumetric pipettes; however, they are not constructed to as strict specifications, and they have larger tolerances. The allowable tolerance for a 5-mL graduated pipette is ±0.02 mL.

**Micropipettes (To-Contain Pipettes).** The **micropipette**, or to-contain pipette, when used properly, is one of the more precise pipettes used in the clinical laboratory. This type of pipette is calibrated to contain a specified amount of liquid. If a pipette contains only 10 $\mu$L (0.1 mL), and 10 $\mu$L of blood is needed for a laboratory determination, then none of the blood can be left inside the pipette. The entire contents of the pipette must be emptied. If this pipette is rinsed well with a diluting solution, then all the blood or similar specimen will be removed from it. The correct way to use a to-contain pipette is to rinse it with a suitable diluent. Thus, a to-contain pipette cannot be used properly unless the receiving vessel contains a diluent; that is, a to-contain pipette should not be used to deliver a specimen into an empty receiving vessel. Since all the liquid in a to-contain pipette is rinsed out and used, there is only one graduation mark.

Micropipettes are used when small amounts of blood or specimen are needed. Many procedures require only a small amount of blood, and a micropipette is used for this measurement. Because even a minute volume remaining in the pipette can cause a significant error in micro work, most micropipettes are calibrated to contain the stated volume rather than to deliver it. They are generally available in small sizes, from 1 to 500 $\mu$L.

*Unopette.* A special disposable micropipette used in the hematology laboratory is a self-filling pipette accompanied by a polyethylene reagent reservoir (see also Chapter 12). This unit is called a Unopette* and is used by many labo-

---

*Becton, Dickinson & Co, Franklin Lakes, NJ.

ratories. A glass capillary pipette is fitted in a plastic holder and fills automatically with blood by means of capillary action. The plastic reagent bottle (called the reservoir) is squeezed slightly while the pipette is inserted. On release of pressure, the sample is drawn into the diluent in the reservoir. Intermittent squeezing fills and empties the pipette to rinse out the contents. This type of unit has been adapted for several chemical and hematologic determinations.

*Capillary pipettes.* An inexpensive, disposable micropipette is one made of capillary tubing with a calibration line marking a specified volume. This micropipette is filled to the line by capillary action, and the measured liquid is delivered by positive pressure, as with a medicine dropper. These **capillary pipettes** are usually calibrated TC and require rinsing to obtain the stated accuracy.

*Automatic micropipettors.* These are **automatic pipetting devices,** which allow rapid, repetitive measurements and delivery of equivalent volumes of reagents or solutions. The most common type of micropipette used in many laboratories is one that is automatic or semiautomatic, called a micropipettor. These are piston-operated devices that allow repeated, accurate, reproducible delivery of specimens, reagents, and other liquids needing measurement in small amounts (see Fig. 4-10). Many pipettors are continuously adjustable so that variable volumes of liquids can be dispensed with the same device. Delivery volume is selected by adjusting the settings on the pipette device. Different types or models are available, which allow volume delivery ranging from 0.5 $\mu$L to 5,000 $\mu$L, for example. The calibration of these micropipettes should be checked periodically.

The piston, usually in the form of a thumb plunger, is depressed to a stop position on the pipetting device, the tip is placed in the liquid to be measured, and then slowly the plunger is allowed to rise back to the original position (see Fig. 4-10). This will fill the tip with the desired volume of liquid. The tips are usually drawn along the inside wall of the vessel from which

the measured volume is drawn, so that any adhering liquid is removed from the end of the tip. These pipette tips are not usually wiped as is done with the manual pipettes, because the plastic surface is considered nonwettable. The tip of the pipette device is then placed against the inside wall of the receiving vessel, and the plunger is depressed. When the manufacturer's directions for the device being used are followed, sample delivery volume is judged to be extremely accurate.

The pipette tips are usually made of disposable plastic, so no cleaning is necessary. Various types of tips are available. Some pipetting devices automatically eject the tip after use. These will also allow the user to insert a new tip as well as remove the used tip without touching it, minimizing infectious biohazard exposures. See Pipetting Technique Using Automatic Pipettes later in this chapter.

**Ostwald Pipettes.** A special type of pipette designed for use in measuring viscous fluids such as whole blood is known as the Ostwald pipette (or the Ostwald-Folin pipette).

**Serologic Pipettes.** Another pipette used in the laboratory, but not often in the chemistry laboratory, is called a **serologic pipette.** It is much like the graduated pipette in appearance (see Fig. 4-2). The orifice, or tip opening, is larger in the serologic pipette than in other pipettes. The rate of fall of liquid is much too fast for great accuracy or precision. For use of the serologic pipette in chemistry, it would be necessary to retard the flow of liquid from the delivery tip. The serologic pipette is graduated to the end of the delivery tip and has an etched band on the suction piece. It is therefore designed to be blown out mechanically. The serologic pipette is less precise than any of the pipettes discussed above. It is designed for use in serology, in which relative values are sought. It is best not to use the serologic pipette for chemistry.

**Burets.** A **buret** is a long cylindrical tube of glassware with graduation divisions on it and a stopcock closing at one end (see Fig. 4-1). The stopcock on the delivery tip of the buret serves to control the flow of liquid. A buret is used to deliver measured quantities of fluids or solutions in the process of **titration**. Like all other volumetric glassware, burets are carefully calibrated according to the specifications set up by the National Bureau of Standards.

Burets also have a specific capacity tolerance depending on their size. Smaller burets are more accurate than larger ones (they have smaller tolerances). Burets with a maximum capacity of 2 mL or less are called microburets. They are usually calibrated with 0.01-mL or smaller divisions. Some common capacities for burets are 5, 10, and 25 mL. The capacity tolerances for burets are similar to those for graduated pipettes, which burets resemble very closely. For a 5-mL buret, the tolerance is ±0.02 mL. This means that the allowable limits for the volume of this particular buret are 4.98 to 5.02 mL. The chief difference between the buret and the graduated pipette is that the buret has a stopcock. The stopcock is made from either glass or Teflon. A glass stopcock requires the use of a lubricant, but a Teflon stopcock does not. Burets are used in titration, a means of quantitative measurement (see under Titration for more information on the use of the buret).

**Calibration of Volumetric Glassware.** Calibration is the means by which glassware or other apparatus used in quantitative measurements is checked to determine its exact volume. To calibrate is to divide the glassware or mark it with graduations (or other indices of quantity) for the purpose of measurement. Calibration marks will be seen on every piece of volumetric glassware used in the laboratory. Specifications for the calibration of glassware are established by the **National Bureau of Standards**.[4] High-quality volumetric glassware is calibrated by the manufacturer; this calibration can be checked by the laboratory using the glassware.

Each piece of volumetric glassware must be checked and must comply with these specifications before it can be accurately used in the clinical laboratory. Pipettes, burets, volumetric flasks, and other types of volumetric glassware are supposed to hold, deliver, or contain a specific amount of liquid. This specified amount, or volume, is known as the units of capacity and is indicated by the manufacturer directly on each piece of glassware.

Volumetric glassware is usually calibrated by weight, using distilled water. Water is commonly used as the liquid for calibration because it is readily available and because it is similar in viscosity and speed of drainage to the solutions and reagents ordinarily used in the clinical laboratory. The units of capacity determined will therefore be the volume of water contained in, or delivered by, the glassware at a particular temperature. The manufacturer knows what the weights of various amounts of distilled water are at specific temperatures. This information is used in the manual calibration of volumetric glassware. If a manufacturer wants a volumetric flask to contain 100 mL, a sensitive balance such as an analytical balance is used. Weights corresponding to what 100 mL of distilled water weighs at a specific temperature are placed on one side of the balance. The flask to be calibrated is placed on the other side of the balance, and distilled water is gradually added to it until equilibrium is achieved. The manufacturer then makes a permanent calibration mark on the neck of the flask at the bottom of the water meniscus level. This flask is then calibrated to contain 100 mL. Other sizes and types of volumetric glassware are similarly calibrated.

The volume of a particular piece of glassware varies with the temperature. For this reason it is necessary to specify the temperature at which the glassware was calibrated. Glass will swell or shrink with changes in temperature, and the volume of the glassware will therefore vary. Most volumetric glassware for routine clinical use is calibrated at 20° C. This means that the calibration process and checking took place at a controlled temperature of 20° C. On all volumetric glassware the inscription 20° C will be seen.

Although 20° C has been almost universally adopted as the standard temperature for calibration of volumetric glassware, each piece of glassware will have the temperature of calibration inscribed on it. The volume of a volumetric flask is smaller at a low temperature than at a high temperature. A 50-mL volumetric flask that was calibrated at 20° C would contain less than 50 mL at 10° C.

Since the laboratory depends to such a great extent on the quality of its glassware in order to produce reliable results, it is necessary to be certain that the glassware is of the very best quality. The glass used for volumetric glassware must meet certain standards of quality. It must be transparent and free from striations and other surface irregularities. It should have no defects that would distort the appearance of the liquid surface or portion of the calibration line seen through the glass.

The design and workmanship for volumetric glassware are also specified by the National Bureau of Standards. The shape of the glassware must permit complete emptying and thorough cleaning, and it must stand solidly on a level surface.

## Plastic Ware

The clinical laboratory has benefited greatly from the introduction of plastic ware. In many cases, plastic ware designed for laboratory use has replaced glassware. Much of the laboratory ware in general use, such as beakers, graduated cylinders, reagent bottles, capillary tubing for pipettes, and test tubes, can be manufactured from plastic as well as from glass. Plastic ware is cheaper and more durable, but glassware is frequently preferred because of its chemical stability and clarity. Plastic is unbreakable, which is its greatest advantage. Plastic is preferred for certain analyses in which glass can be damaged by chemicals used in the testing. Alkaline solutions must be stored in plastic.

The disadvantages of plastic are that there is some leaching of surface-bound constituents into solutions, some permeability to water va-

por, some evaporation through breathing of the plastic, and some absorption of dyes, stains, or proteins. Because evaporation is a significant factor in using plastic ware, small volumes of reagent should never be stored in oversized plastic bottles for long periods of time.

Polymerized organic monomers are used to manufacture plastics for laboratory use. The most commonly used plastics include the polyolefins (polyethylene, polypropylene), polytetrafluoroethylene (Teflon, a fluorinated hydrocarbon), polystyrene, polycarbonate, and polyvinylchloride. These plastics are relatively chemically inert and as a group are unaffected by acids, alkalis, salt solutions, and most aqueous solutions. Most disposable plastic ware is made from polyethylene; it is very resistant to high temperatures, but can absorb some pigments and become discolored. Polyvinylchlorides are soft and flexible and are used to manufacture tubing. Some of the plastics can be autoclaved—Teflon, polycarbonate, and some of the polyolefin plastics. Polycarbonate plastic ware is clear and is ideal for graduated cylinders. Teflon is useful because it is almost totally chemically inert and is also resistant to a wide range of temperatures. Polyolefins are useful, in general, for their strength and their resistance to high temperatures. Specific physical properties for each type of plastic ware can be obtained from the manufacturer of the product. Materials used should be tested under the conditions present in the individual laboratory setting.

## Automatic Measuring Devices
### Automatic Pipettes

Automatic and semiautomatic pipettes are useful in many areas of laboratory work. Several different types are available, and each must be carefully calibrated before use. The problems encountered with automatic pipetting depend to a large degree on the nature of the solution to be pipetted. Some reagents cause more bubbles than others, and some are more viscous. Bubbles and viscous solutions can cause problems with measurement and delivery of samples and solutions.

Automatic pipetting devices permit rapid, repetitive measurement and delivery of predefined volumes of reagent or sample. With the use of these devices, efficient delivery of equal volumes of specific liquids is ensured. Specimens can be measured efficiently, followed by the addition of the necessary reagents or diluents. Some devices can measure the sample and then follow with a diluting reagent dispensed with the same apparatus. Other devices have tip-ejector capabilities, variable digital settings, or repetitive dispensing capabilities for added convenience. The capillary tips into which the sample is drawn can be made from glass or plastic. These are usually disposable. This eliminates cleaning and promotes proper discard techniques for infection control. Proper care, calibration, and maintenance are necessary to ensure precise, accurate sampling when these automatic pipetting devices are used. It is important to read and follow the manufacturer's instructions for each device (see also under Automatic Micropipettors in this chapter).

### Automatic Dispensers or Syringes

Many types of automatic dispensers or syringes are used in the laboratory for repetitive adding of multiple doses of the same reagent or diluent. These devices are used for measuring serial amounts of relatively small volumes of the same liquid. The volume to be dispensed is determined by the pipettor setting. Dispensers are available with varieties of volume settings. Some are available as syringes and others as bottle top devices. Most of these dispensers can be cleaned by autoclaving.

### Diluter-Dispensers

In automated instruments, diluter-dispensers are used to prepare a number of different samples for analysis. These devices pipette a selected aliquot of sample and diluent into the instrument or receiving vessel. These devices are mostly of the dual-piston type, one being used for the sample and the other for the diluent or reagent.

## Cleaning Laboratory Glassware and Plastic Ware

Among the many factors that ensure accurate results in laboratory determinations is the use of clean, unbroken glassware. There is no point in exercising care in obtaining specimens, handling the specimens, and making the laboratory determination if the laboratory ware used is not extremely clean. Plastic ware must also be clean.

There are various methods of cleaning glassware, the one chosen depending on the glassware's use. In all cases, glassware for the clinical laboratory must be physically clean, in most cases it must be chemically clean, and in some cases it must be bacteriologically clean, or sterile.

Laboratory ware that cannot be cleaned immediately after use should be rinsed with tap water and left to soak in a basin or pail of water to which a small amount of detergent has been added. Never allow dirty glassware or plastic ware to dry out. Once dried out on the surface, it is difficult to remove most soil by ordinary means. For this reason it is important to have a soaking bucket available in the working area. Glassware that is new is often slightly alkaline and should be soaked for several hours in a dilute hydrochloric acid or nitric acid solution (about 1 mL/dL is satisfactory). This glassware should then be washed in the usual manner.

Glassware that is contaminated, as by use with patient specimens, must be decontaminated before it is washed. This can be done by presoaking in 5% bleach, or by boiling, autoclaving, or some similar procedure.

General cleaning methods involve the use of a soap, detergent, or cleaning powder. In most laboratories, detergents are used. If the dirty glassware has been soaking in a solution of the detergent water, the cleaning job will be much easier.

### General Cleaning Procedure

There are various methods of cleaning laboratory ware. Most glassware and plastic ware (with the exception of pipettes) can be cleaned manually as described in Procedure 4-1.

## PROCEDURE 4-1

### Cleaning Glassware (Manual Method)

1. Put the specified amount of detergent into a dishpan or washing bucket containing moderately hot water. Allow the detergent to dissolve thoroughly.

2. Rinse glassware (or other items that can be washed) in tap water before placing it in the detergent solution. Never allow dirty glassware to dry out; always place it in a soaking bucket. Glassware should be completely submerged in the bucket or pan. Fill large pieces with detergent water and set aside to soak. Soaking glassware for at least 1 hour before washing makes the washing procedure much more efficient.

3. Using a cleaning brush, thoroughly scrub the glassware, being certain to clean all parts. Brushes of various sizes should be available to fit the different-sized test tubes, flasks, funnels, and bottles. Excessive brushing and improper use of brushes may cause scratching of the glassware. Avoid the use of abrasive cleaners on glassware.

4. Rinse glassware under running tap water; allow the water to run into each piece of glassware, pour it out, and repeat several times (seven to ten times is sufficient). Rinse the outside of the glassware, too. It is especially important to remove all the detergent from the glassware before use; if detergent remains, the alkali in it may interfere with laboratory determinations.

5. After thoroughly rinsing the glassware with tap water, rinse it with deionized water (type I or II) three to five times. Certain glassware used for microbiologic studies requires even longer rinsing with deionized water. Use deionized water (or distilled water in some instances) in the final rinsing of all laboratory glassware.

6. Glassware may be dried in a hot oven (no hotter than 100° C) or at room temperature. If a higher temperature is used, the glassware can become distorted. Always dry glassware or other equipment in an inverted position to ensure complete drainage of water as it dries. Never dry laboratory ware with a towel. Do not dry plastic ware or rubber items in an oven.

7. Check the glassware for cleanliness by observing the water drainage. Chemically clean glassware will drain uniformly; dirty glassware will leave water droplets adhering to the walls of the glass.

### Cleaning Plastic Ware

Most plastic ware can be cleaned in the same manner as glassware and using ordinary glassware washing machines, but the use of any abrasive cleaning materials should be avoided.

Plastic ware should be well cleaned and rinsed with deionized water prior to any necessary autoclaving, since some chemical reactions can occur at autoclaving temperatures that do not occur when the plastics are at room temperature. These reactions can cause deterioration of the plastic.

Some of the transparent plastics, such as polystyrene or polycarbonate, may absorb small quantities of water vapor during autoclaving and appear cloudy. This clouding effect will disappear as the plastic dries, and the plastic becomes transparent again. Drying the plastic ware in a 110° C oven can enhance the clearing effect.

## Cleaning Pipettes

Nondisposable pipettes used in the laboratory are cleaned in a special way. Immediately after use, the pipettes should be placed in a special pipette container or cylinder containing water; the water should be high enough to completely cover the pipettes. Pipettes should be placed in the container carefully with the tip up to avoid breakage. When the pipettes are to be cleaned, they are removed from the cylinder and placed in another cylinder containing a cleaning solution. This cleaning solution can be a detergent or a commercial analytical cleaning product. The pipettes are allowed to soak in the cleaning solution for 30 minutes.

The next step involves thorough rinsing of the pipettes. This can be accomplished by hand, but more often it is done with the aid of an automatic pipette washer. The pipettes are rinsed with tap water, by use of the automatic pipette washer, for 1 to 2 hours. They are then rinsed in deionized or distilled water two or three times and dried in a hot oven.

## Cleaning Photometry Cuvettes

Cuvettes must be scrupulously clean and free from grease smudges or scratches. If non-disposable cuvettes are used, they should be rinsed with tap water, filled with a mild detergent solution, and placed in a rubberized test tube rack as soon as possible after use. It is best not to put them into a regular dishwashing bucket, where they would rub against one another and be scratched. After standing with the detergent solution, the cuvettes are rinsed several times with tap water and two or three times with distilled or deionized water. When cuvettes are dried, high temperatures and unclean air should be avoided. A low to medium oven (not above 100° C) can be used for rapid drying. In some laboratories, there are special dishwashing machines that can adequately handle cuvettes.

## Glass Breakage

It is important in the clinical laboratory to check all glassware periodically to determine its condition. No broken or chipped glassware should be used. Many laboratory accidents are caused by the use of broken glassware. Serious cuts may result, and infections may set in.

Each time a laboratory procedure is carried out, the glassware used should be checked; equipment such as beakers, pipettes, test tubes, and flasks should not have broken edges or cracks. To prevent breakage, glassware should be handled carefully; carrying too much glassware at one time from one place to another in the laboratory is to be avoided.

# LABORATORY REAGENT WATER

The quality of water used in the laboratory is very important. Its use in reagent and solution preparation, reconstitution of lyophilized materials, and dilution of samples demands specific requirements for its level of purity. All water used in the clinical laboratory should be free from substances that could interfere with the tests being performed. It is important that the persons involved in doing the analyses understand the reasons for the special emphasis placed on the kinds of water used and the difficulties involved in obtaining and maintaining a pure reagent water supply. Significant error can be introduced into a laboratory assay if inorganic or organic impurities in the water supply have not been removed prior to analysis.

## Levels of Water Purity

Three levels of laboratory water quality have been recommended by the National Committee for Clinical Laboratory Standards and the College of American Pathologists: type I, type II, and type III.[1,5]

### Type I Reagent Water

This type of reagent water is the most pure and should be used for procedures that require maximum water purity. For preparation of standard solutions, buffers, and controls, in quantitative analytic procedures (especially when nanograms or subnanogram measurements are required), in electrophoresis, in toxicology screening tests, and in high-performance liquid chromatography, type I reagent water must be used.

### Type II Reagent Water

For qualitative chemistry procedures and for most procedures carried out in hematology, immunology, microbiology, and other clinical test areas, type II water is suitable. Type II water can be used when the presence of bacteria can be tolerated.

### Type III Reagent Water

This type of water can be used for some qualitative laboratory tests, such as those done in general urinalysis. Type III water can be used as a water source for preparation of type I or type II water and for washing and rinsing laboratory glassware. Any glassware should be given a final rinse with either type I or type II water, depending on the intended use for the glassware.

## Criteria for Water Purity

The presence of ionizable contaminants in distilled or deionized water is most easily determined by measuring the conductance, or electrical resistance, of the water. This is the basis for having purity meters or conductivity warning lights on distillation and deionization apparatus.

There are several ways to test for water purity. With regard to the presence of inorganic ionized materials, as the purity of the water increases, the amount of dissolved ionized substances decreases and the ability of the water to conduct an electrical current decreases. This principle is used in commercially available resistance test analyzers for water purity. As the ability of the water to conduct an electrical current decreases, the resistance increases.

Water of the highest purity will vary with the method of preparation and may be referred to as nitrogen-free water, double-distilled water, or conductivity water, depending on the actual method used. However, a measure of conductance does not consider the presence of nonionized substances (organic contaminants) such as dissolved gases. Especially important in the clinical laboratory is dissolved carbon dioxide. Water free of such dissolved gases may be obtained by boiling it immediately before use and is often referred to as gas-free, or carbon dioxide–free, water. Such water may be necessary for the preparation of strongly alkaline solutions. Another contaminant of water may be substances dissolved from the storage container.

Accreditation or certification requirements for clinical laboratories, set up by state and federal agencies, have resulted in specific, well-defined criteria for water purity. The classification of and specifications for water purity are designed to enable laboratory personnel to specify the quality of the water needed for particular laboratory analyses and reagent preparation, for example. Each test performed in the laboratory must be evaluated as to the type of water needed, to avoid potential interference with specificity, accuracy, and precision. It is well known, for example, that water contaminated with metal, when used in analyses of enzymes, can have a dramatic effect on the values obtained.

## Storage of Reagent Water

It is important to store reagent water appropriately. Type I water must be used immediately after its production, to prevent carbon dioxide from being absorbed into it. There are no specified storage guidelines for Type I water, because it is not possible to maintain its high level of purity for any length of time. Types II and III water can be stored in borosilicate glass or polyethylene bottles but should be used as soon as possible to prevent contamination with airborne microbes. Containers should be tightly stoppered to prevent absorption of gases. It is also important to keep the delivery system for the water protected from chemical or microbiologic contamination.

## Methods of Purifying Water

The original source of water varies greatly with the health care facility. Water originating from rivers, lakes, springs, or wells contains a variety of inorganic, organic, and microbiologic contaminants. No single purification system can remove all the contaminants. For this reason, a variety of methods, in differing combinations, are used to obtain the particular types of water used in a single laboratory facility. Two general methods are employed to prepare water for laboratory use: deionization and distillation. Sometimes it is necessary to further treat distilled water with a deionization process to obtain water with the degree of purity needed.

### Deionized Water

In the process of **deionization**, water is passed through a resin column containing positively (+) and negatively (−) charged particles. These particles combine with ions present in the water to remove them—this water is known as **deionized water**. Therefore, only substances that can ionize will be removed in the process of deionization; organic substances and other substances that do not ionize are not removed. Further treatment with membrane filtration and activated charcoal is necessary to remove organic impurities, particulate matter, and microorganisms to produce Type I water from deionized water.

### Distilled Water

In the process of distillation, water is boiled, and the resulting steam is cooled; condensed steam is distilled water. Many minerals are found in natural water. Among those commonly found are iron, magnesium, and calcium. Water from which these minerals and others have been removed by distillation is known as **distilled water**. The process of distillation also removes microbiologic organisms, but volatile impurities such as carbon dioxide, chlorine, and ammonia are not removed. Water that has been distilled meets the specifications for type II and type III water.

**Double-Distilled Water.** Distilled or deionized water is not necessarily pure water. There may be contamination by dissolved gases, by nonvolatile substances carried over by steam in the distillation process, or by dissolved substances from storage containers. For example, in tests for nitrogen compounds (such as urea nitrogen, a common clinical chemistry determination) it is important to use ammonia-free (nitrogen-free) water. This may be specially purchased by the laboratory for such determinations or prepared in the laboratory by a specific method, double distillation, to remove the contaminating ammonia.

### Combinations of Deionization and Distillation

Water of higher purity is also produced by special distillation units in which the water is first deionized and then distilled; this eliminates the need for double distillation. Other systems may first distill the water, then deionize it.

### Reverse Osmosis

The process of reverse osmosis passes water under pressure through a semipermeable membrane made of cellulose acetate, or other materials. This treatment removes approximately 90% of dissolved solids, 98% of organic impurities, insoluble matter, and microbiologic organisms. It does not remove dissolved gases and only about 10% of ionized particles.

### Other Processes of Purification

Filtration of water through semipermeable membranes will remove insoluble matter, pyrogens, and microorganisms if the pore size of the membrane is small enough. Adsorption by activated charcoal, clays, silicates, or metal oxides can remove organic matter. Type I water can be processed through a combination of deionization, filtration, and adsorption.

### Tap Water

Rarely is tap water used in the clinical laboratory, the exception being for the initial cleaning of laboratory glassware. Plain tap water is not used in any laboratory analyses or in the preparation of any reagents.

# REAGENTS USED IN LABORATORY ASSAYS

The validity of the laboratory data obtained by analysis of patient specimens is dependent on the use of specific laboratory measuring apparatus and also on the use of specific reagents and materials or products devised for that apparatus. Analytic procedures require the use of properly prepared solutions or reagents. The accuracy of the determinations depends to a large extent on the accuracy of the reagents used.

A **reagent** is defined as any substance employed to produce a chemical reaction. In preparing reagents, instructions should be followed exactly. Often certain reagents will be purchased in a fully prepared state; in this case it is important that they be obtained only from reputable chemical companies. When preprepared reagents are used, manufacturers' instructions must always be followed. When a reagent is prepared, the set of instructions or directions provided for the preparation of the reagent must be followed explicitly.

## Reagent Preparation

Instructions for preparing a reagent resemble a cooking recipe in that they tell what quantities of ingredients to mix together. They tell the names of the chemicals needed, the number of grams or milligrams needed, and the total volume to which the particular reagent should be diluted. The solvent most commonly used for dilution is deionized or distilled water.

### Measurement of Mass and Volume

To prepare reagents, either measurement of mass by use of a balance for weighing or reconstitution of a freeze-dried or otherwise concentrated reagent product is necessary.

Preparation of reagents in the traditional way involves the use of a balance (the analytical, triple-beam, or torsion balance, for example) and other special volumetric measuring devices (such as volumetric flasks and graduated cylinders). The types of volumetric glassware available are discussed under Laboratory Glassware and Plastic Ware.

Since chemicals are used in the preparation of reagents and the accuracy of laboratory determinations depends on the quality of the reagents employed, it is essential that only chemicals from reliable manufacturers be used.

## Concentrations of Solutions

Using solutions of the correct concentrations is of the greatest importance in attaining good results in the laboratory. Quantitative transfer, along with accurate initial measurement of a chemical, helps to ensure that a solution will be of the correct concentration.

The **concentration of a solution** may be expressed in different ways. With the use of SI units, traditional expression of concentration in terms of mass of solute per volume of solution has been replaced by the use of moles of solute per volume of solution for analyte analyses whenever possible, and the use of the liter as the reference value.

In the clinical chemistry laboratory, where the vast majority of the total laboratory analyses are performed, most measurements are concerned with the concentrations of substances in solutions. The solution is usually blood, serum, urine, cerebrospinal fluid, or other body fluid, and the substance to be measured is dissolved in the solution. This substance is known as the **solute**. Therefore, the substances being measured in the analyses (whether they are organic or inorganic, or of high or low molecular weight) are solutes. The substance in which the solute is dissolved is known as the **solvent**.

When a reagent is being prepared, and the solution is being diluted with water, its volume is increased and its concentration decreased, but the amount of solute remains unchanged.

## Laboratory Chemicals

A chemical is a substance that occurs naturally or is obtained through a chemical process; it is used to produce a chemical effect or reaction.

Chemicals are produced in various purities or grades.

**Standards of Purity.** There are many **grades of chemicals** available, and it is essential to understand which grade or type should be used for which reagent.

When quantitative determinations are to be performed and accurate standard solutions prepared, it is necessary to use pure chemicals. In such cases, the more costly, reagent-grade chemicals are necessary for accuracy. Different companies have their own descriptions for the various degrees of purity, and there is no official designation. The label on the bottle and the supplier's catalog may give important information, such as the maximum limits of impurities or an actual analysis of the chemical. Directions for reagent preparation usually specify the grade, and in many instances state the particular brand of chemical. These directions must be followed to ensure reliable results.

The purity of organic chemicals is generally inferior to that of inorganic chemicals. This is due both to the manner in which they are prepared or synthesized and to changes that occur as they stand or are stored.

**Grades of Chemicals.** The following is a general description of the various grades of chemicals available for the clinical laboratory.

1. Reagent grade or analytic reagent (AR) grade. These chemicals are of a high degree of purity and are used often in the preparation of reagents in the clinical laboratory. The American Chemical Society has developed specifications for many reagent-grade or AR chemicals, and those that meet their standards are designated by the letters ACS.
2. Chemically pure (CP) grade. These chemicals are sufficiently pure to be used in many analyses in the clinical laboratory. However, the designation does not reveal the limits of impurities that are tolerated,

and so they may not be acceptable for research and various clinical laboratory techniques unless they have been specifically analyzed for the desired procedure. It may be necessary to use this grade when higher-purity biochemicals are not available.
3. USP and NF grade. These reagents meet the specifications stated in the *United States Pharmacopeia (USP)* or the *National Formulary (NF)*. They are generally less pure than CP grade, as the tolerances specified are such that they are not injurious to health rather than chemically pure.
4. Purified, practical, or pure grade. These chemicals may be used as starting materials for synthesis of chemicals of greater purity but generally should not be used in the clinical laboratory.
5. Technical or commercial grade. These chemicals are used only for industrial purposes and are generally not used in the preparation of reagents for the clinical laboratory.
6. National Bureau of Standards, the College of American Pathologists (CAP), and the National Committee for Clinical Laboratory Standards (NCCLS).[3] These agencies or bureaus all supply certified clinical laboratory standards. The highest grade or purest chemicals are available from the National Bureau of Standards. However, very few such compounds are available to the clinical laboratory, and they are known as standards, clinical type.

**Physical Forms of Chemicals.** Chemicals used in the laboratory have various physical forms. Persons using these chemicals must know the various forms and which form should be used in the preparation of a specific reagent. Some of the common forms are lumps, sticks, pellets, granules, fine granules, crystalline powder, crystals, fine crystals, powder, and liquid. There are some special forms, such as chips, scales, and flakes, but these are not frequently used in reagent preparation.

**Hazardous Chemicals Communication Policies.** Information and training regarding hazardous chemicals must be provided to all persons working with them in the clinical laboratory. The Occupational Safety and Health Administration (OSHA) regulations ensure that all sites where hazardous chemicals are used comply with the necessary safety precautions. Any information about signs and symptoms associated with exposures to hazardous chemicals used in the laboratory must be communicated to all persons. Reference materials about the individual chemicals are provided by all chemical manufacturers and suppliers by means of the **material safety data sheet (MSDS)**. This information accompanies the shipment of all hazardous chemicals and should be available in the laboratory for anyone to review. The MSDS contains information about possible hazards, safe handling, storage, and disposal of the particular chemical it accompanies (see Chemical Hazards in Chapter 2).

**Storage of Chemicals.** It is important that chemicals kept in the laboratory be stored properly, as described in Chapter 2. Chemicals that require refrigeration should be refrigerated immediately. Solids should be kept in a cool, dry place. Acids and bases should be stored separately and in well-ventilated storage units. Flammable solvents (e.g., alcohol, chloroform) should be stored in specially constructed well-ventilated storage units with appropriate labeling in accordance with OSHA regulations. Flammable solvents such as acetone and ether should always be stored in special safety cans or other appropriate storage devices in appropriate storage units. Fuming and volatile chemicals, such as solvents, strong acids, and strong bases, should be opened, and reagent preparation resulting in fumes should be done, only under a fume hood so that the vapors will not escape into the room. Chemicals that absorb water should be weighed only after desiccation or drying in a hot oven; otherwise the weights will not be accurate.

It is very important that the label on a chemical be read for instructions about storage details. Most chemicals are stable at room temperature without desiccation. Some must be stored at refrigeration temperature, some must be frozen, and some that are light sensitive must be stored in brown bottles.

**Chemicals Used to Prepare Standard Solutions.** Chemicals used to prepare **standard solutions** are the most highly purified types of chemicals available. The group includes primary, reference, and certified standards. Primary standards meet specifications set by the Committee on Analytical Reagents of the American Chemical Society. Each lot of these chemicals is assayed, and the chemicals must be stable substances of definite composition. Reference standards are chemicals whose purity has been ensured by the National Bureau of Standards list of standard reference materials (SRM). Certified standards are also available.[3] For example, the CAP certifies bilirubin and cyanmethemoglobin standards, and the NCCLS certifies a standardized protein solution.

### Quantitative Transfer and Dilution of Chemicals for Reagents

In preparing any solution in the clinical laboratory, it is necessary to utilize the practice known as quantitative transfer (Procedure 4-2). It is essential that the entire amount of the weighed or measured substance be used in preparing the solution. In **quantitative transfer**, the entire amount of the measured substance is transferred from one vessel to another for dilution. The usual practice in preparing most laboratory reagents is to weigh the chemical in a beaker (or other suitable vessel, such as a disposable weighing boat) and quantitatively transfer the chemical to a volumetric flask for dilution with deionized or distilled water. The volumetric flask chosen must be of the correct size; that is, it must hold the amount of solution that is desired for the total volume of the reagent being prepared.

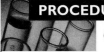

## PROCEDURE 4-2

### Quantitative Transfer

1. Place a clean, dry funnel in the mouth of the volumetric flask.

2. Carefully transfer the chemical in the measuring vessel into the funnel.

3. Wash the chemical into the flask with small amounts of deionized water or the required solvent for the reagent.

4. Rinse the measuring vessel (beaker) three to five times with small portions of deionized water or the required solvent until all of the chemical has been transferred from the vessel into the volumetric flask (add each rinsing to the flask).

5. Rinse the funnel with deionized water or the required solvent, and remove the funnel from the volumetric flask.

6. Dissolve the chemical in the flask by swirling or shaking it. Some chemicals are more difficult to dissolve than others. On occasion, more special attention must be given to the problem of dissolving the chemical.

7. Add deionized water or the required solvent to about 0.5 in. below the calibration line on the flask, allow a few seconds for drainage of fluid above the calibration line, and then carefully add deionized water or the required solvent to the calibration line (the bottom of the meniscus must be exactly on the calibration mark).

8. Stopper the flask with a ground-glass stopper, and mix well by inverting at least 20 times.

9. Rinse a properly labeled reagent bottle with a small amount of the mixed reagent in the volumetric flask. Transfer the prepared reagent to the labeled reagent bottle for storage.

---

The most common amount of solution prepared at one time is 1 L. If 1 L of reagent is needed, the measured chemical must be transferred quantitatively to a 1-L volumetric flask and diluted to the calibration mark with deionized water or the required solvent. The method of quantitative transfer requires a great deal of care and accuracy.

**Dissolving the Chemical into Solution.** There are several methods by which the dissolution of solid materials can be hastened. Heating usually increases the solubility of a chemical, and heat also causes the fluid to move (the currents help in dissolving). Even mild heat, however, will decompose some chemicals, and therefore heat must be used with caution. Agitation by a stirring rod or swirling by means of a mechanical shaker increases solubility by removing the saturated solution from contact with the chemical. Rapid addition of the solvent is another means of hastening the solution of solid materials. Some chemicals tend to cake and form aggregates as soon as the solvent is added. By adding the solvent quickly and keeping the solids in motion, aggregation may be prevented. Since the flask is calibrated at 20° C, the solution must be returned to room temperature before final adjustment is made.

### Labeling the Reagent Container

Containers for storage of reagents (usually reagent bottles) should be labeled before the material is added. A reagent should never be placed in an unlabeled bottle or container. If an unlabeled container is found, the reagent in it must

```
┌─────────────────────────────────────────┐
│  Test Used For              ✓ O.K.       │
│                                          │
│          Name of Reagent                 │
│                                          │
│  Date Prepared         Initial of Maker  │
└─────────────────────────────────────────┘
```

**FIG 4-3.** Sample label.

be discarded. Proper labeling of reagent bottles is of the greatest importance. All labels should include the name and concentration of the reagent, the date on which the reagent was prepared, and the initials of the person who made the reagent (Fig. 4-3).

### Checking the Reagent Before Use

After the prepared reagent is in the reagent bottle, it must be checked by some means before it is put into actual use in any procedure. This can be done in one of several ways, depending on the reagent itself. After the reagent has been checked, this is noted on the label, and the solution can then be put into active use in the laboratory.

### Ready-Made Reagents

In many laboratories, ready-made reagents are used, especially where large automated instruments are utilized. The manufacturers of these instruments usually provide the necessary specific reagents for use with their instruments. These reagents must be handled with extreme care and always must be used according to the manufacturers' directions.

### Immunoreagents

Special commercial reagent kits are commonly used for clinical immunology and radioimmunoassay tests. A typical test kit will contain all necessary reagents, including standards, labeled antigen, and antibody, plus any other associated reagents needed. The laboratory must maintain strict evaluation policies for these kits, to ensure their reliability. The disadvantage of these kits is that the laboratory is dependent on the supplier to produce and maintain components, which must meet the necessary standards. Each new kit must be evaluated by the laboratory according to a strict protocol, and then a periodic monitoring program must be maintained to ensure the reliability of the results produced.

## MEASUREMENT OF MASS: WEIGHING AND THE USE OF BALANCES

### General Use of Balances

Probably some of the most important measurement devices are the various types of balances used in the **measurement of mass or weight (gravimetric analysis)** in preparing the reagents and standard solutions used in the laboratory. This is one method of **quantitative analysis** in the clinical laboratory. Almost every procedure performed in the laboratory depends to some extent on the use of a balance. Laboratory balances function by either mechanical or electronic means.

In the traditional clinical laboratory, gravimetric analysis (analysis by measurement of mass or weight) is used in the preparation of some reagents and standard solutions. Most procedures depend on the use of an accurately prepared standard solution. In many laboratories today, however, reagents, standard solutions, and control solutions are purchased ready to use, and the actual laboratory preparation of these reagents and solutions is not done. Since measurement of mass remains fundamental to all analyses, the technique of weighing should continue to be fundamental to the base of knowledge for all persons working in a clinical laboratory. Even with the use of purchased laboratory solutions, it is likely that a balance will be needed for preparing reagents or standards for certain laboratory determinations. Because of the added cost of purchasing prepared standards, some laboratories routinely prepare their own standard solutions. Another use for weighing is the calibration of volumetric equipment.

The measurement of mass continues to be the quantitative means by which this equipment is calibrated.

Some solutions require more accurately weighed chemicals than others. The accuracy needed depends on what the solution is to be used for. One must decide what type of balance (or scale) is most appropriate for the precision or reproducibility required in weighing the chemicals to be used for a particular solution. The different kinds of balances are suited to particular needs. A balance that sacrifices precision for speed should not be used when precision is needed.

## Types of Balances Used in the Laboratory

The balance considered to be the backbone of the clinical laboratory, especially clinical chemistry, is the analytical balance. This balance and other types—namely, the triple-beam balance, the Cent-O-Gram, and the torsion balance—are discussed in this section. A single laboratory is likely to have all of these types, and for this rea-

son persons working in a laboratory should understand how the various balances are used. Every laboratory should have some type of analytical balance and at least one other, less sensitive type of balance. These are the minimum requirements for weighing devices.

### Analytical Balance

Many different types of analytical balances are made by different companies, and they have various degrees of automatic operation. In this discussion, analytical balances are divided into two types: manually operated (mechanical) analytical (Fig. 4-4) and automatic or electronic analytical (Fig. 4-5) balances. Each company that manufactures analytical balances has its own trade name for each of the analytical balances produced. Some of the fine analytical balances used in the clinical laboratory are the Ainsworth, Voland, Christian-Becker, Mettler, Ohaus, and Sartorius balances. Others are also available. It is important to investigate carefully several different analytical balances before deciding on one for use in a particular laboratory.

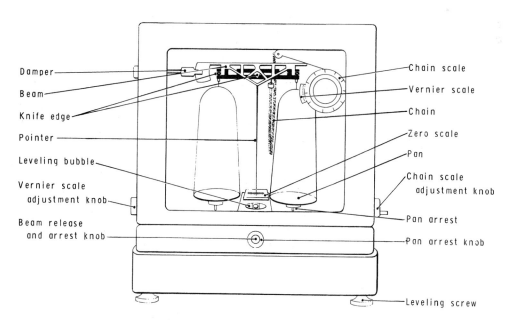

**FIG 4-4.** Manual (mechanical) analytical balance.

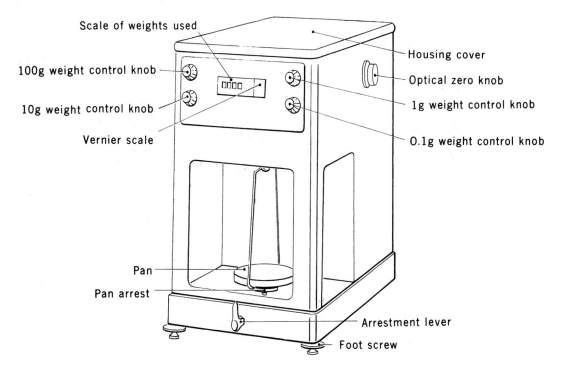

**FIG 4-5.** Electronic analytical balance.

**General Principles of Analytical Balances.** The basic principle in the quantitative measurement of mass is to balance an unknown mass (the substance being weighed) with a known mass. The **analytical balance** uses the basic concept of a simple lever or beam that pivots on a knife-edge fulcrum placed at the center of gravity of the lever. By use of this principle, balances are designed in different ways.

In the traditional mechanical analytical balance, two pans of equal mass are suspended from the ends of the lever or beam and calibrated weights are placed on one pan to counterbalance an object of unknown mass on the other pan. A rider or chain weight device is utilized for fractional weights.

The electronic analytical balance is a single-pan balance that uses an electromagnetic force to counterbalance the load placed on the pan. This pan is mechanically connected to a coil that is suspended in the field of a permanent cylin-drical electromagnet. When a load is placed on the pan, a force is produced that displaces the coil within the magnetic field. A photoelectric cell scanning device changes position and generates a current just sufficient to return the coil to its original position; this is called electromagnetic force compensation. This current is proportional to the weight of the load on the pan and is displayed for the person using the balance to see visually, or it can be interfaced with a data output device. The greater the mass placed on the pan, the greater the deflecting force and the stronger the compensating current required to return the coil to its original position. There is a direct linear relationship between the compensation current and the force produced by the load placed on the pan. Electronic balances permit fast, accurate weighings, with a high degree of resolution. They are easy to use and have replaced the traditional mechanically operated analytical balance in most clinical laboratories.

**Uses for the Analytical Balance.** All analytical balances are used to weigh very small amounts of substances with a high degree of accuracy, but how this is accomplished differs slightly from one balance to another. Some require little or no manual operation, and some are more time consuming and require much more manipulation on the part of the operator.

Almost every procedure performed in the traditional clinical laboratory depends on the use of balances, the most important one being the analytical balance. Before any procedure is started, reagents and standard solutions are prepared. Standard solutions are always very accurately prepared, and the analytical balance is used to weigh the chemicals for these solutions. The analytical balance might be called the starting point of each method used in the laboratory. Its accuracy determines the accuracy of many clinical determinations. An instrument that is so sensitive and so essential must be made with great skill and treated very carefully by those using it.

The analytical balance should be cleaned and adjusted at least once a year to ensure its continued accuracy and sensitivity. Its accuracy is what makes this instrument so essential in the clinical laboratory. The accuracy to which most analytical balances used in the clinical laboratory should weigh chemicals is commonly 0.1 mg, or 0.0001 g. Whenever this accuracy is needed, the analytical balance must be used. Differences between electronic and manual analytical balances lie mainly in the manner in which the weights are added in the weighing procedure. With the manual balance the weights are physically placed on one of the balance pans by the user. With the electronic balance the weights are added by manipulating a series of dials.

**General Rules for Weighing With an Analytical Balance.** Weighing errors will occur if the balance is not properly positioned. It is therefore very important that the balance be located and mounted in an optimal position. The balance must be level. This is usually accomplished by adjusting the movable screws on the legs of the balance. The firmness of support is also important. The bench or table on which the balance rests must be rigid and free from vibrations. Preferably the room in which the balance is set up should have constant temperature and humidity. Ideally, the analytical balance should be in an air-conditioned room. The temperature factor is most important. The balance should not be placed near hot objects such as radiators, flames, stills, or electric ovens. Likewise, it should not be placed near cold objects, especially not near an open window. Sunlight or illumination from high-power lamps should be avoided in choosing a good location for the analytical balance.

The analytical balance is a delicate precision instrument, which will not function properly if abused. When learning to use an analytical balance, one should be responsible for knowing and adhering to the rules for the use of that particular balance. The following general rules apply:

1. Set up the balance where it will be free from vibration.
2. Load and unload the balance only when the pans are arrested; if the pans are not arrested, the delicate knife edges can be damaged.
3. Close the balance case before observing the reading; any air currents present will affect the weighing process.
4. Never weigh any chemical directly on the pan; a container of some type must be used for the chemical.
5. Never place a hot object on the balance pan. If an object is warm, the weight determined will be too little because of convection currents set up by the rising heated air.
6. Whenever the shape of the object to be weighed permits, handle it with tongs or forceps. Round objects such as weighing bottles may be handled with the fingers, but take care to prevent weight changes caused by moisture from the hand. Do not hold any object longer than necessary.

## PROCEDURE 4-3

### Weighing With an Electronic Analytical Balance

1. Before doing any weighing, make certain that the balance is properly leveled. Observe the spirit level (leveling bubble), and adjust the leveling screws on the legs of the balance if necessary.

2. To check the zero point adjustment, fully release the balance and turn the adjustment knob clockwise as far as it will go. The optical scale zero should indicate three divisions below zero on the vernier scale. Using the same adjustment knob, adjust the optical scale zero so that it aligns exactly with the zero line on the vernier scale. Arrest the balance.

3. With the balance arrested, place the weighing vessel on the pan, using tongs if possible, so that no humidity or heat is brought into the weighing chamber by the hands. Close the balance window.

4. Weigh the vessel in the following manner: Partially release the balance and turn the 100-g weight control knob clockwise. When the scale moves up, turn the knob back one step. Repeat this operation with the 10-g, 1.0-g, and 0.1-g knobs, in that order. Arrest the balance. After a short pause, release the balance, and allow the scale to come to rest. Read the result and arrest the balance. With the balance arrested, unload the pan and bring all knobs back to zero.

5. Add the weight of the sample desired to the weight of the vessel just weighed to get the total to be weighed. Set the knobs (100, 10, 1.0, and 0.1 g) to the correct total weight needed. When the 0.1-g knob has been set at its proper reading, the balance should be placed in partial release. Slowly add the chemical to the vessel until the optical scale begins to move downward. When the optical scale starts downward, fully release the beam, and continue to add the chemical until the optical scale registers the exact position desired. To obtain the reading to the nearest 0.1 mg (the sensitivity of most analytical balances), the vernier scale must be used in conjunction with the chain scale.

6. With the balance arrested, unload the pan, and bring all the knobs back to zero. Clean up any spilled chemical in the balance area.

7. On completion of weighing, remove all objects and clean up any chemical spilled on the pans or within the balance area. Close the balance case.

8. Weighed materials should be transferred to labeled containers or made into solutions immediately.

Speed in weighing is obtained only through practice (Procedure 4-3).

**Basic Parts of the Analytical Balance.** It is essential that the parts of the analytical balance be thoroughly understood, so that the weighing process can be carried out to the degree of accuracy necessary. Once the correct use of an analytical balance has been mastered, one should be able to use any of the available types, as they all have the same basic parts. Each manufacturer supplies a complete manual of operating directions, as well as information on the general use and care of the balance, with each balance purchased. These directions should be followed. The following parts are common to most analytical balances, electronic or mechanical (manually operated):

1. *Glass enclosure.* The analytical balance is enclosed in glass to prevent currents of air and collection of dust from disturbing the process of weighing.

2. *Balancing screws.* Before any weighing is done on the balance, it must be properly leveled. This is done by observing the leveling bubbles, or spirit level, located near the bottom of the balance. If necessary, adjust the balancing screws located on the bottom of the balance case (usually found on each leg of the balance).

3. *Beam.* This is the structure from which the pans are suspended.

4. *Knife edges.* These support the beam at the fulcrum during weighing and give sensitivity to the balance. Knife edges are vital parts and are constructed of hard metals to give a minimum amount of friction.

5. *Pans for weighing.* In the manually operated analytical balance, there are two pans: the weights are placed on the right-hand pan, and the object to be weighed is placed on the left-hand pan. In the electronic analytical balance, there is only one pan. The object to be weighed is placed on this pan. The pans are suspended from the ends of the beam.

6. *Weights.* In the manual balance, the weights are found in a separate weight box. These weights are never handled with the fingers but are removed from the box and placed on the balance pan by using special forceps. Mishandling of weights, either by using the fingers or by dropping, can result in an alteration of the actual and true mass of the weight. Weights come in units ranging from 50 g to 100 mg. The values of the weights are stamped directly on top of them. In the electronic analytical balance, the weights are inside the instrument and are not seen by the operator unless there is a need to remove the casing for repair or adjustment. With the electronic analytical balance, the weights are added by manipulating specific dials calibrated for the weighing process. The built-in weights are on the same end of the beam as the sample pan and are counterbalanced by a fixed weight at the opposite end. There is always a constant load on the beam, and the projected scale has the same weight regardless of the load. The total weight of an object is registered automatically by a digital counter or in conjunction with an optical scale.

7. *Pan arrest.* This is a means of arresting the pan so that sudden movement or addition of weights or chemical will not injure the delicate knife edges. The pan arrests (usually found under the pans) can absorb any shock due to weight inequalities, so that the knife edges are not subjected to this shock. The pan must be released to swing freely during actual weighing. In the electronic analytical balance, the arresting mechanism for both the pan and the beam is operated by a single lever. Partial release or full release can be obtained, depending on how the lever is moved.

8. *Damping device.* This is necessary to arrest the swing of the beam in the shortest practical time, thus cutting down the time consumed in the weighing process.

9. *Vernier scale.* This is the small scale used to obtain precise readings to the nearest 0.1 mg. It is used in conjunction with the large reading scale to obtain the necessary readings (Fig. 4-6).

10. *Reading scale.* In the manual analytical balance, this scale is actually the reading scale for the chain that is used for weighing 100 mg or less. It is used in conjunction with the vernier scale to obtain readings to the nearest 0.1 mg. In the electronic analytical balance, this is usually a lighted optical scale, giving a high magnification and sharp definition for easier reading. The total weight of the object in question is registered automatically on this viewing scale.

### Torsion Balance

**Torsion balances** are mechanical and are used mainly for weighing chemicals in the laboratory.

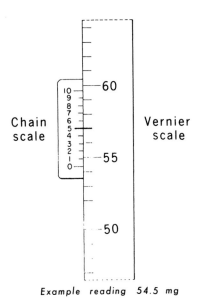

Chain scale    Vernier scale

*Example reading 54.5 mg*

**FIG 4-6.** Reading obtained with a vernier scale.

They are sensitive, responsive instruments with an exceptionally long service life, during which there is no significant deterioration in performance. In normal use, they require very little maintenance. The unique attribute of the torsion balance movement, which is assembled as a single flexible structure by means of highly tensed torsion bands of watch-spring alloy, is that the use of knife edges, bearings, and other loose parts that would become dull, misaligned, and soiled is eliminated. Having no knife edges to dull or other loose parts to be adjusted accounts for the popularity of the torsion balance. Little or no adjustment is required, and this is important in a laboratory, where time is important (Procedure 4-4). Most balances currently in use are a type of torsion balance.

**Use and Basic Parts.** The torsion balance has high sensitivity under a heavy load, permits fast weighing, and is relatively inexpensive. Care must be taken to avoid overloading these balances. Some models have a dial-controlled torque spring to eliminate the use of smaller loose weights. Other models are offered

with dial-controlled built-in weights, which may further reduce the number of loose weights required. Many weighing determinations can be completed in about one-fifth the time formerly required. A sliding tare weight is provided to counterbalance the weighing vessel used. The beam is operated by a lever on the balance case. Some torsion balances are enclosed completely in glass or metal cases. Several of these balances have a damping feature, which brings the balance to equilibrium quickly. One such damping device is an oil dashpot, which is filled at the factory with silicone oil. Weighing can be done more rapidly on torsion balances with damping devices than on those lacking them.

There is usually a means by which the torsion balance can be arrested. This needs to be done only when the balance is to be moved to a new location or otherwise transported.

The sensitivity of the torsion balance varies with the model chosen. For most clinical laboratories, however, balances with a sensitivity of readings to the nearest 0.01 g are satisfactory. The manufacturer supplies a complete manual with directions for setting up, proper use, and care of the particular torsion balance. These directions should be followed closely.

### Top-Loading Balance

A single-pan top-loading balance is one of the most commonly used balances in the laboratory. It is usually electronic and is self-balancing. It is much faster and easier to use than some of the balances described above. A substance can be weighed in just a few seconds. These balances are usually modified torsion or substitution balances. Top-loading balances are used when the substance being weighed does not require as much analytic precision, as when reagents of a large volume are being prepared.

### Triple-Beam Balance

Another piece of laboratory apparatus used for weighing is the **triple-beam** or "trip" **balance**

## PROCEDURE 4-4

### Weighing With a Torsion Balance

1. Check to be sure that the balance is level, and adjust the leveling screws if necessary.

2. Check the zero adjustment. The optical reading scale should read zero with the pan empty and clean; adjust the optical zero with the small control knob if necessary.

3. Place the weighing vessel on the pan. Turn the weight control knob until the optical reading scale reads zero.

4. Add the chemical to the vessel until the desired weight registers on the optical scale. A vernier scale is present on most models so that the weight may be read to the accuracy needed.

5. Remove the vessel with the weighed chemical from the pan. Turn the control knob to zero, and wipe up any spilled chemical immediately.

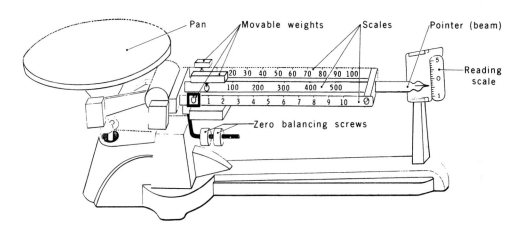

**FIG 4-7.** Triple-beam balance.

(Fig. 4-7). This mechanical balance is less sensitive, with an accuracy to the nearest 0.1 g. Whenever reagents are to be prepared with an accuracy of 0.1 g or less, the triple-beam balance can be used. As the words triple-beam and trip suggest, three beams are present on the balance. Each beam provides a different weighing scale. Scales reading from 0 to 100 g, 0 to 500 g, and 0 to 10 g are usually provided on the triple-beam balance. These scales are provided with movable weights. The two larger scales have weights that lock into accurately milled notches at each

calibration to ensure absolute accuracy at each position.

Some models of the triple-beam balance (called the Harvard triple-beam balance) have two pans, and some have a single pan. The principle of the weighing process is the same whether there are two pans or only one. Two-pan balances are used when two objects must be balanced against each other, as in balancing tubes for use in a centrifuge. One-pan balances are used a great deal in the laboratory for preparing reagents and chemical solutions.

## PROCEDURE 4-5

### Weighing With a Triple-Beam Balance

1. Place the weighing vessel on the balance pan without previously bringing the balance to zero.

2. With the weighing vessel on the pan, bring the balance to zero by adjusting the movable weights on the three scales. Record the sum of the weights required for balance.

3. To the recorded weight add the amount of chemical to be weighed. For example, if the reagent to be prepared requires 10.5 g of NaCl and the weighing vessel weighs 35.5 g, the total weight is 46.0 g. Move the movable weights on the scales to give this total weight.

4. Gradually add the chemical until the pointer of the balance rests exactly at the zero mark on the vertical reading scale. Remove the weighing vessel, and return the movable weights to their zero positions. Transfer the chemical quantitatively to the flask for dilution.

5. Wipe up any spilled chemical immediately from the balance area.

On any type of triple-beam balance, the balance position of an object on the pan can be determined by observing the swing of the pointer. A swing of an equal number of divisions on either side of the zero mark on the dial indicates that the scale is balanced. It is not necessary to wait for the oscillation to stop to determine the correct weight. This observation enables the weighing process to be simple and rapid (Procedure 4-5).

**Use and Basic Parts.** Some type of less sensitive balance, such as the triple-beam or torsion balance, is an essential piece of equipment for every clinical laboratory, as many reagents are prepared that do not need the accuracy of the analytical balance. When an accuracy of 0.1 g or less is acceptable, the triple-beam balance can be used. It can be operated simply and rapidly and gives accurate weighings when used properly. However, even a balance with less sensitivity must be used carefully and according to the directions provided with the particular model.

The triple-beam balance should be placed on a reasonably flat and level surface. The beam should be near zero balance, with all the movable weights at their zero points. A final zero balance is attained by adjusting the balancing screws. It is advisable to check the zero balance periodically, especially if the balance has been moved. If an object is to be weighed, the balance must be set at zero before the weighing is begun. If a vessel is weighed in preparation for the addition of a chemical, it is not necessary to set the balance at the exact zero reading.

Parts basic to triple-beam balances are as follows:

1. *Pan:* where the object or weighing vessel holding the substance to be weighed is placed.

2. *Beam:* a lever supported by a knife plane bearing at the center post. The length of beam to the right of the knife plane is graduated for placement of a sliding weight and ends in a pointer. The other end of the beam is attached to the pan guide with a knife-edge contact.

3. *Movable weights or poises:* sliding weights attached to the beam, which are moved to bring the balance into equilibrium. The trip balance has three beams, and various weight increments are added as the poises are advanced toward the pointer ends of the beams.

4. *Reading scale:* a scale located at the end of the beam pointer that shows when the balance is in equilibrium.

5. *Balancing screws or spindle:* a pair of threaded weights that are used to bring the empty balance into equilibrium.

# MEASUREMENT OF VOLUME: PIPETTING AND TITRATION

## Pipetting

### Pipettes: An Overview and Uses

Pipettes are a type of volumetric glassware used extensively in the laboratory. Many kinds are available. Care and discretion should be used in selecting pipettes for clinical laboratory use, since their accuracy is one of the determining factors in the accuracy of the procedures carried out. A pipette is a cylindrical glass tube used in measuring fluids. It is calibrated to deliver, or transfer, a specified volume from one vessel to another.

Pipettes used in volumetric measurement in the laboratory must be free from all grease and dirt. For that reason, a special analytic cleaning solution is used. For a description of cleaning solutions, see Cleaning Laboratory Glassware and Plastic Ware.

Since the accuracy of laboratory determinations depends to such a large extent on the equipment used and since pipetting is a principal means of volume measurement, it is imperative that any pipettes used in the clinical laboratory be of the finest quality and be manufactured and calibrated by a reputable company. Care and discretion should be used in the selection of laboratory pipettes, whether manual or automatic.

Several types of pipettes are used commonly in the laboratory. It is necessary that their uses be understood and experience in how to handle them in clinical determinations be gained (see Pipettes, under Laboratory Glassware and Plastic ware). Practice, again, is the key to success in the use of laboratory pipettes; only through practice will anyone become proficient in pipetting.

There are two categories of manual pipettes: to-contain (TC) and to-deliver (TD). TC pipettes are calibrated to contain a specified amount of liquid but are not necessarily calibrated to deliver that exact amount. A small amount of fluid will cling to the inside wall of the TC pipette, and when these pipettes are used, they should be rinsed out with a diluting fluid to ensure that the entire contents has been emptied. TD pipettes are calibrated to deliver the amount of fluid designated on the pipette; this volume will flow out of the pipette by gravity when the pipette is held in a vertical position with its tip against the inside wall of the receiving vessel. A small amount of fluid will remain in the tip of the pipette; this amount is to be left in the tip, as the calibrated portion has been delivered into the receiving vessel. There is another category of pipette, called blowout. The calibration of these pipettes is similar to that of TD pipettes, except that the drop remaining in the tip of the pipette must be blown out into the receiving vessel. If a pipette is to be blown out, an etched ring will be seen near the suction opening (see discussions of serologic and Ostwald pipettes above). A mechanical device must be used to blow out the entire contents of the pipette.

### Pipetting Technique Using Manual Pipettes

It is important to develop a good technique for handling pipettes (Fig. 4-8). It is only through practice that this is accomplished, however (Procedure 4-6). With few exceptions, the same general steps apply to pipetting with any of the manual pipettes described under Laboratory Glassware and Plastic Ware.

Laboratory accidents frequently result from improper pipetting techniques. The greatest potential hazard is when mouth pipetting is done instead of mechanical suction. Mouth pipetting is never acceptable in the clinical laboratory. Caustic reagents, contaminated specimens, and poisonous solutions are all pipetted at one time or another in the laboratory, and every precaution must be taken to ensure the safety of the person doing the work (see Chapter 2).

After the pipette has been filled above the top graduation mark, removed from the vessel, and held in a vertical position, the meniscus must be adjusted (Fig. 4-9). The **meniscus** is the curvature in the top surface of a liquid. The pipette should be held in such a way that the calibration mark is

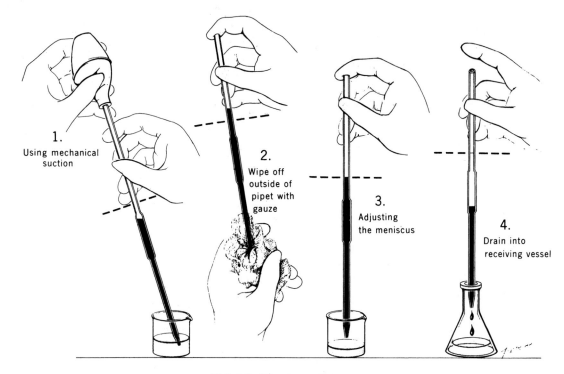

1. Using mechanical suction

2. Wipe off outside of pipet with gauze

3. Adjusting the meniscus

4. Drain into receiving vessel

**FIG 4-8.** Pipetting technique.

at eye level. The delivery tip is touched to the inside wall of the original vessel, not the liquid, and the meniscus of the liquid in the pipette is eased, or adjusted, down to the calibration mark.

When clear solutions are used, the bottom of the meniscus is read. For colored or viscous solutions, the top of the meniscus is read. All readings must be made with the eye at the level of the meniscus (Fig. 4-9).

Before the measured liquid in the pipette is allowed to drain into the receiving vessel, any liquid adhering to the outside of the pipette must be wiped off with a clean piece of gauze or tissue. If this is not done, any drops present on the outside of the pipette might drain into the receiving vessel along with the measured volume. This would make the volume greater than that specified, and an error would result.

### Pipetting Technique Using Automatic Pipettes

**Automatic pipettes** allow fast, repetitive measurement and delivery of solutions of equal volumes. There are several commercially available

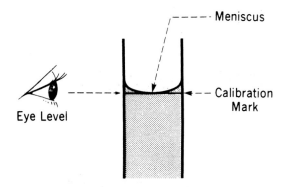

**FIG 4-9.** Reading the meniscus.

types of automatic pipettes, either of the sampling type or of the sampling-diluting type (see Automatic Measuring Devices, under Laboratory Glassware and Plastic Ware). The sampling type measures the substance in question; the sampling-diluting type measures the substance and then adds the desired diluent. The sampling type of automatic pipette is mechanically operated and uses a piston-operated plunger. These

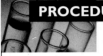

### PROCEDURE 4-6

*Pipetting With Manual Pipettes*

1. Check the pipette to ascertain its correct size, being careful also to check for broken delivery or suction tips.

2. Wearing protective gloves, hold the pipette lightly between the thumb and the last three fingers, leaving the index finger free.

3. Place the tip of the pipette well below the surface of the liquid to be pipetted.

4. Using mechanical suction or an aspirator bulb, carefully draw the liquid up into the pipette until the level of liquid is well above the calibration mark.

5. Quickly cover the suction opening at the top of the pipette with the index finger.

6. Wipe the outside of the pipette dry with a piece of gauze or tissue to remove excess fluid.

7. Hold the pipette in a vertical position with the delivery tip against the inside of the original vessel. Carefully allow the liquid in the pipette to drain by gravity until the bottom of the meniscus is exactly at the calibration mark. (The meniscus is the concave or convex surface of a column of liquid as seen in a laboratory pipette, buret, or other measuring device.) To do this, do not entirely remove the index finger from the suction-hole end of the pipette, but, by rolling the finger slightly over the opening, allow a slow drainage to take place.

8. While still holding the pipette in a vertical position, touch the tip of the pipette to the inside wall of the receiving vessel. Remove the index finger from the top of the pipette to permit free drainage. Remember to keep the pipette in a vertical position for correct drainage. In TD pipettes, a small amount of fluid will remain in the delivery tip.

9. To be certain that the drainage is as complete as possible, touch the delivery tip of the pipette to another area on the inside wall of the receiving vessel.

10. Remove the pipette from the receiving vessel, and place it in the appropriate place for washing (see under Cleaning Laboratory Glassware and Plastic Ware).

are adjustable so that varying amounts of reagent or sample can be delivered with the same device. Disposable and exchangeable tips are available for these pipettes. Automatic pipettes or micropipettors must be calibrated before use.

**Micropipettors.** Micropipettors contain or deliver from 1 to 500 $\mu$L. It is important to follow the manufacturer's instructions for the device being used, as each one may be slightly different. In general, the following steps apply for use of a micropipettor (Fig. 4-10):

1. Attach the proper tip to the pipettor, and set the delivery volume.

2. Depress the piston to a stop position on the pipettor.

3. Place the tip into the solution, and allow the piston to slowly rise back to its original position (this fills the pipettor tip with the desired volume of solution).

4. Some tips are wiped with a dry gauze at this step, and some are not. Follow the manufacturer's directions.

5. Place the tip on the wall of the receiving vessel and depress the piston, first to a stop position where the liquid is allowed to drain, and then to a second stop position where the full dispensing of the liquid takes place.

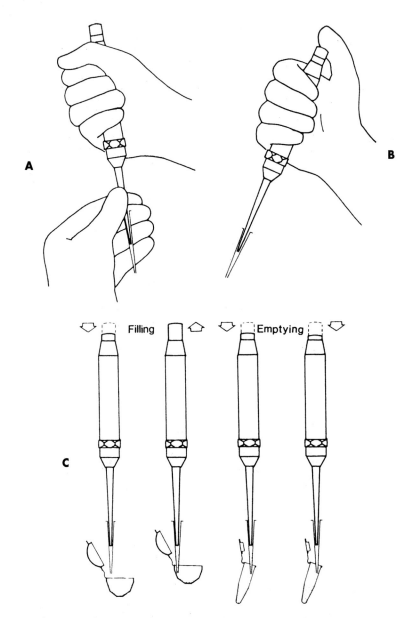

**FIG 4-10.** Steps in using piston-type automatic micropipette. **A,** Attaching proper tip size for range of pipette volume and twisting tip as it is pushed onto pipette to give an airtight, continuous seal. **B,** Holding pipette before use. **C,** Detailed instructions for filling and emptying pipette tip. (From Kaplan LA, Pesce A: *Clinical Chemistry: Theory, Analysis, and Correlation*, ed 3. St Louis, Mosby, 1996, p 16.)

6. Dispose of the tip in the waste disposal receptacle. Some pipettors automatically eject the used tips, thus minimizing biohazard exposure.

**Repipettors.** Several types of repipettors or dispensers are available; they allow repeated volumes of a specific reagent to be delivered to a solution or receiving vessel. These devices are useful for serial dispensing of relatively small volumes of the same liquid (reagent). The volume to be delivered is adjusted on the pipettor dispensing device, which generally is attached by tubing to a reagent bottle containing the reagent to be dispensed. The dispensing device consists of a plunger, a valve system, and the dispensing tip. Once the dispensing device has been primed with liquid, pressing on the plunger allows the selected volume of liquid to be dispensed into the receiving vessel. When the plunger returns to the original position, usually by means of a spring-activated device, the dispenser chamber is refilled with the liquid being measured.

## Titration

Titration is a method of quantitative analysis, a volumetric technique in which the concentration of one solution is determined by comparing it with a measured volume of a solution whose concentration is known. If the concentration of a solution is unknown, it can be found by measuring the volume of the unknown solution that will react with a measured amount of the solution of known concentration (called a standard solution). This process is known as titration.

### Use

In the clinical laboratory, titration is used to determine the concentrations of acids and bases, as the analytic tool for certain laboratory procedures, and in the preparation of some reagents.

This technique is often used to determine the concentration of an unknown acid or an unknown base by means of comparison with a known base or a known acid. In this case the quantity of hydronium ions that react with hydroxyl ions to form water is measured. However, numerous reactions, other than the neutralization reaction between an acid and a base, are used in titrations to determine the concentration of a solution.

The titration technique has numerous other uses in the clinical laboratory. It is the means of checking the concentrations of new reagents before they are used in the clinical laboratory. When weaker acids or bases are prepared from more concentrated solutions, the actual normality of the new solution must be determined by titration (Procedure 4-7).

### Expression of Normality or Equivalents

When titration is used to determine concentration, the concentration is traditionally expressed in terms of normality or equivalents. Normality is employed because it provides a basis for direct comparison of strength for all solutions. Normality is the number of gram-equivalents per liter of solution. A gram-equivalent is the amount of a compound that will liberate, combine with, or replace one gram-atom of hydrogen. Therefore, 1 equivalent of any compound will react with exactly 1 equivalent of any other compound. For example, 1 equivalent of any acid will exactly neutralize 1 equivalent of any base. It is very convenient to have laboratory solutions of such concentrations that any chosen volume of one reagent reacts with an equal volume of another reagent. The system of equivalents or equivalent weights provides this useful tool. The equivalent weight of a substance is calculated by dividing the gram-molecular weight of the substance by the sum of the positive valences. A solution that contains 1 gram-equivalent weight of substance in 1 L of solution is called a normal (1N) solution (see also Chapter 7).

### Essential Components for Titration

In any titration procedure, certain components must always be present:

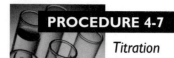

## PROCEDURE 4-7

*Titration*

1. Use the buret clamp to fasten the buret, which must be clean and free from chips or cracks, to the buret stand, which will support it during the titration procedure. Fasten the clamp to the stand about halfway up the rod.

2. Grease the buret stopcock lightly. The stopcock should turn easily and smoothly, but an excess of lubricant will plug the stopcock capillary bore and prevent emptying of the buret. To grease a clean stopcock properly, apply a bit of grease with the fingertip down the two sides of the stopcock away from the capillary bore. Then insert the stopcock in the buret and rotate it until a smooth covering of the whole stopcock is obtained. If the buret is equipped with a Teflon plug, the stopcock need not be lubricated.

3. Rinse the buret with the titrant. In the case of an acid-base titration with phenolphthalein as the indicator, the titrant (or solution to be added and measured by means of the buret) will always be the base. In rinsing the buret, fill it completely with the titrant, and then let it drain. Discard the rinse solution. Fill the buret slowly and carefully to prevent air bubbles from forming in the narrow buret tube. It is essential that the buret be absolutely clean if the results are to be accurate. A clean buret will drain without any solution clinging to its sides; if the buret is dirty, there will be droplets of liquid clinging to the sides. After rinsing the buret several times with the titrant solution, fill it past the zero mark, and then bring the meniscus exactly to the zero mark by draining, using the stopcock to control the flow (see Fig. 4-11).

4. Into an Erlenmeyer flask, pipette the stated amount of the second solution to be employed in the titration. Pipette this solution with a volumetric pipette, using great care to ensure maximal accuracy.

5. Add the required amount of the indicator solution employed to show when the titration reaction has reached completion. (At this point, approximately 5 to 10 mL of water is often added to the Erlenmeyer flask to dilute the indicator and make the end point more visible. The volume of this diluent is not critical, since it does not enter into the reaction or affect the volumes of the solutions that are being titrated.)

6. Titrate each flask in the following manner:

   a. Inspect the buret to be sure that there are no air bubbles trapped in the capillary tube or tip. Air bubbles will add to the apparent volume required to reach the end point, leading to erroneous results. If bubbles are present, drain the buret and refill it with the titrant until there are no bubbles.

   b. Inspect to see that the meniscus is exactly at zero, or record the actual buret reading immediately before beginning the titration.

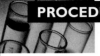

## PROCEDURE 4-7

*Titration—cont'd*

c. Add the solution in the buret to the flask by rotating the stopcock carefully. A right-handed person encircles the buret stopcock with the left hand, using the right hand to swirl the flask during the titration (see Fig. 4-11). This will be awkward at first, but when mastered it will become natural.

d. With the buret tip well within the titration flask, the titrant may be added fairly rapidly at first, but as the reaction nears completion, the titrant is added drop by drop and finally by only portions of drops (split drops). Clues that the reaction is nearing completion depend on the particular reaction and indicator being employed. In the case of an acid-base titration with phenolphthalein as the indicator, there is a change from a colorless to a red solution. The phenolphthalein is colorless in acid solutions and red in alkaline solutions. In the neutralization reaction itself, hydronium ions react with hydroxyl ions to form water. The reaction begins with an excess of hydronium ions in the Erlenmeyer flask, and the titration is performed until all the hydronium ions have been neutralized by the hydroxyl ions added from the buret. The titration should be stopped at the actual point of neutralization, or as close to it as possible.

In practice, a pink color will appear when the alkali is added to the acid. This color will disappear on shaking. As the titration nears completion, the pink color will remain for a longer time. The base is then added slowly, by split drops, until a faint pink color remains. When the pink color no longer disappears but remains for more than 30 seconds, the end point (or neutralization) has been achieved. It is essential that any titration, using any indicator, be stopped at the actual end point, which is the first faint but permanent color change, or the results will be inaccurate.

e. Immediately on reaching the end point, record the buret reading. Be sure to record a figure that is significant, considering the tolerance of the particular buret being used.

7. Clean the buret by rinsing thoroughly with tap water and then with deionized water. Remove any grease from the stopcock. The titrant should not be left standing in the buret. Alkali will "freeze" the stopcock to the buret, and the concentration of the titrant will increase because of evaporation. When the buret is clean, it can be stored either in an inverted position on the buret clamp or in an upright position filled with deionized water.

8. Use the buret readings obtained in the titration procedure to determine the concentration of the unknown solution.

1. A standard solution of known concentration
2. An accurately measured volume of the standard solution or unknown
3. An indicator to show when the reaction has reached completion
4. A buret (or similar device) to measure the volume of solution required to reach the end point

**Standard Solutions.** Standard solutions of a desired normality may be prepared by weighing on the analytical balance the exact amount of substance calculated to give that normality, dissolving it in a small amount of deionized water, and then diluting the solution to the number of liters required in the original calculation. Standard solutions prepared in this way (by direct weighing on the analytical balance) are known as primary standards. The chemical substances used in the preparation of standard solutions must be pure, must have a high molecular weight, and must not take up or give off moisture. Oxalic acid meets these requirements and is often used as a primary standard. A solution of hydrochloric acid prepared from constant-boiling HCl is also often used as a primary standard. Bases are not often used as primary standards because they take up moisture when exposed to the air, which makes the measurement inaccurate.

**Indicator for Reaction.** The point at which equal concentrations of the standard and the unknown are present is called the end point of the titration. In the case of acid-base titrations, the end point is where neutralization occurs. Various means of detecting the end point are used, depending on the procedure. Sometimes the formation of a precipitate indicates that the end point has been reached. A change in color of one of the reacting solutions can also indicate the end point. The most common method of detecting the end point is through the use of an indicator solution. An indicator solution is a third solution added in the titration procedure (in addition to the standard solution and the unknown solution). The indicator solution is added in measured amounts to the titration flask. Most indicators are solids dissolved in water or alcohol. Phenolphthalein (0.1%) is commonly used as the indicator in acid-base titrations. Phenolphthalein is made up in a solution of alcohol. It is generally best to arrange the titration procedure so that one titrates from a colorless solution to the first sign of a permanent color rather than from a colored to a colorless solution. Phenolphthalein is colorless in an acid solution and red in an alkaline solution. When one is near the end point, the addition of a single drop from the buret may overrun the true end point considerably. This can cause significant error in the titration of small amounts of solutions. To avoid this drop error, the titrating solution should be added in split drops as the end point approaches. It is possible to control the flow from the buret with careful manipulation of the stopcock so that only part of a drop goes into the titration flask.

**Burets.** The device that is most often employed to measure the volume required to reach completion of the reaction in a particular titration procedure is the buret. The buret is basically a graduated pipette with a stopcock near the delivery tip to facilitate better control and delivery of the solution (see Figs. 4-1 and 4-11). Burets may be obtained in many different capacities and tolerances. The particular buret capacity and tolerance used in a particular procedure are determined by the degree of accuracy that is desired. To ensure that the buret used is employed with maximum accuracy, a very specific technique or procedure must be followed. Mastery of this technique will come only with practice. It is essential that chemically clean, well-calibrated volumetric equipment be used throughout the procedure to ensure reliable results (see Burets, under Laboratory Glassware and Plastic Ware).

### Calculations

To find the concentration of a solution, the following must be available: a standard solution of known concentration, the volume of the standard solution, and the volume of the undetermined solution required to reach completion in the particular reaction. As mentioned previously, the concentration is usually expressed in terms of normality, which permits direct comparison of solutions. Normality is the number of gram-equivalents per liter of solution, or milliequivalents per milliliter of solution. However, in practice, 1 L of a solution is rarely used; instead, parts of 1 L are used. Therefore, the number of equivalents is actually the normality of the solution times the volume that is used in the titration. All the ingredients required for the equation to determine the concentration of a solution in any titration are now present. If the equivalents of solution 1 are equal to the equivalents of solution 2, and if the number of equivalents of a particular solution is actually the normality of the solution times the volume, it follows that the normality of solution 1 times the volume of solution 1 is equal to the normality of

solution 2 times the volume of solution 2. Or in equation form:

Equivalents of solution 1 = Equivalents of solution 2

or

$$N_1 \times V_1 = N_2 \times V_2$$

In the case of a typical acid-base titration, assume that 2 mL of a standard 0.1000N HCl solution required 1.50 mL of NaOH, added from a buret, to reach the first permanent pink color. What is the normality of the NaOH?

$$N_{acid} \times V_{acid} = N_{base} \times V_{base}$$
$$0.1000N \times 2 \text{ mL} = N_{base} \times 1.50 \text{ mL}$$
$$N_{base} = \frac{0.1000N \times 2 \text{ mL}}{1.50 \text{ mL}} = 0.1333$$

That is, the normality of the sodium hydroxide is 0.1333.

### General Considerations for Titration

Chemically clean, well-calibrated volumetric equipment, including flasks, pipettes, and burets, must be used in every titration procedure. Accurately prepared standard solutions are essential for accurate results. These are weighed analytically and diluted volumetrically. Indicators must be employed to show when the particular reaction has reached completion. These are often color indicators, which change from colorless to a faint permanent color when the reaction has reached completion. However, such instruments as pH meters may also be employed, in which case the end point is a particular hydronium ion concentration as recorded on the pH meter.

### Acid-Base Titration

In acid-base titrations in the clinical laboratory, the most commonly used alkali is 0.1N sodium hydroxide (NaOH). This is relatively stable and can be used to determine the concentration of an acid. However, NaOH is not absolutely stable, and it should be checked daily against a standard acid to be considered reliable.

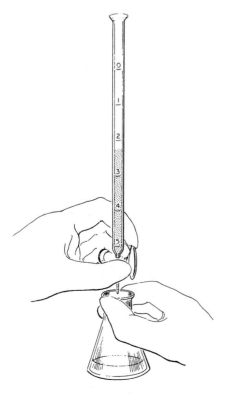

**FIG 4-11.** Method of manual titration.

# LABORATORY CENTRIFUGES

**Centrifugation** is used in the separation of a solid material from a liquid by application of increased gravitational force by rapid rotating or spinning. It is also used in recovering solid materials from suspensions, as in the microscopic examination of urine. The solid material or sediment packed at the bottom of the centrifuge tube is sometimes called the precipitate, and the liquid or top portion is called the supernatant. Another important use for the centrifuge is in the separation of serum or plasma from cells in blood specimens. The suspended particles, solid material, or blood cells usually collect at the bottom of the centrifuge tube because the particles are heavier than the liquid. Occasionally the particles are lighter than the liquid and will collect on the surface of the liquid when it is centrifuged. Centrifugation is employed in many areas of the clinical laboratory—in chemistry, urinalysis, hematology, and blood banking, among others. Proper use of the centrifuge is important for anyone engaged in laboratory work.

## Types of Centrifuges

Centrifuges facilitate the separation of particles in suspension by the application of centrifugal force. Several types of centrifuges will usually be found in the same laboratory; each is designed for special uses. There are table-model and floor-model centrifuges, some small and others very large; there are refrigerated centrifuges, ultracentrifuges, cytocentrifuges, and other centrifuges adapted for special procedures.

Two traditional types of centrifuges are used in routine laboratory determinations. One is a conventional **horizontal-head centrifuge** with swinging buckets, and the other is a **fixed angle-head centrifuge.**

With the horizontal-head centrifuge, the cups holding the tubes of material to be centrifuged occupy a vertical position when the centrifuge is at rest, but assume a horizontal position when the centrifuge revolves (Fig. 4-12). The horizontal-head, or swinging-bucket, centrifuge rotors hold the tubes being centrifuged in a vertical position when the centrifuge is at rest. When the rotor is in motion, the tubes move and remain in a horizontal position. During the process of centrifugation, when the tube is in the horizontal position, the particles being centrifuged constantly move along the tube and any sediment is distributed evenly against the bottom of the tube. When centrifugation is complete and the rotor is no longer turning, the surface of the sediment is flat with the column of liquid resting above it.

For the fixed angle-head centrifuge, the cups are held in a rigid position at a fixed angle. This position makes the process of centrifuging more rapid than it is with the horizontal-head centrifuge. There is also less chance that the sediment will be disturbed when the centrifuge stops. During centrifugation, particles travel along the side of the tube to form a sediment that packs against the bottom and side of the tube. Fixed angle-head centrifuges are used when rapid centrifugation of solutions containing small particles is needed—an example is the microhematocrit centrifuge. The microhematocrit centrifuge used in many hematology laboratories for packing red blood cells attains a speed of about 10,000 to 15,000 rpm with an RCF of up to 14,000 g.

A **cytocentrifuge** utilizes a very-high-torque and low-inertia motor to rapidly spread monolayers of cells across a special slide for critical morphologic studies. This type of preparation can be used for blood, urine, body fluid, or any other liquid specimen that can be spread on a slide. An advantage of this technology is that only a small amount of sample is used, producing evenly distributed cells that can then be stained for microscopic study. The slide produced can be saved and examined at a later time—in contrast to "wet" preparations, which must be examined immediately.

Refrigerated centrifuges are available, with internal refrigeration temperatures ranging from –15 to –25° C during centrifugation. This

## Balanced Load

Top view of
Partially-Filled Rotor

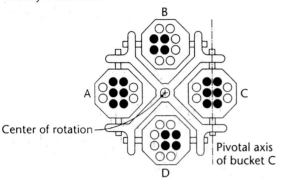

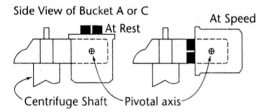

## Unbalanced Load

Top view of
Partially-Filled Rotor

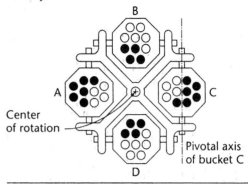

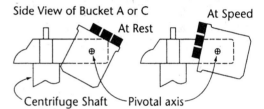

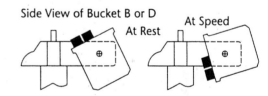

**FIG 4-12.** Examples of balanced and unbalanced loads in a horizontal-head centrifuge. **A,** Assuming all tubes have been filled with an equal amount of liquid, this rotor load is balanced. The opposing bucket sets A-C and B-D are loaded with equal numbers of tubes and are balanced across the center of rotation. Each bucket is also balanced with respect to its pivotal axis. **B,** Even if all the tubes are filled equally, this rotor is improperly loaded. None of the bucket loads are balanced with respect to their pivotal axes. At operating speed, buckets A and C will not reach the horizontal position. Buckets B and D will pivot past the horizontal. Also note that the tube arrangement in the opposing buckets B and D is not symmetrical across the center of rotation. (From *A Centrifuge Primer.* Palo Alto, Calif, Spinco Division of Beckman Instruments, 1980.)

permits centrifugation at higher speeds, because the specimens are protected from the heat that is generated by the rotors of the centrifuge. The temperature of any refrigerated centrifuge should be checked regularly, and the thermometers should be checked periodically for accuracy.

### Centrifuge Speed

Directions for use of a centrifuge are most frequently given in terms of speed, or revolutions per minute. The number of revolutions per minute (rpm) and the centrifugal force generated are expressed as **relative centrifugal force**

**(RCF).** The number of revolutions per minute is related to the relative centrifugal force by the following formula:

$$RCF = 1.12 \times 10^{-5} \times r \times (rpm)^2$$

where $r$ is the radius of the centrifuge expressed in centimeters. This is equal to the distance from the center of the centrifuge head to the bottom of the tube holder in the centrifuge bucket.

General laboratory centrifuges operate at speeds of up to 6,000 rpm, generating RCF up to 7,300 times the force of gravity (g). The top speed of most conventional centrifuges is about 3,000 rpm. Conventional laboratory centrifuges of the horizontal type attain speeds of up to 3,000 rpm—about 1,700 g—without excessive heat production caused by friction between the head of the centrifuge and the air. Angle-head centrifuges produce less heat and may attain speeds of 7,000 rpm (about 9,000 g).

**Ultracentrifuges** are high-speed centrifuges generally used for research projects, but for certain clinical uses, a small air-driven ultracentrifuge is available that operates at 90,000 to 100,000 rpm and generates a maximum RCF of 178,000 g. Ultracentrifuges are often refrigerated.

A rheostat is used to set the desired speed; the setting on the rheostat dial does not necessarily correspond directly to revolutions per minute. The setting speeds on the rheostat can also change with variations in weight load and general aging of the centrifuge.

The College of American Pathologists recommends that the number of revolutions per minute for a centrifuge used in chemistry laboratories be checked every 3 months. This periodic check can be done most easily by using a photoelectric tachometer or strobe tachometer. Timers and speed controls must also be checked on a periodic basis, with any corrections posted near the controls for the centrifuge.

### Uses for Centrifuges

A primary use for centrifuges in clinical laboratories is to process blood specimens. Separation of cells or clotted blood from plasma or serum is done on an ongoing basis in the handling and processing of the many specimens needed for the various divisions of the clinical laboratory. The relative centrifugal force is not critical for the separation of serum from clot for most laboratory determinations; a force of at least 1,000 g for 10 minutes will usually give a good separation. When serum separator collection tubes are used that contain a silicone gel needing displacement up the side of the tube, a greater centrifugal force is needed to displace this gel—1,000 to 1,300 g for 10 minutes. An RCF less than 1,000 g may result in an incomplete displacement of the gel. It is always important to follow the manufacturer's directions when special collection tubes or serum separator devices are being used. These may require different conditions for centrifugation (see Serum Separator Devices under Laboratory Processing of Blood Specimens, in Chapter 3).

In the hematology laboratory, a table-top version of the centrifuge has been specially adapted for determination of microhematocrit values. This centrifuge accelerates rapidly and can be stopped in seconds. Centrifugation is needed to prepare urinary sediment for microscopic examination. The urine specimen is centrifuged, the supernatant decanted, and the remaining sediment examined. Refrigerated centrifuges are utilized in the blood bank and for other temperature-sensitive laboratory procedures. Ultracentrifuges, which can generate G forces in the hundreds of thousands, are used in laboratories where tissue receptor assays and other assays requiring high-speed centrifugation are needed.

### Technical Factors in Using Centrifuges

The most important rule to remember in using any centrifuge is: always balance the tubes placed in the centrifuge. To **balance the centrifuge**, in the centrifuge cup opposite the material to be centrifuged, a container of equivalent size and shape with an equal volume of liquid of the same specific gravity as the load must be placed. (To see examples of a properly balanced centrifuge and one that is unbalanced, see Fig.

4-12.) For most laboratory determinations, water may be placed in the balance load.

Tubes being centrifuged must be capped. Open tubes of blood should never be centrifuged, because of the risk of aerosol spread of infection (see under Protection from Aerosols, in Chapter 2). Aerosols produced from the heat and vibration generated during the centrifugation process can increase the risk of infection to the laboratory personnel. Some evaporation of the sample can occur during centrifugation in uncapped specimen tubes.

Special centrifuge tubes can be used. These tubes are constructed to withstand the force exerted by the centrifuge. They have thicker glass walls or are made of a stronger, more resistant glass or plastic. Some of these tubes are conical, and some have round bottoms.

Before placing the centrifuge tubes in the cups or holders, check the cups to make certain that the rubber cushions are in place. If some cushions are missing, the centrifuge will not be properly balanced. In addition, without the cushions, the tubes are more likely to break.

Whenever a tube breaks in the centrifuge cup, it is most important that both the cup and the rubber cushion in the cup be cleaned well to prevent further breakage by glass particles left behind.

Covers specially made for the centrifuge should be used, except in certain specified instances. Using the cover prevents possible danger from aerosol spread and from flying glass should tubes break in the centrifuge. Keep the centrifuge cover closed at all times, even when not using the machine. In addition to the danger from broken glass, using the centrifuge without the cover in place may cause the revolving parts of the centrifuge to vibrate, which causes excessive wear of the machine.

Do not try to stop the centrifuge with your hands. It is generally best to let the machine stop by itself. A brake may be applied if the centrifuge is equipped with one. The brake should be used with caution, as braking may cause some resuspension of the sediment. Many laboratories discourage use of the brake except when it is evident that a tube or tubes have broken in the centrifuge.

Centrifuges should be checked, cleaned, and lubricated regularly to ensure proper operation. Centrifuges that are used routinely must be checked periodically with a photoelectric or strobe tachometer to comply with quality assurance guidelines set by the CAP.

## REFERENCES

1. *Commission on Laboratory Inspection and Accreditation: Reagent Water Specifications.* Chicago, College of American Pathologists, 1985.
2. *International System of Units.* Washington, DC, National Bureau of Standards, 1972, special publication No. 330.
3. National Bureau of Standards: *Standard Reference Materials: Summary of the Clinical Laboratory Standards.* Washington, DC, US Department of Commerce, 1981, NBS special publication.
4. National Bureau of Standards: *Testing of Glass Volumetric Apparatus.* Washington, DC, US Department of Commerce, 1959, NBS circ 602.
5. *Preparation and Testing of Reagent Water in the Clinical Laboratory: Approved Guideline,* ed 2. Villanova, Pa, National Committee for Clinical Laboratory Standards, 1997, NCCLS document C3-A3.
6. *Quantities and Units (SI): Committee Report.* Villanova, Pa, National Committee for Clinical Laboratory Standards, 1983, NCCLS document C11-CR.

## BIBLIOGRAPHY

Burtis CA, Ashwood ER (eds): *Tietz Fundamentals of Clinical Chemistry,* ed 4. Philadelphia, WB Saunders Co, 1996.

Campbell JM, Campbell JB: *Laboratory Mathematics: Medical and Biological Applications,* ed 4. St Louis, Mosby, 1997.

Henry JB (ed): *Clinical Diagnosis and Management by Laboratory Methods,* ed 19. Philadelphia, WB Saunders Co, 1996.

Kaplan LA, Pesce AJ: *Clinical Chemistry: Theory, Analysis, and Correlation,* ed 3. St Louis, Mosby, 1996.

## STUDY QUESTIONS

1. Match the following measurements (1 to 3) with their standard metric units (A to C) and complete the metric units by filling in their accepted abbreviations:

   1. Volume
   2. Length
   3. Mass
      _____ A. Meter _____ (abbreviation)
      _____ B. Gram _____ (abbreviation)
      _____ C. Liter _____ (abbreviation)

2. Convert the following measurements of length from units listed to units requested:

   Example: 50 mm = _____ m (answer = 0.050 m)

   A. 100 mm = _____ m
   B. 20 cm   = _____ mm
   C. 0.5 m   = _____ cm
   D. 200 mm = _____ cm
   E. 10 mm  = _____ m

3. Convert the following measurements of mass from units listed to units requested:

   A. 25 mg   = _____ g
   B. 500 mg = _____ g
   C. 100 g   = _____ kg
   D. 2.0 kg  = _____ g
   E. 10 g    = _____ mg

4. Convert the following measurements of volume from units listed to units requested:

   A. 200 mL = _____ L
   B. 0.2 L   = _____ mL
   C. 500 $\mu$L = _____ mL
   D. 600 mL = _____ L
   E. 5 mL    = _____ $\mu$L

5. Convert 25° C to degrees Fahrenheit.

6. Convert 40° F to degrees Celsius.

7. If a 100-mL volumetric flask has a capacity tolerance of ±0.05 mL, what is the allowable range of volume for this flask?

8. Match each of the following types of volumetric glassware (1 to 3) with its primary use (A to C):

   1. 1-mL volumetric pipette
   2. 10-mL graduated pipette
   3. 100-mL volumetric flask
      _____ A. To prepare a reagent of specific total volume
      _____ B. To measure an unknown serum sample
      _____ C. To add a reagent to a reaction tube

9. In what form is the manufacturer's information about a chemical provided to the purchaser of the chemical?

10. What is meant by "quantitative transfer" in the preparation of a reagent?

11. Match each of the following types of balances (1 to 3) with its appropriate use (A to C):

    1. Analytical balance
    2. Torsion balance
    3. Triple-beam balance
       _____ A. To weigh chemicals to accuracy of 0.1 g or less
       _____ B. To weigh very small amounts of a substance to a high degree of accuracy
       _____ C. To weigh chemicals to accuracy of 0.01 g or less

12. Answer the following titration problem. What is the normality of an NaOH solution if 1.0 mL of a standard HCl solution (0.1000N) requires titration using 0.50 mL of the NaOH to reach the end point?

# CHAPTER 5

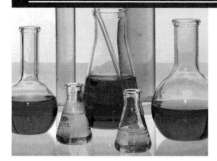

# Use of the Microscope

## Learning Objectives

*From study of this chapter, the reader will be able to:*

➤ Identify the parts of the microscope.

➤ Explain the difference between magnification and resolution.

➤ Explain what is meant by the term parfocal and how it is used in microscopy.

➤ Define alignment and describe the process of aligning a microscope.

➤ Describe the procedure for correct light adjustment to obtain maximum resolution with sufficient contrast.

➤ Describe the components of a phase-contrast microscope and tell how they differ from those of a brightfield microscope.

➤ Define the components of the compensated polarizing microscope and describe their locations and functions.

The microscope is probably the piece of equipment that receives the most use (and misuse) in the clinical laboratory. Microscopy is a basic part of the work in many areas of the laboratory—hematology, urinalysis, and microbiology, to name a few. Because the microscope is such an important piece of equipment and is a precision instrument, it must be kept in excellent condition, optically and mechanically. It must be kept clean, and it must be kept aligned.

## DESCRIPTION

In simple terms, a microscope is a magnifying glass. The compound light microscope (or the **brightfield microscope,** the type used in most clinical laboratories) consists of two magnifying lenses, the objective and the eyepiece (ocular). It is used to magnify an object to a point where it can be seen with the human eye.

The total magnification observed is the product of the magnifications of these two lenses. In other words, the magnification of the objective times the magnification of the ocular equals the total magnification. For example, the total magnification of an object seen with a 10× ocular and a 10× objective is 100 times (100×). These magnification units are in terms of diameters; thus, 10× means that the diameter of an object is magnified to ten times its original size. (The object itself or its area is not magnified ten times; only the diameter of the object is magnified.) The magnification is inscribed on each lens as a number.

Because of the manner in which light travels through the compound microscope, the image that is seen is upside down and reversed. The right side appears as the left, the top as the bottom, and vice versa. This should be kept in mind when one is moving the slide (or object) being observed.

Besides magnification, resolution is a term that is basic in microscopy. **Resolution** tells how small and how close individual objects (dots) can be and still be recognizable. Practically, the resolving power is the limit of usable magnification. Further magnification of two dots that are

no longer resolvable would be "empty magnification" and would result in a dumbbell appearance, as shown in Fig. 5-1.

The relative resolving powers of the human eye, the light microscope, and the electron microscope are shown below.

| | | | |
|---|---|---|---|
| Human eye | 0.25 mm | $0.25 \times 10^3$ m | 0.00025 m |
| Light microscope | 0.25 $\mu$m | $0.25 \times 10^6$ m | 0.00000025 m |
| Electron microscope | 0.5 nm | $0.5 \times 10^9$ m | 0.0000000005 m |

Another term encountered in microscopy is **numerical aperture (NA).** The NA of a lens can be thought of as an index or measurement of the resolving power. As the numerical aperture increases, the closer objects can be positioned and still be distinguished from each other. Or, the greater the numerical aperture, the greater the resolving power of a lens. The numerical aperture can also be thought of as an index of the light-gathering power of a lens—a means of describing the amount of light entering the objective. Any particular lens has a constant rated numerical aperture, and this value is dependent on the radius of the lens and its focal length (the distance from the object being viewed to the lens or the objective); however, decreasing the amount of light passing through a lens will decrease the actual numerical aperture. The importance of this will become apparent when we discuss proper light adjustments with the microscope. The rated numerical aperture is inscribed on each objective lens.

The structures basic to all types of compound microscopes fall into four main categories: (1) the framework, (2) the illumination system, (3)

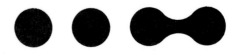

**FIG 5-1.** Resolution versus empty magnification.

the magnification system, and (4) the focusing system (Fig. 5-2).

## PARTS OF THE MICROSCOPE

The framework of the microscope consists of several units. The base is a firm, horseshoe-shaped foot on which the microscope rests. The arm is the structure that supports the magnifying and adjusting systems. It is also the handle by which the microscope can be carried without damaging the delicate parts. The stage is the horizontal platform, or shelf, on which the object being observed is placed. Most microscopes have a mechanical stage, which makes it much easier to manipulate the object being observed.

Good microscope work cannot be accomplished without proper illumination. The illumination system is an important part of the compound light microscope. Different illumination techniques or systems that are useful in the clinical laboratory include: (1) brightfield, (2) phase contrast, (3) interference contrast, (4) polarized and compensated polarized, (5) fluorescence, and (6) darkfield. The electron microscope is also useful but requires a more specialized laboratory than the routine clinical laboratory.

## BRIGHTFIELD MICROSCOPE: GENERAL DESCRIPTION

The brightfield microscope is the type of illumination system most commonly employed in the clinical laboratory. It consists of an illumination system, a magnifying system, and a focusing system.

### Illumination System
#### Light Source and Intensity Control

The illumination system begins with a source of light. The clinical microscope most often has a

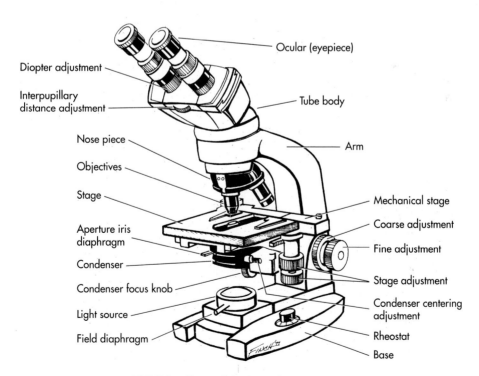

Diopter adjustment
Interpupillary distance adjustment
Nose piece
Objectives
Stage
Aperture iris diaphragm
Condenser
Condenser focus knob
Light source
Field diaphragm
Ocular (eyepiece)
Tube body
Arm
Mechanical stage
Coarse adjustment
Fine adjustment
Stage adjustment
Condenser centering adjustment
Rheostat
Base

**FIG 5-2.**  Parts of the binocular microscope.

built-in light source (or bulb). The bulb is turned on with an on-off switch (or in some cases by a rheostat, which turns on the bulb and adjusts the intensity of light). The light intensity is controlled by a rheostat, dimmer switch or slide, ensuring both adequate illumination and comfort for the microscopist. When there is a separate on-off switch, the light intensity should be lowered before the bulb is turned off, to lengthen the life of the bulb. The light source is located at the base of the microscope, and the light is directed up through the condenser system. It is important that the bulb be positioned correctly for proper alignment of the microscope. (Proper alignment means that the parts of the microscope are adjusted so that the light path from the source of light through the microscope and the ocular is physically correct.) Microscopes are designed so that the light bulb filament will be centered if the bulb is installed properly. Many styles or types of bulbs are available (generally tungsten or tungsten-halogen), and it is important that the bulb designed for a particular microscope be used.

### Condenser

Another part of the illumination system is the **condenser.** Microscopes generally use a substage Abbé-type condenser. The condenser directs and focuses the beam of light from the bulb onto the material under examination. The Abbé condenser is a conical lens system (actually consisting of two lenses) with the point planed off (Fig. 5-3). The condenser position is adjustable; it can be raised and lowered beneath the stage by means of an adjustment knob. It must be correctly positioned to correctly focus the light on the material being viewed. When it is correctly positioned, the image field is evenly lighted. The condenser body must be positioned, because, containing lenses, it has a fixed rated NA. When the microscope is properly used, the apparent NA of the condenser should be equal to or slightly less than the rated NA of the objective being used. The apparent or actual NA of the condenser can be varied by changing its position; as it is lowered, the apparent NA is re-

duced. Thus the condenser position must be adjusted with each objective used in order to maximize the light focus and the resolving power of the microscope. When the apparent NA of the condenser is decreased below that of the rated NA of the objective, contrast and depth of field are gained and resolution is lost. This manipulation is often necessary in the clinical laboratory when wet, unstained preparations are being observed, such as urinary sediment. In this case, when a specimen is being scanned, in order to gain contrast, the condenser is lowered (or the aperture iris diaphragm partially closed), thus reducing the apparent NA of the condenser. Preferably, the condenser should be left in a generally uppermost position, at most only 1 or 2 mm below the specimen, and the light adjusted primarily by opening or closing the aperture iris diaphragm located in the condenser. The old procedure of "racking down" the condenser when one is looking at wet preparations is not acceptable.

Some microscopes are equipped with a condenser element, which is used in place for low-power work and swings out for high power. Others employ an element that swings out for low-power work and is used in place for higher magnification. This changes the apparent NA of the condenser, matching it with that of the objective. Other illumination systems employ different types of condensers, such as phase-contrast, differential interference-contrast, and darkfield condensers.

### Aperture Iris Diaphragm

The **aperture iris diaphragm** also controls the amount of light passing through the material under observation. It is located at the bottom of the condenser, under the lenses but within the condenser body as shown in Fig. 5-3. This aperture diaphragm consists of a series of horizontally arranged interlocking plates with a central aperture (Fig. 5-4). It can be opened or closed as necessary, to adjust the intensity of the light, by means of a lever or dial. The size of the aperture, and consequently the amount of light permitted to pass, is regulated by the micros-

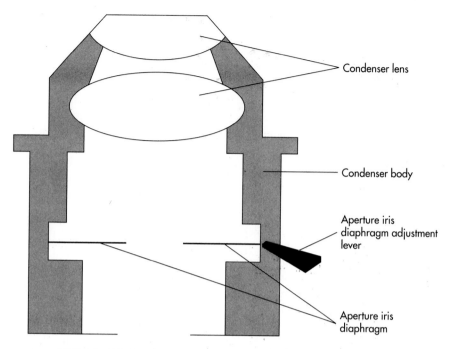

**FIG 5-3.** Abbé-type substage condenser with aperture iris diaphram.

copist. Such regulation of the light affects the apparent NA of the condenser; decreasing the size of the field under observation with the iris diaphragm decreases the apparent NA of the condenser. Thus, proper illumination techniques involve a combination of proper light intensity regulation, condenser position, and field size regulation.

### Field Diaphragm

Better microscopes have a field iris diaphragm, located in the light port in the base of the microscope, through which light passes up to the condenser. The **field diaphragm** controls the area of the circle of light in the field of view when the specimen and condenser have been properly focused. It is also used in the alignment of the microscope.

## Magnification System

The magnification system contains several important parts. It plays an extremely important role in the use of the microscope.

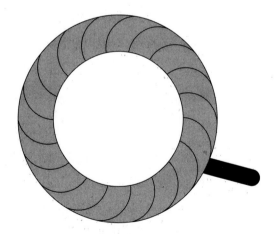

**FIG 5-4.** Aperture iris diaphragm.

### Ocular (Eyepiece)

The **ocular,** or **eyepiece,** is a lens that magnifies the image formed by the objective. The usual magnification of the ocular is 10 (10×); however, 5× and 20× oculars are also generally available. Most microscopes have two oculars and are called binocular microscopes. Some microscopes have only one ocular, and these are called monocular microscopes. The magnification produced by the ocular, when multiplied by the magnification produced by the objective, gives the total magnification of the object being viewed. The distance between the two oculars **(interpupillary distance)** is adjustable, as is the focus on one of the oculars **(diopter adjustment)**.

### Objectives

The **objectives** are the major part of the magnification system. There are usually three objectives on each microscope, with magnifying powers of 10×, 40×, and 100×. The objectives are mounted on the **nosepiece,** which is a pivot that enables a quick change of objectives. Objectives are also described or rated according to **focal length,** which is inscribed on the outside of the objective. Microscopes used in the clinical laboratory most commonly have 16-mm, 4-mm, and 1.8-mm objectives. The focal length is a physical property of the objective lens and is slightly less than the distance from the object being examined to the center of the objective lens. Practically speaking, then, the focal length of a lens is very close in value to the **working distance**—the distance from the bottom of the objective to the material being studied. The greater the magnifying power of a lens, the smaller the focal length and hence the working distance. This becomes very important when the microscope is being used, as the working distance is very short for the 40× (4-mm) and 100× (1.8-mm) objectives. For this reason, correct focusing habits are necessary to prevent damaging the objectives against the slide on the stage.

There are generally two types of objectives available in clinical microscopes: achromats and planachromats. Standard lenses in most microscopes are achromats, which correct for color (chromatic) aberrations. Although achromats are adequate for most laboratory work, the center of the field of view will be in sharp focus, while the edges appear out of focus and the field

does not appear to be flat. Planachromat objectives, while more expensive, are more appropriate for high-magnification work using a 40× or 100× objective, as the field of view is in focus and flat throughout. Apochromatic objectives are also available, which correct for chromatic and spherical aberrations. These are the finest lenses available, and may be necessary for photomicroscopy, but they are significantly more expensive and are not necessary for routine clinical work.

Objective lenses are inscribed with certain information, including type of lens, magnification, rated numerical aperture (NA), body tube length, and cover glass thickness or requirement for immersion oil.

Other terms that are commonly used to describe microscope objectives are *low power, high power* (also *high dry*), and *oil immersion.*

**Low-Power Objective.** The **low-power objective** is usually a 10× magnification, 16-mm objective. This objective is used for the initial scanning and observation in most microscope work. For example, blood films and urinary sediment are routinely examined by using the low-power objective first. This is also the lens employed for the initial focusing and light adjustment of the microscope. Some routine microscopes also have a very low-power 4× magnification lens. This is used in the initial scanning in the morphologic examination of histologic sections.

Often the term *parfocal* is used in speaking about a microscope. It means that if one objective is in focus and a change is made to another objective, the focus will not be lost. Thus the microscope can be focused under low power and then changed to the high-power or oil-immersion objective (by rotating the nosepiece), and it will still be in focus except for fine adjustment.

The rated NA of the low-power objective is significantly less than that of the condenser on most microscopes (for the 10× objective the NA is approximately 0.25; for the condenser it is approximately 0.9). Therefore, to achieve focus, the

NAs must be more closely matched by reducing the light to the specimen; this is done by focusing or lowering the condenser slightly (1 or 2 mm below the specimen) and then reducing the size of the field of light, with the aperture iris diaphragm, to about 70% to 80%.

**High-Power Objective.** The **high-power objective,** or high-dry objective, is usually a 40× magnification lens with a 4-mm working distance. This objective is used for more detailed study, as the total magnification with a 10× eyepiece is 400× rather than the 100× magnification of the low-power system. The high-power objective is used to study histology sections, and to study wet preparations such as urinary sediment in more detail. The working distance of the 4-mm lens is quite short; therefore, care must be taken in focusing. The NA of the high-power lens is fairly close to (although slightly less than) that of most commonly used condensers (for most high-power objectives, NA = 0.85; for the condenser, NA = 0.9). Therefore, the condenser should generally be all the way up (or very slightly lowered) and the light field slightly closed with the aperture iris diaphragm for maximum focus.

**Oil-Immersion Objective.** The **oil-immersion objective** is generally a 100× lens with a 1.8-mm working distance. This is a very short focal length and working distance. In fact, the objective lens almost rests on the microscope slide when the microscope is in use. An oil-immersion lens requires that a special grade of oil, called immersion oil, be placed between the objective and the slide or coverglass. Oil is used to increase the NA and thus the resolving power of the objective. Since the focal length of this lens is so small, there is a problem in getting enough light from the microscope field to the objective. Light travels through air at a greater speed than through glass, and it travels through immersion oil at the same speed as through glass. Thus, to increase the effective NA of the objective, oil is used to slow down the speed at which light

travels, increasing the gathering power of the lens.*

Since the NA of the oil-immersion objective is greater than that of the condenser in most systems (for the 100× objective, NA = 1.2; for the condenser, NA = 0.9), the condenser should be used in the uppermost position and the aperture iris diaphragm should generally be open; practically speaking, however, partial closing of the iris diaphragm may be necessary. The oil-immersion lens, with a total magnification of 1,000× when used with a 10× eyepiece, is generally the limit of magnification with the light microscope.

The oil-immersion lens is routinely used for morphologic examination of blood films and microbes. The short working distance requires dry films, so wet preparations such as urinary sediment cannot be examined under an oil-immersion lens.

The high-power lens is also referred to as a high-dry lens because it does not require the use of immersion oil. Other objectives that might be present on a microscope in the clinical laboratory are a lower-power 4× scanning lens and a 50× or 63× low oil-immersion lens.

## Focusing System

The **body tube** is the part of the microscope through which the light passes to the ocular. The tube length from the eyepiece to the objective lens is generally 160 mm. This is the tube that actually conducts the image. The required body tube length is also inscribed on each objective.

The adjustment system enables the body tube to move up or down for focusing the objectives. This usually consists of two adjustments, one coarse and the other fine. The coarse adjustment gives rapid movement over a wide range and is used to obtain an approximate focus. The fine

---

*The speed at which light travels through a substance is measured in terms of the refractive index. The refractive index is calculated as the speed at which light travels through air divided by the speed at which it travels through the substance. The refractive index of air is therefore 1.00. The refractive index of glass is 1.515; immersion oil, 1.515; and water, 1.33.

adjustment gives very slow movement over a limited range and is used to obtain exact focus after coarse adjustment.

## CARE AND CLEANING OF THE MICROSCOPE

The microscope is a precision instrument and must be handled with great care. When it is necessary to transport the microscope, it should always be carried with both hands; it should be carried by the arm and supported under the base with the other hand. When not in use, the microscope should be covered and put away in a microscope case, or in a desk or cupboard. It should be left with the low-power (10×) objective in place, and the body tube barrel adjusted to the lowest possible position.

### Cleaning the Microscope Exterior

The surface of most microscopes is finished with a black or gray enamel and metal plating that is resistant to most laboratory chemicals. It may be kept clean by washing with a neutral soap and water. To clean the metal and enamel, a gauze or soft cloth should be moistened with the cleaning agent and rubbed over the surface with a circular motion. The surface should be dried immediately with a clean, dry piece of gauze or cloth. Gauze should never be used to clean any of the optical parts of the microscope.

### Cleaning Optical Lenses: General Comments

The glass surfaces of the ocular, the objectives, and the condenser are hand-ground optical lenses. These lenses must be kept meticulously clean. Optical glass is softer than ordinary glass and should never be cleaned with paper tissue or gauze. These materials will scratch the lens. To clean the lenses of the microscope, use lens paper. Before polishing with lens paper, take care that nothing is present that will scratch the optical glass in the polishing process. Such potentially abrasive dirt, dust, or lint can easily be blown away before polishing. Cans of compressed air are commercially available, or an air syringe can be made simply by fitting a plastic eyedropper or a 1-mL plastic tuberculin syringe with the tip cut off into a rubber bulb of the type used for pipetting (Fig. 5-5). This air syringe is used to blow away dust or lint that might otherwise scratch the optical glass in the polishing process.

### Cleaning the Objectives

Oil must be removed from the oil-immersion (100×) objective immediately after use, by wiping with clean lens paper. If not removed, oil may seep inside the lens, or dry on the outside surface of the objective. The high-dry (40×) objective should never be used with oil; however, if this or any other objective or microscope part comes into contact with oil, it should be cleaned immediately. If a lens is especially dirty, it may be cleaned with a small amount of commercial lens cleaner, methanol, or a solution recommended by the manufacturer, applied to lens paper. Xylene should not be used, because it can damage the lens mounting if it is allowed to get beyond the front seal and because its fumes are toxic.

To properly clean the oil-immersion lens, first lower the stage; then rotate the objective to the front and wipe gently with clean lens paper. Then clean off the immersion oil with lens paper dampened with special lens cleaner or methanol. Alternatively, the cleaning agent may be applied to a wooden applicator stick wrapped with cotton or lens paper and moistened with the cleaning agent. Do not use a plastic applicator stick, as it will be dissolved by the solvent, ruining the objective. Apply the cleaning agent by blotting and in a circular motion, beginning at the center and moving outward. Repeat with new dampened

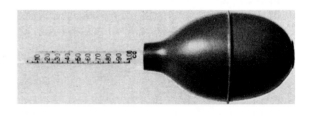

**FIG 5-5.** Air syringe.

lens paper as necessary. Finally, blot dry with clean lens paper. Do not rub, as this may scratch the surface of the lens.

Lenses should never be touched with the fingers. Objectives must not be taken apart, as even a slight alteration of the lens setting may ruin the objective. Merely clean the outer surface of the lens as described. An especially dirty objective may be removed (unscrewed) from the nosepiece, then held upside down and checked for cleanliness by using the ocular (removed from the body tube) as a magnifying glass. Dust or lint can also be removed from the rear lens of the objective by blowing it away with an air syringe. Such removal of the objective from the nosepiece is not a routine cleaning procedure. The final step after using the microscope should always be to wipe off all objectives with clean lens paper.

## Cleaning the Ocular

The ocular or eyepiece is especially vulnerable to dirt because of its location on the microscope and contact with the observer's eye. Mascara presents a constant cleaning problem. Dust can be removed from the lens of the ocular with an air syringe (or camel's hair brush). Air is probably easier to use and more efficient. The lens should then be polished with lens paper. The ocular can be checked for additional dirt by holding it up to a light and looking through it. When one is looking into the microscope, dirt on any part of the ocular will rotate with the ocular when it is turned. The ocular should not be removed for more than a few minutes, as dust can collect in the body tube and settle on the rear lens of an objective.

## Cleaning the Condenser

The light source and condenser should also be free of dust, lint, and dirt. First blow away the dust with an air syringe or camel's hair brush; then polish the light source and condenser with lens paper. It may be necessary to clean them further with lens paper moistened with a commercial lens cleaner or methanol before polishing them with lens paper.

## Cleaning the Stage; Coarse and Fine Adjustments

The stage of the microscope should be cleaned after each use by wiping with gauze or a tissue. After it has been cleaned thoroughly, the stage should be wiped dry.

The coarse and fine adjustments occasionally need attention, as does the mechanical stage adjustment mechanism. When there is unusual resistance to any manipulation of these knobs, force must not be used to overcome the resistance. Such force might damage the screw or rack-and-pinion mechanism. Instead, the cause of the problem must be found. A small drop of oil may be needed. It is best to call in a specialist to repair the microscope when a serious problem occurs. In addition, the microscope should be cleaned at least once a year by a professional microscope service company.

# USE OF THE MICROSCOPE

When a microscope is being used, two conditions must be met: (1) the microscope must be clean, and (2) it must be aligned. The cleaning procedure has been described; alignment will now be discussed.

## Alignment

When properly aligned, the microscope is adjusted in such a way that the light path through the microscope, from the light source to the eye of the observer, is correct. This is referred to as Kohler illumination. If a microscope is misaligned, the field of view will seem to swing—a very uncomfortable situation, often described as making the observer feel seasick. This can be corrected by properly aligning or adjusting the light path through the microscope. Many microscopes that are produced for student use are aligned by the manufacturer, and realignment requires special knowledge and experience, as the field diaphragm, condenser-centering adjustment screws, and removable eyepieces are not present. In such microscopes, realignment should be done by a professional microscope service company.

If the microscope has a field diaphragm, it is utilized in the alignment procedure. A field diaphragm is an iris diaphragm that is part of the built-in illuminator. With the low-power objective in place, close down the field diaphragm to a minimum. Then focus the condenser by adjusting the condenser height with the condenser focus knob, until the image of the field diaphragm is sharply visible in the field of view (Fig. 5-6, *A*). Next bring the image of the field diaphragm into the center of the field by means of the centering screws located on the condenser (Fig. 5-6, *B*). Now open the field diaphragm until it is just contained within the field of view (Fig. 5-6, *C*). At this point, it may be necessary to repeat the centering procedure. Finally, open the diaphragm until the leaves are just out of view.

### Light Adjustment

With the low-power objective in position, the object to be examined, usually on a glass microscope slide, is placed on the stage and secured. Care must be taken to avoid damaging the objective when the specimen is placed on the stage. The slide is positioned so that the portion of the slide containing the specimen to be examined is in the light path, directly over the condenser lens.

The biggest concern in learning how to use a microscope for the first time is the lighting and fine adjustment maneuvers. One must be certain that the light source, condenser, and aperture iris diaphragm are in correct adjustment. Light adjustment is made before any focusing is done. The power supply is turned on and the light intensity adjusted to a bright but comfortable level. Light adjustment will be further accomplished by raising and lowering the condenser and opening and closing the aperture iris diaphragm. At the start of this initial light adjustment, the low-power (10×) objective should be in place. The condenser should be near its highest position, no more than 1 to 2 mm below the slide, with the aperture and field diaphragms open all the way and the body tube down so that the lens is approximately 16 mm from the slide (the working distance for the low-power lens). If the microscope is equipped with a field diaphragm, the condenser height should be adjusted so as to bring the field diaphragm into sharp focus, as described in the alignment procedure.

To adjust the aperture iris diaphragm, while looking through the ocular, close the diaphragm until the light just begins to be reduced. Or, if possible, remove the eyepiece and darken out approximately 20% to 30% of the light by closing the iris diaphragm while looking down the body tube (Fig. 5-7). Further closing of the iris diaphragm (or lowering of the condenser), while it may increase contrast and depth of focus, will reduce resolution.

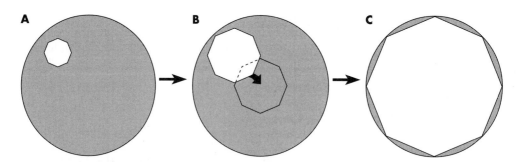

**FIG 5-6.** Microscope alignment; condenser centration. **A,** Stopped down field diaphragm image, off center or misaligned. **B,** Field diaphragm image widened and moved toward center by means of condenser adjustment knobs. **C,** Field diaphragm image diameter widened and centered.

## Focusing

Focusing is the next technique to be mastered. If using a binocular microscope, adjust the interpupillary distance between the oculars so that the left and right fields merge into one. With the object to be examined on the stage, and while watching from the side, bring the low-power (10×) objective down as far as it will go, so that it almost meets the top of the specimen. Use the coarse adjustment for this procedure. The objective must not be in direct contact with the specimen. Watch from the side to avoid damaging the objective. Once the objective is just at the top of the specimen, slowly focus upward, using the coarse adjustment knob and looking through the ocular. When the object is nearly in focus, bring it into clear focus by use of the fine adjustment knob. Do this procedure with the right eye; then set the ocular diopter to the left eye, by rotating until the left eye is in clear focus, so that the object will be in focus with both eyes.

Further light adjustment should now be made to ensure maximum focus and resolution. Adjust the light intensity with the brightness control so that the background light is sufficiently bright (white) but comfortable. Next adjust the iris diaphragm by opening it completely and then slowly closing it until the light intensity just begins to be reduced. Alternatively, remove the eyepiece and close the aperture iris diaphragm until about 80% of the body tube is filled with light.

When one is changing to another objective, the barrel distance need not be changed. As stated previously, most microscopes are parfocal. The only adjustment necessary should be made with the fine adjustment knob. It is essential to remember that fine adjustment is used continuously during microscopic examination, especially when wet preparations such as urine sediment are being examined.

When greater magnification is needed, more light is necessary. It is obtained by repositioning the condenser and aperture iris diaphragm in the manner previously described. In general, the condenser will be raised and the aperture iris diaphragm opened as the objective magnification increases. When the oil-immersion lens is used, the condenser should be raised to its maximum position.

Additional light is provided by the use of immersion oil, which is placed on the viewing slide when the oil-immersion (100×) objective is used. The oil directs the light rays to a finer point, reducing spherical aberration. When the oil-immersion lens is to be used, first find the desired area on the slide by using the low-power (10×) objective. Once this area is located, pivot the objective out of position, place a drop of immersion oil on the slide, and pivot the oil-immersion lens into the oil while observing it from the side. Next, move the objective from side to side to ensure contact with the oil and avoid the presence of air bubbles. The nosepiece, rather than the objective itself, should be grasped when lenses are being changed, to prevent damage to the objective. The ocular should not be looked through during this adjustment procedure. After the initial adjustment has been made, adjust the fine focus while looking through the ocular. After the study has been completed, clean off the oil remaining on the

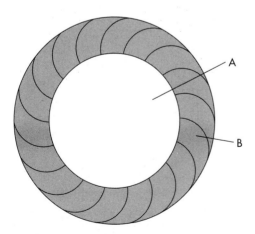

**FIG 5-7.** Adjusting the aperture iris diaphragm. **A,** 70% to 80% of light presented to objective. **B,** 20% to 30% of light restricted by stopping down the aperture iris diaphragm.

objective with lens paper as described previously.

## OTHER TYPES OF MICROSCOPES (ILLUMINATION SYSTEMS)

Until recently, brightfield illumination has, with few exceptions, been the primary type of microscope illumination system used in the routine clinical laboratory. Now other illumination systems are becoming increasingly popular as refinements in microscope design have made them more reliable and easier to use in a clinical situation. These other types of illumination systems—phase contrast, interference contrast, polarizing, darkfield, fluorescence, and electron—will now be briefly described. The basic principles of microscopy and rules for usage apply with all of these variations; the primary difference is the character of light delivered to the specimen and illuminating the microscope.

### Phase-Contrast Microscope

Another extremely useful illumination system is the phase-contrast microscope. A disadvantage of brightfield illumination is that it is necessary to stain (or dye) many objects to give sufficient contrast and detail. **Phase contrast** facilitates the study of unstained structures, which can even be alive, since wet preparations of cells or organisms are observed without prior dehydration and staining. As the name of the technique implies, the structures observed with this system show added contrast compared with the brightfield microscope. The phase-contrast microscope is basically a brightfield microscope with changes in the objective and the condenser. An annular diaphragm, or ring, is put into (or below) the condenser. This condenser annulus is designed to let a hollow cone or "doughnut" of light pass through the condenser to the specimen. A corresponding absorption ring is fitted into the objective. Each phase objective must have a corresponding condenser annulus (Fig. 5-8). In microscopes with multiple phase objectives, the annular diaphragms are usually placed in a rotating condenser arrangement (Fig. 5-9). Use of each phase objective requires an adjustment of the condenser to "match" the annular diaphragm and the phase absorption

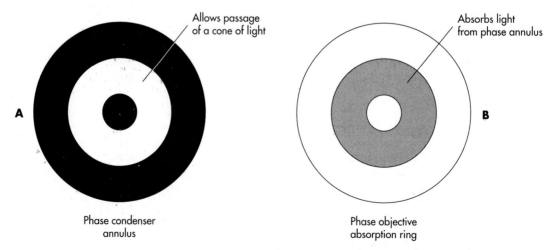

**FIG 5-8.** Phase annulus and absorption ring. **A,** Phase condenser annulus. **B,** Phase objective absorption ring.

ring. The phase microscope may also be used as a brightfield microscope by setting the condenser to a standard brightfield (or open) position, which contains no annulus. However, since the phase objective blocks out a ring of light, the resolution or detail that can be achieved when phase objectives are used for brightfield examination is compromised. For more exact work, an additional brightfield objective should be employed in the microscope.

The annulus and the absorption ring must be perfectly aligned or adjusted so that they are concentric and superimposed. Therefore, a problem with the phase-contrast microscope is the necessity for perfect alignment. First the microscope must be aligned for brightfield work. To align the phase annulus, match the phase objective to the corresponding phase annulus in the condenser by rotating the phase turret. Insert the aperture viewing unit, either by inser-

tion into the body tube or by inserting a phase telescope into an ocular tube. Focus the viewing apparatus until the phase annulus (seen as a white ring of light) is in focus. There will be a bright (white) ring and a dark ring, which should be superimposed (Fig. 5-10). If not perfectly superimposed, the phase annulus can be repositioned by means of the annulus-centering knobs, located on the condenser. Each microscope will have a slightly different means of adjustment, and the operation directions for that microscope should be followed. However, all phase microscopes require alignment as for brightfield plus alignment of the phase annulus to the matching phase objective.

The net effect of phase contrast is to slow down the speed of light by one fourth of a wavelength. This diminution of the speed of light makes the system very sensitive to differences in refractive index. Objects with differ-

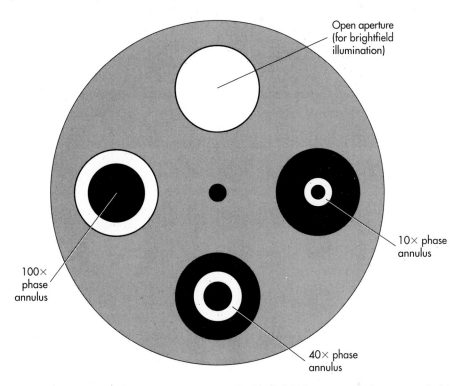

Open aperture (for brightfield illumination)

10× phase annulus

100× phase annulus

40× phase annulus

**FIG 5-9.** Rotating phase condenser with settings for brightfield, low power, high power, and oil immersion.

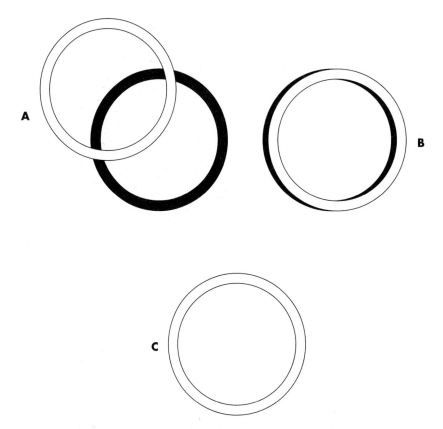

**FIG 5-10.** Alignment of phase annulus to phase absorption ring. **A,** Before alignment: phase annulus is out of phase adjustment. **B,** Phase annulus moved so that it is nearly aligned. **C,** Alignment: phase annulus is superimposed on phase absorption ring.

ences in refractive index, shape, and absorption characteristics show added differences in the intensity and shade of light passing through them. The end result is that one can observe unstained wet preparations with good resolution and detail, as shown in Fig. 5-11. In the clinical laboratory, phase contrast is especially useful for counting platelets and for observing cellular structures and casts in wet preparations of urinary sediment and vaginal smears. Owing to its superior visualization and ease of operation, the phase-contrast microscope has become a common tool in routine urinalysis. However, the microscopist must be proficient in changing from brightfield to phase contrast,

as in a given specimen some structures are better visualized with phase contrast and others with brightfield.

## Interference-Contrast Microscope

Another illumination technique gaining in clinical use is interference-contrast illumination. This technique gives the viewer a three-dimensional image of the object under study. Like phase contrast, it is especially useful for wet preparations such as urinary sediment, showing finer details without the need for special staining techniques. The brightfield microscope is modified by the addition of a special beam-splitting (Wollaston) prism to the condenser. The

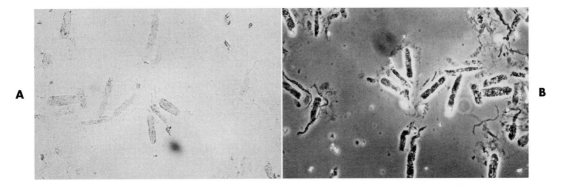

**FIG 5-11.** Brightfield versus phase-contrast illumination. **A,** Several casts with brightfield illumination. **B,** Same field with phase-contrast illumination. Casts are now clearly visible.

two split beams are then polarized; one passes through the specimen, which alters the amplitude (or height) of the light wave, and the other (which serves as a reference) does not pass through the specimen. The two dissimilar light beams then pass separately through the objective and are recombined by a second Wollaston (beam-combining) prism. This recombination of light waves gives the three-dimensional image to the additive or subtractive effects of the light waves as they are combined.

## Polarizing Microscope

Another useful adaptation of the brightfield microscope is the polarizing microscope. A **polarizer** (or polarizing filter) may be thought of as a sieve that takes ordinary light waves, which vibrate in all orientations (or directions), and allows only light waves of one orientation (say north-south or east-west) to pass through the filter (Fig. 5-12, *A*). In a polarizing microscope, a polarizing filter is placed between the light source (bulb) and the specimen. A second polarizing filter (called an **analyzer**) is placed above the specimen, between the objective and the eyepiece (either at some point in the microscope tube or in the eyepiece). One of the polarizers is then rotated until the two are at right angles to each other (Fig. 5-12, *B*). When one is looking through the eyepieces, this will be seen as the extinction of light (one sees a dark or

black field), since all light is blocked out of the light path when the polarizing filters are at right angles to each other. However, certain objects have a property termed **birefringence,** which means that they rotate (or polarize) light. An object that polarizes bends light, so that it can be visualized when viewed through crossed polarizers. Objects that do not bend light will not be observed in the microscope. An object that polarizes light (or is birefringent) will appear light against a dark background (Fig. 5-13).

A further modification of the polarizing microscope involves the use of **compensated polarized light.** A compensator, also referred to as a first-order red plate (filter) or full-wave retardation plate, is placed between the two crossed polarizing filters and positioned at 45 degrees to the crossed polarizer and analyzer (Fig. 5-12, *C* and *D*). With this addition the field background appears red or magenta, while objects that are birefringent (polarize light) appear yellow or blue in relation to their orientation to the compensator and their optical properties.

The compensated polarized microscope is especially useful clinically for differentiating between monosodium urate (MSU) and calcium pyrophosphate dihydrate (CPPD) crystals in synovial fluid. It is also becoming useful in the routine study of urinary sediment and in some

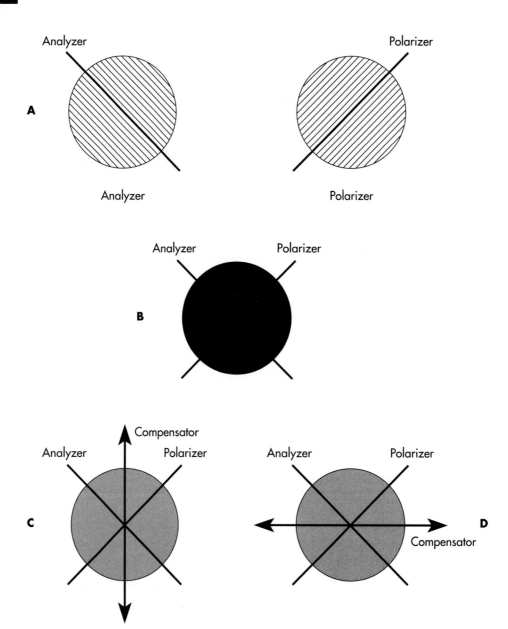

**FIG 5-12.** Principle of polarized light and compensated polarized light. **A,** Polarizing lenses or filters. Polarizer is placed between light source and specimen; analyzer is placed between specimen and eye of the observer. **B,** Polarized light. This is obtained by placing analyzer and polarizer at right angles to each other. The position of the analyzer is fixed, and the polarizer is rotated until light is extinguished (seen as a black or dark background). **C,** Compensated polarized light. The compensator is placed at 45 degrees to the crossed polarizers, resulting in a red or magenta background color. In this case, the direction of the slow wave of compensation is in a north-south (N-S) orientation. **D,** Compensated polarized light. In this case, the direction of the slow wave of compensation is in an east-west (E-W) orientation.

**FIG 5-13.** Brightfield versus polarized light. **A,** Starch granules viewed with brightfield illumination. **B,** Starch granules viewed with polarized light (crossed polarizing filters). Starch is birefringent; therefore it is visible with polarized light.

histologic work. Polarizing microscopy is commonly used in geology for particle analysis, and clinically in forensic medicine. With the polarizing microscope the optical properties of an object can be determined.

### Darkfield Microscope

With darkfield microscopy, a special substage condenser is used that causes light waves to cross on the specimen rather than pass in parallel waves through the specimen. Thus, when one looks through the microscope, the field in view will be black, or dark, as no light passes from the condenser to the objective. However, when an object is present on the stage, light will be deflected as it hits the object and will pass through the objective and be seen by the viewer. As a result, the object under study appears light against a dark background. Any brightfield microscope may be converted to a darkfield microscope by use of a special darkfield condenser in place of the usual condenser.

The darkfield microscope has long been used in the routine clinical laboratory to observe spirochetes in the exudates from leptospiral or syphilitic infections. A more recent use, facilitated by newer microscope design technology, is as a low-power scanner for urinary sediment. A darkfield effect may be achieved by using a mismatched phase annulus and phase objective, such as a low-power phase objective with a high-power phase annulus.

### Fluorescence Microscope

The transmitted light fluorescence microscope is a further refinement of the darkfield microscope. It is basically a darkfield microscope with wavelength selection. Certain objects have the ability to fluoresce. This means that they absorb light of certain very short (ultraviolet) wavelengths and emit light of longer (visible) wavelengths. In fluorescence microscopy with transmitted light and a compound microscope, the darkfield condenser is preceded by a special exciter filter, which allows only shorter-wavelength blue light to pass and cross on the specimen plane. If the specimen contains an object that fluoresces (either naturally or because of staining or labeling with certain fluorescent dyes), it will absorb the blue light and emit light of a longer yellow or green wavelength. A special barrier filter is placed in the microscope tube or eyepiece. This barrier filter will pass only the desired wavelength of emitted light for the particular fluorescent system. Thus, the fluorescence technique shows only the presence or absence of the fluorescing object. The barrier filter used must be carefully chosen so that only light of the desired wavelength will be passed through the microscope to the observer. Objects in the specimen that do not fluoresce will not emit light of that wavelength and will not be seen.

Fluorescence techniques, in particular fluorescent antibody (FA) techniques, are especially useful in the clinical laboratory. They are used particularly in the clinical microbiology laboratory and for various immunologic studies. Different fluorescent antibody techniques may be used in the primary identification of microorganisms, or in the final identification of bacteria (such as group A streptococci), replacing older serologic methods. Such techniques have the advantage of saving time, which results in earlier diagnosis for the patient, and they are often more sensitive than other techniques. They may also be useful in the identification of organisms that cannot be cultured, such as *Treponema pallidum*.

## Electron Microscope

The limit of magnification with any of the variations of the light microscope is about 1,500× to 2,000×. Above this, there is decreased resolving power. However, for magnification up to about 50,000× the electron microscope may be used with good resolution.

In general, the principle of the electron microscope is the same as for the light microscope. Rather than a beam of light, the specimen is illuminated with a beam of electrons, produced by an electron gun. The electrons are accelerated by a high-voltage potential and pass through a condenser lens system, usually composed of two magnetic lenses. The electron beam is concentrated onto the specimen, and the objective lens provides the primary magnification. The final image is not visible and cannot be viewed directly; rather it is projected onto a fluorescent screen or a photographic plate. This is the principle of the **transmission electron microscope (TEM).**

Another variation is the **scanning electron microscope (SEM).** It looks at the surface of the specimen and produces a three-dimensional image by striking the sample with a focused beam of electrons. Electrons emitted from the surface of the sample, in addition to deflected electrons from the focused beam of electrons, are focused onto a cathode ray tube or photographic plate and are visualized as a three-dimensional image.

In both cases, specimens need special preparation that is not done in routine clinical laboratories. Specimens must be extremely thin; with TEM the electron beam must pass through the specimen, and electrons have a very poor penetrating power. With SEM the specimen is thicker, since the beam of electrons does not pass through the specimen. In either case, it is impossible to study living cells with electron microscopy because of the high vacuum to which the specimen is subjected and because the electron beam itself is highly damaging to living tissue. However, much of the knowledge of cell structure and function has come from electron microscopy.

## BIBLIOGRAPHY

Brown BA: *Hematology: Principles and Procedures*, ed 6. Philadelphia, Lea & Febiger, 1993.

Freeman JA, Beeler MF: *Laboratory Medicine/Urinalysis and Medical Microscopy*, ed 2. Philadelphia, Lea & Febiger, 1983.

*Physician's Office Laboratory Procedure Manual: Tentative Guidelines*, Villanova, Pa, National Committee for Clinical Laboratory Standards, 1995, POL 1/2-T3 and POL 3-R.

## STUDY QUESTIONS

1. **Which is the preferred method of obtaining maximum resolution with sufficient contrast when one is observing a wet preparation using the high-power objective?**

   a. Focus the condenser, utilizing the field diaphragm; then reduce the amount of light presented to the objective to 70% to 80% by closing the aperture iris diaphragm.

   b. Adjust the condenser position to be as far from the specimen slide as possible, and close the field diaphragm.

   c. Keep the condenser height as close to the slide as possible, and open the aperture iris diaphragm as far as possible; then reduce the amount of light to the objective with the intensity-control device.

2. **What is the total magnification of an item under study with a 10× ocular and a 40× objective?**

3. **Where is the aperture iris diaphragm located, and what is its function?**

4. **Where is the field diaphragm located, and what is its function?**

5. **Match the following common working distances (1 to 3) with their objectives (A to C).**

   1. 4 mm
   2. 1.8 mm
   3. 16 mm
      _____ A. Oil-immersion objective
      _____ B. High-power objective
      _____ C. Low-power objective

6. **Match the following objectives (1 to 3) with their common numerical apertures (A to C), and tell how the condenser should be positioned (D to F), assuming the NA of the condenser is 0.85.**

   1. Oil-immersion objective
   2. High-power objective
   3. Low-power objective
      _____ A. 0.25 NA
      _____ B. 0.85 NA
      _____ C. 1.2 NA
      _____ D. Highest possible position or very slightly decreased
      _____ E. Highest possible position
      _____ F. Decreased to 1 or 2 mm below the slide

# CHAPTER 6

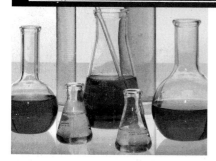

# Photometry

## Learning Objectives

*From study of this chapter, the reader will be able to:*

➤ Compare and contrast components of the filter photometer, the absorbance spectrophotometer, and the reflectance spectrophotometer.

➤ Describe light and explain how the observed color of a solution is related to the wavelengths of light absorbed.

➤ Explain how the intensity of color in a substance can be used to measure its concentration.

➤ Define Beer's Law.

➤ Discuss the differences between plotting concentration against percent transmittance and plotting concentration against absorbance and between the use of linear graph paper and the use of semilogarithmic paper.

➤ Use a standard curve to obtain the concentration of an unknown.

➤ Describe the components of a flame photometer.

# INTRODUCTION TO PHOTOMETRY

In the clinical laboratory there is a continual need for the use of quantitative techniques. By use of a quantitative method, the exact amount of an unknown substance can be determined accurately, and this is the basis for many laboratory determinations, especially in the chemistry department. Various methods for measuring substances quantitatively are discussed in Chapter 4. One of the techniques used most frequently in the clinical laboratory is photometry, or, specifically, absorbance or reflectance spectrophotometry. **Photometry**, or **colorimetry**, employs color and color variation to determine the concentrations of substances. A photometric component is employed in many of the automated analyzers currently in use in the clinical laboratory, and any person doing clinical laboratory techniques should know and understand thoroughly the principles of photometry in general.

# ABSORBANCE SPECTROPHOTOMETRY

## Principle of Absorbance Spectrophotometry

The use of **spectrophotometry**, or colorimetry, as a means of quantitative measurement depends primarily on two factors, the color itself and the intensity of the color. Any substance to be measured by spectrophotometry must be colored to begin with or must be capable of being colored. An example of a substance that is colored to begin with is hemoglobin (determined by use of spectrophotometry in the hematology laboratory). Sugar, specifically glucose, is an example of a substance that is not colored to begin with but is capable of being colored by the use of certain reagents and reactions. Sugar content can therefore be measured by spectrophotometry.

When spectrophotometry is used as a method for quantitative measurement, the unknown colored substance is compared with a similar substance of known strength (a standard solution), according to the principle that the intensity of the color is directly proportional to the concentration of the substance present.

In **absorbance spectrophotometry**, the absorbance units or values for several different concentrations of a standard solution are determined by spectrophotometry and are plotted on graph paper. The resulting graph is known as a **standard calibration curve** or a Beer's law plot. Unknown specimens can then be read in the spectrophotometer and, by use of their absorbance values, their concentrations determined from the calibration curve. Standard solutions are also discussed in Chapter 8.

### The Nature of Light

To understand the use of absorbance spectrophotometry (and photometry in general), one must first understand the fundamentals of color. To understand color, one must also understand the nature of light and its effect on color as we see it. Light is a type of radiant energy, and it travels in the form of waves. The distance between waves is the **wavelength of light**. The term light is used to describe radiant energy with wavelengths visible to the human eye or with wavelengths bordering on those visible to the human eye. The human eye responds to radiant energy, or light, with wavelengths between about 380 and 750 nm. A nanometer is $1 \times 10^{-9}$ m. With modern photometric apparatus, shorter (ultraviolet) or longer (infrared) wavelengths can be measured.

The wavelength of light determines the color of the light seen by the human eye. Every color that is seen is light of a particular wavelength. A combination, or mixture, of light energy of different wavelengths is known as daylight, or white light. When light is passed through a filter, a prism, or a diffraction grating, it can be broken into a spectrum of visible colors ranging from violet to red. The **visible spectrum** consists of the following range of colors: violet, blue, green, yellow, orange, and red. If white light is diffracted or partially absorbed by a filter or a prism, it becomes visible as certain colors. The different portions of the spectrum may be identified by wavelengths ranging from 380 to 750 nm for the visible colors. Wavelengths below approximately 380 nm are ultraviolet, and those above 750 nm are infrared; these light waves are not visible to the human eye. To compare and contrast the colors of the visible spectrum in terms of their respective wavelengths, see Table 6-1.

The color of light seen in the visible spectrum depends on the wavelength that is not absorbed. When light is not absorbed, it is transmitted. A colored solution has color because of its physical properties, which result in its absorbing certain wavelengths and transmitting others. When white light is passed through a solution, part of the light is absorbed and that remaining is transmitted light. A rainbow is seen when there are droplets of moisture in the air that refract or filter certain rays of the sun and allow others to pass through. The colors of the rainbow range from red to violet—the visible spectrum.

### Absorbance and Transmittance of Light: Beer's Law

Many solutions contain particles that absorb certain wavelengths and transmit others. Solutions appear to the human eye to have characteristic colors. The wavelength of light transmitted by the solution is recognized as color by the eye. See Table 6-1 for the visible colors of the spectrum and their respective approximate wavelength ranges.[1] A blue solution appears blue because particles in the solution absorb all the wavelengths except blue; the blue is the color transmitted and seen. A red solution appears red because all other wavelengths except red have been absorbed by the solution, while the red wavelength passes through.

Measurement by spectrophotometry is based on the reaction between the substance to be measured and a reagent, or chemical, used to

### TABLE 6-1

Observed Colors of the Visible Spectrum and Their Corresponding Wavelengths[1]

| Approximate Wavelength (in nm) | Color Observed |
| --- | --- |
| <380 | Not visible (ultraviolet light) |
| 380-440 | Violet |
| 440-500 | Blue |
| 500-580 | Green |
| 580-600 | Yellow |
| 600-620 | Orange |
| 620-750 | Red |
| >750 | Not visible (infrared light) |

produce color. The amount of color produced in a reaction between the substance to be measured and the reagent depends on the concentration of the substance. Therefore, the intensity of the color is proportional to the concentration of the substance. **Beer's law** states this relationship: color intensity at a constant depth is directly proportional to concentration. Beer's law is the basis for the use of photometry in quantitative measurement. If one saw a solution with a very intense red color, one would be correct in assuming that the solution had a high concentration of the substance that made it red. Another way of stating Beer's law is that any increase in the concentration of a color-producing substance will increase the amount of color seen.

As the law states, the depth at which the color is determined must be constant. The depth of the solution is regulated by the **cuvette** or container used to hold it. Increasing the depth of the solution through which the light must pass (by using a cuvette with a larger diameter) is the same as placing more particles between the light and the eye, thereby creating an apparent increase in the concentration, or intensity, of color. To avoid this alteration of the actual concentration, only cuvettes with a constant diameter can

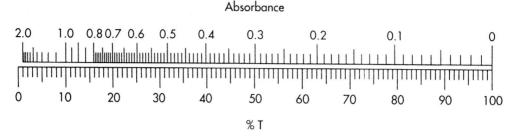

**FIG 6-1.** Viewing scales showing divisions for reading percent transmittance versus absorbance. Absorbance is the measure of light stopped or absorbed. Percent transmittance is the measure of light transmitted through the solution. (From Campbell JB, Campbell JM: *Laboratory Mathematics: Medical and Biological Applications,* ed 5. St Louis, Mosby, 1997, p. 211.)

be used—or a flow-through apparatus, which eliminates the use of cuvettes.

### Expressions of Light Transmitted or Absorbed

There are two common methods of expressing the amount of **light transmitted** or **light absorbed** by a solution. The units used to express the readings obtained by the electronic measuring device (see under Parts Essential to All Spectrophotometers) are either **absorbance (A) units** or **percent transmittance (%T) units**. Another term for absorbed light is **optical density (OD)**; this term is generally not used. Most spectrophotometers give the readings in both units. Absorbance units are sometimes more difficult to read directly from the reading scale because it is divided logarithmically rather than in equal divisions (Fig. 6-1). **Absorbance** is an expression of the amount of light absorbed by a solution. Absorbance values are directly proportional to the concentration of the solution, and therefore they may be plotted on **linear graph paper** to give a straight line (Fig. 6-2, *A*). Most spectrophotometers also give the percent transmittance readings on the viewing scale. **Percent transmittance** is the amount of light that passes through a colored solution compared with the amount of light that passes through a blank or standard solution. The blank solution contains all the reagents used in the procedure, but it does not contain the unknown substance being measured (see also under Ensuring Reliable Results: The Quality Control Program, in Chapter 8). Standard solutions will be discussed later in this chapter. Percent transmittance varies from 0 to 100 (it is usually abbreviated %T), with equal divisions on the viewing scale (see Fig. 6-1). As the concentration of the colored solution increases, the amount of light absorbed increases and the percentage of the light transmitted decreases. The transmitted light does not decrease in direct proportion to the concentration or color intensity of the solution being measured. Percent transmittance readings plotted against concentration will not give a straight line on linear graph paper (see Fig. 6-2, *B*). There is a logarithmic relationship between percent transmittance and concentration, so when percent transmittance is plotted against concentration, **semilogarithmic graph paper** is used to obtain a straight line (Fig. 6-3). Absorbance and percent transmittance are related in the following way:

Absorbance = 2 minus the logarithm of the percent transmittance

or

$$A = 2 - \log \%T$$

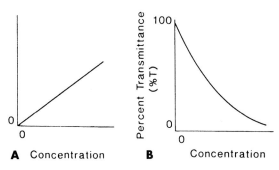

**FIG 6-2.** Relationships of absorbance **(A)** and percent transmittance **(B)** to concentration when plotted using linear graph paper. (From Kaplan LA, Pesce AJ: *Clinical Chemistry: Theory, Analysis, and Correlation*, ed 3. St Louis, Mosby, 1996, p 88.)

Therefore, 2 is the logarithm of 100%T. It is possible to obtain a convenient conversion table for transmittance and absorbance from a standard chemistry reference textbook.

## Preparation of a Standard Curve (Standardizing a Procedure)

The use of standard curves in today's clinical laboratory has declined with the advent of computerized instrumentation, which includes the steps formerly done with graph paper to calculate the relationship between any spectrophotometer readings for the standards and those for the unknowns. It is nevertheless important to understand how standard curves are constructed and used.

For each analytic method utilizing photometry, specific standard solutions must be prepared and used in the procedure. **Standard solutions** of varying concentrations are prepared using high levels of accuracy in their preparation (high-grade chemicals, analytical weighing, and volumetric dilution). Once a series of standard tubes have been read in the spectrophotometer, the galvanometer readings and standard concentrations are plotted on graph paper. The readings for the unknown solutions are then compared with those of the standard solution by use of the **standard curve**. The preparation of a standard curve is also an important component

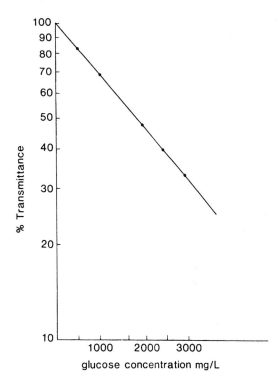

**FIG 6-3.** Use of semilogarithmic graph paper showing percent transmittance plotted against concentration. (From Kaplan LA, Pesce AJ: *Clinical Chemistry: Theory, Analysis, and Correlation*, ed 3. St Louis, Mosby, 1996, p 42.)

of examining laboratory data for validity. It can indicate abnormalities or variations in the analytic systems being used by the laboratory (see also Ensuring Reliable Results: The Quality Control Program, in Chapter 8).

### Types of Graph Paper

**Linear graph paper** can be used to plot absorbance readings, since absorbance of wavelengths of light is directly proportional to the concentration of the colored solution being read. **Semilogarithmic graph paper** is used to plot percent transmittance readings from the photometer, since there is a logarithmic relationship between percent and concentration, as described. The horizontal axis of semilogarithmic graph paper is a linear scale, and the vertical axis is a logarithmic scale (Fig. 6-3). The concentrations of the standard solutions being used are plotted on the horizontal axis. The transmittance or absorbance readings from the photometer are plotted along the vertical axis. When percent transmittance readings are used, these can be plotted directly on the logarithmic scale of the semilogarithmic graph paper (the horizontal axis), as the concentration is proportional to the logarithm of the galvanometer reading. In this way, percent transmittance readings are converted to the appropriate numbers on the logarithmic scale. Using semilogarithmic graph paper is simple and convenient for most laboratory purposes. When percentages are plotted against concentrations on semilogarithmic graph paper, the proportional relationship is direct, and the necessary straight-line graph is obtained when the individual standard points are connected.

The criteria for a good standard curve are that the line is straight, that the line connects all points, and that the line goes through the origin, or intersect, of the two axes. The origin of the graph paper is the point on the vertical and horizontal axes where there is 100%T and zero concentration (see Fig. 6-3).

Another type of graph paper, called linear graph paper, is available for plotting standard curves. This graph paper has linear scales on both the horizontal and vertical axes. If linear graph paper is used to construct a standard curve and only percent transmittance readings are available, these readings must first be converted to logarithmic values and the logarithmic values plotted on the vertical axis. Absorbance units can be plotted directly against the concentration on the linear graph paper to obtain a straight-line graph (Beer's law is followed). To eliminate the conversion of percent transmittance to absorbance in order to obtain the necessary straight-line graph, the use of semilogarithmic graph paper is suggested.

### Plotting a Standard Curve

When points are plotted on graph paper, whether they represent concentrations or galvanometer readings, care must be taken to

note the intervals on the graph paper. Many errors result from carelessness in the initial plotting of points on the graph paper. When a standard curve is prepared, the axes must also be properly labeled, as well as other information labeling or defining the graph specifics (see Fig. 6-4).

### Using a Standard Curve

Once the standard curve has been plotted, it is used to calculate the concentrations of any unknowns that were included in the same batch as the standards used to make the graph. To find the concentration of a solution, there must be some way of comparing it with a solution of known concentration.

A simplified example of the construction and use of a standard curve is given in Figure 6-4. In

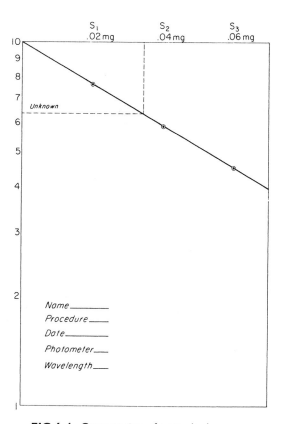

**FIG 6-4.** Construction of a standard curve.

the example shown, three standard solutions are prepared with the following concentrations: standard 1 (S1), 0.02 mg; standard 2 (S2), 0.04 mg; and standard 3 (S3), 0.06 mg. These concentrations are plotted on the linear, horizontal, scale of the semi-logarithmic graph paper. The three standard tubes are read in a photometer, giving the following readings in percent transmittance: S1, $76^2$; $S^2$, $58^3$, and S3, $45^1$%T. The percent transmittance readings are plotted under their respective concentrations on the logarithmic, vertical, scale of the paper. The points are connected, using a ruler. An undetermined substance gives a reading of $63^2$%T. Using the graph in Figure 6-4, the $63^2$%T point on the vertical scale is found, followed horizontally to the graph line just drawn, and then followed vertically to the concentration scale. The degree of accuracy with which an unknown concentration can be read depends on the concentrations of the standards used. The accuracy of the unknown can be no greater than the accuracy of the standard solutions used. Standard solutions are usually weighed to the fourth decimal place. In this example, if the graph lines were present, the unknown concentration would be read as 0.0343 mg (the figure in the fourth decimal place is approximate).

Using standard solutions to standardize the analyses of each batch, rather than relying on a permanently established calibration curve, allows the clinical laboratory to produce more reliable results. It compensates for variables such as time, temperature, the age of the reagents, and the condition of the instruments. It is always best to use several different concentrations of the standard solution, not just one. To obtain reliable photometric information about the concentration of a substance, standard solutions must be used as the basis for comparison.

## Instruments Used in Spectrophotometry

The instrument used to show the quantitative relationship between the colors of the undetermined solution and the standard solution is called a **spectrophotometer**, or **colorimeter**.

Most of the instruments used in photometry have some means of isolating a narrow wavelength, or range, of the color spectrum for mea-surements. Instruments using filters for this purpose are referred to as filter photometers, while those using prisms or gratings are called spectrophotometers or photoelectric colorimeters. Both types are used frequently in the clinical laboratory. In older colorimetric procedures, visual comparison of the color of an unknown with that of a standard was used. In general, visual colorimetry has been replaced by the more specific and accurate photoelectric methods.

One current application of visual colorimetry is employed in the various dry reagent strip tests, which are so prevalent in many clinical chemistry tests—dry reagent strip tests used in urinalysis, for example. These strips can be read visually, although instruments are also available to electronically read the color developed.

There are many types of spectrophotometers in common use in the clinical laboratory. The principle of most of these instruments is the same, in that the amount of light transmitted by the standard solution is compared with the amount of light transmitted by the solution of unknown concentration.

Precise, accurate methods are needed to accomplish the numerous determinations required in today's clinical laboratory. The spectrophotometer is one piece of equipment that is essential and can be considered to be of prime importance in quantitative analysis. Spectrophotometers are also known as photoelectric colorimeters or photometers. The many available spectrophotometers have their own technical variations, but all operate according to the same general principles. For teaching purposes, the Coleman Junior Spectrophotometer has proved to be very satisfactory (Fig. 6-5). In general, photometers employing filters are called filter photometers, and those with diffraction gratings are called spectrophotometers. Photometers utilize an electronic device to compare the actual color intensities of the solutions measured. As the name implies, a spectrophotometer is really two instruments in a single case: a spectrometer, a device for producing light of a

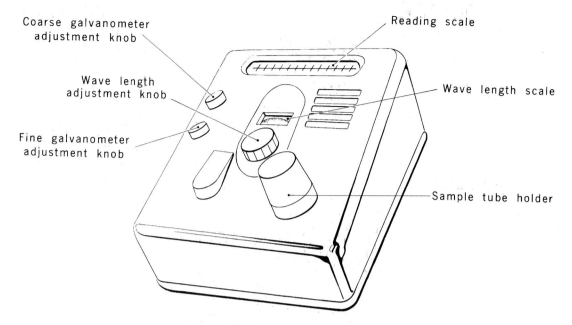

**FIG 6-5.** Coleman Junior Spectrophotometer.

specific wavelength, the monochromator; and a photometer, a device for measuring light intensity. Because of its common use, the operation of the Coleman Junior Spectrophotometer is described in Procedure 6-1. Any spectrophotometric instrument should be used only by following the manufacturer's instructions.

In the automated analyzing instruments used in many laboratories, a photometer is still a necessary component, so that absorbance values for unknown and standard solutions can be determined. Some instruments contain a filter wheel, which allows for the measurement of absorbance at any wavelength for which there is a filter on the wheel. Microprocessors control the location of the correct filter for the particular analyte being measured. From the absorbance information, the computer microprocessor calculates the unknown concentration.

### Parts Essential to All Spectrophotometers

There are parts necessary to all spectrophotometers (Fig 6-6). These are as follows:

1. *Light source.* Each spectrophotometer must have a light source. This can be a light bulb constructed to give the optimum amount of light. The light source must be steady and constant; therefore, use of a voltage regulator or an electronic power supply is recommended. The light source may be movable or stationary.

2. *Wavelength isolator.* Before the light from the light source reaches the sample of solution to be measured, the interfering wavelengths must be removed. A system of isolating a desired wavelength and excluding others is called a monochromator; the light is actually being reduced to a particular wavelength. Filters can be used to accomplish this. Some are very simple, composed of one or two pieces of colored glass. Some are more complicated. The more complicated filters are found in the better spectrophotometers. The filter must transmit a color that the solution can absorb. A red filter transmits red, and a green filter transmits green. Filters are available to cover almost any point in the visible spectrum, and each filter has inscribed on it a number that indicates the wavelength of light that it transmits.

## PROCEDURE 6-1

### Operation of the Coleman Junior Spectrophotometer

1. Mount the selected scale panel in the galvanometer viewing window. A general purpose scale panel is usually used. There are several types of scale panels available, depending on the use to which the spectrophotometer is to be put. The scale panel is calibrated both in percent transmittance and in absorbance (optical density).

2. Insert into the cuvette well the cuvette adapter of the proper size to accommodate the type of cuvette specified in the analytic procedure.

3. Turn on the switch located on the back of the instrument. Allow the instrument to warm up for 5 minutes.

4. Verify the galvanometer zero setting, and readjust if necessary. The indicator line on the galvanometer spot should register at zero on the percent transmittance scale. The zero adjustment level for this instrument is located under the raised housing just to the left of the cuvette well. If the spectrophotometer is not disturbed and its position is not altered, this galvanometer adjustment remains very stable.
   a. To check the zero position, darken the photoelectric cell by inserting into the cuvette well a cuvette adapter turned 90 degrees from the calibration marker. In this position, the body of the adapter completely blocks the pathway of light. A piece of opaque paper may also be slipped into the adapter well; in this way the light pathway is also completely stopped.
   b. Cover the well with the light shield or other suitable cover.
   c. With a pencil point move the galvanometer adjusting lever so that the indicator line on the galvanometer spot reads zero on the left zero index of the selected scale panel.
   d. Complete the adjustment by sliding the scale panel until the index is exactly at zero on the scale.

5. Adjust the wavelength control so that the specific wavelength is set. Different procedures will call for different wavelengths. The wavelength to be used will be specified in the procedure.

6. Cuvettes used for reading in the spectrophotometer must be free from scratches. Before the cuvette is placed in the adapter for reading, it must be free of finger marks and bubbles; the spectrophotometer does not recognize the cause of light impediment and will respond similarly to a scratched tube, lint, bubbles, finger marks, and the absorbance of the solution being examined. Therefore, wipe the cuvettes with a clean, dry, soft cloth or gauze before reading. All cuvettes must contain a certain volume of solution, called the minimum volume. Different sizes of cuvettes need different minimum volumes to ensure that the light passes through the solution rather than through the empty space in the tube.

7. Place the cuvette containing the reagent blank in the adapter first. For more information on the use of blank solutions, see Chapter 8. The calibration mark (or trademark, if precalibrated Coleman cuvettes are used) must face the light source to ensure constancy of the light path. Adjust the galvanometer control knobs (labeled *GALV Coarse* and *GALV Fine*) until the galvanometer index on the viewing scale reads 100%T for the "blank" tube.

8. Remove the blank tube.

*Continued*

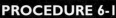

## PROCEDURE 6-1

### Operation of the Coleman Junior Spectrophotometer—cont'd

9. Place the next polished cuvette containing the solution to be read in the adapter well, again taking note of the calibration mark. Place this mark in a position facing the light source.

10. Record the galvanometer reading to the nearest ¼%T reading.

11. Remove the cuvette, and reinsert the blank tube.

12. Observe the reading for the blank tube on the galvanometer scale. It should still read 100%T. If it does, remove the blank tube and proceed with the next tube to be read. If the blank tube does not read exactly 100%T, adjust it to read 100%T with the GALV Coarse and GALV Fine knobs. Then read the next tube. The blank tube should be reinserted between all readings, and it should always read 100%T.

13. Read all tubes, and record results to the nearest ¼%T reading. Fractional parts (in fourths) of percent transmittance readings are recorded with the numerator figure only. For example, if a reading is 75½ (= 75²⁄₄), the result is recorded as 75²%T. For a reading of 75¾ the result is recorded as 75³, and for a reading of 75¼ the result is recorded as 75¹.

14. When finished, return the galvanometer index to the original position by turning both the *GALV Coarse* and *GALV Fine* knobs completely counterclockwise, and turn off the machine switch.

15. Clean up the area around the instrument, wipe up anything spilled on the machine, and cover the spectrophotometer with the protective cover provided. For cleaning cuvettes, see under Cleaning Laboratory Glassware and Plastic Ware, discussed previously in Chapter 4.

*From Operating Directions for the Coleman Model 6A and 6C Junior Spectrophotometer. Maywood, Ill, Coleman Instruments Corp, September 1966.*

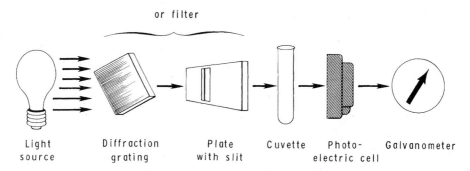

**FIG 6-6.** Parts essential to all spectrophotometers.

For example, a filter inscribed with 540 nm absorbs all light except that of wavelengths around 540 nm. Since the filter must transmit a color that the solution can absorb, for a red solution the filter chosen should not be red (all colors except red are absorbed). The wavelength of light transmitted is, then, the important thing to consider in choosing the correct filter for a procedure.

Light of a desired wavelength can also be provided by other means. One of the more commonly used instruments employs a diffraction grating with a special plate and slit to reduce the spectrum to the desired wavelength. The grating consists of a highly polished surface with numerous lines on it that break up white light into the spectrum. By moving the spectrum behind a slit (the light source must be movable), only one particular portion of the spectrum is allowed to pass through the narrow slit. The particular band of light, or wavelength, that is transmitted through the slit is indicated on a viewing scale on the machine. Certain wavelengths are more desirable than others for a particular color and procedure. The wavelength chosen is determined by running an absorption curve and selecting the correct wavelength after inspecting the curve obtained. Only when new methods are being developed is it necessary to run an absorption curve.

3. *Cuvettes, absorption cells, or photometer tubes.* Any light (of the wavelength selected) coming from the filter or diffraction grating will next pass on to the solution in the cuvette. Glass cuvettes are relatively inexpensive and are satisfactory, provided they are matched or calibrated. **Calibrated cuvettes** are tubes that have been optically matched so that the same solution in each will give the same reading on the photometer. In using calibrated cuvettes, the depth factor of Beer's law is kept constant. Depending on the concentration and thus the color of the solution, a certain amount of light will be absorbed by the solution and the remainder will be transmitted. The light not absorbed by the solution is transmitted. This light next passes on to an electronic measuring device of some type.

Alternatively, to eliminate the cuvette entirely, a flow-through apparatus can be used.

4. *Electronic measuring device.* In the more common spectrophotometers, the electronic measuring device consists of a photoelectric cell and a galvanometer. The amount of light transmitted by the solution in the cuvette is measured by a **photoelectric cell**. This cell is a most sensitive instrument, producing electrons in proportion to the amount of light hitting it. The electrons are passed on to a **galvanometer**, where they are measured. The galvanometer records the amount of current (in the form of electrons) that it receives from the photoelectric cell on a special viewing scale on the spectrophotometer (see Fig. 6-1). The results are reported in terms of percent transmittance. In some cases, the readings are made in terms of absorbance. The percent transmittance is dependent on the concentration of the solution and its depth. If the solution is very concentrated (the color appearing intense), less light will be transmitted than if it is dilute (pale). Therefore, the reading on the galvanometer viewing scale will be lower for a more concentrated solution than for a dilute solution. This is the basis for the comparison of color intensity with the spectrophotometer.

### Flow-Through Adaptation

A special adaptation available for Coleman Junior Spectrophotometers is called a Coleman Vacuvette Cell Assembly. This is designed to increase the speed with which samples can be introduced into and discharged from the photometer. Another name for an assembly of this kind is a flow-through apparatus. Instead of separate cuvettes being used for each sample read in the photometer, the sample is poured directly into a specially designed cuvette incorporating a funnel for easy pouring. The sample is read in the same way as in the regular cuvette method and is then evacuated from the photometer by means of a capillary tubing attached to a discard bottle. When a suitable vacuum system is attached to the cuvette-capillary tubing assembly, rapid and automatic discarding of the sample is possible. This assembly apparatus must be periodically cleaned to maintain its proper operation. A flow-through apparatus can be used for reading samples when the sample can be discarded. It cannot be used to read multiple values on the same sample because the sample is lost once it is poured into the special cuvette. The Coleman Instruments Corporation manufactures this specially designed cuvette in various sizes so that varying amounts of sample may be read in the photometer. This device is another example of how many laboratory functions have been made more efficient so that time can be saved and results can be obtained and reported more quickly.

### Care and Handling of Spectrophotometers

In the use of a spectrophotometer, error caused by color in the reagents used must be eliminated. Since color is so important and since the color produced by the undetermined substance is the desired one, any color resulting from the reagents themselves or from interactions between the reagents could cause confusion and error. By use of a blank solution, a correction can be made for any color resulting from the reagents used. The blank solution contains the same reagents as the unknown and standard tubes, with the exception of the substance being measured. The use of blank solutions is discussed further in Chapter 8.

A spectrophotometer, as is the case with any expensive, delicate instrument, must be handled with care. The manufacturer supplies a manual of complete instructions on the care and use of a particular machine. Care should be taken not to spill reagents on the spectrophotometer. Spillage could damage the delicate instrument, especially the photoelectric cell. Any reagents spilled must be wiped up immediately. Spectrophotometers with filters should not be operated without the filter in place, since the unfiltered light from the light source may damage the photoelectric cell and the galvanometer. A spectrophotometer should be placed on a table with good support, where it will not be bumped or jarred.

### Tests of Quality Control for Spectrophotometers

The spectrophotometer must be tested periodically to ensure that it is functioning properly. Wavelength calibration can be checked by use of a rare-earth glass filter such as didymium. The wavelength calibration can also be checked by use of a stable chromogen solution. Calibration at two wavelengths is necessary for instruments with diffraction gratings and at three wavelengths for instruments with prisms.

Photoelectric accuracy can be checked by reading standard solutions of potassium dichromate or potassium nitrate. As an alternative, the National Bureau of Standards (NBS) has sets of three neutral-density glass filters that have known absorbance at four wavelengths for each filter. These filters are not completely stable, however, and require periodic recalibration.

### Calibration of Cuvettes for the Spectrophotometer

If cuvettes are used, it is essential that their diameters be uniform; that is, it is necessary that the depth of the cuvettes or tubes used in the spectrophotometer be constant for Beer's law to apply. Cuvettes for the spectrophotometer can be purchased precalibrated. Precalibrated cuvettes must be checked before being put into actual use in the laboratory. Calibrated cuvettes are optically matched so that the same solution in each will give the same percent transmittance reading on the galvanometer viewing scale.

In checking cuvettes for use in spectrophotometry, the cuvette is carefully observed to see that the solution in it gives the same reading in that cuvette as it did in other calibrated cuvettes. To check cuvettes for uniformity, the same solution, such as a stable solution of copper sulfate or cyanmethemoglobin, is read in many cuvettes. Readings are taken, and cuvettes that match within an established tolerance are used.

If new plain glass tubes are being calibrated to be used as cuvettes, since all tubes may not be perfectly round, the tubes are rotated in the cuvette well to observe any changes in reading with the position in the well. The cuvette is etched at the point where the reading corresponds with the established tolerance for the absorption reading. Cuvettes that do not agree or do not correspond are not used for spectrophotometry.

Different sizes of cuvettes can be used, depending on the spectrophotometer. The Coleman Junior Spectrophotometer can be adapted to use several different sizes cuvettes in the same machine. For each size, a special cuvette adapter is used, enabling the cuvette to fit securely in the cuvette holder. Only when the cuvette fits securely will the readings obtained be precise and accurate.

## REFLECTANCE SPECTROPHOTOMETRY

Reflectance spectrophotometry is another quantitative spectrophotometric technique; the light reflected from the surface of a colorimetric reaction is used to measure the amount of unknown colored product generated in the reaction. A beam of light is directed at a flat surface, and the amount of light reflected is measured. A photodetector measures the amount of reflected light directed to it. This technology has been employed in many of the handheld instruments for bedside testing and smaller instruments used in physicians' offices and clinics.

### Principle of Technology Employed in Reflectance Spectrophotometry

Different surfaces have different optical properties. The optical properties of plastic strips or test paper are different from those of dry film. To use a reflectance spectrophotometer, the system must use a standard with the same specific surface optical properties as the specific surface used in the test system. The use of reflectance spectrophotometry provides the quantitative measurement of reactions on surfaces such as strips, cartridges, and dry film.

The amount of light reflected and then measured depends on the specific instrumentation

employed. Variables are: angles at which the reflected light is measured and the area of the surface being used for the measurement. Since employment of this technology depends on the use of products manufactured for use in the specific instrumentation, manufacturing processes (quality-control considerations) or shipping and handling or storage problems can affect the resulting measurements.

Quality control for single test instruments—using instrument-based systems—has been integrated into the instruments by the manufacturers. As long as the reagent packs or tabs have been properly stored and are used within the stated outdate, the manufacturer assures the user that calibration of the instrument will function automatically, crucial quality-control information has been encoded via the bar code on the unit packs, and real-time processing is monitored. Use of the usual quality-control measures in place for the laboratory can be problematic for this technology, because when the single-test, instrument-based systems are used, each time a new cartridge, pack, or strip is inserted into the instrument, a new test system is created.

### Parts of a Reflectance Spectrophotometer

The instrumentation necessary for a reflectance spectrophotometer is similar to that of a filter photometer, in which the filter serves to direct the selected wavelength for the methodology. A lamp generates light, which passes through the filter and a series of slits and is focused on the test surface (Fig. 6-7). As in the case of a filter photometer, some light is absorbed by the filter; in the reflectance spectrophotometer, the remaining light is reflected. The light that is reflected is analogous to the light transmitted by the filter spectrophotometer. The reflected light passes next through a series of slits and lenses and on to the photodetector device, where the amount of light is measured and recorded as a signal. The signal is then converted to an appropriate readout.

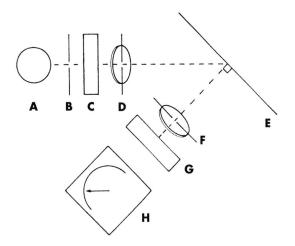

**FIG. 6-7.** Diagram of reflectance spectrophotometer. **A,** Light source; **B,** slit; **C,** filter or wavelength selector; **D,** lens or slit; **E,** test surface; **F,** lens or slit; **G,** detector/photodetector device; **H,** readout device. (From Kaplan LA, Pesce AJ: *Clinical Chemistry: Theory, Analysis, and Correlation,* ed 3. St Louis, Mosby, 1996, p 94.)

## Instruments Used in Reflectance Spectrophotometry

A major use for reflectance spectrophotometry is for the many instruments now available for point-of-care testing (POCT), including analyzers used in physicians' offices and clinics. Common bedside testing and self-testing instruments used for quantitation of blood glucose (employing a single-test methodology) for maintaining good diabetic control are one example. Chemistry and therapeutic drug monitoring analyzer systems also employ this technology, an example being the Reflotron,* for which reagents have been integrated into disposable unit-dose devices. The Reflotron system uses dry reagent tabs containing a magnetic code to identify the tests, reaction parameters, and calibration curve for each assay done. These reagent tabs have a long shelf-life—up to two years in some cases. In this system, blood is placed on a glass-fiber pad, the plasma is separated from the red cells and the plasma transported away from the red cells by capillary action, the required plasma sample volume is added to the reagent at a temperature of 37° C, excess plasma is removed, and the concentration of the desired analyte is determined by reflectance spectrophotometry. The Reflotron system is a single-test system, and blood used for it can be obtained by capillary puncture of the finger or heel. The ability to perform quantitative analyses on only a few microliters of whole blood is a significant benefit of the use of this technology.

In urinalysis testing, the Clinitek Atlas* uses dry reagent reflectance spectrophotometry technology.

## FLAME EMISSION PHOTOMETRY

### Use and Principle of Flame Emission Photometry

**Flame emission photometry** is used most commonly for the quantitative measurement of lithium, sodium, and potassium in body fluids. In flame emission analysis by emission photometry, a solution containing metal ions is sprayed into a flame. The metal ions are energized to emit light of a characteristic color. Atoms of many metallic elements, when given sufficient energy (such as that supplied by a hot flame), will emit this energy at wavelengths characteristic of the elements. Lithium produces a red, sodium a yellow, potassium a violet, and magnesium a blue color in a flame. Sodium and potassium are the metal ions most commonly measured in biological specimens, but lithium, which is not normally present in serum, may also be measured in connection with the use of lithium salts in the treatment of some psychiatric disorders. The intensity of the color is proportional to the amount of the element burned in the flame. **Flame photometers** are laboratory instruments that make use of this principle. Details of the operation of a specific flame photometer should be obtained from the manufac-

---

*Boehringer Mannheim Diagnostics, Indianapolis, Ind.

*Bayer Corp, Diagnostic Division, Tarrytown, NY.

FILTER AND PLATES WITH SLITS

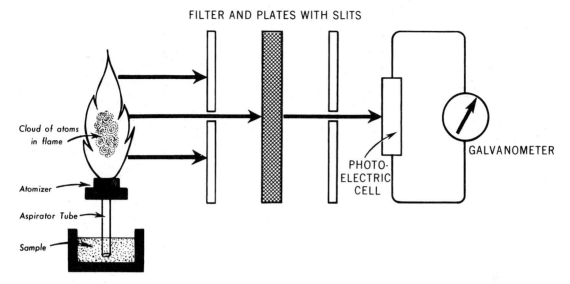

**FIG 6-8.** Essential parts of a flame emission photometer.

turer, but a few general principles and components are common to most instruments.

## Essential Parts of Flame Photometer

An atomizer is needed to spray the sample as fine droplets into the flame. Another name for atomizer is nebulizer (Fig. 6-8). The atomizer creates a fine spray of the sample and feeds this spray into a burner. The fine spray is produced by combining a stream of sample with a stream of air. A total-consumption burner feeds the entire sample directly into the flame. A premix atomizer mixes the fuel gases and the sample in a mixing chamber before sending this mixture to the flame. Both types of atomizers are available.

In most flame photometers the fuel usually consists of various combinations of acetylene, propane, oxygen, natural gas, and compressed air. The combinations and types of fuel used determine the temperature of the flame. For sodium and potassium determinations, a propane–compressed air flame appears entirely adequate. The atomizer and the flame are critical components of a flame photometer. The most important variable in the flame itself is the temperature, since the energy emitted by the metal

ions is measured and the number of energized metal ions is dependent on the temperature of the flame. Frequent standardization of flame photometers is essential, because thermal changes occur and affect the operation of the instrument and subsequent measurements with it.

Flame photometers must also have a filter, prism, grating, or other device for selecting light of the appropriate wavelength for the element to be measured. These devices spread or disperse the light into its spectral components. The desired wavelength is selected by means of a narrow slit. In this respect the flame photometer is similar to the spectrophotometer. However, the light source described for the spectrophotometer has been replaced with an atomizer-flame combination in the flame photometer. The flame photometer must also have an electronic measuring device to detect the intensity of the emitted light. Photocells or photo tubes are used to detect the light intensity by converting the light into an electrical current. The amount of current generated is proportional to the quantity of light that reaches the detector. The amount of current is measured by a galvanometer or other recording device (see under Absorbance Spectrophotometry).

## Types of Flame Photometers

An example of a flame photometer that operates according to an absolute or direct principle is one in which the intensity of color is proportional to the amount of the element burned in the flame. When an unknown sample is being measured, its intensity of color is compared with that of a standard solution of the element being measured. For example, a standard solution of potassium is used for measuring potassium.

In another commonly used method of flame photometry, the principle of the **internal standard** is applied. Most currently used flame photometers employ an internal standard. In this method, another element, usually lithium, is added to all solutions analyzed—blanks, standards, and unknowns. Lithium is usually absent from biological fluids, and it has a high emission intensity. It also emits at a wavelength sufficiently distant from that of potassium or sodium to permit spectral isolation. In flame photometry using the internal standard principle, the emission of the unknown element (sodium or potassium) is compared with that of the reference element lithium. By measuring the ratios of the emissions, any change in gas or air pressure, line voltage, flame temperature, rate of atomization, or other small variable will be minimized because both the unknown element and the reference element are affected simultaneously. A specially designed adaptation of the machine is used for this purpose, and the ratio of the reference lithium and unknown metal emissions is measured by two detectors. Two filter systems are set up, one for the unknown and one for the lithium reference. Lithium does not function as a "true" standard in its use as a reference solution. Therefore, various known concentrations of potassium or sodium are prepared and used to establish calibration curves. The use of lithium as the reference solution can cause problems, however, because lithium salts are given to patients being treated for manic-depressive states. In these patients, the lithium level must be measured.

## REFERENCES

1. Burtis CA, Ashwood ER (eds): *Tietz Fundamentals of Clinical Chemistry*, ed 4. Philadelphia, WB Saunders Co, 1996, p 55.

## BIBLIOGRAPHY

Campbell JB, Campbell JM: *Laboratory Mathematics: Medical and Biological Applications*, ed 5, St Louis, Mosby, 1997.

Henry JB (ed): *Clinical Diagnosis and Management by Laboratory Methods*, ed 19. Philadelphia, WB Saunders Co, 1996.

Kaplan LA, Pesce AJ: *Clinical Chemistry: Theory, Analysis, and Correlation*, ed 3. St Louis, Mosby, 1996.

## STUDY QUESTIONS

1. A. Complete the following: In a colored solution, the intensity of the color at a constant depth is directly proportional to the _____ of the substance present.
   B. What is this principle called?

2. What is the approximate range of wavelengths of light that is visible to the human eye?

3. For a substance to be measured by photometry, what physical capability must be present in the substance?

4. What determines the color of light seen by the human eye?

5. If a solution appears green in absorbance spectrophotometry, which colors are being absorbed and which are being transmitted?

6. **Match each of the following photometry instruments (1 to 3) with its most general use (A to C):**

   1. Absorbance spectrophotometer
   2. Flame photometer
   3. Reflectance spectrophotometer

   _____ A. To measure the concentration of sodium or potassium in a body fluid or serum

   _____ B. To measure the concentration of glucose in blood by using dry film technology

   _____ C. To measure the concentration of hemoglobin in a solution

7. **Match each of the following ways of plotting the concentration of a substance (1 and 2) with the type of graph paper used to obtain a straight line on the graph (A and B):**

   1. Concentration plotted against percent transmittance
   2. Concentration plotted against absorbance

   _____ A. Linear graph paper; plot is a linear relationship

   _____ B. Semilogarithmic graph paper; plot is not a linear relationship

8. **List two or three uses for reflectance spectrophotometric technology.**

# CHAPTER 7

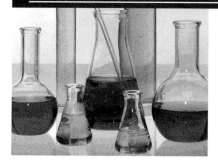

# Laboratory Mathematics

## Learning Objectives

*From study of this chapter, the reader will be able to:*

➤ Use proportions and ratios.
➤ Know the rules for rounding off numbers and for the use of significant figures.
➤ Use exponents.
➤ Describe the procedures for making a single dilution and a serial dilution.
➤ Calculate the amount of one solution needed to make a solution of a lesser concentration from it.
➤ Differentiate the expressions of solution concentration weight per unit weight, weight per unit volume, and volume per unit volume.
➤ Know how to prepare a percent solution.
➤ Describe the differences between molar and normal solutions and be able to calculate how to prepare solutions of a given volume and normality or molarity.

## IMPORTANCE OF LABORATORY CALCULATIONS

With the advent of computerized instrumentation in many laboratories, the formerly repetitious calculations that were necessary are now done via the computer interfaced with the analytic instrument. It remains important for the persons using these instruments, however, to know the way mathematics is applied to obtain the results achieved. It is important for any person involved in doing clinical laboratory analyses to understand not only how the necessary calculations are done but also why the mathematical concepts work as they do. The principles on which a particular formula is based must be understood and not only the formula itself. If principles are understood thoroughly, modifications can be made, when necessary.

A sound background in basic mathematics (including algebra), an understanding of the units in which quantities are expressed, and a knowledge of the methods of analysis are all necessary in performing laboratory calculations. There are no simple formulas for solving all such problems, but certain fundamentals are a part of many of the problems encountered in a clinical laboratory.

## PROPORTIONS AND RATIOS

The use of proportions involves a commonsense approach to problem solving. **Proportions** are used to determine a quantity from a given ratio. A **ratio** is an amount of something compared to an amount of something else.

Ratios always describe a relative amount, and at least two values are always involved. For example, 5 g of something dissolved in 100 mL of something else can be expressed by the ratio 5/100, 5:100, or 5 ÷ 100, or by the decimal 0.05. Proportion is a means of saying that two ratios are equal. Thus, the ratio 5:100 is equal, or proportional to, the ratio 1/20. This proportion can be expressed as 5:100 = 1:20. In the laboratory, proportions and ratios are useful when it is necessary to make more (or less) of the same thing.

However, ratios and proportions can be used only when the concentration (or any other kind of relationship) does not change.

The following is an example of a proportion or ratio problem: A formula calls for 5 g of sodium chloride (NaCl) in 1000 mL of solution. If only 500 mL of solution is needed, how much NaCl is required?

$$\frac{5\ g}{1{,}000\ mL} = \frac{x\ g}{500\ mL}$$

$$x = \frac{5\ g \times 500\ mL}{1{,}000\ mL}$$

$$x = 2.5\ g\ NaCl$$

In setting up ratio and proportion problems, the two ratios being compared must be written in the same order and they must be in the same units.

When specimens are diluted in the various laboratory analyses, the ratio principle is applied. This use of dilutions is described later in this section.

### Relating Concentrations of Solutions

To relate different concentrations of solutions that contain the same amount of substance (or solute), a basic relationship, or ratio, is used. The volume of one solution ($V_1$) times the concentration of that solution ($C_1$) equals the volume of the second solution ($V_2$) times the concentration of the second solution ($C_2$), or:

$$V_1 \times C_1 = V_2 \times C_2$$

If any three of the values are known, the fourth may be determined. This relationship shows that when a solution is diluted, the volume is increased as the concentration is decreased. However, the total amount of substance (or solute) remains unchanged. Several applications of this relationship are used in the clinical laboratory, some of them being in titrations (see under Titration in Chapter 4), in dilution of specimens, and in the preparation of weaker solutions from stronger solutions.

An example of making a less concentrated solution from one more concentrated is as follows: A sodium hydroxide (NaOH) solution is available that has a concentration of 10 g of NaOH per deciliter (dL) of solution (1 dL = 100 mL). To calculate the volume of the 10 g/dL NaOH solution required to prepare 1,000 mL of 2 g/dL NaOH:

$$V_1 \times C_1 = V_2 \times C_2$$
$$x \text{ mL} \times 10 \text{ g/dL} = 1,000 \text{ mL} \times 2 \text{ g/dL}$$
$$x = \frac{2 \text{ g/dL} \times 1,000 \text{ mL}}{10 \text{ g/dL}} = 200 \text{ mL}$$

Note that this relationship is not a direct proportion; instead, it is an inverse proportion. As this is a proportion problem, it is important to remember that the concentrations and volumes on both sides of the equation must be expressed in the same units.

## DILUTIONS

It is often necessary **to make dilutions** of specimens being analyzed or to make weaker solutions from stronger solutions in various laboratory procedures. It is therefore necessary to be capable of working with various dilution problems and **dilution factors.** In these problems one must often be able to determine the concentration of material in each solution, the actual amount of material in each solution, and the total volume of each solution. All dilutions are a kind of ratio. Dilution is an indication of relative concentration.

### Diluting Specimens

In most laboratory determinations, a small sample is taken for analysis, and the final result is expressed as concentration per some convenient standard volume. In a certain procedure, 0.5 mL of blood is diluted to a total of 10 mL with various reagents, and 1 mL of this dilution is then analyzed for a particular chemical constituent. The final result is to be expressed in terms of the concentration of that substance per 100 mL of blood.

### Dilution Factor

A dilution factor is used to correct for having used a diluted sample in a determination rather than the undiluted sample. The result (answer) using the dilution must be multiplied by the reciprocal of the dilution made.

For example, a dilution factor by which all determination answers are multiplied to give the concentration per 100 mL of sample (blood) may be calculated as follows:

First determine the volume of blood that is actually analyzed in the procedure. By use of a simple proportion, it is evident that 0.5 mL of blood diluted to 10 mL is equivalent to 1 mL of blood diluted to 20 mL.

$$\frac{0.5 \text{ mL blood}}{10 \text{ mL solution}} = \frac{1 \text{ mL blood}}{x \text{ mL solution}}$$
$$x = \frac{1 \text{ mL} \times 10 \text{ mL}}{0.5 \text{ mL}} = 20 \text{ mL}$$

In other words, there is a 1:20 dilution of blood in this procedure—that is, 1 mL of blood diluted to a total volume of 20 mL with the desired diluent (usually saline or deionized water) or reagents. This is the same as 1 mL of blood plus 19 mL of diluent.

The concentration of specimen (blood) in each milliliter of solution may be determined, by the use of another simple proportion, to be 0.05 mL of blood per milliliter of solution:

$$\frac{1 \text{ mL blood}}{20 \text{ mL solution}} = \frac{x \text{ mL blood}}{1 \text{ mL solution}}$$
$$x = \frac{1 \text{ mL} \times 1 \text{ mL}}{20 \text{ mL}} = 0.05 \text{ mL}$$

Since 1 mL of the 1:20 dilution of blood is analyzed in the remaining steps of the procedure, 0.05 mL of blood is actually analyzed (1 mL of the dilution used × 0.05 mL/mL = 0.05 mL of blood analyzed).

To relate the concentration of the substance measured in the procedure to the concentration in 100 mL of blood (the units in which the result is to be expressed), another proportion may be used:

$$\frac{100\ mL\ (volume\ of\ blood\ desired)}{0.05\ mL\ (volume\ of\ blood\ used)} =$$

$$\frac{Concentration\ desired}{Concentration\ used\ or\ determined}$$

Concentration desired =

$$\frac{100\ mL \times Concentration\ determined}{0.05\ mL}$$

Concentration desired = 2,000 × Value determined

In other words, the concentration of the substance being measured in the volume of blood actually tested (0.05 mL) must be multiplied by 2,000 in order to report the concentration per 100 mL of blood.

The preceding material may be summarized by the following statement and equations. In reporting results obtained from laboratory determinations, one must first determine the amount of specimen actually analyzed in the procedure and then calculate the factor that will express the concentration in the desired terms of measurement. Thus, in the previous example the following equations may be used:

$$\frac{0.5\ mL\ (volume\ of\ blood\ used)}{10\ mL\ (volume\ of\ total\ dilution)} =$$

$$\frac{x\ mL\ (volume\ of\ blood\ analyzed)}{1\ mL\ (volume\ of\ dilution\ used)}$$

x = 0.05 mL (volume of blood actually analyzed)

$$\frac{100\ mL\ (volume\ of\ blood\ required\ for\ expression\ of\ result)}{0.05\ mL\ (volume\ of\ blood\ actually\ analyzed)}$$

$$= 2,000\ (dilution\ factor)$$

## Single Dilutions

When the concentration of a particular substance in a specimen is too great to be accurately determined, or when there is less specimen available for analysis than the procedure requires, it may be necessary to dilute the original specimen, or to further dilute the initial dilution (or filtrate). Such **single dilutions** are usually expressed as a ratio, such as 1:2, 1:5, or 1:10, or

as a fraction, ½, ⅕, or ⅒. These ratios or fractions refer to 1 unit of the original specimen diluted to a final volume of 2, 5, or 10 units, respectively. A **dilution** therefore refers to the volume or number of parts of the substance to be diluted in the total volume, or parts, of the final solution. A dilution is an expression of concentration; it indicates the relative amount of substance in solution—not an expression of volume. Dilutions can be made singly or in series.

To calculate the concentration of a single dilution, multiply the original concentration by the dilution expressed as a fraction.

### Calculation of the Concentration of a Single Dilution

A specimen contains 500 mg of substance per deciliter of blood. A 1:5 dilution of this specimen is prepared by volumetrically measuring 1 mL of the specimen and adding 4 mL of diluent (usually distilled water or saline). The concentration of substance in the dilution is:

$$500\ mg/dL \times \tfrac{1}{5} = 100\ mg/dL$$

Note that the concentration of the final solution (or dilution) is expressed in the same units as that of the original solution.

To obtain a dilution factor that can be applied to the determination answer in order to express it as a concentration per standard volume, proceed as follows. Rather than multiply by the dilution expressed as a fraction, multiply the determination value by the reciprocal of the dilution fraction. In the case of a 1:5 dilution, the dilution factor that would be applied to values obtained in the procedure would be 5, since the original specimen was five times more concentrated than the diluted specimen tested in the procedure.

### Use of Dilution Factors

A 1:5 dilution of a specimen is prepared, and an **aliquot** (one of a number of equal parts) of the dilution is analyzed for a particular substance. The concentration of the substance in the aliquot is multiplied by 5 to determine its concentration in the original specimen. If the concentration of the dilution is 100 mg/dL, the concentration of the original specimen is:

100 mg/dL × 5 (the dilution factor) = 500 mg/dL in blood

## Serial Dilutions

As mentioned previously, dilutions can be made singly or in series, in which case the original solution is further diluted. A general rule for calculating the concentrations of solutions obtained by dilution in series is to multiply the original concentration by the first dilution (expressed as a fraction), this by the second dilution, and so on until the desired concentration is known.

Several laboratory procedures, especially serologic ones, make use of a dilution series in which all dilutions, including or following the first one, are the same. Such dilutions are re-ferred to as **serial dilutions.** A complete dilution series usually contains five or ten tubes, although any single dilution may be made directly from an undiluted specimen or substance. In calculating the dilution or concentration of substance or serum in each tube of the dilution series, the rules previously discussed apply.

A five-tube twofold dilution may be prepared as follows (see Fig. 7-1): A serum specimen is diluted 1:2 with buffer. A series of five tubes are prepared, in which each succeeding tube is rediluted 1:2. This is accomplished by placing 1 mL of diluent into each of four tubes (tubes 2 to 5). Tube 1 contains 1 mL of undiluted serum. Tube 2 contains 1 mL of undiluted serum plus 1 mL of diluent, resulting in a 1:2 dilution of serum. A 1-mL portion of the 1:2 dilution of serum is placed in tube 3, resulting in a 1:4 dilution of serum ($\frac{1}{2} \times \frac{1}{2} = \frac{1}{4}$). A 1-mL portion of the 1:4 dilution from tube 3 is placed in tube 4, resulting in a 1:8 dilution ($\frac{1}{4} \times \frac{1}{2} = \frac{1}{8}$). Finally, 1 mL of

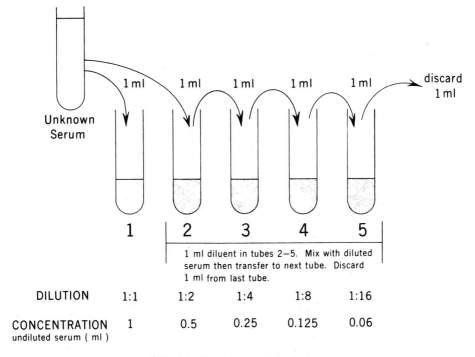

**FIG 7-1.** Five-tube twofold dilution.

the 1:8 dilution from tube 4 is added to tube 5, resulting in a 1:16 dilution ($\frac{1}{8} \times \frac{1}{2} = \frac{1}{16}$). One milliliter of the final dilution is discarded so that the volumes in all the tubes are equal. Note that each tube is diluted twice as much as the previous tube and that the final volume in each tube is the same. The undiluted serum may also be given a dilution value, namely 1:1.

The concentration of serum in terms of milliliters in each tube is calculated by multiplying the previous concentration (mL) by the succeeding dilution. In this example tube 1 contains 1 mL of serum, tube 2 contains 1 mL $\times \frac{1}{2} = 0.5$ mL of serum, and tubes 3 to 5 contain 0.25, 0.125, and 0.06 mL of serum, respectively.

Other serial dilutions might be fivefold or tenfold; that is, each succeeding tube is diluted five or ten times. A fivefold series would begin with 1 mL of serum in 4 mL of diluent and a total volume of 5 mL in each tube, while a tenfold series would begin with 1 mL of serum in 9 mL of diluent and a total volume of 10 mL in each tube. Other systems might begin with a 1:2 dilution and then dilute five succeeding tubes 1:10. The dilutions in such a series would be 1:2, 1:20 ($\frac{1}{2} \times \frac{1}{10} = \frac{1}{20}$), 1:200 ($\frac{1}{20} \times \frac{1}{10} = \frac{1}{200}$), 1:2,000, 1:20,000, and 1:200,000.

### Calculation of the Concentration After a Series of Dilutions

A working solution is prepared from a stock solution. In so doing, a stock solution with a concentration of 100 mg/dL is diluted 1:10 by volumetrically adding 1 mL of it to 9 mL of diluent. The diluted solution (intermediate solution) is further diluted 1:100 by volumetrically measuring 1 mL of intermediate solution and diluting to the mark in a 100-mL volumetric flask. The concentration of the final or working solution is:

$$100 \text{ mg/dL} \times \frac{1}{10} \times \frac{1}{100} = 0.1 \text{ mg/dL}$$

# SIGNIFICANT FIGURES

Using more digits than are necessary to calculate and report the results of a laboratory determina-

tion has several disadvantages. It is important that the number used contain only the digits necessary for the precision of the determination. Using more digits than necessary is misleading in that it ascribes more accuracy to the determination than is actually the case. There is also the danger of overlooking a decimal point and making an error in judging the magnitude of the answer. Digits in a number that are needed to express the precision of the measurement from which the number is derived are known as **significant figures.** A significant figure is one that is known to be reasonably reliable. Judgment must be exercised in determining how many figures should be used. Some rules to assist in making such decisions are as follows:

1. Use the known accuracy of the method to determine the number of digits that are significant in the answer, and, as a general rule, retain one more figure than this. An example is: A urea nitrogen result was reported as 11.2 mg/dL. This would indicate that the result is accurate to the nearest tenth and that the exact value lies between 11.15 and 11.25. In reality, the accuracy of most urea nitrogen methods is ±10%, so that the result reported as 11.2 mg/dL could actually vary from 10 to 12 mg/dL and should be reported as 11 mg/dL. In addition, if the decimal point were omitted or overlooked, the result could be taken as 112 mg/dL.

2. Take the accuracy of the least accurate measurement, or the measurement with the least number of significant figures, as the accuracy of the final result. In doing so, certain things must be done in the addition and subtraction or multiplication and division of numerals. An example of addition or subtraction is as follows: In order to add

$$\begin{array}{r} 206.1 \\ 7.56 \\ \underline{0.8764} \end{array}$$

rewrite it as

$$\begin{array}{r} 206.1 \\ 7.6 \\ \underline{0.9} \end{array}$$

In this example, the least accurate figure is accurate to one decimal place; this is therefore the determining factor. In determining the least accurate figure, the following rule is utilized: in a column of addition or subtraction, in which the decimal points are placed one above the other, the number of significant figures in the final answer is determined by the first digit encountered going from left to right that terminates any one numeral.

An example of multiplication or division is as follows: In the division of

$$32.973 \div 4.3 =$$

the result should be reported as 7.7. This is determined by utilizing the following general rule: the number of significant figures in the final product or quotient should not exceed the smallest number of significant figures in any one factor.

## Rounding Off Numbers

Test results sometimes produce insignificant digits. It is then necessary to **round off the numbers** to a chosen number of significant value in order not to imply an accuracy of precision greater than the test is capable of delivering.

The following general rule may be used in rounding off decimal values to the proper place: When the digit next to the last one to be retained is less than 5, the last digit should be left unchanged. When the digit next to the last one to be retained is greater than 5, the last digit is increased by 1. If the additional digit is 5, the last digit reported is changed to the nearest even number. Examples are as follows:

2.31463 g is rounded off to 2.3146 g.
5.34659 g is rounded off to 5.3466 g.
23.5 mg is rounded off to 24 mg.
24.5 mg is rounded off to 24 mg.

## EXPONENTS

**Exponents** are used to indicate that a number must be multiplied by itself as many times as is indicated by the exponent. The number that is to be multiplied by itself is called the base. Usually the exponent is written as a small superscript figure to the immediate right of the base figure and is sometimes referred to as the power of the base. The exponent figure can have either a plus sign or a minus sign before it. The plus sign is usually implied and does not actually appear.

A **positive exponent** indicates the number of times the base is to be multiplied by itself.

Examples of exponents with no sign or a plus sign (positive exponents) are as follows:

$$10^2 = 10 \times 10 = 100$$
$$10^5 = 10 \times 10 \times 10 \times 10 \times 10 = 100,000$$
$$5^3 = 5 \times 5 \times 5 = 125$$

A **negative exponent** indicates the number of times the reciprocal of the base is to be multiplied by itself—in other words, a negative exponent indicates a fraction.

Examples of exponents with a minus sign (negative exponents) are as follows:

$$10^{-1} = \frac{1}{10} = 0.1$$

$$10^{-4} = \frac{1}{10} \times \frac{1}{10} \times \frac{1}{10} \times \frac{1}{10} \times \frac{1}{10,000} = 0.0001$$

## EXPRESSIONS OF SOLUTION CONCENTRATION

Solutions are made up of a mixture of substances. In making up a solution, there usually are two main parts, the substance that is being dissolved (the **solute**) and the substance into which the solute is being dissolved (the **solvent**). In working with solutions, it is necessary to know, or to be able to measure, the relative amounts of the substance in solution—known as the **concentration of the solution**. Concentration is the amount of one substance relative to the amounts of the other substances in the solution.

Solution concentration is expressed in several different ways. The most common methods used in clinical laboratories involve either weight per unit weight (w/w), also known as mass per unit mass (m/m); weight per unit volume (w/v), also known as mass per unit volume (m/v); or volume per unit volume (v/v). Weight is the term commonly used, although mass is really what is being measured. Mass is the amount of matter in something, and weight is the force of gravity on something. The most accurate measurement is weight per unit weight, since weight (or mass) does not vary with temperature as does volume. Probably the most common measurement is weight per unit volume. The least accurate measurement is volume per unit volume, because of the changes in volume resulting from temperature changes. Volume per unit volume is used in the preparation of a liquid solution from another liquid substance. A few concentrations are expressed as a proper name, such as Wright's stain (used in hematology) or the Sudan III stain (used to demonstrate fat).

### Proper Name

There are very few instances in which a solution is described by a proper name as far as its concentration is concerned. In Chapter 12 (Hematology), the use of Wright's stain is discussed. This solution is prepared with specific amounts of ingredients according to a series of instructions or directions. When Wright's stain is needed, one knows exactly what is meant and what chemicals in which amounts are used in its preparation.

### Weight (Mass) per Unit Volume (w/v)

The most common way of expressing concentration is by **weight (mass) per unit volume (w/v).** When weight (mass) per unit volume is used, the amount of solute (the substance that goes into solution) per volume of solution is expressed. Weight per unit volume is used most often when a solid chemical is diluted in a liquid. The usual way to express weight per unit volume is as grams per liter (g/L) or milligrams per milliliter (mg/mL). If a concentration of a certain solution is given as 10 g/L, it means that

there are 10 g of solute for every liter of solution. If a solution with a concentration of 10 mg/mL is desired and 100 mL of this solution is to be prepared, the use of a proportion formula can be applied. An example follows:

$$\frac{10 \text{ mg}}{1 \text{ mL}} = \frac{x \text{ mg}}{100 \text{ mL}} = 1{,}000 \text{ mg, or } 1 \text{ g}$$

One gram of the desired solute is weighed and diluted to 100 mL (see under Reagents Used in Laboratory Assays, in Chapter 4).

In working with standard solutions, it will be seen that their concentrations, almost without exception, are expressed as milligrams per milliliter (mg/mL).

### Volume per Unit Volume (v/v)

Another way of expressing concentration is by **volume per unit volume (v/v).** Volume per unit volume is used to express concentration when a liquid chemical is diluted with another liquid; the concentration is expressed as the number of milliliters of liquid chemical per unit volume of solution. The usual way to express volume per unit volume is as milliliters per milliliter (mL/mL) or milliliters per liter (mL/L). The number of milliliters of liquid chemical in 1 mL or 1 L of solution utilizes the volume per unit volume expression of concentration. If 10 mL of alcohol is diluted to 100 mL with water, the concentration is expressed as 10 mL/100 mL, or 10 mL/dl, or 0.1 mL/mL, or 100 mL/L. If a solution with a concentration of 0.5 mL/mL is desired and 1 L is to be prepared, a proportion can again be used to solve the problem. An example follows:

$$\frac{0.5 \text{ mL}}{1 \text{ mL}} = \frac{x \text{ mL}}{1{,}000 \text{ mL}}$$
$$x = 500 \text{ mL}$$

Thus 500 mL of the liquid chemical is measured accurately and diluted to 1,000 mL (1 L).

To express concentration in milliliters per liter, one needs to know how many milliliters of liquid chemical there are in 1 L of the solution.

Any chemical (liquid or solid) can be made into a solution by diluting it with a solvent. The usual solvent is deionized or distilled water (see under Laboratory Reagent Water, in Chapter 4). If the desired chemical is a liquid, the amount needed is measured in milliliters or liters (on occasion liquids are weighed, but the usual method is to measure their volume); if the desired chemical is a solid, the amount needed is weighed in grams or milligrams.

## Weight per Unit Weight (w/w)

Another way of expressing concentration is by **weight per unit weight** or **mass per unit mass (m/m)**. This expression is not commonly used. Not many reagents are prepared by using only solid chemicals and no liquid solvent. When the desired chemical is a solid and it is mixed with, or diluted with, another solid, the expression of concentration is mass per unit mass. The usual way to express mass per unit mass is as milligrams per milligram (mg/mg), grams per gram (g/g), or grams per kilogram (g/kg). The number of milligrams or grams of one solid in the total number of milligrams or grams of the dry mixture is the mass per unit mass.

## Percent

Another expression of concentration is the percent solution (%), although in the SI system the preferred units are kilograms (or fractions thereof) per liter (w/v) or milliliters per liter (v/v). A description of the percent solution follows, as this expression of concentration is still used in some instances. **Percent** is defined as parts per hundred parts (the part can be any particular unit). Unless otherwise stated, a percent solution usually means grams or milliliters of solute per 100 mL of solution (g/100 mL or mL/100 mL). Recall that 100 mL is equal to 1 deciliter (dL). Percent solutions can be prepared by using either liquid or solid chemicals. Percent solutions can be expressed either as weight per unit volume percent (w/v%) or as volume per unit volume percent (v/v%), depending on the state of the solute (chemical) used—that is, whether it is a solid or a liquid. When a solid chemical is dissolved in a liquid, percent means grams of solid in 100 mL of solution. If 10 g of NaCl is diluted to 100 mL with deionized water, the concentration is expressed as 10% (10 g/dL). If 2.5 g is diluted to 100 mL, the concentration is 2.5% (2.5 g/dL).

The following is an example of concentration expressed in percent: Ten grams of NaOH is diluted to 200 mL with water. What is the concentration in percent? A proportion can be set up to solve this problem:

$$\frac{10\,g}{200\,mL} = \frac{x\,g}{100\,mL}$$

$$x = 5\% \text{ solution (preferably expressed as 5 g/dL)}$$

Remember that the percent expression is based on how much solute is present in 100 mL (or 1 dL) of the solution.

Some concentrations of solutions are expressed as milligrams of solute in 100 mL of solution (mg%). When this method of expression is used, mg% is always specifically stated. If 25 mg of a chemical is diluted to 100 mL, the concentration in milligrams percent would be 25 mg% (preferably expressed as 25 mg/dL).

If a liquid chemical is used to prepare a percent solution, the concentration is expressed as volume per unit volume percent, or milliliters of solute per 100 mL of solution. If 10 mL of hydrochloric acid (HCl) is diluted to 100 mL with water, the concentration is 10% (preferably expressed as 10 ml/dL). If 10 mL of the same acid is diluted to 1 L (1,000 mL), the concentration is 1% (preferably expressed as 1 mL/dL).

## Molarity

The **molarity of a solution** is defined as the gram-molecular mass (or weight) of a compound per liter of solution. This is a weight per unit volume method of expressing concentration. A basic formula follows:

Molecular weight × Molarity = Grams/liter

Another way to define molarity is as the number of moles per liter (mol/L) of solution. A mole is the molecular weight of a compound in grams (1 mole equals 1 gram-molecular weight). The number of moles of a compound equals the number of grams divided by the gram-molecular weight of that compound. One **gram-molecular weight** equals the sum of all atomic weights in a molecule of the compound, expressed in grams.

To determine the gram-molecular weight of a compound, the correct chemical formula must be known. When this formula is known, the sum of all the atomic weights in the compound can be found by consulting a periodic table of the elements or a chart with the atomic masses of the elements.

### Examples of Molarity Calculations

1. Sodium chloride has one sodium ion and one chloride ion; the correct formula is written as NaCl. The gram-molecular weight is derived by finding the sum of the atomic weights:

$$Na = 23$$
$$Cl = 35.5$$
$$Gram\text{-}molecular\ weight = 58.5$$

If the gram-molecular weight of NaCl is 58.5 g, a 1 molar (1M) solution of NaCl would contain 58.5 g of NaCl per liter of solution, because molarity equals moles per liter, and 1 mol of NaCl equals 58.5 g.

2. For barium sulfate ($BaSO_4$), the gram-molecular weight equals 233 (the formula indicates that there are one barium, one sulfur, and four oxygen ions).

$$1\ Ba = 137 \times 1 = 137$$
$$1\ S = 32 \times 1 = 32$$
$$4\ O = 16 \times 4 = \frac{64}{233}$$

Since the gram-molecular weight is 233, a 1M solution of $BaSO_4$ would contain 233 g of $BaSO_4$ per liter of solution.

The quantities of solutions needed will not always be in units of whole liters, and often fractions or multiples of a 1M concentration will be desired. Parts of a molar solution are expressed as decimals. If a 1M solution of NaCl contains 58.5 g of NaCl per liter of solution, a 0.5M solution would contain one half of 58.5 g, or 29 g/L, and a 3M solution would contain 3 times 58.5 g, or 175.5 g/L.

What is the molarity of a solution containing 30 g of NaCl per liter? Molarity equals the number of moles per liter, and the number of moles equals the grams divided by the gram-molecular weight.

*Step 1:* Find the gram-molecular weight of NaCl. It is 58.5 g (Na = 23 and Cl = 35.5).

*Step 2:* Find the moles per liter.

$$\frac{30\ g/L}{x} = \frac{58.5\ g/L}{1\ mol}$$

$$x = \frac{30\ g/L \times 1\ mol}{58.5\ g/L} = 0.513\ mol\ NaCl$$

*Step 3:* The number of moles per liter of solution equals the molarity; the solution in the example is therefore 0.513M, rounded off to 0.5M.

Equations might prove useful to some in working with molarity solutions. However, all of these equations can be derived by applying a common sense proportion approach to molarity problems, as described above under Proportions and Ratios. Some of these equations are listed below.

$$Molarity = \frac{Moles\ of\ solute}{Liters\ of\ solution}$$

$$Molarity = \frac{Grams\ of\ solute}{Gram\text{-}molecular\ weight} \times \frac{1}{Liters\ of\ solution}$$

$$Moles\ of\ solute = Molarity \times Liters\ of\ solution$$

Grams of solute =
Molarity × Gram-molecular weight × Liters of solution

*Note:* These equations are all on the basis of 1 L of solution; if something other than 1 L is used, refer back to the 1-L basis (500 mL = 0.5 L, or 2,000 mL = 2 L, for example).

Molarity does not provide a basis for direct comparison of strength for all solutions. For example, 1 L of 1M NaOH will exactly neutralize 1 L of 1M HCl, but it will neutralize only 0.5 L of 1M sulfuric acid ($H_2SO_4$). It is therefore more convenient to choose a unit of concentration that will provide a basis for direct comparison of strengths of solutions. Such a unit is referred to as an equivalent (or equivalent weight or mass), and this term is used in describing normality.

### Millimolarity

A **milligram molecular weight** (the molecular weight expressed in milligrams) is a **millimole (mmole)**. This is in contrast to the molarity described above, which is the number of moles per liter. The following formulas compare the two:

$$\text{Molarity (moles/liter)} = \frac{\text{g/L}}{\text{Molecular weight}}$$

$$\text{Millimoles/liter} = \frac{\text{mg/L}}{\text{Molecular weight}}$$

## Normality

**Normality** is defined as the number of equivalent weights per liter of solution. The **equivalent (equiv) weight** is the mass in grams that will liberate, combine, or replace one gram-atom (g atom) of hydrogen ion ($H^+$). By using equivalents, the numbers of units of all substances involved in a reaction are made numerically equal. Normality is expressed as a weight per unit volume concentration.

### Examples of Normality Calculations

*Reaction 1:*

I equiv NaOH + I equiv HCl →
    I equiv $H_2O$ + I equiv NaCl

*Reaction 2:*

I equiv NaOH + I equiv $H_2SO_4$ →
    I equiv $H_2O$ + I equiv $Na_2SO_4$

The balanced equation for this reaction is:

$$2NaOH + IH_2SO_4 \rightarrow 2H_2O + INa_2SO_4$$

This same reaction expressed using moles is:

I mol NaOH + 0.5 mol $H_2SO_4$ →
    I mol $H_2O$ + 0.5 mol $NaSO_4$

One equivalent of any acid will neutralize one equivalent of any base.

In discussing molarity, the term moles per liter (mol/L) is used; in units of normality, the terms equivalents per liter (equiv/L), milliequivalents per milliliter (mEq/mL), and milliequivalents per liter (mEq/L) are used. The normality of a solution is defined as the number of gram-equivalents (or equivalent weights) per liter of solution, or the number of milliequivalents per milliliter of solution.

### Equivalent Weight

The **equivalent weight** (or **mass**) is the weight in grams that will liberate, combine with, or replace one gram-atom of hydrogen. The equivalent weight may be found by dividing the gram-molecular weight (GMW) by the total combining power, or **valence,** of the positive ion (ions) of the substance. As a general rule, the equivalent weight of a compound or substance (element) is equal to the molecular weight divided by the valence. The SI system prefers the use of molarity (mol/L) to express the amount of substance in chemical units. A disadvantage of the concept of normality is that a particular solution may have more than one normality, depending on the reaction in which it is used, while it will always have the same molarity, since there is only one molecular weight for any substance.

**Examples of Equivalent Weights.** Hydrochloric acid has one atom of $H^+$ and one atom of $Cl^-$; therefore, the gram-equivalent weight equals the molecular weight.

Hydrogen sulfide ($H_2S$) has two atoms of $H^+$ and only one atom of $S^{2-}$, or one atom of

$H^+$ and one-half atom of $S^{2-}$; therefore, the equivalent weight equals one-half the molecular weight, or:

$$\frac{\text{Molecular weight}}{\text{Total positive valence}} = \frac{34}{2} = 17$$

NaCl has one atom of $Cl^-$ and one atom of $Na^+$ ($Na^+$ replaces $H^+$); therefore, the gram-equivalent weight equals the gram-molecular weight.

A liter of a 1N solution of $H_2SO_4$ contains the same number of equivalents as 1 L of 1N HCl, or 1N NaOH, or 1N barium hydroxide ($Ba[OH]_2$). Again, equations might prove useful in working with normality solutions. Some of these are:

$$\text{Normality} = \frac{\text{Equivalents of solute}}{\text{Liters of solution}}$$

$$\text{Normality} = \frac{\text{Grams of solute}}{\text{GMW/combining power (valence)}} \times \frac{1}{\text{Liters of solution}}$$

where GMW is gram-molecular weight.

$$\text{Normality} = \frac{\text{Moles}}{\text{Combining power}} \times \frac{1}{\text{Liters of solution}}$$

$$\text{Normality} = \frac{\text{Grams of solute}}{\text{Equivalent weight}} \times \frac{1}{\text{Liters of solution}}$$

$$\text{Normality} = \frac{\text{Equivalents}}{\text{Liters}}$$

$$\text{Normality} = \frac{\text{Milliequivalents}}{\text{Milliliters}}$$

**Milliequivalent Weight.** Just as a millimole relates to a mole, the milliequivalent (mEq) relates to the equivalent. A **milliequivalent weight** (the equivalent weight in milligrams) = 1 mEq. The following formulas apply:

$$\frac{\text{mg}}{\text{eq. wt.}} = \text{mEq}$$

$$1 \text{ eq} = 1,000 \text{ mEq}$$

$$1 \text{ mEq} = \frac{1}{1000} \text{ eq}$$

## Interconversion of Molarity and Normality

On occasion, it is necessary to convert an expression of concentration in molarity to one in normality and vice versa. Two simple formulas are available for this purpose:

$$\text{Molarity} = \frac{\text{Normality}}{\text{Total positive combining power (valence)}}$$

$$\text{or } \frac{N}{\text{Valence}}$$

$$\text{Normality} = \text{Molarity} \times \text{Total positive power (valence)}$$

$$\text{or M} \times \text{valence}$$

To prepare 1 L of a 2N NaCl solution, first calculate the gram-molecular weight, using the known formula for the compound: Na = 23; Cl = 35.5; the gram-molecular weight thus is 58.5 g. In working with normality problems, the gram-equivalent weight is used; therefore, the next step is to calculate this. The gram-equivalent weight equals the gram-molecular weight divided by the valence, or 58.5 g divided by 1; the gram-equivalent weight is therefore 58.5 g. For 1 L of a 1N solution of this compound, 58.5 g would be weighed; for 1 L of a 2N solution, 58.5 g × 2, or 117 g, of NaCl is needed per liter. An example of another such problem follows.

Prepare 200 mL of a 0.5N calcium chloride ($CaCl_2$) solution.

*Step 1:* Calculate the gram-molecular weight.

$$Ca = 40 \times 1 = 40$$
$$Cl = 35.5 \times 2 = \frac{71}{111 \text{ g}} = \text{Total gram-molecular weight}$$

*Step 2:* Calculate the gram-equivalent weight.

$$\text{Equivalent weight} = \frac{\text{GMW}}{\text{Valence}} = \frac{111}{2} = 55.5 \text{ g}$$

*Step 3:* Solve for normality. A 1N solution would contain 55.5 g/L. A 0.5N solution would contain only half as much chemical per liter of solution, or 27.8 g. A proportion could be set up to solve this:

$$\frac{55.5 \text{ g}}{1N \text{ solution}} = \frac{x \text{ g}}{0.5N \text{ solution}} = 27.8 \text{ g}$$

However, only 200 mL of this solution is needed. Therefore another proportion could be set up for this:

$$\frac{27.8 \text{ g}}{1,000 \text{ mL}} = \frac{x \text{ g}}{200 \text{ mL}} = 5.6 \text{ g}$$

*Step 4:* In the actual preparation of solution, 5.6 g of $CaCl_2$ is weighed and diluted to 200 mL volumetrically (see under Reagents Used in Laboratory Assays, in Chapter 4).

## Osmolarity

**Osmolarity** is defined as the number of osmoles of solute per liter of solution. An osmole (osm) is the amount of a substance that will produce 1 mol of particles having osmotic activity. An osmole of any substance is equal to 1 gram-molecular weight (1 mol) of the substance divided by the number of particles formed by the dissociation of the molecules of the substance. For materials that do not ionize, 1 osm is equal to 1 mol. This gives an estimate of the osmotic activity of the solution—the relative number of particles dissolved in the solution. Osmolarity is an expression of weight per unit volume concentration.

For a solution of glucose, a substance that does not ionize or dissociate in aqueous solution, 1 osm of glucose is equal to 1 mol of glucose For a solution of sodium chloride, which does ionize, 1 osm of sodium chloride is equal to 1 gram-molecular weight divided by the number of particles formed upon ionization. Sodium chloride completely ionizes in water to form one sodium ion and one chloride ion, or a total of two particles. The molecular weight of NaCl is 58.5. To calculate the osmolarity of NaCl, the following formula is used:

$$1 \text{ osm NaCl} = \frac{58.5}{2} = 29.25 \text{ g}$$

## Density

**Density** is defined as the amount of matter per unit volume of a substance. All substances have this property, not only solutions. An example of the expression of density is the specific gravity of a substance. Specific gravity is defined as the ratio between the mass of a substance and the mass of an equal volume of water, or:

$$\text{Specific gravity} = \frac{\text{Mass of substance}}{\text{Mass of equal volume of water}}$$

See under Specific Gravity, in Chapter 14.

## BIBLIOGRAPHY

Campbell JB, Campbell JM: *Laboratory Mathematics: Medical and Biological Applications*, ed 5. St Louis, Mosby, 1997.

## STUDY QUESTIONS

1. **Match the following terms (1 to 5) with their definitions (A to E):**

   1. Ratio
   2. Concentration
   3. Normality
   4. Molarity
   5. Dilution

   _____ A. The amount of one substance relative to the amounts of other substances in the solution

   _____ B. An indication of relative concentration

   _____ C. The gram-molecular mass (or weight) of a compound per liter of solution

   _____ D. An amount of something compared with an amount of something else

   _____ E. The number of equivalent weights per liter of solution

2. How would each of the following numbers be rounded off to 1 fewer decimal place?

   A. 63.24
   B. 15.568
   C. 10.021
   D. 25.5
   E. 24.5

3. How much of a 5 g/dL (dL = 100mL) solution of NaCl is needed to prepare 1,000 mL (1 L) of a 2 g/dL solution?

4. Express each of the following as the corresponding whole number, decimal, or fraction.

   A. $4^5$
   B. $3^{-3}$
   C. $10^3$

5. How would you dilute a serum specimen 1:10?

6. How would you prepare 100 mL of a 5% (w/v) solution of NaCl?

7. If there are 20 g of NaCl per liter of solution, what is the molarity of the solution?

8. How would you prepare 1000 mL of a 0.5M solution of NaCl?

9. How much of a 2M solution can be made from 50 mL of a 5M solution?

10. How would you prepare 500 mL of a 0.5N solution of $CaCl_2$?

# CHAPTER 8

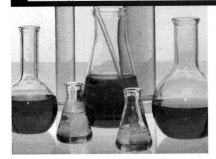

# Quality Assurance in the Clinical Laboratory

## Learning Objectives

*From study of this chapter, the reader will be able to:*

➤ Understand how federal, state, and local regulations require the implementation of quality assurance programs in the clinical laboratory, to ensure that the results reported are of medical use to the physician.

➤ Identify the components necessary to a laboratory's quality assurance program, including its quality control program and the use of control specimens.

➤ Assess the diagnostic usefulness of results reported, which requires an understanding of accuracy and precision, and specificity and sensitivity, for laboratory tests and methodologies.

➤ Understand the sources of variance or error in a laboratory procedure.

➤ Appreciate the use of reference values, including the use of the mean and the standard deviation in determination of the reference range.

➤ Appreciate the importance of a quality control program, including the use of control samples, the determination of the control range, and the use of quality control charts.

# INTRODUCTION

Quality can be defined as satisfaction of the needs and expectations of the users of a service. In a clinical laboratory, the assurance of quality results for the various analyses is critical and is an important component of the operation of every good laboratory. Analytic results obtained through laboratory determinations are used by the physician both to discover the existence of disease in a patient and to follow the progress of treatment. It is the responsibility of the clinical laboratory, to both patient and physician, to ensure that the results reported are reliable and to give the physician an estimate of what constitutes "normal." The dimension of quality assurance (QA) and the improvement of quality—quality improvement, total quality improvement (TQI)—are driven by both public and private pressures and by the need to contain the cost of the service.

# STANDARDS SET BY THE JOINT COMMISSION ON ACCREDITATION OF HEALTHCARE ORGANIZATIONS

The public's focus on health care delivery is relevant to most areas of work done in clinical laboratories. Agencies from public and medical communities, as well as from the government, are continually reexamining health care facilities. Standards have been set by the **Joint Commission on Accreditation of Healthcare Organizations (JCAHO)**, reflecting the commission's focus on **quality assurance programs.** These standards require the monitoring and evaluation of quality and appropriateness of services to patients and the resolution of any identified problems. The JCAHO has published a ten-step monitoring process for quality assurance programs.[1] These steps are:

1. Assign responsibility for a quality assurance plan.
2. Define the scope of patient care.
3. Identify the important aspects of care.
4. Construct indicators.
5. Define the thresholds for evaluation.
6. Collect and organize the data.
7. Evaluate the data.
8. Develop a corrective action plan.
9. Assess actions; document improvement.
10. Communicate relevant information.

No concern is of greater importance than quality assurance. As defined by the JCAHO ten-step plan, **quality assurance** is an overall and continuing process by which the hospital or health care facility monitors all areas that contribute to providing the highest quality and most appropriate care for the patient. Quality assurance requires a planned, systematic process of monitoring all aspects of patient care. As part of the health care team, the clinical laboratory must also have an ongoing quality assurance process for monitoring its analytic results. The analytic results of the test or tests done on a clinical specimen must be as accurate as possible so that the physician can rely on the data and use the information in the diagnostic and treatment plan for the patient. This is the service provided by the clinical laboratory to the total health care plan for the patient. An ongoing, active, comprehensive quality assurance program is an essential component for hospital accreditation. Because quality assurance has become so important, other regulatory groups, such as the College of American Pathologists (CAP), have included quality assurance activities as necessary components of accreditation standards.[6]

# COMPONENTS OF QUALITY ASSURANCE PROGRAMS

The documentation of an ongoing quality assurance program in clinical laboratories is mandated by the CLIA '88 regulations.[3]

## Commitment

It is essential that all persons working in the clinical laboratory be totally committed to the concepts of the quality assurance process as it is defined by the specific health care facility. The dedication of sufficient planning time to quality assurance and the implementation of the program in the total laboratory operation are critical. All persons working in the clinical laboratory must be willing to work together to make the quality of service to the patient their top priority. Because the total laboratory staff must be involved in carrying out any quality assurance process, it is important to develop a comprehensive program to include all levels of laboratorians.

## Facilities and Resources

The physical location and layout of the laboratory are an important aspect of quality assurance. Since the product of the laboratory is the analytic result for the patient's specimen, it is vital that the physical laboratory site be conducive to good performance by the laboratorians working there. A safe working site with adequate, properly maintained equipment and supplies is essential to ensure that high-quality analytic results are a reasonable expectation.

## Technical Competence

The competence of personnel is an important determinant of the quality of the laboratory result. Crucial to any quality assurance process is the maintenance of a high level of performance by the laboratorians doing the analyses. Only well-trained, competent personnel should be carrying out the testing processes. CLIA '88 requirements for laboratory personnel in regard to levels of education and experience or training must be followed for laboratories doing moderately complex or highly complex testing (see under Regulation of the Clinical Laboratory, in Chapter 1). In addition to the actual performance of analytic procedures, competent laboratory personnel must be able to perform quality control activities, maintain instruments, and keep accurate and systematic records of reagents and control specimens, equipment maintenance, and patient and analytic data. For new laboratory personnel, a thorough orientation to the laboratory procedures and policies is vital.

Periodic opportunities for personal upgrading of technical skills and for obtaining new relevant information should be made available to all persons working in the laboratory. This can be accomplished through in-service training classes, opportunities to attend continuing education courses, and by encouraging independent study habits by means of scientific journals and audiovisual materials.

Personnel performance should be monitored with periodic evaluations and reports. Quality assurance demands that the results of daily work be monitored by a supervisor and that all analytic reports produced during a particular shift be evaluated for errors and omissions. Quality control measures are used to monitor possible human error in performing laboratory analyses. Quality control is one aspect of the quality assurance process and is discussed in more detail below.

## Quality Assurance Procedures

Quality assurance programs monitor test requesting procedures; patient identification, specimen procurement, and labeling; specimen transportation and processing procedures; laboratory personnel performance; laboratory instrumentation, reagents, and analytic test procedures; turnaround times; and the accuracy of the final result. Complete documentation of all procedures involved in obtaining the final analytic result for the patient sample must be maintained and monitored in a systematic manner. Some of these procedures are described in the following sections.

### Test Requesting

The request form for each patient's laboratory work must be completed by the physician directing the patient's care. The form must include the patient identification data, the time and date of specimen collection, the source of the specimen, and the analyses requested to be done. The complete request form must accompany the specimen. It is of interest to the laboratory to note the time of receipt of the specimen. This information is necessary for the monitoring of turnaround times—the interval between receipt of the specimen in the laboratory and release of the analytic result when the test has been completed and the result verified. The request form must be clean and legible. The information on the accompanying specimen container must match exactly the patient identification on the request slip. The information needed by the physician to assist in ordering tests is included in a database or handbook described in the following section.

### Patient Identification, Specimen Procurement, and Labeling

A process of educating physicians, nurses, laboratorians, and other health care personnel who are involved in collecting clinical specimens is extremely important. A computerized (electronic) database or handbook of specimen requirement information, in an easily accessible format and location, is one of the first steps in establishing a quality assurance program for the clinical laboratory. This information must be made available on the patient care units or any other place where patient specimens are collected, and it must be kept current. Information about obtaining appropriate specimens, special collection requirements for special kinds of tests, ordering tests correctly, and transporting and processing specimens appropriately is included in this information. Any changes in content must be communicated to those persons needing the information.

Patients must be carefully identified. For hospitalized patients, the most convenient way to do so is to have the patient wear a wristband with the necessary information printed on it.

Using established specimen requirement information, the clinical specimens must be properly labeled or identified once they have been obtained from the patient. The practice of using standard precautions in collecting specimens cannot be overemphasized. All specimens should be handled as though they contained a hazardous agent or pathogen (see also Standard Precautions, in Chapter 2).

The laboratory can accept only properly labeled specimens. Computer-generated labels assist in making certain that proper patient identification is noted on each specimen container sent to the laboratory. Improperly labeled or unlabeled specimens cannot be accepted by the laboratory. All containers must be labeled by the person doing the collection, to make certain that each specimen has been collected from the patient whose identification is noted on the label. An important rule to remember is that the analytic result can only be as good as the specimen received (see also Specimen Collection, in Chapter 3).

### Specimen Transportation and Processing

Specimens must be transported to the laboratory in a safe, timely, and efficient manner. It is important that a central receiving and processing area be set aside in the laboratory to monitor and record all incoming specimens and the request forms accompanying them. The documentation of specimen arrival times in the laboratory as well as other specific test request data is an important aspect of laboratory organization and an essential part of the quality assurance process. It is important that the specimen status can be determined at any time—that is, where in the laboratory processing system a given specimen can be found. Turnaround time is an important factor; specimen processing, analyses, and reporting of results within an acceptable time frame constitute a part of the quality assurance process as a whole (see also Specimen Collection, in Chapter 3).

### Quality Control

**Quality control** activities include monitoring the performance of laboratory instruments, reagents, other testing products, and equipment. In the process of quality assurance, it is important to document the effectiveness of quality control measures. The written record of quality control activities for each procedure or function should also include details of deviation from the usual results, problems, or failures in functioning or in the analytic procedure, as well as any corrective action taken in response to these problems.

Instruments for quality control can include preventive maintenance records, temperature charts, and other records of performance such as quality control charts for specific analytic procedures. All products and reagents used in the analytic procedures must be carefully checked before actual use in testing patient samples. Use of quality control specimens, proficiency testing, and standards depends upon the specific requirements of the accrediting agency of the health care facility. General use of control specimens, proficiency testing programs, and reference values is described later in this chapter.

Sometimes laboratories are asked to assist other departments in the health care facility in their quality control measures. This could include checking the effectiveness of autoclaves in surgery or in the laundry, or providing aseptic checks for the pharmacy, blood bank, or dialysis service.

External quality control activities include periodic inspections by the various accrediting agencies involved in the regulation of clinical laboratories. It is for these inspections that well-monitored, well-documented quality assurance records are maintained.

### Laboratory Procedure Manuals

A complete **laboratory procedure manual** for all analytic procedures performed within the laboratory must be provided. The National Committee for Clinical Laboratory Standards (NCCLS) recommends that these procedure manuals follow a specific pattern in how the procedures in the manual are organized. Each assay done in the laboratory must be included in the manual, beginning with the title of the test, or the test name, along with the principle of the procedure. The manual should also contain the following: specimen requirements such as patient preparation (if needed) and special collection or processing details; test request information; other criteria for performing the test; procedural information (how to perform the test),

including the reagents and control specimens used and the calibration of instruments and maintenance checks performed; quality control data; limitations of the procedure; details about reference values; and information about reporting of results. These manuals must be reviewed regularly by the supervisory staff and updated, as needed. In the process of quality assurance, the documentation of laboratory procedural information is as important as documentation of quality control activities, specimen receiving data, or reporting of the laboratory result itself. The NCCLS has set guidelines for writing laboratory procedure manuals.[2]

### Problem-Solving Mechanisms

Since an important aspect of quality assurance is **documentation,** CLIA '88 regulations mandate that any problem or situation that might affect the outcome of a test result must be recorded and reported. All such incidents must be documented in writing, including the changes proposed and their implementation, and follow-up monitored. These incidents can involve specimens that are improperly collected, labeled, or transported to the laboratory, or problems concerning prolonged turnaround times for test results. There must be a reasonable attempt to correct the problems or situation, and all steps in this process must be documented.

### Continuous Quality Improvement

The ongoing process of making certain that the correct laboratory result is reported for the right patient in a timely manner and cost is known as **continuous quality improvement,** or **CQI.** This is a process of assuring the clinician ordering the test that the testing process has been done in the best possible way to provide the most useful information in diagnosing or managing the particular patient in question. **Quality assurance indicators** are evaluated as part of the CQI process. These indicators monitor the performance of the laboratory. Each laboratory will set its own indicators, depending on the specific goals of the laboratory. Any quality assurance indicators should be appreciated as a tool to ensure that reported results are of the highest quality.

### Test Result and Information Processing Systems

With the use of laboratory computer systems and information processing, record keeping can be done in a fast, efficient manner. Quality assurance programs require documentation, and computer record-keeping capability assists in doing this. Patient test results, by dates performed, as well as quality control data for the same dates, must be recorded. When control results are within the acceptable limits established by the laboratory, these data provide the necessary link between the control and patient data, thus giving reassurance that the patient results are reliable, valid, and reportable. This information is necessary in order to document that uniform protocols have been established and that they are being followed. The data can also support the proper functioning capabilities of the test systems being used at the time patient results are produced.

### CAP Quality Assurance Programs

The College of American Pathologists (CAP) provides assistance to the clinical laboratory in organizing and managing its **CAP quality assurance program.** As described in the CAP's *Physician Office Laboratory Policy and Procedure Manual,* "All laboratories must have a quality assurance program with the proper documentation defining the goals of the program, the procedures necessary to achieve the goals, and specific records showing that procedures have been carried out. A comprehensive quality assurance program must be designed to monitor and evaluate the ongoing and overall quality of the total testing process (preanalytic, analytic, and postanalytic). The laboratory's quality assurance program must evaluate the effectiveness of its policies and procedures; identify and

correct problems; assure the accurate, reliable and prompt reporting of test results; and assure the adequacy and competency of the staff."[5] Quality assurance programs are not without cost, but they are an essential part of health care.

### Components of a CAP Quality Assurance Program

According to the College of American Pathologists, a comprehensive quality assurance program should include the following components:

Patient test management
Procedure manuals
Quality control assessment
Proficiency testing
Comparison of test results
Relationship of patient information to test results
Personnel assessment
Communications

## DIAGNOSTIC VALUE OF RESULTS REPORTED: DESCRIPTORS USED

The ability of the laboratory results reported to substantiate a diagnosis, lead to a change in diagnosis, or follow the management for a diagnosis already made is what makes the laboratory test useful to the clinician. The diagnostic usefulness of a test and its procedure is assessed by using statistical evaluations such as description of the accuracy and reliability of the test and its methodology. To describe the reliability of a particular procedure, two terms are commonly used: **accuracy** and **precision.** The **reliability of a procedure** depends on a combination of these two factors, although they are different and are not dependent on each other. **Variance** is another general term that describes the factors or fluctuations that affect the measurement of the substance in question. Statistical methods available also can assess the usefulness of a test result in terms of its **sensitivity,** its **specificity,** and its **predictive value.**

## Accuracy versus Precision

The **accuracy** of a procedure refers to the closeness of the result obtained to the true or actual value, while **precision** refers to repeatability or reproducibility—that is, the ability to get the same value in subsequent tests on the same sample. It is possible to have great precision, with all laboratory personnel who perform the same procedure arriving at the same answer, but without accuracy if the answer does not represent the actual value being tested for. The precision of a test, its **reproducibility,** may be expressed as **standard deviations (SD)** or the **derived coefficient of variation (CV).** A procedure may be extremely accurate, yet so difficult to perform that individual laboratory personnel are unable to arrive at values that are close enough to be clinically meaningful.

In very general terms, accuracy can be aided by the use of properly standardized procedures, statistically valid comparisons of new methods with established reference methods, the use of samples of known values (controls), and participation in proficiency testing programs.

Precision can be ensured by the proper inclusion of standards, reference samples, or control solutions; statistically valid replicate determinations of a single sample; or duplicate determinations of sufficient numbers of unknown samples. Day-to-day and between-run precision is measured by inclusion of blind samples and control specimens.

### Coefficient of Variation

The coefficient of variation can be used to compare the standard deviations of two samples. Standard deviations cannot be compared directly without considering the mean. The CV can be used to compare one day's work with that of a similar day or to compare test results from one laboratory with the same type of test results from another laboratory. The coefficient of variation in percent is equal to the standard deviation divided by the mean:

$$CV\% = \frac{SD}{Mean} \times 100$$

## Sources of Variance or Error

In general, it is impossible to obtain exactly the same result each time a determination is performed on a particular specimen. This may be described as the **variance (or error) of a procedure.** These factors include limitations of the procedure itself and limitations related to the sampling mechanism used.

### Sampling Factors

One of the major difficulties in guaranteeing reliable results involves the **sampling procedure.** Only a very small amount of sample is taken—for example, 5 to 10 mL of a total blood volume of 5 to 6 L, approximately one thousandth of the total blood volume. Other sources of variance that involve the sample include the time of day when the sample is obtained, the patient's position (lying down or seated), the patient's state of physical activity (in bed, ambulatory, or physically active), the interval since last eating (fasting or not), and the time interval and storage conditions between the obtaining of the specimen and its processing by the laboratory. The aging of the sample is another source of error.

### Procedural Factors

Still other sources of variance involve aging of chemicals or reagents; personal bias or limited experience of the person performing the determination; and laboratory bias because of variations in standards, reagents, environment, methods, or apparatus. There may also be experimental error resulting from changes in the method used for a particular determination, changes in instruments, or changes in personnel.

## Sensitivity and Specificity of a Test

Laboratory results that give medically useful information, including the specificity and sensitivity of the tests being ordered and reported, are important. Both specificity and sensitivity are desirable characteristics for a test, but in different clinical situations, one is generally preferred over the other. For assessing the sensitivity and specificity of a test, four entities are needed: tests positive, tests negative, disease present (positive), or disease absent (negative). **True positives** are those subjects who have a positive test result and who also have the disease in question. **True negatives** represent those subjects who have a negative test result and who do not have the disease. **False positives** are those subjects who have a positive test result yet do not have the disease. **False negatives** are those subjects who have a negative test result yet do have the disease.

### Sensitivity

The **sensitivity** of a test is defined as the proportion of cases with a specific disease or condition that give a positive test result (that is, the assay correctly predicts with a positive result):

$$\text{Sensitivity \%} = \frac{\text{True positives}}{\text{True positives} + \text{False negatives}} \times 100$$

Practically, sensitivity represents how much of a given substance is measured; the more sensitive the test, the smaller the amount of assayed substance that is measured.

### Specificity

The **specificity** of a test is defined as the proportion of cases with absence of the specific disease or condition that gives a negative test result (that is, the assay correctly excludes with a negative result):

$$\text{Specificity \%} = \frac{\text{True negatives}}{\text{False positives} + \text{True negatives}} \times 100$$

Practically, specificity represents what is being measured. A highly specific test measures only the assay substance in question; it does not measure interfering or similar substances.

### Predictive Values

To assess the predictive value (PV) for a test, the sensitivity, specificity, and prevalence of the disease in the population being studied must be known. The **prevalence** of a disease is the pro-

portion of a population that has the disease. This is in contrast to the **incidence** of a disease, which is the number of subjects found to have the disease within a defined time period, such as a year, in a population of 100,000.

A **positive predictive value** for a test indicates the number of patients with an abnormal test result who have the disease, compared with all patients with an abnormal result:

$$\text{Positive PV} = \\ \frac{\text{Number of patients with disease and with abnormal test results}}{\text{Total number of patients with abnormal test results}}$$

$$\text{Positive PV} = \frac{\text{True positives}}{\text{True positives} + \text{False positives}}$$

A **negative predictive value** for a test indicates the number of patients with a normal test result who do not have the disease, compared with all patients with a normal (negative) result:

$$\text{Negative PV} = \frac{\text{True negatives}}{\text{True negatives} + \text{False negatives}}$$

## Reference Values
### Definition of "Normal"

Before physicians can determine whether a patient is diseased, they must have an idea of what is normal. This is not an easy task, yet it is the responsibility of the clinical laboratory to supply the physician with this information. Much attention is being paid to the description of what constitutes normal, yet our knowledge remains quite limited. Many factors enter into this determination. There are variations because of such factors as age, sex, race, geographic location, and ethnic, cultural, and economic characteristics, plus internal factors related to the actual analytic methods and practices used by a particular laboratory. To complicate matters, an individual may show daily physiologic variations within his or her normal range, to say nothing of normal changes with age. **Biometrics** (the science of statistics applied to biological observations) is a rapidly expanding field that attempts to describe these variations. The selection of a group on which to base "normals" is another problem confronting the individual laboratory. Traditionally, normals have been defined by testing such groups as blood donors, persons who are working and "feeling healthy," medical students, student nurses, and medical technologists. Many of the old established normals reported in the medical literature have questionable validity because of such factors as poor sampling techniques, questionable selection of the normal group, and questionable use of clinical methods. In developing normal values or reference values, the proper statistical tools of sampling, selection of the normal comparison group, and analysis of data must be used. Such statistical tools are relatively well defined, but a discussion of them here is beyond the scope of this book.

### Reference Range Statistics

Statistically, the **reference range** for a particular measurement is in most cases related to a normal bell-shaped curve (Fig. 8-1). This **gaussian curve** or **distribution** has been shown to be correct for virtually all types of biological, chemical, and physical measurements. A statistically valid series of individuals who are thought to represent a normal healthy group are measured, and the average value is calculated. This mathematical average is defined as the **mean ($\overline{X}$, called the X-bar).** The distribution of all values around the average

for the particular group measured is described statistically by the standard deviation (SD).

**Mean.** The mean is a term used often in laboratory measurements—it is a mathematical average calculated by dividing the sum of all individual values by the number of values.

**Median.** The median is the middle value of a body of data. In a body of data, if all the variables are arranged in order of increasing magnitude, the median is that variable which falls halfway between the highest and the lowest.

**Mode.** The mode is the value that occurs most commonly in a mass of data.

How the mean, the median, and the mode are used is explained in the following example: A series of results reported for a laboratory test done on 7 different specimens is: 7, 2, 3, 6, 5, 4, and 2.

The mean is the mathematical average and is calculated by taking the sum of the values (29) and dividing by the number of values (7) in the list. The mean is 4.1 (rounded off to 4).

The median equals the middle value. To find the median, the list of numbers must first be ranked according to magnitude: 2, 2, 3, 4, 5, 6, 7. There are seven values in the list, and the median is the middle value in the list. In this example, the median is 4.

The mode is the value most frequently occurring, or 2 in this example.

**Standard Deviation.** The **standard deviation (SD)** is the square root of the variance of the values in any one observation or in a series of test results. In any normal population, 68% of the values will be clustered above and below the average and defined statistically as falling within the first standard deviation (±1 SD) (see Fig. 8-1). The second standard deviation represents 95% of the values falling equally above and below the average, while 99.7% will be included within the third standard deviation (±3 SD). (Again, variations occur equally above and below the average value [or mean] for any measurement.)

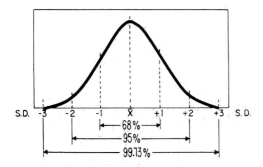

**FIG 8-1.** Normal bell-shaped gaussian curve.

Thus, in determining reference values for a particular measurement, a statistically valid series of people are chosen and assumed to represent a healthy population. These people are then tested, and the results are averaged. The term **reference range** therefore means the range of values that includes 95% of the test results for a healthy reference population. The term replaces "normal values" or "normal range." The limits (or range) of normal are defined in terms of the standard deviation from the average value.

In evaluating an individual's state of health, values outside the third standard deviation value are considered clearly abnormal. When the distribution is gaussian, the reference range closely approximates the mean ±2 SD. Values within the first (68%) and second (95%) standard deviation limits are considered normal, while those between the second (95%) and third (99.7%) standard deviation limits are questionable. Thus, **normal** or **reference values** are stated as a range of values. This stated range is in terms of standard deviation units.

**Confidence Intervals.** When the reference range is expressed using 2 SD on either side of the mean, with 95% of the values falling above and below the mean (see Fig. 8-1), the term **confidence interval** or **confidence limits** is used. This interval should be kept in mind when there are day-to-day shifts in values for a particular analytic procedure. The **95% confidence interval** is used, in part, to account for certain unavoidable error due to sampling variability and imprecision of the methods themselves.

As an example, for a population study, the 95% confidence interval can be interpreted in the following way: if the procedure or experiment is repeated many times and a 95% confidence interval is constructed each time for the parameter being studied, then 95% of these intervals will actually include the true population parameter and 5% will not.

### Reference Values for a Specific Laboratory

It is important to realize that reference values will vary with innumerable factors, but especially between laboratories and between geographic locations. Thus, it is necessary for each laboratory to give the physician information concerning the range of reference values for that particular laboratory. The values will be related to an overall normal, yet they may be more refined or narrow and they may be skewed in the particular situation in question. Although several textbooks are available that describe reference values for virtually all laboratory measurements, and generally accepted reference values are given in such books, the most important indicator of disease is the situation in the clinician's particular institution and locale.

It is hoped that increasing standards and improving the quality of all clinical laboratories will bring all of these reference values closer to an overall value, while parameters describing what constitutes a physiologically normal situation will become established as biometry is further advanced.

## ENSURING RELIABLE RESULTS: THE QUALITY CONTROL PROGRAM

Some type of control system to ensure reliable results in the clinical laboratory is essential, a fact that has been proved by numerous laboratory accuracy surveys. A means of ensuring that a particular procedure is performed in such a way that the day-to-day results are within the established precision for the procedure and that the values reported to the physician represent the true clinical condition of the patient is essential for quality assurance. According to CLIA '88, "The laboratory must establish and follow written quality control procedures for monitoring and evaluating the quality of the analytical testing process of each method to assure the accuracy and reliability of patient test results and reports."[3]

Control of laboratory error is influenced and maintained by several factors. The physician depends on the laboratory values and might be misled if these values are not those expected from the clinical diagnosis. Thus, the laboratory must be sure that the results it gives for any analysis are clinically correct. This is done primarily through the use of a **quality control program,** which makes use of standards and control samples. Other factors influencing the control of laboratory variance are expanding state and federal regulations and participation in various proficiency testing programs, either voluntarily or because of legal mandate.

The control system that is used in most laboratories is the quality control program. The quality control program for the laboratory makes use of a **control specimen,** which is similar in composition to the unknown specimen and is included in every batch or run. It must be carried through the entire test procedure and be treated in exactly the same way as any unknown specimen; it is affected by any or all of the variables that affect the unknown specimen. Control specimens have long been routinely included in the clinical chemistry laboratory as well as in routine hemoglobin determinations. All clinical laboratory departments, such as the chemistry or urinalysis laboratories, recognize the need for quality control programs and the use of control specimens as a part of the quality assurance process as mandated by CLIA '88.[3,4]

The quality control program established by a laboratory involves more than only the use of control samples. The use of standards, blanks, duplicates, and recoveries is a part of the quality control program, and they are discussed separately. The use of automated procedures in place of manual methods often requires the inclusion of additional standards and controls, both between specimens and at the end of the run.

In controlling the reliability of laboratory determinations, the objective is to reject results when there is evidence that more than the permitted amount of error has occurred. The clinical laboratory has several ways of controlling the reliability of the results it turns out. When chemical determinations are performed, the term batch or run is often used. A **batch** or **run** is a collection of any number of specimens to be analyzed plus any or all of the following aids for ensuring reliable results (that is, controlling the variance of the procedure): standard solutions,

blanks (these are used only for photometric procedures), control specimens, duplicates, and recoveries (these are used only occasionally).

**Proficiency testing programs** are still another means for verification of laboratory accuracy. Periodically a specimen is tested which has been provided by a government agency, a professional society, or a commercial company. Identical samples are sent to a group of laboratories participating in the proficiency testing program; each laboratory analyzes the specimen, reports the results to the agency, and is evaluated and graded on those results in comparison to results from other laboratories. In this way, quality control between laboratories is monitored (see also Quality Assurance Under CLIA Regulations, in Chapter 1).

## Standard Solutions

To determine the concentration of a substance in a specimen, there must be a basis of comparison. For analyses that result in a colored solution, a spectrophotometer is used to make this comparison (see also under Chapter 6). The buret is also used in the clinical laboratory in titration for volumetric analysis (see Measurement of Volume: Pipetting and Titration, in Chapter 4).

A **standard solution** is one that contains a known, exact amount of the substance being measured. It is prepared from high-quality reference material with measured, known amounts of a fixed and known chemical composition that can be obtained in a pure form. The standard solution is measured accurately and then treated in the testing procedure as if it were a specimen whose concentration is to be determined. Standard solutions are purchased "ready-made," already prepared from high-quality chemicals, or they can be prepared in the laboratory from high-quality chemicals that have been dried and stored in a desiccator. The standard chemical is weighed on the analytical balance and diluted volumetrically. This standard solution is usually most stable in a concentrated form, in which case it is usually referred to as a stock standard. Working standards are prepared from the stock, and sometimes an intermediate form is prepared. The working standard (a more dilute form of the stock standard) is the one employed in the actual determination. Stock and working standards are usually stored in the refrigerator. The accuracy of a procedure is absolutely dependent on the standard solution used; therefore extreme care must be taken whenever these solutions are prepared or used in a clinical laboratory.

### Standards Used in Spectrophotometry

To use the standard solution as a basis of comparison in quantitative analysis with the spectrophotometer, a series of calibrated cuvettes (or tubes) are prepared. Each cuvette contains a known different amount of the standard solution. In this way, a series of cuvettes is available containing various known amounts of the standard. Standard cuvettes are carried through the same developmental steps as cuvettes containing specimens to be measured. This set of standard cuvettes is read in the spectrophotometer, and the galvanometer readings are recorded. These readings can be recorded in percent transmittance or in absorbance units (see Chapter 6). Standard solutions are also included in automated analytic methods.

### Blanks

For every procedure using the spectrophotometer, a blank solution must be included in the batch. The **blank solution** contains reagents used in the procedure, but it does not contain the substance to be measured. It is treated with the same reagents and processed along with the unknown specimens and the standards. The blank solution is set to read 100% T on the galvanometer viewing scale. In other words, the blank tube is set to transmit 100% of the light. The other cuvettes in the same batch (unknown specimens and standards, for example) transmit only a fraction of this light, because they contain particles that absorb light (particles of the unknown substance), and thus only part of the

100% is transmitted (see also Chapter 6). Using a blank solution corrects for any color that may be present because of the reagents used or an interaction between those reagents.

### Control Specimens

The use of control specimens is based on the fact that repeated determinations on the same or different portions (or aliquots) of the same sample will not, as a rule, give identical values for any particular constituent. Many factors can produce variations in laboratory analyses. However, with a properly designed control system, it is possible to be aware of the variables and to keep them under control.

A **control specimen** is a material or solution with a known concentration of the analyte being measured in the testing procedure. For the control specimen to have meaning in terms of the reliability of all results reported by the laboratory, it must be treated exactly like any unknown specimen. It is of no value to the patient and the physician to have the control specimen within the allowable range if the value reported for the unknown is not accurate and precise. The use of quality control specimens is an indication of the overall reliability (both accuracy and precision) of the results reported by the laboratory, a part of the quality assurance process. According to CLIA '88 regulations, a minimum of two control specimens (negative or normal and positive or increased) must be run in every 24-hour period when patient specimens are being run; or, when automated analyzers are in use, the bi-level controls are run once every eight hours of operation (or once per shift).[3]

If the value of the **quality control specimen** for a particular method is not within the predetermined acceptable range, it must be assumed that the values obtained for the unknown specimens are also incorrect, and the results are not reported. After the procedure has been reviewed for any indication of error, and the error has been found and corrected, the batch must be repeated until the control value falls within the acceptable range.

If the control value in a determination is out of the acceptable range (out of control), one or more of the following factors may be responsible: (1) deterioration of reagents or standards, (2) faulty instrument or equipment, (3) dirty glassware, (4) lack of attention to timing or incubation temperature, (5) use of a method not suited to the needs and facilities of the laboratory, (6) use of poor technique by the person doing the test, owing to carelessness or lack of proper training, and (7) statistics: a certain percentage of all determinations will be statistically out of control.

The control sample may be obtained commercially or may be prepared by the individual laboratory. The most important consideration is that control samples be routinely included with each group of laboratory determinations as previously described and mandated by CLIA '88.

### Commercial Control Specimens

Commercially prepared controls can be purchased from a manufacturer. These control solutions are obtained in small samples, called aliquots, prepared originally from a large pooled supply of serum or plasma. Commercial controls are usually obtained in a lyophilized (or dried) form. Care must be taken in reconstituting the material to add exactly the correct amount of diluent (usually deionized or distilled water) and to make certain that the material is completely dissolved and well mixed. Commercial control solutions generally have an expiration date, the date by which they must be used in order to give reliable results. Controls should not be used after the expiration date. Reconstituted control solutions must be used within a relatively short period of time, which is generally specified by the manufacturer.

Commercial control material may be purchased either assayed or unassayed. Assayed control preparations have been tested by the manufacturer, and stated values are given for each of the constituents. The manufacturer should provide information concerning the analytic method and statistical procedures used in arriving at the stated values, so that the labora-

tory can determine the appropriateness of the material for its particular methods and practices. If unassayed control preparations are used, the laboratory will have to establish its own range of acceptable results for each constituent being measured. The method of arriving at this acceptable range is the same as that used in establishing limits for "laboratory-made" control solutions, to be described next. Tentative standards for manufacturers of control preparations were established in 1972 by the NCCLS.

### Control Solutions Prepared by the Laboratory

In rare circumstances, control solutions can also be prepared by the individual laboratory. In the case of control specimens for certain chemistry determinations, serum or plasma is pooled using blood obtained from known donors. The blood is tested for hepatitis B and human immunodeficiency virus (HIV) pathogens. Only disease-free blood is used. Blood is processed and serum frozen. In most laboratories, the commercially prepared product is preferable. After a sufficient pool of the serum or plasma has accumulated, the control specimens for daily use can be made. Only normal serum or plasma is used (i.e., not lipemic or hemolyzed). When enough serum has been saved, it is thawed and mixed thoroughly. After thorough mixing, the pool is divided into aliquots of a convenient size. Aliquots of 2 to 3 mL in a small tube or vial are satisfactory. These samples are then stored in a freezer. Every effort must be made to exclude from the pool serum from patients with blood-borne diseases.

### Determination of Control Range

Once a control solution has been prepared or if purchased unassayed, it is necessary for the laboratory to determine the **acceptable control range** for a particular analysis. There are various ways of establishing such a range, and one commonly employed method will be described; however, any method must adhere to statistically acceptable methods. In establishing the control range, an aliquot of the control serum being tested is processed along with the regular batch of tests for 15 to 25 days. It is imperative to thoroughly mix the thawed aliquot, since the sample layers as it freezes. In testing the control sample, it is important that it be treated exactly like an unknown specimen; it must not be treated any more or less carefully than the unknown specimen.

As described previously, repeated determinations on different aliquots of the same sample will often not give identical values for any particular constituent. However, it has been shown that if a sufficient number of repeated determinations are made, the values obtained will fall into a normal bell-shaped curve, as described above (see Fig. 8-1). When a statistically sufficient number of determinations have been run (the number is different for averaged duplicate determinations and single tests), the mathematical mean ($\overline{X}$) or average value can be calculated. The acceptable limits or variation from the mean for the control solution are then calculated on the basis of the standard deviation from the mean, using statistical formulas. Most laboratories use 2 SD above and below the mean as the allowable range of the control specimen, while others use this range as a warning limit. According to the normal bell-shaped curve (see Fig. 8-1), setting 2 SD as the allowable range for the control sample means that 95% of all determinations on that sample will fall within the allowable range, while 5% will be out of control. It may not be desirable to disallow this many batches, so the third standard deviation may be chosen as the limit of control, or the action limit. Once the range of acceptable results has been established, one of the control specimens is included in each batch of determinations. If the control value is not within the limits established, the procedure must be repeated, and no patient results may be reported to the physician until the control value is within the allowable range.

### Quality Control Chart

It is conventional in most laboratories to plot the daily control specimen values on a **quality con-**trol chart,** such as the Levy-Jennings control chart (Fig. 8-2). The control chart is made on a rectangular sheet of linear graph paper. Monthly control charts are prepared, with the days of the month marked on the horizontal axis and units of concentration for the determination in question marked on the vertical axis. The mean value for the determination in question is then indicated on the chart, in addition to the limits of acceptable error. Control limits are generally set at ±2 SD or ±3 SD on either side of the mean. The 2- and 3-SD values might be indicated, with the 2-SD value as a warning limit and the 3-SD value as an action limit. Each day the control value is plotted on the chart, and any value falling out of control can easily be seen. The control chart serves as visual documentation of the information derived from using control specimens. A different control chart is plotted for each substance being determined. It is possible to observe trends leading toward trouble by plotting the control values daily. When procedural changes, such as the addition of new reagents, standards, or instruments, are made, they are also noted on the control chart. Such a chart can assist in preventing difficulties and can aid in troubleshooting. If all is going well, the plotted control values should be distributed equally above and below the established mean value. A regular weekly visual inspection of the control chart is particularly useful for observing trends before control specimen values are actually out of the established acceptable limits. Generally, an excess of more than five control value results on one side of the mean indicates a trend, although not all such trends need action. The use of quality control programs, including the control chart, is a part of the process of laboratory quality assurance.

### Duplicate Determinations

In each batch of determinations, one of the specimens is measured in duplicate. This specimen is chosen at random from those to be tested. Often control specimens are measured in duplicate. If this is done, the allowable range for duplicates is

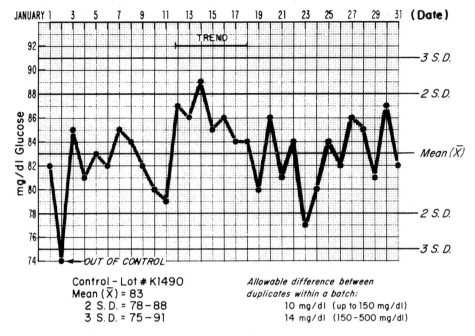

**FIG 8-2.** Quality control chart for glucose (Levy-Jennings type).

less than that for single determinations. The use of **duplicate determinations** checks the technique used—that is, the precision, or repeatability, of the method. Duplicates do not measure accuracy. It is possible to have grossly inaccurate duplicate results that agree perfectly. The allowable difference between duplicate determinations varies and must be established for each determination performed by the laboratory. This is done by using statistical formulas; the standard deviation is calculated from the differences between a set number of duplicate determinations. Duplicate determinations are also part of a quality control and assurance program.

### Recovery Solutions

**Recovery solutions** are used as an indicator of the accuracy of a particular determination. To a specimen in the batch (or to a control solution), in addition to the regular specimens, a measured amount of the pure substance being ana-lyzed is added. Theoretically, the amount of substance added should be recovered at the end of the determination if the method is an accurate one. Recoveries are not used routinely with most procedures, but are often used to evaluate new procedures. Recovery solutions are another part of quality control programs.

### Other Components of Quality Control
#### Specimen Appearance

First, consider the specimen itself—how it is collected, transported to the laboratory, received, identified, processed, and stored. The specimen should be visually inspected for hemolysis or lipemia, as these might affect or invalidate certain determinations. The presence of an abnormal appearance in the specimen should be recorded with the final result. In photometric procedures, the laboratorian should observe the final solution in the cuvette for turbidity or inappropriate color development.

### Validating New Procedures

Another part of the quality control program concerns the way new procedures are validated before they are included among the methods routinely used by the laboratory. Each laboratory must determine the reproducibility (or confidence limits) for each procedure used and establish acceptable limits of variation for control specimens. The quality control program includes calculation of the mean (or average value) and standard deviation and the preparation of control charts for each procedure.

### Control of Human Error

The quality control program should include a means of independent monitoring to minimize bias on the part of the person doing the tests. This may be done by using blind controls, such as commercial control solutions labeled as patient unknowns, or by dividing patient specimens into different aliquots to be processed blindly and independently on the same day, or carried over to another day if the constituent is stable.

### Correlation of Test Results

Another valuable quality control technique is to look at the data generated for each patient and inspect them for relationships between them. There are many relationships, such as the mathematical relationship between anions and cations in the electrolyte report, the correlation between protein and casts in urine, and the relationship between hemoglobin and hematocrit and the appearance of the blood smear in hematologic studies.

### Evaluation of Procedures

Each laboratory must have an assessment routine for all procedures, to be done on a daily, weekly, and monthly basis to detect problems such as trends and shifts in the established mean values. When such problems are indicated, it is most important that they be corrected as soon as possible. Many of the components of the quality control program are the responsibility of the laboratory supervisor or director. However, every person working in the laboratory has an important role in ensuring reliable laboratory results, by carefully doing the analysis itself, including control samples, and by calling potential problems to the attention of the supervisor.

### Proficiency Testing

In addition to the use of internal quality control programs, each laboratory should participate in at least one external control program. These are known as proficiency testing programs and are a required provision of the CLIA '88 regulations.[3,4]

**Proficiency surveys** are a means of establishing quality control between laboratories. Both state and national agencies have established programs to help laboratories maintain their quality control programs. Proficiency testing programs are available through the CAP, the Centers for Disease Control and Prevention (CDC), and various state health departments. These programs periodically send specimens to laboratories that participate in them. Each laboratory analyzes its sample, using its routine procedures, and sends the results to the program administrator. Each participating laboratory is furnished with an evaluation of its results that compares them with those of all other laboratories participating in the survey. Participation in at least one proficiency survey is an important part of a laboratory's quality control program.

## REFERENCES

1. *Accreditation Manual for Pathology and Clinical Laboratory Services: Standards and Scoring Guidelines.* Chicago, Joint Commission on Accreditation of Healthcare Organizations, 1993.
2. *Clinical Laboratory Technical Procedure Manual: Approved Guideline,* ed 3. Villanova, Pa, National Committee for Clinical Laboratory Standards, 1996, NCCLS Document GP2-A3.
3. Department of Health and Human Services, Health Care Financing Administration: Clinical Laboratory Improvement Amendments of 1988. *Federal Register,* February 28, 1992. CLIA '88, Final Rule. 42 CFR. Subpart K, 493.1201.

4. Department of Health and Human Services, Health Care Financing Administration: Clinical Laboratory Improvement Amendments of 1988. *Federal Register*, vol 60, no 78, April 24, 1995. Final rules with comment period.

5. *Physician Office Laboratory Policy and Procedure Manual.* Northfield, Ill, 1993, College of American Pathologists, Section 4, p 1.

6. *Standards for Laboratory Accreditation, Laboratory Accreditation Program,* Northfield, Ill, College of American Pathologists, 1996.

## BIBLIOGRAPHY

Burtis CA, Ashwood ER (eds.): *Tietz Textbook of Clinical Chemistry*, ed 4. Philadelphia, WB Saunders Co, 1996.

Campbell JB, Campbell JM: *Laboratory Mathematics: Medical and Biological Applications*, ed 5. St Louis, Mosby, 1997.

Henry JB (ed): *Clinical Diagnosis and Management by Laboratory Methods*, ed 19. Philadelphia, WB Saunders Co., 1996.

Meisenheimer CG: *Quality Assurance: A Complete Guide to Effective Programs*. Rockville, Md, Aspen Publications, 1985.

NCCLS: *Continuous Quality Improvement: Essential Management Approaches and Their Use in Proficiency Testing: Proposed Guideline*. Villanova, Pa, National Committee for Clinical Laboratory Stan-dards, 1997, Document GP22-P.

Revision of the laboratory regulations for Medicare, Medicaid and Clinical Laboratories Improvement Act of 1967 programs, final rule. *Federal Register* 1990; 55(March 14):50.

## STUDY QUESTIONS

1. **Define quality assurance.**

2. **Which regulations mandate the inclusion of a quality assurance program in the clinical laboratory?**

3. **Which activities of the laboratory are to be included in a quality assurance program?**

4. **Match each of the following terms (1 to 6) with the best definition (A to F):**

   1. Accuracy
   2. Precision
   3. Sensitivity
   4. Specificity
   5. Prevalence
   6. Proficiency testing program
      _____ A. Repeatability or reproducibility of a procedure
      _____ B. Allows monitoring of quality control between laboratories
      _____ C. The proportion of cases with a specific disease that gives a positive test result
      _____ D. Closeness of a result to the true or actual value
      _____ E. The proportion of a population that has the disease being studied
      _____ F. The proportion of cases without disease that gives a negative test result

5. **A new pregnancy screening test (test A) is being compared with the test now in use (test B). Ten known pregnant women and ten known nonpregnant women participate in the testing. The following are the test results for these women:**

   |  | Test A | Test B |
   | --- | --- | --- |
   | **Pregnant women** | 7 of 10 positive | 9 of 10 positive |
   | **Nonpregnant women** | 1 of 10 positive | 3 of 10 positive |

   A. What would be the sensitivity of tests A and B?
   B. What would be the specificity of tests A and B?

6. **For the following numbers: 10, 12, 15, 18, 20, 18, 14**

   A. Calculate the mean.
   B. Calculate the median.
   C. Calculate the mode.

7. **According to a gaussian curve, if the reference range for a test result is expressed as 2 SD on either side of the mean, what percentage of values would fall within that range?**

8. **Define "standard solution."**

9. **Match each of the following terms (1 to 3) with the best definition (A to C):**

    1. Standard solution
    2. Blank solution
    3. Control specimen

    _____ A. Material or solution with a known concentration of the analyte being measured

    _____ B. Reference material that is prepared with measured, known amounts of a fixed and known chemical composition that can be obtained in a pure form

    _____ C. Contains reagents used in the procedure, but does not contain the substance to be measured

10. **What is the use for a quality control chart?**

# CHAPTER 9

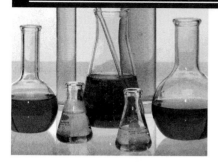

# Automation in the Clinical Laboratory

## Learning Objectives

*From study of this chapter, the reader will be able to:*

➤ Compare and contrast the various types of automated instruments available for chemistry, hematology, and urinalysis.

➤ Outline the steps involved in the process of general automation of laboratory testing.

➤ Define terms used in describing the various automated analytical systems and their methodologies.

➤ Appreciate both the benefits and the potential problems resulting from the use of automated instruments.

# INTRODUCTION TO AUTOMATION

More and more laboratory tests per patient are ordered every year; the variety of tests available has also increased, and test results are generated more quickly, providing the physician with medically useful information. The fast turn-around time required in today's medical practices has affected the instrumentation required, including the devices used for point-of-care testing (POCT). One of the major technologic changes in the clinical laboratory has been the introduction of automated analysis. An automated analytic instrument provides a means of transfer of a specimen within its complex assembly to a series of self-acting components, each of which carries out a specific process or stage of the process, ending in the analytic result being produced.

# USE OF AUTOMATION

In general, laboratory automation has centered on handling the sample after it has been received in the laboratory. Laboratory automation actually begins with the physician ordering the test and ends when the results are reported back to the physician. The sequence of the process includes test ordering, sample collection and transport to the laboratory, sample processing and analysis by the laboratory, quantitating the result, and test reporting (Fig. 9-1). The discussion in this chapter will center primarily on the steps in the sequence from the receipt of the specimen in the laboratory to the results being reported back to the physician. Automation of specimen transfer from patient care units to the laboratory is accomplished in many health care facilities by means of a vacuum tube transport system.

The demand for medically useful laboratory data has grown to such an extent that automation has become essential to process the increasing number of requests for laboratory determinations. Automation provides a means by which an increased workload can be processed rapidly and reproducibly. It does not necessarily im-

prove the accuracy of the results. Ideally, automated testing would use whole blood for analysis, as it would eliminate the need for centrifugation and the problems associated with it. Whether whole blood, serum, or plasma is used, the specimen should be pipetted directly from the primary collection tube. This would prevent specimen mix-ups when samples are transferred from the tube to the sample cups for analysis. Closed-tube sampling is also best—it eliminates possible splashing of the biologic material being tested. Centrifugation and the aliquoting of specimens are manual, time-consuming tasks, which are best automated if possible.

The first practical automated system was introduced into the clinical laboratory in 1957. Numerous other instruments for automation have been devised since that first system, employing the continuous-flow principle, was conceived by L.T. Skeggs.[3] This system was introduced commercially as the AutoAnalyzer* and has since been used extensively by many laboratories. It has undergone several refinements and modifications, so that the latest units have much more versatility than the original instrument. In the **continuous-flow analyzer,** samples flow in sequence through a channel; each sample in the batch or run is subjected to the same analytic reaction. Another group of instruments employs the principle of discrete-sample processing. The **discrete-sample analyzer** processes each specimen separately, generally in steps, somewhat as in a conventional manual method. In the discrete analyzer, each sample undergoes analysis on a discretionary basis; only selected tests are run on each sample. A third group makes use of centrifugal force to transfer and mix samples and reagents.

Originally, automation was used for the tests done most frequently in the clinical laboratory. Automation is now used in many areas of the laboratory, and in many larger laboratories very few procedures are done manually. Perhaps the chemistry department is the area in which the ad-

---

*Technicon Instruments Corp, Tarrytown, NY.

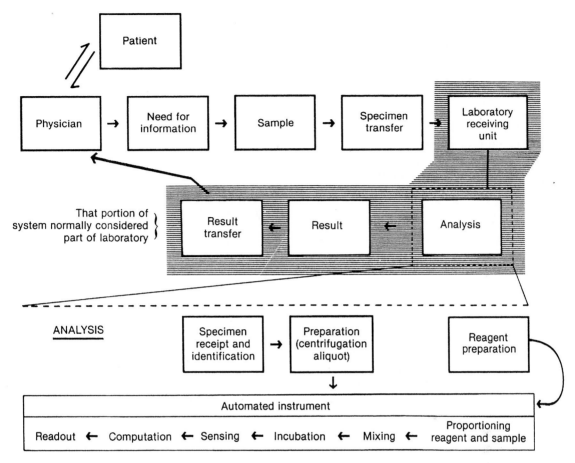

**FIG 9-1.** Example of a sequence for specimen and information flow between the patient/physician and the clinical laboratory. Lower portion shows the steps in sample processing and analysis in the laboratory. (From Kaplan LA, Pesce AJ: *Clinical Chemistry: Theory, Analysis, and Correlation*, ed 3. St Louis, Mosby, 1996, p 294.)

vent of automation has made the greatest difference. In hematology, automation has also made a great change in the way work is done. Electronic cell counters have replaced manual counting of blood cells even in clinics and physicians' office laboratories. There is an automated system for Wright's staining of blood smears. For coagulation studies several automated and semiautomated systems are available. Prothrombin time and activated partial thromboplastin time determinations can be done automatically on various instruments. Semiautomatic instruments are also used, especially for dilution steps. Several instruments are available for precise and convenient diluting, which both aspirate the sample and wash it out with the diluent. Some automatic diluters dispense and dilute in separate processes. There also are automated instruments for performing routine urinalysis determinations, for identification of bacterial organisms, and for setting up and reading blood cultures in the microbiology laboratory.

If an automated system is basically sound and in good working order, there are many advantages to its use: large numbers of samples may be processed with minimal personnel time, two or more methods may be performed simultaneously, precision is superior to that of a manual method, and calculations may not be required. Sometimes the automatic systems are so impressive in their appearance that laboratory personnel put too much faith in them and are misled about their shortcomings. These machines must be appreciated, and yet their potential problems must be noted.

The fact that automation has found its way into the clinical laboratory does not mean that the laboratorian responsible for the work is no longer important. There still are many laboratories in which manual procedures are used, especially in smaller hospitals, where the number of laboratory determinations does not always justify the purchase of an automated system. Many smaller hospital laboratories do lease these units, however, and so the size of the hospital does not always limit the use of automated equipment. Back-up manual procedures are always necessary in case of equipment failure, and these procedures must be set up and ready to use when needed. The emphasis in the laboratory has turned to faster turnaround times for results, with accuracy and precision being maintained. Automation has enabled the laboratory to accommodate the increased demand for increased numbers of tests.

### Disadvantages of Automation

Some problems that may arise with many automated units are as follows: (1) there may be limitations in the methodology that can be used (sometimes a compromise must be made that results in less accurate, although often more precise, values than are obtained with manual methods); (2) with automation, laboratorians are often discouraged from making observations and using their own judgment about potential problems; (3) many systems are impractical for small numbers of samples, and therefore man-

ual methods are still necessary as back-up procedures for emergency individual analyses; (4) back-up procedures must be available in case of instrument failures; (5) automated systems are expensive to purchase and maintain—regular maintenance requires personnel time as well as the time of trained service personnel; and (6) there is often an accumulation of irrelevant data because it is so easy to produce the results—tests are run that are not always necessary.

## COMPONENTS OF AN AUTOMATED LABORATORY ANALYZER

Automation can be applied to any or all of the steps used to perform any manual assay. Automated systems include some kind of device for sampling the patient's specimen or other samples to be tested (such as blanks, controls, and standard solutions), a mechanism to add the necessary amounts of reagents in the proper sequence, incubation modules when needed for the specific reaction, monitoring or measuring devices such as photometric technology to quantitate the extent of the reaction, and a recording mechanism to provide the final reading or permanent record of the analytic result. Most analyzers are capable of processing serum, plasma, urine, and cerebrospinal fluid, but not whole blood. A few instruments are designed to process whole blood.

The steps included in the analytic process can be performed manually or with automated instruments. Generally the automated analyzers employ the same steps as the manual methods, using the same reagents and principles. The precision is greater in automated systems, however, because the operation of the instrument is under better control and manual intervention has been replaced by mechanical intervention. Automated systems perform essentially the same types of analyses as the manual methods do. Almost any manual method can be adapted to one that is automated. As with any piece of laboratory apparatus, the manufacturer's directions must always be followed carefully. Automation of analyses generates test results rapidly and accurately and provides data that can be sent to the requesting physician in a timely manner to affect the medical decisions concerning the patient.

## GENERAL FUNCTIONS PERFORMED BY AUTOMATED ANALYZERS

Whether a laboratory determination is done manually or automatically, certain individual steps are necessary. It is generally advisable to perform as many steps as possible without manual intervention, to increase efficiency. Several of these steps can be automated for faster and more accurate results. Some methods and procedures have been partially automated, or semiautomated, by use of mechanical pipetting and diluting devices. Full automation reduces the possibility of human errors that arise from repetitive and boring manipulations done by laboratorians, such as pipetting errors in routine procedures.

### Collection, Identification, and Preparation of the Sample

The specimen must be collected properly, labeled, and transported to the laboratory for analysis. Specimen handling and processing are a vital step in the total analytic process (see Chapter 3). Automation of specimen preparation steps can include the use of bar-coded labels on samples, which allow electronic identification of the samples and the tests requested. **Bar coding** is a sample or product recognition system that, when coupled with a bar-code reader, can identify a sample and the reagents or analyses needed and relay this information to the automated analyzer. This can prevent clerical errors that could result in improperly entering patient data for analysis.

### Sample and Reagent Measurements and Mixing: Proportioning

Automated instruments measure, aspirate, and introduce samples into the analyzer reagents. Automation combines reagents and sample in a prescribed manner to yield a specific final concentration. This combination of predetermined amounts of reagent and sample is termed **proportioning.** It is important that the proper amounts of reagents be introduced to the sample and in specific sequences for the analysis to be carried through correctly. In most systems, the sample is introduced into the analyzer with a thin probe made from stainless steel. The probe passes into the sample either by directly penetrating the primary collection tube cap/stopper or after the stopper is removed from the tube. Mixing of reagents and sample can be done by stirring, agitation, or some other device.

### Incubation

In automated analyzers, incubation is simply a waiting period in which the test mixture is allowed time to react. This is done at a specified, constant temperature controlled by the analyzer.

### Monitoring or Sensing the Reaction Result

This can be done by optical, thermal, or electrical means. Chemical reactions can be monitored either at one time point or at many. Some measurements can be done in the vessel, cell, or cuvette where the reaction has taken place; this is known as **in situ monitoring.** If the sample has been transferred from the reaction vessel to the sensing device, the monitoring is external. Different instruments employ different monitoring mechanisms.

### Quantitating the Reaction Result: Computation

Quantitating by automated computation can be done by either the digital or the analog format.

#### Analog Computation

In analog computation, the microprocessor uses an electrical signal from the sensor, as from the photoelectric cell, and compares it with a reference signal, as for the blank solution. It then compares the two signals and takes the logarithm of the result as the final result for the unknown sample. **Analog computation** is derived directly from a signal from the instrument, usually in a graphic form.

### Digital Computation

**Digital computation** is usually restricted to certain mathematical functions (such as addition or subtraction). A digital computer needs an analog-to-digital converter in order to process the signals received from the many types of sensing or monitoring devices used in the automated instruments. This converter changes the voltage or current signal into a digital form, which can then be processed by the computer so that the data are available in discrete units or from calculations made from these data.

### Visualizing the Result: Results Reporting

A common and easy way to visualize an instrument readout is with the use of a television monitor **(cathode-ray tube)** or **light-emitting diodes.** Data can be visualized before results are accepted. This visualized readout can be converted to hard copy by means of a paper or tape printout. This data printout information must then be transferred or transcribed to laboratory report slips or other permanent records. If the **data** (results) are **interfaced** with, or connected to, a laboratory computer, this transcription process is done quickly and without errors, which may occur when transcription is done manually. If this interfacing is available, when the laboratorian has verified the results, they are immediately available electronically to the ordering physician.

### Standardization of Methods and Use of Controls

To ensure the accuracy of results obtained with automated systems, there must be frequent standardization of methods. Once the standardization has been done, a well-designed automated system maintains or reproduces the prescribed conditions with great precision. Frequent standardization and running of control specimens are essential to ensure this accuracy and precision. CLIA '88 regulations have mandated the use of control specimens for certain tests. For laboratories doing moderately complex or highly complex testing using automated analyzers, a minimum of two control specimens (negative or normal and positive or increased) must be run once every eight hours of operation or once per shift when patient specimens are being run[1] (see also Chapter 8).

## KINDS OF AUTOMATED ANALYZERS

Many analyzers are being manufactured for use in the clinical laboratory. The choice of which type of instrument to use is dependent on several factors: the volume of determinations done in the laboratory, the type of data profile to be generated, the level of staffing, the initial cost of the instrument, the cost of its upkeep and operation, and the amount of time it takes for each analysis. Automated instruments have been designed to perform the most frequently ordered tests because it is known that six tests make up 50% of the workload of the average chemistry laboratory and that another 14 tests make up an additional 40%.[2] Versatility and flexibility are often just as important as high volume and speed of testing, however, as automation is also desirable for the more rarely ordered tests. Automated chemistry analyzer systems can be based on chemistry reactions and methodologies along with their appropriate quantitating systems, or on immunoassay systems. Some of the most common automated instruments or categories of automated instruments are described in the following paragraphs.

### Automated Chemistry
#### Automated Batch Analyzers

**Batch analyzers** can test a batch of samples simultaneously for one particular analyte at a time. Batch analyzers can also be designed to analyze a number of different analytes. They are controlled by a microprocessor that can change the program for each different analyte to be measured. It is possible to have a batch analyzer capable of measuring 30 or more analytes, one analyte at a time. For these systems, generally there is a reagent delivery apparatus for each reagent needed. This type of analyzer does not require that every sample be tested for every analyte.

### Random Access or Selective Analyzers

The **random access analyzer** does all the selected determinations on a patient sample before it goes on to the next sample. These analyzers can process different assay combinations for individual specimens. The microprocessor enables the analyzer to perform up to 30 determinations. The selected tests are ordered from the menu, and the testing is begun, with the unordered tests being left undone. A sampling device begins the process by measuring the exact amount of sample into the required cells. The microprocessor controls the addition of the necessary diluents and reagents to each cell. After the proper reacting period, the microprocessor begins the spectrophotometric measurements of the various cells, the reaction results are calculated, control values are checked, and the results are reported. Some analyzers of this type have a circular configuration utilizing an analytic turntable device for the various cells. Other random access analyzers have a parallel configuration.

### Discrete Analyzers

Instruments that compartmentalize each sample reaction are **discrete analyzers.** In these analyzers, the sample aliquot and the reagent are contained in a single cuvette that is physically separated from all other cuvettes. Most of the commonly used laboratory chemistry analyzers are of the discrete type.

### Du Pont Automated Clinical Analyzers

The automated clinical analyzers (ACA) introduced by Du Pont* are designed to perform analyses in prepackaged plastic bags. They are discrete, selective analyzers. The sample is automatically discharged into the pack, the reagents that are compartmentalized in the pack are released and mixed with the sample, and the functions that are necessary to carry out a particular analysis are carried out. Samples can be serum, plasma, urine, or cerebrospinal fluid. For some methods, measurement is made photoelectrically; for end-point methods, the measurement is done bichromatically. A Du Pont ACA requires a separate reagent pack for each test, which also serves as the reaction cuvette. The reagent packs allow introduction of the sample into various reagent compartments, where different stages of reagent mixing and reactions occur, depending on the analysis to be done. The pack moves to the photometer, where the amount of absorbance for the particular constituent being measured is noted electronically. The instrument's computer calculates the concentration for the unknown along with the concentrations for the necessary controls and standards.

A Du Pont ACA can serve as a general chemistry analyzer in small hospital laboratories. It can also be used in medium-sized laboratories as a specialty analyzer. Any combination of tests can be run on any sample at any time.

### Vitros Clinical Chemistry Analyzer

There are various models of the Vitros Clinical Chemistry Analyzer*; they are generally discrete, selective analyzers that use a random access design. This instrument was formerly known as Ektachem, an Eastman Kodak product. The Vitros Clinical Chemistry Analyzer utilizes dry film technology, in which the dry reagents are impregnated into Vitros Clinical Chemistry Slides. A thin layer of gelatin is mounted on plastic slides to which the dry reagent is added. The addition of the sample provides the necessary solvent (water) to rehydrate the dry reagents. The slides are composed of multiple layers of film, some of which serve as ultrafilters for the sample. Others provide reactive reagents for the particular analysis being performed.

---

*Du Pont Medical Products, Wilmington, Del.

*Johnson & Johnson Clinical Diagnostics, Rochester, NY.

Samples are pipetted from bar-coded primary collection tubes or from sample cups on a turntable. The sample cups are covered with a top that can be penetrated by the automatic robotic device attached to a disposable pipette. This robotic device applies the measured sample to the selected dry reagent slide. Slides are automatically dispensed from method-specific cartridges. Slides are incubated while color development takes place. For methods utilizing reflectance photometry, after the reaction has taken place on the slide and incubation has occurred, reflected radiant energy is read, with the measured energy being relayed to a microprocessor. The reflected energy is converted into concentration units. Used slides are automatically dropped into containers for disposal. Printouts are available with results for unknown samples and controls.

### Abbott IMx

The IMx* is a bench top immunoassay system capable of producing 40 results per hour. It combines two assay technologies in one system: **latex-microparticle enzyme immunoassay (MEIA) technology** and fluorescence polarization immunoassay. A robotic probe assembly dispenses the sample into either a predilution well for some assays or a reaction well for others. Diluent and reagent with a latex particle suspension are also dispensed into the reaction well by the probe. A bar-code reader scans the reagent pack to select the assay chosen to be done. During the incubation step that follows, an immunocomplex forms. The incubation time is assay specific. After incubation, the reaction mixture (the immunocomplex) is transferred to a capture surface, where the microparticles, together with the bound analyte, adhere to the inert glass-fiber matrix, where they are bound irreversibly to the matrix. After a washing step, an alkaline phosphatase conjugate and substrate are added and the reaction is allowed to continue. The fluorescence of the product formed is measured and related to quantitation of the analyte being assayed.

### Automated Analyzers for the Physician's Office

Since physicians' office laboratories are performing many tests, and since the number of these laboratories is expected to increase over the next few years, many automated or semiautomated analyzers have been introduced for use outside the traditional hospital laboratory setting. The criteria used by the physician to select the appropriate instrument(s) for a particular laboratory include the type of practice or specialty, the volume of tests to be done, whether single tests or chemistry profiles are needed, the turnaround time available, and the cost of the analyzer and its reagents.

In a physician's office laboratory, ideally the specimen to be tested would be whole blood and the automatic pipetting of the specimen and necessary reagents would be done by the analyzer, eliminating as much interaction by laboratory personnel as possible. The use of instruments with stable calibration curves is important, and a quality control program should be available from the manufacturer. Data computation from the analyzing instruments should be interfaced with a computer, if possible, to provide the necessary documentation of laboratory results. Quality control information can also be stored in the computer. The instrument should be easy to use, and, because in many physicians' office laboratories there will be persons working who have little or no laboratory training, the instrument should require only a limited user training period. The reagents, whether wet or dry, should be bar coded, prepackaged, and stable for at least 6 months.

**Dry Reagent Systems.** In **dry-film technology systems,** the reagents are already proportioned in the required amounts and only the sample must be added. The sample may be added volumetrically or by saturation addition, in which an excess of the sample is exposed to

---

*Abbott Laboratories, Diagnostics Division, Irving, Tex.

the dry-film reagent and the pores of the film allow only a fixed amount of sample to be absorbed—this is its proportioning mechanism. Several systems are available for physicians' offices that use this technology. They include the Seralyzer[*]; the DT System,[†] which is similar to the larger Vitros technology; the i-STAT[‡]; the Analyst system[§]; and the Reflotron system.[¶] Each has slightly different testing reagents, but the principle of use is similar. The Reflotron system is described here.

**Reflotron System.** The solid-phase reagent test tabs used in this system are bar coded to identify the tests, the reaction parameters, and the calibration curves for each assay. The manufacturer establishes the calibration curve for each lot of reagent strips, eliminating the need for calibration by the laboratory. The reagent strips have a shelf life of from 1 to 2 years. In this system, whole blood from a finger or heel stick can be used for analysis. The blood is placed on the reagent strip, made up of a glass fiber pad that separates the plasma from the red cells. The separation of cells from plasma is accomplished by capillary action, leaving the required plasma to react with the reagent in the strip at a temperature of 37° C. Excess plasma is removed from the reaction site. The analyte concentration is determined by reflectance photometry and recorded visually or interfaced with a laboratory computer.

**Wet Chemistry Reagent Systems.** One system utilizing wet reagent chemistry is the Vision system,[‖] which is described in this section.

**Vision System.** This automated system uses specially designed reagent packs, which are disposable. The reagent pack is a self-contained unit with a cuvette, liquid reagents, and bar codes to identify the assay to be done. Blood can be obtained by finger or heel stick and placed in a special tube provided by the manufacturer. This special tube can then be inserted directly into the reagent pack, eliminating the step of pipetting the sample from the capillary tube into the analyzer. Two drops of blood, serum, or plasma are placed in the multichambered reagent pack, and the packs are placed in the ten-position rotor in the analyzer. The red cells, if whole blood is used, are separated from plasma by centrifugal force. Next the packs are rotated to a 90-degree angle, allowing the premeasured amount of sample and the reagents to be transferred into the cuvette. The reaction occurs at 37° C; it is monitored, and the absorbances are measured bichromatically. The reagents for this system are stable for several months, and one to ten analytes can be measured. The Vision system is suitable for doing batches of tests, profiles, or stat procedures.

## Automated Hematology

The best source of information about the various instruments available is the manufacturers' product information literature. The continual advances in commercial instruments for hematologic use and their variety preclude an adequate description of them in this chapter. Some basic, general information follows, however.

### Automated Cell Counters

**Automated cell counters** are used extensively in hematology to identify and enumerate the blood cells in a given patient sample. Even the simplest instruments can identify and count red blood cells, white blood cells, and platelets. In more sophisticated instruments, the types of white blood cells can be identified and counted. These instruments are known as **flow cytometers.**

Most automated cell counters can be classified as one of two types, those using electrical resistance and those using optical methods with focused laser beams, in which cells cause a change in the deflection of a beam of light. In the cell counters using **optical methods,** the deflec-

---

[*]Bayer Corp, Diagnostics Division, Tarrytown, NY.
[†]Johnson & Johnson Clinical Diagnostics, Rochester, NY.
[‡]i-STAT Corp, Princeton, NJ.
[§]Du Pont Medical Products, Wilmington, Del.
[¶]Boehringer Mannheim Diagnostics, Indianapolis, Ind.
[‖]Abbott Laboratories, Diagnostics Division, Irving, Tex.

tions are converted to measurable pulses by a photo multiplier tube. Both types of instruments count thousands of cells in a few seconds, and both decrease the coefficient of variation and increase the precision of cell counts as compared with manual methods (see Automated Cell Counting Methods, in Chapter 12).

In the **electrical resistance cell counters,** blood cells passing through an aperture through which a current is flowing cause a change in electrical resistance that is counted as voltage pulses. The voltage pulses are amplified and can be displayed on an oscilloscope screen. Each spike indicates a cell. Several manufacturers employ this principle in instruments for cell counting; these include Coulter,* Abbott,[†] and Nova.[‡]

Alternative systems using **capillary tube density gradient** methodology are available; these systems measure red blood cells, white blood cells, and platelets in a manner similar to the way in which microhematocrits are measured after centrifugation, in which cell layers are noted. One system employing this methodology is the QBC II Plus.[§] In this methodology, the different types of blood cells have different densities, so after centrifugation, they will settle in separate layers. By use of further mechanical expansion and optical magnification, augmented by supravital fluorochrome staining, other measurements are derived.

### Automated Differential Counters

Automated differential counters utilize the impedance method to construct a size-distributed histogram of white blood cells. In most of these instruments, three subpopulations of white cells are counted: lymphocytes, other mononuclear cells, and granulocytes. A computer calculates the number of particles in each area as a percentage of the total white blood cell count histogram. Any abnormal histograms are flagged for review.

### Automated Urinalysis

Instruments are available to automate the routine urinalysis (UA), or parts of it, and most can be interfaced with laboratory computers. One automated system is the Yellow IRIS Urinalysis Workstation,* which includes a slideless sediment examination. Other systems include the Clinitek,[†] the Chemstrip Urine Analyzer,[‡] and the Rapimat.[§] These systems all utilize reflectance photometers for reading their respective reagent strips. Once the strip is placed in the analyzer, the microprocessor mechanically moves the strip into the reflectometer, turns on the light source needed, records the reflectance data, calculates the results, and removes the strip for disposal. (See Chapter 14.)

More recently available, the Clinitek Atlas is an automated urine chemistry analyzer that aspirates the specimen directly from the sample tube, which is then also centrifuged for the microscopic examination of the urine specimen. For chemical analyses, the specimen is aspirated from the sample tube and added to a strip containing nine reactive reagent pads (for chemical and physicochemical tests) and one nonreactive pad (for color) per specimen, supplied on a roll of plastic film to which are affixed 490 reagent strips. Use of this reflectance spectrophotometric instrument eliminates the need for "dipping" the reagent strip into the patient's urine specimen. It measures clarity, color, and specific gravity by refractive index. Samples are identified by bar code, and results may be interfaced to the laboratory computer for reporting.

---

*Coulter Electronics, Hialeah, Fla.
[†]Abbott Laboratories, Diagnostics Division, Irving, Tex.
[‡]Nova Biomedical, Waltham, Mass.
[§]Becton, Dickinson & Co, Franklin Lakes, NJ.

---

*International Remote Imaging Systems, Inc., Chatsworth, Calif.
[†]Bayer Corp, Diagnostics Division, Tarrytown, NY.
[‡]Boehringer Mannheim Diagnostics, Indianapolis, Ind.
[§]Behring Diagnostics, Inc, Somerville, NJ.

# REFERENCES

1. Department of Health and Human Services, Health Care Financing Administration: Clinical Laboratory Improvement Amendments of 1988. *Federal Register,* vol 60, no 78, April 24, 1995. Final rules with comment period.
2. Kaplan LA, Pesce AJ: *Clinical Chemistry: Theory, Analysis, and Correlation,* ed 3. St Louis, Mosby, 1996.
3. Skeggs LT Jr: An automated method for colorimetric analysis. *Am J Clin Pathol* 1957; 28:311.

# BIBLIOGRAPHY

Bender GT: *Principles of Clinical Instrumentation.* Philadelphia, WB Saunders Co, 1987.

Burtis, CA, Ashwood ER (eds): *Tietz Fundamentals of Clinical Chemistry,* ed 4. Philadelphia, WB Saunders Co, 1996.

*Physician's Office Laboratory Guidelines: Tentative Guidelines, ed 3.* Villanova, Pa, National Committee for Clinical Laboratory Standards, 1995, POL ½-T3 and POL 3-R.

## STUDY QUESTIONS

1. **Match each of the following terms (1 to 5) with its definition (A to E):**

   1. Discrete selective analyzer
   2. Continuous-flow analyzer
   3. Proportioning
   4. Dry-film technology
   5. Random access analyzer

   _____ A. Analyzer in which samples flow in sequence through a channel; each sample in the batch or run is subjected to the same analytic reaction.

   _____ B. A combining of predetermined amounts of reagent and sample.

   _____ C. Technology in which the reagents are already proportioned in the required amounts on slides and only the sample must be added.

   _____ D. Analyzer in which each sample undergoes analysis on a discretionary basis and only selected tests are run on each sample.

   _____ E. Analyzer that does all the selected determinations on a patient sample before it goes on to the next sample.

2. **List the sequence of the automation process for laboratory testing, beginning with test ordering by the physician.**

3. **What are the CLIA '88 regulations regarding use of control specimens in automated laboratory testing?**

# CHAPTER 10

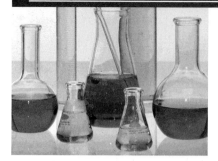

# Introduction to Laboratory Computers

## Learning Objectives

*From study of this chapter, the reader will be able to:*

➤ Be familiar with the terminology used to describe the components of a laboratory information system.

➤ Describe the parts of and uses for laboratory computers.

# PURPOSE OF THE LABORATORY COMPUTER

Because the number of tests performed in the clinical laboratory has grown so dramatically over the years and because so much analytic information has been produced by these tests, the ability to process this information efficiently and accurately has become essential. This information is, of course, utilized for the benefit of the patient. We have seen that the quality assurance process requires the documentation of all work involved in patient care. The laboratory computer provides this service. It is a powerful tool for improvement of the quality of the work done as well as the productivity of the laboratorians employed to do the work. The advent of the microcomputer, under the control of microprocessors, has been responsible for the many changes in the design of laboratory analyzers and their interfaces with laboratory information systems (LIS).

The number of laboratory tests has increased in part as a result of the development of new diagnostic tests and also because of the increased use of automated analyzers. Many **laboratory information systems (LIS)** have been developed to assist in the delivery of the data. The laboratory computer system must be capable of delivering this information to the physician, the billing department, the patient record department, and other administrative support sites, and of ensuring that the data are communicated in a timely manner. In this way, the laboratory computer greatly influences the work done in the laboratory but also aids the users of the results outside the laboratory setting.

# FUNCTIONS AND USES OF THE LABORATORY COMPUTER

An important function of the laboratory computer is to organize the various pieces of information and provide ready access to this information when it is needed. The information provided by each laboratory procedure should be maximized so that the patient receives the greatest benefit at the lowest cost. The functions of

laboratory computers include three categories: preanalytical, analytical, and postanalytical. Test ordering, printing specimen labels, and collecting the required specimens are included in the **preanalytical functions.** Generating work lists, doing the analyses, automatic entering of results via interfaces, quality control measures, and results verification are done as part of the **analytical functions** (process). **Postanalytical functions** include generating chart reports, printing result reports as needed, archiving patient results, workload recording, and billing.

## Preanalytical Functions

Identifying and defining the patient in the computer system must take place before any testing is done. Most health care institutions assign a unique identification number to each patient and also enter other demographic information about the patient in the information database—information such as name, gender, age or birth date, and referring or attending physician. This is known as the **patient demographics.** This information is collected at the time of admission to the facility and entered into the hospital information system (HIS). The information is then transferred automatically and electronically from the HIS to the LIS.

Test ordering, or **order entry,** is an important first step in use of the laboratory information system. Specific data are needed during the order entry process: a patient number and a patient name, name of ordering physician or physicians, name of physician(s) to receive the report, test request time and date, time the specimen was or will be collected, name of person entering the request, tests to be performed, priority of the test request (such as stat or routine), and any other specimen comments pertaining to the request. Orders can be received most efficiently by the LIS through a computer-to-computer interface with the hospital information system, whereby physicians or nursing personnel directly order the test electronically. The laboratory can also receive a paper copy of the tests requested—the test request form or requisition, from which laboratory personnel enter the test request into the laboratory information system. The same data are needed on the paper form as are needed on the electronic order. The computer will generate collection lists, work lists, or logs with patient demographics and any necessary collection or analysis information. Work lists generated may include a loading list for a particular analyzer, for example. The LIS has numerous checks and balances built into it as a part of the order entry process.

Computerized order entry triggers the generation of specimen labels and prints those needed for the collection process. The patient demographic information will be printed on the labels (Fig. 10-1), along with special accession numbers in some institutions. These accession numbers will be represented in the bar-coding format for each of the patient's specimen labels. Bar coding greatly limits errors in specimen handling and improves productivity. For the greatest benefit, the specimen bar coding is also coordinated with the automated instruments used for testing, in which case the sampling is done directly from the primary collection tube (see Chapter 9).

After the specimen has been collected, it is sent to the laboratory for analysis.

## Analytical Functions

The automated analyzers used must link each specimen to its specific test request; this is best

VALIDATION PATIENT
**9-999-999-3**
PLC        02/28/94 11:05
DIGOXIN
**398291**
**AUPS**

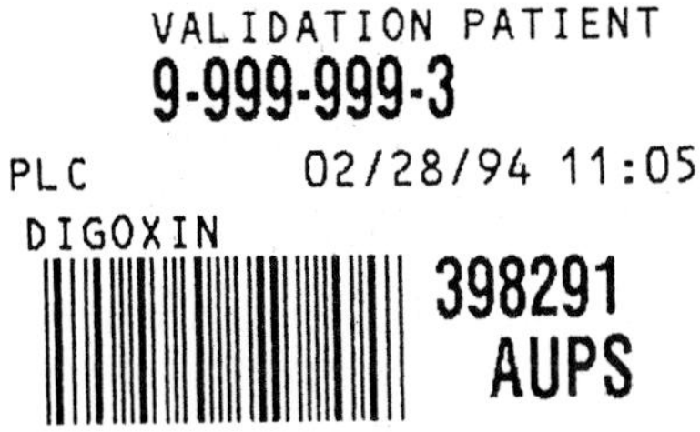

**FIG 10-1.** An example of a bar-coded specimen label. The six-digit specimen number (398291) is bar coded. The patient number, patient demographics, time/date, and test are written in human readable letters. (From Kaplan LA, Pesce AJ: *Clinical Chemistry: Theory, Analysis, and Correlation,* ed 3. St. Louis, Mosby, 1996, p 326.)

done automatically through the use of bar codes on the specimen label but can be done manually by the laboratorian, who can link the sample at the instrument to the specimen number in the computer. Any results generated must be **verified** (approved or reviewed) by the laboratorian before the data are released to the patient report. Data useful to the laboratorian for this verification process include the display of "flags" signifying results that are outside the reference range values, the presence of **critical** or **panic values** (possible life-threatening values), values out of the technical range for the analyzer, or by failing other checks and balances built into the system. The use of automated analyzers is discussed in Chapter 9.

Quality assurance procedures, including the use of quality control solutions, are part of the analytical functions of the analyzer and its interfaced computer. CLIA '88 regulations require the documentation of all quality control data associated with any test results reported.

## Postanalytical Functions

The end product of the work done by the clinical laboratory consists of the testing results produced by the particular methodology used, which are provided in the **laboratory report.** The data can be electronically transmitted to printers, computer terminals, or hand held pager terminals, giving rapid access to the test information for the user.

### The Laboratory Report

An important use for the laboratory computer is to provide the physician with one comprehensive laboratory report that contains all the test information generated by the various laboratories that have performed analyses for a single patient. A paper report is still required by most accreditation agencies and by current medical practice. CLIA '88 regulations require that an LIS have the capacity to print or reprint reports easily when needed. The format of the report should be such that the test results are clear and unambiguous. Many questions need answering to establish or rule out a particular diagnosis, and the report should facilitate this process. The report should indicate any abnormality. It should answer these questions: What is the predictive value of the test for the disease in question? Is the result meaningful? What other factors could produce the result? What should be done next?

If the diagnosis has already been made, other uses can be made for the information on the report form, such as the management of the treatment plan for the patient. The physician must know the result of the most recent laboratory test, what clinically significant changes have occurred since the last test (through the retrieval of current and historical data), whether changes in therapy are indicated, and when the test should next be performed. This information constitutes what is known as an **interpretive report.**

An interpretive report form should give information about the range of reference values, flag any abnormal values, and provide these data in a readily accessible format.

### Other Uses

The laboratory computer system also provides data for the hospital billing department, sends patient laboratory test data to the record room, and provides lists of available laboratory tests for the physician.

Special reports and lists can be generated by the computer. Lists of samples waiting to be tested, quality control data, lists of abnormal test results, and maintenance records all can be generated by the computer with considerable efficiency. The storage of preexisting data—all available tests, specimen requirements, quality control information (means, standard deviations, information included on report forms), instrument parameters—makes up the **database.**

### Intralaboratory Communication

The computer stores information about laboratory policies, mission statements and specific objectives for the particular laboratory facility, and statements about laboratory medicine phi-losophy, in general. Procedure manuals with information about each test procedure, reference range statistics, the quality control systems used, test procedure reference materials, dates of adoption of new test methods, and evidence of other periodic review measures can be stored in the laboratory information system. The College of American Pathologists (CAP) accreditation standards, for example, require that laboratories establish methods for communication of needed information to ensure prompt, reliable reporting of results and that they have appropriate data storage and retrieval capacity.[1]

### Extralaboratory Communication

Information regarding specimen requirements —procurement, transport, and processing—can be stored in an accessible form. Physicians ordering a test, nurses assisting in specimen collection, and others involved with the transport or handling of the specimen must have this information readily available.

Laboratory information systems often are interfaced with other information systems, most commonly the **hospital information system (HIS). Interfacing** is the use of a program allowing electronic communication between two computers. The HIS manages patient census information and demographics and systems for billing, and the more complex systems process and store patient medical information. The interfacing of the HIS and the laboratory computer facilitates the exchange of test request orders, information about the patient (patient census), the return of analytic results (the laboratory report), and the charges for the tests ordered and reported. When the data are verified, results can be retrieved by nurses or physicians in the patient care areas by use of terminals and printers. This linking of hospital and laboratory computer systems is not easy, and totally integrated systems require an institutional commitment to the process. A well-designed, easily accessible HIS-LIS database offers significant improvements in medical record keeping, patient care planning, budget planning, and general operations management tasks.

# MAJOR COMPONENTS OF THE LABORATORY COMPUTER

Electronic computer systems are made up of **hardware,** the physical or "hard" parts of the computer, and **software,** the instructions that tell the computer what to do.

## Hardware

Hardware for the computer consists of the physical components of the computer system. Central processing units, printers, and other terminals used for information input and output are examples of computer hardware.

### Central Processing Unit

The **central processing unit (CPU)** is the central component of the computer. It functions as the brains of the system. The CPU is made up of a control unit, an **arithmetic logic unit (ALU),** and the **central memory.** The CPU carries out the instructions (program) given by the user.

### Data Storage Devices

An important component is the data, or memory, storage section. This contains all the necessary instructions and data needed to operate the computer system. In addition, any short-term information, such as patient records and laboratory data, may also be stored temporarily in the memory. In addition to central memory, magnetic tapes and disks are used to store less frequently accessed data. These require more time for data retrieval but are considerably less expensive than central memory.

**Central Memory, Random Access Memory.** Central memory provides storage and rapid access. **Random access memory (RAM)** is a type of central memory and is commonly used to store data that are frequently altered, changed, or updated.

**Magnetic Tapes.** Magnetic tapes are the least expensive form of data storage. Access to information is generally slow. Data stored on tapes are sequential; all information, whether it is needed or not, must be serially passed over to find the needed information. Access time can be minutes, not seconds. The use of tapes is very common, however, for archival storage of data no longer needed on-line to the computer. Tapes are also used as a standard method for transporting information between computers.

**Hard Disks. Hard disks,** or a **hard drive,** are revolving disks, small record-like plates, with a magnetic surface that can be easily accessed. Data are stored in tracks, a series of concentric circles on the disk. Data are retrieved by positioning the reading head over the desired portion of the track, allowing a given piece of information to rotate under the head. Accessing information from disks takes milliseconds, not minutes. The transfer of information stored on a hard disk to another computer is usually not possible, and the cost of the disks and associated hardware is usually considerably higher than that of magnetic tape.

**Floppy Disks. Floppy disks,** also called **diskettes,** are used in many microcomputer-based instruments and word processors because of their low cost.

### Input Devices

**Input devices** allow communication between the user and the CPU. There are several peripheral devices that allow this communication to take place. Some of these also function as output devices. The exchange of information between the computer and the user is called interfacing. Interfacing is accomplished through one of several kinds of devices. Most often the computer information is displayed on a video screen—the display screen.

Data input and output can be accomplished either by command line entry, also known as string entry, or by menu selection. Command line entry is the inputting of a series of individual commands or pieces of information in a single step to instruct the computer about the task to be done. Information about a patient identification number and a specific piece of information about a test result for that patient are examples of data that could be inputted by string entry. Instead of each piece of information being entered separately, the data are entered together ("strung" together). Individual command lines are separated from each other by commas. By entering a series of related commands, or inputs, as a single command, the user spends less time at the keyboard, the usual input device.

**Menus** are lists of programs or functions or other options offered by the system. A cursor is moved to the point on the list—for example, a list of tests—that is the option of choice and placed on the test desired. The use of a menu for data input is best when there are a limited number of choices to be made and also for persons who are new to the use of the computer.

**Keyboard.** Standardized codes called **ASCII (American Standard Code for Information Interchange)** allow the entire keyboard to be used to enter alphanumeric (letters and numerical symbols) as well as numerical data into the computer. More complex systems use function keys, which enter a series of commands, reducing the number of keystrokes required to carry out a function such as returning to a previous screen or terminating the data entry.

**Cathode-Ray Tube.** The **cathode-ray tube (CRT)** allows exchange of information between the user and the CPU on a specially designed television tube. The user can view on the display screen the commands given as well as the data exchanged.

**Bar-Code Reader.** Bar-code readers read a series of black lines (bars) on a label and convert these data to a sequence of numbers representing specific information (Fig. 10-1). This information can be patient identification, tests requested, or identification of a reagent for a test. Bar codes are being used on identification wristbands and hopefully will allow for better control of accuracy for patient identification purposes and for labels for specimen containers and test requests.

**Interfacing.** Much laboratory time has been saved by the interfacing of the laboratory computer with the analytic testing instrument so that the test result can be entered directly into the computer information system. A port is used to permit the main computer to interface with the computer of the analytic instrument. The test result data are transferred directly over a single wire. The port is a memory location in the CPU that is connected to a series of wires. The wires are, in turn, connected to the instrument computer.

**Other Input Devices.** Additional input devices can enhance the exchange of information between user and computer. Touch screens allow interaction with the CPU through a menu. The position of touch on the screen determines the choice. A light pen (stylus) can be used to interact with a light-sensitive screen to indicate a menu choice. A mouse is a manual device that moves a cursor when the device is rolled along a flat surface. It also interacts with the computer through a menu.

### Output Devices

**Output** is any information that the computer generates as a result of its calculations or processing. The CRT, printers, and instrument computers all can function as **output devices.** The computer directs the needed data from its central memory or from a storage device (magnetic tape or disk) to the specific output device. For the CRT, the output of the data generated is displayed on the screen. The printer is the usual output device of the computer system and produces a paper copy.

As laboratory results are entered and verified, a documented trail can be produced by the computer system. The organization of the data in the computer is called the database.

The computer has stored the data on when a test was ordered, when the specimen was collected, when the test was done in the laboratory, and when the test result was entered and verified. In addition, data are available about who ordered the test, who collected the specimen, and who ran the test in the laboratory. The names of the persons involved in the process are stored in the database of the computer. This documentation of data is an important part of the quality assurance program of the laboratory.

**Printers.** When the computer-generated data are printed on paper, they are called **hard copy.** The printed output data are placed on the patient's chart and added to the official (legal) medical record of the patient. The format or style of the printed report is determined by the kind of software program used. This allows for changes when needed.

One specific output function utilizing the printer is the generating of printed labels for specimen containers at the time of order entry for a test. Another use for printed output is the generation of a printed list of test requests along with their accession numbers. This list defines the workload for the laboratory for a given time period and thus is called a **work list.** This work list can be used in planning the day's work for specific areas within the laboratory. Computer-generated lists showing test results flagged for critical values or abnormal results can alert the laboratorian to transmit critical results to the physician or to ask to have a test repeated. Some computer systems will compare a patient result with a previous result for that patient. This is called a **difference check,** which serves to alert the laboratorian to an otherwise undetected error in analysis. This difference check can also signify a change in the condition of the patient and can alert the physician to this change.

## Software

Instructions that direct the computer to perform its specific tasks are called the software or **program.** These instructions direct the various tasks to be done, using a predetermined order. Instructions that direct the collection of the data, their assimilation, the various tasks that make use of the data, and the transfer of data are all included in the software program. The program also contains the information needed to communicate with the input and output devices being used.

Software programs are written in a specific language so that the computer can understand or accept it. Only by changing the program can any modification be made in the predetermined instructions for the operation of the laboratory information system.

## FUTURE CONSIDERATIONS FOR LABORATORY COMPUTERS

New technologies for computers in the laboratory include the use of voice-recognition devices and portable electronic handwriting notebooks or tablets. Using voice recognition as input for the computer requires considerable computer power. These devices could be potentially easier to use than keyboards, but most are still in the developmental stage.

With the increased use of POCT, it has been difficult to interface results with the LIS; because many POCT devices are currently limited in their ability to interact with the LIS, results cannot be documented as regulations mandate. Often results are needed quickly, however, and the POCT results are utilized by clinicians without the proper documentation. When results are not in the LIS, they are not available for use by all clinical personnel. Interfacing POCT instrumentation with the LIS remains a problem.

Another challenge for computer technology is that of providing more information to the physician about the utilization of the various tests or interpretive data. Access to more clinical information and medical decision-making processes would also be beneficial to the physician.

Proposals have been made to utilize computerized medical charts as an effective cost-reduction scheme. By use of computerized medical charts, information pertaining to the patient could be transferred between users much more efficiently. This activity could be coupled with order entry and guidelines for medical practice. To date, the challenge of accomplishing this task is ongoing.

## REFERENCES

1. Commission on Laboratory Accreditation: Laboratory Accreditation Manual, Inspection Checklist, Section 1, Laboratory general-computer services. Northfield, Ill,. College of American Pathologists, 1996.

## BIBLIOGRAPHY

Aller RD, Elevitch FR (eds): *Clinics in Laboratory Medicine Symposium on Computers in the Clinical Laboratory*, vol 3. Philadelphia, WB Saunders Co, 1983.

Burtis CA, Ashwood ER (eds): *Tietz Textbook of Clinical Chemistry*, ed 4, Philadelphia, WB Saunders Co, 1996.

College of American Pathologists: Standards for laboratory accreditation. *Pathologist* 1982; 36:641.

Henry JB (ed): *Clinical Diagnosis and Management by Laboratory Methods*, ed 19. Philadelphia, WB Saunders Co, 1996.

Kaplan LA, Pesce AJ: *Clinical Chemistry: Theory, Analysis, and Correlation*, ed 3. St Louis, Mosby, 1996.

## STUDY QUESTIONS

1. **Match the following terms (1 to 6) with their definitions (A to F):**

   1. Hardware
   2. Software
   3. Interface
   4. Database
   5. Program
   6. Difference check

   _____ A. Comparison of a patient result with a previous result for that same patient.

   _____ B. The physical or "hard" parts of the computer.

   _____ C. Instructions directing the computer hardware to do specific functions.

   _____ D. The instructions that tell the computer what to do.

   _____ E. Program allowing two computers to interchange data electronically.

   _____ F. Organization of the data in the computer.

2. **What are two common types of output devices?**

3. **What are four input devices?**

4. **Identify the following abbreviations:**
   A. CPU
   B. RAM
   C. LIS
   D. HIS

5. **What are three preanalytical functions of a laboratory computer?**

6. **What are three postanalytical functions of a laboratory computer?**

# PART II

# Divisions of the Clinical Laboratory

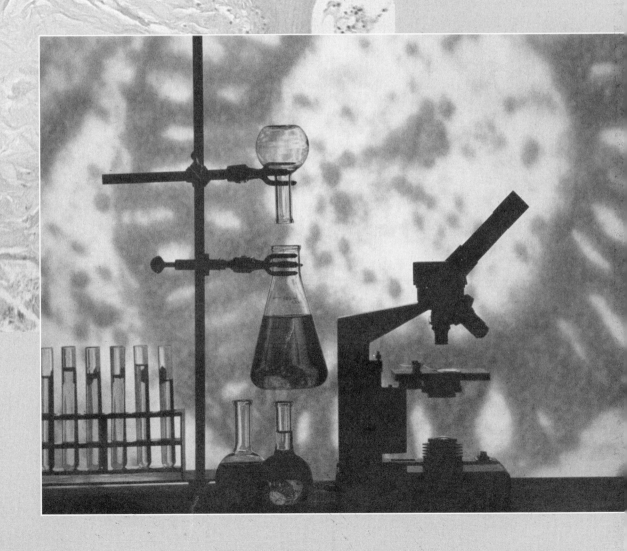

# CHAPTER 11

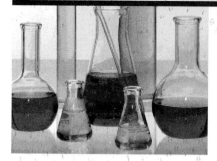

# *Chemistry*

## Learning Objectives

*From study of this chapter, the reader will be able to:*

➤ Describe briefly some of the general instrumentation and methodologies used for chemistry assays.

➤ Appreciate the importance of specimen collection requirements for chemistry assays.

➤ Differentiate between type I diabetes mellitus (insulin-dependent diabetes mellitus [IDDM]) and type II diabetes mellitus (non–insulin-dependent diabetes mellitus [NIDDM]) and understand the pathophysiology of glucose metabolism as it affects the various types of diabetes mellitus.

➤ Describe the tests for electrolytes and explain how their altered concentrations affect the physiologic state of the body.

➤ Describe the two tests that can be used to assess renal function—urea/urea nitrogen and creatinine—and explain how they are different.

➤ State the purpose of the creatinine clearance test and explain how it is calculated.

➤ Describe tests for lipids in serum and plasma and explain the importance of their presence and measurement.

➤ Discuss the risk factors for atherosclerosis.

➤ Describe the metabolism of bilirubin by the liver and define the types of jaundice in terms of their corresponding pathophysiologic states.

➤ Describe tests for liver function.

## INTRODUCTION TO CLINICAL CHEMISTRY

The field of laboratory medicine continues to expand rapidly, and with it the specialty of clinical chemistry. Chemistry is an area in which changes have occurred rapidly, because of the variety of automated instrumentation available. The uses and general principles of selected tests and methodologies in the clinical chemistry laboratory are discussed in this chapter (see also Chapter 9).

The techniques of most chemical procedures performed in the laboratory are not in themselves difficult, but their proper execution requires a good background in the principles involved. It is essential, therefore, that the basic principles as well as the techniques used in clinical chemistry be mastered by the laboratorian. These include the basic theory of chemical determinations, use and care of laboratory equipment and apparatus, application of quantitative measurement, proper preparation of reagents, recognition of problems when they arise, proper collection and handling of laboratory specimens, reporting of results obtained, and, perhaps most important, the use of quality assurance protocol in the performance of any procedure in the laboratory.

If one's basic knowledge is adequate, new chemistry determinations can be learned more easily. The methods described in this chapter illustrate only some of the many procedures used in the clinical chemistry laboratory today. Principles involved in other laboratory assays can be applied by using the methods illustrated. It is inevitable that the medical laboratorian will be called on to perform chemistry tests other than those described in this textbook, and one should be able to apply the basic knowledge to each new laboratory test.

Each new procedure should be approached in a systematic manner. The laboratorian should be aware of the type of specimen required for the test and should make certain that it is collected, prepared, and preserved properly. Any reagents needed for the procedure must be prepared by following the directions carefully. The procedure should be reviewed beforehand, and it is worthwhile to consult clinical chemistry textbooks for the clinical implications and any important background material for the determination. The principle of the test, why the reagents are used and what they do in the reactions that occur, the stepwise method to be followed, technical factors and sources of error for the particular method, calculations, reporting of results to the physician, and reference values for the substance to be measured are all essential information for performing the test. In automated analyzers, these considerations are incorporated into the instrumentation used.

To attain any degree of proficiency, practice and experience are necessary. Repeated practice with the laboratory tools discussed in this chapter and in preceding chapters will result in a much better understanding of clinical chemistry and in an appreciation for reliable and accurate testing in the chemistry laboratory.

Clinical applications are discussed throughout this chapter. In this way it is hoped that the laboratorian will not lose sight of the most important aspect of the chemistry determinations performed and the reason for doing them in the first place—benefit to the patient.

# INSTRUMENTATION AND GENERAL METHODOLOGIES USED IN THE CHEMISTRY LABORATORY

Techniques used in the clinical chemistry laboratory are based on quantitative analytic procedures or analytic chemistry. The kinds of analytic methods and some general types of instruments used to carry out these procedures have been discussed in Chapters 4, 6, and 9. Because there have been such great strides in technology, there have been equally rapid changes in the evolution of analyzing equipment used in the clinical chemistry laboratory. Changes have also taken place because of improvement in chemistry methodologies, changes in testing sites used by health care facilities, including a movement toward more point-of-care testing (POCT) and clinic-based and physician office laboratories, and the increasing awareness of the need for cost-effectiveness in the use of clinical laboratory tests.

The methodologies used in the technologically sophisticated automated analyzers are based on traditional technologies and methodologies. General methods for most assays in the chemistry laboratory, automated and manual, include the use of spectrophotometry, flame emission (or ionization) photometry, atomic absorption spectrometry, fluorometry, ion-selective electrodes, electrophoresis, nephelometry or light scattering, and immunoassays utilizing radionuclides, enzymes, or fluorescing materials as markers or tags. Some of these methods are discussed in the following section and others are discussed later under specific chemistry assays. (See also Chapter 9.)

## Spectrophotometry
### Absorbance Spectrophotometry

In **absorbance spectrophotometry,** the concentration of an unknown sample is determined by measuring its absorption of light at a particular wavelength and comparing it with the absorption of light by known standard solutions measured at the same time and with the same wavelength. The instrument used to perform this measurement is the absorbance spectrophotometer. The application of this kind of analysis is dependent on Beer's law, which states that the concentration of a solution at a constant light path length and at a constant wavelength and temperature is directly proportional to the amount of light absorbed (see also Absorbance Spectrophotometry, in Chapter 6).

**Ultraviolet and Visible Spectrophotometry.**
If the wavelength of light absorbed is in the ultraviolet part of the spectrum (nonvisible), short wavelengths of between 200 and 380 nm, the analysis is called ultraviolet (UV) spectrophotometry. If the wavelength of light absorbed is in the visible part of the spectrum, wavelengths of between 380 and 750 nm, the analysis is called visible (VIS) spectrophotometry. The wavelength used for the analysis depends on the wavelength at which there is significant absorption by the substance to be measured (see also under The Nature of Light, in Chapter 6).

### Reflectance Spectrophotometry

In **reflectance spectrophotometry,** the light reflected from the surface of a colorimetric reaction is used to measure the amount of unknown colored product generated in the reaction. A beam of light is directed at a flat surface, and the amount of light reflected is measured in a reflectance spectrophotometer. This technology is used in many of the bedside or point-of-care tests using smaller handheld instruments as well as for home testing done by patients themselves, an example being diabetics who test their blood glucose concentrations (see also Reflectance Spectrophotometry, in Chapter 6).

### Fluorescence Spectrophotometry

Upon receiving UV radiation, the electrons of some substances absorb the radiation and become excited. After about 7 to 10 seconds (the electron has returned to its ground state), this energy is given up as a photon of light. Fluorescent light is the result of the absorbance of a photon of radiant energy by a molecule.

Once the photon is absorbed by the molecule, the molecule has an increased level of energy. It will seek to eject this excess energy because the energy of the molecule is greater than the energy of its environment. When this excess energy is ejected as a photon, the result is fluorescence emission. Generally, this emitted light is in the visible part of the spectrum. The intensity of the fluorescence is determined by using a fluorometer, sometimes called a spectrofluorometer or fluorescence spectrophotometer. This measurement is governed by the same factors that affect the absorption of light (i.e., the light path through the solution, the concentration of the solution, the wavelength of light being used) and also by the intensity of the UV exciting light. Only a few compounds can fluoresce, and of those that do, not all photons absorbed will be converted to fluorescent light.

## Flame Emission Photometry

When some elements are heated—for example, sprayed into a flame—the atoms of the element become excited and re-emit their energy at wavelengths characteristic of the element. In **flame emission photometry,** the excited elements produce their characteristic flame colors at an intensity that is directly proportional to the concentration of atoms in the solution. The elements that are most often measured in this way are sodium (giving a yellow emission in a flame), potassium (red-violet), and lithium (red). Flame emission photometers are used for this determination (see also Flame Emission Photometry, in Chapter 6).

## Light Scattering and Nephelometry

Light can be absorbed, reflected, scattered, or transmitted when it strikes a particle in a liquid. **Nephelometry** is the measurement of light that has been scattered. Turbidimetry is the measurement of a loss in the intensity of light transmitted through a solution because of the light being scattered (the solution becomes turbid). **Turbidimetry** will measure light that is scattered, not absorbed or reflected by the particles in the suspension. Nephelometers are used to detect the amount of light scattered.

## Electrophoresis

When charged particles are made to move, differences in molecular structure can be seen because different molecules have different velocities in an electric field. The assay utilizing electrophoresis involves the movement of charged particles when an external electrical current is produced in a liquid environment. The electric field is applied to the solution through oppositely charged electrodes placed in the solution. Specific ions then travel through the solution toward the electrode of the opposite charge. Cations (positively charged particles) move toward the negatively charged electrode (cathode), and anions (negatively charged particles) move toward the positively charged electrode (anode).

**Electrophoresis** is a technique for separation and purification of ions, proteins, and other molecules of biochemical interest. It is used frequently in the clinical chemistry laboratory to separate serum proteins. The equipment needed for electrophoresis generally consists of a sample applicator; a solid medium (such as an agar gel); a buffer system; an electrophoresis chamber, which houses the solid medium and the sample; electrodes and wicks; a timer; and a power supply. Additional supplies might be stains for proteins or other substances being assayed and reagents used to remove the stains and to transform the solid media into a stable carrier for further densitometry studies or for preservation needs, depending on the requirements of the laboratory.

## Immunoassays

**Immunoassays** utilize antigen-antibody reactions. When foreign material (called antigens or immunogens) is introduced into the body, protein molecules called antibodies are formed in response. For example, certain bacteria, when introduced into the body, elicit the production of specific antibodies. These antibodies combine specifically with the substance that stimulated the body to produce them in the first place, producing an antigen-antibody complex. In the laboratory, an antigen may be used as a reagent to detect the presence of antibodies in the serum of a patient. If the antibody is present, it shows that the person's body has responded to that specific antigen before. This response can be elicited by exposure to a specific microorganism or by the presence of a drug or medication in the patient's serum. Antigens and antibodies are used as very specific reagents. In the clinical chemistry laboratory, antibodies are used to detect and measure an antigen, such as a drug or medication, present in the serum of the patient.

Antibodies are immunoglobulins (Ig), which occur in one of five groups: IgA, IgD, IgM, IgG, and IgE. These immunoglobulins are proteins with antibody activity and are synthesized by certain types of lymphocytes (see also Chapters 17 and 18). IgG is the immunoglobulin that is most often used in immunoassays. In the serum there are many different immunoglobulins, which are directed toward different antigens. Antibodies (immunoglobulins) can be monoclonal (derived from a single clone or a single ancestral antibody-producing parent cell) or polyclonal (derived from multiple ancestral clones of antibody-producing cells). (See also Monoclonal and Polyclonal Antibodies, in Chapter 17.)

The number of attachment sites on the antibody varies according to the type of immunoglobulin. IgG antibodies have two sites for attachment to antigens. The number of attachment sites on the antigen available to the antibody also varies. The type of antigen-antibody complex that forms is dependent on the proportion of antibody to antigen in the immunochemical reaction. The size and nature of the complex are dependent on this proportion. When an antigen and an antibody form a complex under optimal proportions, one observed reaction can be formation of a precipitate. A precipitate forms because a critical mass has been reached by these complexes. Precipitation is one means of detecting the formation of an antigen-antibody complex. The complex precipitates out of solution. The term flocculation is used to describe a precipitation reaction that produces large, loosely bound precipitate. When antibodies react with large, particulate multivalent antigens, the antigen is said to agglutinate.

Other means of detecting antigen-antibody reactions are used in quantitative immunoassays in the laboratory. Some of these are quantitative radial immunodiffusion, electroimmunoassay (rocket electrophoresis), enzyme-linked immunosorbent assay (ELISA), enzyme-multiplied immunoassay technique (EMIT), radioimmunoassay (RIA), immunoradiometric assay (IRMA), and substrate-labeled fluorescent immunoassay (SLFIA).

## Chromatography

The word chromatography comes from the Greek words *chromatos*, color, and *graphein*, to write. In **chromatography,** mixtures of solutes dissolved in a common solvent are separated from one another by a differential distribution of the solutes between two phases. The solvent, one phase, is mobile and carries the mixture of solutes through the second phase. The second phase is a fixed or stationary phase. There are a number of variations in chromatographic techniques, in which the mobile phase ranges from liquids to gases and the stationary phase from sheets of cellulose paper to internally coated fine capillary glass tubes. The varieties of chromatographic techniques as well as their applications to clinical assays have grown rapidly.

Chromatographic methods are usually classified according to the physical state of the solute carrier phase. The two main categories of chromatography are gas chromatography, in which the solute phase is in a gaseous state, and liquid chromatography, in which the solute phase is a solution or liquid. The methods are further classified according to how the stationary phase matrix is contained. For example, liquid chromatography is subdivided into flat and column methods. In flat chromatography, the stationary phase

is supported on a flat sheet such as cellulose paper (paper chromatography) or in a thin layer on a mechanical backing such as glass or plastic (thin-layer chromatography). Column methods are classically liquid chromatography. Gas chromatography is done by a column method.

The chromatographic method is used to separate the components of a given sample within a reasonable amount of time. The purpose of this separation technique is to detect or quantitate the particular component or group of components to be assayed in a pure form. By convention, the concentrations of solutes in a chromatographic system are plotted versus time or distance. The bands or zones of the various analytes separated in the technique are usually termed peaks.

## Electrochemical Methods

When chemical energy is converted to an electrical current (a flow of electrons) in a galvanic cell, the term electrochemistry is used. Electrochemical reactions are characterized by a loss of electrons (oxidation) at the positive pole (anode) and a simultaneous gain of electrons (reduction) at the negative pole (cathode). The galvanic cell is made up of two parts called half-cells, each containing a metal in a solution of one of its salts. These methods involve the measurement of electrical signals associated with chemical systems that are within an electrochemical cell. Electroanalytic chemistry uses electrochemistry for analysis purposes. The magnitude of the voltage or signal current originating from an electrochemical cell is related to the activity or concentration of the particular chemical constituent being assayed. Measurements can usually be done on very small amounts of sample.

In the clinical laboratory, electroanalytic methods are used to measure ions, drugs, hormones, metals, and gases. Methods are available for the rapid analysis of analytes, such as blood electrolytes ($Na^+$, $K^+$, $Cl^-$, $HCO_3^-$), present in relatively high concentrations, and other analytes, such as heavy metals and drug metabolites, that are present in very low concentrations in blood and urine. There are three general electrochemical techniques used in the clinical laboratory: potentiometric, voltametric, and coulometric.

### Potentiometry

Potentiometry measures the potential of an electrode compared with the potential of another electrode. The method is based on the measurement of a voltage potential difference between two electrodes immersed in a solution under zero current conditions. This difference in voltage between the two electrodes is usually measured on a pH or voltage meter. One electrode is called the indicator electrode; the other is the reference electrode. The reference electrode is an electrochemical half-cell that is used as a fixed reference for the cell potential measurements. One of the most common reference electrodes used for potentiometry is the silver or silver chloride electrode. The indicator electrode is the main component of potentiometric techniques. It is important that the indicator electrode be able to respond selectively to analyte species. The most commonly used indicator electrode in clinical chemistry is the ion-selective electrode (ISE).

The use of **ion-selective electrodes** is based on the measurement of a potential that develops across a selective membrane. The electrochemical cell response is based on an interaction between the membrane and the analyte being measured that alters the potential across the membrane. The specificity of the membrane interaction for the analyte determines the selectivity of the potential response to an analyte.

### Coulometry

Coulometry measures the amount of current passing between two electrodes in an electrochemical cell. The principle of coulometry involves the application of a constant current to generate a titrating agent; the time required to titrate a sample at constant current is measured and is related to the amount of analyte in the sample. The amount of current is directly proportional to the amount of substance produced or consumed by the electrode. The most common clinical application of coulometry is in the measurement of chloride ions in serum, plasma, urine, and other body fluids (see Chloride, under Electrolytes and Electrolyte Balance, below).

## SPECIMENS: GENERAL PREPARATION

Accurate chemical analysis of biological fluids depends on proper collection, preservation, and preparation of the sample, in addition to the technique and method of analysis used. The most quantitatively perfect determination is of no use if the specimen is not properly handled in the initial steps of the procedure. Each chemical method has unique problems of its own, but in general the collection, means of preservation, and initial preparation or processing of samples follow a similar pattern, regardless of what the final analysis is to be (see Chapter 3). The majority of chemistry tests are done on serum, and many use plasma; both are processed from whole blood obtained by venipuncture. Microsamples are sometimes collected from patients, and their processing and handling follow a particular protocol.

### Collecting Microspecimens for Chemistry

There are instances when only small amounts of capillary blood can be collected, and many laboratory determinations have been devised for testing small amounts of sample. In general, the same procedure is followed as for any other drawing of capillary blood (see under Peripheral or Capillary Blood, in Chapter 3). For chemistry procedures, blood can be collected in a capillary tube or microcontainer by touching the tip of the tube to a large drop of blood while the tube is held in a slightly downward position (Figs. 11-1 and 11-2). The blood enters the collection unit by capillary action. Several tubes can be filled from a single skin puncture, if needed. Tubes are capped and brought to the laboratory for testing. Careful centrifugation technique must be used.

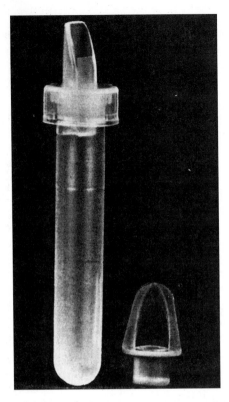

**FIG 11-1.** Microtainer tube system. (Courtesy Becton Dickinson Vacutainer Systems, Franklin Lakes, NJ.)

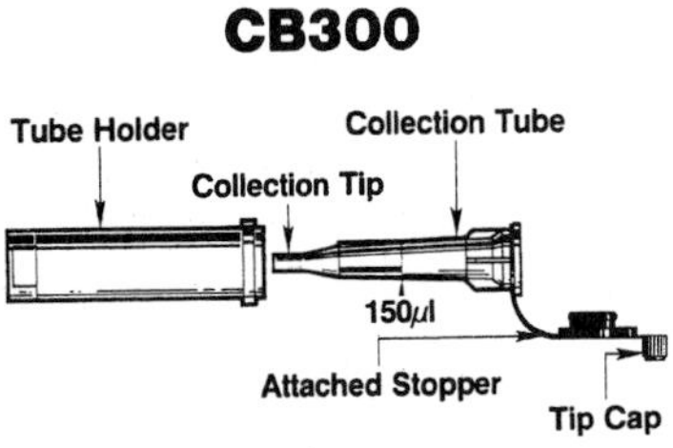

## CB300

Tube Holder          Collection Tube

Collection Tip

150μl

Attached Stopper

Tip Cap

**FIG 11-2.** Microvette capillary blood collection system. (Courtesy Sarstedt, Inc, Newton, NC.)

### Processing the Specimens

Once the blood has been collected and brought to the laboratory, a series of steps is carried out before the analysis is done. Ideally, all laboratory measurements should be performed within 1 hour after collection. When this is not practical,

the specimens should be processed to the point where they can be properly stored so that the constituents to be measured will not be altered. Additional reasons for properly storing specimens include the following: samples should be retained long enough after analysis to permit a repeat analysis if necessary, specimens collected in a timed sequence should be stored until they can be analyzed at the same time, and proper storage and transportation of specimens are necessary when the specimen is being sent to an alternative site for testing—a reference laboratory, for example.

Processing includes separation of cells from serum or plasma, observation of specimen color, refrigeration, and freezing if necessary.

Most chemical determinations are done with venous blood—serum or plasma. Arterial blood is primarily used for blood gas determinations. Plasma is the liquid portion of the circulating blood, and it contains fibrinogen. Serum is plasma with the fibrinogen removed, which is usually accomplished by the clotting mechanism. To obtain serum, the blood is collected in a plain tube or a serum-separator gel tube, using no anticoagulant, and allowed to clot for a minimum of 30 minutes at room temperature before centrifuging and removal of the serum for testing. Vacuum tubes used to collect the blood are usually siliconized to minimize hemolysis and to prevent the clot from adhering to the wall of the tube. By allowing the clot to retract for longer than 30 minutes, hemolysis is minimized and the yield of serum is greater. However, if the serum remains on the clot for too long, glycolysis can occur and other constituents are altered; there can be a shift of substances from the cells to the serum, for instance. Therefore, the time to allow for clot retraction depends on the determination to be done. Serum separator tubes are commonly used to assist in procurement of a serum sample (see Serum Separator Devices, in Chapter 3).

### Use of Serum Separator Tubes

With many of the automated methods being used, processing the blood often takes longer than the actual analysis. A fast, efficient way of separating serum from cells is needed. Special serum separator tubes, which resemble ordinary vacuum tubes but contain inert silicone gel, can be used. The gel is displaced up inside the tube during centrifugation and forms a barrier between the serum and the cells. The serum can easily be removed to the appropriate container or can be aspirated directly into the analyzer used for testing (see Laboratory Processing of Blood Specimens, in Chapter 3). By directly aspirating the centrifuged specimen in the primary collection tube into the analyzer, one step is saved and the possibility of transmission of biohazardous material lessened. Direct use of the primary tube in testing also lessens the risk of mislabeling the specimen during its transfer to an additional tube. Special specimen collection products are designed to save time and to provide a safer mechanism for processing blood specimens.

## Centrifuging the Specimens

After clotting has taken place, the tube is centrifuged with its cap on. It is important to remind persons handling blood specimens in all steps of the laboratory analysis to handle them by using standard precautions. Standard precautions require all persons handling specimens to wear gloves. When necessary, stoppers must be carefully removed from blood collection tubes to prevent aerosolization of the specimen. Centrifuges must be covered and placed in a shielded area. When serum or plasma samples must be removed from the blood cells or clot, mechanical suction is used for pipetting and all specimen tubes and supplies must be discarded properly in biohazard containers.

The use of automated analyzers in many cases allows the use of the primary collection tube for the analysis itself. In these instances, the primary blood tube is centrifuged with its cap on and the serum aspirated directly into the analyzer.

## Hemolyzed Specimens

Hemolyzed serum or plasma is unfit as a specimen for several chemistry determinations.

Hemolyzed serum appears red, usually clear red. Several constituents, such as potassium and the enzymes acid phosphatase, lactate dehydrogenase (LDH), and aspartate aminotransferase (AST, GOT), are present in large amounts in red blood cells, so that hemolysis of red cells will significantly elevate the value obtained for these substances in serum. Hemoglobin is released during hemolysis and may directly interfere with a reaction, or its color may interfere with photometric analysis of the specimen. The procedure to be done should always be checked to see whether abnormal-looking specimens can be used. A determination of whether the hemolysis is in vitro or in vivo is also useful. Although relatively rare, in vivo hemolysis is a clinically significant finding.

## Jaundiced Specimens

Jaundiced serum or plasma takes on a brownish yellow or "vivid" yellow color. One should be especially careful in handling such a specimen. Gloves must be worn, and the hands should be washed frequently. Jaundiced serum is a good indication of the presence of hepatitis, which can be infectious. The abnormal color of the serum can interfere with photometric measurements. The use of standard precautions has significantly reduced the incidence of hepatitis B infections in laboratory workers (see also under Safety in the Clinical Laboratory, in Chapter 2).

## Lipemic Specimens

Lipemic serum takes on a milky white color. The presence of lipids in serum or plasma can cause this abnormal appearance. Often, however, the lipemia results from collecting the blood from the patient too soon after a meal. Lipemic serum interferes with photometric readings for some tests.

## Drug Effect on Specimens

Blood drawn from patients on certain types of medication can give invalid chemistry results for some constituents. Drugs can alter several chemical reactions. Drugs can affect laboratory results in two general ways: some action of the drug or its metabolite can cause an alteration (in vivo) in the concentration of the substance being measured, or some physical or chemical property of the drug can alter the analysis directly (in vitro). The number of drugs that affect laboratory measurements is increasing.

### Logging and Reporting Processes

As part of the processing and handling of laboratory specimens, a careful, accurate logging and recording process must be in place in the laboratory, regardless of the size of the facility. A log sheet and a printed report form are vital to the operation of any laboratory. The log sheet documents on a daily basis the various patient specimens received in the laboratory. Log sheets and result reports are generated by laboratory information systems, when used (see Chapter 10).

Items to be listed on the log sheet are the patient's name, identification number, kind of specimen collected (description of the specimen and its source), date and time of specimen collection, and laboratory tests to be done. The log sheet should also indicate the time when the specimen arrived in the laboratory. The log sheet can also include a column for test results and the date when the tests are completed. Results can be documented by hand, by use of laboratory instrument printed reports, or by computer printouts. The log sheet data are part of the permanent record of the laboratory and must be stored and available for future reference (see also Chapter 10).

A printed report is often sent to the physician with the vital data pertaining to the test results. Result reports are also available electronically in many facilities. The following information should be included in the report: patient's name, identification number, date and time of specimen collection, description and source of specimen, the initials of the person who collected the specimen, tests requested, the name of the physician requesting the tests, the test results, and the initials or signature of the person who performed the test. Much of this documentation of data is being done with the use of laboratory computerized information systems. Copies of this laboratory report may be sent to the medical records department and to the accounting office for patient billing purposes (see also Chapter 10).

## Preserving and Storing the Specimens

Some chemical constituents change rapidly after the blood is removed from the vein. The best policy is to perform tests on fresh specimens. When the specimen must be preserved until the test can be done, there are ways to retard alteration. For example, sodium fluoride can be used to preserve blood glucose specimens, since it prevents glycolysis.

With few exceptions, the lower the temperature, the greater the stability of the chemical constituents. Furthermore, the growth of bacteria is considerably inhibited by refrigeration and is completely inhibited by freezing. Room temperature is generally considered to be 18° to 30° C, the refrigerator temperature about 4° C, and freezing about –5° C or less. Refrigeration is a simple and reliable means of retarding alterations, including bacteriologic action and glycolysis, although some changes still take place. Refrigerated specimens must be brought to room temperature before chemical analysis. Removing cells from plasma and serum is another means of preventing some changes. Some specimens needed for certain assays, such as bilirubin, must be shielded from the light or tested immediately. Bilirubin is a light-sensitive substance.

Serum or plasma may be preserved by freezing. Whole blood cannot be frozen satisfactorily because freezing ruptures the red cells (hemolysis). Freezing preserves enzyme activities in serum and plasma. Serum and plasma freeze in layers with different concentrations, and for this reason these specimens must be well mixed before they are used in a chemical determination.

Every precaution must be taken to preserve the chemical constituents in the specimen from the time of collection to the time of testing in the laboratory, if the results are to be meaningful. In general, tubes for collecting blood for chemical determinations do not have to be sterile, but they should be chemically clean. Serum is usually preferred to whole blood or plasma when the constituents to be measured are relatively evenly distributed between the intracellular and extracellular portions of the blood.

## Removing Interfering Substances

Biological fluids are very complex in their composition. There are hundreds of detectable substances in urine and blood, for instance. Chemical analysis would be impossible if it were necessary to completely isolate each substance before it could be measured. An optimal method is one that can test for a specific substance while the other substances remain. A test is said to be specific when none of the other substances interfere. In chemical analysis, however, almost all determinations are subject to some interference. Sometimes the interference is small enough or constant enough that it does not significantly alter the accuracy or precision of the test results. Sometimes the interference does affect the results, and in such cases the specimen must be specially treated before the analysis can take place. That is, the substances causing the interference must be isolated, or removed, from the specimen.

### Removing Protein

Whole blood is made up of cells and plasma. The red cells are largely composed of protein, and the plasma also contains a significant amount of protein. Protein molecules tend to have many electrically charged areas, and since chemical reactions involve the transfer of charges, the presence of so many charged protein molecules may interfere with reactions. It therefore may be necessary to remove the proteins before beginning the analysis. Removing proteins also has the effect of preserving the specimen, since it removes enzymes, which are proteins.

If proteins are left in the specimen, they can interfere with the analysis by causing turbidity,

foaming, or precipitation, or by directly interfering with color reactions. Any of these effects can lead to errors in many clinical determinations. Therefore many analyses require preliminary treatment to remove proteins. Proteins may be removed by precipitation with chemicals (acids or salts of heavy metals) or by passing the serum through a dialyzing membrane that allows only the smaller particles to pass through. The acids often used to precipitate proteins are trichloroacetic, tungstic, and picric. Salts of heavy metals that can be used to precipitate proteins are sodium sulfate, ammonium sulfate, and zinc sulfate. Ethyl alcohol and methyl alcohol are two organic chemicals used in protein precipitation. The dialyzing membrane is used in many automated methods, but the chemical filtrate methods are used for most manual laboratory analyses. Chemistry procedures requiring initial removal of protein will specify how it should be done.

**Preparation of a Protein-Free Filtrate.** The term **protein-free filtrate** or protein-free supernatant is used to describe the solution left after treatment of a specimen to remove the protein. Many separations of protein are accomplished by means of precipitation. Either the substance being measured is removed by precipitation, or the interfering materials are precipitated. The precipitate is isolated by filtration or centrifugation. Chemical precipitation of serum, plasma, whole blood, urine, or cerebrospinal fluid is thus followed by either filtration or centrifugation and subsequent decantation of the crystal-clear protein-free filtrate. Proteins are easily precipitated, and the techniques used include the use of heat, acids, bases, organic solvents, alcohols, salts, metal ions, or a combination of these. Specific methodologies can be found in a basic clinical chemistry textbook.

It is important in all methods for protein precipitation that the filtrate or supernate not show any foaming or cloudiness, which would indicate incomplete removal of protein. Two variables are important for maximal precipitation:

the pH of the reaction mixture and the concentration of the precipitant. There must be sufficient reagent to combine with the protein in the blood. Ordinarily a safe excess is used.

## QUALITY CONTROL IN THE CHEMISTRY LABORATORY

The purpose of quality control of analytic testing is to ensure the reliability of the measurements performed on the samples for each patient. A quality control program is useful and effective if it can be used to ascertain that the biochemical data generated are consistently precise and accurate. The data can then be used in the medical decision-making process on both a short-term and a long-term basis. As mandated by CLIA '88 regulations, quality control is part of the comprehensive set of policies, procedures, and practices that makes up the quality assurance program for the facility (see also Chapter 8).

Both control samples and patient samples must be assayed with the same testing system so that results of both reflect changes occurring in the system itself. Quality control specimens are also run to ensure that the usefulness of the test result has not been compromised by any changes occurring in the testing system. The use of controls and the recording of their values each time they are used constitute documentation for regulatory agencies that the laboratory routinely performs at a suitable level of competence. The assay results of the control specimen must be recorded or logged (this documentation is needed for accreditation agencies), along with dates. If the values are out-of-control, action must be taken to remedy the problem and the corrective action must be documented in writing. Results of the patient assays are also logged, along with the dates. This provides the necessary link between the control assay and patient assay. It is assumed that when the control values are within the established limits at the time of the patient assay, the patient results are reliable, valid, and reportable. Results for patient samples are not reported if the control values are out of the acceptable range established for the assay. All data are retained in the laboratory's records, whether the data be out-of-control or within the acceptable range. The length of time for retaining these data varies from laboratory to laboratory. This documentation is part of the quality assurance record of the laboratory.

## REPORTING RESULTS AND RECORDING LABORATORY DATA

Results are reported only when values for the quality control specimens or measures are acceptable. It is important that all testing be done by using the quality control protocol established by the individual laboratory and within CLIA regulations. The use of control specimens is included in all testing assays. A control specimen is handled in the assay in exactly the same way as any unknown specimen. When the control value is within the established range for that assay, it is an indication of the overall reliability of the assay values for the unknown specimen (see Chapter 8). The laboratory retains for some time the standard graphs, the galvanometer readings obtained for a particular procedure using manual methods, the results generated by the automated instruments, and all quality control records for the assay. The results themselves are retained by the laboratory indefinitely (see above). The reporting process is done with the use of computer systems in many laboratories.

With the use of computerized information systems, the information generated from the multitude of laboratory tests can be processed and used efficiently. Utilization of laboratory data for the benefit of the patient is the prime goal of the clinical laboratory in the health care facility (see also Chapter 10).

The laboratory may include not only the specific assay value for the test in question but also information as to whether the test result is abnormal and any other pertinent information of interpretive value. Reference ranges are of interest to the physician in interpreting the result.

Each laboratory sets its own reference ranges, using resources available from traditional clinical chemistry reference books, from manufacturers of the various laboratory instruments and products used in the laboratory, and from in-house laboratory procedure manuals.

## GLUCOSE AND GLUCOSE METABOLISM

One of the most commonly performed procedures in the clinical chemistry laboratory is the assay of blood glucose. Blood glucose tests are performed in all types of clinical laboratories, in hospitals, independent laboratories, clinics, and physicians' offices, and by bedside or point-of-care testing (POCT). These tests are used primarily for the diagnosis and treatment (or management) of diabetes mellitus. Although several different methods are used to quantitatively measure the amount of glucose in a blood specimen, most methods depend on the formation or disappearance of color in a solution and employ a photometer for this measurement. Most of the methods have been automated, but the same principles apply as for the nonautomated methods. Self-tests for blood glucose are also being done routinely by many diabetics to better manage their disease.

Glucose determinations may be performed on specimens taken from patients in a **fasting state** (in which no food or drink, other than water, has been consumed for 8 to 12 hours), on specimens taken 2 hours after the patient has had a meal **(postprandial),** or as part of a glucose tolerance test, in which the patient has consumed a high-glucose drink or meal, depending on the physician's instructions. The methods used for glucose determinations can be divided into three categories: the classic oxidation methods, which depend on the reducing ability of glucose; aromatic amine methods, which involve a reaction between the aldehyde group of glucose and the amino group of o-toluidine, an aromatic amine; and enzymatic methods, which are based on the enzymes glucose oxidase and

hexokinase. Since many additional substances that normally occur in the blood can be measured as glucose or can interfere with various tests, the term *true blood glucose* is often encountered when tests of blood glucose are described. The enzyme methods are more specific for glucose and are widely used for that reason.

### Clinical Significance

Glucose is one of the few chemical constituents of the blood that can change rapidly and dramatically in its concentration. Many diseases cause a change in glucose metabolism, but the most frequent cause of an increase in blood glucose **(hyperglycemia)** is diabetes mellitus.

#### Diabetes Mellitus

**Diabetes mellitus** is associated with a relative or absolute deficiency of insulin. This deficiency results in an inability of the body to handle glucose. Diabetes mellitus is a chronic metabolic disorder with deficiencies in carbohydrate, lipid, and protein metabolism. Changes in fat metabolism resulting from diabetes mellitus can be life threatening when they result in **ketoacidosis,** a condition in which there is an increased concentration of ketone bodies (which are derived from fat catabolism) in the blood and an accompanying decrease in blood pH, or **acidosis.** As the disease progresses, other specific complications can include atherosclerosis, a vascular disease with deposits of fat in the blood vessels, which can result in stroke, gangrene, or coronary disease; retinopathy leading to blindness; neuropathy (nerve damage); and renal disease. A person with diabetes has a twofold greater risk of myocardial infarction compared with a nondiabetic person of the same age and sex. There are approximately 8 million recognized diabetes patients in the United States, which is probably only half of the overall incidence, or a prevalence of about 6.6%.[8] There is a strong family tendency to the disease, although the exact mechanism of acquisition is unknown.

Research has shown that a complex interaction between genetic and environmental factors affects the development of diabetes mellitus. Some animal studies have shown a link between viruses and the development of diabetes.

Of the 8 million Americans with diagnosed diabetes mellitus, **type 1,** or **insulin-dependent, diabetes mellitus (IDDM)** afflicts more than 2 million. Insulin injection is required to control this disease. This type of diabetes mellitus is caused by absolute insulin deficiency due to destruction of beta cells in the pancreas. It is usually abrupt in its onset, often being triggered by a viral infection. The remaining diabetes patients have **type 2,** or **non–insulin-dependent, diabetes mellitus (NIDDM),** which has less correlation with blood insulin levels and more correlation with the activity of the insulin present, ranging from insulin resistance to a secretory defect, both resulting in a relative insulin deficiency. These patients usually are not dependent on insulin injections at early stages of their disease. Type 2 diabetes mellitus usually has a gradual onset over many years (increasing with age) and is often associated with obesity. Early diagnosis is important for both types of diabetes mellitus, as proper treatment may delay or minimize the complications of the disease.

The primary symptoms of diabetes mellitus are excessive urination **(polyuria),** abnormally high blood and urine glucose levels **(hyperglycemia** and **glycosuria,** respectively), excessive thirst **(polydipsia),** constant hunger **(polyphagia),** sudden weight loss, and, during acute episodes of the disease, excessive blood and urinary ketones **(ketonemia** and **ketonuria,** respectively). These symptoms result from the body's inability to metabolize glucose and the resulting consequences of the presence of high glucose levels.

Diabetes mellitus is controlled clinically through a number of factors. These include various dosages of insulin, oral drugs, and the composition of the diet. The result of uncontrolled diabetes mellitus is a high blood glucose level, with glucose subsequently appearing in the urine, the **renal threshold** having been surpassed.

In a diabetes patient, the glucose concentration can be very high or very low. At either extreme the patient may be in a state of unconsciousness. It is therefore necessary to know whether the unconsciousness results from a high glucose concentration **(diabetic coma)** or a low glucose concentration **(insulin shock).** It is often not obvious from the physical appearance of the patient which condition exists; however, prompt and appropriate treatment is mandatory. The increased use of POCT provides this information quickly so that immediate treatment may begin.

### Other Causes of Altered Glucose Metabolism

In some cases, high blood glucose values are caused by conditions other than diabetes mellitus. Some of these are traumatic injury to the brain; febrile disease; certain liver diseases; overactivity of the adrenal, pituitary, and thyroid glands, which produce hormones that increase blood glucose levels; and the ingestion of a heavy meal.

A significant number of people have **impaired glucose tolerance.** These persons have an abnormal glucose tolerance test but no measured hyperglycemia. **Gestational diabetes** occurs with some pregnancies, and consequently women are tested regularly during their pregnancies for this condition. Studies have shown that a significant number of women with gestational diabetes will go on to a type 2 diabetes mellitus 20 years after delivery. It is important to screen pregnant women for gestational diabetes to prevent perinatal complications associated with the hyperglycemia of the mother.

There are also conditions that cause low blood sugar, or **hypoglycemia.** These include liver disease in which the metabolism of glycogen is impaired and conditions that result in an increased concentration of insulin in the blood (hyperinsulinemia). A decrease in blood glucose is life-threatening because the brain and cardiac cells are dependent on glucose in the blood and interstitial fluids. Hypoglycemia may result in muscle spasms, unconsciousness, and death. High concentrations of insulin and hypoglycemia can result from an overdose of insulin or from certain pancreatic tumors.

## Glucose Concentration in the Body

Under ordinary conditions, the concentration of glucose in the blood is kept within a narrow range by an elaborate system of mechanisms collectively called carbohydrate metabolism. Some of the mechanisms used by the body to keep the glucose within this range are absorption of glucose by the intestine, storage and breakdown of glycogen (the form in which glucose is stored in the body) by the liver, storage of glucose as glycogen by the mass of skeletal muscles, and production and release of the hormone insulin by the pancreas. Other hormones that affect the blood glucose level are produced by the adrenal cortex and by the pituitary and thyroid glands.

Glucose is the ultimate source of energy for all body cells. Energy is provided by the oxidation of glucose, ultimately to carbon dioxide and water, through the process called glycolysis. Glycolysis, or glucose oxidation, depends on the presence of insulin. Therefore the absence of insulin will result in an increased concentration of glucose in the blood (clinically, the condition diabetes mellitus). Insulin is responsible for maintaining a healthy level of glucose in the blood. This is done in a variety of ways, including the processes of glycogenesis and glycolysis. **Glycolysis** is the breakdown or oxidation of glucose. Other forms of glucose utilization, or breakdown, that are also dependent on insulin are the synthesis of fatty acids and amino acids (the building blocks of protein). **Glycogenesis** is the formation of glycogen from glucose. Glycogen is the form in which glucose is stored in the body, primarily in the liver. Thus, insulin regulates the concentration of blood glucose by either oxidation (glycolysis) or storage (glycogenesis). The secretion of insulin is stimulated by increased blood glucose concentrations.

Glucose can also be provided to the blood by the process of **gluconeogenesis,** the production of glucose from fat and protein. This takes place in the liver, where glucose is derived from certain amino acids (protein) and glycerol (from fat) by glucocorticoid hormones produced by the adrenal cortex. Decreased blood glucose and decreased glycogen storage in cells stimulate this process.

Only a certain amount of glucose can be stored as glycogen. The excess glucose is converted to fatty acids and stored as triglycerides in body fat. Insulin is also necessary for the formation of fat (lipogenesis) in the liver and the adipose tissue, or body fat.

After a period of fasting, the usual amount of glucose in the blood is between 70 and 105 mg/dL of blood, depending on the method of analysis.[2] The blood glucose level usually increases rapidly after carbohydrates are ingested, but returns to normal in 1.5 to 2.0 hours (see Fig. 11-3). Aside from this increase after eating, the level of glucose in the blood is kept within a remarkably narrow range. This regulation of the blood glucose level is largely dependent on the activity of the liver. After a heavy meal, the glucose produced from digested carbohydrates is absorbed and the blood sugar rises. Some of this glucose may be oxidized at once for energy. However, the liver removes a large portion and stores it as glycogen, while some is carried to muscles, where it is also stored as glycogen for later use for immediate energy by the muscles. Some of the glucose diffuses into the tissue fluids and provides a direct source of energy for cell activity. After these immediate needs of the body have been supplied, the remainder is converted to fat and stored in the adipose tissue of the body. If the blood glucose level is so great that these control mechanisms cannot remove the excess glucose, the kidneys exert a regulating effect by excreting glucose in the urine. The blood glucose concentration above which glucose is excreted in the urine is called the renal threshold. For most persons the renal threshold for glucose is 160 to 170 mg/dL.

As a result of these metabolic processes, the blood glucose gradually returns to its fasting level. Since the body continues to utilize glucose for energy during normal activity, the blood glucose has a tendency to drop. This stimulates the liver to convert stored glycogen to glucose (glycogenolysis), maintaining the normal level of blood glucose.

Several hormones have the effect of raising the blood glucose concentration. The actions of growth hormone and adrenocorticotropic hormone (ACTH), which are secreted by the anterior pituitary, are opposite (antagonistic) to that of insulin and tend to raise the blood glucose level. Hydrocortisone and other steroids produced by the adrenal cortex stimulate gluconeogenesis. Epinephrine, which is secreted by the adrenal medulla, stimulates glycogenolysis. Glucagon is secreted by the alpha cells of the pancreas and acts to increase blood glucose by stimulating glycogenolysis in the liver. Finally, thyroxine, which is secreted by the thyroid, also stimulates glycogenolysis and contributes to an increased blood glucose level, besides increasing the rate of absorption of glucose from the intestine.

## Specimens

Glucose determinations may be performed on specimens of fasting whole blood, plasma, or serum, but serum or plasma, free of hemolysis, is the preferred choice. The specimen should be centrifuged and separated from the clot or cells as soon as possible. Glucose testing may be requested on other body fluids, especially urine and cerebrospinal fluid. In the past, glucose determinations were usually performed on whole blood; however, for several reasons, plasma or serum is now preferred. The glucose concentration in whole blood is not identical to that in plasma or serum. There is a uniform concentration of glucose throughout the water portion of plasma and red blood cells, but there is more water in the plasma than in the red cells, which also contain hemoglobin. Since plasma (or serum) contains approximately 10% to 15% more water than whole blood, the total glucose in plasma (or serum) is about 10% to 15% greater than in whole blood. The exact value can be calculated for any specimen; however, it is dependent on the method of analysis used and the hematocrit, or percentage of packed red blood cells per unit volume of blood.

There are other reasons for using plasma (or serum) rather than whole blood. It is easier to interpret values obtained from a single-component system such as plasma than from a two-component system such as whole blood. It is necessary to mix whole blood thoroughly before sampling. This is a particular problem with automated methods, where samples stand in the sample tray for a period of time before being tested. There are several substances in blood that interfere with tests for blood glucose, either because they are measured as glucose or because they interfere in enzyme procedures. These substances are more concentrated within red blood cells, so tests on plasma or serum tend to be more specific for glucose. As indicated above, values based on whole blood tend to vary with the hematocrit. Glucose is more stable in plasma or serum than in whole blood, as many glycolytic enzymes are present in the red blood cell. Finally, plasma or serum is easier to handle, to pipette precisely, and to store than is whole blood.

Because the amount of glucose in the blood increases after a meal, it is important that the principal tests to monitor glucose metabolism be done on fasting blood specimens or on specimens drawn 2 hours after a meal (postprandial). A random sample of blood is of limited value for a glucose determination.

### Fasting Blood Specimen

The blood should be drawn long enough after the last meal that the food has been completely digested and absorbed and any excess has been stored. The specimen for a blood glucose test is usually drawn in the morning before breakfast and is called a **fasting blood glucose.** The term fasting in this case means that the patient has had no food or drink for 8 to 12 hours—no breakfast, no cream or sugar, no coffee, tea, or other caffeinated drink, no drugs that might affect the blood glucose level, and no emotional disturbances that might cause liberation of glucose into the blood.

## Two-Hour Postprandial Specimen

A blood specimen drawn 2 hours after a meal is known as a **two-hour postprandial specimen.** To more completely detect diabetes mellitus, carbohydrate metabolic capacity is tested by stressing the system with a defined glucose load. To do this, a high-carbohydrate drink or meal is given to the patient, blood is collected 2 hours after ingestion, and the glucose concentration is determined (see also under Glucose Tolerance Tests).

## Capillary Blood Specimens

An advantage of using whole blood is the convenience of measuring glucose directly on capillary blood, such as that taken from infants, in mass screening programs for the detection of diabetes mellitus, or in the home monitoring being done by so many diabetes patients. Capillary blood must be thought of as essentially arterial rather than venous. In the fasting state the arterial (capillary) blood glucose concentration is 5 mg/dL higher than the venous concentration.

## Effects of Glycolysis

Another factor that must be taken into account in considering specimens for glucose determinations is the stability of glucose in body fluids. Many enzymes present in the blood, particularly in the red cells, affect glucose. As whole blood is allowed to stand at room temperature in a test tube, these enzymes destroy glucose. This action is called glycolysis, and it occurs at an average rate of approximately 10 mg/dL/hr, or 5% per hour. Plasma that is removed from the red cells after only moderate centrifugation (in-sufficient centrifugation time) still contains leukocytes, which also metabolize glucose. However, cell-free plasma, prepared by adequate centrifugation, shows no glycolytic activity. When unhemolyzed serum or plasma is separated from the cells, the glucose concentration is generally stable for up to 8 hours at room temperature, and up to 72 hours at 4° C. Cerebrospinal fluids are frequently contaminated with bacteria or other cellular constituents, such as leukocytes, that may cause the breakdown of glucose. Thus, cerebrospinal fluids should be analyzed for glucose without delay. Refrigeration or the addition of a small amount of sodium fluoride to the fluid may retard glycolysis for a few hours.

Keeping these considerations in mind, there are several ways to prevent or retard glycolysis in a specimen to be analyzed. Samples for glucose analysis should be delivered to the laboratory as soon as possible after being drawn from the patient. If plasma or serum is to be used for the glucose determination, it must be separated from the cells or clot within 30 minutes after the blood is drawn unless a specific additive is used (such as fluoride).

Using a special anticoagulant, usually sodium fluoride, seems to be the best way to preserve blood glucose specimens. Sodium fluoride acts in two ways to preserve glucose: as an anticoagulant, by tying up calcium and thus preventing clotting, and as an enzyme inhibitor that prevents glycolytic enzymes from destroying the glucose. However, with use of only sodium fluoride, clotting may occur after several hours, so it is advisable to use a combined fluoride-oxalate mixture. When the blood sample is placed in fluoride-oxalate tubes, it must be thoroughly mixed to ensure the proper effect. When certain enzymatic glucose methods are used, fluoride-anticoagulated blood should not be used, as the enzyme might be inhibited by the fluoride. Use of serum separator gel tubes, processed as quickly as possible—within thirty minutes if possible—is preferred for these methods.

## Measurements of Glucose Metabolism
### Fasting and Two-Hour Postprandial Tests

When glucose metabolism is being monitored, glucose is commonly determined on fasting blood specimens and on 2-hour postprandial specimens. For nonpregnant adults, the fasting serum or plasma glucose concentration should normally be less than 110 mg/dL and the serum or plasma glucose taken 2 hours after a meal (postprandial) should normally be less than 126 mg/dL. Included in the new criteria from The Expert Committee on the Diagnosis and Classification of Diabetes Mellitus are three diagnostic criteria for diabetes mellitus: (1) a fasting serum or plasma glucose level equal to or greater than 126 mg/dL; or (2) a random blood glucose (on blood drawn without consideration to time since the last meal) equal to or greater than 200 mg/dL, along with symptoms of diabetes (polyuria, polydipsia, and unexplained weight loss); or (3) a 2-hour postload glucose level equal to or greater than 200 mg/dL during an oral glucose tolerance test.[6] Impaired glucose tolerance (IGT) is indicated if the fasting glucose is between 110 and 126 mg/dL and one postprandial glucose level is greater than 200 mg/dL.[13]

### Glucose Tolerance Tests

In the detection and treatment of diabetes it is sometimes necessary to have more information than can be obtained from only testing the fasting specimen for glucose. Patients with mild or diet-controlled diabetes may have fasting serum or plasma glucose levels within the normal range, but they may be unable to produce sufficient insulin for prompt metabolism of ingested carbohydrates. As a result, the serum or plasma glucose rises to abnormally high levels and the return to normal levels is delayed. One glucose tolerance test commonly done employs a recommended level for adults of a 75-g glucose drink to be consumed within a 5-minute time period. The timing begins when the drink has been consumed. This test is known as the **oral glucose tolerance test (OGTT).**

The glucose tolerance test is usually performed when a person has been found to have a fasting serum or plasma glucose concentration above that of most nondiabetic persons (about 110 mg/dL). It can also be done to identify hypoglycemia, an abnormal response to a glucose load that results in a serum or plasma glucose concentration much below the normally accepted range. Since early detection and management of diabetes are important to avoid the many complications of the disease, it is desirable to detect these early cases of diabetes or prediabetes. For these reasons, the physician may request a glucose tolerance test. The OGTT is rarely necessary for the routine diagnosis of diabetes mellitus, however.

The glucose tolerance test measures the ability of a person to respond appropriately to a heavy load of glucose. Normally, when such a dose is received by the body, the pancreas responds by excreting insulin in the amount necessary for metabolism of the glucose. The degree and timing of the rising and falling of the serum or plasma glucose concentration after administration of glucose indicate how well the person can respond. The test has been standardized by the Committee on Statistics of the American Diabetes Association.

There are many glucose tolerance tests, but all are based on the same basic principles. The test begins with the patient in a fasting state, and blood is sampled and tested as a baseline control. Glucose is then administered, by either ingestion or injection, and samples are obtained at timed intervals—the postload samples. The amount of glucose administered and the collection intervals depend on the tolerance test used. Urine specimens may also be tested at fasting and timed intervals coinciding with the blood sampling. In most tolerance tests, samples are taken at intervals of 30, 60, 120, and 180 minutes. Normal oral glucose tolerance results for a 2-hour postload specimen are less than 140 mg/dL. Imperial glucose tolerance for a 2-hour postload specimen is greater than 140 and less than 200 mg/dL.[6] See Fig. 11-3 for oral glucose

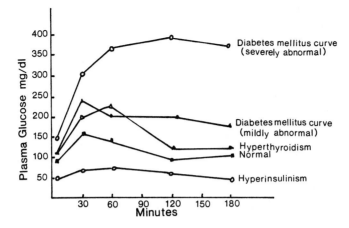

**FIG 11-3.** Oral glucose tolerance test results. (From Becan-McBride K, Ross DL: *Essentials for the Small Laboratory and Physician's Office.* St Louis, Mosby, 1988, p 250.)

tolerance test results for normal persons, for diabetes mellitus, and for other disorders showing glucose intolerance.

### Point-of-Care Tests for Glucose

POCT and the use of semiquantitative reagent strips or cartridge microcuvettes for assessing control of blood glucose in management of diabetes are widespread. These systems are used in emergency departments of hospitals, at the patient's bedside, and also by diabetics for home monitoring purposes. When single test reagent strips or cartridges are used for blood glucose measurements, it is essential that the user be trained to properly calibrate the instruments used and to read the results. Reflectance spectrophotometry meters are used to read the strips (see also Chapter 6). Transmittance photometry is used to read the cartridges. Variations in the amounts of blood used, in the time allowed for the reaction in the instrument, and in its calibration can be minimized only through proper and sufficient training programs for persons performing the tests—nurses, physicians, laboratorians, or the patients themselves.

**Self-Monitoring of Glucose.** Many patients (especially those with type 1 [insulin-dependent] diabetes mellitus) now regularly monitor their own blood glucose concentrations on the advice of their physicians, using reagent test strips and reflectance meters. The goal of diabetic therapy is to maintain near-normal blood glucose levels to prevent or minimize long-term complications. Self-monitoring is recommended for several populations of diabetics.[3]

Several companies manufacture reagent test strips for monitoring blood glucose, and most of these companies market reflectance meters to be used to electronically read the test results. Instruments include One Touch,[*] Accu-Chek Easy,[†] and Glucometer Elite.[‡] The strips used for these tests are impregnated with the enzyme glucose oxidase. Any glucose present in the blood is converted to gluconic acid and hydrogen peroxide, with the glucose oxidase being used to catalyze the reaction (see discussion of glucose oxidase below). A second enzyme, peroxidase, is also present on the strip. The peroxidase uses the hydrogen peroxide formed in the first reaction to oxidize an indicator also present on the strip to give a color change that is detectable. The color

*Lifescan, Milpitas, Calif.
†Boehringer Mannheim Diagnostics, Indianapolis, Ind.
‡Bayer Corp, Inc, Diagnostics Division, Tarrytown, NY.

change can be read in a reflectance meter on which the result (in mg/dL) is visualized. Although blood is tested, results are converted to plasma glucose values by the instrument.

Another product, HemoCue Glucose,* utilizes transmittance photometry and single-test cartridges. The cartridge is a microcuvette that draws up 5 $\mu$L of blood (capillary or venous): it is inserted into the photometer, where the analysis takes place and the result is displayed. The reaction is based on the glucose dehydrogenase method. The cartridge/microcuvette is the unique part to this system—it is a self-filling cuvette, disposable, and serves as a pipette, test tube, and measuring vessel, all in one. The reagent is contained in the tip of the microcuvette, where the chemical reaction takes place.

It is important that the users of these bedside or home monitoring methodologies be fully instructed in and informed about their proper use. The instruments must be calibrated with control solutions of glucose of a known concentration or with a calibration strip or cartridge supplied with each lot of test strips or cartridges. The procedure supplied by the manufacturer must always be followed when any of these products are used. The specimens used for these point-of-care tests are generally capillary blood obtained by finger puncture (see Peripheral or Capillary Blood, in Chapter 3).

### Glycated Hemoglobin

When glucose in the blood plasma reaches abnormally high concentrations, glycosylation of many proteins occurs, including hemoglobin. A hemoglobin derivative, hemoglobin $A_{1c}$ or **glycated hemoglobin,** is formed when glucose and hemoglobin combine. Glycated hemoglobin methods include electrophoresis, ion-exchange chromatography, and high-pressure liquid chromatography. Blood levels of glycated hemoglobin depend on the life span of the red blood cell (an average of 120 days ) and the blood glucose

concentration. Values for glycated hemoglobin are usually expressed as a percentage of the total blood hemoglobin. Normal, healthy subjects have values from 5.3% to 7.5%.

Tests for glycated hemoglobin are used to monitor long-term blood glucose concentration in patients with diabetes mellitus. Increased glycated hemoglobin in the blood indicates long-term hyperglycemia—a high glucose concentration over the previous 4 to 8 weeks. For this reason, this test is considered a better measure of diabetes control than a single blood glucose measurement. The patient's glycated hemoglobin should be routinely monitored every 3 to 4 months. The test is not used to diagnose diabetes mellitus, however.

### Methods for Quantitative Determination of Glucose

The various methods for the quantitative determination of glucose can be divided into three general categories: enzymatic methods, oxidation-reduction methods, and aromatic amine methods. Of these, enzymatic methods using hexokinase or glucose oxidase methodology are most commonly used.

### Enzymatic Methods

Almost all currently used glucose methods utilize enzymatic techniques. The use of enzymes is a means of achieving absolute specificity in the determination of glucose concentration. The two most widely used automated enzyme glucose methods are based on the enzymes hexokinase and glucose oxidase. Glucose oxidase is also used in the most common manual methods.

**Hexokinase.** The hexokinase method is the one used most often in automated chemistry analyzers. Hexokinase methods are less subject to interference than the glucose oxidase–peroxidase methods. The Du Pont ACA* is one instru-

*HemoCue, Inc, Mission Viejo, Calif.

*Du Pont Co, Wilmington, Del.

ment utilizing the hexokinase method. This method employs the enzyme hexokinase to catalyze the formation of glucose-6-phosphate from glucose. In the reaction, adenosine triphosphate (ATP) is simultaneously converted to adenosine diphosphate (ADP). The glucose-6-phosphate formed becomes the substrate for a second enzymatic reaction, in which the coenzyme nicotinamide adenine dinucleotide phosphate (NADP) is reduced to NADPH with 6-phosphogluconate being formed. See hexokinase reaction below.

$$\text{Glucose} + \text{ATP} \xrightarrow{\text{hexokinase}} \text{Glucose-6-phosphate} + \text{ADP}$$

$$\text{Glucose-6-phosphate} + \text{NADP} \xrightarrow{\substack{\text{glucose-6-phosphate} \\ \text{dehydrogenase}}}$$
$$\text{6-phosphogluconate} + \text{NADPH} + \text{H}^+$$

**Hexokinase Reaction**

As seen in the above reaction, for each mole of NADPH formed, 1 mol of glucose has been reacted upon. There is a change in absorbance at 340 nm, and this change is used to measure the concentration of glucose. NADPH is formed in direct proportion to the amount of glucose present in the original specimen.

Although other hexoses can react also in the hexokinase procedure, normal serum concentrations of these other sugars do not usually cause significant interference. No interference is observed with fluoride, heparin, oxalate, and ethylenediaminetetraacetic acid (EDTA) anticoagulants at the usual concentrations. Ascorbic acid does not cause interference in this test.

A set of standards must routinely be included to correct for background absorption. Quality control specimens are run with each batch of tests, and their values must be within the established acceptable range for unknown results to be reported out. Daily control charts are maintained and saved to document any trends or problems that may occur.

The hexokinase method is also an excellent method to determine glucose in urine and other biological fluids. This method has been proposed as a basis-of-reference method because of its accuracy and precision.

**Glucose Oxidase.** Glucose oxidase catalyzes the oxidation of glucose to gluconic acid and hydrogen peroxide. See glucose oxidase reaction below.

$$\beta\text{-D-glucose} + \text{H}_2\text{O} \xrightarrow{\text{glucose oxidase}}$$
$$\text{D-gluconic acid} + \text{H}_2\text{O}_2$$

$$2\text{H}_2\text{O}_2 + 4 \text{ aminopyrine} +$$
$$1,7\text{-dehydroxynapthylene} \xrightarrow{\text{peroxidase}} \text{A red dye} + \text{H}_2\text{O}$$

**Glucose Oxidase Reaction (Vitros Method)**

In some methods the amount of hydrogen peroxide produced or oxygen used is measured by an electrode process. In others a second enzyme, peroxidase, catalyzes the oxidation of a chromogen to a colored product; in this case the color that is formed is proportional to the amount of glucose present. When peroxidase is used in these procedures, the test is subject to interference from reducing agents such as ascorbic acid, which react with hydrogen peroxide, resulting in falsely low results.

The glucose oxidase procedure has been adapted to a wide range of various automated products. Vitros Clinical Chemistry Analyzers* use this methodology; these instruments employ dry chemistry reagents, in either a strip or a film form. In the Vitros analyzers, the oxidation of an indicator dye is used to form a colored compound, which is due to the action of hydrogen peroxide and peroxidase. The specimen is deposited on the Vitros Clinical Chemistry Slide and is evenly distributed by the spreading layer. Water and any nonprotein components of the serum move to the underlying reagent layer.

---

*Johnson & Johnson Clinical Diagnostics, Rochester, NY.

After the reaction has occurred and after a fixed incubation period, the reflectance density of the red dye formed in the reaction is measured by the spectrophotometer through the transparent polyester support. The result is obtained in about 5 minutes.

Glucose oxidase methods can be used to measure glucose in cerebrospinal fluid but should not be used for urine unless the urine is first pretreated, because urine contains a high concentration of substances that interfere with the peroxidase reaction.

### Oxidation-Reduction Methods

Oxidation methods for blood glucose depend on the fact that glucose contains an aldehyde group as part of its chemical structure. The presence of this aldehyde gives glucose its reducing properties (Fig. 11-4). Other substances in blood also have reducing properties. Some of these nonglucose reducing substances are other sugars and metabolic compounds and materials such as uric acid, creatinine, ascorbic acid, certain amino acids, homogentisic acid, creatine, phenols, and glucuronic acid. The oxidation-reduction methods for determining blood glucose differ primarily in the way they handle the nonglucose reducing substances. When the nonglucose reducing substances are removed as part of a glucose determination, the resulting value is called the true glucose value.

When glucose is analyzed with automated devices such as the AutoAnalyzer,* the protein is separated from the specimen by means of a dialyzer. Of the many methods available for the determination of blood glucose, one reduction method employs potassium ferricyanide and another uses alkaline copper solutions. In either case, the glucose acts to reduce the reagent to a lower oxidation product. This product is then analyzed photometrically.

Alkaline copper reduction methods for glucose depend on the reduction of copper II

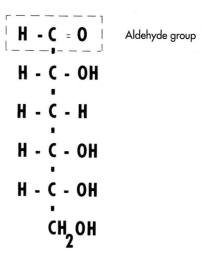

FIG 11-4. Glucose molecule.

($Cu^{2+}$), or cupric ions, to copper I ($Cu^{+}$), or cuprous ions, while the aldehyde group of glucose is oxidized to gluconic acid. These were among the original methods of testing for glucose. Two classic examples of alkaline copper reduction methods are the Folin-Wu method and the Nelson-Somogyi method. A disadvantage of all copper reduction methods is the reoxidation of $Cu^{+}$ ions to $Cu^{2+}$ ions by air. Therefore, steps must be taken to minimize reoxidation in the procedure.

Other procedures that make use of the reducing ability of glucose are the alkaline ferricyanide methods. In these methods, a hot alkaline ferricyanide solution, which is yellow, is reduced by glucose to a ferrocyanide solution, which is colorless. The decrease in the yellow color is proportional to the glucose concentration. The reaction may be followed by measuring the loss of yellow color, or by adding ferric ions, which react with ferrocyanide to form Prussian blue. In this case the formation of a blue color is measured. An advantage of ferricyanide methods is that they are not as subject to reoxidation by air as the copper reduction methods. The ferricyanide method has been automated for

---

*Technicon Instruments Corp, Tarrytown, NY.

use in the AutoAnalyzer. (For specific manual procedures for these oxidation-reduction methods, consult a basic clinical chemistry textbook.)

### Aromatic Amine Methods (the o-Toluidine Test)

Aromatic amine methods depend on the fact that various aromatic amines react with glucose in hot acetic acid to form colored derivatives. The aromatic amine commonly used is *ortho*-toluidine (*o*-toluidine). The methods involve a reaction between the aldehyde group of glucose (see Fig. 11-4) and the amino group ($-NH_2$) of the aromatic amine. A green-colored complex is formed, which is measured spectrophotometrically. The *o*-toluidine method, a nonenzymatic method, is highly specific for glucose, is easily performed, and can be adapted to serum or plasma without deproteinization, but it is not used much anymore because *o*-toluidine is believed to be a carcinogen.

### Reference Values[2]

Reference values for the individual glucose methods can vary significantly. Each laboratory must therefore determine and evaluate the reference range for its particular facility.

There is no significant difference in serum or plasma glucose concentration between males and females or between races. In normal cerebrospinal fluid (CSF), the glucose concentration is about 60% to 70% of the plasma level. It is therefore important to also measure the blood glucose concentration when CSF glucose is tested, so that the CSF glucose results can be evaluated appropriately. (Values in parentheses are in SI units.)

*Glucose, fasting, serum:*

| | | |
|---|---|---|
| Child | 70-105 mg/dL | (3.89-5.83 mmol/L) |
| Adult | 70-105 mg/dL | (3.89-5.83 mmol/L) |

*Glucose, fasting, whole blood:*

| | | |
|---|---|---|
| Adult | 60-95 mg/dL | (3.33-5.27 mmol/L) |

*Glycated hemoglobin, total, blood:* 5.3%-7.5% total blood hemoglobin

*Glucose, CSF:*

| | | |
|---|---|---|
| Infant, child | 60-80 mg/dL | (3.33-4.44 mmol/L) |
| Adult | 40-75 mg/dL | (2.22-4.16 mmol/L) |

There is normally no detectable glucose in urine.

## ELECTROLYTES AND ELECTROLYTE BALANCE

Electrolytes are substances that form or exist as ions or charged particles when dissolved in water. They are either anions or cations, depending on whether they have a negative (an anion) or positive (a cation) charge; cations move toward the cathode and anions toward the anode in an electrical field. Electrolytes include sodium ($Na^+$), potassium ($K^+$), calcium ($Ca^{2+}$), magnesium ($Mg^{2+}$), chloride ($Cl^-$), bicarbonate ($HCO_3^-$), sulfate ($SO_4^{2-}$) and phosphate ($HPO_4^{2-}$). The chief negatively charged constituents (anions) are chloride ($Cl^-$) and bicarbonate ($HCO_3^-$). The chief positively charged constituents (cations) are sodium ($Na^+$) and potassium ($K^+$). There are other electrolytes, but sodium, potassium, chloride, and bicarbonate are the ones most likely to show variation in electrolyte problems. These four electrolytes are often discussed together because changes in the concentration of one of them are almost always accompanied by changes in the concentration of one or more of the others. Collectively, the four charged particles—chloride, bicarbonate, so-dium, and potassium—make up a group of laboratory tests referred to as the **electrolyte battery**. These electrolytes are found throughout the body, but their concentrations or activities vary from one body compartment to another. Assays are usually done on plasma or serum. One example of an electrolyte is sodium chloride, which forms $Na^+$ and $Cl^-$ in water. The sodium and chloride ions are also called electrolytes.

It is essential that the positively charged particles balance, or electrically neutralize, the negatively charged particles. When this balance is not achieved, electrolyte imbalance occurs; this is extremely harmful for the patient and can be fatal, because most of the body's essential metabolic processes are affected by or dependent on electrolyte balance. The assessment of electrolyte balance is an important laboratory assay, and the tests often are done as emergency procedures—electrolyte imbalance cannot be tolerated by the patient for long. Treatment to remedy the imbalance must be started as quickly as possible. Assay of electrolytes in general is done because many important metabolic body functions depend on the maintenance of their proper concentrations—maintenance of water in the various body compartments, maintenance of pH, activity of blood coagulation and enzyme cofactors, control of neuromuscular excitability, and involvement in oxidation-reduction processes. When the body is unable to maintain normal control over the concentrations of the electrolytes, by either excretion or conservation, one or more of the electrolyte constituents will have an abnormal concentration. The kidneys and the lungs are the organs that exert most control over electrolyte concentration.

## Clinical Significance
### Sodium

Sodium ($Na^+$) is the cation, or positively charged particle, found in the highest concentration in extracellular fluid. It is important in maintaining the osmotic pressure and in electrolyte balance. Sodium is associated with the levels of chloride and bicarbonate ions, and for this reason it has a major role in maintaining the **acid-base balance** of the body cells. A low serum sodium level is called **hyponatremia,** and a high one is called **hypernatremia.** Low sodium levels are found in a variety of conditions, including severe polyuria (as in diabetes insipidus), metabolic acidosis (as in diabetic acidosis), Addison's disease (in which the supply of adrenocortical hormones is inadequate; these

hormones have a strong influence on the level of sodium), diarrhea, and some renal tubular diseases. An increased sodium level is found in Cushing's syndrome (in which there is hyperactivity of the adrenal cortex and more hormones than normal are produced), severe dehydration caused by primary water loss, certain types of brain injury, and diabetic coma after therapy with insulin, and after excess treatment with sodium salts.

### Potassium

Potassium ($K^+$) is the chief intracellular cation, but it is also found extracellularly. It has an important influence on the muscle activity of the heart. Since potassium is largely excreted by the kidney, it becomes elevated in kidney failure and shock. Like sodium, potassium is influenced by the presence of the adrenocortical hormones and is associated with acid-base balance. An elevated potassium level in serum is called **hyperkalemia,** and a decreased level is called **hypokalemia.** High serum potassium levels are generally seen in cases of oliguria, anuria, or urinary obstruction. In renal tubular acidosis, there is increased retention of potassium in the serum. One important purpose of renal dialysis is the removal of accumulated potassium from the plasma. Low serum potassium levels can result from prolonged diarrhea or vomiting, or from inadequate intake of dietary potassium. Even in potassium deficiency, the kidney continues to excrete potassium. The body has no effective mechanism to protect itself from excessive loss of potassium, so a regular daily intake of potassium is essential.

### Chloride

The chloride ion ($Cl^-$) is the most important anion of the extracellular fluids in the body. It is the major anion that counterbalances the major cation, sodium, to maintain the electrical neutrality of the body fluids. Electrical neutrality must be maintained at all times in the body fluids. This means that the sum of all the cations (positively charged particles) equals the sum of all the anions (negatively charged particles).

Chloride has two main functions in the body: it is important in determining the osmotic pressure, which controls the distribution of water between cells, plasma, and interstitial fluid, and it is important in maintaining the acid-base balance. Chloride also plays an important role in the buffering action when oxygen and carbon dioxide exchange takes place in the red blood cells. This activity is known as the chloride shift. When blood is oxygenated, chloride travels from the red blood cells to the plasma, and at the same time bicarbonate leaves the plasma and enters the red cells. Water travels in the same direction as chloride, and the red blood cells become dehydrated when the blood is oxygenated. Whenever bicarbonate goes from the red blood cells to the plasma, as it must during carbon dioxide transport, the bicarbonate anions are replaced by an equivalent amount of chloride anions.

An example of the **chloride shift** in the laboratory is the replacement action that occurs when a specimen for a chloride determination is allowed to stand for a while before the cells and plasma are separated. When whole blood comes into contact with air, carbon dioxide (and thus bicarbonate) escapes from the blood. As carbon dioxide leaves the plasma, chloride diffuses (or shifts) out of the red cells to replace it. The contact between whole blood and air, therefore, has the effect of lowering the plasma carbon dioxide and raising the plasma chloride. Specimens of whole blood left in contact with air may therefore give falsely high plasma or serum chloride values. The proper general handling of blood specimens is discussed in Chapter 3. The cells must be removed from the plasma by centrifugation as quickly as possible. Once separated from the cells, the serum or plasma has a very stable chloride concentration.

The other important function of chloride is to regulate the fluid content of the body and its influence on the kidney. The kidney maintains the electrolyte concentration of the plasma within very narrow limits. This regulation is necessary for life. Renal function is set to regulate the composition of the extracellular fluid first and then the volume. Consequently, if the body loses salt (sodium chloride), it loses water.

Low serum or plasma chloride values may be seen in nephritis in which salt is lost, as in chronic pyelonephritis. A low chloride value may also be seen in the types of metabolic acidotic conditions that are caused by excessive production or diminished excretion of acids, as in diabetic acidosis and renal failure. Prolonged vomiting, from any cause, may ultimately result in a decrease in serum and body chloride. High serum or plasma chloride values are seen in dehydration and in conditions that cause decreased renal blood flow, such as congestive heart failure. Excessive treatment with or dietary intake of chloride ions also results in high serum levels.

Chloride is found in serum, plasma, cerebrospinal fluid, tissue fluid, and urine. There is very little chloride inside the cells of the body, with the exception of the red cells, which contain some chloride. The chief extracellular anions are chloride and bicarbonate, and there is a reciprocal relationship between them; that is, when there is a decrease in the amount of one, there is an increase in the amount of the other. In the blood, two thirds of the chloride is found in the plasma and only one third in the red cells. Because of the difference in chloride concentration between the red cells and the plasma, the test for chloride is routinely performed on plasma (or serum) and not on whole blood. Physiologically, only the concentration of chloride in the extracellular fluid is important. This is another reason why plasma or serum is chosen as the specimen for this determination.

### Bicarbonate

Bicarbonate ($HCO_3^-$), along with chloride, is one of the major extracellular anions in body fluids. As the blood perfuses the lungs, carbon dioxide ($CO_2$) and $H_2O$ are formed. During the metabolic processes, carbonic acid ($H_2CO_3$) dissociates and forms bicarbonate. This is reconverted to carbonic acid, followed by the formation of $H_2O$ and $CO_2$. These reactions are as follows:

$$CO_2 \text{ (gas)} \leftrightarrow CO_2 \text{ (dissolved)} + H_2O \leftrightarrow$$
$$H_2CO_3 \leftrightarrow H^+ + HCO_3^-$$

Bicarbonate is filtered by the kidney, and little or no bicarbonate is found in the urine. The proximal tubules reabsorb 85% of these ions, and the remaining 15% are reabsorbed by the distal tubules. Bicarbonate is most commonly measured with other combined forms of $CO_2$ ($CO_2$, $H_2CO_3$, carbamino groups) as total $CO_2$. Since about 90% of all the $CO_2$ in serum is in the form of bicarbonate, this combined form approximates the actual bicarbonate very closely. Total carbon dioxide is the total of carbonic acid and bicarbonate. Bicarbonate is usually reported rather than total $CO_2$ because of potential sample-handling errors with a possible loss of carbonic acid as a result.

Along with pH and carbon dioxide pressure ($Pco_2$) determinations, the total carbon dioxide concentration is a useful measurement in evaluating acid-base disorders. The bicarbonate or carbon dioxide value in itself is not as significant as the value in the context of the other electrolytes assayed. Total carbon dioxide assays are performed volumetrically, manometrically, or colorimetrically, or by using a $Pco_2$ electrode to measure the rate of released carbon dioxide being formed. Most assays are now performed using automated instruments.

### Anion Gap

The calculation of the mathematical difference between the anions ($Cl^-$ and $HCO_3^-$) and the cations ($Na^+$ and $K^+$) is known as the **anion gap.** If the chloride and bicarbonate ions are summed and subtracted from the sum of the sodium and potassium ion concentrations, the difference should be less than 16 mmol/L (with a range of 10 to 20). If the anion gap exceeds 16 mmol/L, this is usually an indication of increased concentrations of the unmeasured anions ($PO_4^{3-}$, $SO_4^{2-}$, protein ions). Increased anion gaps can result from ketotic states, lactic acidosis, toxin ingestion, uremia, or increased plasma proteins. Decreased anion gaps of less than 10 mmol/L can result from either an increase in unmeasured cations ($Ca^{2+}$, $Mg^{2+}$) or a decrease in the unmeasured anions.

The anion gap is also useful as a quality control measure for electrolyte results. If an increased anion gap is found for electrolytes in a healthy person, there is reason to suspect that one or more of the test results is erroneous, and the tests should be repeated.

### Specimens

Plasma can be assayed for electrolyte concentration after use of lithium or sodium heparin as the anticoagulant, except in testing for sodium, in which case sodium heparin cannot be used. Electrolyte testing can also be done on serum. Capillary samples can be collected into microcontainers or capillary tubes. Centrifugation should be done using the unopened primary collection tubes, and the plasma or serum should be separated from the cells promptly. Each assay has specific concerns to note regarding specimen requirements and technical factors relating to the specimen collection and handling.

### Sodium

Lithium heparinized plasma, serum, urine, and other body fluids are suitable specimens. Sodium heparin should not be used, because the presence of sodium will interfere with the assay for sodium. Cells must be separated from serum or plasma as soon as possible.

Sodium is stable in serum for at least one week at room or refrigerator temperature, or it can be frozen for up to one year. If flame photometry is used to analyze sodium levels, scrupulous care is necessary. The slightest contamination of specimens or equipment will drastically alter the results. Sodium can be measured in 24-hour urine specimens and in cerebrospinal fluid.

## Potassium

Lithium or sodium heparin is the preferred anti-coagulant for plasma specimens; an anticoagulant containing potassium cannot be used. Serum can also be tested. The collection of blood for potassium studies requires special attention and technique. Since the concentration of potassium in the red blood cell is about 20 times that in serum or plasma, it is imperative that hemolysis be avoided. To avoid a shift of potassium from the red cells to the plasma or serum, it is important to separate the cells from the plasma or serum within 3 hours of collection. When blood is collected for a potassium test, opening and closing of the fist before venipuncture should be avoided, since this muscle action may result in an increase in plasma potassium levels of 10% to 20%. Potassium levels in plasma are about 0.1 to 0.2 mmol/L lower than those in serum because of the release of potassium from ruptured platelets during the coagulation process. Potassium in serum is stable for at least 1 week at room or refrigerator temperature. Specimens may be frozen for up to one year. Potassium levels in urine vary with dietary intake and are measured in a 24-hour collection.

## Chloride

The anticoagulant used most frequently is lithium or sodium heparin. Serum separator gel tubes are also commonly used for specimens for chloride testing. Chloride is commonly assayed in serum, plasma, urine, or sweat and in other body fluids. Because two thirds of the chloride in blood is found in the plasma, plasma or serum is routinely used for analysis of chloride. When flame photometry methodologies are used, sodium fluoride cannot be used for the chloride determination, because the fluoride is a halogen (as is chloride), and the two react in the same way in these assays. If sodium fluoride is used, a falsely high chloride value is obtained because the fluoride is also measured. The plasma or serum should be removed from the red cells as soon as possible after the blood is drawn, to prevent the chloride shift from occurring. Loss of gaseous carbon dioxide alters the distribution of chloride ions between the cells and plasma (see also under Clinical Significance). Moderate hemolysis does not significantly affect the concentration of chloride in the serum.

**Sweat Chloride.** The chloride content of sweat is useful in diagnosing cystic fibrosis, a disease of the exocrine glands. Affected infants usually have concentrations of sweat chloride greater than 60 mmol/L, adults greater than 70 mmol/L (reference values average about 40 mol/L). In 98% of patients with cystic fibrosis, the secretion of chloride in sweat is two to five times normal. The determination of increased chloride in sweat, as well as an increase of other electrolytes, is useful in the diagnosis of cystic fibrosis. The chloride content of normal sweat varies with age. To collect the sample, the patient is induced to sweat, and the sweat can be measured directly by use of ion-specific electrodes.

## Bicarbonate

Lithium or sodium heparinized plasma or serum may be used for the bicarbonate assay. Venous blood is generally collected, but capillary blood collected in microcontainers or capillary tubes may also be used for this assay. The bicarbonate concentration is most accurately determined immediately when the tube is opened and as quickly as possible after collection and centrifugation of the unopened tube has taken place. A specimen to be assayed for total $CO_2$ must be handled anaerobically to minimize losses of $CO_2$ and $HCO_3^-$ (converted to $CO_2$) into the atmosphere. A falsely low total $CO_2$ would result if this loss has occurred. In the laboratory, the specimen can be protected by covering the specimen container with plastic wrap.

## Methods for Quantitative Measurement

Four electrolytes—sodium, potassium, chloride, and bicarbonate (as total $CO_2$)—are generally grouped together for testing and called an electrolyte profile or electrolyte battery. The determination of electrolyte battery concentrations is an important function of the clinical chemistry laboratory. Most electrolyte testing today is done by use of automatic assay instrumentation. Results are reported only when quality control measures meet the established criteria for the laboratory.

### Sodium and Potassium

There are two usual methods for determination of sodium and potassium levels in serum or plasma, ion-selective electrode (ISE) potentiometry and flame emission photometry. Potentiometric instrumentation gives values approximately 1% to 3% higher than flame emission instrumentation. Automated analyzers using flame photometry and ion-selective electrode potentiometry methods are employed. Basic information on flame photometry as a quantitative technique in the laboratory may be found under Flame Emission Photometry, in Chapter 6.

**Ion-Selective Electrode Potentiometry.** Ion-selective electrode (ISE) methods use a glass ion-exchange membrane for sodium assay and a valinomycin neutral-carrier membrane for potassium assay and have been incorporated into many automated chemistry analyzers. Ion-selective electrode methods measure the activity of an ion in the water-volume fraction in which it is dissolved. Generally, two types of ISE measurements are made on biologic samples, "direct" and "indirect"; direct measurements are becoming more common. Direct measurement is done on undiluted samples; indirect measurement requires prediluted samples for measurement of ion activity.

One model of the Johnson & Johnson Vitros Clinical Chemistry Analyzer uses this method. This instrument uses a dry, multilayered slide with a self-contained analytic element coated on a polyester support. Each slide contains a pair of ion-selective electrodes, one being used as a reference electrode and the other as a measuring electrode. Depending upon which slide-electrode is selected, the instrument can assay sodium or potassium. Another ion-selective electrode is also available for chloride assay using this same instrument. In this method, 10 μL of specimen and reference standard is applied to the appropriate Vitros Clinical Chemistry Slide, and the slide is introduced into the instrument. An electrometer in the instrument measures the potential difference between the two half-cells of the reference and the sample, and the result is calculated.

**Flame Emission Photometry.** Flame emission photometry is based on the principle that when atoms of many metallic elements, especially sodium and potassium, are given sufficient energy in one form or another, they will emit this energy at wavelengths that are characteristic for the element. Dilute solutions of serum or another biological fluid (such as urine) are atomized into a flame and burned; in automated analyzers, the sample is automatically diluted and presented to a flame photometer equipped with a recorder or readout device. The elements in these solutions are excited by the flame and emit characteristic spectra. With the use of appropriate filters, the emission from potassium or sodium may be isolated and focused on a photocell, which responds linearly to the light energy directed on it. Since light is emitted in direct proportion to the concentration of sodium or potassium in the unknown fluid, the response of the photocell is directly related to the concentration, and unknowns may be determined by comparing the response with those of known standard solutions.

Sodium always produces a yellow color in a flame, and potassium produces a violet color. The amount of color is measured with a detector and read with a meter (see Fig. 6-7). In most cases, the internal standard method of flame photometry is used: an exact amount of lithium is added to each sample, and the intensity of the sodium or potassium color in the flame is compared by the instrument with the intensity of the red color from the lithium internal standard. The use of an internal standard (lithium) helps to compensate for changes in the condition of the flame and in the levels of interfering substances in the sample being measured. Standard solutions should be analyzed with the unknown samples.

### Chloride

Analyses for chloride include coulometric titration procedures, ion-selective electrodes, and colorimetry. Coulometry and the use of chloridometers, or titrators, have replaced manual titration methods for most chloride determinations. The classic manual titration method is that of Schales and Schales.[15] Advances in technology have provided Cl⁻ selective electrodes for automation of the analysis. Chloride can also be measured colorimetrically by automated analyzer methods. For chloride measurement in urine and sweat, since there is potentially such a wide variation in possible concentration, a coulometric or ion-selective electrode method is usually used.

**Coulometric Titration.** One assay method measures chloride by coulometric titration with silver ions. **Coulometry** measures the amount of electricity passing between two electrodes in an electrochemical cell. The amount of electricity is directly proportional to the amount of substance produced or consumed by the oxidation-reduction process at the electrode.

With the use of a chloridometer, silver ions are generated at a constant voltage from a silver electrode. These silver ions react with chloride ions in the specimen being analyzed to form insoluble silver chloride. The end point is detected amperometrically by a second pair of electrodes. These electrodes can specifically measure the free silver ions that result when all the chloride ions are consumed. The time required to titrate a chloride standard solution or the unknown sample, using a constant current, is measured. The unknown concentration

is calculated with the following proportion formula:

$$\frac{\text{Chloride concentration (standard)}}{\text{Titration time (standard)}} =$$
$$\frac{\text{Chloride concentration (unknown)}}{\text{Titration time (unknown)}}$$

By use of the Cotlove Chloridometer or titrator, silver ions are released from a silver wire when a current is generated in an electrode.[4] The silver ions combine with chloride in the specimen to form insoluble silver chloride. The potential of the solution being titrated changes at the equivalence point, since the solution goes from having an excess of chloride ions to having an excess of silver ions. There must be a sufficient volume of sample that the electrodes are fully immersed in the solution. A small stirrer attached to the electrode assembly thoroughly mixes the specimen as it is being analyzed.

When all the chloride is used, the change in potential shuts off the instrument—in this way the end point is detected automatically. The lapsed time for each titration is automatically recorded on a timer. Since the rate of release of silver ions is constant, the amount of time during which they are released is directly proportional to the amount of chloride in the sample. That is, the more chloride present in the sample, the longer it takes to generate enough silver ions to combine with all of it. In the calculations, the titration time for the unknown is compared with the titration time for a standard sodium chloride solution. Currently used instruments read directly in millimoles per liter.

The chloridometer method is one of the most accurate methods available for determining chloride. Other halogens interfere with this method, just as they do with other methods for chloride. No anticoagulant containing a halogen (chloride, bromide, fluoride, or iodide) can be used in the determination, because it would give falsely high results. The chloridometer can be used with plasma, serum, cerebrospinal fluid, sweat, and urine specimens.

**Ion-Selective Electrode Potentiometry.** The most common methods for chloride assays now use ion-selective electrode-based technology. The sensing element is usually silver–silver chloride or silver sulfide. "Indirect" ISE measurement of chloride is done in the Spectrum.* The Vitros Clinical Chemistry Analyzer[†] and the Dimension Clinical Chemistry System[‡] utilize the "direct" ISE measurement (see above, under Methods for Quantitative Measurement). See also under Ion-Selective Electrode Potentiometry for sodium and potassium.

**Colorimetric Method.** Another common method for chloride assay employs a quantitative displacement of thiocyanate by chloride from mercuric thiocyanate and formation of a red ferric thiocyanate complex. This amount of the colored compound is measured with a spectrophotometer, the amount of color being proportional to the amount of chloride present in the specimen. In this method, chloride first combines with free mercury ions to form a colorless compound; it then displaces any thiocyanate from mercuric thiocyanate. The free thiocyanate ions react with iron to produce the red-colored end product.

### Bicarbonate

The routine bicarbonate (reported rather than total $CO_2$) assay is automated. The first step in automated methods in general is the acidification of the sample to convert the various forms of bicarbonate present to gaseous $CO_2$. Another important consideration for automated procedures for bicarbonate assays is the need to include several standard solutions with the assay of the unknowns, to keep the automated methods in control.

One common automated bicarbonate assay is that utilizing the continuous-flow procedure of the Technicon AutoAnalyzer.[§] The gas formed in the acidification step is quantitatively converted to $HCO_3^-$ and $H^+$. A change in pH results in a change in the color intensity of the phenolphthalein indicator. This is detected quantitatively with a spectrophotometer. The use of standard solutions is vital to keep the instrument in control.

The Synchron CX3* method uses a $P_{CO_2}$ electrode to quantitate the gaseous $CO_2$ produced in the first acidification step. The $CO_2$ gas diffuses through the membrane of the measuring electrode, and this changes the pH of a bicarbonate electrode buffer. The rate of change of pH of the buffer indicates the concentration of $CO_2$ in the sample.

An enzymatic method is used by discrete analyzers such as the Du Pont ACA,[†] in which all $CO_2$ in the specimen is converted to $HCO_3^-$ by addition of alkali. The $HCO_3^-$ formed is then converted enzymatically to oxaloacetic acid. This is measured by an NADH consumption reaction and quantified spectrophotometrically.

### Reference Values[2]

Reference values are generally instrument-specific. Manufacturers' manuals must be consulted for specific reference values for a particular instrument and specimen type.

*Sodium:*

| | |
|---|---|
| 136-145 mmol/L | Serum or plasma (infancy through adulthood) |
| 40-220 mmol/24 hr | Urine (on an average diet; sodium varies with dietary intake) |
| 70% of value determined simultaneously for plasma or serum sodium | CSF |
| 10-40 mmol/L | Sweat |
| >70 mmol/L | Sweat (suggests cystic fibrosis) |

---

*Abbott Diagnostics, Abbott Laboratories, Irving, Tex.
[†]Johnson & Johnson Clinical Diagnostics, Rochester, NY.
[‡]Du Pont Co, Wilmington, Del.
[§]Technicon Instruments Corp, Tarrytown, NY.

---

*Beckman Instruments, Brea, Calif.
[†]Du Pont, Inc, Wilmington, Del.

*Potassium:*

| | |
|---|---|
| 3.5-5.1 mmol/L | Serum, adults |
| 3.7-5.9 mmol/L | Newborns (serum values for newborns are higher than for adults) |
| 3.5-4.5 mmol/L | Plasma, adults |
| 25-125 mmol/24 hr | Urine, on average diet (urinary potassium varies with dietary intake) |

*Chloride:*

| | |
|---|---|
| 98-107 mmol/L | Serum or plasma, adult (upper limit to 110 mmol/L for both full term and premature neonates) |
| 118-132 mmol/L | CSF |
| 110-250 mmol/24 h | Urine (varies with dietary intake) |
| 5-35 mmol/L | Sweat, normal adult |
| 30-70 mmol/L | Sweat, marginal |
| 60-200 mmol/L | Sweat, cystic fibrosis (>60 mmol/l for 98% of persons with cystic fibrosis) |

*Bicarbonate:*

| | |
|---|---|
| 22-29 mmol/L | Serum, venous, adults (values for newborns and infants are lower) |
| 21-28 mmol/L | Arterial, adults |

## UREA NITROGEN AND CREATININE: NONPROTEIN NITROGEN COMPOUNDS

Nitrogen (N) exists in the body in many forms, mostly in components of complex substances. Nitrogen-containing substances are classified into two main groups: protein nitrogen (protein substances containing nitrogen) and nonprotein nitrogen (NPN). Urea is the major NPN constituent and accounts for more than 75% of the total nonprotein nitrogen excreted by the body; other NPNs are amino acids, uric acid, creatinine, creatine, and ammonia, listed in the order of their quantitative importance. Normally, more than 90% of the urea is excreted through

the kidneys. Urea nitrogen, uric acid, and creatinine occur in increased levels as a consequence of decreased renal function, but increased concentrations of several of the major constituents of NPN are used as indicators of diminished renal function. Most laboratories perform serum urea nitrogen measurements in conjunction with creatinine tests when tests for renal function are needed, since, together, they are more specific indicators of renal function disorders. The usefulness of the serum urea nitrogen test alone to determine kidney function is limited because of its variable blood levels, which are due to nonrenal factors. It is common practice to calculate a **urea nitrogen/creatinine ratio**, which is a useful relationship:

$$\frac{\text{Serum urea nitrogen (mg/dL)}}{\text{Serum creatinine (mg/dL)}}$$

The normal ratio for a person on a normal diet is between 12 and 20. Significantly lower ratios indicate acute tubular necrosis, low protein intake, starvation, or severe liver disease. High ratios with normal creatinine values indicate tissue breakdown, prerenal azotemia, or high protein intake. High ratios with increased creatinine may indicate a postrenal obstruction or prerenal azotemia associated with a renal disease.

### Urea/Urea Nitrogen

Urea (urea nitrogen) is the chief component of the NPN material in the blood; it is distributed throughout the body water, and it is equal in concentration in intracellular and extracellular fluid. Gross alterations in NPN usually reflect a change in the concentration of urea. The liver is the sole site of urea formation. As protein breaks down (as amino acids undergo deamination, for example), ammonia is formed in increased amounts. This potentially toxic substance is removed in the liver, where the ammonia combines with other amino acids and is converted to urea by enzymes present in the liver. Urea is, therefore, a waste product of protein metabolism, normally being removed from the blood in the kidneys. The amount of urea in the blood is determined by the amount of dietary protein and by the kidney's ability to excrete urea. If the kidney is impaired, urea is not removed from the blood and it accumulates in the blood. An increased concentration of serum or plasma urea thus may indicate a flaw in the filtering system of the kidneys.

In the past, it was common practice in the laboratory to determine urea as urea nitrogen, using whole blood; this determination was called blood urea nitrogen, or BUN. Methodologies in automated analyzers now can measure urea directly using serum or plasma. The terms blood urea nitrogen (BUN), urea nitrogen, and urea are still used by many. The chemical formula for urea is $NH_2CONH_2$. Since urea nitrogen is a measure of nitrogen and not of urea, one can convert milligrams of urea nitrogen to milligrams of urea by multiplying the urea nitrogen value by 2.14, or 60/28. The molecular weight of urea is 60, and it contains two nitrogen atoms with a combined weight of 28.

The amount of urea in the blood is determined by the amount of dietary protein and by the kidney's ability to excrete urea. If the kidney is impaired, the urea is not removed from the blood, and as it accumulates, the urea level increases. Since the urea concentration is also influenced by diet, people who are undernourished or who are on low-protein diets may have urea levels that are not accurate indications of kidney function. Therefore, tests for urea/urea nitrogen and creatinine are done; creatinine is sometimes considered a better single test for kidney function than urea nitrogen alone.

### Clinical Significance

The assay for urea is only a rough estimate of renal function. The urea will not show any significant level of increased concentration until the glomerular filtration is decreased by at least 50%. As mentioned, a more reliable single index of renal function is the test for serum creatinine. Contrary to urea concentration, creatinine concentration is relatively independent of protein intake (from the diet), degree of hydration, and protein metabolism.

Because the concentration of urea is directly related to protein metabolism, the protein content of the diet will affect the amount of urea in the blood. The ability of the kidneys to remove urea from the blood will also affect the urea content. However, the urea concentration is primarily influenced by the protein intake. In the normal kidney, urea is removed from the blood and excreted in the urine. If kidney function is impaired, urea will not be removed from the blood and the result will be a high urea concentration in the blood. Considerable deterioration must usually be present before the urea level rises above the reference range. The condition of abnormally high urea nitrogen in the blood is called **uremia.** A significant increase in the plasma concentrations of urea and creatinine, in kidney insufficiency, is known as **azotemia.** Decreased levels are usually not clinically significant, unless liver damage is suspected. During pregnancy, lower-than-normal urea levels are often seen.

Azotemia can result from prerenal, renal, or postrenal causes. **Prerenal azotemia** is the result of poor perfusion of the kidneys and, therefore, diminished glomerular filtration. The kidneys are otherwise normal in their functioning capabilities. Poor perfusion can result from dehydration, shock, diminished blood volume, or congestive heart failure. Another cause of prerenal azotemia is increased protein breakdown, as in fever, stress, or severe burns. **Renal azotemia** is due primarily to diminished glomerular filtration as a consequence of acute or chronic renal disease. Such diseases include acute glomerulonephritis, chronic glomerulonephritis, polycystic kidney disease, and nephrosclerosis. **Postrenal azotemia** is usually the result of any type of obstruction in which the urea is reabsorbed into the circulation. Obstruction can be caused by stones, an enlarged prostate gland, or tumors.

### Specimens

Urea may be determined directly from serum, heparinized (sodium or lithium heparin) plasma, urine, or other biological specimens.

Ammonium heparin cannot be used for methods measuring urea nitrogen, as it contains nitrogen. Anti-coagulants containing fluoride will also interfere with methods using urease, because fluoride inhibits the urease reaction. Since urea can be lost through bacterial action, the specimen should be analyzed within a few hours after collection or should be preserved by refrigeration. Refrigeration at 4° to 8° C preserves the urea without measurable change for up to 72 hours.

Urine urea is particularly susceptible to bacterial action, so in addition to refrigeration of the urine specimen at 4° to 8° C, the pH can be maintained at less than 4 to help reduce the loss of urea. If protein-free filtrates are prepared, they are stable for long periods of time, so if a manual test is to be done, the filtrate can be prepared and stored indefinitely until the analysis is done.

### Methods for Quantitative Determination

**Manual Methods.** A group of manual methods used to determine the urea nitrogen concentration, which are very reliable, require the addition of the enzyme urease to whole blood, serum, or plasma. During incubation with urease, urea is converted to ammonium carbonate ($[NH_4]_2CO_3$) by the urease. The ammonia in the ammonium carbonate is analyzed in one of several ways. One classic manual method, devised by Gentzkow, measures the amount of ammonium carbonate formed by having it react with Nessler's solution.[7]

Before nesslerization, a protein-free filtrate is prepared by the modified Folin-Wu method. Nessler's reagent converts the ammonium carbonate to ammonia and carbon dioxide. The reagent then reacts with the ammonia to produce a yellow color, which can be measured colorimetrically. The intensity of the yellow color is directly proportional to the amount of urea present in the specimen. Manual methods have been replaced, by and large, by automated analyzers.

**Automated Methods.** The most common automated methods in use today are indirect methods based on a preliminary hydrolysis step, in which the urea present is converted to ammonia ($NH_3$) by the enzyme urease. How the ammonia is measured differs according to specific instrumentation. In one commonly used analyzer, an enzymatic measurement of the $NH_3$ formed is accomplished by use of an indicator reaction using glutamate dehydrogenase (GLDH) to oxidize NADH to $NAD^+$. It is a very specific, rapid test for urea. The reaction follows:

$$\text{Urea} + H_2O \xrightarrow{\text{urease}} (NH_4)_2CO_3$$

$$NH_4^+ + \alpha\text{-Ketoglutaric acid} + \text{NADH} \xrightarrow{\text{GLDH}}$$
$$ADP + H^+ + NAD^+ + \text{Glutamic acid}$$

Another automated method uses the reaction between the $NH_3$ formed by the action of urease on urea and a pH indicator dye to produce a color change. This methodology has been employed with analyzers that utilize dry reagent technology using either thin-film or reagent strips.

**Use of Recovery for Enzyme Methods.** Since there are many variables in methods utilizing enzymes as reagents, it is advisable to periodically check the accuracy of a method through the use of a recovery solution. An accurately measured amount of recovery solution is added to one of the samples in a batch. It is best to choose a sample that is known to be in the normal range for the substance being assayed. The **recovery solution** is a quantitatively prepared solution of the substance that is being measured in the unknown patient samples. For example, the recovery solution for a urea determination is a solution of urea. Theoretically, the amount of urea in the recovery solution added to the sample should be recovered at the end of the procedure; none should be lost or gained along the way. The use of a recovery solution checks the accuracy of the method. The acceptable recovery range is 90% to 110%. If the recovery is outside these limits, the procedure must be repeated and the results not reported out until the recovery is within the limits established. The use of a recovery solution tells just how good an enzyme method really is.

### Reference Values[2]

Values in parentheses are in SI units.

*Urea nitrogen, serum:*

| | |
|---|---|
| Adult | 7-18 mg/dL (2.5-6.4 mmol urea/L) |
| >60 yr | 8-21 mg/dL (2.9-7.5 mmol urea/L) |
| Infant/child | 5-18 mg/dL (1.8-6.4 mmol urea/L) |

*Urea, serum:*

| | |
|---|---|
| Adult | 5-39 mg/dL (2.5-6.4 mmol/L) |

*Urea nitrogen, urine:* 12-20 g/24 hr (428-714 mmol urea/24 hr)

## Creatinine

Creatinine in the blood is a product of creatine metabolism in the muscles. Its formation and release into the body fluids occur at a constant rate and have a direct relationship to muscle mass. Its concentration varies, therefore, with age and gender. The clearance of creatinine from the plasma by the kidney is measured as an indicator of the glomerular filtration rate (GFR). Serum or plasma specimens are preferred over whole blood, since there are considerable noncreatinine chromogens present in red cells, which can cause falsely elevated creatinine assay results.

Most methods for creatinine employ the Jaffe reaction (first described in 1886).[9] This reaction is noted to be the oldest clinical chemistry method still in common use. Creatinine reacts with alkaline picrate to form an orange-red solution that is measured in the spectrophotometer. To improve the specificity of the reaction and to eliminate interference from the many noncreatinine substances in blood that can also react with the alkaline picrate solution, an acidification step is added. These noncreatinine Jaffe-reacting chromogens include proteins, glucose,

ascorbic acid, and pyruvate. The color from true creatinine is less resistant to acidification than the color from the noncreatinine substances. The difference between the two colors is measured photometrically.

### Clinical Significance

Creatinine in the blood results from the metabolism of creatine in the muscles of the body. Creatinine is freely filtered by the glomeruli of the kidney and is not reabsorbed under normal circumstances. There is a relatively constant excretion of creatinine in the urine, which parallels creatinine production. In renal disease, the creatinine excretion is impaired, and this is reflected in an increase in creatinine in the blood.

The serum creatinine concentration is relatively constant and is somewhat higher in males than in females. The constancy of concentration and excretion makes creatinine a good measure of renal function, especially of glomerular filtration. The concentration of creatinine is not affected by dietary intake, degree of dehydration in the body, or protein metabolism, which makes the assay a more reliable single screening index of renal function than the urea assay.

A useful index relates creatinine excretion to muscle mass or lean body weight, taking into consideration variables in individual body sizes. This index is known as the **creatinine clearance.**

**Creatinine Clearance.** The creatinine clearance is defined as the milliliters of plasma that are cleared of creatinine by the kidneys per minute. The result is normalized to a standard person's surface area by using the height and weight of the patient. The creatinine clearance is used to assess the glomerular filtration functioning capabilities of the kidneys.

To perform this test for creatinine clearance, timed specimens of both blood and urine must be collected (see Collection Procedure for Timed Urine Specimens, in Chapter 3). All voided urine must be carefully collected for 24 hours. The urine specimen is preserved by refrigeration between collections. Blood is collected at about

12 hours into the urine collection period. Creatinine is measured in the blood (serum or plasma) and in the timed urine specimen (24-hour). The creatinine clearance is calculated as follows:

$$U/P \times V \times 1.73/A = mL \text{ plasma cleared/min}$$

where U is the urine creatinine concentration (mg/dL), P is the plasma creatinine concentration (mg/dL), V is the volume in milliliters of urine excreted per minute, A is the patient's body surface area in square meters, and 1.73 is the standard body surface area in square meters. A nomogram is used to find the patient's body surface area (see Fig. 11-5). Most automated analyzers have calculating capabilities for this value if the specific patient height and weight data are entered into the system.

### Specimens

Serum, heparinized plasma, or diluted urine can be assayed for creatinine. Ammonium heparinized plasma should not be used for methods that measure ammonia production. Usually urine is diluted 1:100 or 1:200. Creatinine is stable in serum or plasma for up to one week if the specimen has been refrigerated. It is important to separate the cells promptly to prevent hemolysis and to minimize ammonia production. Hemolysis causes falsely elevated creatinine values.

### Methods for Quantitative Determination

Most of the commonly used methods for creatinine assay are based on the Jaffe reaction, in which the creatinine present in the specimen is treated with an alkaline picrate reagent to yield a bright orange-red complex. Noncreatinine chromogens (nonspecific) in the specimen can also react, which results in falsely elevated values. Kinetic alkaline picrate methods and enzymatic creatinine methods are commonly used in automated analyzers. Kinetic methods have reduced some of the interferences caused by noncreatinine chromogens. Enzymatic methods

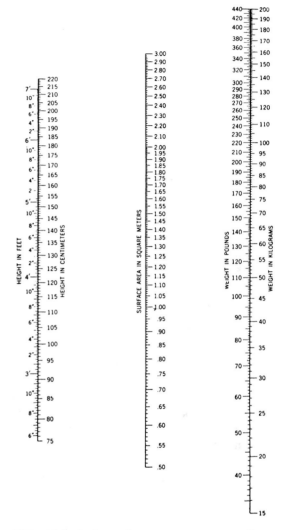

**FIG 11-5.** Body surface area nomogram. (From Boothby W, Sandford RB: N Engl J Med 1921; 185:337.)

make the reaction more specific and sensitive for creatinine.

### Reference Values[2]

Values in parentheses are in SI units.

*Creatinine, serum or plasma* (Jaffe kinetic or enzymatic method):

| Adult men | 0.7-1.3 mg/dL (62-115 $\mu$mmol/L) |
| Adult women | 0.6-1.1 mg/dL (53-97 $\mu$mmol/L) |

*Creatinine, urine:*

| Adult men | 14-26 mg/kg/24 hr (124-230 $\mu$mmol/kg/24 h) |
| Adult women | 11-20 mg/kg/24 hr (97-177 $\mu$mmol/kg/24 h) |

Creatinine excretion decreases with age.

*Creatinine clearance:*

| Male (under 40 yr) | 90-139 mL/min/1.73 m$^2$ |
| Female (under 40 yr) | 80-125 mL/min/1.73 m$^2$ |

Creatinine clearance values decrease approximately 6.5 mL/min/1.73m$^2$ per decade.

## CHOLESTEROL, TRIGLYCERIDES: LIPIDS (FAT)

Lipids play an important role in many of the body's processes; they act as hormones or precursors to hormones that aid in digestion, provide energy storage and fuels for metabolic processes, provide structural and functional components in biomembranes, and form insulation to allow conduction of nerve impulses or to prevent loss of heat. The causative relationship between levels of plasma lipids and lipoproteins and the development of atherosclerosis has been well established, and large programs have been developed by public health agencies to detect, evaluate, and treat certain of these lipid elevations.

Lipids are stored, primarily as triglyceride, in subcutaneous fat and in the liver, where they serve as an energy reservoir. Triglycerides enter the mucosal cells of the intestine, where the triglyceride is incorporated into chylomicrons. **Chylomicrons** give serum its characteristic milky appearance (lipemia) when blood is drawn following a meal (postprandial specimen). Triglycerides make up most of the fat found in food, about 98% to 99%; this is neutral fat. The rest of the lipids (fat) in food include cholesterol, phospholipids, diglycerides, and fat-soluble vitamins. Cholesterol is found in all animal fats; it is not found in fats in plants. The amount of cholesterol absorbed from the diet is self-regulating, and increased levels of dietary triglycerides tend to promote cholesterol absorption for some people. There is great individual variation in cholesterol absorption, and this may account for the variability in how persons respond to diet-induced hypercholesterolemia. About 30% to 60% of cholesterol is absorbed daily, and increased amounts of fat in the diet (because that fat is 98% triglycerides) result in greater absorption of cholesterol. Once cholesterol is synthesized, it is transported in lipoprotein complexes. These include chylomicrons, very low-density lipoproteins (VLDLs), low-density lipoproteins (LDLs), and high-density lipoproteins (HDLs). The level of cholesterol reflects the rate of synthesis of the cholesterol-carrying lipoproteins and how well the mechanism for their breakdown is working in the body. Only a portion of the body's cholesterol is derived from dietary intake; most is synthesized by the liver.

The liver can synthesize lipoprotein particles from dietary constituents recently absorbed. The liver serves as a temporary storage site for lipids as they are synthesized in the liver or absorbed from the intestine after a meal. The liver is the major organ that can synthesize cholesterol—about 70% of the daily cholesterol production comes from the liver. Increases in cholesterol have been implicated in increased atherosclerotic diseases, but cholesterol is also an essential component for normal biological functions. It serves as an essential structural component of animal cell membranes and subcellular particles and as a precursor of bile acids and all steroid hormones, including sex and adrenal hormones.

### Clinical Significance of Hyperlipidemia (Including Increased Cholesterol)

When a hyperlipidemic condition exists for a sufficient length of time, it may be associated with the development of **atherosclerosis,** or hardening of the arteries, and its resulting complications. Coronary artery disease (CAD) is almost always the result of atherosclerosis. Coronary atherosclerosis is primarily a result of the accumulation of fatty deposits in the walls of the arteries, leading to formation of fibrous plaques in the walls of the vessels. CAD is a common cause of heart disease and the leading cause of death in the United States and other parts of the western world. The incidence of coronary heart disease in general increases with age. The majority of coronary-related mortalities are the result of atherosclerosis.

Several factors have been associated with an increase in the likelihood of developing a heart attack later in life. The risk factors listed below correlate with the presence of coronary heart disease (CHD) and are grouped as primary or secondary factors[10]:

*Primary:*

    Genetic predisposition for CHD
    Hypertension
    Cigarette smoking
    Elevated total cholesterol (LDL cholesterol)
    Decreased HDL cholesterol
    Age
    Male sex

*Secondary:*

    Lack of exercise
    Obesity
    Stress
    Diabetes mellitus
    Gout and hyperuricemia
    Renal failure patients receiving hemodialysis
    Postmenopausal state
    Hypothyroidism
    Certain thrombogenic disorders

Some of the risk factors are unavoidable (such as genetic predisposition and age), but many can be modified by a change in behavior or lifestyle.

### National Cholesterol Education Program

In the late 1980s, the federal government, along with a broad range of professional health care groups, formulated guidelines and recommendations with the intent of reducing the occurrence of coronary heart disease in the United States. This campaign resulted in a national educational drive to standardize the approach to the detection and classification of individuals at high risk for CHD and to standardize the treatment and monitoring of these individuals. The establishment of the **National Cholesterol Education Program (NCEP)** was the result of this effort. From the NCEP guidelines, cutoff levels for total cholesterol and LDL cholesterol were established that apply to all adults, 20 years or older (Table 11-1). The goal of this program is to establish criteria to define high-risk persons for medical intervention, in order to treat and monitor these persons over time. Other work is being done to establish guidelines for children and adolescents.

As a result of the NCEP, ongoing studies have been done and modifications have been made to the original guidelines, including the addition of testing for HDL cholesterol as a potential risk factor. An HDL cholesterol level of greater than 60 mg/dL is now considered a beneficial, or a negative, risk factor, while a level less than 35 mg/dL is a significant, or a positive, risk factor. There is also now an increased emphasis on physical activity and weight loss as components of the dietary therapy for high blood cholesterol.

Treatment of patients with hyperlipidemias is initially dietary, with restriction of dietary lipid intake. NCEP cholesterol guidelines recommend

### TABLE 11-1

Classification of adults at risk based on total cholesterol and low-density cholesterol[14,16]

| Total Cholesterol (mg/dL) | Classification of Risk | LDL Cholesterol (mg/dL) |
|---|---|---|
| <200 | Desirable | <130 |
| 200-239 | Borderline high | 130-159 |
| >240 | High | >160 |

screening adults 20 years and older for total blood cholesterol; low-density lipoprotein (LDL) cholesterol and high-density lipoprotein (HDL) cholesterol measurements are also now recommended. Treatment focuses on lowering high levels of LDL cholesterol, since it is the LDL cholesterol and not the total cholesterol that more strongly increases a person's risk for developing coronary heart disease.

## Specimens

Cholesterol determinations may be done using serum or heparinized or EDTA-anticoagulated plasma. The NCEP cholesterol coronary heart disease guidelines are based on serum determinations of cholesterol. If cholesterol alone is to be measured, a fasting specimen is not necessary, but if triglycerides or LDL cholesterol are also to be measured, the specimen must be collected after a minimum 12-hour fast. A fasting specimen for HDL cholesterol is also preferred because some methods for assay of HDL are affected by high triglycerides. Once the blood is collected, the specimen must be processed as soon as possible to separate the serum from the cells to prevent an exchange of cholesterol between red blood cell membranes and the serum or plasma. If analysis needs to be delayed, the serum can be refrigerated at 4° C for several days.

The appearance of the plasma or serum can be observed and noted. If the plasma is clear, the triglyceride level is more than likely less than 200 mg/dL. When the plasma appears hazy-turbid, the triglyceride level has increased to greater than 300 mg/dL, and if the specimen appears opaque and milky (lipemic, due to chylomicrons), the triglyceride level is probably greater than 600 mg/dL. Findings on appearance must only be made if the specimen is collected after a minimum 12-hour fast.

## Methods for Quantitative Determination of Lipids
### Total Cholesterol

In routine laboratories, the most common methodology used to determine cholesterol is by an enzymatic assay. The reference method for cholesterol is a modification of the procedure of Abell et al, which involves the hydrolysis of cholesterol esters, followed by extraction of the free cholesterol into petroleum ether and color development using an acetic acid.[1]

In most common automated enzymatic methods, the enzyme cholesterol esterase hydrolyzes cholesterol esters to free cholesterol. The free cholesterol produced, along with free cholesterol that was initially present in the sample, is then oxidized in a reaction catalyzed by cholesterol oxidase. The hydrogen peroxide ($H_2O_2$) formed oxidizes various compounds to form a colored product that is measured photometrically, the magnitude of the colored compound formed being proportional to the amount of cholesterol present in the sample. Some interferences are noted with lipemic samples when direct methods are used.

The NCEP recommends that cholesterol methods be calibrated to the reference method at the Centers for Disease Control and Prevention (the Abell method; see above).

### Triglycerides

Triglyceride methods are commonly enzymatic. In most automated enzymatic methods, hydrolysis of the triglyceride present in the sample is usually achieved by lipase (triacylglycerol acylhydrolase). The resulting glycerol produced is assayed by various coupled-enzyme methods. The presence of free glycerol in the samples can interfere with the analysis. Reagents must be carefully checked in automated methodologies, as some reagents have a short stability period after reconstitution.

The triglyceride measurement is needed in order to calculate the LDL cholesterol, using the following equation:

LDL cholesterol = Total cholesterol −
        (VLDL cholesterol + HDL cholesterol)

where very low-density lipoprotein (VLDL) cholesterol equals triglycerides divided by 5.

Automated analyzers calculate this finding.

### HDL Cholesterol

To quantify HDL cholesterol, the major lipo-proteins must first be precipitated, leaving the HDL fraction in the supernatant. After centrifugation, the HDL cholesterol can be quantified by using a total cholesterol methodology.

### Reference Values[2]

Values in parentheses are in SI Units.

*Cholesterol, serum, adults* (NCEP guideline recommendations for adults in terms of risk for coronary heart disease[14]):

| | |
|---|---|
| Desirable | <200 mg/dL (<5.18 mmol/L) |
| Borderline/ moderate risk | 200-239 mg/dL (5.18-6.19 mmol/L) |
| High risk | >240 mg/dL (>6.22 mmol/L) |

*Triglycerides, serum* (recommended desirable levels for adults, after a 12-hour fast):

| | |
|---|---|
| Male | 40-160 mg/dL |
| Female | 35-135 mg/dL |

Note: Reference values for triglycerides vary for females and males, with females having values slightly lower. Specific age-related reference value tables are available in clinical chemistry textbooks, if needed. The triglyceride values also increase with age until age 60, when they decrease slightly. Levels for blacks are 10 to 20 mg/dL lower than for Caucasians. The NCEP recommendations have eliminated the use of reference values for triglycerides, but include a few cutoff values (as used for total cholesterols) to simplify the decision-making process.

*HDL cholesterol:*

| | |
|---|---|
| Negative risk factor for CHD | >60 mg/dL |
| Positive risk factor for CHD | <35 mg/dL |

## BILIRUBIN METABOLISM AND LIVER FUNCTION

Bilirubin is derived from the heme portion of hemoglobin, after the breakdown of aged red cells (with an average 120-day life span). Bilirubin is transported to the liver tightly complexed to albumin. This bilirubin is called **unconjugated bilirubin,** and it is not water soluble. In the liver, this bilirubin-bound-to-albumin is released by the albumin, to be conjugated with glucuronide by the liver cells and therefore made water soluble. This bilirubin is thus called **conjugated bilirubin,** and it is in this form that it enters the bile fluid for transport to the small intestine. In the small intestine, most of the conjugated bilirubin is converted to urobilinogens (see also Bilirubin, in Chapter 14).

One frequently used assay for assessment of the excretory function of the liver is the measurement of the serum bilirubin concentration. The classic clinical manifestation of liver disease is jaundice, the yellow discoloration of the plasma, skin, and mucous membranes, specifically the sclera of the eye. **Jaundice,** or **icterus,** is caused by the abnormal metabolism, accumulation, or retention of bilirubin. There are three types of jaundice: prehepatic, hepatic, and posthepatic. Initial evaluation of hyperbilirubinemia depends, in part, on whether there is a predominance of the unconjugated form of bilirubin or a significant increase in the conjugated form of bilirubin in the blood.

### Clinical Significance of Bilirubin

The clinical finding of jaundice is not specific and can be caused by a variety of diseases. Specific diseases involving bilirubin metabolism each represent a defect in the way the liver processes the bilirubin. These can be transport defects, that is, defects of releasing the bilirubin bound to plasma albumin to the liver cell for conjugation with glucuronide (a prehepatic function); impairment in the conjugation step in the liver itself (a hepatic function); or a defect in the excretory function of getting the conjugated bilirubin-glucuronide from the liver cells into the canaliculi of the liver and into the bile fluid (a posthepatic function). Increased hemolysis of red cells, as in a hemolytic anemia, can result in prehepatic jaundice. Hepatitis and cirrhosis of the liver can result in hepatic jaundice. Obstruction of the biliary tract caused by strictures, neoplasms, or stones can result in posthepatic jaundice.

An increased serum bilirubin concentration may indicate increased destruction (hemolysis) of red blood cells, impaired excretory function of liver cells, or obstruction of the bile flow. In obstructive jaundice there is an increase in total bilirubin; however, this is primarily in the form of conjugated bilirubin, measured as "direct" bilirubin, giving an increased value for direct bilirubin. In hemolytic jaundice there is an increase in total bilirubin, primarily unconjugated bilirubin, measured as "indirect" bilirubin (the indirect fraction is increased). With liver damage such as viral hepatitis, both the unconjugated bilirubin and the conjugated bilirubin increase, and total, direct, and indirect fractions are elevated.

### Neonatal Jaundice

Elevations in serum bilirubin occur in some infants in the first few days of life, an example of **physiologic jaundice.** This is especially true of premature infants. Such neonatal jaundice may involve either a deficiency of the enzyme that transfers glucuronate groups onto bilirubin or liver immaturity. In some premature births, infants are born without the necessary enzyme activity of glucuronosyltransferase. This enzyme normally assists in the conjugation of bilirubin glucuronide, and when it is not present, bilirubin will not be conjugated and there will be a rapid build-up of the unconjugated bilirubin. This can be life threatening to the newborn. The unconjugated bilirubin readily passes into the brain and nerve cells and is deposited in the nuclei of these cells. The result is called **kernicterus,** which can result in cell damage and death. Neonatal jaundice can persist until the enzyme glucuronosyltransferase is produced by the liver of the newborn. The blood of the newborn must be monitored frequently to detect any dangerously high levels of unconjugated bilirubin.

Neonatal jaundice is generally a temporary deficiency, which lasts only a few days, until bilirubin metabolism matures. All newborns have serum unconjugated bilirubin values greater than the reference values in a healthy adult, and 50% of newborns will be clinically jaundiced during the first 5 days of life; this jaundice is known as physiologic jaundice. In normal, healthy, full-term newborns, unconjugated bilirubin values can rise to 4 to 5 mg/dL, and in a small percentage of newborns, this value can rise as high as 10 mg/dL. These elevated values usually decrease to normal levels in 7 to 10 days.

If toxic levels do occur, exceeding 20 mg/dL, which is most likely to happen in cases of incompatibility between the blood groups of the mother and the infant and which has been largely alleviated through the use of Rh immune globulin, treatment must be initiated. Treatment of infants with enzyme deficiency involves phototherapy (use of lights). Blood incompatibility or bilirubin levels approaching 20 mg/dL may require exchange transfusion.

### Specimens

Bilirubin analyses may be done on serum or plasma, although serum is preferred. The blood should be drawn when the patient is in a fasting state to avoid alimentary lipemia, which can result in falsely increased bilirubin values because of the turbidity of the specimen. Exposure of serum to heat and light, especially that of wavelengths at the lower end of the visible region, results in oxidation of bilirubin. For this reason, specimens for bilirubin assays must be protected from the light. The procedure should be carried out as soon as possible, at least within 2 or 3 hours after the blood has clotted. Specimens can be stored in the dark in a refrigerator for up to 1 week or in the freezer for 3 months without significant loss of bilirubin. The presence of hemoglobin results in the measurement of an erroneously low value for bilirubin by a diazo method. It is difficult to see hemoglobin in the presence of increased amounts of bilirubin, however.

## Methods for Quantitative Determination of Bilirubin

Most tests for serum bilirubin used in the clinical laboratory are based on a diazo reaction, in which the bilirubin reacts with diazotized sulfanilic acid to form azobilirubin, which has a red-purple color. This reaction was first described by Ehrlich in 1883, and the diazo reagent is also referred to as Ehrlich's reagent. This basic reaction was modified in 1916 by van den Bergh and Muller by the addition of alcohol, usually methanol, which accelerated the reaction of unconjugated bilirubin, called indirect bilirubin. They called the reacting substance, in the absence of alcohol, the direct fraction of bilirubin, or conjugated bilirubin. Total bilirubin is the combination of conjugated and unconjugated bilirubin. The azobilirubin formed in the diazo reactions has indicator properties in strongly acid or strongly alkaline solutions. Thus, some modifications of the diazo reaction measure the amount of red dye in an acid medium, while others measure the blue color in a strongly alkaline medium. Many procedures involve a modification of the Malloy-Evelyn technique, carried out in an acid solution, which utilizes a diazo reaction with methanol added.[12] Another commonly used procedure is the Jendrassik-Grof modification.[11] This is carried out in an alkaline solution. Both the Malloy-Evelyn and Jendrassik-Grof modifications have been automated, and they are currently the most frequently used bilirubin assays.

As described earlier, bilirubin is present in serum in two forms: unconjugated and conjugated to glucuronic acid. Since the glucuronide form of bilirubin is freely soluble in water, it reacts rapidly with Ehrlich's reagent. A reading made at a specific time (usually 1 minute) after the addition of Ehrlich's reagent is generally taken as a measure of the bilirubin glucuronide (conjugated bilirubin or direct bilirubin) concentration. Unconjugated bilirubin is not soluble in water and reacts with Ehrlich's reagent only after the addition of methanol. A reading made after the addition of methanol and a sufficient waiting period, usually 10 or 20 minutes, is a measure of the concentration of the two forms of bilirubin combined. The concentration of unconjugated bilirubin (also referred to as indirect bilirubin) is the difference between the total concentration of bilirubin and the concentration of direct or 1-minute bilirubin.

Conjugated and unconjugated bilirubin are differentiated by the amount of time needed for the reaction and the solubility of the various fractions of bilirubin. Bilirubin that reacts quickly, in the absence of a solvent, is called direct or conjugated bilirubin. It is also known that a portion of the unconjugated bilirubin is also available to react in the absence of a solvent. The extent of this reaction is determined by the time and temperature of the reaction and the final concentration of the reagents used. The extent of the reaction of the unconjugated bilirubin, or indirect bilirubin, in the presence of a solvent is also dependent on the final concentration of the solvent used.

Chromatography, open-column and high-performance liquid chromatography (HPLC), have shown that there is a third fraction of bilirubin, called delta bilirubin.[5] The delta bilirubin fraction reacts like conjugated bilirubin and is normally found in very small amounts in serum. When the levels of unconjugated bilirubin are increased, the levels of delta bilirubin are also increased, resulting in an apparent increase in the conjugated bilirubin fraction when most bilirubin assay methods are used.

The method used as a reference method for total bilirubin is a modified Jendrassik-Grof procedure.[11] The American Association for Clinical Chemistry (AACC) and the National Bureau of Standards have both published this as the recommended reference method.

### Automated Bilirubin Assays

In the Johnson & Johnson Vitros Clinical Chemistry Analyzers,* bilirubin is separated from the protein matrix by means of thin-film technology. Dry reagents are within the multilayered slides, and the reaction occurs within the layers as the serum passes through. Total bilirubin is determined by diazotization after unconjugated bilirubin and conjugated bilirubin have been dissociated from albumin. The bilirubin diffuses into a polymer layer that complexes with the bilirubin. The reaction that occurs is monitored with a reflectance spectrophotometer. This method provides for the measurement of direct bilirubin, which is the sum of the delta and conjugated bilirubin.

In the Ames Seralyzer,[†] plastic strips with a matrix of reagents at one end are used. For the bilirubin assay, the van den Bergh diazo reaction is employed. Results are read using reflectance photometry, which gives a good correlation coefficient with the manual Jendrassik-Grof method. This is a rapid, accurate assay.

### Reference Values[2]

*Total serum bilirubin, adult:* 0.3-1.2 mg/dL
*Direct (conjugated) serum bilirubin:* 0-0.2 mg/dL
*Total serum bilirubin in infants:*

| Age | Premature | Full Term |
|---|---|---|
| Cord | <2.0 mg/dL | <2.0 mg/dL |
| 0-1 day | <8.0 mg/dL | 2.0-6.0 mg/dL |
| 1-2 days | <12.0 mg/dL | 6.0-10.0 mg/dL |
| 3-5 days | <16.0 mg/dL | 1.5-12.0 mg/dL |

Conjugated bilirubin levels up to 2 mg/dL are found in infants by 1 month of age, and this level remains through adulthood.

### Other Liver Function Tests

Tests for several serum enzymes are used in the differential diagnosis of liver diseases. These tests include alkaline phosphatase, gamma-glutamyl-transferase, lactate dehydrogenase, aspartate aminotransferase and alanine aminotransferase, and 5'-nucleotidase. Bile acids, triglycerides, cholesterol, serum proteins, coagulation proteins, and urea and ammonia assays are also used in the diagnosis of liver disease. Results from several laboratory procedures must be evaluated by the physician before an accurate diagnosis can be made. The physician or institution may have a preferred battery of tests to determine liver function. Brief descriptions of some of the tests most often included in such a liver profile follow.

### Aspartate Aminotransferase and Alanine Aminotransferase

These are transaminases that catalyze the conversion of aspartate and alanine to oxaloacetate and pyruvate, respectively. The highest level of alanine aminotransferase (ALT) is found primarily in the liver. Aspartate aminotransferase (AST) is found in the liver, heart, kidney, and muscle tissue. Acute destruction of tissue in any of these areas results in rapid release of the enzymes into the serum. ALT and AST are elevated in the onset of viral jaundice; they are both elevated in chronic active hepatitis. With the onset of acute liver necrosis, both enzymes are increased, but the increase in ALT is higher. Information from these tests is best utilized in conjunction with that from other liver function tests.

### Gamma-glutamyltransferase

Gamma-glutamyltransferase (GGT) is normally in the highest concentration in the renal tissue, but it is also generally elevated in liver disease. Serum GGT is usually elevated earlier than the other liver enzymes in diseases such as acute cholecystitis, acute pancreatitis, acute and subacute liver necrosis, and neoplasms of sites where liver metastases are present. Increased levels of GGT are found in the blood when there is obstruction to bile flow, or cholestasis.

### Alkaline Phosphatase

This enzyme may be produced in many tissues, and it is generally localized in the membranes

---

*Johnson & Johnson, Rochester, NY.
[†]Bayer Corp, Diagnostics Division, Tarrytown, NY.

of cells. It is found in its highest activity in the liver, bone, intestine, kidney, and placenta. It is normally produced in the liver by the bile duct epithelium and in the bone by osteoblasts. The enzyme appears to facilitate the transfer of metabolites across cell membranes and is associated with lipid transport and with the calcification process in bone synthesis. Serum alkaline phosphatase is particularly useful in differentiating hepatobiliary disease from bone disease associated with increased osteoblastic activity. Increased levels are found in the blood when there is obstruction to bile flow, or cholestasis.

### Protein Electrophoresis

In normal healthy individuals, the various plasma proteins are present in delicately balanced concentrations, with a normal ratio of albumin to globulin. Albumin is made only in the liver. In liver disease this ratio may be altered. A number of tests for liver function are therefore based on the albumin-globulin ratio. Protein electrophoresis is the most effective way to demonstrate significant alterations in the protein fractions. Electrophoretic separation of serum proteins is also of value in following the course of liver disease after diagnosis.

### Coagulation Proteins

Another protein formed in the liver is prothrombin, which is necessary for the normal coagulation of blood. If liver function is impaired, less-than-normal amounts of prothrombin are formed and blood clotting is delayed. A determination of the prothrombin time can be used to test for abnormal liver function. Other coagulation proteins are also synthesized in the liver and can be affected if the liver is diseased.

## REFERENCES

1. Abell LL, Levy BB, et al.: Simplified methods for the estimation of the total cholesterol in serum and demonstration of its specificity. *J Biol Chem* 1952; 195:357-366.

2. Burtis CA, Ashwood ER (eds): *Tietz Fundamentals of Clinical Chemistry*, ed 4. Philadelphia, WB Saunders Co, 1996, pp 363, 670, 777, 778, 780, 782, 785, 809, 814, 818, 819.

3. Consensus Development Panel: Consensus statement on self-monitoring of blood glucosse. *Diabetes Care* 1987; 10:95-99.

4. Cotlove E, Trantham HV, Bowman RL: An instrument and method for automatic, rapid, accurate and sensitive titration of chloride in biological samples. *J Lab Clin Med* 1958; 50:461.

5. Doumas BT, Wu TW, Jendrzejczak B: The reaction of bilirubin firmly bound to protein (delta-bilirubin) with the diazo reagent, *Clin Chem* 1984; 30:971.

6. The Expert Committee on the Diagnosis and Classification of Diabetes Mellitus: Report of the Expert Committee on the Diagnosis and Classification of Diabetes Mellitus. *Diabetes Care* 1997; 20(7):1183-1201.

7. Gentzkow CJ: Accurate method for determination of blood urea nitrogen by direct nesslerization. *J Biol Chem* 1942; 143:531.

8. Harris MR, Hadden WC, Knowler WC, et al: Prevalence of diabetes and impaired glucose tolerance and plasma levels in the US population aged 20-74 yr. *Diabetes* 1987; 36:523.

9. Jaffe M: Uber den Niederschlag welchen Pikrinsaure in normalen Harn erzeugt und uber eine neue Reaktion des Kreatininins. *Z Physiol Chem* 1886; 10:391.

10. Kaplan LA, Pesce AJ: *Clinical Chemistry: Theory, Analysis, and Correlation*, ed 3. St Louis, Mosby, 1996, p 664.

11. Koch TR, Doumas DT, Elser RC, et al: Bilirubin, total and conjugated, modified Jendrassik-Grof method. In Faulkner WR, Meites S (eds): *Selected Methods of Clinical Chemistry*, vol 9. Washington, DC, American Association for Clinical Chemistry Press, 1982, pp 113-118.

12. Malloy HT, Evelyn KA: The determination of bilirubin with the photoelectric colorimeter. *J Biol Chem* 1937; 119:481.

13. National Diabetes Data Group: Classification and diagnosis of diabetes mellitus and other categories of glucose intolerance. *Diabetes* 1979; 28:1039-1057.

14. Report of the National Cholesterol Education Program Expert Panel on Detection, Evaluation, and Treatment of High Blood Cholesterol in Adults. *Arch Intern Med* 1988; 148:36-39.

15. Schales O, Schales SS: Simple and accurate method for determination of chloride in biological fluids. *J Biol Chem* 1949; 140:879.
16. Second Expert Panel: Detection, evaluation, and treatment of high blood cholesterol in adults (Adult Treatment Panel II). *Circulation* 1994; 89: 1329-1445.

## BIBLIOGRAPHY

Becan-McBride K, Ross D: *Essentials for the Small Laboratory and Physician's Office*. St Louis, Mosby, 1988.

Henry JB (ed): *Clinical Diagnosis and Management by Laboratory Methods*, ed 19. Philadelphia, WB Saunders Co., 1996.

Jacobs DS, DeMott WR, Grady HJ, et al (eds): *Laboratory Test Handb00k*. Hudson, Ohio, Lexi-Comp, Inc, 1996.

Kaplan LA, Pesce AJ: *Clinical Chemistry: Theory, Analysis, and Correlation*, ed 3. St Louis, Mosby, 1996.

NCCLS: *Ancillary (Bedside) Blood Glucose Testing in Acute and Chronic Care Facilities: Approved Guideline*. Villanova, Pa, National Committee for Clinical Laboratory Standards, 1994, document C30-A.

NCCLS: *Blood Glucose Testing in Settings Without Laboratory Support: Proposed Guideline*. Villanova, Pa, National Committee for Clinical Laboratory Standards, 1996, document AST4-P.

NCCLS: *Physician's Office Laboratory Manual: Tentative Guideline*. Villanova, Pa, National Committee for Clinical Laboratory Standards, 1995, document POL1/2-T3.

NCCLS: *Standardization of Sodium and Potassium Ion-Selective Electrode Systems to the Flame Photometric Reference Method: Approved Standard*. Villanova, Pa, National Committee for Clinical Laboratory Standards, 1995, document C29-A.

NCCLS: *Sweat Testing: Sample Collection and Quantitative Analysis, Approved Guideline*. Villanova, Pa, National Committee for Clinical Laboratory Standards, 1994, document C34-A.

Ravel R: *Clinical Laboratory Medicine*, ed 6. St Louis, Mosby, 1995.

## STUDY QUESTIONS

### GENERAL CHEMISTRY METHODOLOGIES

1. **Match each of the following descriptions of common methodologies employed in analytic chemistry instrumentation (1 to 5) with the name of the analytic technique (A to E).**

   1. The measurement of light scattered by particles in a solution
   2. The measurement of the amount of electricity passing between two electrodes in an electric field
   3. The measurement of the amount of light reflected from the surface of a colorimetric reaction
   4. The measurement of emitted energy produced by some elements when sprayed into a flame
   5. Measurement after a mixture of solvents dissolved in a common solvent have been separated from one another by a differential distribution of the solutes between two phases.
      _____ A. Chromatography
      _____ B. Reflectance spectrophotometry
      _____ C. Flame emission photometry
      _____ D. Electrophoresis
      _____ E. Nephelometry

2. **The most common application of coulometry is in which of the following assays?**

   A. Chloride
   B. Glucose
   C. Sodium
   D. Cholesterol

### GLUCOSE

1. **The level of glycated hemoglobin in a diabetic patient reflects which of the following?**

   A. Blood glucose concentration at the time the blood was collected
   B. The average blood glucose concentration over the past week
   C. The average blood glucose concentration over the past 2 to 3 months (the life span of a red cell)

D. More than one of the above

2. **Sodium fluoride additive used in a specimen collected for glucose:**

   A. Inhibits glycolytic enzymes from destroying the glucose.
   B. Precipitates the protein present.
   C. Prevents nonglucose reducing substances from interfering with the testing.
   D. None of the above

3. **In a person with normal glucose metabolism, the blood glucose level usually increases rapidly after carbohydrates are ingested, but returns to a normal level after:**

   A. 30 minutes
   B. 60 minutes
   C. 90 minutes
   D. 120 minutes

4. **Which of the following organs uses glucose from digested carbohydrates and stores it as glycogen for later use as a source of immediate energy by the muscles?**

   A. Kidneys
   B. Liver
   C. Pancreas
   D. Thyroid

5. **In a person with impaired glucose metabolism, such as in type 1 (insulin-dependent) diabetes mellitus, what is true about the blood glucose level?**

   A. It increases rapidly after carbohydrates are ingested, but returns to a normal level after 120 minutes.
   B. It increases rapidly after carbohydrates are ingested and stays greatly elevated even after 120 minutes.
   C. It does not increase after carbohydrates are ingested and stays at a low level until the next meal.
   D. It increases rapidly after carbohydrates are ingested, but returns to a normal level after 30 minutes.

6. **Which of the following is not a classic symptom of diabetes mellitus?**

   A. Polyuria
   B. Polydipsia
   C. Polyphagia
   D. Proteinuria

7. **Which of the following statements is true about type 1 (insulin-dependent) diabetes mellitus?**

   A. It is associated with an insufficient amount of insulin secreted by the pancreas.
   B. It is associated with inefficient activity of the insulin secreted by the pancreas.
   C. It is a more frequent type of diabetes mellitus than the non–insulin-dependent type (type 2).
   D. Good control of this disease will eliminate complications in the future.

8. **What can be the result of uncontrolled elevated blood glucose?**

   A. Coma from insulin shock
   B. Diabetic coma

9. **Gestational diabetes can occur during pregnancy in some women. Which of the following can occur at a later date for a significant number of these women?**

   A. They can develop type 1 (insulin-dependent) diabetes mellitus.
   B. They can develop type 2 (non–insulin-dependent) diabetes mellitus.

## ELECTROLYTES

1. **Use of the sodium fluoride additive to the collection tube for blood to be tested for chloride will give falsely elevated results in methodologies in which:**

   A. Halogens are measured (chloride, fluoride, etc.).
   B. Coulometric titration is employed.
   C. Silver ions are used in the titration.
   D. Colorimetry is used in automated analyzers.

2. **Ninety percent of the carbon dioxide present in the blood is in the form of:**

   A. Bicarbonate ions
   B. Carbonate
   C. Dissolved $CO_2$
   D. Carbonic acid

3. **The calculation of the anion gap is useful for quality control for:**

A. Calcium
B. Tests in the electrolyte profile (sodium, potassium, chloride, and bicarbonate)
C. Phosphorus
D. Magnesium

4. **The anion gap can be increased in patients with:**

A. Lactic acidosis
B. Toxin ingestion
C. Uremia
D. More than one of the above

5. **A common assay method for chloride that generates silver ions in the reaction is:**

A. Chromatography
B. Coulometric titration
C. Nephelometry
D. Flame emission photometry

6. **Lithium is used in flame emission photometric methods for sodium as a (an):**

A. Internal standard
B. Stabilizer for the flame
C. Quality control specimen
D. Enhancer of the color seen in the flame

7. **The concentration of potassium as measured by flame emission photometry is determined by measuring the light:**

A. Scattered by the atoms of potassium in the unknown specimen.
B. Transmitted by the atoms of potassium in the unknown specimen.
C. Absorbed by the atoms of potassium in the unknown specimen.
D. Emitted by the atoms of potassium in the unknown specimen.

8. **A sweat chloride result of 50 mmol/L is obtained for an adult patient who has a history of respiratory problems. What would be the best interpretation of these results, on the basis of known reference values?**

A. Normal sweat chloride, not consistent with cystic fibrosis
B. Marginally elevated results, borderline for cystic fibrosis
C. Elevated results, diagnostic of cystic fibrosis

9. **Which of the following electrolytes is the chief cation in the plasma, is found in the highest concentration in the extravascular fluid, and has the main function of maintaining osmotic pressure?**

A. Potassium
B. Sodium
C. Calcium
D. Magnesium

10. **Analysis of a serum specimen gives a potassium result of 6.0 mmol/L. Before the result is reported to the physician, what additional step should be taken?**

A. The serum should be observed for hemolysis; hemolysis of the red cells will shift potassium from the cells into the serun, resulting in a falsely elevated potassium value.
B. The serum should be observed for evidence of jaundice; jaundiced serum will result in a falsely elevated potassium value.
C. The test should be run again on the same specimen.
D. Nothing needs to be done; simply report out the result.

## UREA NITROGEN AND CREATININE

1. **Nitrogen is excreted principally in the form of:**

A. Creatinine
B. Creatine
C. Uric acid
D. Urea

2. **The main waste product of protein metabolism is:**

A. Creatinine
B. Creatine
C. Uric acid
D. Urea

3. **The protein content of the diet will affect primarily which of the following test results?**

A. Creatinine
B. Creatine
C. Uric acid
D. Urea or urea nitrogen

4. **Use of the sodium fluoride additive in the collection tube for blood will likely give a falsely low result when blood is tested for:**

A. Sodium, using flame emission photometry methodologyy.

B. Chloride, using coulometric methodology.

C. Urea, when the method employs urease.

D. Glucose, using glucose oxidase methodology.

5. **Creatinine concentration in the blood has a direct relationship to:**

A. Muscle mass

B. Dietary protein intake

C. Age and gender

D. More than one of the above

6. **The creatinine clearance is used to assess the:**

A. Glomerular filtration capabilities of the kidneys

B. Tubular secretion of creatinine

C. Dietary intake of protein

D. Glomerular and tubular mass

7. **The expected creatinine clearance for a patient with chronic renal disease would be:**

A. Very low; renal glomerular filtration is functioning normally

B. Normal; renal glomerular filtration is functioning normally

C. Very high; renal glomerular filtration is not functioning normally

D. Very low; renal glomerular filtration is not functioning normally

8. **A serum creatinine result of 6.6 mg/dL is most likely to be found in conjunction with which one of the following other laboratory results?**

A. Urea, 15 mg/dL

B. Urea, 85 mg/dL

C. Urea nitrogen, 10 mg/dL

D. Urea nitrogen/creatinine ratio, 15

9. **A urea nitrogen result for a serum sample is reported as 10 mg/dL. Calculate the concentration of urea for this sample, using the following information: the chemical formula for urea is $NH_2CONH_2$ (atomic weights: carbon = 12, oxygen = 16, nitrogen = 14, hydrogen = 1). The urea concentration for this sample is:**

A. 28 mg/dL

B. 21 mg/dL

C. 92 mg/dL

D. 43 mg/dL

10. **Testing blood from a patient with acute glomerulonephritis would most likely result in which of the following laboratory findings?**

A. Decreased creatinine

B. Decreased urea

C. Increased glucose

D. Increased creatinine

## LIPIDS

1. **Which of the following lipid results would be expected to be falsely elevated in a blood specimen drawn from a nonfasting patient?**

A Total cholesterol

B. Triglycerides

C. HDL cholesterol

D. More than one of the above

2. **Blood is collected from a patient who has been fasting since midnight; the collection time is 7:00 a.m. Which of the following tests would not give a valid test result?**

A. Cholesterol

B. Triglycerides

C. Total bilirubin

D. Potassium

3. **Which of the following laboratory values is considered a positive risk factor for the occurrence of coronary heart disease?**

A. HDL cholesterol greater than 60 mg/dL

B. HDL cholesterol under 35 mg/dL

C. LDL cholesterol under 130 mg/dL

D. Total cholesterol under 200 mg/dL

4. **The appearance of the plasma or serum can be noted and can give important preliminary findings about lipid levels in the blood when it is collected from a fasting patient. When the specimen appears opaque and milky (lipemic), what is the approximate expected level of triglycerides in the sample?**

A. Within the normal range; test is unaffected by meals

B. From 200 to 300 mg/dL

C. Greater than 600 mg/dL

D. No preliminary findings can be made from observation of the serum.

5. Which of the following is considered a primary risk factor for the development of coronary heart disease later in life?

   A. Cigarette smoking
   B. Stress
   C. Diabetes mellitus
   D. Lack of exercise

6. Which of the following is considered a secondary risk factor for the development of coronary heart disease later in life?

   A. Cigarette smoking
   B. Increased HDL cholesterol
   C. Decreased HDL cholesterol
   D. Obesity

7. When a hyperlipidemic condition exists for a sufficient length of time, it may be associated with the development of which of the following conditions?

   A. Obesity
   B. Diabetes mellitus
   C. Atherosclerosis
   D. Viral hepatitis

8. In what major organ of the body is the majority of the body's cholesterol synthesized?

   A. Heart
   B. Pancreas
   C. Gall Bladder
   D. Liver

9. The National Cholesterol Education Program (NCEP) has established cutoffs for total cholesterol and LDL cholesterol to define persons at high risk for coronary heart disease later in life. What is the cutoff for a desirable LDL cholesterol concentration?

   A. <130 mg/dL
   B. <160 mg/dL
   C. <200 mg/dL
   D. >130 mg/dL

## BILIRUBIN

1. In an adult, if the total bilirubin value is 3.1 mg/dL and the conjugated bilirubin is 1.1 mg/dL, the unconjugated bilirubin value is:

   A. 2.0 mg/dL
   B. 4.2 mg/dL
   C. 1.0 mg/dL
   D. 3.4 mg/dL

2. A rapid buildup of unconjugated bilirubin in a newborn infant can result in kernicterus, which is an accumulation of bilirubin in the:

   A. Heart tissue
   B. Liver cells
   C. Brain tissue
   D. Kidney tissue

3. In which of the following conditions resulting in jaundice is there an increase primarily in unconjugated bilirubin?

   A. Increased hemolysis of red cells
   B. Viral hepatitis
   C. Biliary obstruction
   D. Cirrhosis of the liver

4. In which of the following conditions resulting in jaundice is there an increase in both conjugated and unconjugated bilirubin?

   A. Hemolysis of red cells
   B. Viral hepatitis
   C. Obstruction from gallstones
   D. Constriction of the biliary tract due to a neoplasm

5. What is the classical symptom or manifestation of liver disease?

   A. Hemolysis of red cells
   B. Jaundice
   C. Kernicterus
   D. Formation of gallstones

6. Match each of the following defects of bilirubin metabolism (1 to 3) with the corresponding type of jaundice (A to C):

   1. Impairment of conjugation of bilirubin by the liver cells.
   2. Transport defects involving release of the bilirubin bound to plasma albumin to the liver cell for conjugation with glucuronide.
   3. Defect in getting the conjugated bilirubin out of the liver cells and into the bile fluid.
   _____ A. Prehepatic jaundice
   _____ B. Hepatic jaundice
   _____ C. Posthepatic jaundice

7. In a premature newborn infant, a deficiency of which of the following enzymes can affect the conjugation of bilirubin glucuronide in the liver?

A. Glucuronosyltransferase
B. Aspartate aminotransferase
C. Alanine aminotransferase
D. Gamma-glutamyltransferase

8. Which of the following types of bilirubin is water soluble?

A. Unconjugated bilirubin
B. Conjugated bilirubin (bilirubin glucuronide)

9. Which of the following enzymes is found primarily in the liver?

A. Aspartate aminotransferase
B. Alkaline phosphatase
C. Alanine aminotransferase
D. Gamma-glutamyltransferase

# CASE HISTORIES

## ■ CASE I

A 35-year-old man (height 67 inches; weight 73.3 kg) with known chronic renal disease for 6 months has blood drawn for serum creatinine and urea tests. Urine is collected for a 24-hour quantitative creatinine test; the total volume of urine collected is 1139 mL. The following laboratory results are obtained for the testing done:

| | |
|---|---|
| Urine creatinine | 56 mg/dL |
| Serum creatinine | 9.6 mg/dL |
| Serum urea | 75 mg/dL |

1. Given the above data, calculate the patient's standardized creatinine clearance, in mL/min. Standardized creatinine clearance for this patient is:

A. 4.3 mL/min
B. 4.6 mL/min
C. 6.2 mL/min
D. 5.8 mL/min

2. What is the normal range for creatinine clearance for this patient?

## ■ CASE 2

As part of a lipid screening profile, the following results were obtained for a blood specimen drawn from a 30-year-old woman directly after she had eaten breakfast:

| | |
|---|---|
| Triglycerides | 200 mg/dL |
| Cholesterol | 180 mg/dL |

Which of the following would be a reasonable explanation for these results?

A. The results fall within the reference values for the two tests; they are not affected by the recent meal.
B. The cholesterol is normal; the triglyceride test is elevated; retest using a 12-hour fasting speci-

men, as the triglyceride test is affected by the recent meal.
C. The results are elevated for the two tests; retest for both using a 12-hour fasting specimen, as both cholesterol and triglyceride tests are affected by the recent meal.
D. The results for both tests are below the normal reference values despite the recent meal.

## ■ CASE 3

An adult male patient with jaundice complains of fatigue. He has a decreased blood hemoglobin level (he is anemic) and an elevated serum bilirubin value, most of which represents unconjugated bilirubin. His liver enzyme tests are within the normal reference ranges. The most likely disease process for this patient is:

A. A gallstone obstructing the common bile duct
B. Hemolytic anemia in which his red blood cells are being destroyed
C. Infectious (viral) hepatitis
D. Cirrhosis of the liver

## ■ CASE 4

An 8-year-old boy comes to see his family physician with his mother. He has been urinating excessively and has also has been drinking an excessive quantity of water. He recently recovered from a viral upper respiratory infection, he has lost some weight since his last visit to the clinic six months ago, and he has a slight fever (100° F). Laboratory tests are ordered, fasting blood is drawn for testing, and a urinalysis is done. The following laboratory results are reported:

| | |
|---|---|
| Serum creatinine | 0.8 mg/dL |
| Serum glucose | 180 mg/dL |

White blood count          $15 \times 10^9/L$
Hemoglobin                 14.0 g/dL
Urinalysis:
    Specific gravity         1.025
    Glucose                  1000 mg/dL
    Ketones                  Moderate
    Protein, nitrite, blood  Negative
    Sediment                 No abnormal findings

On the basis of the case history and the laboratory findings, what is a likely diagnosis of this patient's disease?

A. Diabetes mellitus
B. Hyperthyroidism
C. Acute glomerulonephritis
D. Recurring upper respiratory infection

## ■ CASE 5

A 40-year-old woman with nausea, vomiting, and jaundice is seen in a clinic. Laboratory tests are ordered on blood and urine. The following laboratory results are reported:

Hemoglobin                      Normal
White blood cell count          Normal
Total serum bilirubin           6.5 mg/dL
Conjugated (direct)             5.0 mg/dL
  serum bilirubin
Serum enzymes:
  Aspartate amino-              300 U/L (normal:
    transferase (AST)            0-45 U/L)
  Gamma-glutamyl-               70 U/L (normal:
    transferase (GGT)            0-45 U/L)
  Alkaline phosphatase          180 U/L (normal:
                                 0-150 U/L)
Urine (appearance is dark brown):
  Urobilinogen                  Normal/decreased
  Bilirubin                     Positive

These results can best be interpreted as representing which of the following?

A. Unconjugated hyperbilirubinemia, probably from hemolysis
B. Unconjugated hyperbilirubinemia, probably from an injury to the liver cells themselves
C. Conjugated hyperbilirubinemia, probably due to biliary tract disease
D. Conjugated hyperbilirubinemia, probably due to an obstruction such as gallstones

## ■ CASE 6

A 35-year-old man is admitted to the ER with chest pain; past history reveals other episodes of this same pain but of a shorter duration. Inquiry into his personal habits reveals that he is a cigarette smoker and that he follows a modified low-fat diet and engages in some regular exercise. His father died of ischemic heart disease at age 45, and other members of his family have had lipid-related disorders. Fasting blood is drawn for chemistry and hematology tests, and urine is collected for examination. Laboratory results follow:

Hemoglobin                      15.0 g/dL
White blood cell count          Mildly elevated
Serum glucose                   120 mg/dL
Serum triglycerides             300 mg/dL
Serum LDL cholesterol           150 mg/dL
Serum total cholesterol         275 mg/dL
Enzymes, serum (for             All mildly increased
  assessing damage to
  heart muscle)
Urinalysis                      Normal findings

1. Which of the information in the history and laboratory findings is considered the most important risk factor influencing the development of life-threatening coronary heart disease in this patient?
   A. LDL cholesterol level
   B. Triglyceride level
   C. Family history
   D. Cigarette smoking

2. Treatment focuses on which of the risk factors noted in this patient?
   A. Lowering the LDL cholesterol
   B. Lowering the total cholesterol
   C. Giving up smoking cigarettes
   D. Engaging in a more strenuous exercise program

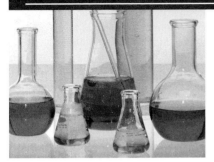

# CHAPTER 12

# *Hematology*

## Learning Objectives

*From study of this chapter, the reader will be able to:*

- Describe the three cell types or formed elements of the blood and, for each, describe their enumeration and routine testing methods.
- For routine hematologic tests, describe the basic theory or principle of the determination, the use and care of equipment used to perform the tests, the proper preparation of reagents, the calculation of results, the use of quality control solutions and precautions, technical factors, and sources of error.
- Be able to recognize problems that may be encountered in hematologic testing and propose problem-solving strategies.
- Describe proper collection techniques for blood specimens for hematologic testing and tell when specimens are unacceptable for testing.
- Describe common clinical application of the hematologic techniques included in this chapter.
- Calculate the red cell indices and correlate them with red cell morphology on the peripheral blood film.
- Explain the general principle of each of the three types of automated cell counters, namely Coulter principle, flow cytometry, and electro-optical measurement of cell layers.
- Describe and recognize the five types of white blood cells encountered in normal peripheral blood and stained with Wright stain, including maturation and function of each.

➤ Describe, in general terms, the method for examination of the blood film, including examination with low power (10×) and oil immersion (100×).

➤ Describe and recognize the various red cell alterations, including alterations in color (staining reaction), size, shape, structure, and inclusions.

➤ Describe the various morphologic leukocyte alterations seen in granulocytes and lymphocytes and classify them as toxic or reactive, anomalous, or leukemic or malignant.

## INTRODUCTION AND DEFINITION OF HEMATOLOGY

The word hematology comes from the Greek *haima*, blood, and *logos*, discourse; therefore, the study of hematology is the science, or study, of blood. In a hematology course, one is concerned with the main constituents of the blood. Blood is composed of plasma and cells; the plasma is the fluid portion of the blood.

The total volume of blood in an average adult is about 6 L, or 7% to 8% of the body weight. About 45% of this amount is composed of the formed elements of the blood (i.e., cells), and the remaining 55% is the plasma. Approximately 90% of the plasma is water; the remaining 10% consists of proteins (albumin, globulin, fibrinogen), carbohydrates, vitamins, hormones, enzymes, lipids, and salts.

Blood is part of the circulatory system of the body and has several functions. It carries nutrients to the tissues, the most important nutrient being oxygen, which is carried by the red cells. Waste products (end products of metabolism) are carried by the blood to the organs of excretion. Many natural defense agents circulate continuously with the blood supply. Much valuable information can be readily obtained from hematologic tests, and certain routine measurements and examinations are useful in the evaluation of the wellness or illness of a patient.

The blood cells, or formed elements, to be discussed in this chapter are the red blood cells **(erythrocytes),** the white blood cells **(leukocytes),** and the platelets **(thrombocytes).** The laboratory tests performed in the area of hematology center around the cells and some of their constituents: their number or concentration, the relative distribution of various types of cells, and their structural or biochemical abnormalities that contribute to disease. The entire range of types of disease is seen: hereditary, immunologic, nutritional, metabolic, traumatic, and inflammatory (including infectious, hormonal, and neoplastic). In many instances the hematologic examination is virtually diagnostic, and in many instances it is a major contribution to the eventual solution of a diagnostic problem.

Diseases with a primary hematologic cause are not common, but hematologic manifestations secondary to other diseases are quite common. A wide variety of diseases may show signs or symptoms of a hematologic nature. Many diseases produce anemia, and others produce enlarged lymph nodes. Additional examination will usually indicate the primary involvement of some system besides the blood and lymph nodes.

The major source of the blood cells is the bone marrow, although the lymph nodes and the spleen contribute some of the white blood cells. Many other sources make contributions to the blood.

### The Complete Blood Count

Several hematologic tests are basic to the initial evaluation and follow-up of the patient. Many of these tests are considered routine and can be done by a laboratorian with limited training. These tests are referred to as the **complete blood count (CBC).** According to the NCCLS, the CBC "...consists of measurement of the hemoglobin, hematocrit, red blood cell count with morphology, white blood cell count with differential, and platelet estimate."[7] With the prevalence of electronic cell counters, other values or tests are also considered routine. The meaning of CBC may vary depending on the institution or laboratory. The term may refer to the complete hematology profile generated by the instrument in use. The RBC count and calculated RBC indices are a part of the routine CBC in laboratories that employ electronic cell counters. In addition to their use for screening, the CBC results are helpful in the diagnosis of many diseases. They can reflect the body's ability to fight disease and may be used to determine how the patient is progressing in certain disease states such as infection or anemia. That these tests are done frequently does not mean that they are unimportant. Valuable information about a patient's physical condition can be obtained from accurately performed routine hematologic determinations.

## SPECIMENS

Since samples for hematologic study are usually obtained by skin puncture or venipuncture, the collection of specimens and the approach to the patient in general should be reviewed (see under Types of Specimens Collected, in Chapter 3).

### Capillary Blood

Capillary blood can be used with good results for morphologic studies in hematology. For doing differential blood counts and for enumerating cellular elements, capillary or peripheral blood can be obtained from the fingertip, heel, or big toe. This kind of sampling is sometimes called micro sampling. In newborn infants, blood is generally obtained from the plantar surface of the big toe or heel, since these areas are more accessible than the fingertip (see Fig. 3-2). Newborns have a small blood supply, and removing blood by venipuncture would deplete too much of their total blood volume. If blood is needed from very young children, the third or fourth fingertip is generally punctured. In adults who have very poor veins or whose veins cannot be used because intravenous solutions are being administered, the tip of the third or fourth finger is punctured to obtain the blood sample. A free flow of blood is needed for the results obtained with capillary blood to agree with those from venous blood.

### Tests Using Capillary Blood

Tests for hemoglobin, microhematocrit, red cell, white cell, and platelet counts, and evaluation of blood films may all be done from capillary blood. When capillary blood is used, the tip of the sampling device is placed in the drop of blood; the sampling device (pipet, microcuvette, or slide) is not touched to the skin. The order of collection is an important consideration. Usually, blood for the hemoglobin test is taken first. Cell counts are collected next, followed by the microhematocrit, and finally blood films (smears) are prepared. If platelet counts are done, they are taken off first, however. Knowledge of correct collection techniques and preparation for testing, such as adequate mixing of blood with diluting fluid, is essential for reliable results.

### Venous Blood

Because it is not always practical to obtain capillary blood for hematology, venous blood is often used. More tests can be done with a tube of venous blood, including measurement of the erythrocyte sedimentation rate, which requires more blood than some of the other hematology determinations. There must be some means of preventing coagulation, as clotted blood cannot be used. The types of anticoagulants available and their use are discussed under Additives and Anticoagulants, in Chapter 3. For most hematologic studies the anticoagulant used is ethylenediaminetetraacetic acid (EDTA). This preserves the morphology of the cellular elements and prevents coagulation. It is important that the blood be mixed well with the anticoagulant immediately after it is collected, to ensure proper antico-

agulation. Liquid EDTA mixes more easily than the dry form. Not even small clots are acceptable for hematology. When refrigerated properly, EDTA specimens can be preserved for several hours until the work can be done. White cell counts, microhematocrit, platelet counts, and sedimentation rates can be determined up to 24 hours after blood is collected in EDTA if it is refrigerated at 4° C. The EDTA binds the calcium ions in the blood and thus inhibits coagulation.

In addition to keeping the blood in a liquid form (preventing clotting), the anticoagulant must maintain the natural appearance of the RBCs, WBCs, and platelets. EDTA is the anticoagulant in general use that can do all these things.

Immediately after the blood has been properly drawn and placed in the tube containing the anticoagulant, it should be gently mixed by gentle inversion 5 to 10 times. This is necessary to ensure thorough contact with the anticoagulant. Clotted specimens are absolutely unacceptable for most tests done in the hematology laboratory, especially cell counts. If there is even a tiny clot in a specimen, the cell count will be grossly inaccurate.

### Processing and Testing the Specimen

After the blood specimen has been collected from the patient, it must be transported to the laboratory for analysis. Assuming that the specimen was properly labeled when it was drawn and that it has been handled properly, it is examined in the laboratory as quickly as possible to prevent deterioration. Laboratory tests are done on fresh specimens whenever possible. Special handling of specimens for the various hematologic determinations is discussed later in this chapter in connection with specific tests.

To comply with standard precautions, gloves must be worn during all laboratory handling and testing using blood specimens. All samples are to be considered as potentially infectious, and the proper use of barrier-protective apparel and devices is essential.

Immediately before a test is performed on a blood specimen, the blood sample must be mixed by repeated gentle inversion at least 15 times. This can be accomplished by hand or with a mechanical tube inverter. If the blood sample has stood for a few minutes, it should be mixed again.

When a preserved blood specimen is allowed to stand for a period of time, the components will settle into three distinct layers: (1) the plasma, or top layer, (2) the buffy coat, a grayish-white cellular layer composed of WBCs and platelets, and (3) the RBCs, the bottom layer (Fig. 12-1). Some hematologic procedures are based on the ability of the blood specimen to settle into layers when it has been preserved by use of an anticoagulant.

## Appearance of Specimens

When the blood specimen has been properly drawn and preserved in the prescribed manner, the plasma will have its natural color, a very light yellow or straw hue. There are occasions when the plasma may have an altered color because of a disease process, but color changes can also result from improper handling of the specimen by the laboratory worker.

### Hemolysis

The color change most often seen is the appearance of red in the plasma, caused by the release of hemoglobin into the solution when the RBCs are broken up. This breakup, or rupturing, of red cells is called **hemolysis.** Hemolysis is one of the changes resulting from alterations in osmotic pressure in the solution surrounding the red cells. It can also occur when the membrane surrounding the red cells has been mechanically ruptured either in vivo, as the result of a disease process, or in vitro, as the result of difficult collection of poor handling.

### Unsuitable Hematologic Specimens

Two types of blood samples are unsuitable for hematology tests: clotted samples and samples that are hemolyzed in the process of collection or handling. Clotted specimens are not suitable for cell counts because the cells are trapped in the clot and are therefore not counted. A cell count on a clotted sample will be falsely low. In hemolyzed specimens the red cells are no longer intact, and red cell counts on hemolyzed samples will also give falsely low results. Although hemolyzed specimens are generally considered unacceptable for testing, it must be remembered that there are cases of intravascular hemolysis when hemolysis is a clinically significant finding and not cause for rejection of the specimen for testing.

### Layers of Normal Anticoagulated Blood

If blood is collected, anticoagulated, and allowed to settle, or be centrifuged, three layers will separate and be observed (see Fig. 12-1).

The bottom layer will consist of packed red blood cells and will normally make up about 45% of the total blood volume (the percentage differs in males and females). On top of this layer a thin grayish-white layer called the **buffy**

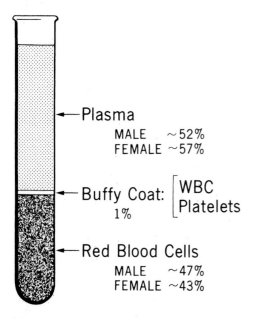

**FIG 12-1.** Layers of normal blood (after centrifugation).

coat will be seen. This consists of the leukocytes and platelets and normally makes up about 1% of the total blood volume. The uppermost layer is a colloidal liquid called plasma. The plasma layer normally represents about 55% of the total blood volume.

## Homeostasis

All of the fluid and cellular elements that make up the blood are in a constant state of exchange. The overall effect is a state of equilibrium in which the supply is equal to the demand for normal body function. This state of equilibrium is termed **homeostasis,** and various tests that are done on blood measure the overall state of homeostasis within the body. Many of the constituents of plasma (or serum, if the blood is allowed to clot) are measured in the clinical chemistry laboratory.

### Osmosis and Osmotic Pressure

The principle of osmotic pressure and osmosis is very important whenever a solution or diluent is used as part of a procedure, as they are in many hematologic procedures. In simple terms, **osmosis** is the passage of a solvent through a membrane from a dilute solution into a more concentrated one. The difference in concentration between the solutions on either side of the membrane causes the phenomenon called **osmotic pressure.** If the concentrations of these solutions are the same, there will not be any pressure.

### Isotonic, Hypotonic, and Hypertonic Solutions

When the concentration is the same in the diluent solution as it is inside the RBC, the diluent is called an **isotonic** solution. If the diluent is less concentrated than the inside of the RBC, the solution is called **hypotonic.** From the definition of osmosis it can be seen that in the case of a hypotonic (dilute) solution, the passage of diluent will be from outside the red cell into the red cell, causing the cell to swell and eventually to rupture, or hemolyze.

If the solution outside the RBC is more concentrated than that inside it, the outside solution is called **hypertonic.** In the case of a hypertonic solution, the osmosis of the solvent is from the inside of the red cell to the surrounding solution. When this happens, the red cell will shrink from loss of liquid and will become crenated.

When red cells are in plasma, they are in an isotonic solution. For this reason, any diluent used to dilute blood for hematology tests must have the same ionic concentration as plasma. When a solution has the same concentration as, or is isotonic with, plasma, it is called a physiologic solution. One very common physiologic solution is isotonic saline solution, a 0.85 g/dL solution of sodium chloride (NaCl). If RBCs are placed in an isotonic saline solution, their size is preserved. Hypotonic and hypertonic solutions are unsatisfactory as diluents for hematologic studies.

## FORMATION AND FUNCTION OF BLOOD CELLS AND COMPONENTS

### Hematopoiesis

During early fetal life, blood cells are formed in many of the body tissues. During this period, the liver and spleen are the most active sites of blood cell production, or **hematopoiesis.** At about the fourth month of fetal life, the bone marrow begins functioning as a blood cell producer. Shortly after birth, under normal conditions, the marrow is the only tissue that continues to produce red cells, granular leukocytes (granulocytes), monocytes, and platelets. Until the age of 5 years, the marrow in all the bones is red and cellular, and actively produces cells. Between 5 and 7 years, the long bones become inactive and fat cells appear to replace the active marrow. Red marrow is gradually displaced by fat cells in the other bones through the maturing years. In other words, red marrow is transformed to yellow marrow. After age 18 to 20 years, red marrow remains only in the vertebrae, the ribs, the sternum, the skull, and partially in the femur and the humerus.

However, the marrow is able to become active again when necessary, as in hemolytic anemias or chronic hemorrhage, when there is an increased loss of RBCs from the body and a demand for increased RBC production. Such increased marrow activity is helpful to normal body function. This is not the case in other instances, as in **leukemia** or other malignancies, in which increased marrow activity of one cell type is detrimental to the body as a whole. Another situation that is incompatible with life occurs when the marrow is suppressed or unable to function normally in cell production. In this case the marrow is said to be **aplastic.** Bone marrow aspirations may therefore be necessary to detect abnormal changes in the newly formed cells or in their quantity. Early blood disease may be detected by an examination of the bone marrow before changes are seen in the peripheral blood.

The leukocytes found in normal circulating peripheral blood consist of the granulocytes (neutrophils, eosinophils, basophils), monocytes, and lymphocytes. The bone marrow produces the myeloid cells, namely erythrocytes, granulocytes (neutrophils, eosinophils, and basophils), monocytes, and platelets. Lymphocytes are produced primarily by the lymphoid tissue (lymph nodes and nodules, thymus, and spleen); some are also produced in the bone marrow.

These formed elements of the blood go through a normal series of developmental steps or stages in the marrow or lymphoid tissue and are found in the general peripheral blood circulation only when they are sufficiently developed or mature. However, immature cells, or cells in early developmental stages, may appear in the peripheral blood in certain disease states. Each cell type has a normal life span and function. This is summarized in Table 12-1. When their normal life spans are complete, the formed elements are eliminated from the body by processes in which parts of the cells are reused and parts are eliminated from the body.

When the body is functioning normally, the production and destruction of the formed ele-

### TABLE 12-1

Approximate Life Spans of Various Cell Types in Peripheral Blood

| Cell Type | Life Span in Peripheral Blood |
|---|---|
| Erythrocytes | 120 days |
| Neutrophils (PMNs) | About 10 hours |
| Eosinophils | Less than 8 hours |
| Basophils | Unknown; assume like PMNs and eosinophils |
| Monocytes | Variable: 1 to 3 days |
| B Lymphocytes | Days |
| T Lymphocytes | Months to years |

ments of the blood are balanced so that a constant supply is available. When one of the steps in these processes is not functioning properly or is occurring too rapidly, a blood disorder will result, and this will cause alterations in the other steps as well, since they are all closely related. These alterations might reflect diseases of the blood formation system or diseases of nonhematologic origin. For example, chronic bleeding resulting from a nonhematologic cause such as gastric ulcer or carcinoma results in hypochromic microcytic anemia because of loss of iron. A similar condition of hematologic origin results from simple dietary iron deficiency. When tests are performed in the hematology laboratory, changes in the appearance of the red blood cells or other formed elements, or changes in the manner in which whole blood or various components react under certain test conditions, are noted to determine whether alterations in function have occurred.

## Normal Red Blood Cells (Erythrocytes)
### Formation of Red Blood Cells

In adults, erythrocytes are formed in the bone marrow. The mature RBC is often described as a biconcave disk—that is, it is doughnut-shaped, with a depressed area rather than a hole in the center, as shown in Fig. 12-2. It does not contain a nucleus (it is nonnucleated) and is about 7 to 8 $\mu$m in diameter.

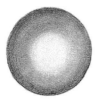 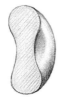

**Normal
Red Cell**

**Side View
of Normal
Red Cell**

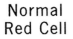

**FIG 12-2.** Normal red blood cell.

The RBC begins as a nucleated cell within the bone marrow. As the cell matures in the bone marrow, its diameter decreases and the nucleus becomes denser and smaller and is finally released from the cell (extruded). While this occurs, the concentration of hemoglobin increases. This is seen as a progressive change in color of the cytoplasm (cell material other than the nucleus) from blue to orange on a Wright-stained blood film. The whole sequence of maturation from an early cell precursor to a circulating red cell takes 3 to 5 days.

**Reticulocytes.** The young RBC that has just extruded its nucleus is referred to as a **reticulocyte.** It is about the same size as or slightly larger than a mature RBC. Reticulocytes differ from mature RBCs morphologically because they contain a fine basophilic reticulum or network of RNA (ribonucleic acid), a cytoplasmic remnant that decreases as the cell matures. When stained with Wright stain, reticulocytes appear pink-gray or pale purple—they have a slight bluish tinge. This **polychromasia** (many colors) represents the presence of RNA within the cell. With a special stain, such as brilliant cresyl blue or new methylene blue, the basophilic reticulum of RNA appears blue (see under Counting Reticulocytes). Under normal conditions, reticulocytes remain and mature further in the bone marrow for a day or two before they are released into the peripheral blood. RBCs are released into the peripheral blood as reticulocytes by squeezing (or insinuating) through openings in the endothelial cells lining the marrow cavity. These reticulocytes become fully mature—that is, they lose all RNA—within a day or two. Therefore, the number of reticulocytes in the peripheral blood is an indication of the degree of RBC production by the marrow. Normally about 1% of the circulating RBCs are reticulocytes.

### Function of Red Blood Cells

The main function of the RBC is to carry oxygen to the cells of the body. The oxygen is transported in a chemical combination with hemoglobin. Thus, the concentration of hemoglobin in the blood is a measure of its capacity to carry oxygen, on which all cells are absolutely dependent for energy and therefore life. At the tissues, the oxygen is exchanged for carbon dioxide, which is carried to the lungs for excretion in exchange for oxygen. To combine with and therefore transport oxygen, the hemoglobin molecule must have a certain combination of substances, namely heme (which contains iron) and globin. Deficiencies in the presence or metabolism of any of these substances will result in a decrease in hemoglobin and oxygen-carrying capacity.

### Destruction of RBC by the Reticuloendothelial System

Red blood cells have a total life span of about 120 days, and the body releases new red cells into the circulatory system every day. When red cells are worn out, the body stores the cell components that are reusable, including iron (from the heme portion of the hemoglobin molecule) and protein (from the globin portion of the hemoglobin molecule) and eliminates the nonreusable components. The remaining heme portion of the hemoglobin molecule (with iron removed) is such a waste product. It is converted to bilirubin, concentrated in the bile, and eliminated from the body by way of the feces, and to a much smaller extent the urine, as urobilin and urobilinogen. The metabolism and elimination of bilirubin are described in Chapters 11 and 14. A schematic representation of the red blood cell formation and destruction process is shown in Fig. 12-3.

Worn out red cells are broken down by the **reticuloendothelial system (RES).** The RES is composed of connective tissue cells that carry on **phagocytosis,** a process in which a cell engulfs, or eats, foreign material. The RES cells are located in the blood sinusoids (tiny blood vessels) in the liver, spleen, and bone marrow, and the lining of the lymph channels in the lymph nodes. They are important in the body's defense mechanism and in the breakdown of globin to amino acids, which are returned to the protein storage pool of the body. They are also essential for the retention and reuse or storage of iron, which is needed for the formation of hemoglobin and transport of oxygen. A deficiency of iron results in anemia, a condition in which the oxygen-carrying capacity of blood is decreased. Iron deficiency anemia, one of the more common types of anemia, may result from a dietary deficiency of iron or from loss of iron from the body through bleeding.

## Normal White Blood Cells (Leukocytes)

The leukocytes are nucleated and are part of the defense mechanism of the body. Unlike the red cells, white cells use the bloodstream primarily for transportation to their place of function in the body tissues.

### Function of White Blood Cells

The neutrophils, eosinophils, and monocytes act as phagocytic scavengers—they engulf and destroy invading microorganisms and clear the body of unwanted particulate material such as dead or injured tissue cells. This is the first step in the repair of injured tissue. The lymphocytes and plasma cells act as immunocytes, inactivating foreign antigens by antibody production and by delayed hypersensitivity reactions. Plasma cells are not normally found in the peripheral blood. Lymphocytes and plasma cells are produced primarily in the lymphoid tissue (lymph nodes, nodules, and spleen) and secondarily in the marrow.

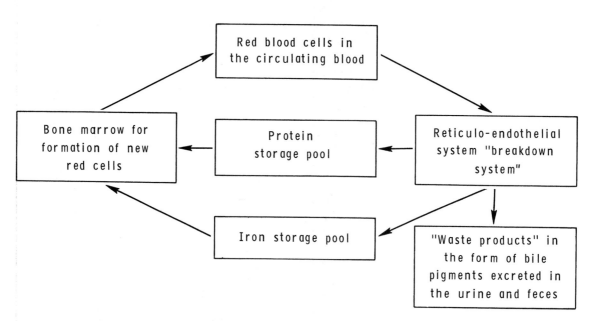

**FIG 12-3.** Red blood cell formation and destruction process.

### Types of Normal White Blood Cells

Under normal conditions, five types of leukocytes are found in the blood: lymphocytes, neutrophils, monocytes, eosinophils, and basophils. When a blood film is stained with Wright (a Romanowsky) stain and examined with the microscope, the majority of the cells seen will be RBCs, which appear as small, rounded, pink, or reddish-orange bodies. Scattered among the red-staining cells are the less numerous leukocytes. There are normally 600 to 800 red cells to each leukocyte. The leukocytes are larger and more complex in appearance than the RBCs. They consist of a nucleus surrounded by cytoplasm. Usually the nucleus is in the center of the cell and is a prominent purple-staining body. It can be round or oval (as in the lymphocyte) or lobulated (as in the neutrophil and eosinophil). The cytoplasm, which gives the cell its shape, stains a variety of colors, depending on its contents. The size of the cell, the shape and size of the nucleus, and the staining reactions of the nucleus and the cytoplasm aid in the identification of leukocytes.

Leukocytes are categorized as granulocytes and nongranulocytes (lymphocytes). Granulocytes are leukocytes that come from the **myeloid** series of cell development. Of these, neutrophils, eosinophils, and basophils contain specific granulation in their cytoplasm. Monocytes are classified as myeloid cells that contain nonspecific granulation. Lymphocytes are cells derived from the lymphoid series of cell development. They are nongranulocytes that may contain nonspecific granulation (see also under Origin and Function of Blood Cells Related to Morphologic Examination; and Leukocyte Alterations).

The five types of leukocytes are discussed more thoroughly under Normal Leukocyte Morphology, but a brief description of each follows.

**Neutrophil.** This cell is normally the most numerous and most prominent of the white cells seen in an adult blood film. The nucleus is lobulated (with three to five lobes), and the cytoplasm stains a faint pink or is colorless and contains numerous fine lilac neutrophilic granules.

**Lymphocyte.** This cell is the next most numerous in adult blood samples (usually about three neutrophils are seen to each lymphocyte). The nucleus is round or oval, and the cytoplasm stains light blue and is usually free from any granules, although it may contain a few pink, azurophilic granules that are unevenly distributed. Lymphocytes are further classified as small or large.

**Monocyte.** This is the largest white cell and is often confused with the lymphocyte. It usually has an indented or horseshoe-shaped nucleus (although it may be oval, lobular, notched, or polymorphic). The abundant cytoplasm stains gray or gray-blue and can be vacuolated. Extremely fine azurophilic granules called azure dust may be present in the cytoplasm.

**Eosinophil.** This cell is easily recognized by the large, red, beadlike granules seen in the cytoplasm. The nucleus is usually bilobed. Normally, few eosinophils are present (only about 3 per 100 total white cells counted).

**Basophil.** This cell is the one least likely to be seen (only 0.5 per 100 total white cells counted). It is easily distinguished, however, by the dark purple or black beadlike granules seen in the cytoplasm. The nucleus is indistinctly lobulated and may appear smudged.

## Normal Platelets (Thrombocytes)

Another formed element of the blood is the platelet, or thrombocyte. Platelets are small colorless bodies 1.5 to 4 $\mu$m in diameter. Platelets are generally round or ovoid, although they may have projections called pseudopods. Platelets have a colorless to pale blue background substance containing centrally located, purplish red granules.

## Formation of Platelets

Platelets are produced in the bone marrow by cells called megakaryocytes, which are large and multinucleated. Platelets do not have a nucleus and are not actually cells—they are portions of cytoplasm pinched off from megakaryocytes and released into the bloodstream.

## Function of Platelets

In the bloodstream, platelets are an essential part of the blood clotting mechanism. They act to maintain the structure or integrity of the endothelial cells lining the vascular system by plugging any gaps in the lining. They also function in the clotting process by (1) acting as plugs around the opening of a wound and (2) releasing certain factors that are necessary for the formation of a blood clot.

## Blood Plasma

The formed elements of blood are suspended in a fluid called blood plasma. Plasma is the protein fraction of the blood, and it contains in solution many substances that are necessary for maintenance of the body. It is a complex mixture including water, proteins, carbohydrates, lipids, electrolytes, and clotting factors, plus enzymes, vitamins, hormones, and trace metals.

# CLINICAL HEMATOLOGY

Clinical hematology is primarily concerned with testing the formed elements within the blood. This includes red cells, white cells, and platelets.

The oxygen-carrying capacity of the blood is routinely measured by measuring the hemoglobin concentration and the hematocrit (percentage of total blood volume occupied by the RBCs), counting the RBCs, and observing the morphology or appearance of the RBCs on a peripheral blood film. RBC production by the marrow is assessed by means of a reticulocyte count, and examination of the bone marrow may be necessary in certain disease states.

The leukocytes in the blood are routinely assessed by counting the number of cells present in a particular volume, and observing the morphology and determining the percentage of each cell type present in a peripheral blood film. This is referred to as a **white blood cell differential.** Here again, examination of the bone marrow may be necessary in certain cases; however, this is not a routine procedure.

Platelets are also routinely assessed in clinical hematologic studies by observing their number and morphology in the peripheral blood film. If certain disorders are suspected, platelets may also be counted. The blood clotting mechanism may also be checked, when necessary, by testing for the clotting factors that are present within the plasma.

Since the equilibrium of the blood is affected by a great many factors, hematology tests are useful in the study of all sorts of disease states, of hematologic or nonhematologic origin. Thus, hereditary, nutritional, metabolic, traumatic, inflammatory, infectious, hormonal, immunologic, neoplastic, drug-induced, and other disease states can be assessed by hematologic studies. The physician will depend on such laboratory results, in combination with the clinical history and physical examination, to determine the state of health or disease of the patient.

# HEMOGLOBIN

The determination of hemoglobin (Hb) is the test ordered most frequently in the clinical hematology laboratory. It is part of the routine CBC. Although the meaning of the CBC will vary somewhat from institution to institution, a hemoglobin measurement is standard and is part of the automated instrumentation that includes cells counts and calculated hematocrit. The measurement of hemoglobin is relatively simple and can be done quickly by the laboratory. Single-analyte instruments are also available and are waived under CLIA '88, making this a common laboratory procedure. One such test will be described in this section. Along with the hematocrit measurement, the hemoglobin value is used to follow many disease states, especially the anemias. The measurement of the concentration of hemoglobin in the blood is called *hemoglobinometry*.

## Hemoglobin Synthesis and Structure

Hemoglobin synthesis is a complex process, starting in the bone marrow with the production of the erythrocytes. The heme (iron-containing) portion of the molecule combines with globin (the protein portion) and forms an activated form of hemoglobin that is ready to transport oxygen. Each hemoglobin molecule consists of four heme groups and a globin moiety, which is composed of four polypeptide chains (Fig. 12-4).

### Heme

The **heme** group is an iron complex containing one iron atom. Iron is essential for the primary function of the hemoglobin molecule—that is, carrying oxygen to the tissues. If iron is lacking, because of either inadequate dietary intake or increased loss from the body, anemia results, since hemoglobin is not formed in sufficient quantity. When reduced hemoglobin is exposed to oxygen at increased pressure, oxygen is taken up at the iron atom until each molecule of hemoglobin has bound four oxygen molecules, one molecule at each iron atom. Since this is not a true oxidation-reduction reaction, the hemoglobin molecule carrying oxygen is said to be oxygenated. The molecule fully saturated with oxygen (four oxygen molecules per hemoglobin) is called **oxyhemoglobin.** It contains 1.34 mL of oxygen per gram of hemoglobin.

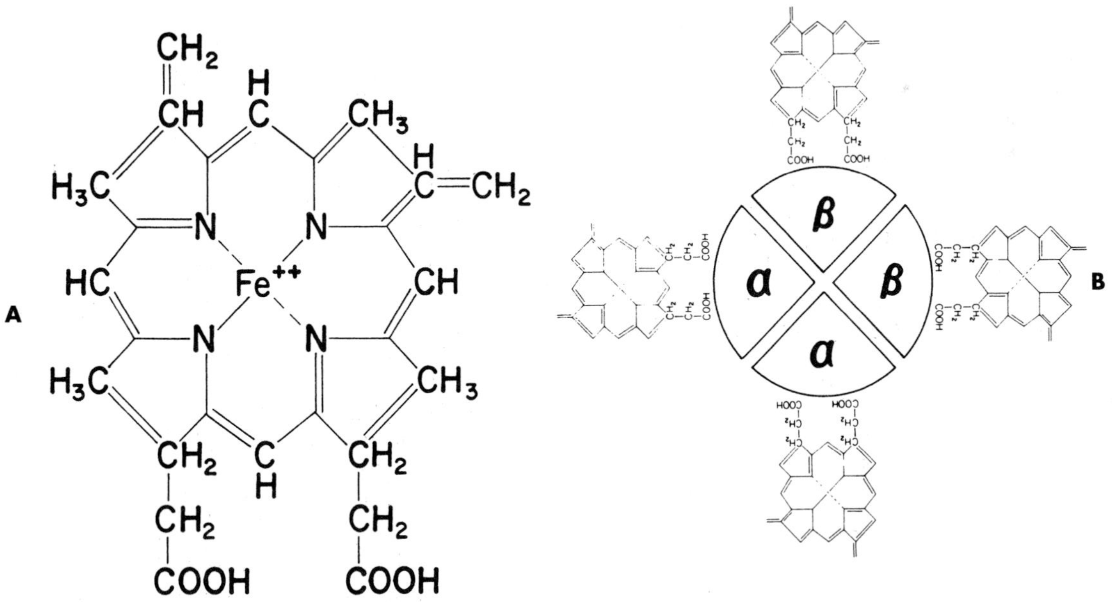

**FIG 12-4.** Hemoglobin molecules. **A,** Heme moiety (one protoporphyrin ring with a single iron atom). **B,** Hemoglobin A molecule (made up of four heme groups with their appropriate globin chains—two alpha and two beta).

Oxyhemoglobin carries oxygen from the lungs to the tissues of the body. Hemoglobin returning to the lungs with carbon dioxide from the tissues is known as reduced hemoglobin.

Heme is itself a complex molecule. It is made up of a series of tetrapyrrole rings, terminating in protoporphyrin, with a central iron, as shown in Fig. 12-4. Since the heme molecule is a porphyrin, a group of diseases called the porphyrias result from certain disorders of heme synthesis. Normally heme is excreted from the body as bilirubin, which is eventually converted to the various bile salts and pigments. The iron is normally removed and retained by the RES, stored, and reused in the production of new hemoglobin.

### Globin

The globin portion of the hemoglobin molecule is a protein substance that consists of four chains of amino acids (polypeptides). Each of the four globin chains is attached to a heme portion to form a single hemoglobin molecule, as shown in Fig. 12-4.

## Hemoglobin Variants

Different structural forms of hemoglobin may occur in the red cells. These **hemoglobin variants** or forms differ in the content and sequence of amino acids in the globin chains. The alpha chain is composed of 141 amino acids in a specific sequence, and the beta chain contains 146 amino acids of a specific sequence. Other polypeptide globin chains that may be encountered include gamma, delta, and possibly epsilon.

### Hemoglobin A

The principal adult hemoglobin, Hb A, contains two alpha ($\alpha$) and two beta ($\beta$) globin chains, as shown in Fig. 12-4. In another form of adult hemoglobin (Hb $A_2$), the alpha chains are paired with two delta polypeptide chains. The delta chains are related to beta chains, but 10 amino acids have been substituted. These are the major normal forms of adult hemoglobin. Other genetically determined forms of hemoglobin may be demonstrated by means of electrophoresis. Many abnormal forms of hemoglobin lead to clinical illness because they interfere with the oxygen-carrying capacity of the blood.

The combination of Hb A and Hb $A_2$ should normally make up 95% of the hemoglobin in an adult, with Hb F making up 5% or less.

### Hemoglobin F

Hemoglobin F is the major form found during intrauterine life and at birth. In fetal hemoglobin (Hb F), the two alpha globin chains are paired with two gamma chains. Adult hemoglobin (Hb A) is formed in small amounts by the fetus and rapidly increases after birth.

### Abnormal Hemoglobin Variants

Disorders in which the presence of structurally abnormal hemoglobins is considered to play an important role pathologically are called **hemoglobinopathies.** In some hemoglobinopathies, all the hemoglobin is in one abnormal form. In others, two abnormal forms may be present. In still others, some normal forms and some abnormal forms are present. The structurally abnormal hemoglobins usually consist of polypeptide chains with a normal number of amino acids but with a single amino acid substitution. These substitutions are under genetic control, and the hemoglobinopathies may be either inherited or the result of genetic mutations. In clinically significant disease either the alpha or the beta chain may be affected; however, most of the hemoglobinopathies are the result of beta chain abnormalities.

The four clinically important abnormal hemoglobins are Hb S, Hb C, Hb D, and Hb E. These are all hereditary, and the disorders affect the protein portion of the hemoglobin molecule, altering the structure of the polypeptide chain. These abnormal hemoglobins, as well as the normal ones, can be distinguished from one another by electrophoresis.

**Hb S.** One fairly common abnormal hemoglobin is Hb S. It occurs almost exclusively in the black population and is responsible for the disease sickle cell anemia. Hemoglobin S has an amino acid substitution in the beta chain, where valine is substituted for glutamic acid at the sixth position in the normal beta chain. It causes sickling of the red cells under conditions of reduced oxygen concentration, resulting in sickle cell anemia when present in the homozygous state.

**Hb C.** Hemoglobin C results from a substitution of the amino acid lysine for glutamic acid on the sixth position of the beta chain. It may be inherited in combination with hemoglobin S and may occur in a homozygous or heterozygous state. The red blood cells may appear as target cells when hemoglobin C is present; less frequently crystals of precipitated hemoglobin C may be seen in the red blood cells.

## Hemoglobin Derivatives

The circulating blood carries a composite of derivatives of hemoglobin. Most of the hemoglobin in circulating blood is oxyhemoglobin and reduced hemoglobin. Other hemoglobin derivatives found in normal circulating blood include carboxyhemoglobin (hemoglobin combined with carbon monoxide), methemoglobin, or hemiglobin, which is oxidized hemoglobin, and minor amounts of other derivatives. When iron in the hemoglobin molecule is converted from the ferrous (++) to the ferric (+++) state, it can combine with other substances besides oxygen and is no longer capable of oxygen transport. When sufficient quantities of these hemoglobin derivatives are present in the circulating blood, **hypoxia** (lack of oxygen) or **cyanosis** (bluish discoloration of the skin and mucous membranes) will be seen clinically.

### Oxyhemoglobin and Reduced Hemoglobin

These are the major forms of circulating hemoglobin. The main function of hemoglobin is to transport oxygen from the lungs, where oxygen tension is high, to the tissues where it is low. At an increased oxygen tension (100 mm Hg), hemoglobin is oxygenated by the reversible association of an oxygen molecule at each iron atom, forming oxyhemoglobin ($HbO_2$). At the reduced oxygen tension of the tissues (down to 20 mm Hg), oxygen is dissociated from the iron in each heme group and replaced by carbon dioxide. This is called reduced hemoglobin (Hb). This is not an oxidation-reduction reaction, because the iron is in the ferrous state in both forms of hemoglobin ($HbO_2$ and Hb).

### Carboxyhemoglobin

The hemoglobin molecule has a much greater affinity for carbon monoxide than for oxygen and will readily combine with carbon monoxide if it is present even in low concentration. The affinity of carbon monoxide for hemoglobin is 200 times greater than the affinity of oxygen. Carboxyhemoglobin (HbCO) cannot bind to and carry oxygen and will result in carbon monoxide poisoning, even at relatively low concentrations of carbon monoxide. The formation of carboxyhemoglobin is reversible, and if carbon monoxide is removed the hemoglobin will once again combine with oxygen. Clinically, with sufficient levels of carboxyhemoglobin the skin will turn bright cherry red, and at high levels (over 50% to 70% of total hemoglobin) the individual can be asphyxiated. Carboxyhemoglobin is found normally in small amounts, especially in the blood of smokers, where concentrations range from 1% to 10% of circulating hemoglobin.

### Methemoglobin (Hemiglobin)

Methemoglobin (also referred to as hemiglobin or Hi) is a hemoglobin derivative in which the iron has been oxidized from the ferrous to the ferric state and is therefore incapable of combining reversibly with oxygen. The formation of methemoglobin is usually an acquired condition resulting from the presence of certain chemicals or drugs, and is reversible. An inherited methemoglobinemia may result from a structurally abnormal globin chain or a red cell enzyme defect. Up to 1.5% of circulating hemoglobin is normally methemoglobin.

The formation of methemoglobin is used as an intermediary in the cyanmethemoglobin (or hemiglobincyanide) method for the quantitation of whole blood hemoglobin.

### Hemiglobincyanide (Cyanmethemoglobin)

To measure total hemoglobin concentration in blood, it is necessary to prepare a stable derivative containing all the hemoglobin forms that are present. All forms of circulating hemoglobin are readily converted to hemiglobincyanide (HiCN), except for sulfhemoglobin, which is rarely present in significant amounts. For this reason, the hemiglobincyanide, or cyanmethemoglobin, method is the standard method for the determination of hemoglobin.

### Sulfhemoglobin

Another abnormal hemoglobin derivative is sulfhemoglobin. The formation of sulfhemoglobin is irreversible, and it remains in the RBC for the cell's entire 120-day life span. Its exact nature is not clear, but it is thought to be formed by the action of some drugs and chemicals, such as sulfonamides. Although sulfhemoglobin is not capable of transporting oxygen, and cannot be converted back to normally functioning hemoglobin, sulfhemoglobinemia hardly ever exceeds 10% of the total hemoglobin. This is not a life-threatening level, although sulfhemoglobinemia may be seen clinically as cyanosis.

### Variations in Reference Values

The reference (or normal) values for hemoglobin in the peripheral blood vary with the age and sex of the individual. Altitude also affects the hemoglobin measurement, in that the normal hemoglobin concentration is higher at high altitudes than at sea level. At birth, the hemoglobin concentration is normally 15 to 20 g/dL. It decreases to 9 to 14 g/dL by about 2 months of age.

By 10 years of age, the normal hemoglobin will be 12 to 15 g/dL. Normal adult values range from 12 to 16 g/dL in women and 13 to 18 g/dL in men. There may be a slight decrease in the hemoglobin level after 50 years of age.[2]

When the hemoglobin value is below normal, the patient is said to be anemic. Anemia is a very common condition and is frequently a complication of other diseases (see under Erythrocyte Alterations in this chapter). In this condition the circulating erythrocytes may be deficient in number, deficient in total hemoglobin content per unit of blood volume, or both. A decrease in hemoglobin can result from bleeding conditions, in which the patient loses erythrocytes. An increase in hemoglobin, usually as a result of an increase in the number of erythrocytes (erythrocytosis), is seen in polycythemia and newborn infants.

## Hemoglobin Measurement in the Laboratory

Hemoglobin is determined as grams of hemoglobin per 100 mL of blood, or grams per deciliter (g/dL). Reporting hemoglobin as a percentage of a normal value is unacceptable. A method for measuring hemoglobin must be chosen that will detect all forms of hemoglobin. The one used by most laboratories is the hemiglobincyanide (HiCN) or cyanmethemoglobin method. This is now the internationally recognized method of choice. All forms of circulating hemoglobin, except for sulfhemoglobin, are readily converted to cyanmethemoglobin. Spectrophotometric hemoglobin determinations are rapid and can give accurate results. The degree of accuracy will also depend on the basic technique used and the accuracy of the equipment, the stability of the reagents, and the cleanliness of the glassware.

### Hemiglobincyanide or Cyanmethemoglobin Method

The hemiglobincyanide (HiCN) or cyanmethemoglobin method uses a modified Drabkin's reagent. The original Drabkin's reagent required at least 10 minutes for color conversion of hemoglobin to hemiglobincyanide and also sometimes produced turbid solutions caused by protein precipitation or incomplete lysis of red blood cells. The modified Drabkin's reagent contains potassium cyanide, potassium ferricyanide, dihydrogen potassium phosphate ($KH_2PO_4$), which shortens the conversion time to 3 minutes, and a nonionic detergent, which minimizes turbidity and enhances red cell lysis. When the cyanmethemoglobin reagent is mixed with the blood specimen, the stable pigment hemiglobincyanide (HiCN) is formed. This pigment can be measured quantitatively in the spectrophotometer.

### Automated Hemoglobinometry

Various automated and semiautomated techniques have been employed to measure hemoglobin. Automatic pipettors and dilutors are used for portions of the measuring and diluting steps in many procedures. A special flow-through apparatus attached to the Coleman Junior Spectrophotometer enables a faster, more efficient spectrophotometric measurement of the unknown hemoglobin solution (see under Flow-through Adaptation, under Absorbance Spectrophotometry in Chapter 6). This apparatus is designed to increase the speed with which samples can be introduced and discharged from the spectrophotometer. Automated cell counters measure hemoglobin as well as determine the white cell count, red cell count, hematocrit, and red cell indices. Automation has made a significant contribution to the efficiency of the hematology laboratory (see under Counting the Formed Elements of the Blood).

Hemoglobin determinations done by an automated instrument generally use the cyanmethemoglobin method. The sample is lysed by using the detergent-modified Drabkin's reagent and light absorbance is measured at 540 nm.

### Specimens

The test for hemoglobin can be done on free-flowing capillary blood obtained from a finger puncture, or on venous blood preserved with an anticoagulant. The anticoagulant of choice for hematologic studies, including hemoglobin determinations, is EDTA. The hemoglobin content of blood remains unchanged for several days when the blood is properly anticoagulated and refrigerated at 4° C.

### Equipment for Nonautomated Hemoglobinometry

**Measuring Device.** Disposable, self-filling, self-measuring dilution micropipettes are commercially available for determination of hemoglobin. One such system is the Unopette* (Fig. 12-5; see also Chapter 3). These systems are easy to use and are available with a series of different diluting fluids for different purposes. The Unopette System for hemoglobin determination consists of a self-filling, self-measuring pipette attached to a plastic holder; the pipette fills with blood automatically by capillary action. A plastic reagent container, called the reservoir, is filled with modified Drabkin's reagent (hemiglobincyanide) in the hemoglobin

*Becton Dickinson VACUTAINER Systems, Franklin Lakes, NJ.

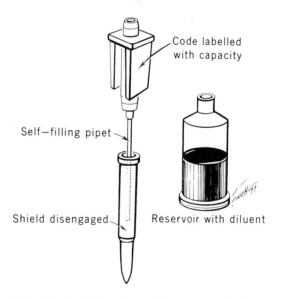

**FIG 12-5.** Self-filling disposable pipette and diluent reservoir.

Unopette system. The pipette containing the blood is inserted into the reagent reservoir, emptied, and rinsed according to the manufacturer's instructions. The blood is mixed well with the reagent and is then ready to be read in the spectrophotometer.

**Spectrophotometer.** Since most hemoglobin determinations employ photometry, a spectrophotometer of good quality and in good working order is essential. Most brands of spectrophotometers give good results if certain precautions are taken. Before a spectrophotometer can be used to determine the hemoglobin concentration, it must be standardized. Since the Coleman Junior Spectrophotometer has been discussed in some detail in Chapter 6, the procedure presented in this section for standardization of the spectrophotometer will deal specifically with this instrument. However, the same general procedure can be followed for any type of spectrophotometer.

### Hemiglobincyanide (Cyanmethemoglobin) Method (See Procedure 12-1)

**Principle.** A 20 $\mu$L (0.02 mL) portion of blood is diluted and hemolyzed in 5 mL of cyanmethemoglobin (HiCN) reagent, which contains potassium ferricyanide and potassium cyanide. The ferricyanide converts the hemoglobin iron from the ferrous state ($Fe^{2+}$) to the ferric state ($Fe^{3+}$) to form hemiglobin (Hi) or methemoglobin. This combines with potassium cyanide to form the stable pigment hemiglobincyanide (HiCN). The chemical reaction that occurs is, briefly:

$$Hb + K_3Fe(CN)_6 \rightarrow Hi$$
$$Hi + KCN \rightarrow HiCN$$

Hemiglobin is hemoglobin in which the iron has been oxidized to the ferric state. Hemiglobincyanide is methemoglobin bonded to cyanide ions. The hemiglobincyanide reagent has three primary purposes: to dilute the blood, to lyse the red cells, and to convert hemoglobin to hemiglobincyanide.

The color reaction takes 3 minutes to reach completion if the reagent contains $KH_2PO_4$ as a buffer (10 minutes if $NaHCO_3$ is used). All derivatives of hemoglobin, except sulfhemoglobin, are measured by using this method. The color intensity of this mixture is measured in a spectrophotometer at a wavelength of 540 nm. Absorbance is directly proportional to the concentration of hemoglobin. The concentration (C) of hemoglobin (g/dL) can be calculated from $C = A/K$, where K is the constant for the spectrophotometer used in the standardization and A is absorbance. The concentration can also be read directly from a standard line or from a hemoglobin table prepared from a standard line. (See Procedure 12-2.)

**Reagents.** A Unopette reservoir with 5 mL of hemiglobincyanide reagent already in it is supplied by the manufacturer. The manufacturer's directions must be followed carefully. Hemiglobincyanide reagent is a clear, pale yellow solution. It should be discarded if it becomes turbid. Although the reagent contains only a small amount of cyanide, it is still regarded as a poison and must be treated with caution.

**Quality Control Solution.** Daily controls should be run by using either a commercial control specimen or one prepared by the laboratory.

A control sample is run in duplicate with each batch of hemoglobins or for the first batch run by each new shift on duty in the laboratory. Controls must be assayed in exactly the same manner as the unknown samples. Control values are plotted on a quality control chart. This chart indicates the previously established acceptable range or limits for the hemoglobin values in grams per deciliter. Each laboratory establishes its own acceptable quality control limits. One acceptability criterion includes the following: replicate hemoglobin values on the same specimen agree within 0.4 g/dL of each other; if a "true" value is known for a control or patient sample, results must agree within ±0.4

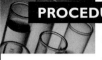

## PROCEDURE 12-1

*Hemoglobin: Hemiglobincyanide Method Using the Unopette Diluting System and Spectrophotometric Measurement*

1. Allow the spectrophotometer to warm up adequately. Set the wavelength scale at 540 nm.

2. Prepare a blank tube with 5 mL of hemiglobincyanide reagent. Use one hemoglobin Unopette reservoir to fill a cuvette.

3. Label cuvettes or tubes for each specimen.

4. Assemble necessary equipment: Unopette 20-μL (0.02-mL) capillary pipette, and reservoir with 5-mL cyanmethemoglobin reagent.

5. Puncture the neck of the reservoir with the shielded pipette to make an opening for the blood sample.

6. Obtain blood sample from a free-flowing finger or heel puncture or from a well-mixed venous blood specimen collected in EDTA.

7. Holding the capillary pipette in an almost horizontal position, touch the tip of the pipette to the blood. Capillary action fills the pipette, and the blood collection into the pipette stops automatically. Wipe any excess blood off the outside of the pipette, making certain to remove no blood from inside the capillary bore.

8. Insert the capillary pipette into the reservoir through the open diaphragm (neck) without seating the pipette firmly in the reservoir neck.

9. Squeeze the reservoir. Cover the upper opening of the pipette (overflow chamber) with the index finger, and then seat the pipette firmly into the reservoir. Remove the finger from the pipette opening. Blood will be drawn into the diluent by suction.

10. Squeeze the reservoir gently two or three times to rinse the capillary bore, forcing diluent up into, but not out of, the overflow chamber, releasing pressure each time to return the mixture to the reservoir.

11. Place the index finger over the upper opening of the pipette, and gently invert a few times to mix blood and diluent.

12. Wait at least 3 minutes for color development to take place.

13. Invert the reservoir tube over the cuvette used for spectrophotometry, and squeeze the entire contents of the reservoir into the cuvette. If a spectrophotometer with a flow-through system is being used, empty the contents of the reservoir directly into the flow-through apparatus.

14. Read the blank solution at 540 nm and adjust to 100%T. Then read the unknown hemoglobin samples, using the same wavelength. Record readings in percent transmittance to the nearest ¼ %T unit.

15. Convert the percent transmittance readings to concentrations by using the calibration curve or table prepared for the photometer (see under Standardization of the Coleman Junior Spectrophotometer).

16. Report hemoglobin results to the first decimal place.

*Continued*

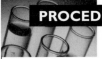

## PROCEDURE 12-1

*Hemoglobin: Hemiglobincyanide Method Using the Unopette Diluting System and Spectrophotometric Measurement—cont'd*

17. Test quality control samples daily, and plot the values on the control chart for the machine. Report patient values only when the control values have checked out.

18. Duplicate determinations should agree within 0.4 g/dL, or the procedure should be repeated.

g/dL of that value; if hemoglobin values do not meet these limits, they will be repeated in duplicate; results will not be reported unless the control values run simultaneously with the unknown batch of patient samples are within the acceptable range.

Daily use of control values gives information about the state of the hemoglobin reagent (whether deterioration has occurred), the accuracy of the pipettes used, the variation and cleanliness of the calibrated photometer cuvettes, and the variation in the photometer used to measure the amount of hemoglobin in the samples. Technical skills are also checked. When the control values for the duplicate control specimens run are not within the acceptable limits, hemoglobin values for the unknown patient blood specimens being measured should not be reported until the reason for the control error is found, the problem corrected, and the sample retested. "Out-of-control" values are seen with deterioration of reagents, faulty equipment (spectrophotometer), dirty glassware, inaccurate standardization of the spectrophotometer, deterioration of the control specimen, inaccurate or broken pipettes, or poor technique (see Chapter 8).

**Precautions, Technical Factors, and Sources of Error.** Several precautions have already been discussed. Photometric methods for the determination of hemoglobin are rapid and give accurate results only when the equipment is in good working condition. The spectrophotometer must be working well, and the pipettes and

calibrated cuvettes must be clean and free from breaks or scratches. Hemiglobincyanide reagent, if prepared by the laboratory, must be prepared fresh each month and stored in a brown bottle to prevent deterioration. Spectrophotometers must be standardized before being used for the hemoglobin determination. They should be re-standardized periodically and the calibrated hemoglobin tables redone when changes occur in the values. Each spectrophotometer must have a calibration table.

Before the unknown samples are read in the spectrophotometer, they must be crystal clear. If there is any turbidity, a falsely high result will be read. Turbidity may result from exceptionally high white blood cell counts, the presence of Hb S or Hb C, the presence of abnormal globulins, or lipemic blood specimens. The use of the modified hemiglobincyanide reagents (with detergents added) has eliminated many of these interferences.

Blood containing carbon monoxide requires 3 hours for the formation of hemiglobincyanide from carboxyhemoglobin with hemiglobincyanide reagent.

One of the greatest causes of error is improper pipetting technique. Using precalibrated, self-filling pipettes (such as the Unopette) helps to eliminate some of this error. If the capillary blood flow is slow and the finger is squeezed to obtain the sample, error can result from the introduction of tissue juice into the blood sample. If venous blood is not mixed well before measurement, gross errors result.

Salts and solutions of cyanide are poisonous, and care should be taken to avoid getting them into the mouth or inhaling their fumes. Hemiglobincyanide reagent contains 50 mg of potassium cyanide per liter, significantly less than the lethal dose for an average 70-kg person. Nevertheless, this reagent must be handled with great care. Many laboratories obtain the reagent commercially, so that handling KCN is not necessary. The salt is potentially very dangerous and must be kept in a secure place if it is used by the laboratory.

Samples and reagents must be discarded carefully and under no circumstances come in contact with acid. Hydrogen cyanide gas (HCN) is released when the hemiglobincyanide reagent is acidified.

The reagent may be inactivated by oxidation with bleach. When inactivated, samples and reagents can be poured down a laboratory sink drain, with large amounts of running tap water being used before, during, and after disposal. Disposal should be in accordance with federal, state, and local codes.

To eliminate error resulting from poorly calibrated cuvettes or cuvettes that are not matched correctly, many photometric instruments are supplied with a flow-through cuvette system. The solution to be read is poured directly into the system. After each reading, the solution is emptied into a discard container by means of a valve in the bottom of the cuvette. Since all readings, standards, controls, and unknowns are taken through the same flow-through cuvette, errors caused by imperfectly matched cuvettes are eliminated.

### Standardization of the Spectrophotometer Hemoglobin Determinations
*(See Procedure 12-2)*

Before any unknown solution can be measured with a spectrophotometer, the instrument must be standardized; that is, a standard curve must be prepared from which to read the unknowns. To do this, samples of known concentration of the substance to be measured (the standard so-

lutions) must be read in the spectrophotometer. The principles of Beer's law are applied (see under Absorbance and Transmittance of Light: Beer's Law, in Chapter 6). When the wavelength of light and its path length are a constant (K factor) for the procedure, the concentration (C) of hemiglobincyanide in each sample is directly proportional to the absorbance (A) obtained.

**Procedure Using ICSH-Certified Standards.** Stable standard hemiglobincyanide solutions representing 1:250 dilutions of whole blood containing 5, 10, and 15 g of hemoglobin per 100 mL of blood are available commercially and are certified by the College of American Pathologists (CAP) and approved by the International Council for Standardization in Haematology (ICSH). This type of hemoglobin standard is commonly used by all clinical laboratories. When a certified standard is used, Procedure 12-2 may be followed in setting up the cuvettes for reading in the spectrophotometer.

### Hemoglobin by HemoCue: Azide Methemoglobin Method *(See Procedure 12-3)*

The HemoCue* is an example of a self-contained instrument that measures hemoglobin only. This methodology represents a method of hemoglobin determination that is waivered under CLIA '88. It gives a reliable quantitative value and can be performed within 45 seconds. The instrument utilizes a microcuvette that serves as a sampling device, a test tube, and a measuring device. It automatically measures precisely 10 $\mu$L of blood, from a capillary puncture or from a tube of anticoagulated blood collected by venipuncture. The microcuvette does not require the mixing or dispensing of reagents. It contains an exact quantity of a dry reagent, which yields a reaction when contact is made with the measured blood sample. Once the blood is sampled, the microcuvette is placed into the HemoCue photometer and the hemoglobin concentration is displayed in g/dL.

*HemoCue, Inc, Mission Viejo, Calif.

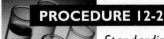

### Standardization of the Coleman Junior Spectrophotometer Using ICSH-Certified Hemoglobin Standards

1. Label 11 cuvettes (test tubes may be used if the flow-through type of apparatus is available for the spectrophotometer) as follows: blank, 1, 1 duplicate; 2, 2 duplicate; 3, 3 duplicate; 4, 4 duplicate; and 5, 5 duplicate. High-quality disposable glass tubes also may be satisfactory for use in the spectrophotometer in place of calibrated cuvettes.

2. Using volumetric pipettes, pipette the following amounts into the cuvettes:

| Tube | Standard (mL) | Hemiglobincyanide Reagent (mL) |
|---|---|---|
| Blank | 0 | 5 |
| 1 | 1 | 4 |
| 1 duplicate | 1 | 4 |
| 2 | 2 | 3 |
| 2 duplicate | 2 | 3 |
| 3 | 3 | 2 |
| 3 duplicate | 3 | 2 |
| 4 | 4 | 1 |
| 4 duplicate | 4 | 1 |
| 5 | 5 | 0 |
| 5 duplicate | 5 | 0 |

3. Mix the contents of the cuvettes well.

4. Read each cuvette in the spectrophotometer, using a wavelength setting of 540 nm.

5. Record absorbance (A) readings directly, or record percent transmittance (%T) readings and convert to absorbance.

6. Calculate the concentration (C) of hemoglobin (mg/dL) for each of the standard cuvettes (see the original concentration of standard solution used).

7. Calculate the concentration of hemoglobin (g/dL) for each of the standard dilutions.

8. Calculate the K value for each standard (K = A/C) and calculate the average K value for the spectrophotometer.

9. Plot the standard line on semilogarithmic graph paper with percent transmittance readings (use linear graph paper for absorbance readings). Draw the straight line through the points that gives the best fit for the graph. Subsequent hemoglobin concentrations can then be read directly from this straight line. Generally, readings between 20%T and 80%T are more accurate than readings at either end of the scale. If a patient sample gives a reading greater than 80%T, the test is repeated with twice as much blood. If a patient sample gives a reading less than 20%T, the blood sample is diluted with twice as much diluent and the test is repeated. Volumes must be taken into account in the calculations.

An alternative method is to calculate the constant factor K (= A/C) for the instrument (see step 8 above). By using the average K value, hemoglobin concentrations corresponding to all the potential galvanometer readings may be calculated and a standard chart may be prepared. The standard chart will show the range of hemoglobin concentrations that can be accurately determined with a particular spectrophotometer. Only hemoglobin values obtained from the linear portion of the graph may be used to prepare the standard chart. The chart prepared from data obtained with one spectrophotometer cannot be used with any other spectrophotometer.

## PROCEDURE 12-3

### Hemoglobin by HemoCue

1. Assemble equipment, wash hands, and put on gloves.

2. Remove the necessary microcuvettes from the HemoCue vial and replace the cap immediately. Hold the cuvette by the winged end.

3. If the instrument has been left "OFF," turn the power switch at the back of the photometer to the "ON" position and pull out the cuvette holder to the insertion position. The correct position will be noted by a distinct stop. The display shows "Hb" and after six seconds, "READY" with three blinking dashes.

4. Obtain a blood sample from thoroughly mixed venous blood collected in EDTA or from a free-flowing finger puncture. Allow the cuvette to completely fill in a continuous process by capillary action. Never "top off" the cuvette after the first filling.

5. Dry off any surplus blood at the tip of the microcuvette, making certain that no blood is drawn out of the cuvette; do not touch the curved end.

6. Place the filled cuvette in the holder and insert it into the photometer to the measuring position—that is, the stop point. The display will read "measuring."

7. The hemoglobin result in g/dL will be displayed in approximately 45 seconds.

8. When the measurement has been completed, remove the cuvette from the holder and discard appropriately. When no more assays are to be performed, turn the photometer power switch to the "POWER OFF" position.

9. Record result.

---

**Principle.** After lysis of red cells, sodium nitrite converts hemoglobin iron from the ferrous to the ferric state to form methemoglobin, which then combines with sodium azide to form azide methemoglobin. The absorbance is measured at two wavelengths (565 and 880nm) in order to compensate for turbidity in the sample.

**Precision.** Three percent (manufacturer's value) with hemoglobin concentration from 5.4 to 18.5 g/dL.

### Equipment
**Measuring Device.** The HemoCue single-purpose photometer.

**Microcuvettes.** Special disposable microcuvettes are used as the device for measuring 10 μL of blood, as the reaction vessel (they contain reagent in dry form), and as the cuvette that is placed in the photometer.

**Specimen collection supplies.** For venipuncture or finger puncture.

**Technical Considerations.** The photometer is calibrated at the factory against the hemiglobincyanide (HiCN) method.

A control cuvette, which is an optical filter, is used to check that the calibration of the photometer is stable from day to day. Before any patient samples are assayed, the calibration check for the instrument must be performed. This is done each day prior to use. The reading should be within ±0.3 g/dL of the assigned value for the calibration cuvette.

The filled cuvette should be analyzed immediately or at the latest, 10 minutes after it has been filled.

Filled cuvettes should be examined for the presence of air bubbles, which, if present, can produce erroneously low readings. Small bubbles around the edge do not influence the result.

Store microcuvettes in the vial in which they are supplied, tightly capped.

Store microcuvettes at room temperature, away from any direct heat source.

### Reference Values*

*For adult male:* 15.7 (14.0-17.5) g/dL
*For adult female:* 13.8 (12.3-15.3) g/dL
*For 12-month-old:* 12.6 (11.1-14.1) g/dL
*For 10-year-old:* 13.4 (11.8-15.0) g/dL

The mean hemoglobin level of blacks of both sexes and all ages is reported to be 0.5 to 1.0 g/dL below the mean for comparable whites.

### Reference Values (HemoCue Methodology)

*Adult males* 13-18 g/dL
*Adult females:* 11-16 g/dL

## HEMATOCRIT (PACKED CELL VOLUME)

The **hematocrit (Hct)** is a macroscopic observation by which the percentage volume of the packed RBCs is measured. Hematocrit is therefore also known as the **packed cell volume,** or **PCV.** More correctly, the test name is the packed cell volume and the equipment is the hematocrit. This test is relatively simple and reliable. It gives useful information about the RBCs, which may be correlated with the number of RBCs and their hemoglobin content (see under Blood Cell Counts and under Hemoglobin). These measurements together enable the red cell indices to be calculated (see under Red Cell Indices). The

*Beutler E, Lichtman MA, Coller BS, Kipps TJ: *Williams Hematology,* ed 5. New York, McGraw-Hill, Inc, 1995, pp 9, 12.

hematocrit measurement is more useful and reliable than the red cell count done manually, because much less error is associated with it. Most laboratories perform hematocrit determinations along with hemoglobin measurements, and some do the hematocrit even more regularly. A fast quality control check on hemoglobin results (in g/dL) is done by comparing them with the hematocrit results (in % units), using the following formula:

$$Hb \times 3 = Hct \pm 3 \text{ units}$$

This rule applies only when red cells are of normal size and color, however.

The hematocrit is used in evaluating and classifying the various types of anemias according to red cell indices. The spun microhematocrit method has generally replaced the Wintrobe method for determining packed cell volume. It takes less time and labor and requires a smaller blood sample than the Wintrobe macrohematocrit. The spun microhematocrit method is well suited to screen for anemia in certain clinics where actual hemoglobin determinations are impractical, such as for potential blood donors or for children for adequate nutritional status, especially for iron deficiency.

When whole blood is centrifuged, the heavier particles fall to the bottom of the tube and the lighter particles settle on top of the heavier cells. The hematocrit is the percentage of red cells in a volume of whole blood. It is expressed as units of percent or as a ratio in the SI system.

When the hematocrit result is read, it is important to take the reading at the top of the RBC layer, particularly when there is an extremely elevated white cell or platelet count. The buffy coat (WBCs and platelets) should not be included in the measurement of red cell volume for the hematocrit result (Fig. 12-6.)

Automated hematology instruments give a calculated hematocrit value and have generally replaced the manual methods.

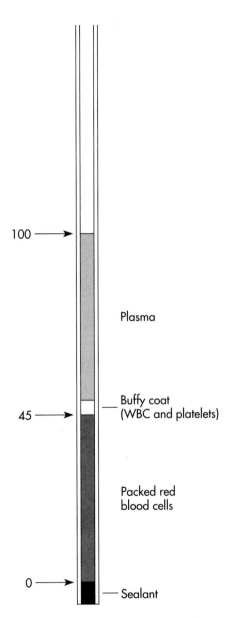

100 ——▶

Plasma

Buffy coat
(WBC and platelets)

45 ——▶

Packed red
blood cells

0 ——▶

Sealant

**FIG 12-6.** Spun microhematocrit tube.

## Methods for Measurement of Packed Cell Volume (Hematocrit)

The **spun microhematocrit method** is used commonly. (See Procedure 12-4.) It can be done with either free-flowing capillary blood from a skin puncture or EDTA-anticoagulated venous blood; a very small amount of blood is needed. The test utilizes a high-speed centrifuge, which yields a relatively short centrifugation time. The microhematocrit is there-

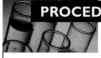

## PROCEDURE 12-4

### *Microhematocrit: Manual Method*

1. Well-mixed EDTA-anticoagulated venous blood or freely flowing blood from a skin puncture may be used.

2. Fill two microhematocrit capillary tubes to approximately two-thirds to three-fourths full.
   *With venous blood:* Use a plain microhematocrit tube, color coded with a blue ring.
   a. Hold the tube of blood as horizontally as possible without pouring the blood out of the tube.
   b. Place the unplugged tip of the self-sealing microhematocrit tube, or either end of the conventional microhematocrit tube, in the blood, and let the tube fill by capillary action two-thirds to three-fourths full.
   *With capillary blood:* Use a heparinized microhematocrit tube, color coded with a red ring.
   a. Massage a generous drop of free-flowing blood from the puncture site.
   b. Place the unplugged tip of the self-sealing microhematocrit tube, or either end of the conventional microhematocrit tube, in the blood, and let the tube fill by capillary action two-thirds to three-fourths full.

3. Seal the capillary tube.
   *With self-sealing tubes:* When the tube is two-thirds to three-fourths full, hold the tube vertically (plug end down) so that the blood runs down the tube. When the blood sample touches the self-sealing plug, the tube seals automatically. Allow blood to contact the self-sealing plug for at least 15 seconds to ensure sealing. Failure to do so may result in leakage of the sample during centrifugation and inaccurate results.
   *With conventional tubes:* Seal the dry end of each tube by inserting at a right angle to a sealing clay for microhematocrit tubes. Place your gloved index finger over the opposite end to prevent blood from leaking onto the sealant.

4. Place the sealed tubes into the radial groove of the microhematocrit centrifuge. Be sure the centrifuge is balanced with another microhematocrit tube in an exactly opposite groove. Place the sealed end of the tube away from the center of the centrifuge, against the peripheral gasket (Fig. 12-7).

fore a quick test, and the results can be ready in a short time.

The **Wintrobe hematocrit method** is a macromethod, which requires more blood and a longer centrifugation time. Blood must be drawn by venipuncture and properly anticoagulated. This method has been generally replaced by the microhematocrit or calculated (automated) hematocrit.

An **automated hematocrit** result is obtained when multiparameter instruments are used. This result is computed from individual red cell volumes (MCV) and the red cell count and is not affected by the trapped plasma that is left in the red cell column for the manual methods. Therefore, the hematocrit value obtained with the automated instruments is lower than the value obtained by the centrifugation methods.

### Specimens

For the spun microhematocrit method, either venous blood anticoagulated with EDTA or freely flowing capillary blood may be used.

## PROCEDURE 12-4

### Microhematocrit: Manual Method—cont'd

5. Follow the directions for the particular microhematocrit centrifuge in use. Generally there is a rotator head cover that is screwed firmly over the tubes. A second lid or top is then lowered and locked securely. Centrifuge the tubes for 5 minutes at 10,000 to 15,000 rpm.

6. As soon as the centrifuge has stopped spinning, remove the tubes, one at a time, and read and record results. If the tubes are left in the centrifuge in a horizontal position for more than 10 minutes, the layers will merge and it will be impossible to get an accurate result.

7. Read the microhematocrit result with a graphic reading device or some other accurate measuring device. The percent of the total volume that is composed of red cells is measured; this is the hematocrit. (See Fig. 12-6.)

8. The general principle of measurement is the same for all readers and includes:
   a. The interface between the clay and the red cells is set at 0%.
   b. The top of the plasma is set as 100%.
   c. The top of the red cell layer is read as a percent from a sliding scale. This is the hematocrit.

9. To calculate the PCV from direct measurements of the red cell and plasma columns, use the following formula:

$$PCV = \frac{\text{Length of red cell column (in mm)}}{\text{Length of cells plus plasma column (in mm)}}$$

10. Results for duplicate tests should agree within 2%.

With capillary blood, microhematocrit tubes coated with heparin are used. With venous blood, plain, uncoated microhematocrit tubes must be used.

Blood that has been properly anticoagulated with EDTA is used for automated analysis.

### Equipment for Spun Microhematocrit
#### Capillary Tubes

Special nongraduated glass capillary tubes are used. These tubes are 1 mm in diameter and 7 cm long. They can be purchased lined with dried heparin for use with capillary blood, or plain (without heparin) for use with previously anticoagulated venous blood. Some type of seal is needed for one end of the tube before it can be centrifuged. A special sealing compound (similar to modeling clay) can be used for this purpose. Or tubes are available that have a self-sealing plug and a multilayered Mylar wrap to ensure safer blood handling by preventing breakage during collection and centrifugation and contamination of the sealant.

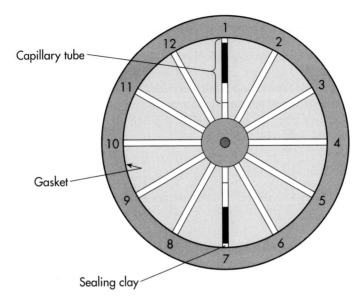

**FIG 12-7.** Placement of capillary tubes in the microhematocrit centrifuge. The centrifuge must be balanced by placing the tubes directly across from each other, as shown for places 1 and 7.

### Centrifuge

A special microhematocrit centrifuge is used, capable of producing centrifugal fields up to 10,000 g.

### Reading Device

Since the capillary tubes are not graduated, a special reading device is used to measure the percentage of packed red blood cells after centrifugation.

## Results

In current laboratory practice, hematocrit values are generally expressed as a percentage. However, according to the SI system, packed cell volume is preferably expressed as a decimal; the units are undesignated, but units of liter per liter are implied. Thus a 45% result is reported as 0.45.

## Precautions and Technical Factors

The blood sample must be properly collected and preserved. Anticoagulated blood samples using EDTA should be centrifuged within 6 hours of collection. EDTA is the anticoagulant of choice. The blood must not be clotted or hemolyzed for any hematocrit test. If clotted blood is used, there will be false packing of the red cells, and the true packing in the tube will not be noted (a falsely high result will be observed). In a hemolyzed specimen some of the red cells have been destroyed, so again the packing of the red cells will not be true (a falsely low result will be observed). Centrifugation must be sufficient to yield maximum packing of the red cells.

The hematocrit value is frequently accompanied by a hemoglobin determination. There should be a correlation between the two results: the hematocrit result in percent units should be approximately three times the hemoglobin result, assuming the red cells are of normal size and color.

Any capillary blood samples collected should be freely flowing. The capillary tubes must be properly sealed so that no leakage occurs. Since these tubes are not calibrated, the level of packed red cells and the total volume of the cells and plasma must be accurately measured by some convenient reading device. The buffy coat layer is not included in the reading for the hematocrit.

Even with adequate centrifugation, providing tightly packed red cells, a small amount of plasma remains trapped around the red cells. This is unavoidable, and in normal blood, with normally shaped and sized red cells, this trapped plasma accounts for 1.5% to 3.0% of the height of the red cell column in a microhematocrit tube. When the red cells have an irregular shape or size, there will be an increase in the amount of plasma being trapped.

When hematocrits are determined by use of automated hematology analyzers, the hematocrit is determined indirectly by determining the average size of the red cell population (the mean corpuscular volume, or MCV) and multiplying it by the total red cell count. The hematocrit value as determined by automation is therefore consistently lower than that done by the spun microhematocrit method.

Unique to the microhematocrit is the error caused by excess EDTA (inadequate blood for the fixed amount of EDTA in the blood collection tube). The microhematocrit will be falsely low because of cell shrinkage. Thus, heparinized capillary tubes must not be used with anticoagulated blood samples.

With good technique, the precision of the hematocrit is ± 1%. Inadequate centrifugation will give falsely high results. If the tubes are not sealed properly, falsely low results will be obtained because more RBCs will be lost than plasma.

## Reference Values*

Reference values are influenced by the age and sex of the individual, as well as by the altitude, and vary among authors (see also under Hemoglobin). According to the NCCLS, generally accepted values at sea level are as follows:

*For adult male:* mean 0.47; 0.40-0.54 (40%-54%)
*For adult female:* mean 0.42; 0.37-0.47 (37%-47%)

## RED BLOOD CELL INDICES

In the classification of anemias, quantitative measurements of the average size, hemoglobin content, and hemoglobin concentration of the RBCs are especially useful (see under Erythrocyte Alterations). These can be calculated from the red cell count, the hemoglobin concentration, and the hematocrit. The indices are the mean corpuscular (cell) volume (MCV), the mean corpuscular (cell) hemoglobin (MCH), and the mean corpuscular (cell) hemoglobin concentration (MCHC).

The MCV represents the volume or size of the average RBC, the MCHC represents the hemoglobin concentration or color of the average RBC, and the MCH represents the weight of hemoglobin in the average RBC.

A derived measurement determined electronically is the red cell distribution width (RDW). This is a measurement of the degree of red cell size variability.

Determination of these indices has become routine with the use of automated multiparameter instruments. These instruments measure the hemoglobin, MCV, and RBC count, and then automatically calculate the hematocrit, MCH, and MCHC.

When the indices are calculated from manually determined values for hemoglobin, hematocrit, and red cell count, the greatest inaccuracy results from errors associated with the red cell count. By electronic counting of the number of RBCs, this error is significantly reduced. Indices calculated by electronic methods have been found to be more accurate by several investigators. It is important to verify all indices against observations of stained blood films. When the red cell indices are used in conjunction with an examination of the stained blood film, a clear picture of red cell morphology is obtained.

---

*NCCLS: *Procedure for Determining Packed Cell Volume by the Microhematocrit Method: Approved Standard,* ed 2. Villanova, Pa, National Committee for Clinical Laboratory Standards, 1993 (August), H7-A2.

Since an RBC is very small and the amount of hemoglobin in a single cell is minute, the units in which the red cells are measured and recorded are micrometers ($\mu$m) and picograms (pg).

With automated hematology instrumentation, reporting the red cell indices is routine and the data are considered highly reliable.

The red cell indices are calculated from the following hematology data (with abbreviations) in units as indicated.

| Test Name | Abbreviation | Units |
|---|---|---|
| Hematocrit | Hct | % |
| Packed cell volume | PCV | L/L |
| Red cell count | RBC | $\times 10^{12}$/L |
| Hemoglobin | Hb | g/dL |

Description and formulas follow.

## Mean Corpuscular Volume

The MCV is the average volume of an RBC in femtoliters. One femtoliter (fL) = $10^{-15}$ L = one cubic micrometer ($\mu$m$^3$). The MCV is calculated manually by dividing the volume of packed red cells (hematocrit) by the number of red cells, using the formula:

$$MCV\ (fL) = \frac{Hct \times 10}{RBC}$$

The factor 10 is introduced to convert the hematocrit reading (in %) from volume of packed red cells per 100 mL to volume per liter. *Example:* If the Hct is 45% and the red cell count is $5 \times 10^{12}$ cells per liter:

$$MCV = \frac{45 \times 10}{5} = 90\ fL$$

When the hematocrit (or PCV) is measured in liter-per-liter units, such as 0.45 L/L:

$$MCV\ (fL) = \frac{PCV \times 1000}{RBC}\ or\ \frac{0.45 \times 1000}{5} = 90\ fL$$

The MCV in normal adults is between 80 and 96 fL.

The MCV indicates whether the RBCs will appear small (microcytic), normal (normocytic), or large (macrocytic). If the MCV is less than 80 fL, the red cells will be microcytic. If it is greater than 100 fL, the red cells will be macrocytic. If it is within the normal range, the red cells will be normocytic. In some macrocytic anemias (for instance, pernicious anemia) the MCV may be as high as 150 fL. In microcytic anemia with marked iron deficiency, it may be 60 to 70 fL. The chief source of error in the MCV is the considerable error in the manual red cell count if it is used.

With the automated cell counters and electronically calculated indices, the MCV is measured directly and the hematocrit is calculated from it and the red cell count (Hct = MCV $\times$ RBC). The MCV is now considered the most reliable automated index and is probably the most effective discriminant for the classification of anemias. Previously, the MCHC was the most reliable index, since it was calculated from the two manual measurements that could be done most accurately, the hematocrit and the hemoglobin.

## Mean Corpuscular Hemoglobin

The MCH is the content (weight) of hemoglobin in the average red cell. It is measured in picograms. One picogram (pg) = $10^{-12}$ g = 1 micromicrogram ($\mu\mu$g). The MCH is obtained by dividing the hemoglobin by the red cell count. A simple formula can be used to calculate this value:

$$MCH\ (pg) = \frac{Hb \times 10}{RBC}$$

The factor 10 is used to convert the hemoglobin from grams per deciliter to grams per liter. *Example:* If the hemoglobin is 15 g/dL and the RBC is $5 \times 10^{12}$ cells per liter:

$$MCH = \frac{15 \times 10}{5} = 30\ pg$$

The normal range for the MCH is 27 to 33 pg. It should always correlate with the MCV and the MCHC. It may be as high as 50 pg in macrocytic anemias or as low as 20 pg or less in hypochromic microcytic anemias.

The chief source of error is the RBC count if it is done manually. However, when the red cell count is determined by electronic cell counters, the MCH is a reliable index.

## Mean Corpuscular Hemoglobin Concentration

The MCHC is the average hemoglobin concentration in a given volume of packed red cells. It is expressed as grams per deciliter. It may be calculated from the MCV and the MCH or from the hemoglobin and hematocrit values by using the following formula:

$$\text{MCHC (g/dL)} = \frac{\text{MCH}}{\text{MCV}} \times 100$$

or

$$\text{MCHC (g/dL)} = \frac{\text{Hb}}{\text{Hct}} \times 100$$

*Example:* If the hemoglobin concentration is 15 g/dL and the Hct is 45%:

$$\text{MCHC} = \frac{15}{45} \times 100 = 33.3 \text{ g/dL}$$

*Or:* If the packed cell volume of 0.45 is used in the above example:

$$\text{MCHC} = \frac{15}{0.45} = 33.3 \text{ g/dL}$$

This measurement tells what percentage of a red cell is hemoglobin. Normal values range from 33 to 36 g/dL, and values below 32 g/dL indicate hypochromasia. An MCHC above 40 g/dL would indicate malfunctioning of the instrument or error in the calculation of the manual measurements used, because an MCHC of 37 g/dL is near the upper limits for hemoglobin solubility, thus limiting the physiologic upper limits for the MCHC. The MCHC typically increases only in spherocytosis. In other anemias it is decreased or normal. In true hypochromic anemias the hemoglobin concentration is re-

duced, and values as low as 20 to 25 g/dL are not uncommon.

With the use of electronic cell counters, the MCHC has become the least useful of the red cell indices. It is most useful in situations when only the hemoglobin and the hematocrit are available.

## Red Cell Distribution Width

This is a measurement of the degree of anisocytosis present, or the degree of red cell size variability in a blood sample. This measurement is derived by the automated multiparameter instruments that can directly measure the MCV as one of the parameters determined. If anisocytosis is present on the peripheral blood film, and the variation in red cell size is prominent, then there is an increase in the standard deviation of the MCV from the mean.

In the Coulter Model S Plus, for example, a red cell histogram is plotted and the RDW (%) is defined as the coefficient of variation of the MCV:

$$\text{RDW (\%)} = \frac{\text{SD of MCV}}{\text{Mean MCV}} \times 100$$

The reference range for RDW is from 11% to 15%, but varies with the instrument used.

## Indices: Precautions, Technical Factors, and General Comments

Any manual RBC count, hematocrit, or hemoglobin concentration used in the calculations must be accurate. It is also essential to check the appearance of the RBCs in a well-stained blood film against the calculated indices. The calculations must agree with the appearance of the red cells in the blood film. For example, a corresponding decrease in hemoglobin color intensity should be observed on the blood film when there is a low MCHC (an increase in the amount of central pallor in the red cells), but often it is difficult to recognize hypochromasia under these circumstances. The MCHC is often below 30 g/dL before hypochromasia is observed on the blood film.

## Reference Values*

*Mean corpuscular volume (MCV):* mean 88.0 fL (range 80-96.1 fL)

*Mean corpuscular hemoglobin (MCH):* mean 30.4 pg (range 27.5-33.2 pg)

*Mean corpuscular hemoglobin concentration (MCHC):* mean 34.4 g/dL (range 33.4-35.5 g/dL)

*Red cell distribution width (RDW):* mean 13.1% (range 11.5%-14.5%)

## BLOOD CELL COUNTS

Counting the various cells found in blood is a fundamental procedure in the hematology laboratory. The procedures used for enumeration include manual counts, which involve microscopic observation of cells in a counting chamber (hemocytometer), and the use of various electronic counting devices. The cells counted in routine practice are RBCs, WBCs, and platelets. Manual techniques lend themselves to enumeration of all cells found in blood and other body fluids, such as cerebrospinal fluid and semen. Practically speaking, most cell counts now done on blood are electronic. Manual counts are rarely performed, and are basically limited to WBC counts and platelet counts. Red blood cell counts are almost never done manually, because of the high degree of error inherent in this procedure and the time required to perform this technique. Electronic counting devices avoid human error, which is significant in manual cell counts, and are statistically more accurate because of sampling; they count many more cells than can be counted manually.

The main principles for cell counts are as follows:

1. Selection of a diluting fluid that will dilute the cells so that manageable numbers may be counted and will either identify them in some manner or destroy cellular elements that are not to be counted

2. Use of a hemocytometer, or electronic cell counter, that will present the cells to the laboratorian or to an electronic counting device in such a way that the number of cells per unit volume of fluid can be counted

Since there are a great many cells per unit volume of blood, it is necessary to dilute the blood before attempting to count them. Methods for counting cells are designed to obtain the number of cells in 1 L of whole blood. This is the unit (SI) of measurement of volume recommended by the International Council for Standardization in Haematology (ICSH). The units formerly used to record cell counts were cells per cubic millimeter.

## Units Reported

Since the enumerated constituents are to be reported in units per liter of blood, the number of cells actually counted (platelets, RBCs, WBCs) must be converted to the number present per liter of blood. Previously, cells were counted and reported as the number of cells per cubic millimeter ($mm^3$). This was a convenient unit of measurement because cells were counted in a hemocytometer, an accurately ruled chamber or device where cells were counted in areas of square millimeters, and the results converted to number per cubic millimeter. However, one cubic millimeter is essentially equal to one microliter. This is summarized as follows:

$$1\ mm^3 = 1\ \mu L = 1 \times 10^{-6}\ L$$

Therefore:

$$1 \times 10^6\ \mu L = 1\ L$$

## General Methods Used to Count Blood Cells

Whether an electronic cell counter or a manual method is used, the steps in the basic proce-

---

*Beutler E, Lichtman MA, Coller BS, Kipps TJ: *Williams Hematology,* ed 5. New York, McGraw-Hill, Inc., 1995, p 9.

dure used to count cells is the same. These include:

1. Diluting the blood sample quantitatively by using special measuring devices (pipettes) and appropriate diluents.
2. Determining the number of cells in the diluted sample.
3. Converting the number of cells in the diluted sample to the final result—the number of cells in 1 L of whole blood.

Blood cell counts are done on minute portions of already small samples of an individual's blood. For this reason, errors are inherent in the best methods, and the steps in the procedure must be performed as carefully as possible to reduce the variation of the final result from the actual or true count.

## Specimens

Free-flowing capillary blood obtained from a skin puncture, or venous blood preserved with an anticoagulant may be used. The anticoagulant of choice is EDTA.

Before using any blood sample, the laboratorian must make certain that it has been preserved with the proper anticoagulant and has been properly labeled, and that its appearance indicates that a good collection technique was used. Each sample should be checked for hemolysis and small clots (known as fibrin clots) as soon as it is received. Clotted blood or samples with fibrin clots are unacceptable for cell counts. Standard precautions must always be used when any blood specimen is handled.

## Diluents Used
### For Red Cell Counts

When RBCs are counted, the most important characteristic of the diluent is isotonicity. The cell integrity must be maintained. Two other necessary characteristics of a diluent for red cell counts are that it prevents clumping or clotting of the cells and that it has the proper specific gravity, so that all the cells will settle as evenly

as possible. Hayem's solution is a diluent commonly used for manual counting of red cells. It contains mercuric chloride ($HgCl_2$) to prevent clumping of the red cells, and sodium sulfate ($Na_2SO_4$) and sodium chloride (NaCl) to provide the proper specific gravity and isotonicity. Other diluents for red cell counts include 0.85 g/dL NaCl (or saline) solution, Gowers' solution, Toison's solution, and Rees-Ecker solution. Automated methods generally use a saline or Isoton* solution, which provides both isotonicity and electrical conductivity.

### For White Cell Counts

In the methods for leukocyte counts, the diluting fluid must meet a very different requirement—it must destroy the more numerous red cells so that the white cells may be counted more readily. (The white cells need not be eliminated when red cells are being counted.) The principle of osmotic pressure is again employed, but in a different way. The diluent used most commonly for white cell counts is 2 mL/dL acetic acid, which (1) darkens the nuclei of the white cells so that they are easier to see and (2) hemolyzes the red cells. When the acetic acid hemolyzes the red cells, it converts the hemoglobin released from the red cells into acid hematin, which gives the resulting solution a brown color. The intensity of the brown color is directly related to the amount of hemoglobin present in the red cells. When the Unopette system is used, the reservoir for white cell counts contains 0.475 mL of 3 mL/dL acetic acid. Another diluting fluid used for white cell counts is 0.1N HCl. The principle is the same with either 2 or 3 mL/dL acetic acid or 0.1N HCl.

## Counting Red and White Blood Cells

The white blood cell (leukocyte) count is a basic procedure in the hematology laboratory. With common use of automated cell counters, the red blood cell (erythrocyte) count is also considered a routine laboratory examination. Before the ad-

---

*Coulter Diagnostics, Hialeah, Fla.

vent of automatic cell counting devices, the red count had been virtually eliminated from most routine laboratory tests because of the large error ($\pm20\%$) in the manual methods of counting red cells. White cells are still counted manually in smaller laboratories, and when carefully done, this is an accurate measurement.

Manual white counts are described in this chapter. Although generally replaced by automated cell counts, they are still done in certain circumstances and are the usual method of counting cells in other body fluids, such as cerebrospinal fluid or synovial fluid, which do not lend themselves to electronic cell counts.

The basic principle of electronic cell counts will be described in general terms in this chapter. The manufacturers of electronic cell counting devices supply the purchaser with details of the use and care of the instruments. When a new instrument is used, the manufacturer's instructions must be followed explicitly.

## The Unopette System for Cell Counts

The standard Unopette system consists of a self-filling glass pipette available in various sizes depending on the procedure to be performed. Each pipette is color coded and marked with its measuring capacity. The end opposite the pipette tip is termed the overflow chamber (see Fig. 12-5). The shield over the pipette tip protects the pipette and is also designed to puncture the diaphragm of the reservoir prior to use.

The reservoir is the other main component of the Unopette system. The reservoir contains a premeasured volume of diluent. The container is sealed with a covering of plastic, the diaphragm, located in the neck of the reservoir. It is this diaphragm that must be opened by puncture with the pipette shield prior to actual use.

The Unopette system is a self-filling, disposable system that has proved extremely useful when manual cell counts must be performed: manual cell counts for eosinophils, platelet counts in thrombocytopenic patients, and leukocyte counts in neutropenic patients.

Special Unopettes are available for platelet counts, leukocyte counts, hemoglobin measurement, erythrocyte counts, reticulocyte counts, eosinophil counts, and erythrocyte fragility tests. Unopette systems are available for various hematologic automated analyzers and for some chemistry determinations (blood lead and sodium and potassium determinations by flame photometry).[5] The use of these disposable, self-filling precalibrated glass capillary pipettes for measuring and diluting blood for cell counts has proved extremely helpful. The Unopette system was described previously under Hemoglobin. It consists of a special glass pipette attached to a holder, and a plastic reservoir containing diluent (see Fig. 12-5). The pipette fills automatically with blood, either capillary or venous, by means of capillary action, and the blood stops automatically when the pipette is filled. This avoids the errors inherent in drawing blood into Thoma pipettes.

## Clinical Significance of Cell Counts
### White Blood Cell Counts

The normal white cell count varies from 4.4 to $11.3 \times 10^9$/L. An increase in the white cell (leukocyte) count above the normal upper limit is termed **leukocytosis**. A decrease below the normal lower limit is termed **leukopenia.**

*Leukopenia* may occur with certain viral infections, with typhoid fever and malaria, after radiation therapy, after the administration of certain drugs, and in pernicious anemia.

*Leukocytosis* may occur in many acute infections, especially bacterial infections, in severe malaria, after hemorrhage, during pregnancy, postoperatively, in some forms of anemia, in some carcinomas, and in leukemia.

Leukemia is characterized by uncontrolled proliferation of one or more of the various hematopoietic cells and is associated with many changes in the circulating cells of the blood. Blood films prepared from leukemia patients should be examined only by a qualified person—a pathologist or an experienced clinical laboratory scientist. There are two main classifications of leukemia, lymphocytic and myelocytic, according to the predominant type of leukocyte seen. Leukemias are further divided into the subclassifications acute and chronic. In the acute condition, the disease progresses rapidly and morphologic changes are marked. In the chronic condition, the changes are neither as rapid nor as marked.

The normal white count varies with age. The white cell count of a newborn baby is 10 to 30 × $10^9$/L at birth and drops to about $10 \times 10^9$/L after the first week of life. By about age 4 years, the white cell count reaches the normal level.

As mentioned earlier, the white count is used to indicate the presence of infection and to follow the progress of certain diseases. It may be elevated in acute bacterial infections, appendicitis, pregnancy, hemolytic disease of the newborn, uremia, and ulcers, and may be decreased in hepatitis, rheumatoid arthritis, cirrhosis of the liver, and lupus erythematosus. A child's leukocyte count usually shows a much greater variation during disease than an adult's. An individual's leukocyte count is subject to some variation during the course of a normal day, being slightly higher in the afternoon than in the morning. There is also an increase in the leukocyte count after strenuous exercise, emotional stress, and anxiety.

### Red Blood Cell Counts

**Anemia** is a term generally applied to a decrease in the number of erythrocytes. There are many types of anemias. Anemia can be caused by excessive blood loss or blood destruction (called hemolytic anemia). Anemias caused by decreased blood cell or hemoglobin formation include pernicious anemia, bone marrow failure anemia, and iron deficiency anemia. **Polycythemia** is a condition in which the number of erythrocytes is increased.

## Manual White Blood Cell (Leukocyte) Counts
### Diluent

Because blood cells are so numerous, they cannot be counted accurately without dilution. For white cell counts the diluent must destroy the more numerous red cells so that the white cells may be counted more readily. The diluent used most commonly for white cell counts is 2 mL/dL acetic acid, which (1) darkens the nuclei of the white cells so that they are easier to see and (2) hemolyzes the red cells.

### Measuring Device for White Cell Counts

**Unopette System.** A 25-μL capillary Unopette pipette is used for white cell counts. It is inserted into the reservoir containing 0.475 mL of 3 mL/dL acetic acid, resulting in a 1:20 dilution of WBCs (0.025 mL to a total of 0.500 mL). The pipette is carefully emptied and rinsed, and the resulting solution in the reservoir is mixed well. The Unopette pipette and reservoir system is easily converted to a dropper assembly for charging the counting chamber. The manufacturer's directions must be followed carefully.

**Thoma Pipettes.** Thoma pipettes require aspirating tubes and suction. They are shown in Fig. 12-8. Because of the importance of standard precautionary techniques and the employment of barrier protective devices, the use of the Thoma pipettes has virtually been replaced by automated analyzers, or the Unopette if manual counting must be done.

**20-μL Pipette.** A 20-μL pipette may be used to prepare a 1:20 dilution of blood. Exactly 0.4

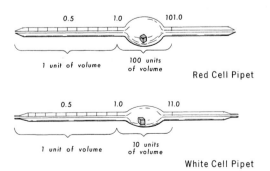

**FIG 12-8.** Thoma diluting pipettes. Red cell (*above*) and white cell (*below*).

mL of diluting fluid (such as 2% acetic acid) is placed in a 10 × 75 mm test tube. Exactly 0.02 mL (20 μL) of diluting fluid is removed from the tube so that 0.38 mL remains. Exactly 0.02 mL of well-mixed whole blood is added to the tube, resulting in a 1:20 dilution (0.02 mL to a total of 0.40 mL).

### Counting Chamber for White Cell Counts

After proper handling of the blood sample and careful dilution by a known amount to obtain a less concentrated solution, the number of cells in a known volume of the diluted sample is determined by counting the number of cells in a special counting chamber. The counting chamber is often called a hemocytometer. Technically, however, a hemocytometer consists of a counting chamber, a special coverglass for the counting chamber, and the diluting pipettes. In this section the terms *counting chamber* and *hemocytometer* are used interchangeably. For a routine count by a manual method, the counting chamber used most often is the Levy-Hausser hemocytometer with Neubauer ruling.

To understand how a counting chamber gives the blood cell count in terms of volume when the chamber is a flat surface, we start with a cube and work backward. Picture a cube 1 mm on each side. The counting chamber allows the cube to be divided into equal units that are 0.1 mm in depth. When the counting chamber is viewed from the side, one can see that when the coverglass is placed on the chamber, it rests on supports (Fig. 12-9). The space between the bottom of the coverglass and the surface of the counting chamber is 0.1 mm. Essentially, the chamber provides a series of "slices" of the cube that are 1 mm² in area and 0.1 mm in depth. The only way to be sure that the depth is 0.1 mm is to use plane-ground coverglasses that have a constant weight and an even surface. The 0.1-mm slices are arranged so that one may count the cells in one of the slices or in portions of one slice by varying the area of the ruled surface of the chamber.

Each counting chamber has two precision-ruled counting areas 3 mm wide and 3 mm long, or 9 square millimeters. One such counting chamber is shown in Fig. 12-10. All hemocytometers used in the hematology laboratory must meet the specifications of the National Bureau of Standards.

When the ruled area of the counting chamber is viewed for the first time under the microscope, it may be difficult to see the nine basic 1-mm squares because each one has been ruled into smaller areas. The 1-mm² sections in the four corners are ruled into 16 equal portions (Figs. 12-10 and 12-11). The square in the center of the ruled area is divided into 25 equal portions (see Fig. 12-11). In turn, each of the $\frac{1}{25}$ mm squares is divided into 16 parts, providing $\frac{1}{400}$ mm squares (see Fig. 12-11). With the surface of the counting chamber ruled in this manner, it is possible to measure aliquots of the diluted

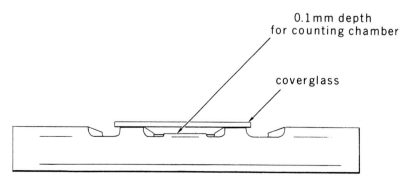

**FIG 12-9.** Counting chamber—side view.

blood sample that are contained in 1-mm, $\frac{1}{16}$ mm, $\frac{1}{25}$ mm, $\frac{1}{80}$ mm, and $\frac{1}{400}$ mm squares, all of which are 0.1 mm in depth. The area to be counted will depend on the type of cell count to be done.

Other types of counting chambers can also be used to count blood cells. Some of these are the Spencer Brightline with Neubauer ruling and the Levy chamber with Fuchs-Rosenthal ruling.

### Mixing and Mounting Samples in the Counting Chamber

The diluted blood must be mixed before the mixture is placed on the counting chamber. It is important that the hemocytometer and its coverglass be carefully cleaned with alcohol and dried before anything is mounted on it. After cleaning, the coverglass must be centered over the ruled areas of the counting chamber, with

care being taken to touch only the edges of the coverglass.

### Using the Unopette System for White Cell Counts

For the Unopette system, the equipment for the initial blood measurement and dilution can be converted to a dropper assembly. In this way, the blood-diluent mixture can be easily mounted on the counting chamber. For doing a white cell count, after the blood has been diluted, a period of about 10 minutes is needed for the red cells to lyse. Diluted samples are stable for 3 hours. The sample must be mixed well just prior to mounting on the counting chamber by means of the easily converted dropper assembly capability incorporated into the Unopette system.

While the pipette is held at an angle of about 40 degrees, the chamber between the ruled area

( 9 square millimeters )

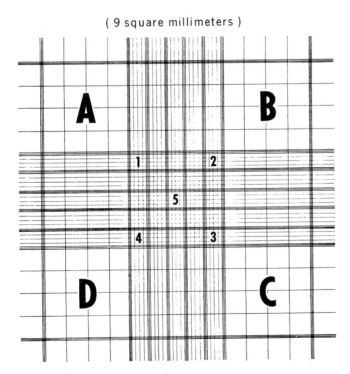

White blood cells are counted in areas A, B, C, and D (4 sq. mm.)

Red blood cells are counted in areas 1, 2, 3, 4, and 5

(80/400 sq. mm.)

**FIG 12-10.** Improved Neubauer ruling for one counting chamber area.

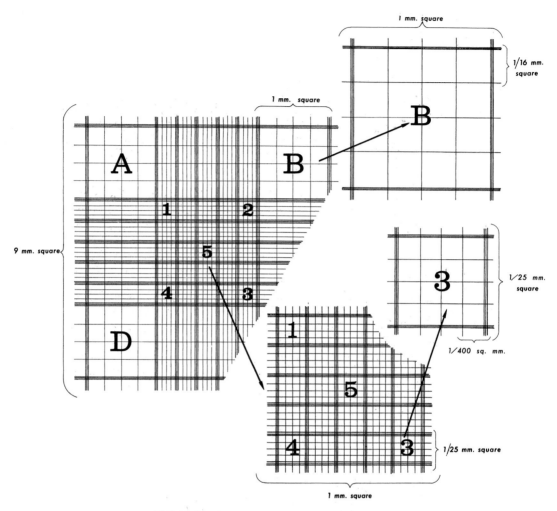

**FIG 12-11.** Counting areas of the hemocytometer.

and the coverglass is filled with a single drop, which should be drawn rapidly into the chamber by capillary action. The pipette is placed at the edge of the coverglass, and the reservoir is gently squeezed so the diluted blood flows evenly under the coverglass. Do not move the coverglass. Both sides of the hemocytometer must be filled. If the fluid spills into the dividing moats or is otherwise distributed unevenly, mounting must be repeated. Only one drop can be used to fill the chamber. It should not be filled partially with a small drop and filled completely with a second drop; this would result in uneven distribution of the cells.

Adequately mixing the diluted blood in the Unopette reservoir, discarding three to four drops, and properly filling the counting chamber are important factors in obtaining a good distribution of cells in the counting areas and in obtaining accurate cell counts.

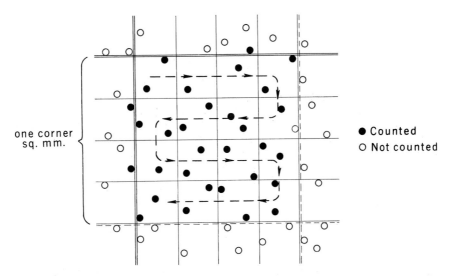

**FIG 12-12.** Examples of white blood cells counted in a representative area.

### Performing and Calculating White Cell Counts

Before any counting is done, the microscope must be properly adjusted (review Chapter 5). It is necessary to know how to adjust the microscope for proper illumination, and how to focus correctly (avoiding damage to the objectives and the object to be viewed).

The filled counting chambers should be allowed to sit for at least 1 minute before any counting is begun. Place the filled counting chamber on the stage of the microscope and fasten securely. Place one of the ruled counting areas of the chamber in position over the condenser. Using the low-power (10×) objective, turn the coarse adjustment knob until the objective is at its lowest position, which is about 0.25 inch above the coverglass. Adjust the light, so that the field is evenly illuminated and comfortable to view, by moving the condenser down slightly and then closing the iris diaphragm and adjusting the light intensity. Turn the coarse adjustment knob slowly until the ruled area comes into focus, and use the fine adjustment knob to bring the area into perfect focus. Use the iris diaphragm to adjust the light. If this technique is used, there is little danger of damaging the coverglass with the objective. If the objective touches the coverglass, the cell distribution is altered and a new mounting must be made. After the ruled area is in focus, scan it quickly to identify the various ruled portions. Approximately one square millimeter can be seen in each field with the low-power (10×) objective.

When the counting chamber is properly in place on the microscope and the various ruled areas are identified and understood, cell counting can begin.

White blood cells are counted under low magnification (10× objective) in the four corner 1-mm squares of the ruled area of the counting chamber. Each 1-mm square is divided into 16 equal parts. Cells touching the lines on the left side or on the top of the squares are included in the count, but cells touching the lines on the right side or on the bottom of the squares are not counted (Fig. 12-12). In this way, every cell is assigned to a square and cells are not counted twice or omitted from the count.

The counts obtained in the 1-mm² sections in the four corners are tabulated separately. These values should not differ by more than 10 cells. Tallying the squares separately provides a check of the distribution of the cells and indicates whether mixing and mounting were adequate. When the values do not agree within 10 cells, another pipette must be used, because remounts from the previously used pipette usually result in progressively higher counts.

In calculating the total count per unit volume of blood, four important facts must be considered:

1. The total number of cells counted in the four 1-mm squares
2. The dilution of the blood sample
3. The area counted
4. The depth of the counting chamber

These four factors are used in the following general formula:

Cells counted in 1-mm² areas × Dilution of blood
× Area counted × Depth of chamber =
White cells per microliter of whole blood (or cells per mm³)
Cells per microliter ($\mu$L) × $10^6$ = Cells × $10^9$/L

The dilution factor for the blood is 1:20, since with the Unopette system 25 $\mu$L of blood is diluted in 0.475 mL of 3 mL/dL acetic acid (giving 0.025 mL blood in a total of 0.500 mL of blood and diluent). This means that to obtain the white cell count for a unit of undiluted blood, the calculation must be multiplied by 20, the dilution factor.

The area and depth can be considered together as the volume factor, since the volume of any solution is the product of its area times its depth. For the routine white cell count, four 1-mm² corners are counted. The depth of the counting area is 0.1 mm. Therefore the volume of the area counted is 0.4 mm³ or 0.4 $\mu$L:

$$4 \text{ mm}^2 \times 0.1 \text{ mm} = 0.4 \ \mu L$$

To obtain the number of white blood cells in 1 $\mu$L of blood, the number of cells counted in 0.4 $\mu$L is multiplied by 1/0.4 or 2.5, the volume factor.

For example, the sum of the cells counted in the four 1-mm² corner areas is 33 + 32 + 40 + 35 = 140. In this case, the calculation would be 140/1 × 20/1 × 1/4 × 1/0.1 = 7,000/$\mu$L. If the square areas and the depth are considered as volume, the general formula is:

$$\frac{\text{Cells counted in 4 squares} \times \text{Dilution of blood}}{\text{Volume}} =$$

White cells/$\mu$L

where volume = area × depth.

The count when a total of 140 cells are counted in the four squares would be calculated as:

$$\frac{140 \times 20}{4 \times 0.1} = 7,000/\mu L \text{ or } 7 \times 10^3/\mu L$$

Because the current units of choice for reporting are cells counted per liter of blood, the WBCs per microliter are multiplied by $10^6$. White cell counts are reported to the nearest 100 cells. Using the example from above, a count of 7,000/$\mu$L is the same as $7 \times 10^3/\mu$L. To report this in cells per liter:

$$7 \times 10^3/\mu L \times 10^6 = 7 \times 10^9/L$$

For each white cell count completed in the routine manner, the dilution of the blood and the volume of diluted blood used for counting remain constant. Therefore, the total cells counted may be multiplied by a constant factor to find the final result. Leaving out the number of cells in the last equation, 20/(4 × 0.1) = 50. Any total number of cells counted in 4 square mm can be converted to the number of white cells per microliter of blood by multiplying by 50. Thus, 50 is the constant factor for counting white cells in the routine manner by the manual method presented.

White cells should be counted in duplicate until accuracy is attained, after which duplicate determinations may be done when appropriate (for low counts or counts of grave clinical importance).

The allowable difference between duplicate pipettes for the same blood sample is $500/\mu L$ for counts within the normal range (4.4 to 11 $\times$ $10^3/\mu L$ or 4.4 to 11 $\times$ $10^9/L$) and 10% of the lowest count when the total count is above or below the normal range. The resulting white cell count is rounded off to the nearest 100 cells, as results are reported to the first decimal place. For example, a white cell count calculated as 8,050 would be reported as $8,100/\mu L$ or 8.1 $\times$ $10^9/L$ and a count calculated as 7,950 would be reported as $8,000/\mu L$ or 8.0 $\times$ $10^9/L$. The general rule for rounding off numbers to the next significant figure is used.

### Precautions and Technical Factors for Manual Cell Counts

Errors in counting blood cells manually are related to the extremely small size of the sample, the nature of the sample, faulty laboratory equipment, faulty technique, and the inherent error of cell distribution in the counting chamber.

The minute size of the blood sample is illustrated by the fact that a variation of even 1 cell in the red cell count changes the final result by 10,000 cells, or 50 cells with the white blood cell count.

Venous blood must be free of clots and mixed well immediately before it is diluted. Peripheral blood or capillary blood must be obtained freely flowing from a puncture and must be diluted rapidly to prevent coagulation.

Thoma pipettes, if used, must be checked against National Bureau of Standards pipettes. Pipettes must be clean and dry and without chipped tips.

The counting chamber must be clean and dry. The usual practice is to clean the chamber and coverglass immediately before each use by flooding them with medicated alcohol and wiping them dry with a piece of gauze. Dirt on the chamber can alter the count.

The blood sample must be measured precisely and diluted properly. The counting chamber must be charged with only one drop of the diluted sample; an excess could raise the coverglass and thus change the depth factor.

Even with excellent technique and equipment, the probable error in manual red cell counts can be 20%, because of the chance error in the distribution of the cells in the counting chamber. The same distribution factor can also affect the WBC count, and the error in this count can be 15%.

In certain conditions, such as leukemia, the WBC count may be extremely high. If it is more than 30 $\times$ $10^9/L$, a greater dilution of the blood, such as 1:100, should be used. When the white cell count drops below 3 $\times$ $10^9/L$, a smaller dilution of blood, such as 1:10, should be used to achieve a more accurate count. The white cell count is determined as usual, using the change in blood dilution in the calculations. Other dilutions may be employed when necessary, and are taken into account when the final calculations are made.

The diluting fluid used for the WBC count destroys or hemolyzes all nonnucleated red cells. In certain disease conditions, nucleated RBCs may be present in the peripheral blood. These cells cannot be distinguished from the white cells and are counted as white cells in the counting chamber. Therefore, whenever there are 5 or more nucleated red cells per 100 white cells in a differential done on a stained blood film, the white cell count must be corrected as follows:

$$\frac{\text{Uncorrected WBC count} \times 100}{100 + \text{Number of nucleated RBCs per 100 WBCs}} = \text{Corrected WBC count}$$

The WBC count is then reported as the corrected count.

Use of electronic cell counters does not relieve the laboratory worker of the responsibility for being constantly alert for sources of error. Unless equipment is properly calibrated and fundamental aspects such as the quality of the sample are considered carefully, electronic counters are merely tools for producing inadequate results faster.

## Platelet Counts

Platelets, or thrombocytes, function in the coagulation of the blood and are therefore associated with the bleeding and clotting, or hemostatic, mechanism of the body. Platelets are formed in the bone marrow from megakaryocytes. They are difficult to count accurately for several reasons: they are small and difficult to discern, they have an adhesive character and become attached readily to glassware or to particles of debris in the diluting fluid, and they clump easily and are probably not evenly distributed in the blood in the first place. Platelets disintegrate easily and are difficult to distinguish from debris. Because of their sticky nature, they also tend to adhere to other platelets in clumps. By using EDTA as an anticoagulant, the clumping tendency of platelets can be decreased.

### Clinical Significance of the Platelet Count

The normal number of platelets, depending in part on the method employed for their enumeration, ranges from 172 to 450 $\times$ 10$^9$/L whole blood. A count lower than normal may be associated with a generalized bleeding tendency and a prolonged bleeding time. A count higher than normal may be associated with a tendency toward thrombosis.

There are several diseases in which a high or low platelet count can result.

*Thrombocytopenia*, or a decrease in platelets, is found in thrombocytopenic purpura, in some infectious diseases, in some acute leukemias, in some anemias (aplastic and pernicious), and when the patient is undergoing radiation treatment or chemotherapy.

*Thrombocytosis*, or an increase in platelets, can be found in rheumatic fever, asphyxiation, following surgical treatment, following splenectomy, with acute blood loss, and with some types of chemotherapy used in the treatment of leukemia.

### Specimens

Capillary blood from a finger puncture can be used, but venous blood generally gives more satisfactory results. Platelet counts on capillary blood are generally lower than those on venous blood because of immediate platelet clumping at the puncture site. EDTA is the anticoagulant of choice for platelet counts, as it lessens the tendency for platelet clumping.

### Methods Used to Count Platelets

With good technique and experience, platelets can be manually counted accurately. One basic manual method, the Brecher-Cronkite method, utilizes phase-contrast microscopy.[1] The Brecher-Cronkite method uses a blood diluent, 1 g/dL ammonium oxalate, that completely hemolyzes the red cells. A Unopette system is also available for platelet counts, which uses the same diluent.

The diluent used for counting platelets must meet certain requirements. It must (1) provide fixation to reduce the adhesiveness of the platelets, (2) prevent coagulation, (3) prevent hemolysis (unless the method chosen eliminates the RBCs), and (4) provide a low specific gravity so that the platelets will settle in one plane. A diluent that meets all these requirements is Rees-Ecker solution. Rees-Ecker solution contains sodium citrate, which prevents coagulation, preserves the RBCs, and provides the necessary low specific gravity; formalin, which is a fixative; and brilliant cresyl blue, which is a dye used for the identification of the diluent. This dye does not stain the platelets, and it is not essential for the counting procedure. All diluents used, including Rees-Ecker, must be stored in the refrigerator and filtered before each use.

After adequate dilution, the platelets are counted, generally with a phase hemocytometer and a phase-contrast microscope, to enhance refractiveness of the platelets. An ordinary light microscope may be used to count the platelets, but the differentiation is not as sharp. Manual methods are time consuming, cause eyestrain, and are not recommended for large-volume work. A manual platelet count is always done by using duplicate pipettes. They have generally been replaced by automated techniques.

Some laboratories have discontinued manual platelet counts altogether because the error involved can be very large and a well-prepared blood smear can be used to estimate platelets.

The Unopette system for platelets utilizes a self-measuring dilution system and enumeration of platelets by means of a phase hemocytometer and phase microscopy.

Manual methods are time-consuming and must be verified by performing a platelet estimate on a blood film.

Automated methods for counting platelets have made platelet counts somewhat routine. With impedance methods (Coulter principle), as platelets and red cells pass through the apertures, particles that are between 2 and 20 fL are counted as platelets. A platelet graph is also plotted according to the size distribution of the platelets counted. Questionable results may be verified by an estimate of the platelet count from an examination of the stained blood film.

### Manual Platelet Counts: Using the Unopette System

A Unopette diluting system is available for counting platelets. The platelet Unopette capillary pipette measures 20 $\mu$L of blood, which is diluted in a Unopette reservoir containing 1.98 mL of 1 g/dL ammonium oxalate. This hemolyzes the red cells, leaving white cells and platelets intact. By means of the method described for manual white cell counts using the Unopette system, the diluted sample is mounted on a hemocytometer after a 10-minute waiting period for complete red cell lysis to

take place. The diluted specimen for platelet counts is mounted on both sides of two hemocytometers.

A phase hemocytometer is used, preferably, to enhance platelet refractiveness for an easier microscopic enumeration. After mounting of the dilution on the phase hemocytometer, the unit should be placed in a high-humidity chamber for at least 15 minutes so the platelets come to rest in the same focal plane. If a phase hemocytometer is not available, the dilution is mounted on a Spencer Brightline hemocytometer and the platelets are counted by using a brightfield microscope, with the platelets being allowed to settle to one focal plane as for the phase hemocytometer.

### Counting Platelets in the Counting Chamber

Place the chamber under the microscope, and locate the center ruled area by using the low-power (10×) objective. Carefully change to the high-power (40×) objective, and adjust the light for maximum contrast.

With the use of phase microscopy, platelets should appear as shiny structures with a halo-like area of light around them. Focus up and down on the platelets. Fine projections can be seen on the platelet edges with the phase microscope.

With brightfield microscopy, the platelets appear as small, round, refractile bodies. Platelets are counted in the center square millimeter of each of the four mounted counting areas, using the high-power (40×) objective. (See Fig. 12-11.) The cell counts on the four center squares must agree within $25 \times 10^9$/L for duplicate mounts and within $40 \times 10^9$/L for duplicate pipettes. When the platelet count is below $200 \times 10^9$/L, replicate counts should agree within $30 \times 10^9$/L. When the platelet count is above $200 \times 10^9$/L, replicate counts should agree within $50 \times 10^9$/L. Manual platelet counts should be done by mounting duplicate Unopettes on both sides of a chamber and averaging the replicates, if they are within the acceptable range. Platelet counts are reported to the nearest 1,000/$\mu$L.

### Calculations for Manual Platelet Count

The number of platelets per liter of whole blood must be calculated. The important factors are:

1. The average number of platelets counted in 1 mm$^2$
2. The dilution of the blood (1:100 using the Unopette system)
3. The volume of diluted blood counted, which is equal to the depth of the chamber (0.1 mm) times the area in which the cells are counted (1 mm$^2$), or 0.1 $\mu$L

The following general formula applies:

$$\frac{\text{Average no. of platelets in 4 squares} \times 1 \text{ mm}^2 \times 100}{0.1 \text{ mm}}$$
$$\times 10^6 = \text{Platelets} \times 10^9/\text{L}$$

In this case, a constant factor of 1,000 can be used.

### Precautions and Technical Factors

Many of the precautions described for manually counting erythrocytes and leukocytes also apply to platelet counts. In platelet counts, however, it is imperative that peripheral blood be freely flowing when obtained from a finger puncture. Pipettes and counting chambers must be clean and free from lint, since platelets may be confused with dirt and debris. Rapid dilution of the blood is essential, or the platelets may form clumps and the blood may clot. If clumps of platelets are noted during the platelet count, the procedure should be repeated. Clumping may result from inadequate mixing of the blood with the diluent or from poor technique in obtaining the blood sample.

To minimize the error for manual platelet counts, duplicates are always prepared and duplicate counts done on both sides of two counting chambers. Duplicate counts of a sample should agree within 10% to be acceptable.

Constant focusing of the microscope is necessary to identify the platelets among the larger, more numerous other cells still present (such as WBCs). A blood film is made, stained, and viewed microscopically to check each platelet count.

If a platelet count is requested in combination with other counts for the same patient and one wishes to utilize the same finger puncture, it is necessary to take the blood for the platelet count first before performing the remaining counts. The finger must not be squeezed excessively when the blood is drawn into the pipette.

## Automated Cell Counting Methods

A wide range of automated and semiautomated devices are available for measuring different hematologic parameters. The most useful instruments are those for counting cells. Automated cell counters count larger numbers of cells than manual counting methods and thus allow much greater precision. Thousands of particles pass through the instrument's aperture in a few seconds. The coefficient of variation (CV), or allowable error, in a manual cell counting method varies from 8% to 15%, depending on the type of cell counted. Automated counting methods have been reported as having a CV of 1% to 3%.

Two general methods are used by automated cell counters for hematology: optical methods using focused laser beams and impedance methods utilizing the **Coulter principle.** Impedance counting, or voltage pulse counting, was developed by Coulter in the late 1950s, and because it has been used so extensively, it is referred to as the *Coulter principle.*

A third screening method, which uses centrifugation and electro-optical measurement of cell layers, will also be described.

### Cell Counters Using the Voltage Pulse Counting Principle (Coulter Counters)

In the basic Coulter counter, cells passing through an aperture through which a current is flowing cause changes in electrical resistance

---

*Coulter Diagnostics, Hialeah, Fla.

that are counted as voltage pulses (Fig. 12-13). A reduced pressure system operated by a vacuum unit draws the suspension through the aperture into a system of tubing following a column of mercury. The Coulter counter system is based on the principle that cells are poor electrical conductors, compared with saline or Isoton,* which are good conductors.

The instrument system has a glass aperture tube that can be filled with the conducting fluid (the suspension of diluted cells, for example) and has an electrode (the internal electrode) and an aperture or small orifice that is 100 μm in diameter. Just outside the glass aperture tube is another electrode (the external electrode). The aperture tube is connected to a U-shaped glass tube that is partly filled with mercury and has two electrical contacts—an activating counter and a deactivating counter. The aperture tube is immersed in the cell suspension, filled with conductive solution, and closed by a stopcock valve. A current now flows through the aperture between the internal and external electrodes. As the vacuum unit draws the mercury up the tube, the cell suspension flows through the aperture into the aperture tube.

Each cell that passes through the aperture displaces an equal volume of conductive solution, increasing the electrical resistance and creating a voltage pulse, because its resistance is much greater than that of the conductive solution. The pulses, which are proportional in height to the volume of cells, are counted. The section of tubing between the activating and deactivating counters is calibrated to contain 0.5 mL (see Fig. 12-13). The counting mechanism is started when the mercury reaches the activating counter and is stopped when it reaches the deactivating counter. During this time the cells are counted in a volume of suspension exactly equal to the volume of glass tubing between the two contact wires in the activating and deactivating electrodes.

If two or more cells enter the aperture at the same time, they will be counted as one cell.

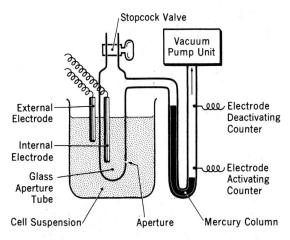

**FIG 12-13.** Schematic diagram of a cell counter based on voltage pulse counting (Coulter principle). Cells flow through an aperture that separates two compartments. The electrical potential between electrodes changes as the cells pass. The number of impulses translates to the cell count, and the amplitude of the pulse depends on the cell volume that displaces the conductive fluid.

This produces a coincidence error for which a correction must be made. The size of the coincidence error may be decreased by decreasing the concentration of the cells and the size of the aperture. However, decreasing the concentration of the cells increases the dilution error and the inherent counting error and makes the error resulting from background "noise" from contaminating particles more critical. When the aperture is decreased, it may become partially or completely plugged with debris. For this reason a compromise is made, and for a count above a certain critical number, a coincidence correction is made by referring to a chart supplied by the manufacturer of the counting instrument.

Variations of the current measured across the aperture make it possible to determine the particle or cell count, cell volume, and particle size. All the cells in 0.5 mL of suspension are counted, and the results are displayed. This pulse or count is amplified, numerically registered by the counter, and visualized on an oscilloscope.

*Coulter Diagnostics, Hialeah, Fla.

**Coulter Counter, Model S.** The Model S Coulter counter uses the voltage pulse counting principle described for general basic models of Coulter counters. It provides seven hematologic parameters: white cell count, red cell count, hemoglobin, hematocrit, MCV, MCH, and MCHC. Hemoglobin is determined photometrically by passing a light beam through the mixture in the white cell aperture bath. The light absorbed by the solution at a specific wavelength is proportional to the hemoglobin concentration and is measured by a photosensitive device. The principle is the same as that of the hemiglobin-cyanide (cyanmethemoglobin) method (see under Hemoglobin).

This instrument has a totally automated diluting system, which aspirates and pipettes approximately 1 mL of whole blood and carries it through the blood sampling valve, where it is diluted. Part of the sample is diluted with Isoton, an isotonic solution that preserves the size and shape of the cells when white and red blood cells are being counted. A lysing reagent is added, causing complete lysis of red cells, and a hemoglobin reference reading is made.

For cell counts, a specific amount of diluted blood is passed through the orifice of the glass aperture tube. Each time a cell passes through this orifice, a change in the current flowing between the external and internal apertures is observed (see Fig. 12-13). This change in current produces a voltage pulse, the magnitude of which is proportional to the size of the cell causing the change. Three WBC counts are done simultaneously, with an average of the three counts being taken and recorded.

Hemoglobin is measured by using the diluted sample used for the white cell count. The amount of light passing through the solution is measured with a photosensitive device, and this reading is converted into a hemoglobin value.

A separate solution diluted for counting RBCs is passed through the orifice of the aperture tube in a manner similar to that for counting WBCs. The changes in current produced by the number of red cells passing through the orifice are recorded in a manner similar to that for white cells. In addition, the red cell MCV is electronically derived and recorded.

The hematocrit is calculated from the values for RBCs counted and the derived MCV. The MCH and the MCHC are also calculated.

**Coulter Counter, Model S Plus.** Another Coulter counter is the model S Plus, which is more computerized and more compact and has a less complicated pneumatic system. In addition to the seven parameters reported by the model S, the S Plus also performs a platelet count and tests the degree of anisocytosis by determining the RDW. This represents the coefficient of variation of the red cell size distribution or shows the degree of variation of the MCV from the mean. The RDW is determined and calculated by using the MCV and the red cell count.

**Coulter Counter, Model STKS.** This instrument includes the features of the Coulter Counter model S Plus and has a five-part leukocyte differential capability.

### Flow Cytometry: Use of a Focused Laser Beam

Cells or particles passing through a focused beam of a laser can be used for counting blood cells. The blood is diluted in isotonic saline and passed through the laser beam as a stream of single cells. The principle of hydrodynamic focusing allows the focusing of the blood cells with a second fluid, forming an outer sheath of liquid moving in the same direction. The instrument accomplishing this task is known as a **flow cytometer.**

Light is scattered at angles proportional to the structural features of a cell as it passes through the light beam (Fig. 12-14). Most laser systems utilize light sensors that detect forward scatter of the beam (180 degrees from the light source) and right-angle (90-degree) scatter.

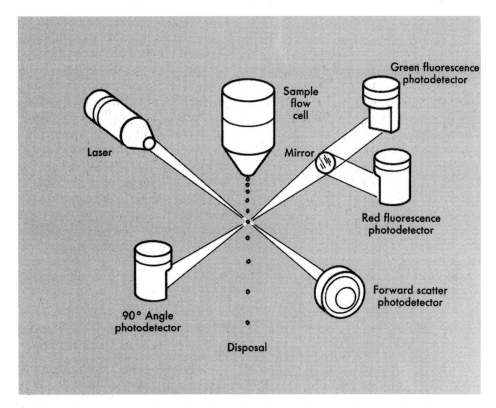

**FIG 12-14.** Flow cytometry: optical detection of cells by a laser-based system. Cells are focused by the laminar flow of a sheath fluid. Cells are counted and partly identified by differential light scatter of a laser beam. (From Powers LW: *Diagnostic Hematology.* St Louis, Mosby, 1989, p 452.)

Forward scatter is correlated with cell volume or density, analogous to the impedance counting of the Coulter principle instruments. Right-angle deflection is dependent on cellular contents, mainly the granularity of the cell cytoplasm. Photodetectors convert the light signals to electrical impulses, which are processed by a computer. The display of data includes cell counts and MCV, but the flow cytometer also can produce simple cell differential counts (granulocytes as compared with nongranulocytes).

A fluorochrome dye can be employed in the cell suspension to enhance the cell identification. This dye can directly stain or tag certain cell components, such as a granule or an enzyme.

The dye can be attached to an immunologic component, such as an antibody to a lymphocyte surface antigen. Different wavelengths of light excite different types of fluorochrome dyes, enabling particular tagged cells to be counted separately. Differential leukocyte counts or reticulocyte counts are done by using two or more laser detection systems in sequence.

For specialized testing, the flow cytometry principle is used to separate cells. Positive or negative electrical charges are applied by a charging collar to the labeled cell as it passes through the laser beam (Fig. 12-15). The charged cell is sorted into a unique stream, providing a sample of specific cells that can be identified by specific cell markers.

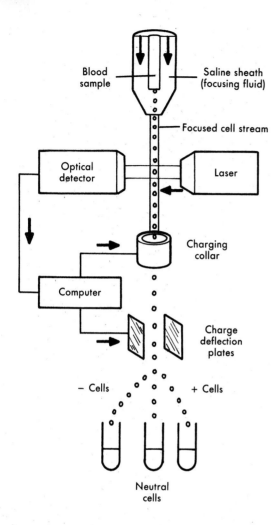

**FIG 12-15.** Flow cytometry: sorting cells. A laser detection system is combined with a computer and a charging collar. Cells of a particular identity (carrying fluorescent tags that react to the laser) are charged and deflected to a collection container. (From Powers LW: *Diagnostic Hematology*. St Louis, Mosby, 1989, p 453.)

### Centrifugation and Electro-optical Measurement of Cell Layers

The QBC II Plus System* is a screening system that utilizes centrifugation and different cell den-

---

*Becton Dickinson & Co, Primary Care Diagnostics, Franklin Lakes, NJ.

sities to assay hemoglobin, hematocrit, platelet count, and white blood cell count, including granulocyte count (percent and number) and lymphocyte/monocyte count (percent and number).

The platelet count, white blood cell count, and counts of granulocyte and mononuclear cell subpopulations are estimates derived from electro-optical measurements of the packed cell volumes in a specially designed QBC blood tube. The system cannot discriminate between normal and abnormal cell types. The hematocrit (or PCV) is measured and the hemoglobin calculated from the hematocrit, along with measurements of cell density by determination of float depth.

The system is based on measurements of the buffy coat, which consists of packed leukocytes and platelets. The platelets are less dense and settle in a separate layer above the leukocytes (see Fig. 12-16). Further subdivision of layering occurs between two subpopulations of leukocytes by virtue of the different specific gravities. The upper layer contains predominantly lymphocytes and monocytes, the lower layer predominantly granulocytes (neutrophils, eosinophils, and basophils), as shown in Fig. 12-16.

The system uses mechanical expansion and optical magnification augmented by supravital staining to derive the platelet count, white cell count, and two white cell subgroups from linear measurements of the packed cell layers in the buffy coat. A hematocrit or PCV is also obtained.

The buffy coat is expanded by use of a precision-molded cylindrical float as part of the test system. This is inserted into a precision bore QBC blood tube before centrifugation. The specific gravity of the float is approximately midway between that of the plasma and that of the red cells, causing part of the float to settle in the buffy coat. Expanded layers of packed white cells and platelets are thereby formed in the annulus between the float and the inner wall of the blood tube.

Under centrifugal force, the float settles into the buffy coat, where it axially expands the formed cell layer by a factor of 10. Part of the float also descends into the red cells (to a vari-

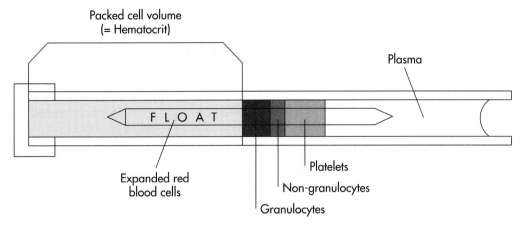

**FIG 12-16.** Centrifugation and electro-optical measurement of cell layers. Blood is shown in a special analyzer centrifuge tube containing a solid plastic float that expands the cell layers so that they can be measured with a special viewer to give the appropriate cell counts.

able depth), similarly expanding the upper portion of the packed erythrocyte column and creating a clearly visible light band of red cells surrounding the bottom portion of the float.

The depth that the float sinks in the packed red blood cells when the tube is centrifuged is a function of red cell density. Since cell density is primarily a function of hemoglobin concentration, the hemoglobin is calculated from measurements of the float depth and the hematocrit.

To separate white cell types, the QBC tube is internally coated with Acridine Orange (AO), a supravital fluorochrome. When excited by blue-violet light, the cells fluoresce differently. The granulocyte cells fluoresce orange-yellow, while lymphocytes and monocytes fluoresce a brilliant green and platelets a pale yellow. Erythrocytes are unaffected by AO and appear their normal dark red.

### Quality Control

All automated methods require the use of quality assurance measures, including the use of quality control solutions to ensure that the instrument is functioning correctly and that valid results are reported.

### Reference Values*

*For red blood cell count* ($\times 10^{12}$/L):

| Men | Mean 5.2 (range 4.5-5.9) |
| Women | Mean 4.6 (range 4.1-5.1) |

*For white blood cell count* ($\times 10^{9}$/L):

| 12 mo | Mean 11.4 (range 6.0-17.5) |
| 10 yr | Mean 8.1 (range 4.5-13.5) |
| 21 yr | Mean 7.4 (range 4.5-11.0) |
| >21 yr | Mean 7.8 (range 4.4-11.3) |

*For platelet counts* ($\times 10^{9}$/L): mean 311 (range 172-450)

## EXAMINATION OF THE PERIPHERAL BLOOD FILM

Microscopic examination of the peripheral blood is most often done by preparing, staining, and examining a thin film (smear) of blood on a glass slide. A great deal of information can be

*Beutler E, Lichtman MA, Coller BS, Kipps TJ: *Williams Hematology,* ed 5. New York, McGraw-Hill, Inc., 1995, pp 9, 12.

obtained from the examination of a blood film (also called a blood smear). With the use of automatic counting devices that determine hemoglobin, hematocrit, red cell, white cell, and platelet counts together with MCV, MCH, MCHC, and RDW, white cell differential, and histograms, there is a tendency to place less emphasis on the routine examination of the peripheral blood film. This is a consideration in the utility and cost-effectiveness debate in our current medical care system. However, these same automated results may also point to the need to examine the blood film microscopically to confirm the presence of disease suggested by the results or for early detection of disease. Of course, in a laboratory without access to such automated information, the microscopic examination of the peripheral blood film is invaluable. Unfortunately, although it is very inexpensive in terms of capital investment, it is expensive in terms of labor or personnel, as this technique is highly labor intensive. The routine examination of the blood film—at least routine preparation of the blood film for possible examination and to confirm abnormal automated results—remains a question of protocol.

Traditionally, the microscopic examination of the peripheral blood film has been used to study the morphology (form and structure) of red cells, white cells, and platelets. The various types of white cells are classified, and the percentage of each is recorded; this is the leukocyte differential count. The blood film can also be used to verify the hemoglobin value, the hematocrit, and the red cell count. It is used to check or estimate the white cell, reticulocyte, and platelet counts and the red cell indices. As such, it is a quality assurance measure to evaluate results from automated devices. Because the blood film has so many uses, a well-made smear is essential. Generally, two good films are prepared. One of these films is stained, and the other is kept in reserve. The blood film is a permanent record of hematologic work that can be retained in the laboratory. It may occasionally be necessary to reexamine a blood film to check for errors or to evaluate changes in the clinical status of the patient.

## Sources of Blood for the Blood Film

Fresh blood from a finger, heel, or big toe puncture can be used for morphologic examination of the white and red cells. The finger must not be squeezed excessively to obtain the drop of blood, and it must not be touched with the glass slide. Only the drop of blood is touched to the glass slide, not the skin. If the slide touches the finger, oils or moisture from the finger will lead to a poorly prepared film.

Most of the work in the hematology laboratory is done on venous blood. EDTA is the anticoagulant of choice. EDTA preserves the morphologic features of the white and red cells and gives a more even distribution of the platelets. If blood is collected in EDTA for morphologic studies, the film should be prepared as soon as possible, certainly within 2 hours.

## Preparation of the Blood Film

Blood is most often examined under the microscope by preparing a thin film or smear of blood on a glass slide or a coverglass, fixing the blood film, and then staining it with a polychromatic stain (Fig. 12-17). Wet films of blood can also be prepared and observed with a phase-contrast microscope or by use of a supravital stain, but these techniques are rarely used in the examination of blood. Smears can also be prepared by centrifugation; centrifugal force is used to spread a monolayer of blood cells over the surface of a glass slide (see Fig. 12-17).

### Coverglass Blood Films

When a coverglass is used to prepare a blood film, more of the prepared film can be examined, which reduces the sampling error. With a glass slide only a relatively small counting area can be examined. In addition, the leukocytes and platelets are more evenly distributed on a coverglass. The disadvantages of the coverglass method are that it is more time consuming and more difficult to learn and perform correctly,

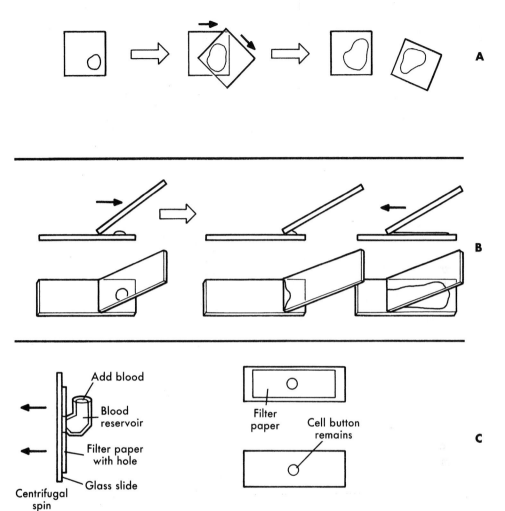

**FIG 12-17.** Preparation of blood smears. **A,** Coverglass preparation. A drop of blood or marrow is spread between two coverglasses as they are pulled in opposite directions. **B,** Wedge smear. A drop of blood is pulled across the slide by another slide at an acute angle, creating a wedge-shaped smear with decreasing cell density. **C,** Centrifugal smear. A drop of blood is spun from a central point, creating an evenly dispersed monolayer of cells. (From Powers LW: *Diagnostic Hematology.* St Louis, Mosby, 1989, p 445.)

and requires more care in handling of the preparations. Automatic staining devices are available for glass slides, but not for coverglasses.

### Wedge Blood Films

Although the coverglass method is recommended by many hematologists, the glass slide wedge method is far more commonly used. It is the method used by the NCCLS for the reference leukocyte differential count to evaluate any leukocyte differential count method.[8] The glass slide (push wedge) blood film method is described in detail in Procedure 12-5. The directions for the examination of the blood film

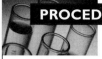

## PROCEDURE 12-5

### *Making a Blood Film (Push Wedge Slide Method)*

1. Place a drop of capillary or well-mixed venous blood preserved with EDTA on one end of a slide, on the midline about 1 cm from the end. The drop should be about 2 mm in diameter (about the size of a match head), as shown in Fig. 12-19. Venous blood must be well mixed by gentle inversion at least 15 times; it should also be checked for clots. If capillary blood is used, touch the top of the drop to the slide, being careful not to let the skin touch the slide. Transfer venous blood to the slide with the aid of two wooden applicator sticks or a plain capillary pipette.

2. Lay the specimen slide on a flat surface, and hold it in position at the left end (these directions are for a right-handed person) with the middle finger or thumb and index finger of the left hand (see Figs. 12-17 and 12-19).

3. Place the smooth clean edge of the spreader slide on the specimen slide just in front (to the left of) the drop of blood (see Figs. 12-17 and 12-19).

4. Using the right hand, balance the spreader slide on one or two fingers (for example, the middle finger or the index and middle fingers) and draw it backward into the drop of blood at an angle of approximately 45 degrees to the specimen slide.

5. Decrease the spreader slide angle to about 25 to 30 degrees, and allow the blood to flow evenly across the edge of the spreader slide (see Fig. 12-19).

6. When the blood has spread evenly across the edge of the spreader slide, quickly push the spreader slide over the entire length of the specimen slide. As the spreader is moved, a thin film of blood will be deposited behind it. The blood film should take up one-half to three-fourths of the slide when properly prepared (Fig. 12-20). The goal is to achieve a wedge-shaped smear with a thin, feathery edge.

7. Turn the spreader slide over (this gives another clean edge) and prepare a second blood film, using the same procedure. Two films should always be prepared for the same blood specimen.

8. Dry the blood film immediately. If it is not dried quickly, the blood cells will shrink and appear distorted.

9. Label the film by writing the name of the patient and the date in the dried blood at the thick end of the film, using a lead pencil (see Fig. 12-20).

also can apply to the coverglass method. In either case, for the correct interpretation of a blood film, (1) the film must be prepared in a technically correct manner, (2) it must be stained correctly, and (3) it must be examined correctly. A film that is not prepared and stained correctly is useless for microscopic examination.

The equipment used for making blood films must be meticulously clean. Precleaned glass slides or slides cleaned with alcohol and wiped dry give the best results. Use of a spreading device is recommended; for example, a margin-free spreader slide with ground-glass edges may be used to spread the film of blood on the clean, lint-free slide. The edges of the spreader slide must be clean and free from chips. Coverglasses held by a suitable clip or holder can also be used as spreading devices (Fig. 12-18). The spreading device must be cleaned thoroughly with alcohol and dried between films, and it must be discarded when chipped or broken.

### Cytocentrifuged Blood Films

With the use of a cytocentrifuge, a monolayer of cells can be prepared. These centrifuges facilitate rapid spreading of the cells across a slide from a central point by virtue of their high torque and low inertia motors (see Fig. 12-17). With a cytocentrifuged preparation, cellular destruction and artifacts present in the glass wedge slide method are eliminated. Only small volumes of a sample are used, and the cells are evenly distributed and less distorted, producing better conditions for critical morphologic studies. They are especially useful for other body fluids, such as cerebrospinal, pleural, or synovial fluid or urine.

### Criteria and Precautions for a Good Blood Film

A blood film should satisfy certain criteria when observed macroscopically, as shown in Fig. 12-20.

The body of the film should be smooth and not interrupted by ridges, waves, or holes.

It should be thickest at the origin and gradually thin out, rather than having alternating thick and thin areas. Pushing the spreader slide with an uneven motion results in thicker and thinner areas in the body of the film.

A good blood film should cover one-half to three-fourths of the length of the slide. All of the initial drop of blood should be incorporated into the film, not just part of it.

The thin end of the smear should have a good feather edge; that is, the film should fade away without a defined border on the end. In some institutions a fairly straight feather edge is sought, while others prefer a more tongue-like edge.

A defined border at the end of a blood film indicates that most of the white cells have piled up

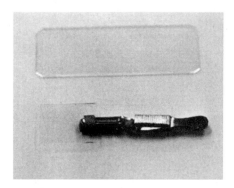

**FIG 12-18.** Spreading devices. *Top*, Notched-corner "spreader slide." *Bottom*, Ground glass coverglass in forceps.

at the end. When this occurs, the heavier neutrophils accumulate at the end to a greater extent than the other types of white cells, giving an incorrect distribution of the types of white cells in the body of the smear. Platelets also tend to accumulate at the end of a smear, decreasing the number in the body of the smear.

This will also result in inaccurate percentages for the cell types within the body of the film, as the relatively stickier neutrophils and platelets tend to concentrate in such tails. Chips in the spreader slide may be detected by running the index finger lightly over the spreading edge. The spreader slide should be cleaned by being rubbed vigorously with a piece of gauze moistened with medicated alcohol. Be sure that all the alcohol is evaporated (the edge is dry) before making the film.

Slides should be made in almost one motion; that is, the drop of blood should be placed on the slide and the smear made immediately. As soon as the blood is placed on the slide it should be spread, because drying of the blood drop will lead to an uneven distribution of cells in the body of the film and the larger white cells will accumulate at the end. Rouleau formation by the red cells and clumping of the platelets will also occur if the blood is not spread immediately. Pressing down on the spreader slide will also lead to an accumulation of white cells and

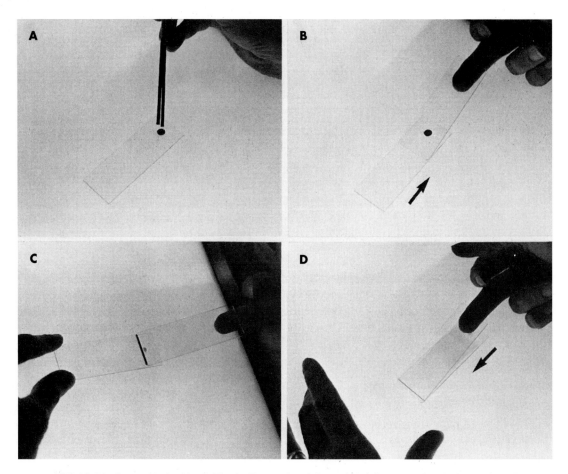

**FIG 12-19.** Preparing the blood film. **A,** Placement of drop of blood on the slide. **B,** Placement of spreading device on the slide in front of the drop of blood. **C,** Spreading device is moved backward into the drop of blood, and the blood is allowed to flow evenly across the edge of the spreading device. **D,** Spreading device is rapidly moved across the length of the microscope slide.

Thick End

Feather
Edge

NAME
DATE

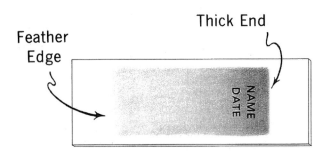

**FIG 12-20.** Good blood film.

platelets at the end. This is why it should be balanced on the finger as the blood is spread, rather than held between the finger and thumb.

The degree of thickness or thinness of the blood film is also important. When a film is too thick, the cells pile up, which makes them difficult to count and obscures their morphology. A very thin film is satisfactory for morphologic studies, but it may be tedious to examine. The thickness of the film is determined by the size of the drop of blood used, the speed of the stroke used to move the spreader slide, and the angle at which the spreader slide is moved. A thick film results when the drop of blood is large, the angle is greater than 45 degrees, and the spreading motion is fast. A thin film results when the drop of blood is small, the angle is less than 30 degrees, and the motion is slow.

Blood films with vacuoles or bubbles result from the use of dirty slides or in some cases from an excess of fat in the specimen (as in a specimen obtained after a fatty meal).

Only a small part of a blood film is actually examined microscopically. This part is referred to as the examination or counting area, as shown in Fig. 12-21. The counting area must be one where the red and white cells are clearly separated and well distributed. It should be about one cell thick and approximately 6 to 7 mm wide.

## Staining the Blood Film

After a blood film has been prepared, the next step is the staining procedure. The blood film should be stained as soon as possible. If it cannot be stained within a few hours, it should be fixed by immersion in absolute methyl alcohol (methanol) for 1 or 2 seconds and air dried. If this is not done, the slides will stain with a pale blue background of dried plasma.

The stain most often used for the examination of blood films is **Wright stain** or a variation of it, the **Wright-Giemsa stain** (Procedure 12-6). Both Wright stain and Wright-Giemsa stain are adaptations of polychrome Romanovsky stains. Such polychrome stains produce multiple colors when applied to cells, since they are made up of

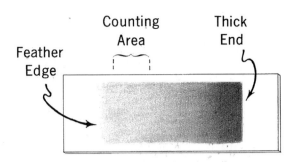

**FIG 12-21.** Blood film: counting area.

both basic and acidic aniline dyes. Romanovsky stains contain methylene blue (a basic dye), eosin (an acidic dye), and methylene azure (an oxidation product of methylene blue also referred to as polychrome methylene blue). Variations of the Romanovsky stains differ in the way the methylene azure is produced or added to the stains.

Polychrome stains produce multiple colors, since they dye both acidic and basic cell components in an acid-base reaction. The acidic cell components such as nuclei (nuclear DNA) and cytoplasmic RNA are stained blue-violet by the basic methylene azure. They are called **basophilic** (base loving), as they stain with the basic dye. The more basic cell components, such as hemoglobin and eosinophilic granules, are stained orange to pink and are called **acidophilic** (acid loving) because they stain with the acidic dye. Some structures within cells stain with both components, such as the neutrophilic granules, while the azurophilic granules stain with methylene azure.

The staining method for blood films fixes dead cells, as opposed to supravital staining, which is used with living cells. Fixation is the process by which the blood is made to adhere to the slide and the cellular proteins are coagulated. Wright stain and Wright-Giemsa stain are used as methanol solutions. The blood cells are fixed by the methanol in the first step of the staining reaction, when the Wright or Wright-Giemsa dye mixture is added to the blood film. Heat can also be used for fixation, but it is not necessary when

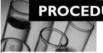

## PROCEDURE 12-6

### Staining Blood Films Using Wright-Giemsa Stain

1. Place the dried blood film on a level staining rack, with the film side up and the feather edge away from you. Allow the dried film to set at least 5 minutes before staining is begun.

2. Fix the film by flooding the slide with the filtered stain. The amount of stain is important. There must be enough to avoid excessive evaporation, which would result in precipitation of stain on the slide.

3. Allow the stain to remain on the slide for 3 to 5 minutes. This is the fixation period. Determine the exact timing for each batch of stain used.

4. Without removing the Wright-Giemsa stain, add phosphate buffer, using about 1 to 1½ times as much buffer as stain on the slide so that a layer piles up but none spills off. Add the buffer dropwise: then blow on the surface to mix the stain and buffer. A metallic greenish sheen should form on the surface when the slide is buffered adequately.

5. Allow the stain and buffer mixture to remain on the slide for 10 to 15 minutes. During this time the staining takes place as a result of the combination of dye and buffer at the correct pH.

6. Wash the slide with a steady stream of deionized water. Precipitation of the metallic scum on the film must be avoided. This is done by first flooding the slide with water, and then washing and tipping the slide simultaneously. If this is not done and the dye is poured off the slide before it is washed, the insoluble metallic scum will settle on the blood film.

7. Wipe the dye from the back of the slide when it is still wet by rubbing with a piece of moist gauze.

8. Place the slide in a vertical position to air dry, with the feather edge (thin edge) up. Never blot a blood film dry. The heaviest part of the film is at the bottom to allow precipitated stain to flow away from the thin edge, which will be used for examination of the blood film.

9. Do not use the slide for microscopic examination until it is dry.

---

the stain contains methanol. The actual polychrome staining of the blood film takes place in the second step of the procedure, when an aqueous phosphate buffer solution with a pH of 6.4 is added to the Wright-Giemsa dye.

Wright stain or Wright-Giemsa stain can be purchased as a dry powder, which is diluted in absolute, anhydrous, acetone-free methyl alcohol (CP), or as a prepared methanol solution. Both powders and solutions are certified by the Biological Stain Commission.[4] The preparation of methylene azure by oxidation of methylene blue and addition of eosin is quite complex, so

Wright stain powder may vary slightly from lot to lot. This necessitates determination of fixing and staining times for each new batch.

### Rapid Staining Methods Using a Dipping Technique

Modification of Wright stain has been incorporated into various commercially available quick staining methods. Blood films are prepared in the classic way, usually by the wedge method, and then stained. Each commercial product is somewhat different, so the manufacturer's instructions must be carefully followed. The advantage of these products is that they are faster to use than the traditional Wright staining method described earlier. Slides are usually dipped into each of the various staining reagents, with only a few seconds being taken for each step. For critical morphologic studies, the traditional Wright stain should be used, as some of the morphologic detail is lost when certain of the quick stains are used.

The traditional Wright staining technique has also been adapted to a "boat" or container staining method, in which slides are placed (feather edge up) in slide holders and moved at specific times to containers filled with (1) acetone-free methyl alcohol, (2) Wright-Giemsa stain, and (3) Wright stain mixed with phosphate buffer, and then rinsed by being dipped five times each in three separate containers of deionized water.

### Characteristics of a Properly Stained Blood Film

If the blood film has been stained properly, it will appear pink when observed with the naked eye. When examined microscopically with the low-power (10×) objective, the film should be thin enough so that the red and white cells are clearly separated. There should not be an excessive accumulation of white cells and platelets at the edge of the film. In addition, there should be no precipitated stain.

The background or space between the cells should be clear. The RBCs should appear red-orange through the microscope. Correctly stained leukocytes should have the following colors under the microscope. The lymphocytes and neutrophils should have dark purple nuclei, while the monocyte nuclei should be a lighter purple. The granules should be bright orange in the eosinophils and dark blue in the basophils. The appearance of the cytoplasm varies with the type of leukocyte. In monocytes, the cytoplasm should be blue-gray or have a faint bluish tinge. The neutrophil cytoplasm should be light pink with lilac granules, and the lymphocyte cytoplasm should be a shade of blue, generally clear blue or robin's-egg blue. The platelets should

stain violet to purple. If the blood film does not meet these criteria, it should be discarded and a new film should be stained and examined.

### Precautions and Comments on Staining Blood Films

When the blood film is being stained, it is important that the staining rack be level so that the stain is uniform throughout the film.

It is important that the stain and buffer be made correctly. When prepared in the laboratory, the stain should stand for 1 month before it is used. There are Wright and Wright-Giemsa stains that can be purchased ready to use. These reagents must be checked out carefully before being used for daily staining needs.

The pH of the buffer must be correct. With every new batch of stain and buffer, the fixing and staining times should be checked by staining a few slides. If staining of the cells is satisfactory, the times used for fixing and staining should be noted and used with that batch of reagents. If the pH is too acid or too alkaline, the stain will give a false color and appearance to the cells.

Adequate fixing time must be allowed. A minimum of 3 minutes is recommended for the initial reaction of the blood film and Wright-Giemsa stain. Since inadequate fixation allows dissolution of the nuclear chromatin, overfixation is preferable. To achieve the proper staining reactions in the cells, the stain and buffer must be prepared correctly, the correct timing must be determined for each batch of stain and buffer, and the correct staining technique must be used.

Properly applied Wright-Giemsa stain dyes both acidic and basic components of the blood cells. The phosphate buffer controls the pH of the staining system. If the pH is *too acid*, the parts of the cell taking up acidic dye will be overstained and will appear too red, while the parts of the cells taking up basic dye will appear pale. If the pH of the staining system is *too alkaline*, the parts of the cells taking up basic dye will be overstained, giving an overall blue effect, with very dark blue to black nuclear chromatin and bluish red cells. The following situations will indicate staining errors.

*A faded or washed-out appearance* of all the cells is caused by overwashing, understaining, or underfixing, leaving water on the slide, or by using improperly made stain.

When the slide has an *excessively blue appearance* on gross examination, the red cells will appear blue-red and the white cells will be darker and more granular microscopically. This may result from overfixing or overstaining, inadequate washing, using a stain or buffer that is too alkaline, or using too thick a film. It may be corrected by decreasing the fixation time (the time before the buffer is added to the dye), or increasing the time during which the buffer and stain mixture stands on the slide. Alternatively, the amount of stain used may be decreased and the amount of buffer increased. Finally, the pH of the buffer may be checked with a pH meter and readjusted to 6.4, or a new Wright-Giemsa stain may be tried.

When the slide has an *excessively red appearance* to the naked eye, the red cells will appear bright red, the white cells will appear indistinct with pale blue rather than purple nuclei, and brilliant red eosinophilic granules will be seen microscopically. This may be caused by understaining; overwashing; or use of stain, buffer, or wash water that is too acid. To correct this situation, the following measures may be tried. The fixation or staining time may be increased. The washing technique may be corrected so that it is adequate but not excessive. The pH of the buffer and water may be checked with a pH meter and adjusted, or a new stain or buffer may be used.

Large amounts of *precipitated stain* on the film result from either improper washing (not washing enough to remove the metallic scum) or using an old stain that has started to precipitate. This may be corrected by using the proper washing technique—first flooding the slide with water and then tipping and washing the slide simultaneously—and making sure that the stain is filtered daily.

## Examination of the Blood Film: General Comments

Since accurate examination of the blood film depends on proper use of the microscope, a general review of the procedure to be used is presented for a person viewing a blood film for the first time (see Chapter 5). The film is first examined with the low-power (10×) objective, with the slide being moved with the mechanical stage to get different areas into the field of view. The difference in appearance of the various areas results from the technique used in preparing the film: the film is relatively thick at the beginning and gradually thins out to a feather edge. Most of the cells seen under the low-power objective are RBCs, which appear as small, round, reddish-orange bodies.

Scattered among the red-staining cells are the less numerous WBCs, which are larger and more complex in appearance than the RBCs. The white cells consist of nuclei surrounded by cytoplasm. The nuclei stain purple, and the cytoplasms stain different colors, depending on their contents. The size of the cell, the shape, size, and chromatin pattern of the nucleus, the presence of nucleoli in the nucleus, and the contents, staining reaction, and relative size of the cytoplasm are used in the identification of WBCs.

With the low-power objective, an area of the film is found where the red cells are just touching and are not overlapping or piled on top of one another, as shown in Fig. 12-22. This area will be found near the feather edge of the film. The color of the cells should be examined at this magnification. When this area has been found, the oil-immersion (100×) objective should be used next. The high-dry (40×) objective is not suitable for examination of blood films, as important morphologic changes cannot be seen at this magnification. To change to the oil-immersion lens, the low-power objective is moved out of position and a drop of immersion oil is placed on the selected area of the blood film (where the red cells are just touching one another). The oil-immersion lens is moved

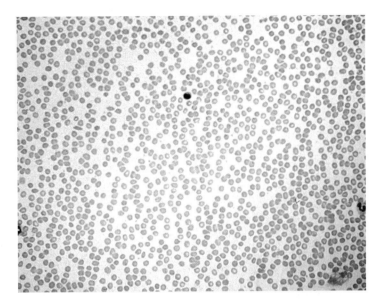

**FIG 12-22.** Good counting area, about 2 to 3 fields in from feather edge. (×100.)

into the oil while you look at it from the side. The oil must be in direct contact with the lens. If necessary, it can be focused with the fine adjustment. If the slide has been placed upside down on the microscope stage, it will be impossible to bring the blood cells into focus. More light will be needed with the oil-immersion lens. It can be obtained by repositioning the condenser (which should be all the way up for maximum resolution under oil immersion), opening the iris diaphragm, and increasing the intensity of the light source.

Under the oil-immersion objective, red cells appear as round, unstructured bodies containing no nuclei, granules, or discrete material. The red color is darker at the edge of the cell than in the center. This variation is caused by the biconcave shape of the red cell, which contains less pigment (hemoglobin) in its thinner center. With oil immersion, most of the red cells in a normal blood film are about the same size, averaging 7.2 μm in diameter. A normal red cell is uniformly round on a dry film, although variations in shape can be produced by poor

spreading technique in the preparation of the blood film.

When experience has been gained in using the microscope to view blood films, a more specific technique is used to observe the morphologic features of the blood cells.

Certain things must be done whenever peripheral blood films are examined. The blood film must first be evaluated for acceptable gross appearance and staining, as previously described. It must be evaluated for acceptable white cell distribution by observing the feather edge under low power. The numbers of erythrocytes, leukocytes, and platelets should be estimated, and the erythrocyte and platelet morphology should be described. Finally, the percentage of each type of leukocyte should be estimated.

### Microscopic Examination of the Blood Film

After the initial preparations, manipulations of the microscope and the observations described above, the following steps are taken in the examination of every blood film. These steps will be described in detail; however, in more general terms the blood film will be examined under low power and oil immersion. The general steps are outlined below and are described in the following section. Low-power examination (10× objective) includes:

1. An evaluation of the overall quality of the blood film
2. An estimate of the red cell count and the leukocyte count
3. A scan of the blood film for abnormal cells and clumps of platelets

Oil-immersion examination (100× objective) includes:

1. An examination of the erythrocytes for alterations and variations in morphology
2. An evaluation of platelet numbers and morphology
3. The differential count of the leukocytes
4. An examination of the leukocytes for morphologic alterations

### Method for Microscopic Examination
#### Low-Power (10×Objective) Examination of the Blood Film

1. *Evaluate the quality of the blood film.* The film should be thin enough that the red and white cells are clearly separated. The space between the cells should be clear. There should be no precipitated dye. The red and white cells should be properly stained, and there should not be a large accumulation of white cells at the feather edge of the blood film. If the blood film does not meet these criteria, it should not be examined further; a new film must be made.

2. *Estimate the red and white cell counts.* A rough estimate of the red cell count as increased, decreased, or normal can be made by noting the number of cells and the space between them. Normally, fewer and fewer intercellular spaces will be seen as one moves into the thicker portion of the blood film. In the optimal counting area, there should be no agglutination (clump-

ing) or rouleaux (cells stacked like coins). The optimal counting area is generally 2 to 3 microscope fields in from the feather edge, as shown in Fig. 12-22.

To find the optimal counting area, focus on the feather edge as shown in Fig. 12-23; then begin moving into the body of the blood film. At the very thin edge of the film (about 1 or 2 microscope fields into the body of the blood film) the red cells flatten out, appear completely filled with hemoglobin (showing no area of central pallor), and are generally distorted and show a cobblestoned appearance (Fig. 12-24). In the thick end of the film, the morphologic characteristics of all cell types are difficult to distinguish and the red cells show an apparent rouleau formation (Fig. 12-25).

The number of white cells is estimated in the optimal counting area of the film. With the low-power (10×) objective and the usual 10 × eyepiece (a total magnification of 100 times), five leukocytes in one low-power field are equal to approximately 1000 cells per microliter, or the number of cells per low-power field times 200 equals the number of cells per microliter. In other words, 5 white blood cells in one low-power field are equal to a white cell count of approximately $1 \times 10^9$/L; thus the number of white cells per low-power field divided by 5 is equal to the number of cells $\times 10^9$ per liter.

As a general observation, approximately 20 to 30 white cells per field are equivalent to a white cell count of approximately $5 \times 10^9$/L. Under the same magnification, 40 to 60 white cells per field are equivalent to a white cell count of approximately $10 \times 10^9$/L.

3. *Scan the blood film for abnormal cells and clumps of platelets.* The slide should also be examined under low power for the presence of immature or abnormal cells. With experience, the cells may be recognizable under low power; however, they are positively identified under oil immersion. If very few such abnormal cells are present, they may be overlooked if the slide is examined under oil immersion alone, in which the examination area is much smaller.

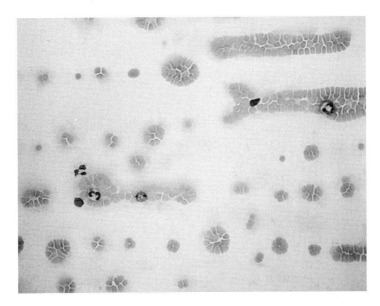

**FIG 12-23.** Feather edge. (×100.)

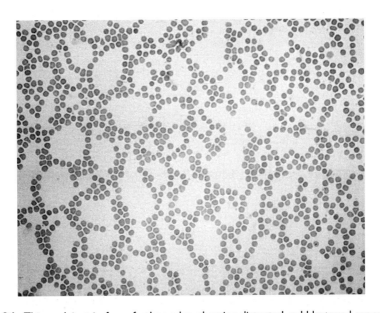

**FIG 12-24.** Thin end, just in from feather edge, showing distorted, cobblestoned appearance of red cells. (×100.)

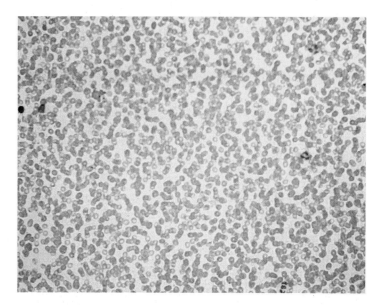

**FIG 12-25.** Thick end, too far in from feather edge, showing rouleaux and overlapping of red cells. This is not a suitable area for morphology of red or white cells. (×100.)

Such abnormal cells should be looked for especially in the feather edge and along the sides of the slide.

The optimal counting area, sides, and feather edge should also be scanned for clumps of platelets. Clumps of platelets should not be seen normally; however, when the platelet count is increased, they may be found along the sides and in the feather edge.

### Oil-Immersion (100× Objective) Examination of the Blood Film

1. *Examine the red cells for alterations and variations in morphologic features.* The normal red cell is a nonnucleated biconcave disk containing hemoglobin. Most red cells measure 7.2 to 7.9 μm on a stained blood film. The normal red cell is approximately 2 μm thick; values of 2.14, 2.05, 1.84, and 1.64 μm have been reported as the normal mean thickness. The mean volume, calculated from the hematocrit and the red cell count, is 87 fL. In estimating the diameters of WBCs or other structures, it is often advantageous to use the red cell as a 7-μm measuring stick.

When normal red cells are studied on dried and stained blood films, they are nearly uniform in size, shape, and color. Such normal-appearing cells are referred to as *normocytic* (normal size) and *normochromic* (normal color).

The normal red cell appears as a disk with a rim of hemoglobin and a clear central area, referred to as central pallor. The area of central pallor is normally less than one-third the diameter of the red cell, although there is some variation within the film. The amount of color in the cell (the staining reaction) and the corresponding amount of central pallor reflect the amount of hemoglobin in the cell. Normal red cells are pink. The staining reaction is referred to in terms of **chromasia,** and red cells with a normal amount of color are referred to as normochromic or, less frequently, orthochromatic. Normochromic, normocytic red cells are shown in Fig. 12-26.

It is important to observe red cell morphology only in the optimal counting area that is found by using the low-power (10×) objective. When red cells are examined morphologically,

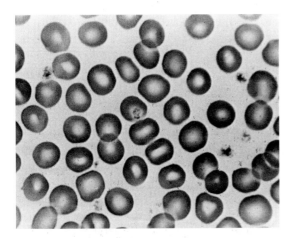

**FIG 12-26.** Normal red blood cells. (×1000.)

the following characteristics must be observed and noted:

a. Variations in color
b. Variations in size (anisocytosis)
c. Variations in shape (poikilocytosis)
d. Variations in structure and inclusions
e. Presence of artifacts and abnormal distribution patterns
f. Presence of nucleated red cells

Various terms are used to describe changes in the red cell size, shape, and staining reaction. The degree of the observed red cell alteration is noted as slight, moderate, or marked. These changes are thoroughly described under Morphologic Alterations in Erythrocytes and are summarized below.

a. *Variations in color or staining reaction.* The normal amount of hemoglobin and normal staining is referred to as **normochromasia** or sometimes as **orthochromasia**. Other terms used to described variations in staining reaction and hemoglobin content include:
Hypochromasia
Polychromasia

b. *Alterations in size.* An overall excessive variation in cell size is referred to as **anisocytosis**. The degree of anisocytosis is reflected by the RDW. Examples of anisocytosis include:
Macrocytosis
Microcytosis

c. *Alterations in shape.* An overall abnormal variation in shape is referred to as **poikilocytosis**. Examples of poikilocytosis include:
Spherocytes
Schiztocytes
Sickle cells, or drepanocytes
Ovalocytes
Target cells

d. *Red cell inclusions.* Several inclusions are also seen under certain conditions in the red cells, and they must be identified. Examples include:
Basophilic stippling
Siderocytes
Howell-Jolly bodies

e. *Abnormal red cell distribution.* This includes:
Rouleaux
Agglutination

f. *Presence of nucleated red cells (necessitates white cell count correction).* When nucleated red cells **(normoblasts)** are seen on the blood film, the number of these cells per 100 white cells is reported. It is necessary to correct the total white cell count when normoblasts are present, since they are not destroyed by the acetic acid diluents used for the white cell count and will be counted along with the white cells. The total white cell count can be corrected in the following way:

$$\text{Corrected white cell count} = \frac{\text{Uncorrected white cell count} \times 100}{100 + \text{Number of nucleated RBCs per 100 WBCs}}$$

2. *Estimate the platelet count and evaluate for morphologic changes.* The blood film is examined

with the oil-immersion objective to estimate the number of platelets and to detect morphologic alterations. The platelet count is estimated as adequate, decreased, or increased.

Platelets generally vary from 2 to 5 $\mu$m in diameter. They are ovoid structures having a colorless to pale-blue background (hyalomere) containing centrally located, reddish to violet granules (chromomere). Platelets are not cells, but portions of cytoplasm pinched off from megakaryocytes, giant cells of the bone marrow. Platelets are often increased in size when the blood is being actively regenerated; their size is also a function of age, with younger cells being generally larger. Bizarre forms are also noted after splenectomy and in myelofibrosis, hemorrhagic thrombocytosis, and polycythemia vera. Giant platelets are characteristic of platelet disorders associated with thrombocytopenia and the megaloblastic anemias.

Normally, 6 to 20 platelets should be seen in each oil-immersion field, representing a normal platelet count of 172 to 450 $\times$ 10$^9$/L. A rough estimate of the platelet count can be made by letting each platelet seen in an oil-immersion field equal approximately 20 $\times$ 10$^9$/L. Values as low as 3 to 5 platelets per oil-immersion field have been considered to represent a normal platelet count. The difference in normal values is probably a result of the use of specimens from different sources: the lower value is more consistent with capillary blood, where some of the platelets are utilized in the clotting mechanism, while the higher value is consistent with anticoagulated venous blood.

Estimate the platelet count as adequate, decreased, or increased and report as follows:

a. Report the platelet estimate as *adequate* if 6 to 20 platelets are seen per oil-immersion field. Several fields should be checked, and the platelets may be estimated while the white cell differential is being done.

b. Report the platelets as *decreased* if the average number of platelets is less than 6, un-

less the blood film was prepared on capillary blood. In this case 3 to 5 platelets per oil-immersion field is normal. Before reporting as decreased, scan the slide for clumps of platelets with the low-power objective, especially at the feather edge. If the blood film is well made, without aggregates at the feather edge, and platelets can be found only with great difficulty, the platelet count is below 20 $\times$ 10$^9$/L and the estimate should be reported as decreased. In addition, the tube of blood should be rechecked for the presence of clots, as platelets would be utilized in the clots and the blood film value artificially decreased.

c. Report the platelets as *increased* if there are more than 20 platelets per oil-immersion field. If there are many masses of platelets at the feather edge and platelets in the body of the film are sufficiently abundant to attract the attention of the observer, it is reasonable to assume that the platelet count is increased.

d. Observe the platelet morphology. Report the presence of large, bizarre, or atypical forms. This may be done while the white cell differential is being done (Fig. 12-27).

*3. Perform the differential count of white cells.* The differential count consists of identifying and counting a minimum of 100 white cells. After the red cells and platelets have been examined, the white cells are classified and counted in the optimal counting area of the blood film under oil immersion.

a. Move the slide in a way that will allow continuous counting and classification of white cells from margin to margin of the film.

b. When a margin is reached, move the slide toward the thicker end (a distance of one or two microscope fields).

c. Count and classify each white blood cell seen in the successive fields from one margin to the other margin of the blood film.

# Normal Platelets

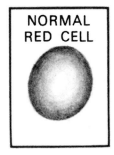

NORMAL RED CELL

## Atypical

## Giant

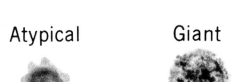

**FIG 12-27.** Platelets. Normal and abnormal forms are shown, with red blood cell for size comparison.

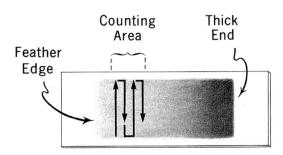

**FIG 12-28.** Pathway for differential cell count.

f. Count any nucleated red cells that are encountered separately; they should not be included in the 100 cells counted. However, the white cell count must be corrected when nucleated red cell forms are noted. This correction was described previously.

Continue this process until the required number of white cells have been counted (Fig. 12-28).

d. Count a minimum of one hundred white blood cells. Classify and tally each basic cell type within the cells counted as:
Neutrophil (including segmented and band forms)
Lymphocyte
Monocyte
Eosinophil
Basophil
Other: use morphologically descriptive terms; avoid eponyms or implication of function or disease process.

e. When exactly 100 white cells have been counted, the numbers of the different types of white cells recorded are estimates of the percentages of these types making up the total white cell count. For example, if 3 of the 100 cells counted are eosinophils, then 3% of the circulating white cells are assumed to be eosinophils. This is of relative value.

In certain situations it may be necessary to count more or fewer than 100 cells. If the relative numbers of specific types of white cells differ markedly from the accepted normal values, it is advisable to count 200 cells or more before recording percentages. Specifically, 200 cells should be counted if more than 5% of the cells are eosinophils, if more than 2% are basophils, if more than 10% are monocytes, or if the percentage of lymphocytes is greater than 50%. If the differential for an adult with a normal white cell count shows fewer than 15 or more than 40 lymphocytes, an additional 100 cells should be counted on another blood film to rule out distribution errors.

In cases of leukopenia, if the white cell count is less than $1 \times 10^9$/L, only 50 cells need to be counted in the white cell differential. When such changes are made, the percentages of the different cell types must be calculated, and the number of cells actually counted in the differential must be noted on the report form—for example, 3% basophils, 200 cells counted. Occasionally, the absolute number of cells of each type is of interest, although values are usually reported as percentages. To calculate the absolute value, multiply the percentage of each cell type, expressed as a decimal, by the total white cell count.

4. *Examine the leukocytes for morphologic alterations.* As the cells are being classified and counted, any morphologic alterations or abnormalities should be noted. These are described later in this section. A white cell cannot be skipped because it cannot be identified. Experience is necessary for morphologic studies of white cells, especially when an immature or abnormal cell is seen. Persons with limited training in hematology should not attempt to identify abnormal white cells. This should be done by a more qualified person, such as a pathologist or a clinical laboratory scientist with special hematologic training. Persons with limited training should be able to identify and classify the normal white cells, but should be encouraged to seek assistance when a questionable cell is seen.

### Reporting Leukocyte Differential Results (Relative and Absolute Counts)

The numbers and types of leukocytes counted are traditionally reported in percent numbers—cells identified while examining and counting 100 WBCs in a systematic fashion. These results are reported in **relative numbers,** or percent. The alternative method is to report the differentials in terms of **absolute numbers.** In using this method, the numbers and types of cells counted are reported in number of cells $\times$ $10^9$/L. Increases or decreases of individual cell lines are reported individually along with the total white cell count. The absolute count provides a much more accurate measure of the actual numbers of cell types present in the peripheral blood.

The absolute cell count by cell type is obtained by multiplying the relative number of white cells (in decimal units) by the total white cell count per liter. For example, if a patient's WBC count is 7.5 $\times$ $10^9$/L and 68% neutrophils are identified in the leukocyte differential, the relative neutrophil count is 68%. The absolute neutrophil count is:

$0.68 \times 7.5 \times 10^9$/L $= 5.1 \times 10^9$ neutrophils/L. The absolute count should be reported to the nearest $0.1 \times 10^9$/L cells. Many laboratories report both the relative and absolute values for leukocyte differentials. According to The National Committee for Clinical Laboratory Standards, "In the future, absolute concentrations of circulating leukocytes will likely become the preferable method of reporting."[8]

### Reference Values*

*For leukocyte differential cell count; relative (%) and absolute ($\times 10^9$/L) counts, age 21 and above:*

| Cell Type | Mean (%) | Absolute Count ($\times 10^9$/L) and Mean (range) |
|---|---|---|
| Neutrophils | | |
| Total | 59 | 4.4 (1.8-7.7) |
| Band | 3.0 | 0.22 (0-0.7) |
| Segmented | 56 | 4.2 (1.8-7.0) |
| Eosinophils | 2.7 | 0.20 (0-0.45) |
| Basophils | 0.5 | 0.04 (0-0.2) |
| Lymphocytes | 34 | 2.5 (1.0-4.8) |
| Monocytes | 4.0 | 0.3 (0-0.8) |

See also reference values for routine hematologic Procedures, Appendix C.

### Leukocyte Differentials Provided by Hematology Analyzers

Many of the multiparameter hematology analyzers provide some degree of differentiation of leukocytes, and many instruments that provide five-cell differentials are available. The major advantage of automated differentiation of leukocytes is that many thousands of cells are analyzed rapidly. This increases the precision of the method. The major disadvantage is that these cells are not actually "seen" by anyone. For this reason, it is possible that an individual's blood may contain a few very abnormal cells, such as blast cells of acute leukemia, that are not

---

*Beutler E, Lichtman MA, Coller BS, Kipps TJ: *Williams Hematology*, ed 5. New York, McGraw-Hill, Inc., 1995, p 12.

recognizable by instrumentation but that would be recognized visually by an experienced hematologist. This might result in failure to treat the disease in a timely manner.

In an environment of cost containment and shortage of laboratorians, together with more and more sophisticated instrumentation, the so-called routine hematologic examination (complete blood count) often uses an automated, rather than a manual, leukocyte differential. Each laboratory needs to develop a policy for the preparation of a blood film and visual examination and counting of cells when the automated results are flagged, so that clinically significant findings will not be missed.

Automated differentials can provide a great amount of useful, cost-efficient information when interpreted by an experienced laboratorian, especially when a manual leukocyte differential or review of the blood film is performed on abnormal results, as determined by the laboratory. The multiparameter analyzers differ in the principle by which leukocytes are differentiated. In general, they employ (1) impedance-related, conductivity, light scattering

measurements of cell volume, (2) automated continuous-flow systems that use cytochemical and light scattering measurements, and (3) automated computer image analysis of a blood film prepared by an instrument. The Coulter principle is utilized to construct a size-distributed histogram of leukocytes. These methods are combined and the electrical signals are further manipulated with computer-assisted synthesis and derivations. Several instruments are available, and none is clearly superior to the others.

## Normal Leukocyte Morphology

The five types of WBCs encountered in normal peripheral blood are shown in Fig. 12-29. Certain characteristics should be kept in mind when cells are to be classified; these are related to size, the nucleus, and the cytoplasm. Cell size (small, medium, or large), especially as it compares to a normal red blood cell, which is approximately 7 µm in diameter, should be noted. Also, cell shape—round, oval, irregular, or spreading with projections—helps in identification. Characteristics of the nucleus that should

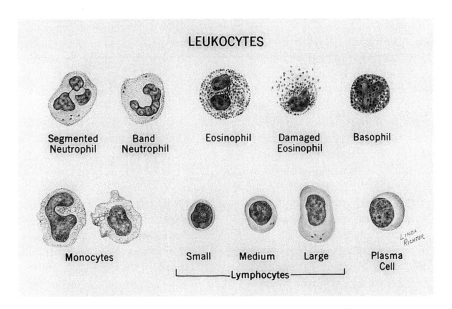

**LEUKOCYTES**

Segmented Neutrophil   Band Neutrophil   Eosinophil   Damaged Eosinophil   Basophil

Monocytes   Small   Medium   Large   Plasma Cell

└──────Lymphocytes──────┘

**FIG 12-29.** Leukocytes.

be considered are the shape, the size compared with the rest of the cell (nuclear/cytoplasmic or N/C ratio), the chromatin pattern (smooth or coarse), and the presence of nucleoli. Characteristics of the cytoplasm that should be considered include the presence or absence of granules, their staining characteristics, and whether they are specific or nonspecific, as well as the staining properties and relative amount of the cytoplasm. Other considerations are the relative amount of cytoplasm (N/C ratio) and the presence of other inclusions. These properties should be noted for all types of cells that may be encountered in the peripheral blood or bone marrow, whether they are of the granulocyte, lymphocyte, erythrocyte, or megakaryocyte series.

### Segmented Neutrophils

The most numerous of the granulocytes are the polymorphonuclear neutrophilic (PMN) leukocytes or segmented neutrophilic leukocytes. Neutrophils make up about 59% of the leukocytes in peripheral blood, with a range of 35% to 71%. Infants and children have fewer neutrophils and more lymphocytes (see Appendix C, which includes reference values for routine hematologic procedures).

Neutrophils are generally round cells, which vary in diameter from about 10 to 15 μm. The nucleus forms a relatively small part of the cell. The nucleus can assume various shapes, but it is usually lobular—that is, the nucleus is usually constricted, forming a series of lobes connected by narrow strands or filaments of chromatin; it may have two to five lobes. The nuclear chromatin is coarse and clumped and stains deep purple. These irregular chromatin masses are distinct and distinguishable from the lighter purple parachromatin. The nuclear membrane is distinct, and no nucleoli are visible. The ratio of nucleus to cytoplasm ratio (N/C ratio) is 1:3. The abundant cytoplasm is colorless or faintly pink and contains a large number of very small, often indiscrete lilac specific neutrophilic granules distributed irregularly throughout it. A

variable number of nonspecific azurophilic granules may be present.

### Band Neutrophils

The band neutrophil is a younger form of the mature neutrophil. Laboratories differ in the reporting of band neutrophils. Some classify and report band and segmented neutrophils separately; others report total neutrophils. Normal adults generally have about 3% band neutrophils in their peripheral blood. An obvious increase of band neutrophils should be reported.

Morphologically, band neutrophils are like segmented cells except for the shape of the nucleus. In band neutrophils the nucleus may be rod- or band-shaped, when distinct lobes have not yet formed, or it may have begun to form lobes. In the latter case, the lobes are connected by wide strips or bands rather than narrow threads or filaments as in segmented neutrophils. The College of American Pathologists defines a band as a connecting strip or isthmus that is wide enough to show two distinct margins with nuclear material in between.[3] A filament, on the other hand, is so narrow that there is no visible nuclear material between the two sides. The differentiation between band and segmented neutrophils may be difficult; if there is doubt, the cell should be classified as segmented (see Fig. 12-29).

Generally, an increased white cell count (leukocytosis) results from an increase in the absolute number of neutrophils present in the blood; in this case it is called **neutrophilia.** Neutrophilia is found in acute infections (especially bacterial infections); metabolic, chemical, and drug intoxications; acute hemorrhage; postoperative states; certain noninflammatory conditions such as coronary thrombosis; malignant neoplasms; and after acute hemolytic episodes. It is usually accompanied by a shift to the left, or an increase in the number of immature cells, and by toxic changes in the cytoplasm. An increase in the number of band forms, which may be accompanied by the presence of more immature neutrophils, is significant. The presence of forms more immature than bands is also termed a **leukoblastotic** reaction. Toxic changes in the neutrophil cytoplasm are indicated by the presence of deeply stained basophilic (or toxic) granules, pale-blue Döhle bodies, and vacuolization. Toxic changes in the nucleus include hypersegmentation (more than five lobes) and degeneration, or pyknosis. The cell size may be increased or decreased.

**Neutropenia** is a reduction of the absolute neutrophil count. Severe neutropenia has been called agranulocytosis. The risk of infection is considerably increased as the neutrophil count falls below about $1 \times 10^9$/L. For this reason, neutrophil counts are important in the care of patients undergoing chemotherapy or other conditions in which the bone marrow is suppressed.

### Eosinophils

Eosinophils are granulocytes and generally make up about 3% of the circulating leukocytes. They are slightly larger than neutrophils, usually 12 to 16 $\mu$m in diameter. The nucleus occupies a relatively small part of the cell. The nucleus is usually bilobed, and occasionally three lobes are seen. The nuclear structure is much like that of the neutrophil, but the lobes are plumper and the chromatin often stains lighter purple than in the neutrophil. The nuclear membrane is distinct, and no nucleoli are visible. The cytoplasm is usually colorless, but it may be faintly basophilic. It is crowded with spherical acidophilic granules, which stain red-orange with eosin and are larger and more distinct than neutrophilic granules. The granules are evenly distributed throughout the cytoplasm but are rarely seen overlying the nucleus. They are hard, firm bodies that are not easily damaged; they remain intact when pressed into the nucleus or even when the whole cell is damaged and the cell membrane is broken. Eosinophilic granules are also highly refractive, a feature that is often a valuable distinguishing characteristic.

**Eosinophilia,** an increase in the number of eosinophils above normal, is associated with a wide variety of conditions, but especially with allergic reactions, drug reactions, certain skin disorders, parasitic infestations, collagen vascular diseases, Hodgkin's disease, and myeloproliferative diseases. **Eosinopenia,** or decreased eosinophils, is seen with hyperadrenalism.

### Basophils

Basophils, which are also granulocytes, normally constitute only 0.5% of the total circulating leukocytes. They are about the same size as neutrophils, 10 to 14 $\mu$m in diameter, but their nuclei usually occupy a relatively greater portion of the cell. The nucleus is often extremely irregular in shape, varying from a lobular form to a form showing indentations that are not deep enough to divide it into definite lobes. The nuclear pattern is indistinct; there appears to be a mixture of chromatin and parachromatin, and this mixture stains purple or blue and shows little structure. The nuclear membrane is fairly distinct, and no nucleoli are visible. The cytoplasm is usually colorless; it contains a variable number of deeply stained, coarse, round, or angular basophilic granules. The granules (metachromatic) stain deep purple or black; occasionally a few smaller, brownish granules may be present. They may overlie and obscure the nucleus. Since the granules are soluble in water, occasionally a few or even most of them may be dissolved during the staining procedure. When this occurs, the cell will contain vacuoles in place of granules, and the cytoplasm may appear grayish or brownish in their vicinity. The cytoplasm of a mature basophil is colorless. An immature basophil has a pale blue cytoplasm and is seen only in myelogenous leukemia.

**Basophilia,** an increase in the number of basophils, is associated with chronic myelogenous leukemia. It is also seen in allergic reactions, myeloid metaplasia, and polycythemia vera. The basophil number may increase temporarily after irradiation, and basophilia may be present in chronic hemolytic anemia and after splenectomy.

Tissue basophils, also called mast cells, are similar but not identical to basophilic granulocytes. They are larger and differ somewhat in their chemical makeup and function.

### Monocytes

Monocytes, like the granulocytes, are derived from the myeloid cell line. They make up about 4% to 6% of normal circulating leukocytes, ranging from 2% to 10% depending on the laboratory or author. They are the largest of the normal leukocytes, usually larger than neutrophils, measuring from 12 to 22 $\mu$m in diameter.

The nucleus is fairly large; it may be round, oval, indented, lobular, notched, or rarely even segmented, but most frequently it is indented or horseshoe shaped. The nuclear chromatin stains light purple and is delicate or lacy. Chromatin and parachromatin are sharply segregated, and the chromatin is distributed in a linear arrangement of delicate strands, which gives the nucleus a stringy appearance. (Occasionally the nuclear pattern resembles that of a lymphocyte, and the cytoplasmic differences must be relied on for identification.) The nuclear membrane is delicate but not distinct, and nucleoli usually are not seen.

The cytoplasm is abundant, and stains gray or gray-blue. It may contain numerous small, poorly defined granules resulting in a "ground glass" like appearance, and is often vacuolated. Extremely fine and abundant azurophilic granules are present; this granulation is called azure dust and is seen only in monocytes. The granules vary in color from light pink to bright purplish red. In addition, phagocytized particles may be seen in the cytoplasm.

### Lymphocytes

Lymphocytes make up about 34% of the leukocytes in the normal adult. Infants and children normally have more lymphocytes and fewer neutrophils than adults. Lymphocytes fall into two general size groups: small (approximately 7 to 10 $\mu$m) and large (up to 20 $\mu$m). Most normal lymphocytes are 7 to 12 $\mu$m in diameter. An intermediate or medium lymphocyte (approximately 10 to 12 $\mu$m) is also described by some authors. There are numerous gradations of size and form from one type to another; some lymphocytes can be as large as monocytes.

The small lymphocyte is composed chiefly of nucleus and is the type of lymphocyte predominating in normal adult blood. It is about the same size as a normocytic red blood cell and is a useful size marker during examination of the peripheral blood film, especially in cases of megaloblastic leukemia, in which all cell forms other than lymphocytes are increased in diameter. The nucleus is round or slightly notched, and the nuclear chromatin is in the form of coarse, dense, deeply staining blocks. There is relatively little parachromatin, and it is not very distinct. Almost the entire nucleus stains deep purple. The nuclear membrane is heavy and distinct, and nucleoli are not usually seen. The cytoplasm appears in the form of a narrow band that stains relatively dark blue, usually free of azure granules.

The large lymphocyte shows a further increase in the size of the nucleus and an increase in the relative amount of cytoplasm. The nucleus contains more parachromatin, and so stains more lightly than the nuclei of the smaller forms. However, the chromatin is still present in clumps, without distinct outlines because of the blending of chromatin and parachromatin. The nuclear membrane is distinct, and nucleoli usually are not seen. The cytoplasm in this form can be abundant and is most frequently smooth; it may, however, be spongy; azure granules are frequently seen. The cytoplasm color varies from colorless to a clear light or medium blue.

Nucleoli are rarely seen in lymphocytes of normal blood, but they may be seen in cells that have been crushed during the spreading of the film. It is possible that blood lymphocytes contain nucleoli but that they are normally obscured by the coarse nuclear chromatin.

It is sometimes difficult to distinguish between nucleated red cells (normoblasts) and small lymphocytes. The staining reaction of the parachromatin of the two cells is an important diagnostic criterion; the parachromatin of the lymphocyte is pale blue or violet, and that of the normoblast is red or pink. In addition, the cytoplasm of nucleated erythrocytes contains hemoglobin, which stains pink in blood films.

**Lymphocytosis,** an increase in the number of lymphocytes, is associated with viral infections. It is characteristic of certain acute infections (infectious mononucleosis, pertusis, mumps, and rubella, or German measles) and of chronic infections such as tuberculosis, brucellosis, and infectious hepatitis. The changes seen in these diseases have been referred to as reactive or atypical changes, and are particularly associated with infectious mononucleosis. The cells are called reactive lymphocytes, as the increased amount and apparent activity of the cytoplasm indicate that it may be reacting to some sort of stimulus (see under Leukocyte Alterations). The NCCLS recommends that these cells be referred to as **variant** forms.[8]

### Plasma Cells

In addition to the five types of white cells that normally appear in the peripheral blood, the plasma cell (plasmacyte) can occur in certain blood specimens. The plasma cell is thought to be a derivative of the B lymphocyte. It is large, with a round or oval nucleus that is usually in an eccentric position. The chromatin consists of deeply stained, heavy masses that may be arranged in a radial pattern. The cytoplasm is strongly basophilic. There may be a pale, clear zone in the cytoplasm to one side of the nucleus, referred to as a hof. Immature forms may occasionally be seen. Plasma cells function in the synthesis of immunoglobulins. They may be found in the peripheral blood in cases of measles, chickenpox, or scarlet fever and in the malignant conditions multiple myeloma and plasmacytic leukemia.

## Blood Cell Alterations

Morphologic changes in the red and white blood cells seen on the stained blood film aid in determining the nature of many blood diseases. Certain diseases produce fairly characteristic alterations of red cells, white cells, and platelets, in addition to other clinical signs. It is important that the laboratory personnel be well acquainted with the appearance of normal blood cells, so that abnormal or immature cell forms will be recognized immediately. Abnormal or immature cells should be identified by someone experienced in cell morphology. The general laboratorian should screen the films and give questionable ones to a pathologist or an experienced clinical laboratory scientist for final evaluation.

Most abnormalities found in white cells are related to the age of the cell. All white cells in the circulating blood should be mature, and the presence of immature white cells in the blood is considered abnormal. Immature white cells may be differentiated from mature ones by size, the appearance of intracellular structure (e.g., the presence of granules or changes in the nucleoli, chromatin, or nucleus), the staining properties, and the cell function.

There is a progressive decrease in cell size with maturity, with the nucleus becoming smaller and the cytoplasmic ratio correspondingly increasing. In granulocytes, granules appear with maturity. In immature white cells the nucleus is round; with age it becomes lobular or indented. Chromatin is fine and lacy in the young cell and eventually becomes coarse and clumped. Nucleoli may be present in young cells and absent in the mature forms. The cytoplasm is basophilic (stains blue) in young granulocytes, and eventually turns pink with maturity. The young nucleus stains reddish violet and becomes strongly basophilic with maturity. The granules in the cytoplasm assume specific staining qualities with increasing cell maturity.

Certain evidence of cell function is observed that is characteristic of specific developmental stages of the white cells. Examples are the presence of nucleoli, which indicate a young cell; mitotic figures, which indicate a young cell; cytoplasmic inclusions, which are characteristic of a mature cell; phagocytosis, which is seen in mature cells; and hemoglobin, which is seen in mature red cells.

The laboratorian should be able to differentiate an immature cell from a mature one. There are many stages of young cells, and it is not necessary for all levels of laboratory personnel to be able to differentiate among these stages; the trained clinical laboratory scientist or pathologist makes this evaluation. The general medical laboratorian should be aware of the various developmental stages of the blood cells, however, and for this reason the following material is presented.

### Origin and Function of Blood Cells Related to Morphologic Examination

It is generally accepted that all types of blood cells are derived in the bone marrow from a common progenitor or an uncommitted pluripotential stem cell, which is designated as **CFU-S (colony forming unit, spleen)**, also known as **CFU-LM (colony forming unit, lymphoid-myeloid)**. Stem cells are able to reproduce themselves and to differentiate into other cell types. The uncommitted pluripotential stem cell is able to differentiate or be committed into the lymphoid stem cell **(CFU-L)** (L refers to lymphoid) and the hematopoietic (or myeloid) stem cell **(CFU-C)** (C refers to culture). The various stem cells cannot be identified morphologically; however, they are thought to look very much like small or intermediate-sized lymphocytes. Their existence has been demonstrated by various culture techniques; hence CFU-C. They are present in the bone marrow in very small numbers; less than 1% of the marrow consists of stem cells. They do have the ability to repopulate the bone marrow after injury or lethal radiation. This is the basis of bone marrow transplantation.

The uncommitted pluripotential stem cell (CFU-S), also called CFU-LM (colony forming unit, lymphoid-myeloid), may become committed to a lymphoid (CFU-L) or hematopoietic cell line (CFU-C).

The lymphoid stem cells leave the bone marrow for differentiation into B lymphocytes in the lymph nodes and into T lymphocytes in the thymus.

The multipotential hematopoietic stem cell (CFU-C) further differentiates or commits to stem cells that form the erythrocyte (BFU-E or burst-erythroid) and then (CFU-E or colony-erythroid); megakaryocyte/platelet (CFU-Meg); and monocyte and granulocyte (neutrophil, eosinophil, basophil) (CFU-GM).

This progression of pluripotential stem cells to multipotential stem cells and then committed progenitor cells is summarized in Fig. 12-30. A general relationship of the mature cell lines and the stem cells is shown in Fig. 12-31.

The hematopoietic stem cells (CFU-C), which will form the red cells, granulocytes and monocytes, and megakaryocytes, require **colony stimulating factor (CSF)** to multiply and differentiate. Further differentiation of each of the cell lines is influenced by local effects in the microenvironment of the bone marrow and by humoral factors.

**Interleukins (IL)** are hematopoietic growth factors, such as erythropoietin, which contribute to the control of hematopoiesis. They are soluble or membrane-bound biochemical growth factors, which have been identified as being associated with genes and then cloned and sequenced; the products are then generated by recombinant DNA methods.

Blood cell differentiation and maturation occur primarily in the bone marrow. There the environment is well organized and complex. Mature cells must migrate across the sinusoidal endothelia of the marrow capillaries to enter the peripheral circulation. The endothelial membrane allows the passage of the more deformable mature cells and holds back the immature cells, which are more rigid and less motile. Pathologic processes can facilitate the release of more immature cells by affecting the cellular composition of the sinusoidal endothelia. The location and relationship of the various

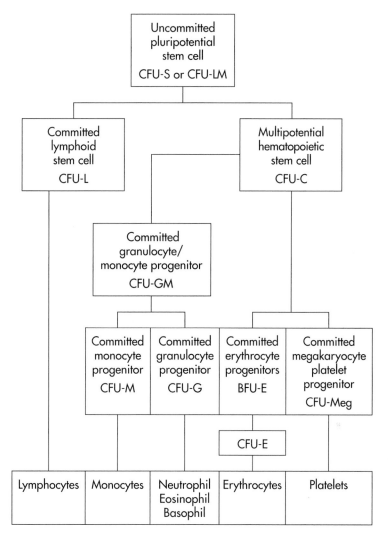

**FIG 12-30.** Progression of stem cells: pluripotential, multipotential, committed progenitor, and mature cell forms. Intermediate stages are not shown.

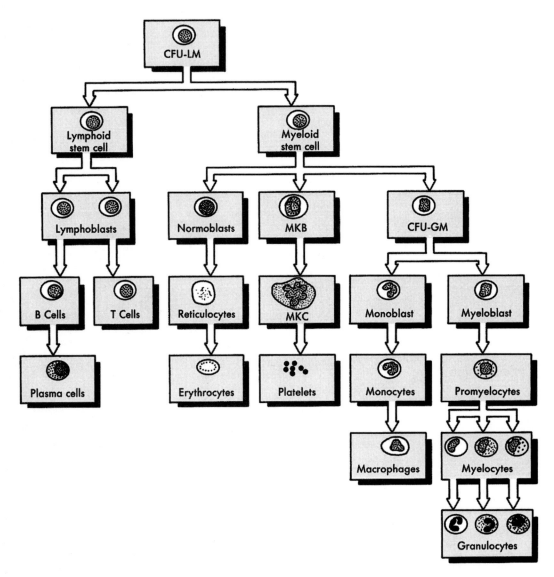

**FIG 12-31.** Blood cell differentiation and maturation. A general model of cellular differentiation and maturation shows the relationships of the mature cell lines and stem cells. Intermediate stages are not shown for all cells. *CFU-LM*, Colony forming unit, lymphoid-myeloid; also called CFU-S (spleen); *CFU-GM*, colony forming unit, granulocyte-monocyte; *MKB*, megakaryoblast; *MKC*, megakaryocyte. (From Powers LW: *Diagnostic Hematology.* St Louis, Mosby, 1989, p 87.)

blood cells in marrow, peripheral blood, and the tissue compartments are summarized in Fig. 12-32.

A diagrammatic representation of one blood cell origin theory, showing the origin and rela- tionships of all blood cell types, is given in Fig. 12-33. It should be remembered that this is theo- retical and that the actual details are unknown. All stages in the maturation process are gradual, and it is often impossible to identify an exact

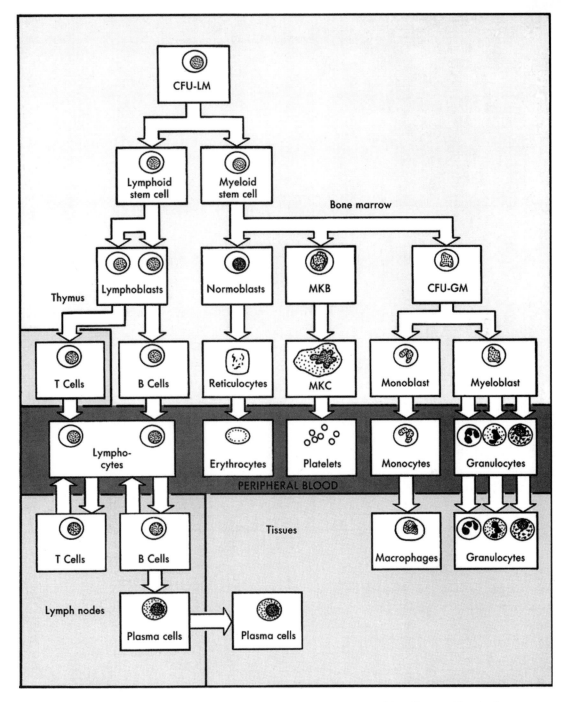

**FIG 12-32.** Blood cells in marrow, blood, and tissue compartments. Not all tissue–blood cell relationships are depicted. Lymphocytes, for example, recirculate between various organs, lymphatic vessels, and the bloodstream. *CFU-LM,* Colony forming unit, lymphoid-myeloid; *CFU-GM,* Colony forming unit, granulocyte-monocyte; *MKB,* megakaryoblast; *MKC,* megakaryocyte. (From Powers LW: *Diagnostic Hematology.* St Louis, Mosby, 1989, p 77.)

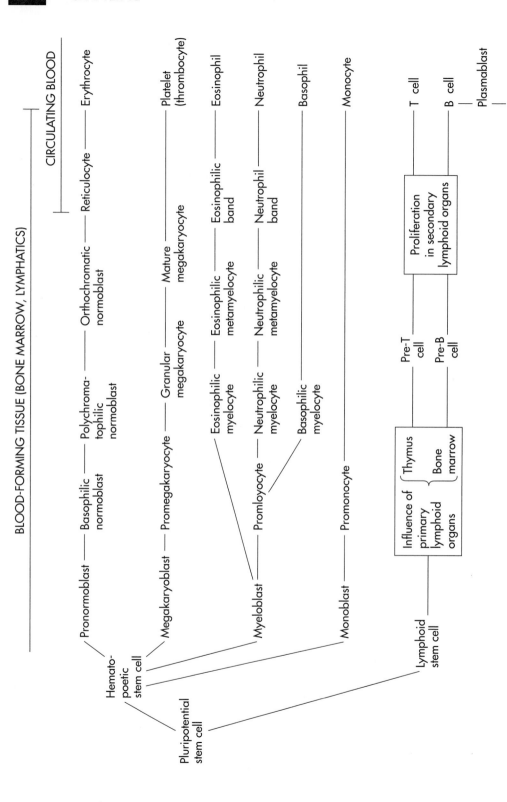

**FIG 12-33.** Origin of blood cells. (Adapted from Henry JB: *Clinical Diagnosis and Management by Laboratory Methods*, ed 19. Philadelphia, WB Saunders Co, 1996, p 598.)

stage with certainty. The most immature forms in all series (pronormoblast, myeloblast, lymphoblast, and plasmablast) appear very similar morphologically, and their identification is often based on surrounding cell types in various stages of development.

### Erythrocyte Maturation

Red blood cells are normally produced in the bone marrow. Their maturation takes 3 to 5 days, and six stages of development have been described. Several systems of nomenclature have been used to describe these stages, two of which will be discussed here. The stages of erythrocyte maturation from the youngest to the mature cell are: pronormoblast (rubriblast), basophilic normoblast (prorubricyte), polychromatophilic normoblast (rubricyte), orthochromic normoblast (metarubricyte), reticulocyte (diffusely basophilic erythrocyte), and mature erythrocyte. These stages are diagrammed in Fig. 12-34.

Remember that cells do not jump from one stage to another; there is a gradual progression, and exact classification is often very difficult. Rather than learning the characteristics of the specific stages, one should understand certain statements that are applicable in general to explain the maturation of the erythroblast to a nonnucleated erythrocyte.

Concerning the cell size and cytoplasm, there is a progressive decrease in size and there is also a decrease in the intensity of the blue color because of loss of RNA. There is an increase in red color, caused by an increased hemoglobin concentration. Finally, there are no granules in the cytoplasm in the mature erythrocyte.

The nucleus is generally round and in the center of the cell. In the early stages the chromatin is fine and lace-like. As the cell matures and the nucleus becomes smaller, the chromatin becomes coarse and more condensed. Finally, the nucleus degenerates into clumps or a solid pyknotic mass, which is eventually released (or extruded) from the cell. At the same time, the color of the nucleus changes from purplish red to dark blue. When the nucleus is extruded, it is phagocytosed and digested by marrow macrophages. The reticulocyte, or early nonnucleated erythrocyte, then squeezes through an opening in the endothelial lining of the marrow cavity and thus enters the peripheral circulatory system.

The earliest normoblast (pronormoblast) appears morphologically very much like the myeloblast or lymphoblast, and it may be impossible to distinguish them. It may be necessary to depend on their association with and transition to hemoglobin-containing cells in the same area of the marrow for identification. Cells

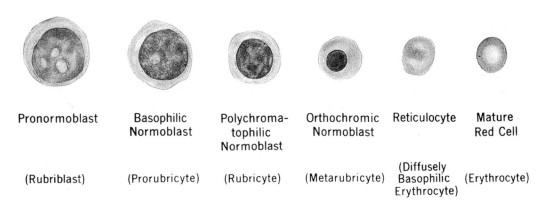

| Pronormoblast | Basophilic Normoblast | Polychroma-tophilic Normoblast | Orthochromic Normoblast | Reticulocyte | Mature Red Cell |
|---|---|---|---|---|---|
| (Rubriblast) | (Prorubricyte) | (Rubricyte) | (Metarubricyte) | (Diffusely Basophilic Erythrocyte) | (Erythrocyte) |

**FIG 12-34.** Maturation of the erythrocyte series.

of the erythrocyte series tend to stain more intensely than myeloblasts or lymphoblasts because of the combination of hemoglobin and RNA in the cytoplasm. The stages are described in terms of the staining reaction of the cytoplasm as it gains in hemoglobin concentration: basophilic cytoplasm is blue, polychromatic cytoplasm shows shades of blue and gray as hemoglobin increases, and orthochromatic cytoplasm is orange-red.

Another erythrocyte developmental series is that of the megaloblastic erythrocytes. It is similar to the sequence of maturation of the normoblasts, but the cells are larger, as the name implies. Megaloblasts are found in certain anemias, called megaloblastic anemias, which are the result of vitamin $B_{12}$ or folic acid deficiency. As they develop, cells of the megaloblastic sequence have a more open or immature chromatin pattern in the nucleus. This is referred to as asynchronous maturation or dyssynchronous development of the nucleus and cytoplasm. In megaloblastic anemia these changes are not limited to the erythrocyte series—all types of cells normally produced in the bone marrow are similarly affected, as evidenced by large hypersegmented neutrophils. This increase in size of all the cells makes it difficult to appreciate the increased red cell volume. However, the lymphocytes are unaffected, and a small lymphocyte at 7 $\mu$m is a useful visual size marker.

### Granulocyte Maturation and Function

Neutrophils normally mature in the bone marrow in the following stages, from the youngest to the most mature: myeloblast, promyelocyte (progranulocyte), myelocyte, metamyelocyte, band, and segmented neutrophils. These maturation stages are similar for all granulocytes and are diagrammed in Fig. 12-35.

Cells of the neutrophil series are generally round with smooth margins or edges. As the cells mature they become progressively smaller. Most immature cells have cytoplasm that stains dark blue, and becomes light pink as the cells mature. As the cells mature from the myeloblast to the promyelocyte stage, nonspecific granules that stain blue to reddish purple appear in the cytoplasm. Eventually, these nonspecific granules are replaced by specific neutrophilic granules. Both types of granules are not produced at the same time, but they may both be seen in the promyelocyte and myelocyte stages.

Nuclear changes also occur as the cells mature. In the myeloblast the nucleus is round or oval and very large in proportion to the rest of the cell. As the cell matures, the nucleus decreases in relative size and begins to contort or form lobes. At the same time, the nuclear chromatin changes from a fine delicate pattern to the more clumped pattern characteristic of the mature cell. The staining of the nucleus also changes from reddish purple to bluish purple as the cell matures. Nucleoli may be apparent in the early forms but gradually disappear as the chromatin thickens and the cell matures.

The term **shift to the left** refers to the release into the peripheral blood of immature cell forms, which are normally present only in the bone marrow. It is derived from the diagram-

Myeloblast　　Promyelocyte　　Myelocyte　　Metamyelocyte　　Band Neutrophil　　Mature (Segmented) Neutrophil

**FIG 12-35.** Maturation of granulocytes.

matic representation of cell maturation, in which the more immature forms are shown on the left side (see Fig. 12-35).

Neutrophils exist in the peripheral blood for about 10 hours after they are released from the marrow. During this time they move back and forth between the general blood circulation and the walls of the blood vessels, where they accumulate. They also leave the blood and enter the tissues, where they carry out their primary functions. In the tissues, they are utilized to fight bacterial infections and are then destroyed or eliminated from the body by the excretory system (intestinal tract, urine, lungs, or saliva).

Metabolically, neutrophils are very active and can carry out both anaerobic and aerobic glycolysis. The neutrophilic granules contain several digestive enzymes that are able to destroy many kinds of bacteria. The cells are capable of random locomotion and can be directed to an area of infection by the process referred to as chemotaxis. Once in the tissues, the neutrophils destroy bacteria by engulfing them and releasing digestive enzymes into the phagocytic vacuole thus formed.

Not as much is known about the other granulocytes, namely the eosinophils and the basophils.

The first recognizable precursor of the eosinophil is the eosinophil myelocyte. Culture studies show that there is a separate eosinophilic committed progenitor cell (CFU-Eo). However, the eosinophil myeloblast cannot be recognized microscopically from the neutrophilic myeloblast. Eosinophils exist in the peripheral blood for less than 8 hours after release from the marrow and have a short survival time in the tissues. The function of eosinophils is not completely understood. They do leave the peripheral blood when adrenal corticosteroid hormones increase and proliferate in response to immunologic stimuli. Eosinophils are capable of locomotion and phagocytosis and respond to foreign proteins They play a role in modulation of hypersensitivity reactions and inactivate fac-

tors such as histamine released by mast cells and basophils. They are active in allergic reactions and certain parasitic infections, especially those involving parasitic invasion of the tissues.

Studies and knowledge of basophils are very limited, because of their very low numbers (less than 1%) in normal peripheral blood. Basophils probably develop from a cell resembling a myeloblast. The first recognizable cell type is the basophilic myeloblast, which contains basophilic granules. Their life span in blood is probably similar to that of neutrophils and eosinophils. The basophils are capable of sluggish locomotion. The granules contain histamine, heparin or a heparin-like substance, and peroxidase. Functionally, little is known about basophils except that they apparently play a role in immediate hypersensitivity reactions such as allergic asthma. They also play a role in delayed hypersensitivity reactions such as contact allergies.

### Monocyte Maturation and Function

Monocytes, like granulocytes, are produced mainly in the bone marrow. The stages of development are myelomonoblast, promonocyte, and monocyte. The myelomonoblast looks very much like the myeloblast or the lymphoblast, and it may be impossible to distinguish them morphologically on films prepared with Wright stain. In such cases, the term blast is used. It may be necessary to classify the type of blast present on the basis of other cell types in the area.

Monocytes remain in the peripheral blood for hours to days after leaving the bone marrow, depending on the reference cited. They are very motile and phagocytic cells. Unlike neutrophils, monocytes do not die after they engage in phagocytic activity. Instead, after 1 to 3 days in the peripheral blood, they move into the body tissues and are transformed into **macrophages;** they may remain for months, depending on location. Macrophages are thought to be derived from both monocytes and histiocytic cells. Cells that have become free are known as **histiocytes,** and a histiocyte that has begun to phagocytose is called a macrophage. The macrophage is the final mature form of the monocyte when it travels through the tissues. Therefore, monohistiocytic cells (histiocytes, monocytes, and macrophages) are considered to be related in terms of function and origin. In addition to phagocytosing bacteria, macrophages appear to make antigens and interact with lymphocytes in the synthesis of antibodies.

The mononuclear phagocytes (monocytes and macrophages) are important in the defense against microorganisms, including mycobacteria, fungi, bacteria, protozoa, and viruses. They play a role in immune response, phagocytic defense, and the inflammatory response. They also secrete hematopoietic growth factors, remove senescent blood cells, and have antitumor activity.

### Lymphocyte Maturation and Function

Lymphocytes are normally produced in the lymphoid tissue (nodes, spleen, and thymus) but may also be produced in the bone marrow. The stages of development are: lymphoid stem cell, lymphoblast, pre-T cell or pre-B cell, and T lymphocyte or B lymphocyte. The number of precursor stages that exist from the lymphoid stem cell to the first identifiable B lymphocytes and T lymphocytes is not known. Lymphoid stem cells are indistinguishable from other undifferentiated stem cells. These stem cells are also called lymphoblasts by many hematologists. Lymphoid stem cells, or lymphoblasts, look very much like myeloblasts, and their morphologic differentiation is beyond the scope of this book.

When observed microscopically, lymphocytes are described on the basis of their size and cytoplasmic granularity. Small lymphocytes are found in the greatest numbers, ranging in size from 6 to 10 $\mu$m. Large granular lymphocytes are also regarded as mature cells. These cells contain additional cytoplasm, which appears typically sky-blue, as does the cytoplasm of the small lymphocyte.

The cytoplasm of the large granular lymphocyte can be deeply basophilic. Mature lymphocytes include different subsets of highly specialized lymphocytes. Morphologically, B and T lymphocytes appear identical on a Wright-stained blood film.

Only when immunologic studies are performed can these cells be identified as belonging to specific subsets of lymphocytes. As lymphocytes mature, their identity and function are specified by the antigenic structures on their external membrane surface.

The cell membranes of B lymphocytes contain immunoglobulins, which can be identified by immunofluorescent techniques. Characteristic antigens and receptors on the B lymphocyte membranes can also be identified and differentiated from T lymphocytes by the use of cell markers employing monoclonal antibodies. The T surface antigens correspond to a set of monoclonal antibodies often referred to as CD or cluster differentiation antigens. T lymphocytes lack immunoglobulins on their membranes but do contain a receptor for sheep erythrocytes. In a test utilizing sheep erythrocytes, the sheep red cells form rosettes with T lymphocytes; three or more sheep red cells attach to the cell membrane of the T lymphocyte.

The lymphatic system consists of a network of vessels throughout most of the body tissues. The smaller vessels unite to form larger and larger vessels, which finally come together in two main trunks, the right lymphatic duct and the thoracic duct. The ducts empty into the circulatory system through veins in the neck. Lymph nodes are located all along the lymphatic vessels, and the lymph (fluid within the system) circulates through the nodes as it progresses through the lymphatic system. Many of the lymphocytes are formed in the lymph nodes and circulate back and forth between the blood, the organs, and the lymphatic tissues. Functionally, there are two types of lymphocytes, T cells, or T lymphocytes, and B cells, or B lymphocytes.

B lymphocytes most likely mature in the bone marrow and function primarily in antibody production or the formation of immunoglobulins. They are related to plasma cells and may transform into plasma cells if appropriately stimulated. B lymphocytes have a short life span, measured in days, and constitute about 10% to 30% of the blood lymphocytes.

T lymphocytes mature in the thymus, an organ found in the anterior mediastinum, and function in cell-mediated immune responses such as delayed hypersensitivity, graft-versus-host reactions, and homograft rejection. They make up the majority of the lymphocytes circulating in the peripheral blood and have a life span of months to years as they continually recirculate from blood to lymph.

Lymphocytes act to direct and effect the immune response system of the body. Maturation of lymphocytes in the bone marrow or thymus results in cells that are immunocompetent. The cells are able to respond to antigenic challenges by directing the immune responses of the host defense. They migrate to various sites in the body to await antigenic stimulus and activation.

After antigenic stimulation, small lymphocytes can undergo transformation. These transformed cells appear large (15 to 25 $\mu$m) on Wright-stained films, with a relatively large amount of deep blue cytoplasn, and are called large granular lymphocytes. The large nucleus has a reticular appearance, with uniform chromatin and prominent nucleoli. Such cells have various names, including reactive, atypical, variant, and reticular lymphocytes.

### Erythrocyte Alterations

**Clinical Significance of Erythrocyte Alterations.** Clinically, alterations in erythrocyte morphology are associated with many diseases and especially with anemia. *Anemia* is not a specific disease, but a condition in which there is a decrease in the oxygen-carrying capacity of the blood and therefore in the amount of oxygen reaching the tissues and organs. Its causes are many and varied, and the type of anemia present and its underlying cause must be determined before treatment can be effectively undertaken. It may or may not be the result of a disorder of the blood or blood-forming tissues.

**Types of Anemias.** Clinically, all patients with anemia have similar symptoms or complaints regardless of the cause of the anemia. The severity is generally dependent on the hemoglobin concentration of the blood, as most symptoms result from the decreased oxygen-carrying capacity. The primary complaints are fatigue and shortness of breath. Other common complaints are faintness, dizziness, heart palpitation, and headache. All of these symptoms are general and can be present without the clinical condition of anemia. Once the existence of anemia has been demonstrated, usually on the basis of the blood hemoglobin concentration, the underlying cause must be determined. Besides the case history and physical examination, various laboratory procedures, including the appearance of the red cells on the peripheral blood film, are helpful in establishing the diagnosis.

Generally, anemias are classified according to either the appearance of the red cells (morphologic classification) or the physiologic cause of the anemia (etiologic or pathogenic classification). A morphologic classification, showing some of the more common types of anemia that result in the alterations in red cell morphology observed on the peripheral blood film, is one classification used. Such morphologic classifications fail to deal effectively with the hemolytic anemias, and these are described separately. Although they are helpful, these observations will be transferred into an etiologic system in determining the appropriate therapy for the patient.

Morphologically, anemias are generally classified as:

1. Normochromic-normocytic
2. Macrocytic
3. Hypochromic-microcytic

These types are discussed in terms of common laboratory changes, especially as reflected by the red blood cell indices, and common examples of each type are given. These changes are summarized in Table 12-2.

**Normochromic-Normocytic Anemias.** These anemias are characterized by normal-looking red cells on the peripheral blood film and normal red cell indices. The cells produced by the marrow are normal, but the number of cells in circulation is reduced for a variety of reasons. Such anemias may result from acute blood loss caused by external trauma such as a wound, or internal trauma such as an acute bleeding ulcer

## TABLE 12-2

Morphologic Classification of Anemias

| Type of Anemia | Changes in Red Cell Indices | | | Common Red Cell Alterations* | Common Examples and Causes |
| | Mean Corpuscular Volume (MCV) | Mean Corpuscular Hemoglobin (MCH) | Mean Corpuscular Hemoglobin Concentration (MCHC) | | |
|---|---|---|---|---|---|
| Normochromic-normocytic | Normal | Normal | Normal | Normal size, shape, and hemoglobin content; decreased cell count | Acute blood loss; aplastic anemia; increased plasma volume; infiltrated bone marrow; some hemolytic diseases; some chronic renal and liver diseases |
| Macrocytic | Increased | Increased | Normal | Macrocytosis (elliptocytes, ovalocytes) | Megaloblastic anemias from vitamin $B^{12}$ or folic acid deficiency; chronic liver disease |
| Hypochromic-microcytic | Decreased | Decreased | Decreased | Microcytosis (cells may appear large because of decreased hemoglobin content and flattening out on the slide); anisocytosis (slight to marked depending on condition and severity); poikilocytosis (changes characteristic of certain diseases); various inclusions, depending on cause | Iron deficiency (from blood loss, dietary deficiency, or iron metabolism error); globulin synthesis disorders (e.g., thalassemia, porphyria); heme synthesis disorders (e.g., sideroblastic anemias, lead poisoning) |

*Seen on films of peripheral blood stained with Wright stain.

or a ruptured organ. Conditions resulting in increased plasma volume, such as pregnancy and overhydration, will also result in normochromic-normocytic anemia. If the bone marrow is suppressed (hypoplastic), as seen in cases of aplastic anemia (a possible result of exposure to various chemicals or drugs), the red cells that remain are normal, although the number is decreased. Suppressed marrow results in a deficiency of the myeloid series and platelets, seen as decreased leukocyte and platelet counts. Likewise, if the marrow is infiltrated with a neoplasm or malignancy, as in leukemia or multiple myeloma, the remaining red cells appear normal, although they are decreased in number. In certain hemolytic diseases and chronic kidney and liver diseases, the red cells also appear normal but are reduced in number.

*Macrocytic Anemias.* Macrocytic anemias are primarily represented by the megaloblastic anemias resulting from vitamin $B_{12}$ or folic acid deficiency, or a combination of the two. The deficiency may be nutritional or may result from a malabsorption syndrome such as pernicious anemia, in which the patient is unable to absorb vitamin $B_{12}$. In either case, the deficiency leads to a nuclear maturation defect and megaloblastic anemia. The marrow shows certain changes in the myeloid series, including the red cells, granulocytes, and megakaryocytes (platelets). Megaloblastic changes are characterized by larger cells having a more open chromatin pattern in the nucleus (asynchronous maturation or dyssynchronous development of nucleus and cytoplasm) and by the presence of larger, hypersegmented neutrophils in the peripheral blood. The enlarged red cells (macrocytes) have MCV values on the order of 120 to 140 fL. Actual hyperchromasia is impossible, but the red cells appear to contain more hemoglobin because of their increased size and therefore thickness. Although the anemia may be severe, the red cell count is decreased more than the hemoglobin concentration, since the cells that are present are large and fairly completely filled with hemoglobin. Other changes seen in the blood film include anisocytosis (erythrocytes varying in size), poikilocytosis (erythrocytes varying in shape), and Howell-Jolly bodies.

Nutritional deficiency of vitamin $B_{12}$ is relatively rare, but nutritional deficiency of folic acid is fairly common. It may be found in chronic alcoholism or other conditions in which the diet is not well balanced. Folate deficiency is also observed when the requirement is increased, as in pregnancy, infancy, certain hemolytic anemias, and hyperthyroidism. Celiac disease, tropical sprue, certain drugs, contraceptives, and liver disease may lead to malabsorption and megaloblastic anemia.

*Hypochromic-Microcytic Anemias.* These anemias are probably the most common types encountered, with iron deficiency anemia being the one most frequently seen. However, iron deficiency is not a simple classification, as there are several possible causes of this clinical condition. In simplified terms, iron deficiency anemia may result from decreased iron intake (either from inadequate diet or impaired absorption), increased iron loss (generally from chronic bleeding from a variety of causes), or an error of iron metabolism. In addition, the increased iron requirements in infancy, pregnancy, and lactation may result in iron deficiency anemia. The cause of the anemia must be determined in order to treat it. If it results from a dietary deficiency of iron, a relatively simple and effective treatment is to administer iron, usually orally as ferrous sulfate tablets. However, if it is caused by another condition, the administration of iron will do no good, and may do harm either in itself (such as in the thalassemias, in which iron overload is a possibility) or because it delays the use of appropriate therapy.

If the iron deficiency anemia results from chronic bleeding, the cause of the bleeding must be determined. The bleeding is most often gastrointestinal, although women with excessive menstrual flow often develop iron deficiency anemia. Gastrointestinal bleeding leading to iron deficiency anemia may result from such causes as ulcer, carcinoma or other neoplasms, hemorrhoids, hookworm, or even the ingestion of salicylate (usually as aspirin). The treatment is different for each of these.

All iron deficiency anemias produce similar changes in red cell morphology. The cells are smaller than normal (microcytic), and the MCV is decreased. Unfortunately, the decreased size is not always as apparent on the blood film as it is in the MCV value. In iron deficiency anemia the amount of hemoglobin within each red cell is significantly decreased; such cells are hypochromic (deficient in color). This shows up in the red cell volume, which is primarily a function of hemoglobin, but may not be evident on the slide because the hypochromic red cell spreads out or flattens and may appear to be of normal size or even larger than normal. The hypochromic cell is extremely pale, showing only a thin rim of color with a significantly increased area of central pallor, which occupies over one third of the cell. The decreased hemoglobin per red cell is measured in the laboratory as decreased MCH and decreased MCHC. Other changes that are characteristic of iron deficiency anemia include anisocytosis and poikilocytosis, which vary in degree with the severity of the disease and are reflected by an increased RDW. Other tests that may be useful in the investigation of iron deficiency anemias include examination of the stool for occult blood, determination of serum iron and total iron-binding capacity, radiographic study of the gastrointestinal tract, and, rarely, bone marrow examination.

Another group of anemias that are microcytic and hypochromic are those that result from disorders in the synthesis of globin, another component of the hemoglobin molecule. These are the thalassemias, a group of inherited disorders of hemoglobin synthesis. The microscopic appearance of the red cells varies with and within the various types of thalassemias. However, microcytosis, hypochromasia, and basophilic stippling are general observations. Anisocytosis, poikilocytosis, and target cells may also be pres-

ent, as well as decreased osmotic fragility. Actual differentiation of various forms of thalassemia requires family studies and fairly sophisticated laboratory tests.

The last group of hypochromic-microcytic anemias that will be discussed are those resulting from disorders of porphyrin and heme synthesis. Again, the hemoglobin molecule is malformed. The sideroblastic anemias are a heterogeneous group of disorders that have in common increased storage of iron, especially in the RES. The bone marrow in these conditions shows sideroblasts, nucleated red cells with granules of iron that can be demonstrated with Prussian blue stain. The granules occur characteristically in a full or partial ring around the nucleus. Besides microcytosis and hypochromasia, the peripheral blood from these patients shows siderocytes, nonnucleated red cells with granules of iron (see also under Alterations in Erythrocyte Structure and Inclusions). Since the body is already overloaded with iron that is not being utilized appropriately, iron therapy in these anemias would be harmful to the patient.

A number of chemicals cause sideroblastic anemias by inhibiting heme synthesis. Lead poisoning produces an anemia that is characteristically mildly microcytic and hypochromic and is often characterized by basophilic stippling of the red cells. It is most often seen in children who have ingested lead paint chips and may be seen in adults as the result of industrial exposure to lead.

***Hemolytic Anemias.*** One problem with a morphologic classification of anemias is that it does not deal conveniently with a broad etiologic class of anemias, namely the hemolytic anemias. They are sometimes classified as normochromic-normocytic on the basis of calculated indices. However, the RDW is very increased because of anisocytosis and poikilocytosis, unlike the other normochromic-normocytic anemias. In addition, because of the increased number of young red cells (reticulocytes), which are larger than mature red cells, the MCV is increased, although not as much as for the megaloblastic anemias.

The hemolytic anemias are generally classified as congenital or acquired. They are characterized by increased destruction or hemolysis of red cells from a variety of causes, accompanied by increased production of red cells by the bone marrow. This is seen as polychromasia and even nucleated forms of red cells on Wright-stained blood films and as increased reticulocyte counts. Anisocytosis and poikilocytosis with increased RDW are characteristic of hemolytic anemias in general. An inherited form of spherocytic anemia, hereditary spherocytosis, results from an inherited red cell abnormality and is characterized by the presence of spherocytes in the peripheral blood. This condition is indistinguishable morphologically from certain acquired disorders that result in spherocytic anemia. In such cases a useful laboratory test is the direct antiglobulin (Coombs) test.

The direct antiglobulin test is used to detect red cells that have been coated, or sensitized, with antibodies. This is one of the most useful procedures for distinguishing immune from nonimmune mechanisms that can underlie hemolytic anemias. When red cells are precoated with an antibody, the direct antiglobulin test usually will be positive; unless the amount of antibody on the cell membrane is too small. Red cells can become sensitized when an autoimmune process is in effect. In this type of disorder, antibodies are produced by the patient's own immune system, which react with specific antigens on the patient's own red cells. These anemias can be temperature induced or drug induced.

Other changes of shape (poikilocytosis) characteristic of certain hemolytic anemias include the following: Elliptocytes are characteristic of hereditary elliptocytosis, a red cell membrane disorder. Sickle cells are characteristic of sickle-cell anemia, an inherited hemoglobin abnormality. Schistocytes, or fragmented cells, are characteristic of the microangiopathic hemolytic anemias, and may be produced by mechanical fragmentation caused by some sort of intravascular pathologic condition or intravascular coagulation.

### Morphologic Alterations in Erythrocytes: Description

The morphologic examination of red cells is very helpful in evaluating and determining the cause of anemia. Therefore, it is important that the clinical laboratorian recognize and report changes in red cell morphology so that the patient can be effectively evaluated and treated. The following must be observed and noted:

1. Color or staining reaction
2. Size
3. Shape
4. Structure and inclusions
5. Artifacts and abnormal distribution pattern
6. Nucleated red cells

Red cells are described as normochromic and normocytic when they are of normal color, size, and shape.

#### Alterations in Erythrocyte Color or Hemoglobin Content

*Normochromasia (See Fig. 12-26).* Red cells are described as **normochromic** when they contain the normal amount of hemoglobin. With Wright stain the cells show a deep orange-red color in the peripheral area, which gradually diminishes toward the center of the cell. The diameter of the pale central area (central pallor) is less than one-third the diameter of a normochromic erythrocyte.

*Hypochromasia (Fig. 12-36).* Red cells that are very pale and show an increased area of central pallor (making up more than one-third that of the cell) are termed **hypochromic**. Hypochromasia is the result of a decrease in the hemoglobin content of the cell, and is often accompanied by a decrease in cell size, seen as a decreased MCV, or microcytosis, evidenced by low MCH and MCHC values. The cells tend to

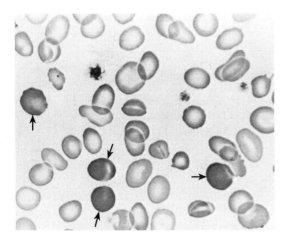

**FIG 12-36.** Hypochromic red blood cells. Compare with the four transfused normal cells *(arrows)*. (×1000.)

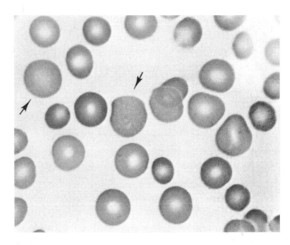

**FIG 12-37.** Polychromatic red cells. These cells are called reticulocytes when stained with supravital dye. (×1000.)

flatten out on the blood film and may appear normal in size. Such cells are particularly characteristic of iron deficiency anemias.

*"Hyperchromasia."* True hyperchromasia cannot exist because normal red cells are filled with hemoglobin and cannot be oversaturated, as the cell membrane would burst. However, certain red cells appear to have an increased hemoglobin content. For example, cells that are larger than normal (macrocytes) are also thicker, and therefore the color intensity appears greater on the blood film. Another abnormally shaped red cell, the spherocyte, which is a round cell without a depression in the center, also appears hyperchromic because it is thicker and stains equally throughout the cell.

*Polychromasia (Fig. 12-37).* Polychromasia refers to red cells that show a faint blue or blue-orange color with Wright stain. Poly refers to a mixed staining reaction (poly = many) due to the presence of both blue RNA and red hemoglobin. Polychromic cells are young cells that have just extruded their nuclei and stain diffusely basophilic because of the presence of small numbers of ribosomes (or cytoplasmic RNA). When such cells enter the bloodstream, they lack 20% of their final hemoglobin content

and retain the ribosomes for hemoglobin synthesis. Polychromatic red cells are generally larger than mature red cells. With supravital dyes such as new methylene blue, the RNA reticulum stains blue, and the cells are called reticulocytes. The presence of polychromasia (or an increased reticulocyte count) is an indication of increased red cell formation by the marrow and is characteristically seen in the various hemolytic anemias.

### Alterations in Erythrocyte Size

*Anisocytosis (Fig. 12-38).* Anisocytosis is a general term indicating increased variation in the size of red cells in the blood film. It is often accompanied by variations in hemoglobin concentration.

*Macrocytosis (Fig. 12-39).* Macrocytes are large red cells. They have a mean cell diameter greater than 9 µm or an MCV greater than 100 fL. They should be differentiated from polychromatic red cells, which are also large. Macrocytes are characteristic of the megaloblastic anemias of folic acid or vitamin $B_{12}$ deficiency.

*Microcytosis.* Microcytes are small red cells, less than 6.5 µm in diameter, with an MCV less than 78 fL. They are often associated with

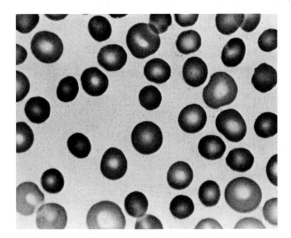

**FIG 12-38.** Anisocytosis. Note abnormal variation in size. (×1000.)

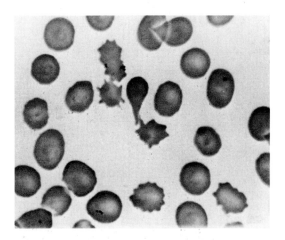

**FIG 12-40.** Poikilocytosis. Note the variation in shape of the red blood cells, including crenated cells. (×1000.)

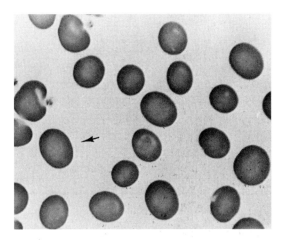

**FIG 12-39.** Macrocytosis. Oval macrocytes *(arrow)* are also present. (×1000.)

hypochromasia, but their decreased size may not be appreciated on the blood film because they tend to flatten out. Microcytosis is characteristic of iron deficiency anemia, thalassemia, lead poisoning, sideroblastic anemia, idiopathic pulmonary hemosiderosis, and anemias of chronic diseases. (See Fig. 12-36.)

### Alterations in Erythrocyte Shape

*Discocyte.* When an RBC is not being subjected to external deforming processes, its nor-

mal shape is that of a smooth biconcave disk. One term used to describe a red cell with a normal shape is discocyte.

*Poikilocytosis (Fig. 12-40).* Poikilocytosis is a general term indicating an increased variation in the shape of red cells. Many different variations in shape are seen in blood films; red cells have been described as appearing pear, oat, teardrop, or helmet shaped, triangular, or fragmented, or as having various numbers and types of membrane projections. The size and hemoglobin content can vary greatly within poikilocytes. They are found in a variety of anemias and hemolytic states, and a particular shape may or may not indicate a specific type of disease.

*Elliptocyte, Ovalocyte (Fig. 12-41).* These red cells are oval, or egg shaped, showing varying degrees of elliptic shaping, from slightly oval to almost a cylindrical form. Large elliptocytes, called macro-ovalocytes, are characteristic of megaloblastic anemias. Because of their increased size and thickness, these cells may not show an area of central pallor on the blood film. More elongated forms may occur in a variety of conditions, the most striking and least pathologic being hereditary elliptocytosis.

*Sickle Cell (Drepanocyte) (Fig. 12-42).* Sickle cells are most typically narrow and shaped like a

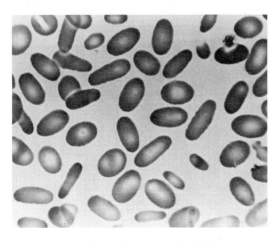

**FIG 12-41.** Elliptocytes. (×1000.)

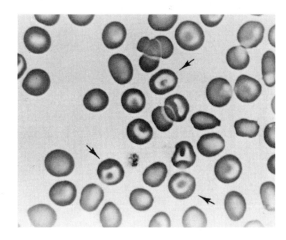

**FIG 12-43.** Target cells (codocytes) at arrows. (×1000.)

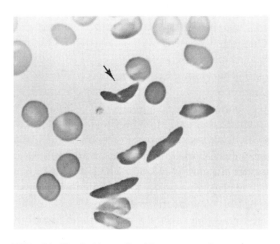

**FIG 12-42.** Sickle cells (drepanocytes) at arrow. (×1000.)

sickle with two pointed ends. They may also vary in shape from crescent-shaped, to bipolar, spiculated forms, to cells with long irregular spicules. They have defective membranes and do not function normally. They are the result of a genetic condition in which abnormal hemoglobin (Hb S) is present in the red cells. Sickle cells may be found in sickle cell disease (Hb SS) or sickle cell trait (including Hb SC, Hb SD, and Hb S beta thalassemia). Sickling of red cells is enhanced by lack of oxygen.

*Target Cell (Codocyte) (Fig. 12-43).* These cells look like targets, showing a peripheral ring of hemoglobin, an area of pallor or clearing, and then a central area of hemoglobin. This cell circulates as a bell-shaped cell, but takes on the target shape when dried on a slide for morphologic examination. Target cells represent another membrane defect; they have excessive cell membrane in relation to the amount of hemoglobin. They are seen in a variety of clinical conditions, especially in various hemoglobin abnormalities and in chronic liver disease.

*Spherocyte (Fig. 12-44).* Spherocytes are red cells that are not biconcave; instead, they appear round or spherical because of the loss of a portion of the cell membrane. As a result, they are small cells, usually less than 6 μm in diameter, and are often called *microspherocytes.* They appear hyperchromic, staining a uniform intense orange-red because of the lack of central pallor, a result of the round shape. Spherocytes are characteristic of certain hemolytic anemias, both hereditary (hereditary spherocytosis) and acquired (e.g., drug induced) and are associated with the presence of polychromasia and an increased reticulocyte count.

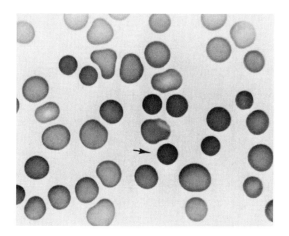

**FIG 12-44.** Spherocytes as at arrow. (×1000.)

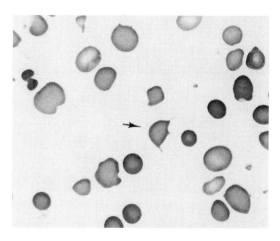

**FIG 12-45.** Schiztocytes (fragmented cells). The arrow indicates a helmet cell. (×1000.)

***Stomatocyte.*** Stomatocytes show a slit-like or mouth-like, rather than round, area of central pallor on the blood film. They are not biconcave, but are bowl shaped, or concave on only one side. They are often found in chronic liver disease.

***Schistocyte (Fragmented Cell, Helmet Cell) (Fig. 12-45).*** Schistocytes have a variety of names and forms, depending on what is left after the cell is physically fragmented. *Helmet cells* are small triangular cells with one or two pointed ends that resemble a helmet. Schistocytosis is a very serious pathologic condition. It may be the result of mechanical fracture of cells as they pass through the circulatory system, as on filaments of fibrin resulting from disseminated intravascular coagulation (DIC) or on artificial heart valves. Schistocytes are also seen in cases of severe burns. The fragmentation may also be the result of toxic or metabolic injury, as seen with certain malignancies. Schistocytes are characteristic of microangiopathic hemolytic anemias, and their presence is a danger signal requiring immediate action by the physician.

***Teardrop Cell (Dacryocyte).*** These are pear-shaped or teardrop-shaped red cells with an elongated point or tail at one end (see Fig. 12-40). They may be the result of the cell squeez-ing and subsequently fracturing as it passes through the spleen.

***Burr Cell, Crenated (Echinocyte).*** Burr cells or echinocytes are red cells with scalloped, spicular, or spiny projections regularly distributed around the cell membrane (see Fig. 12-40). They can usually revert back to normal cells. The term *crenated* is sometimes reserved for artifactual spicular cells, such as artifacts that result when the blood film is not adequately dried.

***Acanthocyte (Spike Cell, Acanthoid Cell).*** Acanthocytes are similar to echinocytes, but their spiny projections are irregularly distributed around the cell membrane. They are not artifacts and cannot revert to normal cells. They are related to and may occur with schistocytes, and represent serious pathologic conditions.

***Keratocyte (Horn Cell).*** Keratocytes are shaped like a half-moon or spindle. They have a relatively normal cell volume but have been deformed so that they appear to have two or more spicules.

### Alterations in Erythrocyte Structure and Inclusions

***Basophilic Stippling (Fig. 12-46).*** The presence of dark blue granules evenly distributed throughout the red cell is called **basophilic stip-**

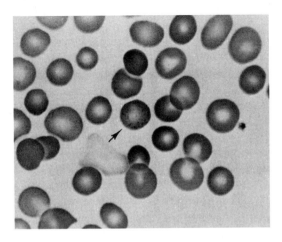

**FIG 12-46.** Basophilic stippling in cell at arrow. (×1000.)

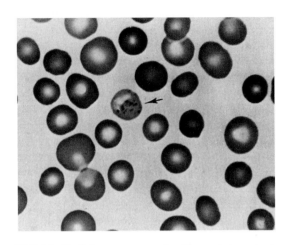

**FIG 12-47.** Siderosome granules (Pappenheimer bodies) in cell at arrow. (×1000.)

**pling.** The stippling may be very fine or dot-like, or it may be coarse and larger. The stippled cell may resemble the polychromatic red cell; however, these are actual granules, not just an overall blueness. Stippling does not exist in the circulating red cell but results from precipitation of ribosomes and RNA in the staining process. However, the stippling is not an artifact in the clinical sense, as it may indicate abnormal red cell formation in the marrow, as in thalassemia minor, megaloblastic anemia, and lead poisoning.

*Siderocytes, Pappenheimer Body (Fig. 12-47).* These are cells containing small, dense, blue-purple granules of free iron, uncombined with hemoglobin. Usually only one or two of these granules are present in a cell, and they are located in the cell periphery. They may be confused with Howell-Jolly bodies and can be distinguished and seen better with a specific stain for iron, such as Prussian blue. When sidero-somes are stained with Wright stain, they are sometimes called *Pappenheimer bodies.* They are rarely seen in peripheral blood except after removal of the spleen.

*Howell-Jolly Body (Fig. 12-48).* Howell-Jolly bodies are round, densely staining purple granules that stain like dense nuclear chromatin.

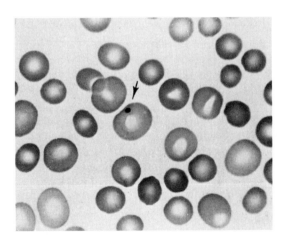

**FIG 12-48.** Howell-Jolly body shown in cell at arrow. (×1000.)

Usually only one or two such bodies are seen in the red cells. They are eccentrically located in the red cell and less than 1 µm in diameter. Howell-Jolly bodies are remnants of the red cell nucleus, and thus are DNA. Under normal conditions they are derived from nuclear fragmentation (karyorrhexis) or incomplete expulsion of the nucleus in the later stages of red cell maturation and are thought to be aberrant chromosomes in certain abnormal conditions. These nuclear remnants are normally removed from the reticulocytes in the peripheral blood by a pitting process as they pass through the spleen. Therefore, they are seen in peripheral blood after removal of the spleen, and also in cases of abnormal red cell formation such as megaloblastic anemias and some hemolytic anemias.

*Cabot's Rings.* These are threadlike red-violet strands occurring in ring, twisted, or figure-of-8 shapes in reticulocytes. Cabot's rings are rare. Their origin is unknown, but they are thought to result from abnormal red cell formation during mitosis and can be seen in megaloblastic anemias and lead poisoning.

*Parasitized Red Cell (Malarial) (Fig. 12-49).* In cases of malaria, various stages of the malaria parasites may be seen in the red cells. Depending on the species of malaria organism present, the parasites may appear as, and be confused with, Cabot's ring bodies, basophilic stippling, or platelets lying on top of red cells (Fig. 12-50).

### Erythrocyte Artifacts and Abnormal Distribution Patterns

*Platelet on Top of Erythrocyte (See Fig. 12-50).* When platelets lie on top of red cells in the blood film, they may be confused with inclusions, especially the trophozoite stage of malaria organisms. In such cases, the overlying platelets should be compared with those in the surrounding field.

*Crenation.* Crenated cells on the blood film appear like echinocytes, with scalloped, spicular, or spiny projections regularly distributed around the cell surface. These crenated cells are an artifact resulting from incorrect preparation of the blood film, usually failure to dry it adequately.

*Punched-Out Red Cells (Fig. 12-51).* Red cells with a punched-out appearance rather than a normal area of central pallor are also drying artifacts. They should not be confused with hypochromic red cells. The remaining cell shows a normal staining reaction with this artifact.

*Rouleaux (Fig. 12-52).* Rouleaux represent an

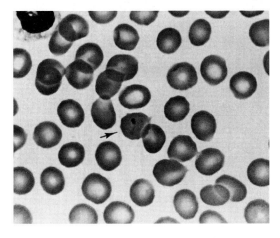

**FIG 12-49.** Parasitized red cell (malarial) shown at arrow. Compare with Fig. 12-50.

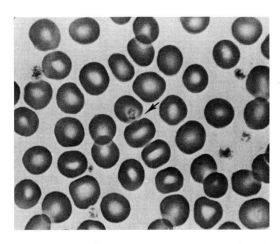

**FIG 12-50.** Platelet on top of red cell *(arrow).* (×1000.)

abnormal distribution pattern of red cells, which stick together or become aligned in aggregates that look like stacks of coins. This arrangement is a typical artifact in the thick area of blood films. It is clinically significant when found in the normal examination area and associated with elevated plasma fibrinogen or globulin with a corresponding increase in the ESR, as in multiple myeloma.

*Agglutination.* Agglutination, irregular or amorphous clumping of red cells in the blood

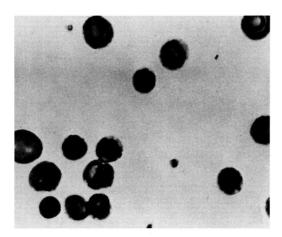

**FIG 12-51.** Drying artifact in red cells showing punched-out appearance. (×1000.)

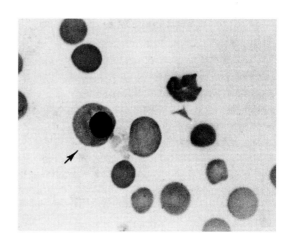

**FIG 12-53.** Nucleated red cell (normoblast) in peripheral blood *(arrow)*. (×1000.)

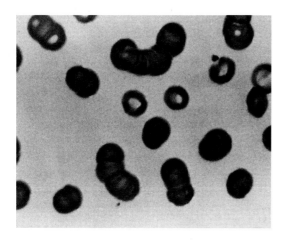

**FIG 12-52.** Rouleau formation, an abnormal distribution pattern. Drying artifact is also present. (×1000.)

film, represents another alteration in red cell distribution. Clinically, this may be caused by the presence of a cold agglutinin (antibody) in the patient's serum and may indicate an autoimmune hemolytic state or anemia.

**Nucleated Red Cells in the Peripheral Blood (Fig. 12-53).** Normally, red cells do not enter the blood until the reticulocyte stage of maturation, just after extrusion of the shrunken nucleus. Therefore, the presence of earlier nucle-

ated forms of red cells in the peripheral blood is abnormal. It indicates intense marrow stimulation, such as that seen in acute blood loss, megaloblastic anemias, or pathologic conditions associated with various malignancies. The presence of nucleated red cells is termed an *erythroblastotic* reaction.

Cells in the later stages of maturation are most often present, so the cytoplasm is orange-red because the cells contain hemoglobin. However, the nucleus is also present, although shrunken and dark blue in color. Earlier forms may occur and may be difficult to distinguish from small lymphocytes or plasma cells; the presence of pink in the red cell cytoplasm is helpful in such cases. The presence of nucleated red cell forms in the peripheral blood is characteristic of megaloblastic anemias. In these cases the young red cells are larger (macrocytic) and tend to have a more open chromatin pattern than corresponding stages of normocytic red cells (dyssynchrony of nucleus and cytoplasm maturation).

It is important to remember that the white cell count must be corrected when nucleated red cells are observed in the peripheral blood film, as these cells are counted as white cells when present.

## Leukocyte Alterations

In the examination of peripheral blood, leukocytes are studied for alterations in both quantity (number) and quality (morphology).

Quantitative changes in leukocytes are measured by the white cell count—the actual number of leukocytes in a certain volume of blood. A white cell count above normal is *leukocytosis*; a count below normal is *leukopenia*. There can also be increases or decreases in number of any of the five types of white cells that are enumerated collectively in the white cell count, and such changes are measured by the white cell differential. Quantitative changes in any of the cell types are described by the following terms: neutrophilia (increase), neutropenia (decrease); eosinophilia, eosinopenia; basophilia, basopenia; lymphocytosis, lymphopenia; and monocytosis, monocytopenia.

In addition, these increases or decreases may be relative or absolute (see Reporting Leukocyte Differential Results (Relative and Absolute Counts). If the change is *absolute*, the particular cell type shows a numerical increase or decrease from its normal concentration in the blood. If it is *relative*, there is an alteration (either high or low) of the percentage of the particular cell type as determined in the leukocyte differential, while the numerical concentration is within normal values. Finally, there may be both an absolute and a relative change when both the percentage and the numerical values are above or below normal.

Qualitative or morphologic alterations in circulating leukocytes may be described in terms of a *shift to the left,* referring to the presence of younger or more immature cell forms than are normally found in the peripheral blood. Such changes may be found within any cell line, including erythrocytes. The presence of younger forms of leukocytes in the blood may be termed a *leukoblastotic reaction.* Since they often occur along with younger or nucleated red cell forms, the term **leukoerythroblastotic reaction** is also used.

Most alterations in leukocyte morphology can be classified as (1) toxic or reactive changes, (2) anomalous changes, or (3) leukemic or other malignant changes.

### Toxic or Reactive Leukocyte Alterations

*Toxic changes.* These changes are seen in neutrophils and are generally associated with a bacterial infection or a toxic reaction. They are seen on a blood film as toxic granulation, vacuolization, hypersegmentation (hyperlobulation), a shift to the left, the presence of Döhle bodies, increased or decreased cell size, degeneration or pyknosis of the nucleus, and karyolysis (dissolution of the nucleus).

*Reactive alterations.* Reactive alterations are particularly characteristic of lymphocytes. **Reactive lymphocytes** can be seen in viral infections and are often associated with infectious mononucleosis, although many other conditions produce reactive cell forms. Changes generally include increased cytoplasmic basophilia with or without radial or peripheral localization, increased or decreased cytoplasmic volume, increased coarse azurophilic granulation, and alterations in the nuclear chromatin, which becomes either loose, delicate, and reticular, or dark, heavy, and clumped. These changes will be defined further later in this section.

**Anomalous Changes.** An anomaly is a deviation from the common rule, or an irregularity. Hematologic deviations from normal may be congenital or acquired. Leukocyte anomalies are described later in this section.

**Malignant or Leukemic Changes.** The hematologic malignancies include a large and varied group of diseases, which are well beyond the scope of this book. However, some general comments and descriptions follow. The hematologic malignancies may be classified as (1) acute myelocytic leukemias, (2) chronic myeloproliferative disorders (which include chronic myelogenous leukemia), (3) acute lymphocytic leukemias, and (4) chronic lymphoproliferative disorders (including chronic lymphocytic leukemia and the lymphomas).

*Leukemia* is a disease of the blood-forming tissues that is an abnormal, uncontrolled proliferation of one or more of the various hematopoietic cells that progressively displaces normal cellular elements. There are usually, but not always, qualitative changes in the affected cells.

The exact cause of leukemia is not known. There is evidence to suggest hereditary factors and genetic predisposition. Environmental causes have also been cited, especially exposure to gamma radiation, producing genetic mutations or chromosome damage such as the Philadelphia chromosome seen in chronic myelogenous leukemia (CML). Various chemicals and drugs have also been implicated, and viruses have been shown to be related to leukemia in mice and other animals. The chronic myeloproliferative disorders are a group of myeloid neoplasms in which there is a malignant clonal proliferation of predominantly myeloid cells in the marrow and blood. These may be cells of the granulocytic, erythrocytic, or megakaryocytic cell lines. Diseases include chronic myelogenous leukemia (neutrophilic), polycythemia vera (erythrocytic), and essential thrombocythemia (megakaryocytic).

Leukemias are classified as acute or chronic on the basis of clinical course (prognosis) and the number of blasts present. Acute leukemias usually occur with sudden onset. There is usually anemia, which is normocytic and normochromic and which increases as the disease progresses. The platelet count is low to markedly decreased. The leukocyte count varies but is usually moderately to markedly elevated—with 50.0 to 100.0 $\times$ 10$^9$/L being not uncommon—although the count may be normal or even decreased. Blast cells are present in the peripheral blood film; generally, more than 60% blasts indicates an acute leukemic process. The bone marrow is hypercellular and consists predominantly of blast cells. Untreated acute leukemias can lead to death within 2 to 3 months. Death is often the result of hemorrhage, which increases in severity as the platelet count falls below 20.0 $\times$ 10$^9$/L, or infection, which re-

sults as the granulocyte count falls below 1.5 $\times$ 10$^9$/L. Treatment includes chemotherapy, transfusion therapy, and bone marrow transplantation.

Chronic leukemias (myeloproliferative or lymphoproliferative disorders) begin slowly and insidiously and may exist for a long time without symptoms. Symptoms develop slowly and include fatigue, night sweats, weight loss, and fever. Anemia usually develops late in the disease, but hemolytic anemia may develop as the disease progresses. The platelet count is usually normal and may even increase in chronic myelogenous leukemia; however, in the later stages both thrombocytopenia and anemia usually occur. The white cell count is usually markedly increased, often higher than 100.0 $\times$ 10$^9$/L, but it can be normal or even decreased. Morphologically, fewer than 10% myeloblasts will be seen in the peripheral blood in chronic myelogenous leukemias, and the blood tends to look like bone marrow, as it contains all granulocyte developmental stages plus basophilia, an important finding. In chronic lymphocytic leukemia (CLL), very few to no lymphoblasts are seen in the peripheral blood. The blood characteristically shows a monotonous picture of lymphocytes that are all similar in size and morphology. In addition, many damaged or basket cells may be present, as the lymphocytes tend to be fragile. The average length of survival for patients with CML is relatively short, 3 to 4 years. CLL has an average survival of about 10 years, although prolonged survival for up to 35 years is possible, and about 30% of the patients die of causes unrelated to the disease. Infection is the most common cause of death related to CLL. CML tends to proceed to an acute or accelerated stage called a blast crisis, and patients eventually die of hemorrhage or infection, as in acute leukemia.

Leukemias are classified morphologically as lymphocytic (or lymphoid) and myelogenous (or myeloid ). The youngest cell forms or blasts common to these leukemias are the lymphoblast and the myeloblast, respectively. It may be impossible to distinguish between the myeloblast and the lymphoblast morphologically, especially in the most serious or acute forms of the disease, when only blast forms are seen in the blood. The presence of *Auer rods* (rods or granules of lysosomal material, an azurophilic substance) in the cytoplasm is diagnostic of the myeloblast. However, Auer rods are not seen in all cases of myelogenous leukemia. Other considerations in the differentiation of myeloblasts and lymphoblasts are the nucleocytoplasmic ratio, the number of nucleoli, and the nuclear chromatin pattern. However, such differences are often inconclusive and may be misleading. If more mature cells are present, they may aid in the morphologic identification.

Although, traditionally, morphologic criteria are used to classify leukemias, the use of cytochemical and histochemical staining techniques and immunologic markers now makes it possible to identify abnormal hematopoietic precursors with more assurance. A testing battery of special studies using staining and immunologic methods is employed as part of the complete workup for a patient with leukemia. Tests for myeloperoxidase activity using Sudan black stain, leukocyte alkaline phosphatase activity, TdT enzyme activity, nonspecific and specific esterase activity, and the periodic acid–Schiff (PAS) reaction for lymphoblast granules are included in these special studies. These tests are used to classify the acute leukemias in the French-American-British (FAB) system.

Leukemia can occur at any age, but certain forms appear to be age related. CLL is generally a disease of later adult years (generally over 50 years of age). Treatment is usually only for complications of the disease. ALL is generally a disease of children under 10 years of age (seldom over 20 years) and peaks between the ages of 3 and 7. ALL is the most prevalent form of malignancy in children. Bone marrow transplantation with chemotherapy is especially useful in treatment of this type of leukemia. Chronic myelogenous leukemia (CML) usually occurs between the ages of 20 and 50. Chemotherapy is com-

monly used to suppress the proliferation of leukemic cells. Other treatment includes symptom-related administration of antibiotics and transfusions. Remissions are usually shorter than in ALL and are more difficult to achieve. Acute myelogenous leukemia (AML) occurs at all ages, but is primarily a disease of middle age. Treatment can include platelet transfusions for thrombocytopenia, antibiotics for infection, chemotherapy to inhibit the proliferation of the leukemic cells, and bone marrow transplantation. Survival rates and prognosis are less encouraging than in ALL.

**Other Malignant Changes.** Malignant hematologic conditions other than leukemia include plasma cell dyscrasias (multiple myeloma, primary macroglobulinemia, and Fc fragment or heavy chain disease), Hodgkin's disease (or malignant lymphoma, Hodgkin's type), non-Hodgkin's malignant lymphomas, and some unusual tumors closely resembling hematologic malignancies.

The laboratory has a significant role in the diagnosis and management or treatment of patients with these various hematologic diseases. Many laboratory procedures will be requested, such as cell and platelet counts, tests for the presence of anemia, coagulation studies, white cell differential count, blood film examination, cytochemical and histochemical stains, immunologic tests, and preparation and selection of appropriate blood products for transfusion therapy.

Again, the actual examination of the blood film in cases of such altered and complex morphology is left to the trained hematologist. Such changes should be recognized as abnormal during routine screening of blood films and referred to the pathologist or technologist with special training.

To identify changes in leukocyte morphology, the cells should be examined for the following features:

1. Nuclear chromatin pattern
2. Nuclear shape

3. Size and number of nucleoli, when present
4. Cytoplasmic inclusions
5. Nucleocytoplasmic ratio

Various alterations in leukocyte morphology are described and illustrated below.

### Morphologic Alterations in Leukocytes: Description

#### Granulocyte Alterations

*Toxic Granulation (Fig. 12-54).* Toxic granules are deeply staining basophilic or blue-black larger-than-normal granules found in the cytoplasm of neutrophils, bands, and metamyelocytes. They resemble the primary granules seen in the promyelocyte, an early developmental stage of the neutrophil. Their presence is associated with acute bacterial infections, drug poisoning, and burns.

*Döhle Bodies.* These are round or oval, small, clear light blue staining areas found in the neutrophil cytoplasm. They are remnants of cytoplasmic RNA from an earlier stage of neutrophil development. They are often seen together with toxic granulation in infections, in burns, after administration of toxic agents, and in pregnancy.

*Toxic Vacuolization.* Vacuoles are also signs of toxic change and imply the occurrence of phagocytosis. Sites of digestion of phagocytized material are seen as vacuoles in the cytoplasm of neutrophils and bands, and vacuoles are often found in association with toxic granulation.

*Hypersegmentation of Nucleus.* Neutrophils that are hypersegmented contain six or more lobes in their nuclei. They are characteristic of the megaloblastic anemias of vitamin $B_{12}$ and folic acid deficiency and have been called pernicious anemia (or PA) neutrophils. The megaloblastic neutrophil is larger than the normal neutrophil (all cell types are larger in the megaloblastic process).

*Barr Bodies.* A Barr body is a small knob attached to or projecting from a lobe of the neutrophil nucleus and consisting of the same nuclear chromatin or substance. It is often referred to as the sex chromatin or sex chromosome, as it is seen in some of the neutrophils of normal females and is thought to be an inactivated X chromosome.

*Auer Rods (Bodies) (Fig. 12-55).* Auer rods or bodies are slender, rod-shaped or needle-shaped bodies found in the cytoplasm that stain reddish purple (like azurophilic gran-

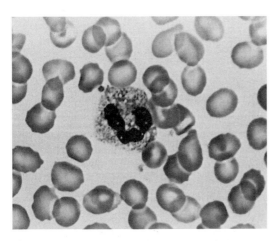

**FIG 12-54.** Neutrophil showing toxic changes (toxic granules, vacuoles, Döhle bodies).

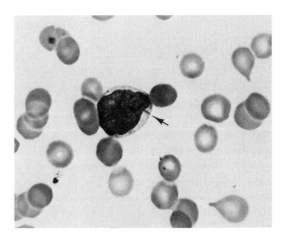

**FIG 12-55.** Auer rod in myeloblast. ($\times$1000.)

ules). They are composed of lysosomal material and fused primary granules. They are found only in the cytoplasm of myeloblasts or promyelocytes and are considered diagnostic in distinguishing myeloblastic from lymphoblastic leukemias.

### Anomalous Changes

***Pelger-Huet Anomaly.*** This anomaly is seen as a failure of the granulocyte nucleus to segment or form lobes normally. The neutrophil nuclei are band shaped or at most have two lobes in this condition. In addition, the chromatin is quite coarsely clumped. This is a benign anomaly that can be inherited or acquired. In its acquired form, it is known as pseudo-Pelger-Huet anomaly.

***Chediak-Higashi Anomaly.*** Large amorphous granules are observed in the neutrophil cytoplasm; granules are also seen in the lymphocyte and monocyte cytoplasm. The disease is inherited and rare. It has been treated with marrow transplantation.

***May-Hegglin Anomaly.*** These blue inclusion bodies are similar to the Döhle bodies present in neutrophils but are usually larger and have more sharply defined borders. Platelets may be decreased in number, but some giant forms can be present. The disorder is inherited, and most patients have no clinical symptoms.

***Alder-Reilly Anomaly.*** Heavy dark azurophilic granulation is observed in neutrophils, eosinophils, basophils, and sometimes lymphocytes and monocytes. This anomaly is inherited and is often associated with mucopolysaccharidoses.

### Lymphocyte Alterations

***Variant Lymphocytes (Reactive or Atypical Lymphocytes) (Fig. 12-56).*** Reactive, atypical, or variant lymphocytes (also called transformed lymphocytes or virocytes) are particularly associated with infectious mononucleosis; however, many other viral infections also show such alterations. They generally show the different stages of immune responsiveness of B and T lymphocytes in the peripheral blood and im-

mune system. In general, the cytoplasm increases in amount and appears to be reacting to a stimulus. Although the cells have been more specifically classified morphologically, they tend to have one or several of the following characteristics:

The cytoplasm tends to become more intensely blue in color (cytoplasmic basophilia). The basophilia tends to be localized, either peripherally, with an increased blue color around the outer edge of the cell, or radially, with areas of blueness radiating from the more central nucleus to the outer edges of the cell like spokes of a wheel. Radial and peripheral basophilia may be combined, in which case the cell is described as resembling a fried egg or a flared skirt. The reactive cell may also show increases or decreases in cytoplasmic volume. Cells with increased cytoplasmic volume, when observed on films prepared with Wright stain, tend to show indentations by adjacent structures, especially RBCs. The cytoplasm appears to be flowing around and almost engulfing such structures. The cells also tend to have an increased number of nonspecific azurophilic granules in the cytoplasm.

Reactive or atypical lymphocytes also show nuclear changes. There is generally a sharper

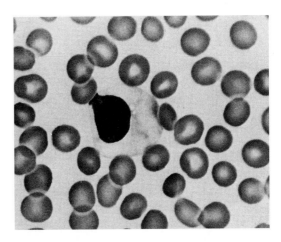

**FIG 12-56.** Reactive, atypical, or variant lymphocyte. (×1000.)

separation of chromatin and parachromatin. The nucleus may become loose and delicate, resembling an earlier developmental stage; this is referred to as a reticular appearance—hence the term reticular lymphocyte. In other cases, the nucleus becomes oval or kidney shaped with heavy clumps of deeply stained chromatin; these are called plasmacytoid changes, since the cells resemble plasma cells.

The reactive lymphocyte may resemble the lymphoblast, and it may be necessary to rule out a leukemic process in such cases of reactive lymphocytosis.

*Turk Cells.* These are darkly staining cells having plasmacytoid characteristics. They are classified as atypical lymphocytes or plasma cells by different authors and are associated with viral infections.

*Smudge or Basket Cells (Fig. 12-57).* These are damaged white cells. They are cellular fragments consisting of battered or frayed nuclei with no cytoplasmic material. Basket cells are not counted as part of the white cell differential, and a few damaged cells are encountered in most peripheral blood films. They are not significant unless present in large numbers. They may be associated with CLL, and in some cases of CLL and acute leukemias the number of basket

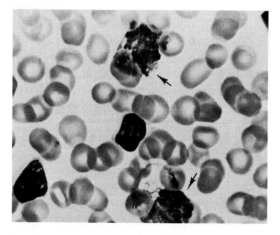

**FIG 12-57.** Smudge or basket cells *(arrows).* Lymphocytes are also present. (×1000.)

cells may be greater than the usual lymphocyte count.

## ADDITIONAL HEMATOLOGY PROCEDURES

Thus far, the procedures and material discussed have been part of what is often included in the so-called complete blood count. Two additional procedures will now be discussed. These are frequently performed in the clinical laboratory, but are not part of the CBC.

### Reticulocyte Counts

Reticulocytes are young red cells that have matured enough to have lost their nuclei but not their cytoplasmic RNA. They do not have the full amount of hemoglobin. The number of reticulocytes is a measure of the regeneration or production of RBCs. Reticulocytes appear in a blood film stained with Wright stain as polychromatic RBCs because of the basophilic cytoplasmic remnant of the immature red cell RNA.

### *Normal Erythropoiesis and Reticulocytes*

In the circulating blood 0.5% to 1.5% of the red cells are usually reticulocytes. This is based on a normal red cell life span of 120 ± 20 days and a normal red cell count necessitating replacement of approximately 1% of the adult circulating red cells each day. The range represents technical or counting errors in the method. A reticulocyte count above this level (reticulocytosis) is clinically significant, indicating that the body is attempting to meet an increased need for red cells. Such an increase in reticulocytes is observed when red cells are being hemolyzed within the body. Thus, increased reticulocyte counts and polychromasia are characteristic of the hemolytic anemias. The bone marrow sends out red cells at an increased rate until only the younger cells are available to be released, although increased red cell production is probably taking place at the same time. The demand may be so great in some instances that nucleated red cells are sent from the bone marrow.

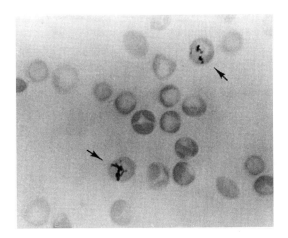

**FIG 12-58.** Reticulocytes stained with new methylene blue *(arrows)*. (×1000.)

## Clinical Uses for Reticulocyte Counts

The reticulocyte count is used to follow therapeutic measures for anemias in which the patient is deficient in, or lacking, one of the substances essential for manufacturing red cells. When the deficiency has been diagnosed, therapy is begun. This consists of supplying the missing essential substances to the body and waiting for the body to react by increasing red cell production. New red cells will be released rapidly into the circulating blood, many before they are fully matured, in response to therapy. The corresponding increase in the reticulocyte count indicates a favorable response to therapy. The response to therapy in iron deficiency anemia (treated with iron) and pernicious anemia (treated with vitamin $B_{12}$) is followed by reticulocyte counts. As the total red cell count and the hemoglobin concentration reach normal levels, red cell regeneration slows to the normal rate, allowing more time for maturation of the red cells in the bone marrow. This is indicated by the presence of fewer reticulocytes in the circulating blood.

## Specimen Requirements

Anticoagulated whole blood or capillary blood from the finger, toe, or heel may be used. Venous blood should be anticoagulated with EDTA. Heparinized blood should be avoided, as the staining quality is poor. If anticoagulated whole blood is used, the test should be performed within 1 or 2 hours after the specimen is drawn, as cells will continue to mature in the test tube, resulting in a decreased percent of reticulocytes seen.

### Manual Methods for Counting Reticulocytes

RNA content can be detected in reticulocytes by exposing the living cells to a supravital stain. Manual methods for preparing reticulocyte slides for counts require supravital staining of the red cells, whether the end result is a dry film or not. In supravital staining the living blood cells are mixed with the stain, as opposed to making a film and staining it. One method consists of spreading the stain on the slide and drying it; the blood is then added to the dried stain and mixed, and the usual blood smear is prepared. Another method uses the same slide preparation, but the stain is mixed with a drop of blood and cover-slipped, and the mixture is sealed on the slide and viewed in the liquid form under the microscope. A third method (described in this book) is to mix blood and stain in a small test tube, allow time for the staining reaction to occur, and then prepare a blood film from the mixture; the prepared blood film is then viewed microscopically (Procedure 12-7). In some procedures the resulting film is counterstained with Wright stain, using the method previously described. This is not an essential step, and it may be omitted, as in the procedure to be described here. Such counterstaining with Wright stain may be helpful in differentiating basophilic stippling and Howell-Jolly bodies from reticular RNA. The first two methods described employ an alcoholic solution of the dye; the third method uses a saline solution.

**Dyes Used to Stain Reticulocytes Using Manual Methods.** New methylene blue (NMB) or brilliant cresyl blue is used for the staining of reticulocytes. New methylene blue dye is pre-

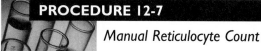

## PROCEDURE 12-7

### *Manual Reticulocyte Count*

1. Add two drops of blood (capillary or venous) to three drops of NMB stain in a small test tube. If the hemoglobin is low, add another drop of blood to ensure proper staining and good films.

2. Mix the blood and dye thoroughly and allow to stand for 15 minutes.

3. Resuspend the cells by mixing well, and prepare at least three thin films on glass microscope slides. Use small drops of the blood-stain mixture, and the usual procedure for making blood films. Dry the films completely and rapidly.

4. When the films are dry, count the reticulocytes.

5. Count a total of 1,000 erythrocytes (500 on each of two slides), using the oil-immersion (100×) objective, in an area of the smear considered to be medium thin, where the erythrocytes are well distributed and not touching (about 100 cells per oil-immersion field).

6. Count 1,000 erythrocytes, including the reticulocytes seen in this count; tally and record reticulocytes separately. Record the number of reticulocytes on each of the slides separately in order to compare the distribution of reticulocytes.

7. Reticulocytes appear as greenish blue cells, with the reticulum showing as a deep blue network of strands or granules within the cells (Fig. 12-58).

8. If the two slides counted do not agree within 5 cells when the reticulocyte count is 3% or less (30 reticulocytes per 1,000 cells), count another 500 cells on a third slide. If agreement within 5 cells cannot be achieved after counting all three slides, repeat the procedure with new slides. If the reticulocyte count is greater than 3%, a reasonable difference between the counts on the two slides is allowable. This will be determined by the quality assurance system of the laboratory and is somewhat dependent on the experience of the person performing the procedure.

9. It is essential to focus the microscope carefully and continually when reticulocytes are being counted. The dye will stain platelet granules and leukocyte granules, and these or precipitated stain may be mistaken for reticulocytes. Inadequate drying will cause the red cells to contain highly refractile areas resembling remnants of RNA. Artifacts in red cells must not be confused with reticulocytes.

10. Report the reticulocyte count as a percentage of the total number of erythrocytes counted. However, more meaningful results are attained by correcting the reticulocyte count for the patient's hematocrit and for red cells prematurely released by the marrow, as indicated by the presence of "shift cells."

ferred. It gives consistent results and a sharp blue staining of the RNA reticulum. In addition to the dye, the stain should contain an ingredient to preserve the red cells (provide an isotonic condition). The method to be described in this section requires that the stain prevent coagulation. Brilliant cresyl blue contains sodium citrate, which prevents coagulation, and sodium chloride, which provides isotonicity. New methylene blue contains sodium oxalate, which prevents coagulation, and sodium chloride. These supravital dyes precipitate the RNA in the reticulocytes, coloring it blue.

### Preparation of New Methylene Blue Stain.
Dilute 0.50 g of new methylene blue (NMB) (color index 52030), 0.70 g of NaCl (CP grade), and 0.13 g of sodium oxalate (CP grade) to 100 mL with deionized water. Mix for at least 15 minutes, filter, and store at room temperature. Filter immediately before using.

### Calculations for Manual Reticulocyte Count.
The reticulocyte count is reported as the percentage of reticulocytes in the total red cells counted. The following general formula can be used:

$$\frac{\text{Reticulocytes}}{\text{RBCs}} \times 100 = \% \text{ reticulocytes}$$

This formula can be derived from a simple proportion relating the number of reticulocytes counted in a given number of red cells to the number of reticulocytes per 100 red cells, which is the percentage of reticulocytes. *Example:* On each of two slides, 500 red cells are counted. The first slide shows 16 reticulocytes, and the second shows 20 reticulocytes. What is the percentage of reticulocytes in the blood?

$$500 + 500 = 1,000 \text{ cells counted}$$
$$20 + 16 = 36 \text{ reticulocytes per 1,000 cells counted}$$
$$\frac{36 \text{ reticulocytes}}{1,000 \text{ cells}} = \frac{x}{100 \text{ cells}}$$
$$x = \frac{36 \times 100}{1,000} = 3.6 \text{ reticulocytes per 100 cells}$$
$$= 3.6\% \text{ reticulocytes}$$

## Reporting Reticulocyte Results

The classic reporting unit for the reticulocyte count is percent reticulocytes, based on counting 1,000 erythrocytes, reticulocytes included. The reference values vary from 0.9% to 2.0% for adults, with a 2% to 10% accuracy for manually counted cells.

**Absolute Reticulocyte Count.** There is a relation between the percentage of reticulocytes calculated and the total erythrocyte count. A meaningful reticulocyte count should indicate the total production of erythrocytes, regardless of the concentration of erythrocytes in the blood. The reticulocyte count can also be reported as an absolute value by multiplying the reticulocyte count in percent by the total red cell count. This reporting method provides a comparable basis for following the progress or treatment of anemias and is the preferred way of reporting reticulocyte values.

**Reticulocyte Count Corrected for a Low Hematocrit (Anemia).** Since a decreased hematocrit and an increased reticulocyte count ratio can exaggerate the red cell production response, the reticulocyte count can be corrected for the degree of anemia present by application of a factor involving hematocrit values. The patient's hematocrit is compared with a normal hematocrit (considered to be 42% for women and 45% for men) and then related to the patient's reticulocyte count as shown below:

$$\text{Corrected reticulocyte count (\%)} =$$
$$\text{Patient's reticulocyte count (\%)} \times \frac{\text{Patient's Hct}}{\text{Normal Hct}}$$

**Reticulocyte Production Index.** The use of this correction compensates for the amount of time it takes for reticulocytes to mature in the peripheral blood, especially for instances in which the anemia is severe and the subsequent erythropoietic response involves early release of red cells from the bone marrow. A reticulocyte production index factor can be applied to correct the reticulocyte count for abnormally early release of red cells from the marrow into the peripheral blood. Premature release of cells from the marrow does not necessarily indicate increased marrow production. Abnormally early release of the red cells from the marrow into the peripheral blood is indicated by the presence of nucleated RBCs or polychromatic macrocytes, also known as **"shift cells,"** on blood films prepared with Wright stain. Reticulocytes normally spend approximately 2 to 3 days in the bone marrow before being released into the blood, and approximately 1% of the circulating red cells are replaced each day. When the hematocrit and the rate of marrow release are normal, the apparent reticulocyte percentage may be considered an index of production, or maturation, and set equal to 1.

Normal reticulocyte production index = 1

However, if reticulocytes are being released directly into the blood before maturation in the marrow, as evidenced by the presence of nucleated forms or shift cells on the blood film, the count is corrected by dividing the apparent reticulocyte count by 2 (the usual number of days of maturation).

If the presence of polychromatic red cells is observed on a Wright-stained blood film, a reticulocyte production index factor must be applied. The maturation time, in days, for the reticulocyte is as follows[6]:

| Maturation Factor (Days) | Hematocrit (% Units) |
|---|---|
| 1 | 45 |
| 1.5 | 35 |
| 2 | 25 |
| 3 | 15 |

The corrected reticulocyte count is referred to as the reticulocyte production index. If no nucleated cells or shift cells are seen in the blood, the reticulocyte count is divided by 1 (i.e., left unchanged).

When there is both an abnormally low hematocrit and shift cells on the blood film, both corrections should be applied to the apparent reticulocyte count. The following general formula can be used:

Reticulocyte production index

$$= \frac{1}{2}\left[\text{Patient's reticulocyte count (\%)} \times \frac{\text{Patient's Hct}}{\text{Normal Hct}}\right]$$

The factor $\frac{1}{2}$ represents division by a maturation factor of 2. The maturation factor can vary, depending on the severity of the anemia. Marrow can respond to anemia by a twofold to fivefold increase in red cell production.

### Precautions and Technical Factors When Counting Reticulocytes Manually

Careful focusing of the microscope is essential when reticulocytes are being counted. Stained platelet granules and leukocyte granules must not be mistaken for reticulocytes. Precipitated stain might also be mistaken for reticulum within the erythrocytes. To minimize this possibility, the dye must be filtered immediately before use. Immediate drying of the film will prevent the formation of the crystalline-like artifacts that sometimes appear in the red cell and resemble remnants of RNA.

The proportions of dye and blood must be altered if the patient is anemic. More blood must be used. If the procedure is followed carefully, the distribution of reticulocytes on the blood films will be good. With experience, the problem of agreement will be primarily a result of the distribution of reticulocytes on the films and not misidentification of reticulocytes. Reticulocytes have a lower specific gravity than mature red cells and rise to the top of a blood-stain mixture. Therefore, the specimen must be well mixed before the incubation period and immediately before the three slides are made. The slides must be made in a uniform fashion to ensure random sampling.

Procedures employed for reticulocyte counts vary in different clinical laboratories, although the principles are the same. Variations include the manner in which the stain and cells are mixed, the total number of red cells counted and the number of slides observed, the use of a

Miller disk in the eyepiece of the microscope to help define the field to be counted, counterstaining of the reticulocyte film with Wright stain, and the use of corrections for the patient's hematocrit and the presence of shift cells.

### Automated Reticulocyte Counts

With the use of an automated procedure, the process of counting reticulocytes is very much enhanced. The flow cytometry principle is employed, cells are stained with a fluorochrome dye that preferentially stains RNA, and the cells are counted by a fluorescent technique. The RNA-containing reticulocytes will fluoresce when exposed to ultraviolet light. The instrument can count thousands of reticulocytes in just a few seconds with an accuracy of about 0.1%.

### Reference Values*

*Reticulocytes:*

| | |
|---|---|
| Adult male | 1.1%-2.1% |
| Adult female | 0.9%-1.9% |

Absolute reticulocyte count: $50 \times 10^9/L$

## Erythrocyte Sedimentation Rate

If blood is prevented from clotting (by using a suitable anticoagulant) and allowed to settle, sedimentation of the erythrocytes will occur. The rate at which the red cells fall is known as the **erythrocyte sedimentation rate (ESR).** This rate depends on three main factors: (1) the number and size of erythrocyte particles, (2) plasma factors, and (3) certain technical and mechanical factors.

The most important factor determining the rate of fall of the RBCs is the size or mass of the falling particle: the larger the particle, the faster it falls. The size of the falling particles depends on the formation of red cell aggregates, which in turn depends on the presence of certain factors in the plasma. The rate of sedimentation

appears to be dependent on the amount of fibrinogen and, to a lesser extent, the amount of globulin present in the plasma. In normal blood, the red cells tend to remain separate from one another because they are negatively charged (zeta potential) and tend to repel one another. In many pathologic conditions the phenomenon of erythrocyte aggregation is caused by alteration of the erythrocyte surface charge by plasma proteins. The protein that is most often involved is fibrinogen, although increases in gamma globulins or abnormal proteins also produce this effect. These factors determine the size of the aggregates of erythrocytes. With increased concentrations of large molecules in the plasma, there is a greater tendency for erythrocytes to pile up in rouleau formation (resembling a stack of coins).

### Stages of Erythrocyte Sedimentation

The sedimentation of erythrocytes in a sample of blood may be plotted as a curve on graph paper, with the millimeters of fall as the ordinate and the time in minutes as the abscissa. Such a curve shows at first a variable period of gradual fall, during which the aggregates of erythrocytes are forming (rouleau formation). Next, very rapid and marked fall of the aggregates occurs, constituting the main portion of the sedimentation of erythrocytes. The last part of the curve represents a more gradual, but relatively slight, falling off of the sedimentation rate as the erythrocyte aggregates are being packed at the bottom of the sedimentation tube. This packing will be more marked in an anemic patient than in a person with the normal number of erythrocytes. In any event, the effect of anemia on the sedimentation rate will be relatively slight. By far the most important factor in determining the rate of sedimentation is the size of the erythrocyte aggregates, or rouleaux.

### Clinical Significance of the Erythrocyte Sedimentation Rate

The ESR is a nonspecific screening test for inflammatory activity. It a measure of the pres-

---

*Williams WJ, Beutler E, Erslev A, et al: *Hematology,* ed 4. New York, McGraw-Hill Book Co, 1990, p 1703.

ence and severity of pathologic processes. In the vast majority of infections there is at least some increase in the ESR; chorea and undulant fever are two exceptions. The ESR also increases in most cases of carcinoma, leukemia and diseases of the bone marrow, degenerative vascular disease, active rheumatic fever, multiple myeloma, systemic lupus, rheumatoid arthritis, and acute gout. As patients recover from infectious diseases, the sedimentation rate slowly returns to normal. It may still be increased long after other clinical manifestations have disappeared, showing that the defense mechanisms of the body continue to be more active than normal.

Changes in the number and shape of erythrocytes also affect the ESR. In anemia, the ESR is increased, more so in megaloblastic than iron deficiency anemias. However, the rate of sedimentation is inhibited by variations in red cell shape, such as spherocytes, acanthocytes, and sickle cell formation.

Increased numbers of erythrocytes, as seen in cases of polycythemia and failure of the right side of the heart, tend to cause a marked slowing of sedimentation (decreased sedimentation rate). When the hematocrit is greater than 48% to 50%, sedimentation is markedly slowed, regardless of any factors present that might otherwise accelerate it.

A decrease in the ESR will result when the plasma fibrinogen level is decreased, as in cases of severe liver disease (e.g., acute yellow atrophy). The ESR is not increased in viral diseases, such as infectious mononucleosis and acute hepatitis, probably because fibrinogen production is not increased in these diseases in spite of a pronounced inflammatory reaction. The ESR is also not usually increased in chronic degenerative joint disease (it is increased, however, in inflammatory joint disease).

### Methods for Determination of the Erythrocyte Sedimentation Rate

There are two traditional methods for determining the sedimentation rate: the Westergren method (See Procedure 12-8) and the Wintrobe method. Normal values for both methods are sedimentation rates of 0 to 20 mm in 1 hour for women and 0 to 15 mm in 1 hour for men. The normal ESR varies with age, sex, and the specific methodology used.

Both methods use venous blood, which must be properly anticoagulated. EDTA is the usual anticoagulant used, although sodium citrate was the anticoagulant used in the original Westergren method. Heparin is unsatisfactory and should not be used for the ESR test.

Semi-automated instruments and various technical modifications of the traditional Westergren method are being introduced that attempt to eliminate or decrease the risk of exposure to potentially infectious material, namely blood. They are less hazardous in that they use self-contained and/or disposable materials. One example, Sediplast, is described in this section.

**Wintrobe Method.** For the Wintrobe method, enough blood is drawn into a Pasteur pipette to fill a Wintrobe hematocrit tube to the 100-mm mark. Bubbles must be avoided. The tube is placed in the support rack in an exactly vertical position so that the cells will sediment properly, and the time is noted. At the end of 1 hour, the ESR is read as the length of the plasma column above the cells. This method is simple and requires a small amount of blood.

**Westergren Method.** The Westergren method is the reference method for the ESR.[10] For this test, the procedure should be carried out within 2 hours after the blood has been drawn. The blood is diluted 4:1 with sodium citrate or NaCl, mixed well, and drawn into a Westergren tube to the zero mark. The tube is placed in a rack in an exactly vertical position at room temperature. Direct drafts, sunlight, and vibrations must be avoided. In most Westergren methods, a liquid sodium citrate solution is added to the blood before it is drawn into the tube. One modification of this method eliminates the addition

## PROCEDURE 12-8

### Erythrocyte Sedimentation Rate Using the Modified Westergren Method

1. Draw 5 milliliters of venous blood into EDTA.

2. Dilute 2 milliliters of well-mixed EDTA blood with 0.5 mL of 3.8 g/dL sodium citrate or 0.5 mL of 0.85 g/dL NaCl. (The original Westergren method used sodium citrate as the anticoagulant. The modified method employs EDTA blood, but this is diluted to give results consistent with the classic Westergren method.)

3. Mix the diluted blood-citrate mixture well.

4. Fill a Westergren tube to the zero mark with the diluted blood, using mechanical suction, and place it vertically in the Westergren rack.

5. At 60 minutes, read the top of the red cell layer in millimeters from the graduation marks on the tube. Adjust results if the top of the plasma level is not exactly at 0 mm.

6. Record results as number of mm at 1 hour.

of the citrate solution and still gives satisfactory results. The time when the tube is placed in the rack is noted, and a reading is taken at 60 minutes. The length of the plasma level above the red cells is measured in millimeters from the markings on the tube. A larger amount of blood is required for the Westergren method. See Procedure 12-8.

One commercial product utilizing the Westergren method for performing the ESR test is the Sediplast System.*

This employs a capped vial prefilled with 3.8% sodium citrate. To this vial is added the amount of blood sample that results in the correct sodium citrate–to–blood ratio of 1:4. This diluted sample is used to fill the Sediplast Autozero tube, which is placed in a vertical position in its special rack on a level surface. The ESR is read after 1 hour. See Procedure 12-9.

**Equipment for the Westergren Method.** The Westergren tube is really an open-ended pipette. The classic tube is 300 mm long, with an inner diameter of 2.5 mm; it is graduated in millimeters, from 0 at the top of the tube to

200 at the bottom. The diameter is important; according to the NCCLS, the diameter of the internal bore should be at least 2.55 mm.[9] The graduated volume of the tube is 1.0 mL. A special rack to hold the Westergren pipettes in a vertical position is needed for this test. The Westergren sedimentation rack is constructed so that rubber stoppers attached to springs close the open ends of the tubes when they are placed properly in the rack. Mechanical suction should be used to fill Westergren tubes.

### Precautions and Technical Factors

An anticoagulant that not only prevents clotting but preserves the shape and volume of the red cells must be used. Anticoagulants that prevent erythrocyte sedimentation are unsuitable for this test. Since erythrocyte numbers influence the rate of fall, the specimen must not be hemolyzed. Fibrin clots must not be present. The tube used for the test must be placed vertically in the rack; an angle different from this position can alter the rate of fall significantly. As the blood specimen stands after the venipuncture, the suspension stability of the erythrocytes increases. The test must be set up

*Polymedco, Inc, Crompond, NY.

## PROCEDURE 12-9

### Erythrocyte Sedimentation Rate Using Sediplast

1. Remove the cap on the vial containing sodium citrate. Using a disposable pipette, fill the vial to the indicated fill line with the well-mixed EDTA blood sample to be tested (approximately 0.8 mL of blood is required). Mix thoroughly using the pipetting device.

2. Insert the Sediplast tube, pushing it into the vial with a slight twisting motion, allowing the blood to rise to the zero mark and the excess blood to flow into the reservoir overflow compartment at the top of the tube. Continue inserting the tube until it rests at the bottom of the vial. The tube must completely touch the bottom of the vial to ensure proper results with this system.

3. Allow the sample to stand vertically for exactly 1 hour, and then read the numerical results of the erythrocyte sedimentation in millimeters. Record results.

in the Westergren tube within 2 hours after the blood has been drawn to ensure a reliable sedimentation rate. Preferably the test should be set up within 1 hour. Specimens may be refrigerated for up to 6 hours. Temperature and vibrations can affect the sedimentation rate, and these factors should be taken into consideration.

### Reporting of Test Results

The RBCs in the ESR tube are allowed to sediment for 1 hour. The results of the test are expressed in millimeters, the distance of fall of the top of the red cell column after 1 hour. Reporting an ESR result in this manner indicates that this test measures a distance of fall after a specified time interval.

### Reference Values*

*Erythrocyte sedimentation rate:*

|  | Less than 50 Years | Over 50 Years | Over 85 Years |
|---|---|---|---|
| Male | 0-15 mm/hr | 0-20 | 0-30 |
| Female | 0-20 mm/hr | 0-30 | 0-42 |

*Henry JB (ed): *Clinical Diagnosis and Management by Laboratory Methods*, ed 19. Philadelphia, WB Saunders Co, 1996, p 590.

## REFERENCES

1. Brecher G, Cronkite EP: Morphology and enumeration of human blood platelets. *J Appl Physiol* 1950; 3:365.

2. Brown B: *Hematology: Principles and Procedures,* ed 6. Philadelphia, Lea & Febiger, 1993, p 83.

3. College of American Pathologists: *Surveys Manual,* Section 2, Appendix 1: Glossary of Terms, Hematology—Coagulation/Clinical Microscopy. Northfield, Ill, College of American Pathologists, 1995.

4. Conn HJ, Darrow MS: *Staining Procedures Used by the Biological Stain Commission,* ed 2. Baltimore, Williams & Wilkins Co, 1960.

5. *Laboratory Procedures Using the UNOPETTE Brand System,* ed 8. Rutherford, NJ, Becton Dickinson VACUTAINER Systems, 1977.

6. NCCLS: *Method for Reticulocyte Counting: Proposed Standard.* Villanova, Pa, National Committee for Clinical Laboratory Standards, 1985, document H16-P, p 229.

7. NCCLS: *Physician's Office Laboratory Guidelines, Procedure Manual: Tentative Guideline,* ed 3. Villanova, Pa, National Committee for Clinical Laboratory Standards, 1995, document POL1/2-T3.

8. NCCLS: *Reference Leukocyte Differential Count (Proportional) and Evaluation of Instrumental Methods: Approved Standard.* Villanova, Pa, National Committee for Clinical Laboratory Standards, 1992 (March), H20-A (vol 12, no 1).

9. NCCLS: *Reference Procedure for Human Erythrocyte Sedimentation Rate (ESR) Test: Approved Standard.* Villanova, Pa, National Committee for Clinical Laboratory Standards, 1993, document H2-A3.

10. Westergren A: The techniques of the red cell sedimentation reaction. *Am Rev Tuberc Pulmonary Dis* 1926; 14:94.

## BIBLIOGRAPHY

Bessman JD: *Automated Blood Counts and Differentials.* Baltimore, Johns Hopkins University Press, 1986.

Beutler E, Lichtman MA, Coller BS, Kipps TJ: *Williams Hematology*, ed 5. New York, McGraw-Hill, Inc., 1995.

Brown B: *Hematology: Principles and Procedures*, ed 6. Philadelphia, Lea & Febiger, 1993.

College of American Pathologists: *Surveys Manual, Section 2, Appendix 1: Glossary of Terms, Hematology—Coagulation/Clinical Microscopy.* Northfield, Ill, College of American Pathologists, 1995.

Henry JB (ed): *Clinical Diagnosis and Management by Laboratory Methods*, ed 19. Philadelphia, WB Saunders Co, 1996.

Jacobs DS et al (eds): *Laboratory Test Handbook: Concise with Disease Index*, Hudson, Ohio, Lexi-Comp Inc, 1996.

Lee GR, Bithell TC, Foerster J, Athens JW, Lukens JN: *Wintrobe's Clinical Hematology*, ed 9. Philadelphia, Lea & Febiger, 1993.

Lotspeich-Steininger CA, Stiene-Martin EA, Koepke JA: *Clinical Hematology: Principles, Procedures, Correlations*, ed 2. Philadelphia, Lippincott-Raven, 1998.

NCCLS: *Method for Reticulocyte Counting: Flow Cytometry and Supravital Dyes, Approved Guideline.* Villanova, Pa, National Committee for Clinical Laboratory Standards, 1997, document H44-A.

NCCLS: *Methods for the Erythrocyte Sedimentation Rate (ESR) Test: Approved Standard*, ed 3. Villanova, Pa, National Committee for Clinical Laboratory Standards, 1993, document H2-A3.

NCCLS: *Procedure for Determining Packed Cell Volume by the Microhematocrit Method: Approved Standard*, ed 2. Villanova, Pa, National Committee for Clinical Laboratory Standards, 1993, document H7-A2.

NCCLS: *Reference Leukocyte Differential Count (Proportional) and Evaluation of Instrumental Methods: Approved Standard.* Villanova, Pa, National Committee for Clinical Laboratory Standards, 1992, document H20-A.

NCCLS: *Reference Procedures for the Quantitative Determination of Hemoglobin in Blood: Approved Standard*, ed 2. Vil-lanova, Pa, National Committee for Clinical Laboratory Standards, 1994, document H15-A2.

Powers L: *Diagnostic Hematology.* St Louis, Mosby, 1989.

## STUDY QUESTIONS

1. Samples for the following tests are to be collected from capillary blood. Arrange the samples in the order they should be collected from a capillary skin puncture.

   A. Blood films (smears)
   B. Hemoglobin
   C. Microhematocrit
   D. Platelet count
   E. White cell count

2. The anticoagulant of choice for most hematologic studies is:

   A. Dry EDTA
   B. Heparin
   C. Liquid EDTA
   D. Oxalate

3. Name two conditions that make hematologic specimens unacceptable for testing.

   A. _____
   B. _____

4. Match each of the following cell types (1 to 7) with its approximate life span in peripheral blood (A to G).

   1. B lymphocyte
   2. Basophil

3. Eosinophil
4. Monocyte
5. Neutrophil (PMN)
6. Red blood cell
7. T lymphocyte

_____ A. Months to years
_____ B. 120 days
_____ C. 1 to 3 days
_____ D. Days
_____ E. About 10 hours
_____ F. Less than 8 hours
_____ G. Unknown

5. A young red cell that has just extruded its nucleus, when seen on a Wright-stained peripheral blood film, is referred to as a:

A. Normoblast
B. Orthochromatic cell
C. Polychromatic cell
D. Reticulocyte

6. Which of the following are classified as Romanowsky stains?

A. Brilliant Cresyl blue stain
B. New methylene blue stain
C. Wright Stain
D. Wright-Giemsa Stain

7. Classify the following cells as myeloid (M) or lymphoid (L).

_____ A. B cells
_____ B. Basophils
_____ C. Eosinophils
_____ D. Erythrocytes
_____ E. Monocytes
_____ F. Neutrophils
_____ G. Platelets
_____ H. T cells

8. Which of the following is essential to the oxygen-carrying capacity of hemoglobin?

A. Globin
B. Heme
C. Iron

9. Match each of the following descriptions (1 to 4) with the correct hemoglobin variant (A to D).

1. A hemoglobin variant associated with the presence of target cells on the blood film

2. A hemoglobin variant resulting in sickle cell anemia in the homozygous state
3. The principal form of hemoglobin found in the blood of normal adults
4. The principal form of hemoglobin in intrauterine life and at birth

_____ A. Hemoglobin A
_____ B. Hemoglobin C
_____ C. Hemoglobin F
_____ D. Hemoglobin S

10. Match each of the following descriptions (1 to 6) with the correct hemoglobin derivative (A to F).

1. A stable derivative of hemoglobin bound to cyanide; used in the standard method of hemoglobin determination
2. An irreversible combination of hemoglobin with a sulf group; incapable of transporting oxygen or reverting to functional hemoglobin
3. Hemoglobin bound to carbon monoxide with an affinity 100 times that of oxygen
4. Hemoglobin containing iron in a ferric, rather than a ferrous, state
5. The form of hemoglobin that normally transports carbon dioxide from the tissues to the lungs
6. The form of hemoglobin that normally transports oxygen from the lungs to the tissues

_____ A. Carboxyhemoglobin
_____ B. Hemiglobincyanide (cyanmethemoglobin)
_____ C. Methemoglobin
_____ D. Oxyhemoglobin
_____ E. Reduced hemoglobin
_____ F. Sulfhemoglobin

11. The use of daily hemoglobin control solutions will detect which of the following? (More than one may apply.)

A. Accuracy of the measuring device used
B. Deterioration of the hemoglobin reagent
C. Dirty or scratched photometer cuvettes
D. Malfunction of the spectrophotometer
E. Technical skill of the laboratorian

12. Turbidity in a sample diluted with hemiglobincyanide reagent for analysis in a spectrometer will result in:

A. Falsely high results

B. Falsely low results

C. No effect on the hemoglobin result

13. **Which of the following situations may result in turbidity in a blood sample diluted with hemiglobincyanide reagent? (More than one may apply.)**

A. Abnormal globulins

B. Exceptionally high white count

C. Hemolysis

D. Lipemia

E. The presence of Hb A or Hb F

F. The presence of Hb S or Hb C

14. **Match the following tests (1 to 6) with the units by which they are normally reported (A to E).**

1. Hematocrit
2. Hemoglobin
3. Packed cell volume
4. Platelet count
5. Red cell count
6. White cell count
     _____ A. Cells $\times$ $10^9$ per liter
     _____ B. Cells $\times$ $10^{12}$ per liter
     _____ C. Grams per deciliter
     _____ D. Liters per liter
     _____ E. Percent

15. **Assuming normochromic and normocytic red cells, a blood sample with a hemoglobin of 15 g/dL would be expected to show a hematocrit of:**

A. 0.45 %

B. 5 %

C. 40 %

D. 45 %

E. 50 %

16. **Match each of the following descriptions of methodology (1 to 4) with the corresponding method for determining packed cell volume (or hematocrit) (A to C).**

1. A centrifugation method that is rarely used; requires anticoagulated venipuncture blood and a relatively long centrifugation time
2. A direct measurement of packed cell volume, which may use capillary or venous blood
3. An indirect measurement of packed cell volume; derived from mean cell volume and red cell count

4. Results may be lower than with centrifugation methods because they are unaffected by plasma trapping.
     _____ A. Automated hematocrit by multiparameter instrument
     _____ B. Spun microhematocrit
     _____ C. Wintrobe hematocrit

17. **Match the following situations regarding spun microhematocrit determinations (1 to 7) with results (A to C). Match all situations that apply to each result.**

1. Capillary blood is drawn into an anticoagulated microhematocrit tube
2. Inadequate sealing of the microhematocrit tube
3. Inclusion of the buffy coat in the measured packed cell volume
4. Red blood cells show marked anisocytosis and poikilocytosis on the blood film
5. Use of a clotted blood sample
6. Use of a hemolyzed blood sample
7. Anticoagulated venous blood is drawn into an anticoagulated microhematocrit tube
     _____ A. Falsely high
     _____ B. Falsely low
     _____ C. Unaffected

18. **Match each of the following definitions of red cell indices (1 to 4) with its common abbreviation (A to D).**

1. Hemoglobin concentration or color of the average RBC
2. Measure of the degree of RBC variability
3. Volume or size of the average RBC
4. Weight of hemoglobin in the average RBC
     _____ A. MCH
     _____ B. MCHC
     _____ C. MCV
     _____ D. RDW

19. **Given the following results, calculate MCV, MCH, and MCHC in units as indicated.**

| | |
|---|---|
| **Hemoglobin (Hb)** | **12.0 g/dL** |
| **Hematocrit (Hct)** | **36%** |
| **RBC** | **$4 \times 10^{12}$/L** |

A. MCV = _____ fl

B. MCH = _____ pg

C MCHC = _____ g/dL

20. **How would you expect the red cells to appear on the blood film from the patient in question 19?**

    A Hypochromic and microcytic
    B. Normochromic and macrocytic
    C. Normochromic and normocytic

21. **Match the following requirements for diluents (1 to 7) with the appropriate manual cell count. (A to C).**

    1. Accentuates cell nucleus
    2. Hemolysis of erythrocytes
    3. Prevents clotting
    4. Provides fixation
    5. Provides isotonicity and prevents hemolysis
    6. Specific gravity sufficient for settling
       _____ A. Platelet count
       _____ B. Red cell count
       _____ C. White cell count

22. **Given the following information, calculate the white cell count in cells × 10⁹/L.**

    **Four square mm are counted. with the following results: 20, 18, 19, 21.**
    **Blood dilution = 10:1**
    **Chamber depth = 0.1 mm**
    **White blood cell count is:**

    A. $0.5 \times 10^9/L$
    B. $1.95 \times 10^9/L$
    C. $3.9 \times 10^9/L$
    D. $1950 \times 10^9/L$
    E. $3900 \times 10^9/L$

23. **If only manual methods are available, which of the following red cell indices is most accurate? Explain your answer.**

    A. MCV
    B. MCH
    C. MCHC

24. **Match the following situations regarding the preparation of the peripheral blood film (1 to 6) with the results seen in the blood film (A to G).**

    1. Blood film covers ½ to ¾ of the length of the slide
    2. Defined border at end of blood film (no feather edge)
    3. Dirty or chipped slides

4. Dirty slides or excess fat in lipemic specimen or very high white cell count
5. Large drop of blood, large angle, and slow stroke
6. Small drop of blood, small angle, and fast stroke
   _____ A. Good blood film
   _____ B. Incorrect distribution of types of white cells in body of film
   _____ C. Neutrophils accumulate in feather edge
   _____ D. Platelets decreased in body of blood film
   _____ E. Unusually thick blood film
   _____ F. Unusually thin blood film
   _____ G. Vacuoles or bubbles in blood film

25. **For blood films stained with a polychrome Romanovsky-type stain, match the cell components (1 to 6) with the dye component (A to C).**

    1. Azurophilic granules
    2. Cytoplasmic RNA
    3. Eosinophilic granules
    4. Hemoglobin
    5. Neutrophilic granules
    6. Nuclear DNA
       _____ A. Acidophilic (eosin)
       _____ B. Basophilic (methylene blue)
       _____ C. Methylene azure (polychrome methylene blue)

26. **Match each of the following alterations in staining (1 to 6) with the most probable cause (A to F). Use only one alteration per cause.**

    1. Faded or washed-out appearance of all cells
    2. Gross appearance of slide excessively blue, with blue-red erythrocytes and dark, granular leukocytes
    3. Gross appearance of slide excessively red, with bright red erythrocytes, white cell pale blue, brilliant red eosinophilic granules
    4. Large amounts of precipitated stain
       _____ A. Improper washing or old stain
       _____ B. Overfixing, overstaining, underwashing; too alkaline stain, buffer, or too thick blood film
       _____ C. Overwashing, understaining, underfixing
       _____ D. Understaining, overwashing; too acid stain, buffer, or water

27. A white blood cell count and a white cell differential are performed and yield the following results: WBC = $7.0 \times 10^9$/L. Of 100 white cells classified, there were 70 neutrophils, 20 lymphocytes, 7 monocytes, 2 eosinophils, and 1 basophil. For each cell type, give the absolute and relative cell counts.

| Cell type | Relative cell count | Absolute cell count $\times 10^9$/L |
|---|---|---|
| Neutrophil | | |
| Lymphocyte | | |
| Monocyte | | |
| Eosinophil | | |
| Basophil | | |

28. Match each of the following stem cells (1 to 4) with its colony forming unit designation (A to E).

   1. The committed progenitor cell for granulocytes and monocytes
   2. The committed stem cell for B and T lymphocytes
   3. The multipotential stem cell for granulocytes, monocytes, erythrocytes, and platelets
   4. The common progenitor or uncommitted pluripotential stem cell
   _____ A. CFU-C
   _____ B. CFU-GM
   _____ C. CFU-L
   _____ D. CFU-LM
   _____ E. CFU-S

29. Match each of the following causes or descriptions of anemia (1 to 6) with the morphologic type (A to C).

   1. Acute blood loss (trauma)
   2. Anemia associated with increased plasma volume (pregnancy and overhydration)
   3. Aplastic anemia from bone marrow suppression
   4. Iron deficiency due to diet or blood loss
   5. Thalassemia and other hemoglobinopathies
   6. Vitamin $B_{12}$ or folate deficiency
   _____ A. Hypochromic-microcytic
   _____ B. Macrocytic
   _____ C. Normochromic-normocytic

30. Erythrocytes that show normal color or staining reaction are referred to as:

   A. Discocytic
   B. Normochromic
   C. Normocytic
   D. Orthochromatic
   E. Polychromatic

31. An increased variation in size of erythrocytes on the blood film is referred to as:

   A. Anisocytosis
   B. Microcytosis
   C. Orthochromasia
   D. Poikilocytosis
   E. Polychromasia

32. An increased variation in the shape of erythrocytes on the blood film is referred to as:

   A. Anisocytosis
   B. Microcytosis
   C. Orthochromasia
   D. Poikilocytosis
   E. Polychromasia

33. The presence of anisocytosis and poikilocytosis is reflected in which of the following red cell indices?

   A. MCV
   B. MCH
   C. MCHC
   D. RDW

34. A patient being treated for metastatic carcinoma was found to have a white cell count of $5 \times 10^9$/L with 5 normoblasts (nucleated red cells) per 100 white WBCs. What is the corrected white cell count for this patient?

   A. $2.1 \times 10^9$/L
   B. $2.4 \times 10^9$/L
   C. $4.8 \times 10^9$/L
   D. $5.2 \times 10^9$/L

35. The presence of young red and white blood cells not normally present in the peripheral blood is termed a (an):

   A. Erythroblastotic reaction
   B. Leukoblastotic reaction
   C. Leukoerythroblastotic reaction
   D. Lymphoblastotic reaction

36. The presence of polychromasia on a Wright-stained peripheral blood film is associated with which of the following *untreated* anemias?

   A. Aplastic anemia
   B. Hemolytic anemia
   C. Iron deficiency anemia
   D. Megaloblastic anemia

37. Toxic changes in neutrophils include all of the following except:

   A. Auer rods or bodies
   B. Hypersegmentation
   C. Shift to the left
   D. Toxic granulation
   E. Vacuolization

38. Which of the following leukemias is associated with the presence of the Philadelphia chromosome?

   A. Acute lymphocytic
   B. Acute myelogenous
   C. Chronic lymphocytic
   D. Chronic myelogenous

39. The presence of Auer rods in the peripheral blood is associated with which of the following cells?

   A. Lymphoblast
   B. Myeloblast
   C. Reactive lymphocyte
   D. Shift cell
   E. Turk cell

40. Which of the following types of leukemia is most associated with infants or young children?

   A. Acute lymphocytic
   B. Acute myelogenous
   C. Chronic lymphocytic
   D. Chronic myelogenous

41. Which of the following hematologic tests is *not* part of the usual complete blood count?

   A. Hematocrit
   B. Hemoglobin
   C. Platelet estimate
   D. Reticulocyte count
   E. White cell count
   F. White cell differential

42. Which of the following is a nonspecific screening test for inflammation?

   A. Erythrocyte morphology
   B. Erythrocyte sedimentation rate
   C. Leukocyte morphology and differential
   D. Platelet count
   E. Reticulocyte count

43. Which of the following tests is used to evaluate the response to therapy in the treatment of iron deficiency anemia?

   A. Erythrocyte sedimentation rate
   B. Leukocyte morphology and differential
   C. Platelet count
   D. Reticulocyte count
   E. T cell count

# CASE HISTORIES

## ■ Case I

A 15-year-old woman has a 2-month history of difficulty in breathing and extreme tiredness (fatigue). In the last 2 days she has experienced heart palpitations and has noticed blood in her stools and urine. She has no enlargement of the spleen or liver. The following laboratory results are obtained:

| | |
|---|---|
| Hemoglobin | 6 g/dL |
| Hematocrit | 18 % |
| White cell count | $3.3 \times 10^9$/L |

| White cell differential | |
|---|---|
| Neutrophils | 10% |
| Lymphocytes | 80% |
| Monocytes | 10% |
| Eosinophils and basophils | 0% |
| Red cell count | $2 \times 10^{12}$/L |
| RDW | 12 |
| Platelet count | $13 \times 10^9$/L |
| Reticulocyte count | 0.6% |

1. Calculate the red cell indices for this patient, and tell if they are increased, decreased, or normal:

MCV =

MCH =

MCHC =

2. How would you classify this anemia morphologically?
   A. Hypochromic-microcytic
   B. Macrocytic
   C. Normochromic-normocytic

3. The blood present in the patient's stool and urine is due to which of the following?
   A. Low hemoglobin
   B. Low platelet count
   C. Low red cell count
   D. Low reticulocyte count
   E. Low white cell count

4. The patient's difficulty in breathing and extreme tiredness are most directly due to which of the following?
   A. Low hemoglobin
   B. Low platelet count
   C. Low reticulocyte count
   D. Low white cell count

5. Calculate the absolute neutrophil and lymphocyte counts for this patient, and tell if these results are normal or low.

Absolute neutrophil count =

Absolute lymphocyte count =

6. The most probable type of anemia seen in this patient is:
   A. Aplastic anemia from bone marrow depletion
   B. Folate deficiency anemia
   C. Hemolytic anemia
   D. Iron deficiency anemia
      Explain:

---

## ■ Case 2

An 80-year-old man is seen for an annual physical examination. He says he is short of breath when he exerts himself and is often tired, but otherwise he feels well. The following laboratory results are obtained.

| | |
|---|---|
| Hemoglobin | 8.2 g/dL (12.4 g/dL one year previously) |
| Hematocrit | 30% |
| White cell count | 4.2 × 10⁹/L |

White cell differential

| | |
|---|---|
| Neutrophils | 60% |
| Lymphocytes | 31% |
| Monocytes | 7% |
| Eosinophils | 2% |
| Basophils | 0% |
| Red cell count | $4.0 \times 10^{12}$/L |
| RDW | 20% |
| Platelet count | $400 \times 10^9$/L |
| Reticulocyte count | 1.2 % |

1. Calculate the red cell indices for this patient, and tell if they are increased, decreased, or normal:

MCV =

MCH =

MCHC =

2. How would you classify this anemia morphologically?
   A Hypochromic-microcytic
   B. Macrocytic
   C. Normochromic-normocytic

3. The most probable type of anemia seen in this patient is:
   A. Aplastic anemia from bone marrow depletion
   B. Folate deficiency anemia
   C. Hemolytic anemia
   D. Iron deficiency anemia

4. The anemia seen in this patient is *most likely* due to which of the following?
   (More than one answer may apply.)
   A. Bleeding due to bone marrow depletion
   B. Blood loss due to gastrointestinal bleeding
   C. Lack of adequate folic acid in the diet
   D. Lack of adequate iron in the diet
   E. Loss of blood due to hemolysis

5. From the hematologic results provided, which of the following erythrocyte changes would you expect to find on a Wright-stained blood film from this patient? (Choose all that apply.)
   A. Anisocytosis
   B. Hyperchromasia
   C. Hypochromasia
   D. Macrocytosis
   E. Microcytosis
   F. Poikilocytosis
   G. Polychromasia

6. Suggest a cost-efficient screening test that would be helpful in determining the cause of anemia in this patient.

---

## ■ Case 3

A 65-year-old woman is seen in clinic. She complains of extreme tiredness (fatigue), difficulty in breathing, and an extremely sore tongue. The following laboratory results are obtained.

| | |
|---|---|
| Hemoglobin | 8.7 g/dL |
| Hematocrit | 25.5% |
| White cell count | $5 \times 10^9$/L |
| White cell differential | |
| Neutrophils | 65% |
| Lymphocytes | 31% |
| Monocytes | 4% |
| Red cell count | $1.97 \times 10^{12}$/L |
| RDW | 19% |
| Platelet count | $134 \times 10^9$/L |
| Reticulocyte count | 0.9 % |

1. Calculate the red cell indices for this patient, and tell if they are increased, decreased, or normal:
   MCV =
   MCH =
   MCHC =
2. How would you classify this anemia morphologically?
   A. Hypochromic-microcytic
   B. Macrocytic
   C. Normochromic-normocyttic
3. The most probable type of anemia seen in this patient is:
   A. Aplastic anemia from bone marrow depletion
   B. Megaloblastic anemia from folate or $B_{12}$ deficiency
   C. Hemolytic anemia
   D. Iron deficiency anemia
4. From the hematologic results provided, which of the following erythrocyte changes would you expect to find on a Wright-stained blood film from this patient? (Choose all that apply.)
   A. Anisocytosis
   B. Hypochromasia
   C. Macrocytosis
   D. Microcytosis
   E. Normochromasia
   F. Poikilocytosis
   G. Polychromasia
5. Which of the following leukocyte changes would you expect to find on a Wright-stained blood film from this patient? (Choose all that apply.)
   A. Cytoplasmic vacuolization of neutrophils
   B. Hypersegmentation of neutrophils
   C. Reactive lymphocytosis
   D. Shift to the left
   E. Toxic granulation of neutrophils

---

## ■ Case 4

A 20-year-old female university student is seen in the student health clinic. She has a general feeling of sickness, an extremely sore throat, and swollen lymph nodes in her neck.

Blood is drawn for a CBC, and her throat is swabbed for a rapid strep test and culture. The following laboratory results are obtained.

| | |
|---|---|
| Hemoglobin | 13.5 g/dL |
| Red cell indices | All within normal limits |
| White cell count | $14.5 \times 10^9$/L |
| White cell differential | |
| Neutrophils | 7% |
| Lymphocytes | 89% |
| Monocytes | 3% |
| Eosinophils | 1% |
| Basophils | 0 % |

Comment: many reactive (variant) lymphocytes and basket cells seen

| | |
|---|---|
| Platelet estimate | Normal, with normal morphology |
| Rapid throat culture test | Negative; culture pending |

1. Does this patient have an anemia? (yes or no)
2. Does this patient have an infection? (yes or no) Explain:
3. Is the infection most likely bacterial or viral?
4. Calculate the absolute neutrophil and lymphocyte counts for this patient, and tell if they are increased, decreased, or normal.
   Absolute neutrophil count =
   Absolute lymphocyte count =
5. From the laboratory results provided, and your calculations, which of the following apply?
   A. Absolute lymphocytosis
   B. Absolute neutropenia

C. Leukocytosis
D. Neutrophilia
E. Reactive lymphocytosis
F. Relative lymphocytosis
G. Relative neutropenia

6. Which of the following leukocyte changes would you expect to find on a Wright-stained blood film from this patient? (Choose all that apply.)
   A. Cytoplasmic vacuolization of neutrophils
   B. Hypersegmentation of neutrophils
   C. Reactive lymphocytosis
   D. Shift to the left
   E. Toxic granulation of neutrophils

7. The disease most likely exhibited by this patient is:
   A. Infectious mononucleosis
   B. Leukemia
   C. Pneumonia
   D. Sore throat due to group A beta-hemolytic streptococcus

## ■ Case 5

A 65-year old man has chills, high spiking fevers, cough, and signs of consolidation in the left lower lobe of his lung. Blood is drawn for a CBC, sputum is collected for gram stain and culture, and a chest x-ray is obtained. The following results are obtained:

| | |
|---|---|
| Hemoglobin | 14.5 g/dL |
| Red cell indices | All within normal limits |
| White cell count | $24 \times 10^9$/L |
| White cell differential | |
| Segmented neutrophils | 33% |
| Band neutrophils | 61% |
| Lymphocytes | 6% |
| Platelet estimate | Normal with normal morphology |
| Sputum gram stain | Many gram-positive cocci in pairs; culture pending |

1. Does this patient have an anemia? (yes or no).
2. Does this patient have an infection? (yes or no) Explain:
3. Is the infection most likely bacterial or viral?
4. Calculate the absolute neutrophil and lymphocyte counts for this patient, and tell if they are increased, decreased, or normal.
   Absolute neutrophil count =
   Absolute lymphocyte count =
5. From the laboratory results provided, and your calculations, which of the following apply?
   A. Absolute lymphocytosis
   B. Absolute neutrophilia
   C. Leukocytosis
   D. Reactive lymphocytosis
   E. Relative lymphopenia
   F. Relative neutrophilia
6. Which of the following leukocyte changes would you expect to find on a Wright-stained blood film from this patient? (Choose all that apply.)
   A. Cytoplasmic vacuolization of neutrophils
   B. Hypersegmentation of neutrophils
   C. Reactive lymphocytosis
   D. Shift to the left
   E. Toxic granulation of neutrophils
7. The disease most likely exhibited by this patient is:
   A. Infectious mononucleosis
   B. Leukemia
   C. Pneumonia
   D. Sore throat due to group A beta-hemolytic streptococcus

# CHAPTER 13

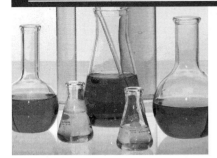

# Coagulation and Hemostasis

## Learning Objectives

*From study of this chapter, the reader will be able to:*

➣ Describe the three components of the hemostatic system.

➣ Describe the role of platelets in hemostasis.

➣ Describe three major steps of the mechanism of coagulation.

➣ Summarize the activity of the extrinsic pathway of coagulation.

➣ Summarize the activity of the intrinsic pathway of coagulation.

➣ Describe the role of the various coagulation factors.

➣ Describe the common laboratory tests used for coagulation and hemostasis.

➣ Describe the use of coagulation point-of-care tests

## INTRODUCTION TO HEMOSTASIS

**Hemostasis** is the cessation of blood flow from an injured blood vessel. It is one of the most important natural defense mechanisms of the body. The result of activation of the hemostatic system is the formation of the **hemostatic plug** or **platelet plug** or **thrombus**—all three terms denoting the same activity—at the site of injury to the vessel. Hemostasis also prevents pathologic or harmful **thrombosis** (the action of formation of a thrombus) by setting limitations on formation of the hemostatic plug. The process of hemostasis involves a balance of numerous interdependent factors that are controlled carefully by the body for the purpose of preventing bleeding—a complex interaction between the blood vessels, the platelets, and the plasma coagulation factors. **Primary hemostasis** involves the platelets and the vascular response to an injury. **Secondary hemostasis** includes the response by the coagulation proteins. When there is an injury to a blood vessel, the hemostatic process is designed to repair the break. Thus, hemostasis is the process whereby the body retains the blood within the vascular system, in spite of the many traumas that injure the blood vessel walls. Activation of both the hemostatic and inflammatory responses are simultaneous after injury to a blood vessel.

The most immediate response of the body to bleeding is **vasoconstriction.** In this process, the damaged blood vessel constricts, decreasing the blood flow through the injured area. A platelet plug can then form, which helps to further inhibit the bleeding; an essential requirement for primary hemostasis is **platelet adhesion.** Platelets must be available in adequate numbers and must be functioning normally for this to occur. Finally, coagulation factors present in the blood interact, forming a fibrin network, the thrombus or **clot,** to stop the bleeding completely. By convention, a "thrombus" is defined as coagulation within the blood vessels during life, an in vivo reaction, while a "clot" is coagulation in a test tube in the laboratory, an in vitro reaction. These terms often are used interchangeably, however. Slow lysis of the thrombus begins, and final repair to the site of the injury takes place.

## HEMOSTATIC MECHANISM

The hemostatic mechanism is the entire process by which bleeding from an injured blood vessel is controlled and finally stopped. It is a series of physical and biochemical changes that are normally initiated by an injury to the blood vessel and tissues and that culminate in the transformation of fluid blood into a thrombus or clot, which effectively seals the injured vessel. The entire hemostatic mechanism can be divided into three components: extravascular effects, vascular effects, and intravascular effects.

A bleeding tendency can result from a defect in any of the phases of repair; that is, (1) the vascular system itself may be prone to injury; (2) the platelets may be inadequate in number to form the temporary platelet plug; (3) the fibrin clotting mechanism may be inadequate; or (4) the fibroblastic repair may be inadequate. Excessive abnormal bleeding is usually the result of a combination of defects.

## Extravascular Effects

The tissue surrounding the blood vessels constitutes the **extravascular component.** Extravascular effects consist of (1) the physical effect of the surrounding tissues, such as muscle, skin, and elastic tissue, which tend to close and seal the tear in the vessel that is injured, and (2) the biochemical effects of certain substances that are released from the injured tissues and react with plasma and platelet factors. The latter factors are called the **extrinsic system of coagulation.**

## Vascular Effects

The blood vessels themselves constitute the **vascular component.** The inner monolayer of cells of the blood vessel, the vascular endothelium, is very important to the hemostatic process. If trauma or injury disrupts this cell layer, the underlying basement membrane of the vessel is exposed. Basement membrane contains collagenous material, and when circulating platelets make contact with this collagenous material, biochemical and structural changes occur that result in the formation of platelet aggregates and fibrin clots. These platelet aggregates—the platelet plug—can plug the gaps in the endothelial lining and thus prevent more stimulation by the collagen layer.

Vascular effects also involve the blood vessels themselves, which constrict almost instantaneously when injured, a process known as vasoconstriction. This vasoconstriction phenomenon tends to last a relatively short time, but it may be enhanced and prolonged by local release of a vasoconstricting substance, **serotonin.** Serotonin is released from the platelets as they adhere to the margins of the injury in the wall of the blood vessel. It promotes local, direct, biochemically stimulated narrowing of the torn blood vessel and of lo-

cally intact blood vessels in the same vicinity as the injury.

## Intravascular Effects

Included in the **intravascular component** are the platelets and plasma coagulation proteins that circulate in the blood vessels. The intravascular factors take part in an extremely complicated sequence of physiochemical reactions that transform the liquid blood into a firm **fibrin clot.** This process requires the initiation of a platelet plug, which is followed by reinforcement with fibrin derived from the activation of the **intrinsic system of coagulation.** All the factors necessary for the intrinsic system are contained within the blood. Many natural inhibitors and accelerators are brought into action during this time.

## The Function of Platelets

Platelets have three important functions: (1) to react to injury of vessels by forming an aggregate plug or platelet mass that can physically slow down or stop blood loss; (2) to help activate and be a participant in plasma coagulation to more effectively serve as a barrier to extensive blood loss; and (3) to maintain the endothelial lining of the blood vessels. To provide normal primary hemostasis, there must be an adequate number of normally functioning platelets. The bleeding time (BT) test is used as a general screening test for platelet function.

### Formation of Platelet Plug

When endothelial cells are damaged, displaced, or become degenerate, the platelets in the bloodstream are exposed to the underlying collagen and to a subendothelial factor, **von Willebrand's factor** VIII:vWF. The contact with collagen results in activation or changes taking place in platelet function, which, in turn, result in **platelet adherence** to the damaged area of the blood vessel. During this process, fibronectin is secreted by the endothelial cells. **Fibronectin** has been shown to assist in bonding platelets to the collagen substrate. The additional protein factor VIII:vWF acts as the glue necessary for optimal platelet-collagen binding to occur. Adherence to the collagen initiates platelet activation. Upon activation, platelets take on a different shape, becoming more spherical, with long, irregular arms. This greatly increases the surface area of the platelet and facilitates interaction with other platelets and proteins in the coagulation cascade process. Platelets also aggregate with one another as a result of changes that take place on their outer coats—a phenomenon known as **platelet aggregation.** The mass of platelets grows and forms the primary hemostatic plug in vivo. This plug must be stabilized by fibrin strands produced during plasma protein coagulation in order for the plug to be anything other than temporary. A bleeding time test can assess platelet plug formation, which is dependent on platelet concentration (the platelet count), platelet qualitative function, and vessel integrity. See Procedure 13-1.

### Platelets in Coagulation

The role of platelets in the coagulation process is varied. They secrete substances that serve to promote coagulation and aggregation and that promote vasoconstriction and vascular repair. During platelet activation, alterations occur that result in the formation of receptors capable of binding several plasma proteins, the most important being fibrinogen. Activation of coagulation factors or enzymes occurs on the surface of the platelets where specific receptor molecules are present.

Platelet factor 3 (PF3) is a phospholipoprotein (phospholipid) that is contained on or within the plasma membrane of the platelets and is needed in activating certain of the coagulation factors. The formation of thrombin is facilitated as one important function of this activation process.

The endothelia of blood vessels are repaired and maintained with help from products that are secreted by the platelets. One such product is platelet-derived growth factor (PDGF).

## COAGULATION

**Coagulation** is the mechanism whereby, when there is injury to a blood vessel, plasma proteins—coagulation factors and tissue factors—and calcium work together on the surface of the platelets to form a fibrin clot. Most of the clinical conditions requiring coagulation studies involve the intrinsic system of coagulation. The coagulation factors, their nomenclature, and procedures for analyzing some of the more important coagulation factors are discussed in this section.

The blood coagulation mechanism is complicated and involves many factors. Knowing which factor is not performing its proper function is of critical importance. This knowledge is gained through the use of several different laboratory tests. The proper formation of a blood clot after a scratch or cut depends on healthy functioning of all the factors. In an individual having a weakness or deficiency in one or several of the factors, severe trauma from a serious injury or from surgical treatment can result in collapse of the clotting mechanism. This in turn will result in a most drastic manifestation—severe hemorrhage. This has been dramatically demonstrated in persons whose clotting mechanism is adequate for everyday living but who, during such common surgical procedures as dental extractions or tonsillectomies, experience severe bleeding. It is of the utmost importance, therefore, that the laboratory tests in this area be accurately performed. Most of these tests employ macroscopic observations.

The topic of blood coagulation is not completely understood, and much research is still in progress in this field. It is generally agreed that all the elements necessary for clot formation are normally present in the circulating blood. The fluidity of the blood, therefore, depends on a balance between the coagulant and anticoagulant factors.

The mechanism of coagulation takes place in three major steps, with the formation of a fibrin thrombus being the major goal: (1) the formation of thromboplastin, (2) the formation of thrombin, and (3) the formation of fibrin. Various clotting factors, or constituents, are involved in this mechanism.

## Coagulation Factors

The **coagulation factors** are fundamentally protein, with the exception of calcium and the phospholipid of the platelets. The factors are divided into three categories: substrate, cofactors, and enzymes. Factor I (fibrinogen) is considered the substrate because the formation of a fibrin clot from fibrinogen is considered the major goal of the process of coagulation in hemostasis. **Cofactors** are proteins that accelerate the reactions of the enzymes involved in the process. Cofactors are factor III (tissue factor), factor V (labile factor), factor VIII (antihemophilic factor, or AHF), and Fitzgerald factor (high-molecular-weight kininogen, or HMWK). Most of the remaining coagulation factors are enzyme precursors—**proenzymes** or **zymogens**—which become active enzymes after proteolytic or structural change. With the exception of factor XIII (fibrin-stabilizing factor), which is a transamidase, the enzyme factors functioning in coagulation are serine proteases. With the possible exception of factor VIII, the coagulation proteins are produced in the liver.

The process of coagulation is a series of biochemical reactions in which inactive proenzymes are converted to active enzyme forms, which then, in turn, activate other proenzymes. The coagulation process is thus a true **coagulation cascade** of factor activities, all interrelated to other factors. It is a carefully controlled process that responds to injury while continuing the maintenance of blood circulation.

### Nomenclature

To standardize the complex nomenclature that is used by those involved in coagulation studies, the **International Committee on Nomenclature of Blood Clotting Factors** was established in 1954 (Table 13-1).[10] Twelve coagulation factors

are described and designated by Roman numerals; other factors are known by name only.

Roman numerals have been assigned to the various coagulation factors in the order of their discovery and do not indicate anything about the sequence of the reactions. No factor has been assigned the Roman numeral VI. The numerals used denote the factors as they exist in the plasma, except for factor III, tissue thromboplastin, which is not normally present in plasma but is found in tissue. Factor III is not a single substance but a variety of substances. The lowercase *a* denotes activated forms and cofactors for the coagulation factors. All coagulation factors, except factor III, circulate in an inactive, or precursor, form. In addition to the factors denoted by Roman numerals, other essential coagulation reactants include phospholipid (or phospholipoprotein), the phospholipoprotein of platelets (PF3); prekallikrein, the active form of kallikrein; kininogen; and protein C, a vitamin K–dependent factor that is an inactivator of thrombin-activated factors V and VIII.

### Factor I (Fibrinogen)

The term fibrinogen has been in use for many years. **Fibrinogen** is the soluble precursor of the clot-forming protein, **fibrin,** and is involved in the common pathway of both the extrinsic and intrinsic clotting pathways. Factor I is a globulin with a molecular weight of 340,000 daltons. It is present in the plasma of normal persons at a concentration of 200 to 400 mg/dL. A minimum of 50 to 100 mg/dL is required for normal coagulation.

Fibrinogen is synthesized by the liver but does not require vitamin K for its production. In severe liver disease a moderate lowering of the plasma fibrinogen level may occur, although rarely to the degree that hemorrhage occurs.

By the action of thrombin, two peptides are split from the fibrinogen molecule, leaving a fibrin monomer. Fibrin monomers aggregate to form the final polymerized fibrin clot.

**TABLE 13-1**

Nomenclature of the Coagulation Factors

| Factor* | Name | Synonym(s) |
|---|---|---|
| I | Fibrinogen | |
| II | Prothrombin | |
| III | Tissue thromboplastin | Tissue factor |
| IV | Calcium | |
| V | Labile factor | Proaccelerin, accelerator globulin (AcG) |
| VI | Not assigned | |
| VII | Stable factor | Proconvertin, serum prothrombin conversion accelerator (SPCA) |
| VIII:C | Antihemophilic factor (AHF) | Antihemophilic globulin (AHG), antihemophilic factor A, subunit VIII:C |
| VIII:vWF | von Willebrand Factor (vWF) | Subunit VIII:vWF |
| IX | Plasma thromboplastin component (PTC) | Antihemophilic factor B (AHB), Christmas factor |
| X | Stuart-Prower factor | Stuart factor |
| XI | Plasma thromboplastin antecedent (PTA) | Antihemophilic factor C |
| XII | Hageman factor | Glass or contact factor |
| XIII | Fibrin stabilizing factor (FSF) | |
| Others | Prekallikrein (PK) | Fletcher factor |
| | High-molecular-weight kininogen (HMWK) | HMW kininogen, Fitzgerald factor |
| | von Willebrand factor | |
| | Fibronectin | |
| | Antithrombin III | |
| | Protein C | |
| | Protein S | |

*When factors have been activated, they have the designation *a* after the Roman numeral.

Fibrinogen is relatively unaffected by heat and storage (is stable), but may be irreversibly precipitated at 56° C. It has a half-life of 120 hours.

### Factor II (Prothrombin)

**Thrombin** is generated from a precursor, **prothrombin,** and is involved in the common pathway of both the extrinsic and intrinsic clotting pathways. Prothrombin is synthesized by the liver through the action of vitamin K. It is a protein (globulin) with a molecular weight of about 70,000 daltons, and is normally present in the plasma in a concentration of approximately 8 to 15 mg/dL. It is utilized in the clotting mechanism to such a degree that little remains in the serum. In normal plasma, there is an excess of prothrombin relative to the amount of thrombin

needed to clot fibrinogen. A wide margin of safety has been provided for this important substance. About 20% to 40% of the normal concentration must be present to ensure hemostasis. Prothrombin is heat stable and has a half-life of 70 to 110 hours.

### Factor III (Tissue Thromboplastin)

**Thromboplastin,** or tissue factor, is the name given to any substance capable of converting prothrombin to thrombin. In coagulation, two separate mechanisms utilize thromboplastin: as intrinsic or blood thromboplastin and as extrinsic or tissue thromboplastin. All injured tissues yield a complex mixture of as yet unclassified substances that possess potential thromboplastic activity. During clotting of whole blood, platelets appear to be the source of thromboplastin. The clot-accelerating activity of tissues has been assigned the name factor III by the International Committee on Nomenclature of Blood Clotting Factors.

Complete thromboplastins and partial thromboplastins are used in different laboratory diagnostic procedures. The term partial thromboplastin is used to designate thromboplastic reagents that are found to clot hemophilic plasma less rapidly than normal plasma. Complete thromboplastins are able to produce clotting as rapidly with hemophilic plasma as with normal plasma.

Tissue thromboplastin is a high-molecular-weight lipoprotein that is found in almost all body tissues; it is found in increased concentrations in the lungs and brain.

The molecular weight depends on the type of tissue from which the particular thromboplastin is derived; it can range from 45,000 to over 1 million daltons. Tissue thromboplastin is found in increased concentrations in red cell membranes, platelets, brain tissue, placenta, and lung.

### Factor IV (Ionized Calcium)

It has been known for many years that calcium in the ionized state is essential for coagulation, and the term **ionized calcium** is now used for calcium when it participates in this process (this was formerly called factor IV). Ionized calcium is necessary to activate thromboplastin and to convert prothrombin to thrombin; the exact mechanism by which calcium acts is not completely understood. Only a small amount of ionized calcium is required for blood coagulation. The fact that it is essential for clotting makes possible the use of anticoagulants that bind calcium; by binding of calcium, fibrin formation cannot take place and clotting does not occur.

Calcium appears to function mainly as a bridge between the phospholipid surface of platelets and several clotting factors. Binding sites on several factors allow bridging with the calcium-phospholipid complex.

### Factor V (Proaccelerin or Labile Factor)

Factor V is essential for the prompt conversion of prothrombin to thrombin in the clotting of whole blood and is involved in the common pathway of both the extrinsic and intrinsic clotting pathways. It is synthesized in the liver; acquired deficiencies have been observed in liver disease. When factor V levels decrease to 5% to 25% of normal, bleeding occurs. Factor V is a globulin with a molecular weight of about 330,000 daltons. It is labile, its activity being destroyed in the clotting process. The activity of factor V in plasma deteriorates even when the plasma is frozen; it is the most unstable of the coagulation factors and is therefore also known as **labile factor.** Its activity decreases within a few hours when human blood or plasma is stored at or above room temperature. It has a half-life of about 25 hours in the plasma.

### Factor VII (Proconvertin or Stable Factor)

Factor VII is not destroyed or consumed in the clotting process and therefore is also known as **stable factor.** Thus it is present in both plasma and serum. It is essential only for the extrinsic clotting pathway. It is a beta globulin with a molecular weight of 60,000 daltons. It is synthesized in the liver and requires vitamin K for its production. For normal coagulation, minimum levels are 5% to 10% of the normal amount. An acquired deficiency of factor VII results from any disorder that decreases its synthesis in the liver. It has a very short biological half-life, 4 to 6 hours, which results in a rapid disappearance from the blood when factor VII production is halted. This may occur during drug therapy with coumarin or in a congenitally deficient patient. Factor VII remains at a high level in stored blood as well as in serum. Factor VII activates tissue thromboplastin and accelerates the production of thrombin from prothrombin. Its presence can be monitored by the prothrombin test.

### Factor VIII (Antihemophilic Factor, Subunit VIII:C, and von Willebrand Factor, Subunit VIII:vWF)

Factor VIII is actually a combination of two functional subunits circulating as a complex: factors VIII:C and VIII:vWF. The entire circulating molecule can be designated VIII/vWF.

**Factor VIII:C.** The subunit designated factor VIII:C acts in the intrinsic clotting pathway as a cofactor to factor IXa in the conversion of X to Xa. Factor VIII:C represents the ability of the factor VIII molecule to correct coagulation abnormalities associated with classic hemophilia A. This unit is measured by the various factor VIII assays and by the activated partial thromboplastin time test used routinely in the laboratory.

**Factor VIII:vWF.** The other subunit, called factor VIII:vWF or von Willebrand's factor, facilitates platelet adherence to subendothelial surfaces. Factor VIII:vWF is necessary for normal platelet adhesion. It is the portion of the molecule responsible for binding platelets to endothelium and thus supports normal platelet adhesion and function. This subunit is not involved in the coagulation pathways. It is present in plasma, platelets, megakaryocytes, and endothelial cells. The larger part of the factor VIII complex is made up of the subunit factor VIII:vWF. It is strongly antigenic, and a portion of the molecule participates in platelet aggregation induced by the antibiotic ristocetin. Laboratory tests utilizing immunoassay are used to measure antigenic activity, while the basis of another test is the portion of the molecule that makes possible platelet aggregation in the presence of ristocetin.

The production site of factor VIII is not certain; possible sites are endothelial cells and megakaryocytes for the VIII:vWF subunits. Factor VIII is a beta globulin with a high molecular weight—over a million daltons. It is lost rapidly from the bloodstream, having a half-life of 6 to 10 hours for the factor VIII:C subunit. This rapid clearance occurs in normal persons as well as in those with a congenital deficiency of the factor (classic hemophilia A).

**Hemophilia A. Hemophilia** refers to a sex-linked recessive coagulation disorder. It has been demonstrated that the coagulation defect can be corrected by the use of normal plasma. The terms antihemophilic factor (AHF) and antihemophilic globulin (AHG) have been used to designate the procoagulant present in normal plasma but deficient in the plasma of patients with hemophilia. The term **hemophilia A,** the classic "bleeder's disease," is adopted to designate the hereditary disease caused by a deficiency in factor VIII:C subunit. Persons with severe hemophilia A will have a history of bleeding into joints and intramuscular hemorrhage. They will generally have normal levels of the von Willebrand factor, VIII:vWF, subunit and a normal bleeding time.

**von Willebrand's Disease. von Willebrand's disease (vWD)** is hereditary and is found in several different subtypes; the clinical manifestations will vary with the severity of the disease. Symptoms can include abnormal bleeding in childhood, easy bruising, bleeding gums, gastrointestinal bleeding, and abnormal bleeding after dental procedures. In von Willebrand's disease there is a deficiency of von Willebrand's factor (the VIII:vWF subunit of factor VIII); this factor is required for normal platelet adhesion to endothelium in the hemostatic process. A prolonged bleeding time is characteristic of vWD because platelet adhesiveness is found to be markedly decreased. Platelet aggregation is also abnormal.

### Factor IX (Plasma Thromboplastin Component)

Factor IX is a stable protein factor, an alpha or beta globulin, with a molecular weight of 55,000 to 62,000 daltons. It has a half-life of about 20 hours, is not consumed during clotting, and is not destroyed by aging. It is present in both serum and plasma, and there is probably no significant loss of the factor in blood or plasma stored at $4°$ C for 2 weeks. Factor IX is an essential component of the intrinsic thromboplastin-generating system. It is synthesized in the liver and requires vitamin K for its production.

**Hemophilia B.** The disease resulting from a deficiency of factor IX is known as **hemophilia B.** Hemophilia B is also inherited as a sex-linked recessive disorder. Its clinical symptoms are identical to those of hemophilia A, and the disorder can be classified as mild, moderate, or severe, paralleling the level of factor IX present.

### Factor X (Stuart-Prower Factor)

This is a relatively stable factor that is not consumed during the clotting process and therefore is found in both serum and plasma. It is an alpha globulin weighing 59,000 daltons that requires vitamin K for its synthesis in the liver. Factor X is essential to the intrinsic pathway, working with other substances to generate thromboplastin that converts prothrombin to thrombin. It helps to form the final common pathway through which products of both the intrinsic and the extrinsic thromboplastin-generating system act. Factor X is stable for several weeks to 2 months when stored at 4° C. It has a half-life of 24 to 65 hours.

### Factor XI (Plasma Thromboplastin Antecedent)

Factor XI is a beta globulin weighing 160,000 to 200,000 daltons. Its synthesis takes place in the liver, and vitamin K is not required for its production. It circulates as a complex with another protein—high-molecular-weight kininogen (HMWK). Only part of factor XI is consumed during the clotting process, so it is present in the serum as well as the plasma. It is essential for the intrinsic thromboplastin-generating mechanism.

### Factor XII (Hageman Factor)

Factor XII is a stable gamma globulin weighing 80,000 daltons. It is not consumed during the clotting process and is therefore found in both serum and plasma. It is synthesized in the liver and does not depend on vitamin K for its synthesis. Factor XII is converted to an active form when it comes in contact with glass and is therefore also known as the contact factor. The natural counterpart of glass is not known, but platelets or damaged endothelium may be involved in this primary activation process. Factor XII is involved in the initial phase of the intrinsic coagulation pathway.

### Factor XIII (Fibrin-Stabilizing Factor, Fibrinase)

Factor XIII is an alpha globulin with a high molecular weight. Its site of production is not fully known, but is believed to be in the liver for the plasma factor. Platelet XIII factor is synthesized by megakaryocytes. There is evidence that factor XIII is an enzyme (fibrinase) that catalyzes the polymerization of fibrin; polymerization of the fine fibrin clots produces a stable fibrin clot. This factor is inhibited by ethylenediaminetetraacetic acid (EDTA)—a common blood anticoagulant used for routine laboratory assays in hematology, specifically. Very little factor XIII is present in the serum, the major portion being used up in the polymerization of fibrin. It acts to stabilize the fibrin clot and also acts further to assist in linking the endothelial cell protein, fibronectin, to collagen and fibrin residues; this is extremely important in tissue growth and repair.

### Prekallikrein (PK, Fletcher Factor)

Prekallikrein is a precursor for a serine protease, kallikrein, which also activates plasminogen. It is involved in the intrinsic coagulation pathway. Kallikrein is a chemotactic factor used to recruit phagocytes and can stimulate the complement cascade. PK is found in the plasma in association with HMWK. It is produced in the liver but it is not dependent on vitamin K for its synthesis.

### High-Molecular-Weight Kininogen (HMWK, Fitzgerald Factor)

High-molecular-weight kininogen can be acted upon to yield kinin. It serves as a cofactor for reactions involving factor XII and activation of factor VII. HMWK is involved in the intrinsic coagulation pathway. It is the precursor molecule of bradykinin, an important inflammatory mediator involving vascular permeability and dilation, pain production at sites of inflammation, and synthesis of prostaglandin. HMWK is produced in the liver and is not dependent on vitamin K for its synthesis.

### Properties of Coagulation Factors

Coagulation factors can be divided into three groups on the basis of their properties:

**Fibrinogen Group.** The fibrinogen group (thrombin sensitive) consists of factors I, V, VIII, and XIII. Thrombin acts on all of these factors. Thrombin enhances factors V and VIII by converting them to active cofactors. It also activates factor XIII and converts fibrinogen (factor I) to fibrin. All of these factors are consumed in the coagulation process. Factors V and VIII are relatively labile and are therefore not present in plasma that has been stored. In addition to the presence of these fibrinogen factors in plasma, these factors are also found within platelets.

**Prothrombin Group.** The prothrombin group (vitamin K dependent) consists of factors II, VII, IX, and X. Vitamin K is essential for synthesis of all these factors. Coumarin-type drugs, which inhibit vitamin K, cause a decrease in these factors. Factors VII, IX, and X are not consumed in the coagulation process and are therefore present in serum as well in plasma. They are stable and are therefore well preserved in plasma that has been stored.

**Contact Group.** The contact group consists of factors XI and XII, prekallikrein (Fletcher factor), and HMWK (Fitzgerald factor). These factors are not consumed in the coagulation process, are not dependent on vitamin K for their synthesis, and are relatively stable.

### Mechanism of Coagulation

The complex mechanism of coagulation takes place in three major stages.

**Stage 1: Generation of Thromboplastic Activity.** The thromboplastic activity necessary to convert prothrombin to thrombin is produced in stage 1 through the interaction of platelets with factors XII, XI, IX, and VIII (the intrinsic pathway), or through the release of tissue thromboplastin from the injured tissues (the extrinsic pathway). Plasma factor VII activates the tissue thromboplastic substances. Various tests will detect stage 1 deficiencies, but the one test of choice for screening purposes and for identification of stage 1 deficiencies is the activated partial thromboplastin time (APTT) test (see Procedure 13-3).

**Stage 2: Generation of Thrombin.** The plasma or tissue thromboplastin, plus factor VII produced in stage 1, in the presence of plasma factors V and X, converts prothrombin to the active enzyme thrombin. Laboratory tests are available to detect deficiencies in stage 2. The one-stage prothrombin time (PT) test detects deficiencies best in stages 2 and 3 (see Procedure 13-2). Abnormal formation of a clot results from a deficiency of any of the coagulation factors or the presence of an inhibitor or anticoagulant. The anticoagulants EDTA, oxalate, and citrate remove calcium to prevent clotting in vitro. Heparin and coumarin drugs prevent the conversion of prothrombin to thrombin, also preventing the clotting mechanism from functioning in vivo.

**Stage 3: Conversion of Fibrinogen to Fibrin.** Thrombin converts fibrinogen to fibrin, and a fibrin clot is formed that is stabilized by the presence of factor XIII. The thrombin time test measures the concentration and activity of fibrinogen in stage 3.

The presence of calcium ions is necessary in all three stages of the clotting mechanism.

## PATHWAYS FOR THE COAGULATION CASCADE

The final product in the clotting process is the production of a stable fibrin clot. A series of events must take place involving many reactions and feedback mechanisms before the clot is formed. By means of the intrinsic or extrinsic pathway, or both, leading to a common pathway, the various precursors, factors, and other reactants respond normally in an orderly, controlled process—the coagulation cascade.

## Intrinsic versus Extrinsic Coagulation Pathway

All factors required for the intrinsic pathway are contained within the blood. The extrinsic pathway uses thromboplastin (factor III), which is released from the damaged cells and tissues outside the circulating blood.

### Intrinsic Pathway (Activation of Factor X)

In the intrinsic pathway, the circulating blood contains all the necessary components that lead to the activation of factor X. It is thought that tissue injury, following exposure to foreign substances such as collagen, activates the intrinsic pathway. Injury to endothelial cells can begin this process. In this pathway, a complex involving factors VIII and IX, in association with calcium and phospholipid on the platelets, ultimately activates factor X. To accomplish this, factor IX is first activated by the action of factor XIa (in the presence of calcium ions), which has previously been activated by factor XII (Fig. 13-1). Factors XI and XII are known as contact factors because their activation is initiated by

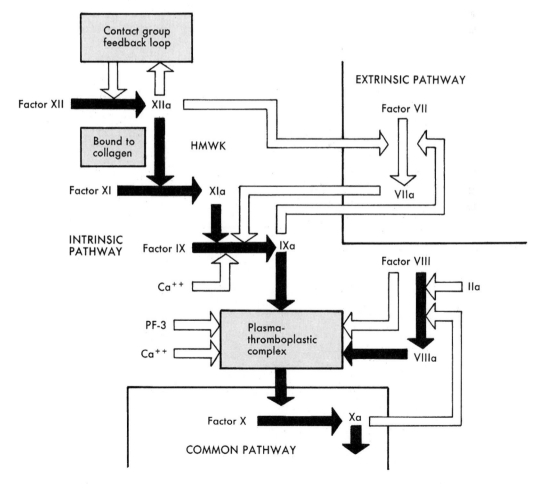

**FIG 13-1.** Major reactions of the intrinsic pathway. Generation of factor IXa and the plasma thromboplastin complex. (From Powers LW: *Diagnostic Hematology.* St Louis, Mosby, 1989, p 170.)

contact with subendothelial basement membrane that is exposed at the time of a tissue or blood vessel injury.

Although the complex reactions that occur in the intrinsic pathway take place relatively slowly, they account for the majority of the coagulation activities in the body. A laboratory test that monitors the intrinsic pathway leading to fibrin clot formation is the activated partial thromboplastin time (APTT) test (see Procedure 13-3). The APTT measures factors XII, XI, X, IX, VIII, V, II, and I.

### Extrinsic Pathway (Activation of Factor X)

The term extrinsic is used to indicate the pathway taken when tissue thromboplastin, a substance not found in the blood, enters the vascular system and, in the presence of calcium, activates factor X. Factor VII is activated to its VIIa form in the presence of calcium (factor IV) and tissue thromboplastin (factor III), which, in turn, activates factor X to Xa. Thromboplastin is released from the injured wall of the blood vessel. Only activated factor VII is needed in the extrinsic pathway, bypassing factors XII, XI, IX, and VIII (used in the intrinsic pathway to activate factor X to its activated form, Xa) (Fig. 13-2). In addition to quickly providing small amounts of thrombin, which leads to fibrin formation, the thrombin generated in the extrinsic pathway can enhance the activity of factors V and VIII in the intrinsic pathway. To monitor the extrinsic pathway leading to fibrin clot formation in the laboratory, the prothrombin time (PT) test is performed (see Procedure 13-2). The PT measures factors VII, X, V, II, and I.

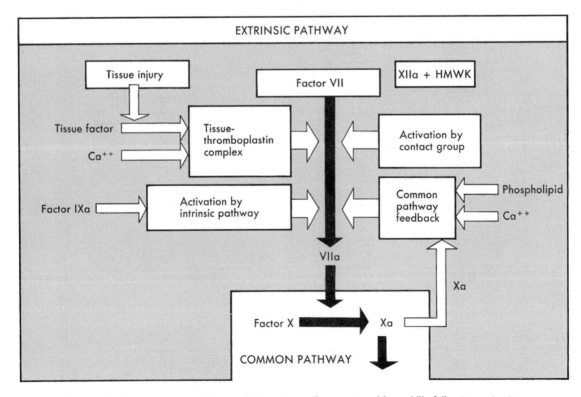

**FIG 13-2.** Major reactions of the extrinsic pathway. Generation of factor VIIa following activation of tissue factors. (From Powers LW: *Diagnostic Hematology.* St Louis, Mosby, 1989, p 168.)

## The Common Pathway (Formation of the Fibrin Clot From Factor X)

By means of either the extrinsic or the intrinsic pathway, or a combination of both pathways, the common pathway, the activation of factor X to Xa occurs. The activation of factor X is the point where the two pathways converge to form the **common pathway.** Once Xa is formed, another cofactor, V, in the presence of calcium and PF3, converts factor II, prothrombin, to the active enzyme, thrombin. The activation of thrombin is slow, but once it is generated, it further amplifies the coagulation process. Thrombin acts to convert fibrinogen to fibrin (Fig. 13-3).

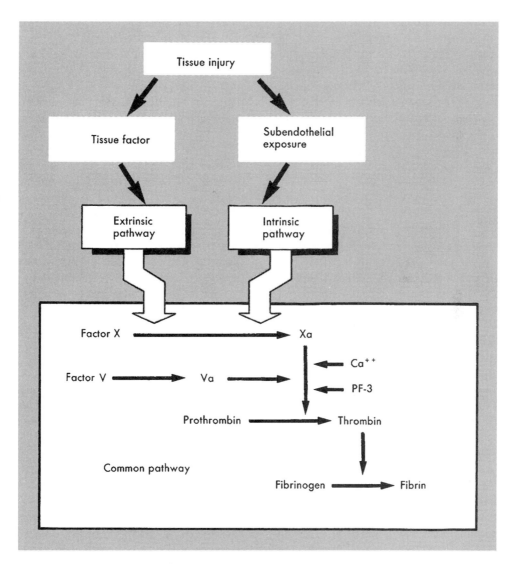

**FIG 13-3.** Overview of coagulation. Relationship between the three pathways, common, extrinsic, and intrinsic, emphasizing the major events of the common pathway. *PF-3,* Platelet factor 3. (From Powers LW: *Diagnostic Hematology.* St Louis, Mosby, 1989, p 162.)

Activation of factor XIII during this process results in the formation of a stronger, more durable clot.

### Fibrin Clot and Clot Retraction

The result of converting fibrinogen to fibrin is a visible fibrin clot. The fibrin clot is formed loosely over the site of injury, reinforcing the platelet plug and closing off the wound. After a period of time, the clot begins to retract and becomes smaller—**clot retraction.** This retraction is attributed to the action of the platelets and other cells that have been trapped in the clot. The fibers of fibrin are pulled closer together by cytoplasmic processes that have been sent out by the platelets. Clot retraction can also be observed in a test tube—in vitro (see Fig. 13-5). The liquid remaining after the clot has retracted is serum. Normal clot retraction in vitro should be complete by 4 hours at 37° C.

## FIBRINOLYSIS

Besides having a system for clot formation, the body also has a means by which the fibrin clot may be removed and the flow of blood reestablished. The mechanism for clot removal is not completely understood.

As soon as the clotting process has begun, **fibrinolysis** is initiated to break down the fibrin clot that is formed. Normally, the **fibrinolytic system** functions to keep the vascular system free of fibrin clots or deposited fibrin. There is evidence that the fibrinolytic system and the coagulation system are in equilibrium in normal persons. As a general rule, fibrinolysis is increased whenever coagulation is increased.

The active enzyme that is responsible for digesting fibrin or fibrinogen is **plasmin.** Plasmin is not normally found in the circulating blood, but is present in an inactive form, plasminogen. Plasminogen is converted to plasmin by certain proteolytic enzymes. These plasminogen activators are found in small amounts in most body tissues, in very low amounts in most body fluids, and in urine. The decomposition products of fibrin formed during fibrinolysis are removed from the blood by the reticuloendothelial system.

## TESTS FOR HEMOSTASIS AND COAGULATION

### Screening Tests for Disorders of the Hemostatic System

Diagnosis of disorders of the hemostatic system should begin with a physical examination and a clinical history of the patient and the family members of the patient. It is important to also include a complete drug history, which will often provide information about the type of disorder that may be affecting the patient. Hemostatic disorders can be secondary to several primary diseases, such as liver disorders, renal failure, and certain carcinomas. Screening tests for hemostasis and coagulation include tests for the condition of the blood vessels (vascular factors), for platelets, and for the coagulation and fibrinolytic systems—divided according to the main lines of defense against hemorrhage (see under Hemostatic Mechanism). A comprehensive and carefully obtained clinical history is considered the single most valuable screening test.

Tests for the vascular factors include the capillary fragility test (also known as the cuff test, tourniquet test, or capillary resistance test) and tests for bleeding time. Tests for the platelet factors include the platelet count, platelet aggregation assays, platelet adhesiveness studies, the bleeding time, and the clot retraction test. There are numerous tests for the plasma factors and whole blood factors involved in coagulation—the venous clotting time, PT, and APPT (see Table 13-2). Selected tests will be discussed in this chapter.

### Tests for Vascular Factors
#### Bleeding Time Tests

**Bleeding time (BT)** tests measure the time required for cessation of bleeding after a standardized capillary puncture to a capillary bed. The time required will depend on capillary integrity, the number of platelets, and the platelet function.

There must be an adequate number of circulating platelets for a normal bleeding time. Below a platelet count of $50 \times 10^9/L$ the bleeding time is almost always prolonged. Platelet dysfunction is better assayed by more specific tests, such as platelet aggregation and clot retraction tests, and the use of the BT test for platelet function is not considered as useful as in the past.

Under the conditions of the BT test, bleeding is believed to be controlled by capillary retraction and the formation of a platelet plug in the wound. Tissue factors are also thought to play a role, especially tissue tonus (contraction). Defects in the clotting mechanism have little effect on the bleeding time. The bleeding time is prolonged when there is a combination of poor capillary retraction and platelet deficiency.

The bleeding time test is positive (bleeding time is prolonged) in thrombocytopenic purpura and in constitutional capillary inferiority. Normal bleeding times are found in hemophilia and other defects of the clotting mechanism.

**Template Bleeding Time Test (Mielke Modification).** A number of different bleeding time tests have been devised. The test now in use is a modification by Mielke et al of the original Ivy bleeding time test; two incisions of a standardized depth are made, and the average of the two bleeding times is reported.[2,3] A blood pressure cuff is used to maintain the blood pressure at 40 mm Hg during the test. The chief difficulty in performing bleeding time tests in general is the production of adequate and standardized skin punctures; a valid test result depends greatly on the way the skin wound is made. Capillary bleeding is tested, and wounds more than 3 mm deep are likely to involve vessels of greater than capillary size, whereas wounds that are shallow are not likely to adequately test the capillaries and the hemostatic factors involved. A standardized, disposable BT test system such as the Simplate* or other similar system is pre-

*General Diagnostics Division of Warner-Lambert Co, Morris Plains, NJ.

ferred, whereby compliance with infection control measures is also achieved. An NCCLS guideline document provides information about performing template bleeding time tests.[7]

**Simplate Bleeding Time Test.** The Simplate lancet device contains dual spring-loaded blades within a plastic holder. When the trigger is depressed, the edge of the blades (each 5 mm in length) will spring forward 1 mm from the housing, making two parallel cuts 1 mm deep and 5 mm long. The incisions made are therefore 5 mm long and 1 mm deep (see Procedure 13-1). This procedure is similar to the Mielke template modification of the Ivy bleeding time test, except that the commercial product includes a disposable lancet device that makes the incisions. With very shallow incisions being made, venules are rarely cut. The normal range for this procedure is from 2.3 to 9.5 minutes. The patient should be bandaged with a butterfly bandage over the puncture site and advised to keep it in place for 24 hours.

**Precautions in Bleeding Time Tests.** Results of bleeding time tests are not always significant, because normal bleeding times are found in patients who have defects in the clotting mechanism. Bleeding time is prolonged in conditions in which there is a combination of poor muscle contraction in the blood vessels and platelet deficiency. Obtaining an adequate bleeding time depends greatly on the depth of the skin puncture. In the original Ivy method and its modifications, the blood pressure cuff must be maintained at 40 mm Hg throughout the test. The commercial template method is considered the best bleeding time test because the skin punctures are uniformly deep.

### Tests for Platelet Factors

Tests for the platelet factors involved in hemostasis include the platelet count (see under Counting Platelets, Chapter 12), assays of platelet aggregation or adhesiveness, the bleeding time tests (described above), the prothrom-

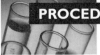

## PROCEDURE 13-1

*Bleeding Time Test Using Simplate\* Device, Based on Mielke Modification of the Ivy Bleeding Time Test[2,3]*

1. Place a blood pressure cuff on the patient's forearm above the elbow. Inflate to 40 mm Hg and maintain this pressure for the duration of the testing procedure.

2. Extend the patient's arm, palm down. Cleanse the site to be used with alcohol.

3. Remove the template device from the package, twist off the white, tear-away tab on the side of the device.

4. Place the template on the forearm, avoiding superficial veins. The template should be placed so that the blades are in a line with the thumb and elbow. The template is pressed firmly against the surface of the skin.

5. Depress the trigger, and remove the device about one second after triggering. Start the stopwatches as soon as bleeding is evident (two cuts are made with this device and two stopwatches can be used). Cuts 5 mm long and 1 mm deep are made. Note that because there is an initial period of vasospasm, there is no bleeding when the cuts are first made (during the first 5 to 15 seconds after the cuts have been made). Stopwatches should not be started until bleeding actually begins.

6. Wick (do not blot) the blood from the puncture site every 30 seconds, using filter paper (Fig. 13-4). The filter paper should not touch the wound at any time. Blood is wicked as necessary from the sides of the cuts to avoid disturbing the clot as it is formed.

7. When bleeding ceases, stop the stopwatches and release the blood pressure cuff. Cleanse the site with an antiseptic solution. Place a butterfly bandage over the site, and have the patient keep the bandage in place for at least 24 hours.

8. Record results. Normal values are up to 9.5 minutes.

\*General Diagnostics Division of Warner-Lambert Co, Morris Plains, NJ.

---

bin consumption test, and the clot retraction test. The bleeding time tests are especially concerned with platelets—the number of platelets present and their ability to form a plug. Prolonged bleeding times will generally be found when the platelet count is below $50 \times 10^9/L$ and when there is platelet dysfunction, and it is recommended that bleeding times not be done in these cases. In any case, a bleeding time test should not be done unless a platelet count has been done shortly before.

### Platelet Aggregation Studies

The response of platelets during the hemostatic process includes a change in shape, increasing surface adhesiveness and the tendency to aggregate with other platelets to form a plug. Measurement of platelet aggregation is an essential part of the investigation of any patient with suspected platelet dysfunction. An aggregating agent is added to a suspension of platelets in plasma—**platelet-rich plasma, PRP**—and the response is measured turbido-

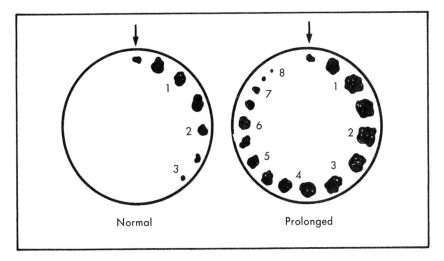

**FIG 13-4.** Bleeding time determination. Appearance of blood spots on filter paper from a patient with a normal bleeding time *(left)* and from a patient with a platelet defect *(right)*. (From Powers LW: *Diagnostic Hematology.* St Louis, Mosby, 1989, p 474.)

metrically as a change in the transmission of light. A variety of commercially available instruments have been devised to conduct this test. These instruments are called **aggregometers.**

When an aggregating reagent (including thrombin, adenosine diphosphate, epinephrine, serotonin, arachidonic acid, ristocetin, snake venoms, collagen) is added to PRP being stirred in a cuvette at a constant temperature, platelets start to aggregate and the transmission of light increases. The PRP appears turbid at the beginning of the test. With the addition of the aggregating reagent, larger platelet aggregates begin to form, and because of this, the PRP begins to clear and there is a corresponding increase in the light being transmitted. The increased change in optical density or transmission of light is recorded as a function of time on a moving strip recording. The platelet response curve consists of distinct phases that will vary with the concentration and type of aggregating reagent used.

### Platelet Retention or Adhesiveness Test

This test measures the ability of platelets to adhere to glass surfaces. When anticoagulated blood is passed at a constant rate through a plastic tube containing glass beads, some platelets will adhere to the glass beads. The percentage difference between the platelet counts done prior to and after passage through the glass bead column is calculated. The normal range is 75% to 95% platelet retention. The platelet adhesiveness test is nonspecific. It is abnormal in several platelet functional disorders.

### Clot Retraction Tests

Normal blood will clot completely and the clot will begin to retract within 1 hour at room temperature. At the end of 18 to 24 hours, the clot should have retracted completely and serum should be expressed (Fig. 13-5). The clot should be tough and elastic and not easily broken with an applicator stick. Retraction is primarily dependent on normal platelet function, but hematocrit level and the fibrinogen level also can affect clot retraction. The extent of the retraction is influenced by the amount of fibrin formed, the presence of intact platelets within the fibrin network, and physical interference from trapped red blood cells. When the platelet count is less

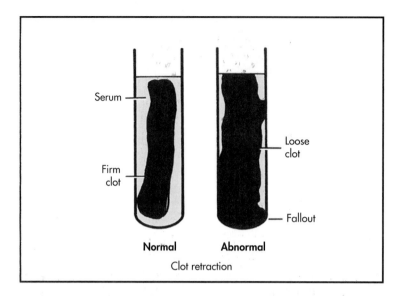

**FIG 13-5.** Clot retraction. Normal and abnormal appearance of a clot after 24 hours' incubation. (From Powers LW: *Diagnostic Hematology.* St Louis, Mosby, 1989, p 476.)

than $100 \times 10^9$/L, poor clot retractility is usually seen.

If the tube of blood is incubated in a water bath at 37° C and observed periodically, clot retraction is complete in 4 hours for a normal subject, but may be poor or absent 24 hours later in a patient with inadequate thrombosthenin (a protein component of platelets, important in a clot reaction) or a low platelet count. This test is not considered to be a very sensitive measure of platelet dysfunction.

### Tests for Plasma Coagulation Factors

To assess potential defects in the coagulation cascade, screening tests are first performed. Common screening tests of the plasma coagulation system are the one-stage **prothrombin time (PT)**, the **activated partial thromboplastin time (APTT),** and the **thrombin time (TT).** Other related tests for coagulation are bleeding time, platelet counts, and clot retraction tests (Table 13-2). Once it has been determined by the coagulation screening tests that the patient has a coagulation disorder, the exact factor, deficiency, or abnormality should be identified.

In the monitoring of anticoagulant therapy, the measurement of prothrombin is most generally employed when the patient is receiving coumarin drugs. Heparin therapy is usually followed by determining the APTT and the thrombin time, although the whole blood coagulation time is occasionally used.

The manual methods for doing coagulation tests have been replaced in most laboratories by automated and semiautomated equipment. Automated methodology is based on manual methods. Several instruments are available that can do coagulation tests for prothrombin and APTTs. Some of these instruments can detect the formation of the clot photoelectrically, thus eliminating the error associated with visual timing of clot formation.

Two nonautomated techniques for performing plasma clotting tests are discussed in this section: the assay for prothrombin and the APTT.

### Specimens For Coagulation Tests

It is most important that specimens for coagulation tests be collected in the least traumatic man-

**TABLE 13-2**

Laboratory Tests for Hemostasis and Coagulation

| Test | Purpose of Test/Test Assesses |
| --- | --- |
| Bleeding time (BT) | Platelet factors: function and number |
| | Vascular factors: capillary integrity |
| Capillary fragility (cuff test/tourniquet test) | Vascular factors (condition of blood vessels) |
| Platelet count | Platelet factors: platelet numbers |
| Platelet aggregation | Platelet factors: platelet function |
| Platelet adhesion (platelet retention) | Platelet factors: platelet function |
| Clot retraction | Platelet factors: platelet function |
| Activated partial thromboplastin time (APTT) | Plasma factors: deficiencies in intrinsic and common pathways; identifies stage I deficiencies (factors XII, XI, IX, VIII, V, II, I); monitors heparin therapy |
| Prothrombin time (PT) | Plasma factors: deficiencies in extrinsic and common pathways; identifies stage II and III deficiencies (factors VII, X, V, II, I); monitors coumarin therapy |
| Thrombin time (TT) | Plasma factors: measures concentration and activity of fibrinogen in stage III; monitors coumarin therapy |
| Fibrinogen | Plasma factors: deficiencies of fibrinogen, alteration of conversion of fibrinogen to fibrin |
| Specific factor assays: | Plasma factors: |
| Factor VIII:C | Deficiency: hemophilia A |
| Factor VIII:vWF | Deficiency: von Willebrand's disease |
| Factor IX | Deficiency: hemophilia B |

ner; the premature activation of the clotting process must be avoided to ensure valid test results. The blood must be drawn carefully, avoiding contamination of the specimen with tissue thromboplastin, contact with the surface of an inappropriate specimen container, use of an inappropriate anticoagulant, improper temperature conditions, and any technique that would produce hemolysis of the specimen. NCCLS guidelines cover the essentials for the proper collection, transport, and processing of blood specimens for coagulation testing.[4]

**Anticoagulants.** Screening coagulation assays are performed on plasma that has been processed from blood anticoagulated with a sodium citrate solution. The citrate reversibly binds calcium ions and prevents the various steps in the coagulation process that begin with the activation of factors IX and VII from taking place.

Binding the calcium does not inhibit the contact phase of coagulation, so it is critical that no activation of this process be made while the blood is being collected or processed. An example of contact phase effects is premature activation of coagulation contact factors XI and XII if blood comes in contact with glass. For this reason, only nonreactive materials can be used for collection tubes or testing steps in doing coagulation tests (see also under Collection Technique). Sodium citrate (3.2%) is the anticoagulant of choice for most coagulation tests, usually a buffered sodium citrate (3.2% or 3.8%). The manufacturer's specifications should be followed for the optimal concentration.

The ratio of blood to anticoagulant is critical for clotting tests, necessitating the use of only evacuated tube systems with the proper vacuum; expiration dates must be observed and outdated tubes not used. By a long-established convention for coagulation tests, nine volumes of carefully drawn blood are mixed with one volume of citrate anticoagulant (1:10 ratio). The standard ratio of anticoagulant to sample is 1:10 for persons with hematocrits between 20% and 60%. Ratios must be changed for persons who are extremely anemic or polycythemic. For example, for specimens with very high hematocrits when there is a reduced plasma volume, the use of a reduced anticoagulant volume is needed.

Clots are unacceptable in the sample because most of the routine coagulation tests are performed on instruments using a turbidometric analyzing methodology for measuring the formation of a clot in the detection process.

**Collection Technique.** A clean, rapid venipuncture is necessary to prevent tissue thromboplastin from contaminating the blood sample. Tissue thromboplastin (in the tissue juices) can be found in blood samples when the vessel has been cut or traumatized, and even a slight amount can alter coagulation test results for both normal and abnormal samples. Hemolyzed red cells act like tissue thromboplastin in activating plasma clotting factors, so for this reason hemolysis of the sample must be avoided. Glass surfaces affect hemostasis; certain of the coagulation contact factors will be prematurely activated by contact with glass. Nonreactive materials and nonwettable surfaces, which will not interact or activate the coagulation mechanism, should be used; silicone-coated glass or plastic containers are recommended for collecting specimens to be used for coagulation tests. Temperature also affects hemostasis; some of the coagulation factors (factors V and VIII) are very labile if left at room temperature for any length of time, and other factors (factors VII and XI) are activated prematurely by cold temperatures.

Either a syringe or an evacuated tube system can be used to collect the specimen. A clean entry into the vein must be made. The blood should flow quickly and smoothly into the container.

***"Two-Syringe" Method.*** The method of collection that ensures the highest quality of specimen for coagulation tests is a "two-syringe" method. This is the best way to prevent contamination of the blood specimen with traces of tissue juices that would activate the coagulation process. Two plastic syringes should be used to prevent activation of the contact phase of coagulation. The first syringe is used to withdraw a few milliliters of blood; then a second syringe is attached and the specimen collected for coagulation testing. The tourniquet should not be left in place for a prolonged time, as extended stasis can result in endothelial injury and the release of plasminogen activators. As soon as the blood is drawn into the syringe, the needle is removed and the blood allowed to flow down the inside of the specimen tube. The tube of blood and anticoagulant should be covered and gently inverted three or four times without shaking or foaming. Shaking the tube will result in activation of platelets and the contact system.

***Evacuated Tube System.*** A more common collection system uses evacuation tubes. Evacuated collection tubes are available with 3.2% buffered citrate anticoagulant in them. There is less direct contact with the actual blood specimen when these tubes are used. In the evacuated tube system, blood should be collected into the citrated tubes for coagulation studies after blood has been drawn for other tests. The coagulation testing specimen should be the second or third tube obtained. If only a single coagulation tube is needed, an extra discard tube of blood is drawn prior to the blood being drawn into the citrate tube. This is done so that the coagulation specimen is not part of the first flow of blood out of the vein. The same precautions in venipuncture technique and handling procedures for the specimen should be used as described for the syringe method, to ensure that the specimen is collected in the best possible way, eliminating invalid coagulation assay results. It is important that the correct ratio of blood to anticoagulant be maintained, so the vacuum citrate tube must be allowed to fill completely and only tubes within their expiration dates should be used.

**Specimen Processing.** Once the sample is drawn, some changes can begin quickly in vitro. For this reason, transportation to the laboratory for testing should be done as quickly and carefully as possible. Specimens should be centrifuged and the plasma separated from the cells within 60 minutes of being drawn. The tubes should be kept stoppered during centrifuging and until the plasma is removed for testing. The cell-free plasma-anticoagulant mixture is separated from the cellular elements unless testing is done immediately; when immediate testing is done, the plasma may remain on the packed cells.

It is important to check the sample for microclot formation. If it is present, specimens are unacceptable for testing, as clotting has been initiated. Specimens that have visible hemolysis are also unacceptable for testing because of possible clotting factor activation and interference in end points for many of the analytic testing instruments being used. Most current instruments using an optical detector may also have problems with end point determinations using samples that are icteric or lipemic. The plasma to be tested should be kept refrigerated in a tightly covered clean tube until it is tested. The screening coagulation tests are performed on plasma.

### Performance of Coagulation Assays

General guidelines apply to most coagulation tests. NCCLS guidelines outline recommendations for determination of factor coagulant activities, specifically assays for measurement of prothrombin and for activated partial thromboplastin time.[5,6] Specific manufacturer's instructions for each instrument must be followed explicitly. For coagulation assays, an ongoing program of quality control should be in place and carefully followed to comply with CLIA '88 regulations. Records must be maintained for documentation purposes.

**Quality Control.** Normal and abnormal controls should be run when testing is begun each day and at the beginning of each new work shift or with each test run of assays. Control specimens are reconstituted daily from a lyophilized aliquot, or frozen controls are used. Controls must be used within their established viability periods (usually 8 to 16 hours). Once a control is thawed or reconstituted, it should not be refrozen or reused. Control samples should be handled and tested under conditions similar or identical to those for the patient samples being tested. Patient values are not reported unless the control values are within the established reference range. NCCLS guidelines cover the essentials in regard to issues of quality control for coagulation testing.[6]

**Reference Ranges.** Laboratories must develop their own reference ranges for control specimens, representing a normal population for the particular facility. Reference values should be reestablished when new reagents are implemented, with major changes in collection techniques, or when new instruments are introduced into the laboratory.

### Prothrombin Assay (Quick's One-Stage Method for Prothrombin Time[9])

The test for prothrombin was devised on the assumption that when an optimal amount of calcium and an excess of thromboplastin are added to decalcified plasma, the rate of coagulation depends on the concentration of prothrombin in the plasma (Procedure 13-2). The prothrombin time (PT) is therefore the time required for the plasma to clot after an excess of thromboplastin and an optimal concentration of calcium have been added. It measures the functional activity of the extrinsic (and common) coagulation pathway. It is a test of generation of thrombin (stage 2) and conversion of fibrinogen to fibrin (stage 3) of the clotting mechanism and screens for deficiencies of factors I, II, V, VII, and X. It is used as a method of choice for monitoring anticoagulant therapy by vitamin K antagonists (coumarin drugs).

A normal prothrombin assay shows that the elements of stages 2 and 3 of the coagulation mechanism are probably not disturbed. This finding, coupled with a prolonged venous clotting

## PROCEDURE 13-2

### Prothrombin Time Assay, Manual Method (Quick's One-Stage Method for Prothrombin Time[6])

1. As soon as possible after collection, centrifuge the blood specimen at 3000 rpm for at least 10 minutes. Separate the plasma from the cells as soon as possible after centrifugation.

2. Pipette 0.2-mL portions of the thromboplastin–calcium chloride reagent into small test tubes or cups.

3. Incubate the tubes containing the thromboplastin–calcium chloride mixture and the tubes containing portions of the plasma for patient and control at 37° C. Allow a minimum of 1 minute for the thromboplastin and plasma to reach 37° C.

4. Add 0.1-mL samples of plasma to the tubes containing the thromboplastin–calcium chloride reagent. Start the stopwatch simultaneously. At this point, automated instruments use mechanical agitation or an optical beam to measure formation of the clot. Automated methods will start the timing process simultaneously as the test plasma is added using automatic pipettes and will stop when the fibrin web or clot is formed.

5. Mix the tubes, and leave them in the water bath (37° C) for a minimum of 7 to 8 seconds. Then remove them and tip them gently back and forth until a clot is formed. The clot is best seen by tilting against a bright light.

6. Stop the stopwatch immediately when a clot is observed, and record the time.

7. Report calculated INR.

8. Manual prothrombin assays should always be done in duplicate for patient specimens and for control samples.

time, places the abnormality within stage 1. The measurement of prothrombin is used to follow the progress of patients treated with coumarin-type oral anticoagulant drugs (warfarin) used to inhibit clotting (especially for preventing postoperative thrombosis and pulmonary embolism) and to screen for factor deficiencies in hemorrhagic diseases. Antithrombotic drugs are commonly used, and they can present some very real hazards to the patient. If the degree of anticoagulation is insufficient, rethrombosis or embolism can occur. If there is too much anticoagulation, fatal hemorrhage can take place. The laboratory tests for coagulation can provide information whereby therapeutic balance is maintained. The laboratory is responsible for advising the physician about the level of anticoagulation achieved.

Two categories of antithrombotic drugs are the coumarins, which act as vitamin K antagonists, and heparin. Therapeutic management of patients being medicated with coumarin drugs is monitored by use of the prothrombin assay.

The reagents necessary for the prothrombin assay are primarily calcium chloride and thromboplastin. Only carefully manufactured reagents can be used—thromboplastin reagents with their assigned ISI (international sensitivity index). (See also under Reporting Prothrombin Results: Use of the International Normalized Ratio.) Each prothrombin control must be prepared before use according to the manufacturer's directions. Control values and limits will vary with the brand of control used. The laboratory will establish its own reference range for the control specimens. Proper use of the control can detect deterioration of the thromboplastin, use of a calcium solution of the wrong concentration, or use of an improper incubation temperature.

Use of automatic pipetting devices is recommended when the prothrombin assays are performed manually. Many of the automated instruments used in laboratories incorporate automatic pipetting as a part of the testing process. All plasma samples are tested at least in duplicate and usually in triplicate. Determinations must agree within the established limits for duplicate or triplicate tests. A control plasma is tested in the same manner as the patient plasma is tested, and the control value is recorded. Laboratories will establish acceptable reference ranges for the control specimens they use. The test must be repeated if the allowable error is exceeded.

**Precautions and Technical Factors.** The prothrombin assays should be done within 4 hours of blood collection because of progressive inactivation of certain coagulation factors. The plasma may be frozen and stored up to 1 week without appreciably affecting the result of the test.

When the thromboplastin-calcium reagent is used, it is important to mix the suspension very well. The blood for this test must be free of clots; if any clots are present, a new specimen must be drawn. The ratio of anticoagulant to blood specimen must be 1:10 (0.5 mL of anticoagulant and 4.5 mL of whole blood).

**Automated Prothrombin Assays.** Automated or semiautomated methods using fibrometers or fully automated methods using optical density readings are employed for screening coagulation tests (prothrombin assays and activated partial thromboplastin time tests) by many laboratories. These instruments automatically pipette all necessary reagents for the testing process. The principle of the test is the same as for the nonautomated (manual) methods described, but the end point of the reaction—the

formation of the fibrin clots—is detected photoelectrically. A sudden change in optical density occurs as the clot is formed, timing automatically is stopped, and the clotting time recorded. The clotting time is recorded to the nearest 0.1 second, and an INR is calculated.

The FibroSystem* is a semiautomated, electromechanical instrument for coagulation assays. It consists of a Fibrometer coagulation timer, a thermal preparation block or incubator, and an automatic pipetting system. The Fibrometer is the main unit of the instrument and consists of a timer, several warming wells, and a clot detector that is a probe arm with electrodes. Most coagulation assays that use a clot as the end point may be performed with this system.

Automated or semiautomated coagulation systems can be one of several variations of an MLA Electra.† Clot formation is timed automatically and is detected by use of a photocell that reads the optical density change when the clot is formed. Contained within the unit is a heating block that maintains the reagents and plasma samples at 37° C before and during the testing process. Certain varieties of this analyzer automatically pipet the necessary reagents and samples; others require manual pipetting prior to analysis. All routine coagulation assays may be performed with these instruments—PT, APTT, specific coagulation factor assays, thrombin time, and fibrinogen tests, among others.

**Reporting Prothrombin Results: Use of the International Normalized Ratio.** For many years, the results of assays to measure prothrombin were reported in seconds and tests were called prothrombin time tests, or PTs. The prothrombin time is not actually a quantitative assay for prothrombin. The international normalized ratio was first used instead of seconds to report results for prothrombin assays when the test was

---

*BBL Microbiology Systems, Division of Becton Dickinson & Co, Cockeysville, Md.
†Medical Laboratory Automation, Inc, Mount Vernon, NY.

being used to monitor patients receiving oral anticoagulant therapy (see earlier in this section).

The **international normalized ratio (INR)** is the PT ratio obtained by using the appropriate World Health Organization (WHO) international reference standard preparation as the source of thromboplastin in the assay for prothrombin time. The INR compares the patient's PT to a mean, normal prothrombin time, using a highly responsive WHO reference thromboplastin, and therefore removes any bias between different methods. The INR is the PT ratio that would have been obtained if a WHO international standard reference thromboplastin had been used in the test methodology. The WHO originally helped devise use of the INR for patients on long-term anticoagulant therapy to ensure that tests done in different laboratories in any part of the country (or worldwide) would yield comparable results. Even though different thromboplastins and different instrumentation are used in various laboratories, the great value of the INR is that it makes standardization of oral anticoagulant therapy possible. The use of the INR effectively calibrates the results of a particular PT reagent and/or instrument system to results of an international reference reagent.[6]

Manufacturers of thromboplastin reagents provide the **international sensitivity index (ISI)** for each lot of reagents. The ISI is a mathematical indicator of the responsiveness of the PT testing system to deficiencies of the vitamin K coagulation factors. The WHO reference thromboplastin is highly responsive and has an assigned ISI of 1.0. The ISI is obtained by comparing the manufacturer's thromboplastin reagent with the WHO international reference thromboplastin. The ISI for a specific test system is used to convert the observed PT ratio to its INR equivalent by means of the following formula[1]:

$$INR = \frac{Patient\ PT^{ISI}}{Normal\ PT}$$

Experience has shown that reporting the INR works better than reporting the PT in seconds for any purpose—not just for patients on oral anticoagulant therapy—and for this reason, in most clinical settings the PT is no longer reported in seconds only.

The INR becomes elevated with deficiencies in factors in the extrinsic pathway. These deficiencies most commonly result from: (1) use of oral anticoagulant therapy, which depletes the vitamin K–dependent factors (II, VII, IX, and X), and (2) liver disease. The reference INR range for persons 1 year and older is 0.85 to 1.15.

**Reporting Prothrombin Results in Seconds.** The normal values for the prothrombin time in seconds range from 10 to 13 seconds.

### Activated Partial Thromboplastin Time

In the activated partial thromboplastin time test (APTT), an activator is mixed with a phospholipid component of thromboplastin (a platelet substitute) before addition to the plasma being tested; only a partial component of thromboplastin is used, thus giving the test its name (Procedure 13-3). The activator used depends on the manufacturer of the reagents—one activator is a kaolin suspension (a finely divided silicate clay). The APTT test is the single most useful procedure available for routine screening for coagulation factor deficiencies of the intrinsic and common pathways. The APTT adds kaolin, an activator of factor XII, which allows more complete activation, shortens the clotting times, and improves reproducibility over the formerly used partial thromboplastin time (PTT) test.

The APTT measures deficiencies mainly in factors VIII, IX, XI, and XII, but can detect deficiencies of all factors except VII and XIII. The tests are based on the observation that when whole thromboplastin is used, as for prothrombin assays, the times obtained for hemophilic plasma are about the same as those for normal plasma. With a partial thromboplastin solution or platelet substitute, the times obtained for hemophilic plasma are much longer than those for normal plasma. One important use of the APTT test is in the management of patients receiving

## PROCEDURE 13-3

### Activated Partial Thromboplastin Time, Manual Method[6]

1. As soon as possible after the blood has been collected, centrifuge the anticoagulated specimen at 3,000 rpm for at least 10 minutes.

2. Remove the plasma from the cells immediately.

3. Warm the calcium reagents at 37° C.

4. Pipette 0.1 mL of activated platelet substitute suspension (kaolin plus partial thromboplastin) into the desired number of tubes (duplicates for patient and control samples), and incubate at 37° C for a minimum of 1 minute.

5. Add 0.1 mL of plasma (patient or control) to the activated thromboplastin mixture already incubating in the tubes. Mix well and allow to incubate for at least 2 minutes. The minimum incubation time for this mixture is 2 minutes. Incubation times over 5 minutes may cause loss of certain factors in the plasma coagulation system being measured.

6. Add 0.1 mL of the calcium chloride reagent to the plasma-thromboplastin reagent mixture, and start the stopwatch immediately (simultaneously).

7. Mix the tube once, immediately after adding the calcium reagent. Allow the tube to remain in the water bath for about 25 seconds.

8. After 25 seconds, remove the tube from the water bath. Wipe off the outside of the tube so that the contents can be clearly seen. Gently tilt the tube back and forth. The clot is best seen by tilting against a bright light. The end point is the appearance of fibrin strands.

9. At the appearance of fibrin strands, stop the stopwatch and note the time.

10. Control and patient plasmas must always be tested in duplicate when manual methods are used; the two results are averaged to obtain the final result. The duplicate results should agree within 1.5 seconds when the APTT is less than 45 seconds. If they do not, another test should be done. When the clotting time is longer, duplication of results is more difficult and the allowable range of variation is wider. If formation of the clot has not started by the end of 2 minutes, the test may be stopped and the results reported as greater than 2 minutes.

heparin therapy. The sensitivity of the thromboplastin reagent must be evaluated before this test is used as a heparin control.

A phospholipid substitute for platelets acts as a partial thromboplastin. It is more sensitive to the absence of factors involved in intrinsic thromboplastin formation than are the more complete tissue thromboplastins used in the assays for prothrombin.

Activation in the procedure is obtained by separate addition of a kaolin suspension.[8] Kaolin ensures maximal activation of the coagulation factors. By addition of kaolin, the slow contact phase of the coagulation cascade is speeded up. Activators used can vary with the manufacturer of the reagents being used. By activation of the contact factors, more consistent and reproducible results are achieved.

The APTT test result will be prolonged in contact factor and intrinsic factor deficiencies. The presence of an inhibitor, such as the lupus anticoagulant, in the patient's plasma may also be the cause of a prolonged APTT. The APTT is used to monitor heparin concentration during intravenous administration. The APTT is not sensitive to minor abnormalities in some common pathway factors, but is useful to screen mild to moderate deficiencies of factors VIII and IX and the contact factors. Deficiencies of these factors represent the most common and potentially serious disorders. If an abnormal APTT is determined, differential studies should be done for specific factor deficiencies.

The principle of this test is the assumption that during anticoagulation, the calcium present in the blood is bound to the anticoagulant. After centrifugation, the plasma contains all the intrinsic coagulation factors except calcium (removed during anticoagulation) and platelets (removed during centrifugation). Under carefully controlled conditions and with properly prepared reagents, calcium, a phospholipid platelet substitute (the partial thromboplastin), and an activator (kaolin) are added to the plasma to be tested by means of the APTT test. The time required for the plasma to clot is the APTT. The normal times proposed by the reagent manufacturer should be followed.

Control specimens are always run along with the patient's specimen. Normal control results must always fall within the normal control range; if they do not, something is wrong with the reagents, the equipment, or the technique being used. When the control is out of range, the entire test must be repeated.

**Precautions and Technical Factors.** Use of kaolin gives maximal activation of the coagulation factors and therefore more consistent and reproducible results. Kaolin in suspension settles out very quickly; when kaolin is used, it is necessary to mix the solutions vigorously before any pipetting is done. If there are enough stopwatches, more than one test can be done at a time by starting the separate incubations at intervals to allow time for the manipulations and observations of the clots.

Citrated blood should be centrifuged within 30 minutes of collection. Plasma allowed to sit longer than the recommended time can give abnormal results.

**Reporting Results of APTT.** APTT tests are reported in seconds to the nearest tenth of a second, along with the control specimen reference values established for the laboratory. Results must be clearly marked for "patient" or "control." Generally, a normal APTT is less than 35 seconds, with a range from 25 to 40 seconds. Control plasmas must be run and their values carefully monitored. Deviations in control results can be due to temperature changes, different reagent lots, the technique being used, or instrument malfunction, if automation or semiautomation is being employed. Patient results are always reported along with control values. All test results must be repeated if the control results do not fall within the established reference range for the control specimens. Each laboratory must determine its own reference range for normal and abnormal controls used for these tests, as values vary greatly depending on the reagents used.

### Point-of-Care Tests for Coagulation Assays

Because turnaround time is of great importance in certain clinical situations, **point-of-care testing (POCT)** for some coagulation assays is used. During surgical procedures for patients receiving heparin anticoagulant therapy, tests for activated clotting time (ACT), prothrombin, activated partial thromboplastin time, fibrinogen, thrombin time, and heparin neutralizing thrombin time can be performed by POCT instruments. There is also an interest in use of home-testing instruments whereby patients on long-term anticoagulant therapy can test their own blood to ensure better control of their medications. Of the many POCT assays being done in today's health care facilities, however, coagulation assays remain among the least commonly performed procedures.

**Analyzers Used for POCT Coagulation Assays.** Hemochron Jr.* and CoaguChek and CoaguChek Plus[†] will be briefly described.

---

*International Technidyne Corp, Edison, NJ.
[†]Boehringer Mannheim Corp, Indianapolis, Ind.

These instruments are hand-held analyzers using fresh, whole blood from a finger puncture or venipuncture. They can be used in surgical suites, intensive care units, dialysis units, or other patient care units. Fresh whole blood is added to a sample well on a test cartridge inserted into the instrument after a prompt signal appears. The blood sample is drawn by capillary action into the test channel, where it mixes with the reagents. An electro-optical system detects the point at which blood flow ceases—the clot forms. This is the end point of the assay. The result appears in a display window. Results with whole blood are higher than for the typical laboratory analyzers, which use plasma. Results are converted to equivalent plasma values, and INRs are given for prothrombin assays. Coagulation POCT results should be included in the patient's chart in the same manner as for traditional coagulation test results.

**Quality Control.** Quality control programs must be used with any POCT coagulation analyzer. CLIA '88 mandates that two levels of control—normal and abnormal—be assayed in each 8-hour shift for automated coagulation systems, traditional methods, and POCT. The manufacturers of these coagulation POCT analyzers are working to improve their electronic QC, but conventional liquid coagulation controls remain the CLIA '88–acceptable type, for the present. Use of liquid controls is expensive for POCT coagulation assays because the control specimen is viable for only a specific period of time (usually 8 to 16 hours), and often only a few patients are tested by POCT during that time, contrary to traditional in-laboratory coagulation testing, in which case many tests are performed during an 8-hour shift. Each time a control specimen or patient specimen is tested, a test cartridge is used, increasing the cost for the testing.

**Problems and Drawbacks.** Reagents for coagulation POCT are considerably more expensive than reagents for conventional coagulation assays. One estimate is that POCT reagents cost three to five times more than conventional coagulation assay reagents. Another potential drawback of coagulation POCT is that with the ease of using these analyzers and with the availability of almost instantaneous data, the advantages of their use may be negated if data are lost or never transferred to the patient's permanent record.

**Training for Users.** It is important that any person who is to use the coagulation POCT analyzers be adequately trained in their use and that the training be documented. Ideally, the users should be trained under the auspices of the laboratory and the quality control measures also carried out by a laboratorian. Some manufacturers of coagulation POCT analyzers provide users—physicians, patients (in their homes), other health care workers—with a system of quality management. This includes in-depth training in the use of the analyzer and technical support, if needed, in the future. Training includes information about the importance of good specimen collection techniques and the use of quality control measures.

### Other Tests for Coagulation

Several other tests for specific coagulation factors are done in a coagulation laboratory. These include the prothrombin consumption test, the thromboplastin generation test, plasma recalcification time (plasma clotting time), thrombin time, fibrinogen titer, quantitative tests for fibrinogen, Russell viper venom time, reptilase time, and various coagulation factor assays. Specific tests for von Willebrand's factor, such as that employing ristocetin reagent, are also performed.

## REFERENCES

1. International Committee for Standardization in Haematology, International Committee on Thrombosis and Haemostasis: ICSH/ICTH recommendations for reporting prothrombin time in oral anticoagulant control. *Thromb Haemost* 1985; 53:155-156.

2. Ivy AC, Shapiro PF, Melnick P: The bleeding tendency in jaundice. *Surg Gynecol Obstet* 1935; 60:781.

3. Mielke CH, Kaneshiro IA, Maher JM, et al: The standardized normal Ivy bleeding time and its prolongation by aspirin. *Blood* 1969; 34:204.

4. NCCLS: *Collection, Transport, and Processing of Blood Specimens for Coagulation Testing and Performance of Coagulation Assays: Approved Guideline,* ed 2. Villanova, Pa, National Committee for Clinical Laboratory Standards, 1991, document H21-A2.

5. NCCLS: *Determination of Factor Coagulant Activities: Approved Guideline.* Villanova, Pa, National Committee for Clinical Laboratory Standards, 1997, document H48-A.

6. NCCLS: *One-Stage Prothrombin Time (PT) Test and Activated Partial Thromboplastin Time Test (APTT): Approved Guideline.* Villanova, Pa, National Committee for Clinical Laboratory Standards, 1996, document H47-A.

7. NCCLS: *Performance of the Bleeding Time Test: Approved Guideline.* Villanova, Pa, National Committee for Clinical Laboratory Standards, 1998, document H45-A.

8. Proctor RR, Rapaport SL: The partial thromboplastin time with kaolin. *Am J Clin Pathol* 1961; 36:212.

9. Quick AJ et al: Study of coagulation defects in hemophilia and jaundice. *Am J Med Sci* 1935; 190:501.

10. Wright IS: The nomenclature of blood clotting factors. *Thromb Diath Haemorrh* 1962; 7:381.

## BIBLIOGRAPHY

Beutler E, Lichtman MA, et al: *Williams Hematology,* ed 5. New York, McGraw-Hill Book Co, 1995.

Brown B: *Hematology: Principles and Procedures,* ed 6. Philadelphia, Lea & Febiger, 1993.

Harmening DM: *Clinical Hematology and Fundamentals of Hemostasis,* ed 3. Philadelphia, FA Davis Co, 1997.

Lotspeich-Steininger C, Stiene-Martin A, Koepke J (eds): *Clinical Hematology: Principles, Procedures, Correlations,* ed 2. Philadelphia, Lippincott-Raven Publishers, 1998.

Turgeon ML: *Clinical Hematology: Theory and Procedures,* ed 3. Philadelphia, Lippincott-Raven Publishers, 1998.

## STUDY QUESTIONS

1. Which of the following is the anticoagulant of choice for routine coagulation assays?

   A. Heparin
   B. Sodium oxalate
   C. Sodium citrate
   D. Sodium fluoride

2. The prothrombin assay requires that the patient's citrated plasma be combined with which one of the following?

   A. Thromboplastin
   B. Calcium and thromboplastin
   C. Calcium
   D. Kaolin

3. Why are plastic or siliconized tubes used for blood specimens for coagulation assays?

4. What does the silicate (kaolin) do in the test system for APTT?

   A. Binds calcium so clotting does not occur
   B. Activates tissue thromboplastin
   C. Facilitates platelet adherence to endothelial surfaces
   D. Allows more complete activation of factor XII, thus shortening the clotting times

5. Which of the following peripheral blood cells is involved in hemostasis?

   A. Thrombocytes
   B. Lymphocytes
   C. Erythrocytes
   D. Granulocytes

6. Which of the following coagulation factors is (are) used only in the extrinsic coagulation pathway? (More than one response may be correct.)

   A. II
   B. V
   C. VII
   D. VIII

7. Which of the following factors is part of the common coagulation pathway? (More than one response may be correct.)

   A. Factor VII
   B. Factor X
   C. Factor XI
   D. Factor XII

8. The bleeding time test is not recommended when there is platelet dysfunction or when the platelet count is:

   A. $<50 \times 10^9/L$
   B. $<100 \times 10^9/L$

9. Which of the following coagulation factors will be inhibited by coumarin-type drugs? (More than one response may be correct.)

   A. II
   B. VII
   C. VIII
   D. X

10. Fibrinogen is synthesized in the:

    A. Liver
    B. Endothelium
    C. Platelets
    D. Plasma

11. What is the ratio of blood to anticoagulant used for the common coagulation assays?

12. Why is sodium citrate anticoagulant used when coagulation tests are performed?

13. An essential requirement for adequate primary hemostasis is:

    A. Formation of a thrombus
    B. Retraction of the clot
    C. Adhesion of platelets
    D. Presence of vitamin K

14. For control of most bleeding, which one of the following statements about platelets is true?

    A. Platelet numbers must be adequate.
    B. Platelet function must be normal.
    C. Both A and B are true.
    D. Neither A nor B is true.

15. Clot removal is accomplished by which of the following systems?

    A. Fibrinolysis
    B. Hemostasis
    C. Thrombosis
    D. Anticoagulation

16. Tests that measure the integrity of the hemostatic system include which of the following? (More than one response may be correct.)

    A. Platelet count
    B. Bleeding time
    C. Prothrombin assay
    D. Activated partial thromboplastin time

17. Hemostasis is defined as a process to:

    A. Localize an injury
    B. Restore normal anatomy
    C. Prevent excessive bleeding following an injury
    D. Facilitate the removal of a clot

18. Hemophilia A is a disorder associated with a deficiency of:

    A. Plasma factor VIII
    B. Plasma factor IX
    C. Circulating platelets
    D. Vitamin K–dependent factors

19. Which of the following coagulation factors is (are) measured only by the assay for prothrombin? (More than one response may be correct.)

    A. Factor VI
    B. Factor VII
    C. Factor VIII
    D. Factor IX

20. The most accurate POCT coagulation test used to monitor heparin activity is that for:

    A. Prothrombin
    B. Activated partial thromboplastin time
    C. Bleeding time
    D. Platelet count

## CASE HISTORIES

### ■ CASE I

The following laboratory data were obtained from a 23-year-old man with a long history of abnormal bleeding into his joints:

| | |
|---|---|
| Prothrombin assay | Normal |
| Activated partial thromboplastin time | Markedly prolonged |
| Factor VIII assay | Markedly decreased |
| Factor IX assay | Normal |
| Platelet count | Normal |
| Template bleeding time | Normal |

Which of the following disorders is the most likely for this patient?
  A. Classic hemophilia A
  B. Classic hemophilia B
  C. von Willebrand's disease
  D. Severe liver disease

### ■ CASE 2

A 45-year-old female patient has severe liver disease with jaundice, purpura (bleeding into the tissues), and a platelet count of between 100 and $120 \times 10^9$/L. Which one of the following profiles is most likely in this situation?
  A. Prolonged prothrombin time (PT), prolonged bleeding time (BT)
  B. Normal PT, prolonged bleeding time
  C. Normal PT, normal bleeding time
  D. Prolonged PT, normal bleeding time

### ■ CASE 3

A 25-year-old man was admitted to the hospital for surgical repair of an abdominal hernia. He was in good physical condition, but his family history included minor bleeding problems among some of his relatives. The following laboratory results were obtained:

| | |
|---|---|
| Prothrombin time | Normal |
| Activated partial thromboplastin time | Prolonged |
| Factor VIII assay | Decreased |
| Factor VIII:C | Decreased 10% |
| Factor VIII:vWF | Decreased |
| Factor IX assay | Normal |
| Platelet count | Normal |
| Platelet aggregation test | Decreased |
| Template bleeding time | Increased |

On the basis of the patient's history and laboratory test results, which of the following disorders is the most likely for this patient?
  A. Classic hemophilia A
  B. Classic hemophilia B
  C. von Willebrand's disease
  D. Severe liver disease

# CHAPTER 14

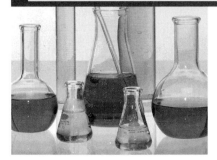

# *Urinalysis*

## Learning Objectives

*From study of this chapter, the reader will be able to:*

➤ Define routine urinalysis and describe its three main components.

➤ Explain the clinical usefulness of urinalysis and classify tests pertaining to diseases or conditions affecting the kidney or urinary tract and metabolic disease.

➤ Describe the basic anatomic components of the urinary system and the function of each.

➤ Discuss the chemical composition of normal urine.

➤ Describe a suitable urine specimen for routine urinalysis, including storage and preservation.

➤ Recognize and describe normal and abnormal physical properties (especially color and transparency) that might be encountered in urine specimens and to correlate physical findings with chemical and microscopic findings.

➤ Discuss the relationship between urine volume, color, and specific gravity.

➤ Define specific gravity and explain the difference between measurement by refractometer and measurement by reagent strip.

➤ Test a urine specimen for chemical constituents by using a multiple-reagent strip with correct technique and with knowledge of the general procedure and precautions necessary for valid results.

➤ For each of the ten analytes discussed in this chapter, describe the following: clinical importance, principle of the test, specificity and sensitivity, interferences, additional considerations, and confirmatory or related follow-up tests.

➤ Discuss the pathophysiology and significance of proteinuria caused by glomerular damage, tubular damage, prerenal disorders, lower urinary tract disorders, asymptomatic proteinuria, and consistent microalbuminuria.

➤ Discuss the pathophysiology of hematuria, hemoglobinuria, and myoglobinuria and how to differentiate between the respective analytes when a positive reagent strip test for blood is seen.

➤ Discuss the pathophysiology and clinical importance of tests for nitrite and leukocyte esterase and how they relate to each other.

➤ Discuss the difference between reagent strip tests for glucose and copper reduction tests for reducing sugars.

➤ Discuss the pathophysiology and clinical importance of bilirubin and urobilinogen and laboratory findings in various types of jaundice.

➤ Discuss the difference between reagent strip tests for Ehrlich-reactive substance and urobilinogen and how to differentiate the presence of urobilinogen from the presence of porphobilinogen.

➤ Explain the significance of the presence of ascorbic acid in urine, how to recognize its presence, and how to resolve discrepancies in laboratory test results due to the presence of ascorbic acid.

➤ Define urine sediment and describe conditions when it must be examined microscopically.

➤ List changes that occur in the urine sediment after it is voided.

➤ Perform a microscopic examination of the urine sediment, using appropriate microscopic and or staining techniques as needed.

➤ Identify, describe, and discuss the various urine sediment constituents that might be encountered, including pathophysiology and clinical importance.

➤ Describe the formation and significance of casts and how they are classified and reported.

➤ List the normal crystals encountered in acid and alkaline urine and describe the most commonly encountered forms of each.

➤ List the abnormal crystals of metabolic and iatrogenic origin and describe the most commonly encountered forms of each.

➤ Discuss the relationship between sediment, chemical, and physical findings in the urine.

➤ Discuss the components of a quality assurance system for urinalysis.

➤ Be able to recognize discrepant results when reviewing urinalysis findings (physical, chemical, and sediment), before results are reported.

# ROUTINE URINALYSIS

Of all the diagnostic procedures performed in the laboratory, the analysis of the urine is perhaps the oldest. Urine samples are readily available, and many of the routine tests are relatively simple to perform using readily available chemical reagent strips. The reagent strip (a plastic strip with one or more chemically impregnated test sites on an absorbant pad) is immersed into the urine specimen, and a color reaction is observed by comparison with a color chart at an appropriate time. Some constituents may be tested with a commercially available tablet test. The simplicity of the tests in no way means that they are unimportant or should be performed sloppily or in haste. It cannot be overemphasized that it is extremely important to do careful, accurate work at all times.

## Definition

The physical, chemical, and microscopic analysis of the urine is known as **urinalysis.** It is made up of a number of different tests and observations. Some of these tests are chemical, and others are not. When the urinalysis is performed in an orderly fashion and the results are recorded accurately, the combination of observations and test results will provide a valuable picture of the patient's general health pattern.

According to The National Committee for Clinical Laboratory Standards (NCCLS), "Urinalysis is defined as the testing of urine with procedures commonly performed in an expeditious, reliable, accurate, safe, and cost effective manner."[4] The purposes for urinalysis as described by the NCCLS are shown in Box 14-1.

## Components of the Routine Urinalysis

Each laboratory needs to determine the exact components and protocol of its routine urinalysis procedure and whether or when to include a microscopic examination of the urine sediment. However, the routine urinalysis generally consists of three parts, as shown in Box 14-2 and described below.

---

**BOX 14-1**

Purposes for Urinalysis

To aid in the diagnosis of disease

To monitor wellness (screening for asymptomatic, congenital, or hereditary disease)

To monitor the progress of disease

To monitor therapy (effectiveness or complications)

---

**BOX 14-2**

Routine Urinalysis Protocol

**Physical properties**
Color
Transparency
Odor
Foam
Specific gravity (refractometer)

**Chemical screening tests (reagent strips)**
pH
Specific gravity
Protein
Blood
Nitrite
Leukocyte esterase
Glucose
Ketones
Bilirubin
Urobilinogen

**Microscopic examination of urinary sediment**
Red blood cells
White blood cells
Epithelial cells
Bacteria and other cellular components
Casts
Crystals
Other Components

## Physical Properties

These include color, transparency, odor, foam, and specific gravity. Abnormalities in any of these must be accounted for in subsequent parts of the urinalysis.

## Chemical Tests

These are generally done by using multiple reagent strips, which measure up to 10 parameters. Tests for protein and glucose are basic to any urinalysis. Other chemical tests have become routine as they have been added to the readily available multiple reagent strips. Different combinations are available for use in different clinical situations. For example, in an obstetric clinic, tests for glucose, protein, blood, and leukocyte esterase are especially desirable. In certain instances, positive findings in the chemical screen may require confirmation with other chemical tests or indicate the likelihood of certain findings in the microscopic examination of the urinary sediment.

## Microscopic Examination of the Urinary Sediment

This is especially helpful in assessing the presence of kidney and urinary tract disease. The presence of certain findings in the microscopic examination will explain abnormal physical and chemical tests.

## Confirmatory Tests

In many cases it is necessary to confirm the presence of a substance in urine that is indicated on the basis of initial screening tests. The confirmatory test is used to establish the accuracy or correctness of another procedure. It is used both to decide if an analyte is actually present in low-level (trace) reactions, and to further estimate the quantity of analyte present. The confirmatory test is not just a repeat test using the same methodology. Rather, it is an alternative method with at least the same or better specificity, is based on a different principle, or has equal or better sensitivity than the original test. Examples of common confirmatory tests in urinalysis when positive results are seen on the chemical screen by reagent strips include: a protein precipitation test for protein; use of another reagent strip for glucose, with greater differentiation of values; testing high specific gravity values with a refractometer; testing with a tablet test for bilirubin; and looking for red cells, leukocytes, and casts in the microscopic analysis of the urine sediment based on the chemical screen. Other confirmatory tests that might be requested by the physician based on routine urinalysis include: quantitative protein or protein electrophoresis; bacterial culture; and cytology using a cytocentrifuged and stained preparation.

## Clinical Usefulness of Urinalysis

In general the urinalysis will provide information concerning (1) the state of the kidney and urinary tract, and (2) information about metabolic or systemic (nonrenal) disorders. Tests for the presence of protein, blood, nitrite, and leukocyte esterase together with the physical properties and the finding of casts, cells, and certain crystals are most helpful in assessing and treating renal and urinary tract disease. On the other hand, tests for glucose, ketone bodies, bilirubin, and urobilinogen are useful indicators in metabolic and systemic disorders such as diabetes and jaundice. This is summarized in Table 14-1.

## Considerations in Performing the Urinalysis

Certain factors must be kept in mind and understood when the routine urinalysis is being performed. These include:

1. The basic principle on which the test is based
2. Limitations of the test; this includes knowledge of test specificity (what substance is being measured), test sensitivity (minimum detectable concentration of the substance being measured), and the range of detectable substance being measured

**TABLE 14-1**

Clinical Usefulness of the Routine Urinalysis

**Indicators of the state of the kidney or urinary tract**
Appearance (color, transparency, odor and foam)
Specific gravity
Chemical tests
    Protein
    Blood
    Nitrite
    Leukocyte esterase
Urinary sediment
    Cells
    Casts
    Certain crystals

**Indicators of metabolic and other conditions or disease**

| | |
|---|---|
| pH | For crystal identification; occasionally for acid-base status |
| Appearance | Pigments, concentration and/or dilution |
| Glucose and ketones | For diabetes mellitus |
| Bilirubin | Jaundice and liver disease |
| Urobilinogen | Hemolytic anemias and some liver diseases |

**Indicators of other systemic (nonrenal) conditions or disease**

| | |
|---|---|
| Hemoglobin | Intravascular hemolysis |
| Myoglobin | Rhabdomyolysis |
| Light-chain proteins | Multiple myeloma or other gammaglobulinopathies |
| Porphobilinogen | Some porphyrias |

3. Knowledge of common interfering substances (false-negative and false-positive reactions)
4. Knowledge of any critical steps or considerations in the procedure
5. A general idea of the clinical application of the substance being tested for and its correlation to other findings in the urinalysis: physical, chemical, and microscopic
6. The need for additional or confirmatory tests, based on results of the physical and chemical screen and microscopic examination

For example, the finding of protein in the urine is an especially helpful indicator of renal or urinary tract disease. Both the amount of protein and the presence or absence of other findings in the sediment will help indicate the site and nature of the disease. Chemical tests for blood, nitrite, and leukocyte esterase are also helpful in assessing the cause of proteinuria.

Urinary glucose may indicate the metabolic disorder diabetes mellitus. This is further indicated when ketone bodies, a reduced pH, and increased output of a pale urine specimen with a high specific gravity when measured with a refractometer are found.

## RENAL ANATOMY AND PHYSIOLOGY[11]

### Renal Anatomy: The Urinary System

In general, urine can be considered a fluid composed of the waste materials of the blood. It is formed in the kidney and excreted from the body by way of the urinary system.

The urinary system consists of two kidneys, two ureters, the bladder, and the urethra. The working unit of the kidney is the **nephron,** where urine is formed. The formed urine flows from the kidney into the ureter and is passed to the bladder for temporary storage. It is eliminated from the body through the urethra. (See Fig. 14-1.)

The nephron consists of the **glomerulus** (made up of a tuft of blood vessels) and the renal tubules, which include the glomerular (Bowman's) capsule, the proximal convoluted tubule, the loop of Henle, and the distal convoluted tubule. Several nephrons flow into the collecting duct, which combine to form the renal papilla and eventually the ureter (Fig. 14-1). Each kidney consists of about 1.2 million nephrons, and the total length of the tubules in each nephron is 30 to 40 mm. The kidney itself has two anatomical portions, the outer **cortex,** which is made up of the glomerular portions of the nephron and the proximal convoluted tubules, and the central **medulla,** consisting of the loop of Henle, the distal convoluted tubules, and the collecting tubes.

Blood enters the kidney through the renal artery. This branches into smaller and smaller units, finally becoming the afferent arterioles entering the glomerular tuft. Blood leaves the glomerulus via the efferent arterioles. These arterioles run close to the corresponding renal tubules of the nephron, so that reabsorption and secretion between the blood and glomerular filtrate can occur. The kidney is a highly vascular organ. Normally, one fourth of the cardiac output is contained within the kidneys at a given time.

## Renal Physiology

The kidney may be described as having the following main functions:

1. Removal of waste products, primarily nitrogenous wastes from protein metabolism, and acids

2. Retention of nutrients, such as electrolytes, protein, water, and glucose
3. Acid-base balance
4. Water and electrolyte balance
5. Hormone synthesis, such as erythropoietin, renin, and vitamin D

These functions are carried out by means of filtration, reabsorption, and secretion.

### Glomerulus

The glomerulus consists of a small knot or tuft of blood capillaries. Blood enters the glomerulus from the renal circulation through the afferent arteriole and leaves through the efferent arteriole. Urine formation begins with the glomerulus, the structure that delivers the blood to the nephron—the working portion of the kidney.

### Glomerular (Bowman's) Capsule

As blood circulates through the glomerulus, it is filtered into Bowman's capsule. The glomerular capillaries are covered by the inner layer of Bowman's capsule, forming a semipermeable membrane that allows passage of all substances with molecular weights less than about 70,000 daltons. The fluid that passes through this membrane is basically blood plasma without proteins and fats. It is an ultrafiltrate of blood, and is called the **glomerular filtrate.** Because it has most of the solutes of plasma, the glomerular filtrate is **iso-osmolar** with plasma. That is, it has about the same osmolality as plasma-232 to 300 mOsm/L, with a specific gravity of ~1.008. The formation of the glomerular filtrate is the first step in urine formation. About 180 liters of glomerular filtrate are produced daily, yet only 1 or 2 liters of urine are eliminated from the body. Therefore, most of the glomerular filtrate is reabsorbed back into the blood.

### Proximal Convoluted Tubule

Reabsorption from the renal tubules back into the blood begins at the proximal convoluted tubule,

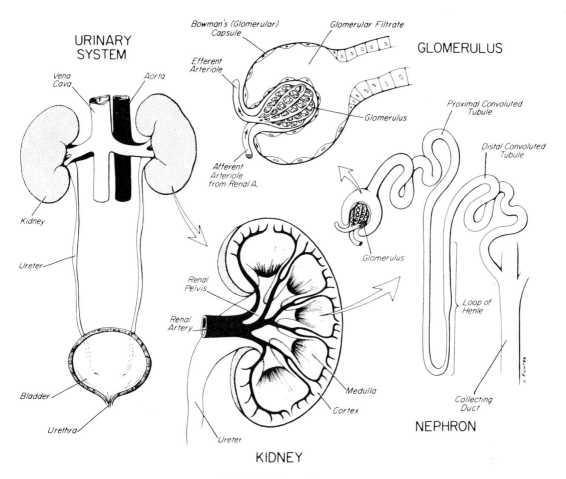

**FIG 14-1.** The urinary system.

where about 80% of the fluid and electrolytes filtered by the glomerulus are reabsorbed.

Reabsorption may be **active reabsorption,** with an expenditure of energy required for the analyte to be reabsorbed—usually against a concentration gradient, from a region of lower to one of higher concentration. Or the reabsorption may be **passive,** in which case an analyte moves passively down a concentration gradient, from a region of higher to a region of lower concentration. In addition, an analyte can move passively along with another analyte that may be actively reabsorbed.

Most of the water in the glomerular filtrate is passively reabsorbed along with sodium ions,

which are actively reabsorbed by the sodium pump mechanism. Chloride, bicarbonate, and potassium ions, together with 40% to 50% of the urea present in the filtrate, are passively reabsorbed with water at the proximal tubules. Other analytes that are actively reabsorbed in the proximal convoluted tubules include glucose, protein as albumin (a small amount of albumin is filtered into Bowman's capsule and subsequently reabsorbed), amino acids, uric acid, calcium, potassium, magnesium, and phosphate.

The proximal tubule has a limit to the amount of an analyte that will be completely reabsorbed from the glomerular filtrate. This is referred to as the **renal plasma threshold.** This differs with each analyte. When the plasma concentration of an analyte is greater than its renal plasma threshold, it will remain in the glomerular filtrate and be excreted in the urine. For example, the renal plasma threshold for glucose is about 180 mg/dL. When a patient with diabetes mellitus has a blood glucose concentration greater than 180 gm/dL, excess glucose will be eliminated in the urine.

The proximal convoluted tubules are also a site of active secretion of body wastes. The secretion includes hydrogen ions, phosphate, organic acids, and certain drugs such as penicillin. Hydrogen ions are secreted in exchange for sodium ions, which are reabsorbed with bicarbonate into the plasma. This exchange is dependent on the presence of the enzyme carbonic anhydrase, which is present in proximal and distal renal tubular cells and red blood cells.

Solutes and water are reabsorbed in equal proportions at the proximal tubules; therefore the tubular fluid is still iso-osmolar with plasma when it leaves the proximal tubules.

### Loop of Henle

The descending and ascending loops of Henle function to reduce the volume of the urine while reabsorbing or recovering sodium and chloride. The descending portion of the loop is the concentrating portion. The interstitial fluid outside the tubules in the medulla of the kidney becomes hypertonic as a result of increased concentrations of sodium, chloride, and urea in the tubules. This occurs because the descending portion is freely permeable to water but not to solutes. As the loop passes further into the medulla, water moves from the loop into the interstitium. This further concentrates the urine in the tubule. The water released into the interstitium is then reabsorbed back into the blood vessels that accompany the tubules. In other words, as the fluid (to be urine) moves down the descending loop, water moves out and into the bloodstream in a so-called **counter-current mechanism.**

The ascending loop of Henle serves as the diluting segment because of the ability to actively secrete sodium and chloride, but prevent water loss. Therefore, the fluid within the tubule loses sodium and chloride and eventually is either hypertonic or isotonic compared to plasma when it reaches the distal convoluted tubule.

### Distal Convoluted Tubule

There are two main functions of the nephron at the distal tubule. The final reabsorption of sodium occurs at this point (maintaining water and electrolyte balance), and excess acid is removed from the body (acid-base balance).

Sodium is actively reabsorbed with some bicarbonate at this point. However, the primary mechanism for sodium reabsorption is by the sodium-potassium pump under the control of the hormone **aldosterone.** Aldosterone is released from the adrenal medulla in response to angiotensin II, which is a product of the renin response to either hypotension or low plasma sodium. Aldosterone stimulates active absorption of sodium ion in exchange for potassium that is excreted by tubular cells (the sodium-potassium pump). Overall there is an increase in plasma sodium and water, with a decrease in body potassium levels.

When it is necessary to retain more sodium ions, ammonia is formed from glutamine and combines with hydrogen ions to form ammonium ions. This allows for a greater exchange of hydrogen ions for sodium ions. The pH of the final urine is affected by the distal tubules, especially by an excretion of hydrogen and ammonium ions in exchange for sodium. In general, the blood pH is maintained within very narrow limits at about 7.4, while urine generally has a pH of 5 or 6. Water is also reabsorbed under the influence of **antidiuretic hormone (ADH).**

### Collecting tubules

This is the site of the final concentration of urine. The fluid that will eventually be urine is still isotonic when it leaves the distal tubule and enters the collecting ducts. Although the collecting ducts are permeable to water, reabsorption is under the control of ADH or vasopressin, a hormone produced by the pituitary gland. ADH is produced in response to increased plasma osmolality and has the effect of preventing excess excretion of water (antidiuresis). A lack of ADH results in production of a more dilute urine (diuresis).

### Ureter

The fluid that leaves the collecting ducts and enters the ureters is now urine. It is temporarily stored in the bladder, and eliminated from the body by way of the urethra.

## Histology

All of the structures that make up the urinary system are lined with epithelial cells—from the glomerular capsule to the terminal portion of the urethra. Each of these portions is characterized by a specific type of epithelial cells. These are generally classified as either renal (meaning from the kidney or nephron itself), transitional, or squamous epithelial cells. These will be described in the section on the microscopic examination of the urinary sediment. A few of these cells are constantly sloughed off into the urine. However, it should be remembered that increased numbers or cytologic changes of any of these cells may have clinical significance and may be important in determining the cause of renal dysfunction.

## ▍COMPOSITION OF URINE

The composition of urine varies a great deal, depending on such factors as diet, nutritional status, metabolic rate, the general state of the body, and the state of the kidney or its ability to function normally.

Urine is a complex aqueous mixture consisting of 96% water and 4% dissolved substances, most of which either are derived from the food eaten or are waste products of metabolism. The dissolved substances consist primarily of *salt* (sodium and some potassium chloride and *urea* (the principal end product of protein metabolism).

In addition to urea, the principal organic substances found in urine are uric acid and creatinine. Urea, uric acid, and creatinine are nitrogenous waste products of protein metabolism, which must be eliminated from the body because increased levels are toxic. Urea makes up about one half of the dissolved substances in urine. It is the end product of amino acid and protein breakdown. The amount of creatinine excretion is related to the muscle mass of the body, not diet. Each individual excretes a constant amount of creatinine daily; therefore, urine creatinine measurements are used to assess the completeness of timed urine collections. Blood (plasma) creatinine levels are used to indicate renal function, because of the fact that creatinine is normally filtered through the glomerulus and none is reabsorbed back into the blood. Therefore, an increase in the plasma creatinine indicates impaired glomerular filtration—impaired renal function. The glomerular filtration rate is calculated from the urine and plasma creatinine levels together with 24-hour urine volume, height, and weight (see also Creatinine Clearance in Chapter 11).

In addition to sodium and chloride, the main inorganic substances present in urine include potassium, calcium, magnesium, and ammonia plus phosphates and sulfates.

## Normal Urine

Any of the substances tested for in routine urinalysis may be present in various disease states. Normal urine contains a few cells from the blood and lining of the urinary tract but little or no protein and no casts (although a few hyaline casts may be present). The reference values shown in Table 14-2 are those established for the Fairview-University Medical Center, University Campus, and are included

## TABLE 14-2

Urine Reference Values (Physical and Chemical)

| | |
|---|---|
| Color | Yellow |
| Transparency | Clear |
| pH | 5-7 |
| Specific gravity | 1.001-1.035 (adult random urine) |
| Protein, albumin | Negative<br>Trace (in a concentrated specimen) |
| Blood (hemoglobin) | Negative |
| Nitrite | Negative |
| Leukocyte esterase | Negative |
| Glucose | Negative |
| Ketones | Negative |
| Bilirubin (conjugated) | Negative |
| Urobilinogens | ≤1 mg/dL |

as an example of what may be "normally" encountered when the urine is examined for physical and chemical properties.

Reference values for the urine sediment are given in the section Examination of the Urine Sediment.

Normal but concentrated urine will commonly crystallize certain chemicals out of solution at room or refrigerator temperature. Therefore, a routine urinalysis will commonly show crystals of uric acid or its salts, the urates, at an acid pH, while phosphates will commonly crystallize out of solution in concentrated urine of an alkaline pH. Such crystallization will show grossly as cloudiness or turbidity of the urine, and the crystals are identified morphologically by microscopic examination. Although they are the primary constituents of urine, urea and sodium chloride do not crystallize out of urine specimens.

### Identification of a Fluid as Urine

It is sometimes necessary to determine if a specimen is urine or a body fluid such as amniotic fluid, or drainage fluid formed after abdominal or pelvic surgery. This is done by measuring urea, creatinine, sodium, and chloride levels, which are all significantly higher in urine than in other body fluids.

## COLLECTION AND PRESERVATION OF URINE SPECIMENS

Important considerations in the proper collection and handling of urine for routine examination include the container used, the collection procedure, and the conditions of storage and preservation from the time of collection until the specimen is tested. A good working relationship and good avenues of communication are necessary between all members of the medical team to ensure that a suitable specimen is collected and delivered to the laboratory for examination.

For routine urinalysis, a freely voided specimen, rather than one obtained by catheterization, is usually suitable. If the specimen is likely to be contaminated by vaginal discharge or hemorrhage, a clean-voided midstream specimen as required for bacteriologic examination (described in Chapter 3) may be necessary. It may be necessary to pack the vagina or use a tampon to avoid vaginal contamination. Although any random urine specimen voided during the day may be used for routine urinalysis, a fairly concentrated specimen is preferable to a dilute one. The first specimen voided in the morning is usually the most concentrated one, as fluids are not taken while the patient is asleep but dissolved substances are still excreted by the kidneys. A concentrated specimen is especially desirable for examining for protein and the contents of the urinary sediment. For testing for the presence of glucose, the best specimen to use is one voided 2 or 3 hours after a meal (postprandial). This is the major exception to the recommended use of the first morning specimen for routine tests.

It is of primary importance that the containers used to collect the urine specimen be clean and dry. Although several types of containers are suitable for this purpose, disposable inert plastic containers, with a secure closure to prevent leaks, are usual.

## TABLE 14-3

Changes in Urine Left at Room Temperature

| Constituent | Observed Change | Mechanism of Change |
|---|---|---|
| pH | Increased (alkaline) | Breakdown of urea to ammonia |
| Cells | Decreased number | Lysis |
| Casts | Decreased number | Lysis-dissolution |
| Glucose | Decreased | Glycolysis (by bacterial action) |
| Ketones | Decreased | Conversion of diacetic acid to acetone and evaporation of acetone from specimen |
| Bilirubin | Decreased (color change from yellow to green) | Oxidation to biliverdin |
| Urobilinogen | Decreased (color change from colorless to orange-red) | Oxidation to urobilin |

Modified from Ringsrud KM, Linne JJ: *Urinalysis and Body Fluids: A ColorText and Atlas*, St Louis, Mosby, 1995, p 23.

Probably the most important consideration is that the urine specimen be fresh or suitably preserved, usually by refrigeration. Ideally, the urine should be examined within 30 minutes of collection, as decomposition begins within this time, urine being an excellent culture medium for bacterial growth. If this is impossible, test the specimen within 1 or 2 hours, but it should be refrigerated at 4° C as soon as possible after voiding. It can generally be preserved in this way for 6 to 8 hours with no gross alterations (with the possible exception of bilirubin and urobilinogen, which are also susceptible to exposure to light). Refrigeration can precipitate amorphous urates or phosphates, which may obscure more important components in the microscopic examination. Specimens left for over 2 hours at room temperature are not acceptable. Chemical preservatives are usually reserved for 24-hour urine collections, as they may interfere with parts of the routine urinalysis.

Decomposition of urine primarily involves the growth of bacteria. At room temperature, bacteria reproduce rapidly. This bacterial growth results in a cloudy-looking specimen. Changes in pH also occur as a result of bacterial growth. These changes interfere markedly with other tests. Other substances, namely phosphates and urates, may precipitate out of solution, adding to the turbidity of the urine specimen. Changes in urine left at room temperature for over 2 hours are shown in Table 14-3.

In summary, for routine urinalysis the urine specimen must be collected in a suitable clean, dry container. In most cases the first specimen freely voided in the morning is preferred, although a specimen collected 2 to 3 hours after eating is preferable for testing for glucose. The specimen must be examined when fresh, ideally within 30 minutes, or suitably preserved, such as by refrigeration for up to 6 to 8 hours.

### Urine Volume for Routine Urinalysis

The minimum volume for routine urinalysis is usually 12 mL, but 50 mL is preferable. Twelve mL is the minimum amount necessary for the usual processing procedure, in which 12 mL of urine is placed in a disposable centrifuge tube, centrifuged, and concentrated 12:1, so that 1 mL of sediment is retained for the microscopic analysis of the sediment. This volume also allows for a convenient, standardized volume of urine for assessment of physical properties, such as color and transparency, which are often observed in the centrifuge tube.

Smaller volumes may be accepted for chemical analysis from oliguric patients or from infants. If only 3 mL of urine is collected, a 12:1 concentration of sediment may still be made. A drop of unconcentrated urine placed on the desired portion of a reagent strip or observed microscopically may be all that is possible in some situations.

## PHYSICAL PROPERTIES OF URINE

The first part of a routine urinalysis usually involves an assessment of physical properties, such as volume, color, transparency, odor, and foam. Another physical property, specific gravity, is discussed in a separate section. Observation of physical properties is probably the easiest part of a urinalysis. However, these simple observations are extremely useful both for the eventual diagnosis of the patient and for the laboratory personnel who perform the complete urinalysis. Such tests often give clues leading to findings in subsequent portions of the urinalysis. For example, if a urine specimen is cloudy and red, the presence of red blood cells will probably be revealed by microscopic analysis of the urinary sediment. If red cells are not found, all parts of the urinalysis must be carefully rechecked for accuracy. Chemical tests for blood (hemoglobin) might be falsely negative when ascorbic acid is present in urine; however, the presence of blood might be indicated by an abnormal red color and confirmed by the presence of red cells in the urinary sediment. If hemoglobin is present without red cells, the only indication of ascorbic acid interference might be the abnormal color of the urine.

Certain tests are performed when abnormal physical properties are observed. For example, a chemical test for the pigment bilirubin is necessary when it is suspected on the basis of abnormal color of the urine. There are several situations in which the complete urinalysis is evaluated by the laboratory for reliability before results are reported to the physician, or abnormal constituents are found in subsequent tests because abnormal physical proper-

ties were noted. The final evaluation of urinalysis results will be described more completely after all parts of the routine urinalysis have been discussed. Physical properties are summarized in Table 14-4.

## VOLUME

### Normal Volume

Although it is a physical property, the volume of the urine is not measured as part of a routine urinalysis. However, in certain conditions the volume of urine excreted in 24 hours is a valuable aid to clinical diagnosis. In normal adults with normal fluid intake, the average 24-hour urine volume is 1200 to 1500 mL. It can, however, normally range from 600 to 1600 mL. The total volume of urine excreted in 24 hours must be measured when quantitative tests are performed, since it enters into the calculation of results in these tests.

Under normal conditions, there is a direct relationship between urine volume and water intake. That is, if water intake is increased, the kidney will protect the body from excessive retention of water by eliminating a larger volume of urine than normal. Conversely, if water intake is decreased, the kidney will protect the body against dehydration by eliminating a smaller amount of urine.

### Abnormal Volume

There are various situations that result in abnormal urine volumes.

#### Polyuria

The term **polyuria** refers to the consistent elimination of an abnormally large volume of urine, over 2,000 mL/24 hr.

#### Diuresis

**Diuresis** refers to any increase in urine volume, even if the increase is only temporary.

#### Oliguria

**Oliguria** refers to the excretion of an abnormally small amount of urine, less than 500 mL/24 hr.

**TABLE 14-4**

Physical Properties of Urine

| Physical Property | Description | Possible Cause |
|---|---|---|
| Normal color | Yellow (straw to amber) | Urochrome, uroerythrin, and urobilin |
| Abnormal color | Pale | Dilute urine |
| | Amber (dark yellow or orange-red) | Concentrated urine or bilirubin |
| | Brown (yellow-brown or green-brown) | Bilirubin or biliverdin |
| | Orange (orange-red or orange-brown) | Urobilin (excreted colorless as urobilinogen) |
| | Bright orange | Azo-containing dyes or compounds |
| | Red | Blood or heme-derived pigment, urates or uric acid, drugs, foodstuffs |
| | Clear red | Hemoglobin |
| | Cloudy red | Red blood cells |
| | Dark red-brown | Myoglobin |
| | Dark red or red-purple | Porphyrins |
| | Black (dark brown and black) | Melanin, homogentisic acid, phenol poisoning |
| | Green, blue, orange | Drugs, medications, foodstuffs |
| Normal Transparency | Clear | Normal or dilute |
| Abnormal Transparency | Hazy, cloudy, turbid | Mucus, phosphates, urates, crystals, bacteria, pus, fat, casts |
| Normal Odor | Aromatic | Normal |
| Abnormal Odor | Ammoniacal, putrid or foul | Breakdown of urea by bacteria (old urine), or urinary tract infection |
| | Sweet or "fruity" | Ketone bodies |
| | Sweaty feet, maple syrup, cabbage or hops, mousy, rotting fish, rancid | Specific amino acid disorder for each |
| Normal Foam | White, small amount | Normal |
| Abnormal foam | White, large amount | Protein |
| | Yellow, large amount | Bilirubin |

### Anuria

The complete absence of urine formation is **anuria**.

### Nocturia

The excretion of over 400 mL urine at night is called **nocturia**.

•  •  •

These terms merely describe abnormalities in urine volume. Each abnormality has several possible causes, reflecting various abnormal conditions. The actual cause and significance of volume changes will be determined with the aid of the routine urinalysis, together with other clinical and laboratory findings.

## COLOR

### Normal Color

The color of normal urine varies considerably, even in one person in a single day. Numerous words have been used to describe the range of normal color. In general, it can be said that normal urine is some shade of yellow. The exact name that is attached is not as important as the recognition that the color is normal. It is advisable for each institution to use precise terms to define normal color. The terms yellow, straw, and amber are often used. Straw is generally used to describe a lighter-colored urine with normal yellow pigment. Amber refers to a darker color, with red or orange pigments in addition to yellow. The term yellow is often used to describe all normal-colored urine.

Urine that is more highly colored has a greater concentration of normal waste products because its volume is diminished. Color, however, is not an adequate measure of concentration. Specific gravity or osmolality values are preferred.

The color of normal urine seems to result from the presence of three pigments: urochrome, uroerythrin, and urobilin. **Urochrome** is a yellow pigment and is present in larger concentrations than the other two. **Uroerythrin** is a red pigment, and **urobilin** is an orange-yellow pigment.

## Abnormal Color

The ability to recognize normal color is necessary to ensure the recognition of abnormal color. Several abnormal colors are of pathologic significance and require special attention. Descriptions follow.

### Pale

Pale urine suggests that the urine is dilute. The paleness results from a large volume with correspondingly low concentrations of normal constituents, as in polyuria. Pale urine is often associated with diabetes mellitus or diabetes insipidus. However, the large sugar content in diabetes mellitus results in a high specific gravity when measured by a refractometer, whereas dilute urine is characterized by low specific gravity. Pale urine specimens are also seen in kidney and urinary tract diseases in which there is a loss of the ability to concentrate urine. Pale, foamy urine specimens are seen, along with large amounts of protein, in the nephrotic syndrome.

### Amber (Dark Yellow or Orange-Red)

Highly colored dark yellow or orange-red urine is indicative of very concentrated constituents and a correspondingly low volume. It is often seen in conditions associated with fever, in which water is eliminated through sweat rather than the kidney. When such concentrated and acid urine is excreted, a pink or red precipitate of urates or uric acid, also referred to as brick dust, is often seen. The color may be similar to specimens containing the pigments bilirubin or urobilin.

### Brown (Yellow-Brown or Green-Brown)

This is a very characteristic and alarming color to the experienced observer, which has also been referred to as "beer-brown." It indicates the presence of bilirubin, a highly colored bile pigment, which is related to the clinical condition jaundice if it is also present in the blood. Urine specimens containing bilirubin will foam considerably when shaken, and the foam will have a vivid yellow color. This is not true of other highly colored urine specimens. Whenever bilirubin is suspected, it is the responsibility of the laboratory worker to perform a chemical test to detect it. This is extremely important, for bilirubin may appear in the urine before clinical jaundice develops, and detection will lead to early treatment of the condition, whatever its cause. On standing, urine containing bilirubin may become green as a result of the oxidation of bilirubin to biliverdin, a green pigment. Unfortunately, this might result in a negative or reduced chemical test for bilirubin.

### Orange (Orange-Red or Orange-Brown)

This color is very similar to that of urine containing bilirubin and results from a related pigment, urobilin. In fact, urines that are tested for bilirubin on the basis of color should also be tested for urobilinogen. The cause of clinical jaundice may be discovered by observing the presence or absence of either or both of these pigments in the urine. When urine is freshly voided, the pigment urobilin is present in a colorless form—urobilinogen. The urine slowly takes on color on standing, because of oxidation of urobilinogen to urobilin. If shaken, urine containing urobilin will not produce a colored foam, and results of chemical tests will be negative or decreased when oxidation to urobilin has taken place.

### Orange (Bright Orange)

This is very similar to the color of urine containing bilirubin or urobilinogen, although it is somewhat more vivid. In this case the color is caused by the presence of the azo-containing phenazopyridine (Pyridium) or other aminopyrine drugs, which are given to patients as a urinary analgesic. Certain azo-containing antibiotics such as Azo Gantrisin, a sulfonamide containing sulfisoxazole, and phenazopyridine cause similar color in urine. The presence of these azo-containing substances presents a problem because they interfere with several reagent strip tests by masking or obscuring the color reaction and thus lead to false-positive results.

### Red or Pink

When a red or pink urine specimen is seen, the presence of blood or a heme-related pigment should be suspected. If the color is due to red blood cells, hemoglobin, or myoglobin, the reagent strip test for blood will be positive.

Other causes of a red or pink urine include a very concentrated urine specimen resulting from the presence of uric acid or urates. This is seen as a pink or orange deposit or precipitate, which has been referred to as "brick dust." Such urine specimens are seen with dehydration and fever. Certain genetically susceptible persons will produce a beet-colored urine after eating beets. Other drugs or foodstuffs that may result in red or pink urine specimens include rhubarb, red or pink dyes (congo red, Bromsulphalein (BSP), phenolsulfonphthalein (PSP), ethoxazene (Serenium), anthraquinone laxatives (senna, cascara), levodopa, methyldopa (Aldomet), and azo-containing compounds.

Pathologic causes of red or pink urine specimens follow.

**Clear Red.** Urine that is clear and red characteristically contains hemoglobin, the pigment of red blood cells. The hemoglobin may result from increased red cell destruction in the body (intravascular hemolysis), which has several causes, such as an incompatible blood transfusion reaction, autoimmune hemolytic anemia, paroxysmal nocturnal hemoglobinuria, march hemoglobinuria, glucose-6-phosphate dehydrogenase deficiency, and certain infections and drugs. The urine may be bright red, red-brown, or even black as a result of the conversion of hemoglobin to methemoglobin. Red urine should be tested chemically for the presence of hemoglobin.

**Cloudy Red.** The presence of red blood cells is suggested when the urine specimen is cloudy and red. It is important to differentiate hematuria (red cells in urine) from hemoglobinuria (hemoglobin in urine). This may be most easily done by observation of red blood cells in the urine sediment. However, if the urine is very dilute (low specific gravity), red blood cells will lyse, resulting in hemoglobinuria. The intensity of the red will depend on the number of red cells present; the urine color ranges from barely pink to smoky red or reddish brown to a frankly bloody specimen. The possibility of menstrual contamination should be considered in urine from a female patient.

**Dark Red-Brown.** Also referred to as cola colored, this is characteristic of myoglobin, the form of hemoglobin contained in muscles. It is especially associated with cases of extensive muscle injury, from trauma or extreme exercise. Reagent strip tests for blood (hemoglobin) also detect myoglobin. Detection is an important finding, as myoglobin is nephrotoxic.

**Dark Red or Red-Purple.** Described as the color of port wine, this is characteristic of the presence of porphyrins in the urine. The urine may be colorless when voided but darkens upon standing, because of the oxidation of porphobilinogen to porphobilin.

### Brown or Black

This color may result from melanin or homogentisic acid. In both cases the urine is colorless when voided and becomes black on standing. Both are the result of serious conditions, and the color must not be overlooked. Melanin is associated with melanoma, a type of tumor. Homogentisic acid is associated with alkaptonuria, a result of an inborn error in the metabolism of tyrosine. Phenol poisoning may also result in an olive-green to black urine. Specific chemical tests for all these possible causes of black urine must be performed, since immediate diagnosis and treatment are imperative in each case. These conditions are rarely encountered. Some patients taking levodopa for parkinsonism may excrete urine that is dark brown or cola colored.

### Miscellaneous Colors

Various bizarre urine colors, such as yellow, orange, red, pink, blue, green, and brown, may result from such causes as vitamins, vegetables, fruits, certain chemicals, and dyes. These have very little clinical significance; for example, the ingestion of chlorophyll in mouth deodorants may color the urine green. Pathologic findings include indicans produced from infections of the small intestine and *Pseudomonas* infections that may result in blue or green specimens.

## TRANSPARENCY

When voided, urine is normally clear; most urines, however, will become cloudy when allowed to stand. Cloudiness of a specimen when voided is usually of clinical significance and should not be disregarded.

The degree of cloudiness is observed in a well-mixed urine specimen at the time of urinalysis. The degree of transparency (clear to turbid) should be assessed on a well-mixed urine speci-

men by looking through the specimen in an optically clear container held in front of a light source against printed material (such as newsprint). All urine specimens should be assessed for color and transparency in similar containers to ensure consistent results. When cloudiness is noted, it must be accounted for in the microscopic analysis of the urinary sediment, since it is caused by solid materials that will be visible under the microscope.

As with color, numerous words have been used in attempts to describe the degree of transparency of a urine specimen. According to the NCCLS, standardized terms such as clear, hazy, cloudy, and turbid should be used to reduce ambiguity and subjectivity. Schweitzer et al advocate the use of a limited number of descriptors, which are clearly defined as follows[12]:

| | |
|---|---|
| Clear | No visible particulate matter present. |
| Hazy | Some visible particulate matter present; newsprint is not distorted or obscured when viewed through the urine. |
| Cloudy | Newsprint can be seen through the urine but letters are distorted or blurry. |
| Turbid | Newsprint cannot be seen through the urine. |

Common constituents that cause cloudiness in urine, both generally normal and possibly significant or pathologic, are summarized in Table 14-5. See the section on the microscopic analysis of the urine sediment for descriptions of each.

## ODOR

### Normal Odor

Normal urine has a characteristic, faintly aromatic odor because of the presence of certain volatile acids. See also Table 14-4.

### Abnormal Odor
#### Bacterial Action

If allowed to stand, urine acquires a strong ammoniacal odor. This is caused by the breakdown

## TABLE 14-5

Common Constituents Causing
Cloudiness in Urine

| Generally Normal | Possibly Pathologic |
|---|---|
| Amorphous phosphates and urates | Amorphous urates |
| Normal crystals | Abnormal crystals |
| | Red blood cells |
| | White blood cells |
| | Casts |
| | Fat (lipids) |
| Epithelial cells (squamous, transitional) | Epithelial cells (renal, transitional, malignant) |
| Bacteria (old urine) | Bacteria (fresh urine) |
| | Other microorganisms (yeast, fungi, parasites) |
| Mucus | |
| Sperm, prostatic fluid | Chyluria (lymph, rare) |
| Powders, antiseptics | Fecal matter (from fistula) |

of urea by bacteria (which are invariably present in the urine specimen), resulting in the formation of ammonia. This odor is important as an indication that the urine specimen is probably too old for the urinalysis to have clinical significance. Along with the breakdown of urea, various other decomposition reactions will have occurred, altering or destroying other components that were present at the time the urine was voided. Urine heavily infected with bacteria may have a particularly unpleasant odor, which may be described as foul or putrid. This is also caused by the action of bacteria on urea, forming ammonia, plus the decay of proteins that are also present in infection. Practically, it cannot be distinguished from the smell of old urine. Therefore, foul-smelling urine will indicate urinary infection only if the specimen is known to be fresh.

### Ketones

Another characteristic odor that is significant clinically is a so-called fruity, or sweet, odor. This results from the presence of acetone and acetoacetic acid, an important finding in the urine of diabetic patients at risk of diabetic coma.

### Amino Acid Metabolism Errors

In certain extremely rare disorders of amino acid metabolism, a characteristic odor has helped in the diagnosis of the condition. These odors are generally observed by the mother or caretaker of a baby who has particularly unusual-smelling diapers. It is not expected that this will be noticed by laboratory personnel. The odors have been described as being like sweaty feet, maple syrup, cabbage or hops, mousy, rotting fish, or rancid. Each has a specific amino acid disorder associated with it.

### Foodstuffs

Finally, the ingestion of certain foodstuffs will result in a characteristic urine odor. Probably the most obvious is the odor of asparagus. This is of no clinical significance.

## FOAM

### Normal Foam

Normal urine will show a small amount of white foam when stoppered and shaken, which dissipates on standing. Foam should be observed, but reported only if abnormal. See also Table 14-4.

### Abnormal Foam
#### Abundant White Foam

When high concentrations of protein are present in the urine, a large amount of white foam may be seen if the urine container is securely closed and shaken. This is especially true of conditions like the nephrotic syndrome, in which large amounts of protein (albumin) are lost from the body into the urine. The foam that is formed looks like beaten egg white; the substance responsible for the foam in both cases is albumin. This observation should be confirmed by the chemical test for protein. In addition, the urine sediment should be observed carefully for the presence of casts and lipids such as oval fat bodies (renal tubular fat) or free fat.

### Abundant Yellow Foam

When certain bile pigments are present, especially bilirubin, the urine will foam significantly and show a vivid yellow color. This is a simple test for the detection of bilirubin, which should be performed on abnormally dark urine specimens. However, it is not a confirmatory test, and all urine specimens suspected of containing bilirubin should be tested chemically whether the foam test is positive or negative.

## SPECIFIC GRAVITY

Urine is a mixture of substances dissolved and suspended in water. In normal urine, these dissolved substances are primarily urea and sodium chloride. **Specific gravity** is a measure of the amount of dissolved substances in a solution. The specific gravity of urine is used as a measure of the ability of the kidney to regulate the composition and osmotic pressure of the extracellular fluid by concentrating or diluting the urine.

Specific gravity is defined as the weight of a solution compared with the weight of an equal volume of water. More specifically, it is the ratio of the density (weight per unit volume) of a solution to the density (weight per unit volume) of an equal volume of water at a constant temperature. From this definition, it is clear that the specific gravity of water is always 1.000. Since it is a ratio, specific gravity has no units. It is always reported to the third decimal place.

### Clinical Aspects

Clinically, the specific gravity of urine may be used to obtain information about two general functions: the state of the kidney and the state of hydration of the patient. If the kidney is performing adequately, it is capable of producing urine with a specific gravity ranging from about 1.003 to 1.035. However, if the renal epithelium is not functioning adequately, it will gradually lose the ability to concentrate and dilute the urine. The ability to concentrate urine is one of the first functions lost when the kidney is impaired. Deficiency or failure to respond to ADH will also result in failure to concentrate urine. The specific gravity of the protein-free glomerular filtrate is about 1.008. Without any active work on the part of the kidney, this will increase to 1.010 as a result of simple diffusion as the filtrate passes through the kidney tubules. Thus, if the kidney has completely lost its ability to concentrate and dilute the urine, the specific gravity will remain at 1.010. If it is known that the kidney is functioning adequately, the state of hydration may be reflected by the specific gravity. For example, if the urine is consistently very concentrated, dehydration is implied.

Although normal specific gravity may range from 1.001 to 1.035, the specific gravity of a 24-hour collection is usually between 1.016 and 1.022 with normal diet and fluid intake. Since the specific gravity is a reflection of the amount of dissolved substances present in solution, it varies inversely with the volume of urine (this is because a fairly constant amount of waste is produced each day). Therefore, if the urinary volume increases because of increased water intake, and the amount of waste produced remains constant, the specific gravity of the urine decreases. In other words, if the urinary volume is high, the specific gravity is low, and vice versa, assuming the kidney is functioning normally. With an individual on a restricted fluid diet for 12 hours, the normal kidney is capable of concentrating urine to a specific gravity of about 1.022 or more. A person without fluids for 24 hours should produce urine with a specific gravity of 1.026 or more. If the individual is placed on a very high-fluid diet, the normal kidney is capable of diluting the urine to a specific gravity of about 1.003. The concentrated first urine specimen passed in the morning should have a specific gravity greater than 1.020 if the kidney is functioning normally.

Two frequently observed cases in which specific gravity does not vary inversely with urinary volume are diabetes mellitus and certain types of renal disease. With diabetes mellitus an abnormally large urinary volume associated with an abnormally high specific gravity is observed. This is caused by the presence of large amounts of dissolved glucose, which raises the specific gravity of the urine. In certain types of renal disease, such as glomerulonephritis, pyelonephritis, and various anomalies, there is a combination of low specific gravity and low urinary volume. This results from the inability of the renal tubular epithelium either to excrete normal amounts of water or to concentrate the waste products. The specific gravity in these cases may eventually be fixed at about 1.010.

The loss of concentrating ability is seen in the disease diabetes insipidus, an impairment of ADH. This rare condition results in extremely large volumes of urine with very low specific gravity, ranging from 1.001 to 1.003.

Abnormally high specific gravity values, usually greater than 1.035 and up to 1.050 or more, may also be encountered after certain diagnostic x-ray procedures in which a radiographic dye is injected intravenously to obtain a pyelogram of the kidney. Such high specific gravity readings will be accompanied by delayed false-positive reactions for protein with the sulfosalicylic acid procedure, and the dye may crystallize out of the urine as an abnormal colorless crystal resembling plates of cholesterol.

### Measures of Urine Solute Concentration (Specific Gravity and Osmolality)

Although specific gravity is a convenient measure of the urine solute concentration, it is not the only one available. Other measures are osmolality, refractive index, and ionic concentration. All of the methods of measuring solute concentration are influenced by the number of molecules present in solution in addition to the size and/or ionic charge.

#### Specific Gravity by Urinometer

**Specific gravity** is a measure of the amount of dissolved substances present in a solution.

Specific gravity in urine was traditionally measured with a urinometer, a specialized hydrometer that is calibrated to measure specific gravity in urine at a given temperature. The urinometer is a glass float weighted with mercury, with an air bulb above the weight and a graduated stem on the top (Fig. 14-2). It is weighted to float at the 1.000 graduation in pure water when placed in a glass urinometer cylinder or appropriate-sized test tube. It is important that the cylinder, or test tube, be of the correct size so that the urinometer can float freely. The specific gravity of the urine is read directly from the graduated scale in the urinometer stem. Specific gravity by urinometer has generally been replaced by the refractometer or reagent strip method. It has the disadvantage of being time consuming and requires a relatively large volume (10 or 15 mL) of urine. According to the NCCLS, urinometers can be inaccurate and require standardization

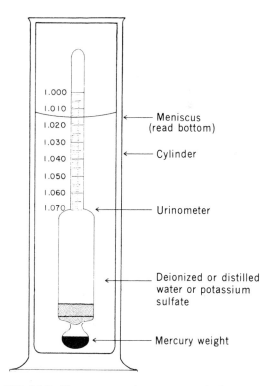

**FIG 14-2.** Urinometer and urinometer cylinder.

after purchase. They are not the method of choice for determining specific gravity.[6]

### Osmolality by Osmometer

This is another method of determining solute concentration. It is a measure of the number of solute particles per unit amount of solvent. Thus it is dependent only on the number of particles in solution. It is determined with an osmometer by measuring the freezing point of a solution, since the freezing point is depressed in proportion to the amount of dissolved substances present. In normal persons with a normal diet and fluid intake, the urine will contain about 500 to 850 mOsm/kg of water. Osmolality is preferred to specific gravity as a measurement of urine concentration. Urine and plasma osmolality as a ratio is used to evaluate renal tubular concentration, which is dependent on the state of hydration of the patient.

### Specific Gravity as Refractive Index by Refractometer

Another measure of solute concentration, reported in the urinalysis laboratory as specific gravity, is **refractive index.** The refractive index of a solution is the ratio of the velocity of light in air to the velocity of light in solution. This ratio varies directly with the number of dissolved particles in solution. Although not identical to specific gravity, refractive index varies and corresponds with specific gravity. Measurement is made with a refractometer that is calibrated to give results in terms of specific gravity (see Fig. 14-3). Results agree well with urinometer readings, although the reading by refractometer is generally about 0.002 lower than by urinometer. The specific gravity scale by refractometer is valid only for urine. It cannot be used to determine the specific gravity of salt or glucose solutions, which have much lower readings on the urine specific gravity scale by refractometer than by urinometer.[3]

The refractometer has the advantage of requiring only a drop of urine, as opposed to 10 to 15 mL for the urinometer. Automated instru-

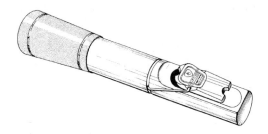

**FIG 14-3.** Refractometer.

ments are available that use pass-through models of refractometers. These use a larger volume of urine (about 2 mL). Refractometer results are valid up to 1.035—results above this should be reported as greater than 1.035. Such values suggest the presence of unusual solutes, such as glucose or radiopaque compounds. (See also Use of the Refractometer.)

### Specific Gravity as Ionic Concentration by Reagent Strip

Reagent strips have been developed to give specific gravity values of urine. These strips actually measure **ionic concentration,** which relates to specific gravity. Values are reported as specific gravity. However, substances that are dissolved in urine must ionize in order to be measured by this method. The waste products that constitute normal urinary constituents and indicate the concentration and dilution ability of the kidney do ionize. Certain substances that may be present in urine, such as glucose or certain radiopaque dyes, do not ionize; therefore, specific gravity results obtained with the urinometer or refractometer will be significantly higher than with the reagent strip if the urine contains significant quantities of a nonionizable, dissolved substance.

### Use of the Refractometer

The refractive index of urine is closely correlated with the specific gravity. Since the development of the Goldberg refractometer, a temperature-compensated small hand-held instrument, measurements of the refractive index have become common in routine urinalysis (Fig. 14-3). They

## PROCEDURE 14-1

### Specific Gravity By Refractometer

1. Clean surface of instrument prism and cover by rinsing with water. Wipe dry.

2. Close the coverplate of the instrument.

3. Apply a drop of urine to the exposed portion of the measuring prism, at the notched bottom of the cover, using a disposable pipette. The liquid will be drawn into the space between the prisms by capillary action.

4. Hold the instrument up to a light source, or position in the refractometer stand so that light passes over the chamber.

5. Looking through the eyepiece, make the reading on the specific gravity scale at the point where the dividing line between the bright and dark fields crosses the scale.

6. Rinse the chamber and cover with water and wipe dry.

have the advantage that they require only a drop of urine, while the urinometer requires 10 to 15 mL of specimen. In addition, the refractometer is simple to operate and rapidly gives reliable results. Its major disadvantage is its cost. The steps involved in measuring specific gravity with a refractometer are given in Procedure 14-1.

Although the refractometer actually measures the refractive index, the scales of the instrument are calibrated in terms of total solids (g/100 mL) for plasma or serum, or in terms of specific gravity for urine. Up to a value of 1.035, the urinary refractive index and specific gravity agree. Few normal urines have values greater than 1.035; higher values suggest the presence of unusual solutes in the specimen, such as glucose, protein, or radiopaque compounds. Beyond a value of 1.035, the refractive index is poorly correlated with the specific gravity and should be reported only as greater than 1.035, rather than extrapolated to a higher value.

The refractive index changes with temperature, but the Goldberg refractometer compensates for temperature changes in the solution being measured. Therefore, it is not necessary to correct for changes in temperature of the urine.

### Quality Control

The refractometer should be checked each day with deionized or distilled water and with a solution of known specific gravity. The distilled water should read $1.000 \pm 0.001$. The instrument contains a zero set screw to adjust the reading to water. Follow the manufacturer's directions. The known solution may be a commercial control solution or one of the following:

| NaCl | 0.513 mol/L | 3% w/v | SG = 1.015 |
| NaCl | 0.856 mol/L | 5% w/v | SG = 1.022 |
| Sucrose | 0.263 mol/L | 9% w/v | SG = 1.034 |

### Corrections for Abnormal Dissolved Substances

Since refractive index is a measure of dissolved particles in solution, the presence of substances such as glucose, protein, or radiopaque dyes will act to raise the specific gravity when measured with the refractometer as compared with reagent strips. It is sometimes desirable to correct refractometer readings for dissolved substances in order to access the concentrating ability of the kidneys.

**Correction for Glucose.** Subtract 0.004 from the refractometer value for each gram of glucose per deciliter of urine. Urine specimens from diabetic patients often contain 3 or 4 grams glucose per deciliter of urine, resulting in a specific gravity value by refractometer 0.012 to 0.016 higher than by reagent strip, on the same specimen.

**Correction for Protein.** Subtract 0.003 from the refractometer value for each gram of protein per deciliter of urine. Urine specimens rarely contain 1 or more grams of protein per deciliter of urine; therefore, correction for protein is rarely necessary.

**Radiopaque Media.** With values greater than 1.035, unusual substances such as radiopaque media or certain antibiotics should be suspected when not explained by other findings, such as high glucose concentration. The presence of unusual crystals of these substances in the microscopic analysis of the urine sediment is often associated with very high specific gravity readings with the refractometer. Or their presence may be indicated by the occurrence of a delayed false-positive sulfosalicylic acid test for urine protein. These substances will not be measured by the reagent strip method. (See also the sulfosalicylic acid test for urine protein.)

## Use of Reagent Strips for Specific Gravity
### Principle

The reagent strips for specific gravity actually measure ionic concentration. Both Multistix* and Chemstrip† have multiple reagent strips with test areas for specific gravity. The test is based on a pKa change of certain pretreated polyelectrolytes in relation to the ionic concentration of the urine. The polyelectrolytes in the reagent strip contain acid groups that dissociate in proportion to the number of ions in solution. This produces hydrogen ions, which reduce the

pH. The pH change is indicated by the color change of an acid-base indicator. The system is buffered so that any change in color is related to pKa change, and not pH of the urine itself.

Readings are made at 0.005 intervals from 1.000 to 1.030 by comparison with a color chart. Therefore, precision is significantly less than by refractometer, which is read at 0.001 intervals. The procedure for measuring urine specific gravity with reagent strips is the same as that used for all reagent strips, as described in Procedure 14-2.

### Corrections and Limitations

Dissolved substances must ionize in order to be detected by the reagent strips for specific gravity. Therefore, substances, like glucose or radiopaque dyes, that do not ionize will not affect the reagent strips, giving different values from those obtained by urinometer or refractometer. Although this may give a better picture of the concentrating ability of the kidney, it is important that the clinician understand which methodology is used by the laboratory for specific gravity, and if the results are "corrected" or not, to adequately interpret the specific gravity results.

Highly buffered alkaline urine may cause low readings, and 0.005 may be added to readings from urines with pH equal to or greater than 6.5. Automated instruments apply this correction. Unlike readings with the urinometer or refractometer, elevated specific gravity readings may be obtained in the presence of only moderate (100 to 750 mg/dL) amounts of protein. Finally, urine specimens containing urea at concentrations over 1 g/dL will cause low readings relative to more traditional methods.

## CHEMICAL TESTS IN ROUTINE URINALYSIS

Most of the chemical tests that are done as part of the routine urinalysis use dry reagent strips. Reagent strips are available both as single tests for a specific chemical substance and as combi-

*Bayer Corp. Diagnostics Division, Tarrytown, NY..
†Boehringer Mannheim Diagnostics Division of Boehringer Mannheim Corp., Indianapolis, Ind.

nations of single tests, referred to as **multiple-reagent strips.** Two commercially available products are described in this section, namely Chemstrip products and Multistix reagent strips and tablet tests, formerly Ames products. Other products exist, but the two described are the most commonly used in the CAP Interlaboratory Comparison Program.* If another product is used, test principle, sensitivity and specificity, and interferences must be considered and understood.

Reagent strips are plastic strips that contain one or more chemically impregnated test sites on an absorbent pad. When the chemicals on the test site come into contact with urine or a control solution, a chemical reaction occurs. The reaction is indicated by a color change, which is compared with a special color chart that is provided with the reagent strip, usually printed on the bottle. Results can be read visually, or in special instruments (usually reflectance meters) that automatically read specific reagent strips.

The intensity of the color formed is generally proportional to the amount of substance present in the specimen or control when observed at a specific time. Some areas are used as screening tests, which tell if a substance is present or absent. Others are used to estimate (semiquantitate) the amount of substance present and are reported in a plus system or in numerical values (e.g., mg/dL, g/dL). The method of reporting results will vary from laboratory to laboratory, but must be consistent for a given laboratory.

There are several advantages to dry reagent strip tests over the more traditional chemical tests on which they are based. These include:

1. Convenience—rapid results with a minimum of time and personnel
2. Cost-effectiveness
3. Stability
4. Relative ease in learning to use
5. Disposability

6. Smaller sample volumes required
7. Space savings—storage, use, and cleanup

Because they are so apparently easy to use, reagent strip tests are candidates for abuse. Reliable, reproducible results depend on correct technique. Manufacturers' directions must be followed. Any person using reagent strips should understand the principle and specificity of each chemical test area, be aware of precautions or limitations and interferences that occur, and know the sensitivity and significance of positive or negative results.

In certain instances, additional confirmatory tests are necessary when positive results are obtained with the reagent strip tests. These may be in the form of tablet tests, or more traditional chemical tests. These are described as necessary in the following sections.

A discussion of each of the test areas present on the commonly used multiple-reagent strips follows. The order of tests is not that found on either of the products described. Rather, tests are arranged in order of clinical utility or physiologic significance. Therefore chemical tests indicating disease of the kidney or urinary tract—pH, specific gravity, protein, blood, nitrite, and leukocyte esterase—are described first. Next are chemical tests indicating metabolic and other disease—glucose, ketones, bilirubin, and urobilinogen. Although many reagent strips include a test for specific gravity, this was described previously.

Each parameter is described in terms of clinical importance, principle of the test, specificity (what is being tested), sensitivity (minimum detectable level), and interferences (false-positive and false-negative reactions).

## REAGENT STRIP TESTS: GENERAL PROCEDURE AND PRECAUTIONS
(See Procedure 14-2)

### Manufacturer's Directions

General directions that apply to all reagent strip tests are included in this section. However, it is imperative that the specific directions of the

---

*College of American Pathologists, 325 Waukegan Rd., Northfield, IL 60093-0800.

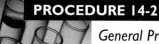

## PROCEDURE 14-2

### General Procedure for Urine Reagent Strips

1. Test fresh, well-mixed, uncentrifuged urine at room temperature.

2. Completely immerse all chemical areas of the reagent strip briefly—not over 1 second.

3. Remove excess urine from the reagent strip. Draw the strip along the lip or rim of the urine container as it is removed; then touch the *edge* of the strip to absorbent paper or gauze.

4. Avoid possible mixing of chemicals from adjacent reagent areas; hold the strip horizontally while waiting and reading results.

5. Read each chemical reaction at the time stated by the manufacturer.

6. Use adequate light. Hold the strip close to the color block on the chart supplied by the manufacturer, and match carefully for each chemical test. Be sure the strip is properly oriented to the color chart. Multistix are held perpendicular to the bottle, while Chemstips are held parallel to the bottle (see Fig. 14-4).

7. Record the results in consistent units as established for your laboratory.

manufacturer be followed for all reagent strip tests. Tests are continually changed and reformulated in this highly competitive market. Each container of reagent strips is supplied with a product insert. This contains the most up-to-date information for the successful performance of the test in question. Inserts include directions for use, warnings, procedure limitations, specimen handling information, storage, and expected values. Information on interfering substances that may produce false-negative or false-positive reactions is also included. For each new lot number of reagent strips, the laboratorian should study the product insert, compare it to the previous insert, noting any changes, and file it with the laboratory procedure manual.

### The Urine Specimen

The specimen to be tested must be fresh, or adequately preserved, well mixed, not centrifuged, and at room temperature.

### Sampling or Wetting

The first step in using the reagent strip is adequately sampling the specimen or wetting the reagent strip. Although this sounds easy, it is a common source of error. The strip must be adequately moistened so that all test areas of the strip are brought into contact with the sample. However, care must be taken not to leave the strip in contact with the sample too long, or chemicals will be leached out of the strip and be unavailable for the chemical reaction to occur. Therefore, the strip is inserted into the specimen only briefly, for 1 second or less. Another problem is runover between chemicals on adjacent pads. This is avoided by drawing the edge of the strip along the edge of the urine container as it is removed, touching the edge of the strip to absorbent paper, and holding the strip horizontally while waiting for and reading results.

### Storage and General Precautions

Reagent strips must be kept in tightly capped containers. They will deteriorate rapidly when exposed to moisture, direct sunlight, heat, or volatile substances. Each container contains a desiccant, or drying agent, to protect it from moisture. It should not be removed. The desiccant is contained within the original stopper in the Chemstrip products. Store containers at recommended temperatures, generally at room temperature, under 30° C, but not refrigerated or frozen. Keep strips in their original containers. Do not mix strips from different containers. Remove only the number of strips needed at a time, and close the container tightly. Do not touch the test areas. Keep the test areas away from detergents or other contaminating substances, such as bleach (hypochlorite), that may be present in the work area.

## Stability

Each container of reagent strips is marked with a lot number and an expiration date. Do not use strips after the expiration date. Write the date opened on each container. Once the container is opened, use strips within 6 months. Watch test areas for possible deterioration by comparing the color of the dry reagent with the color of a negative test block on the color chart. If deterioration is suspected, test the strip with a known control solution. Discard the entire bottle of strips if any reagent pads are discolored or when quality control is consistently out of range.

## Timing

Read the results at the time stated by the manufacturer for each chemical test. This is absolutely necessary if results are to be semiquantitated. Very different results will be seen for the same specimen at different times. In general, the Multistix products are read during the kinetic phase of reactions, and timing is absolutely critical. The Chemstrip products are generally read at an end point or stable phase, allowing all results to be read at 1 minute with results stable for 2 minutes. An advantage of using an automated or semiautomated instrument to read reagent strips is that it controls the exact time at which all of the chemical reactions are read.

## Reading Results: Color Comparison

Whenever results depend on color comparison, individual interpretation is a possible source of error. Adequate light is essential in visual interpretation. Hold the strip next to the most closely matched color block for each chemical test. Be sure to correctly orient the reagent strip to the color chart when reading results. Multistix products are held perpendicular with respect to the bottle; Chemstrip products should be held parallel to the bottle (Fig. 14-4). The use of automated or semiautomated instruments will eliminate individual differences in color interpretation and improve the reproducibility of results. Report results in a consistent manner as established for your institution.

## Control Solutions

Several commercial control products are readily available either lyophilized or as a liquid. Manufacturers' directions for reconstitution and use should be followed. Generally a negative control and a positive control should be used to test every parameter of the reagent strip in use. Reagent strips should be tested at least once each day or shift that the test is performed and whenever a new bottle of reagent strips is opened. Acceptable results are generally within one color block of the assigned target, as stated by manufacturer. The only acceptable result for a negative control solution is negative. According to the NCCLS, quality control should "adhere to all local, state and federal regulation, as well as manufacturers' instructions."[5]

## AUTOMATION IN URINALYSIS

Although multiple-reagent strips were developed to be read visually, instruments have been developed to electronically measure the intensity of the color reactions produced on the reagent strips. The instruments are reflectance photometers. They measure the intensity of light that is produced by the chemical reaction between the analyte in question and the chemicals impregnated on each test portion of the reagent strip. The intensity of light produced is proportional to the amount of analyte in the specimen being tested. The instruments contain a microprocessor that controls and coordinates reflectance measurements at each test area. It mechanically moves the reagent strip through the

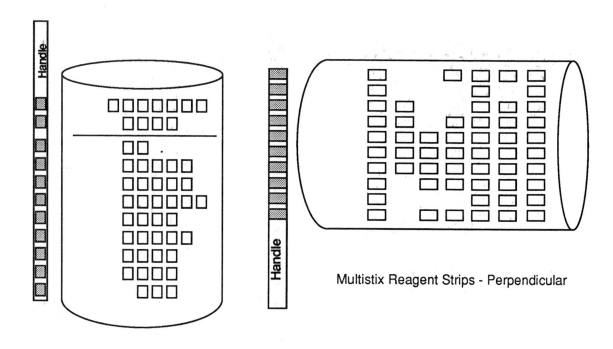

Chemstrip Reagent Strips - Parallel

Multistix Reagent Strips - Perpendicular

**FIG 14-4.** Reading reagent strips (orientation to bottle).

photometer to ensure accurate and consistent timing, and displays or prints out the results for each test area. In addition, it displays error codes when the strips are inserted improperly or otherwise mishandled. Actual instruments vary in the way the strips are inserted into the instrument, the degree of automation, and the manner in which patient specimens are identified and results are displayed or printed.

Some instruments, such as the Clinitek Atlas,* use a reagent pad consisting of a roll of dry chemistry reagent strips affixed to a clear plastic support. The dry chemistry is the same as for the Multistix reagent strips. The specimen is automatically pipetted onto each test pad, rather than dipping a reagent strip into the sample. Specific gravity is measured by refractive index, rather than reagent strip, and color is determined by measuring the color on a special

reagent pad, while clarity (transparency) is determined by measurement of transmitted and scattered light through the sample.

There are many advantages to instrumentation. The readings are more reproducible and unbiased. Visual readings may vary from person to person, especially with respect to color interpretation and timing. The instruments are programmed to read each test area at a specific time, which, although very important, is sometimes difficult to do manually. It is also possible to analyze a greater number of specimens in less time than is possible manually. Printed results decrease the incidence of transcription (clerical) errors. Results can also be interfaced with the laboratory computer system to further minimize clerical errors and save time in reporting results. It should be remembered that the instrument does not alter the chemical methodology of the reagent strip but does increase reproducibility.

*Bayer Corp, Diagnostics Division, Tarrytown, NY.

Before the instrument is used, it must be calibrated. This is done as specified by the manufacturer. After this calibration is done, the reflectance readings are compared with calibration curves that are stored in the microprocessor. These are used to estimate the concentration of each analyte.

Although these instruments are fairly simple and relatively easy to use, several important factors must be kept in mind. The person using the instrument must read the operating manual carefully and follow the directions exactly. Shortcuts cannot be tolerated. The instrument must be maintained on an established, regular schedule. The instrument must be kept clean and free from contamination. One person should be responsible for maintenance.

Although only visual chemical urinalysis by reagent or tablet test was classified as a waived test according to CLIA '88 regulations, an automated instrument, the Clinitek 50 Urine Chemistry Analyzer,* has been given waived status by the FDA.

The microscopic analysis of urine has also been automated by the Yellow IRIS.† This is an integrated system that uses multiple-reagent strips and instrumentation for the chemical analysis of the urine specimen. An aliquot of the urine is presented to a videomicroscope in a single layer of particles, which are analyzed by computer according to size and number. A laboratorian views low-power and high-power digitized images on a color monitor and makes final identification by selecting an appropriate category on the monitor screen.

The use of instrumentation for the chemical analysis of urine should provide time for other parts of the urinalysis, leaving valuable time for careful microscopic analysis of the urinary sediment. Care must be taken with standardization and controls, and the instrument must not be misused. The laboratorian must still be aware of the principles and limitations of the tests. A gross examination of the urine specimen must not be omitted, and the instrumental results must be checked against the gross appearance and correlated with findings in the urinary sediment before final results are reported.

## pH

One function of the kidney is to regulate the acidity of the extracellular fluid. Some information about this function, and other information as well, may be obtained by testing the urinary pH.

pH is the unit that describes the acidity or alkalinity of a solution. In ordinary terms, acidity refers to the sourness of a solution, while alkalinity refers to its bitterness. Lemon juice is an example of a sour, or acidic, solution; baking soda (sodium bicarbonate) is a bitter, or alkaline, substance in solution. In chemical terms, acidity refers to the hydronium ion ($H_3O^+$) concentration of a solution and alkalinity refers to its hydroxyl ion ($OH^-$) concentration. These concentrations are usually expressed in terms of pH.

All solutions can be placed somewhere on a scale of pH values from 0 to 14. Some solutions, however, are neither acidic nor basic. These solutions are neutral and are placed at 7 on the pH scale. Water is an example of a neutral solution; its pH is 7. Water is neutral because the concentration of hydronium ions is equal to the concentration of hydroxyl ions.

A solution with more hydronium ions than hydroxyl ions is an acidic solution. On the pH scale an acidic solution has a value ranging from 0 to 7. The farther it is from 7, the greater the acidity. For instance, solutions of pH 2 and pH 5 are both acidic; however, a solution of pH 2 is more acidic than a solution of pH 5. In simpler terms, a solution of pH 2 is more sour than a solution with a higher pH value. For example, lemon juice has a pH of about 2.3, while orange juice has a pH of about 3.5.

An alkaline solution has a pH value greater than 7. It can be anything from 7 to 14; the farther it is from 7, the greater the alkalinity, or the more bitter the solution.

---

*Bayer Corp, Diagnostics Division, Tarrytown, NY.
†International Remote Imaging Systems, Chatsworth, Calif.

## Clinical Importance

Regulation of the pH of the extracellular fluid is an extremely important function of the kidney. Normally, the pH of blood is about 7.4 and varies no more than ±0.05 pH unit. If the blood pH is 6.8 to 7.3, marked **acidosis** will be seen clinically; if it is 7.5 to 7.8, marked **alkalosis** will be observed. A pH less than 6.8 or greater than 7.8 will result in death. The carbon dioxide produced in normal metabolism results in a tremendous amount of acid, which must be eliminated from the blood and extracellular fluid, or death will result. This acid is normally eliminated from the body by the lungs and the kidneys.

Because the kidney is generally working to eliminate excess acid, the pH of urine is normally between 5 and 7, with a mean of 6. The kidney is capable of producing urine ranging in pH from 4.6 to 8.0. The urine is normally acidified through an exchange of hydrogen ions for sodium ions in the distal convoluted tubules. In renal tubular acidosis this exchange and the ability to form ammonia are impaired, resulting in a relatively alkaline urine. Certain metabolic acid-base disturbances may also be reflected in measurements of urinary pH as the kidney attempts to compensate for changes in blood pH. Such acid-base disturbances are classified as metabolic or respiratory acidosis and alkalosis, and measurements of titratable acidity, ammonium ion, and bicarbonate concentration are used in these distinctions.

Although the kidney is essential in controlling the pH of blood and extracellular fluid, measurements of urinary pH are not necessarily used to obtain information about this role. The routine urinalysis includes a measurement of urinary pH for the following reasons:

1. Freshly voided urine usually has a pH of 5 or 6. However, on standing at room temperature, urea is converted to ammonia by bacterial action. The production of ammonia raises the hydroxyl ion concentration, resulting in an alkaline urine specimen. Therefore, unless it is known that a urine specimen is fresh, an alkaline pH probably indicates an old urine specimen.

2. Alkalinity of freshly voided urine, especially if persistent throughout the day, may indicate a urinary tract infection. Other urinalysis findings in infection include positive reagent strip tests for nitrite and leukocyte esterase and large numbers of bacteria and possibly white cells (neutrophils) in the urine sediment.

3. The urinary pH helps in the identification of crystals of certain chemical compounds that are often seen in the urine sediment. Certain crystals are associated with acid urine, pH under 7, and others with alkaline urine, pH 7 and over. Knowledge of the urine pH is of great importance in the identification of crystals and may be the major reason for testing the pH of a urine specimen.

4. If the urine specimen is dilute and alkaline, various formed elements, such as casts and red blood cells, will rapidly dissolve.

5. Persistently acidic urine may be seen in a variety of metabolic disorders, especially diabetic acidosis resulting from an accumulation of ketone bodies in the blood.

6. Persistently alkaline urine may be seen in some infections, in metabolic disorders, and with the administration of certain drugs.

7. It is sometimes necessary to control the urinary pH in the management of kidney infections, in cases of renal calculi (stones), and during the administration of certain drugs. This is done by regulating the diet; meat diets generally result in acidic urine and vegetable diets in alkaline urine.

## Principle of Reagent Strip Tests for pH

Reagent strip tests utilize a methyl red and bromthymol blue double indicator system that measures urine pH in a range from 5 to 9. They are available as multiple-reagent strips in combination with other tests for urinary constituents. The methyl red is used to indicate a pH change from 4.4 to 6.2 with a color change from red to yellow. Bromthymol blue indicates a pH change from 6.0 to 7.6 as seen by a color change from yellow to blue.

### Interferences

No interferences are known. The pH value is not affected by the buffer concentration of the urine.

### Additional Comments

The specimen must be tested when fresh, since bacterial growth may result in a significant shift to an alkaline pH, giving falsely alkaline values. Be careful not to wet the reagent strip excessively so that the acid buffer from the protein area runs into the pH area, causing an orange discoloration.

### Follow-Up or Confirmatory Tests

In most instances a precise measure of the urinary pH is not necessary. A rough estimate using multiple-reagent strips is sufficient. For more accurate measurements, a pH meter may be used. This is rarely necessary clinically, but may be useful if renal tubular acidosis is suspected.

If the reagent strip value is greater than 9.0 or if results are uncertain, the specimen may be tested with special pH indicator strips. Usual protocol is to merely report such values as ≥9.

### ▌SPECIFIC GRAVITY (See Previous Section on Specific Gravity)

Reagent strip tests for specific gravity are based on a pKa change of certain pretreated polyelectrolytes in relation to the ionic concentration of urine. Therefore, they measure only ionizable substances. In general, reagent strip tests correlate to within 0.005 of the refractometer. However, urines with specific gravity greater than 1.025 are not reliably measured with ionic concentration methodology and should be tested with the refractometer.

## ▌PROTEIN

### Clinical Importance

In the detection and diagnosis of renal disease, probably the most significant single finding is that of urinary protein. The presence of protein when correlated with certain chemical tests, especially tests for blood, nitrite, and leukocyte esterase, and findings in the microscopic analysis of the urinary sediment, is part of the eventual diagnosis.

The occurrence of protein in the urine is termed **proteinuria.** Proteinuria is an abnormal condition, probably the most important pathologic condition found in a routine urinalysis. In general proteinuria may be the result of:

1. Glomerular damage
2. Tubular damage
3. Prerenal disorders or overflow from the excessive production of low-molecular-weight proteins such as hemoglobin, myoglobin, or immunoglobulins
4. Lower urinary tract disorders
5. Asymptomatic disorders

Proteinuria may be classified as to the amount (quantity) or degree of protein excreted per day (24 hours) as follows:

| Amount of Proteinuria | Grams Excreted per Day |
|---|---|
| Mild (minimal) | <1 g/day |
| Moderate | 1 to 3 or 4 g/day |
| Large (heavy) | >3 or 4 g/day |

Note that the amount of protein per 100 mL in a random urine specimen is related to 24-hour urine volume. Thus, heavy proteinuria, with 3 grams of protein eliminated per day and a 24-hour urine volume of 1500 mL, would correspond to 200 mg protein/dL in a random urine specimen. If the 24-hour urine volume were 500 mL, there might be 600 mg protein/dL.

Normally, the glomerular filtrate, the initial stage in the formation of urine, is an ultrafiltrate of blood plasma without cells, larger protein molecules, and certain fatty substances. Normal urine contains less than 10 mg/dL of protein as albumin. This is not detectable by normal tests for urinary protein. The normal glomerular membrane allows the passage of proteins with molecular weights of 50,000 to 60,000 or less. Albumin has a molecular weight of about 67,000. This is a fairly small molecule, and some albumin is normally filtered through the glomerulus. However, this is normally reabsorbed in the convoluted tubules. Therefore, proteinuria (measurable amounts of protein in urine) may be the result of increased permeability of the glomerulus or decreased reabsorption by the renal tubules

**Tamm-Horsfall protein** is a high-molecular-weight glycoprotein (mucoprotein) that is normally secreted by renal tubular epithelial cells. It is a product of the kidney and not present in the blood plasma. This is the protein that forms the basic matrix of most urinary casts. **Casts** are an important pathologic urinary finding and are associated with proteinuria. The occurrence of casts with proteinuria distinguishes an upper urinary tract (kidney) disorder from a disorder of the lower urinary tract (bladder).

The implications of protein in the urine in association with renal disease are extremely serious, and prompt diagnosis and treatment are vitally important. In addition, the loss of protein from the blood plasma will result in severe water balance problems, since the osmotic pressure of the blood is largely dependent on the concentration of plasma proteins. This is readily seen in the edema that is often associated with kidney disorders.

Although proteinuria is indicative of renal disease, additional tests are needed for the final diagnosis. These include observations of the urinary sediment (especially for the presence and types of casts), a determination of the amount of protein excreted per day by quantitative tests, the type of protein by electrophoresis, and the patient's clinical history.

### Glomerular Damage

Proteinuria (generally albuminuria) is a consistent finding in glomerular disease. If the glomerular membrane is damaged, larger protein molecules find their way into the glomerular filtrate and are detected in the urine. This increased glomerular permeability usually begins with the passage of the smaller albumin molecules, and the larger globulin molecules remain in the blood plasma.

A variety of causes, including toxins, infections, vascular disorders, and immunologic reactions, may result in glomerular damage and increased filtration with proteinuria. Poststreptococcal **acute glomerulonephritis (AGN)** is an example of glomerular proteinuria. This is an immunologic sequela of a bacterial infection, usually a throat infection due to group A beta-hemolytic streptococcus. Urinalysis findings include proteinuria, hematuria (red blood cells), and casts (red cell, blood, or granular).

Early in cases of glomerular damage, only the small protein molecules (albumin) are filtered through the glomerulus. As the glomerular damage progresses, virtually all proteins present in the plasma find their way into the urine. In the **nephrotic syndrome,** heavy (massive) proteinuria (>3 or 4 g/day) is seen. So much protein is lost from the body via the urine that the ability of the liver to synthesize sufficient albumin to maintain the normal blood albumin is lost and **albuminemia** results. Albumin is responsible for the osmotic pressure; thus albuminemia results in generalized swelling or edema throughout the body. In addition to massive proteinuria, the nephrotic syndrome is associated with the presence of free fat, tubular epithelial cells containing fat (oval fat bodies), and fatty casts in the urine sediment.

### Tubular Damage

A very small amount of protein (albumin) does find its way into the glomerular filtrate. In normal situations, all of this protein is reabsorbed back into the blood through the renal convoluted tubules. Although the concentration of protein that normally filters into the glomerular filtrate is extremely small and only 1 in 180 parts of the glomerular filtrate is eliminated from the body as urine (the rest is reabsorbed), failure to reabsorb any protein from this large volume of glomerular filtrate will result in fairly large amounts of protein in the urine. In other words, another cause of proteinuria is decreased reabsorption of protein by the renal tubular cells. The amount of proteinuria in tubular damage is generally mild to moderate. Examples of tubular proteinuria include pyelonephritis, acute tubular necrosis, polycystic kidney disease, heavy metal and vitamin D intoxication, phenacetin damage, hypokalemia, Wilson's disease, galactosemia, Fanconi's syndrome, and post-transplantation syndrome.

**Acute pyelonephritis** is an infection of the pelvis and parenchyma of the kidney. It is usually the result of infection ascending from the lower urinary tract into the kidney. In addition to moderate proteinuria, urinalysis findings may include nitrite, leukocyte esterase, white blood cells (neutrophils), and casts (white cell, cellular, granular, or bacterial). The presence of casts in the urine locates the infection in the kidney.

Drug-induced **acute interstitial nephritis** (an allergic response) is also associated with moderate proteinuria. The presence of eosinophils is especially characteristic, together with neutrophils, red cells, and cellular or granular casts.

Only mild proteinuria may be seen with acute renal failure or acute tubular necrosis. However, the sediment may contain renal tubular epithelial cells and casts (epithelial, granular, or waxy).

### Prerenal Disorders

Prerenal or overflow disorders may result in proteinuria from disorders in body sites other than the kidney. Overflow from excessive production of low-molecular-weight proteins such as hemoglobin, myoglobin, or immunoglobulins may result in such proteinuria. The presence of light-chain immunoglobulins (Bence Jones protein) associated with multiple myeloma is an example.

Prerenal proteinuria may also be the result of a change in hydrostatic pressure in the kid-

ney glomerulus. Increased blood pressure may force more proteins than normal through the glomerulus, resulting in the mild proteinuria seem with hypertension, congestive heart failure, and dehydration.

### Lower Urinary Tract Disorders

Infections of the lower urinary tract may result in a mild proteinuria. The proteinuria may result from infection of the ureters or bladder with exudation through the mucosa (lining). Other urinalysis findings include positive chemical tests for nitrite (depending on the infecting organism) and leukocyte esterase, and the presence of white cells and bacteria in the sediment. Casts are not present in lower urinary tract infection—they originate in the kidney.

### Asymptomatic Proteinuria

There are situations in which small amounts of urinary protein may occur transiently in normal persons. In particular, they may be found in young adults after excessive exercise or exposure to cold, or in so-called **orthostatic proteinuria,** which occurs in persons engaged in normal activity but disappears when they lie down.

In general, the proteinuria associated with renal disease is consistent, while that found in normal persons is transient. The long-term significance of asymptomatic proteinuria is unclear. To determine the cause of the proteinuria, it is often necessary to quantitatively determine the amount of protein in a 24-hour urine collection. Tests for orthostatic proteinuria are made on urine collections obtained both when the patient is at rest (first morning, collected immediately after rising) and after the patient has been walking and standing, but not sitting, for about 2 hours.

### Consistent Microalbuminuria

Although screening tests for proteinuria should not be so sensitive that they detect the very small amount of protein that may be normally present in urine, it is sometimes desirable to detect the consistent passage of very small amounts of protein (microproteinuria). This is especially true of patients with diabetes mellitus. In these patients, it is thought that the early development of renal complications can be predicted by the early detection of consistent microalbuminuria. This early detection is desirable, as better control of blood glucose levels may delay the progression of renal disease. The methodology for the detection of microalbuminuria includes nephelometry, radial immunodiffusion, and radioimmunoassay. A relatively simple tablet test, Micro-Bumintest,* has been developed to detect very small amounts of albumin. The principle of this test is analogous to that of the reagent strip tests; however, the sensitivity of Micro-Bumintest is significantly greater at 4 to 8 mg albumin/dL urine.

## Methods of Measurement

Tests for urinary protein are of two major types:

1. Tests that are based on the use of the protein error of pH indicators. This is the methodology employed in the various reagent strip tests. They are more sensitive to the presence of albumin than to other proteins.
2. Tests that are based on the precipitation of protein by a chemical or coagulation by heat. These tests will detect all proteins, including albumin, glycoproteins, globulins (light-chain immunoglobulin or Bence Jones protein), and hemoglobin.

In some laboratories, all urine specimens are tested both with reagent strips and precipitation tests; in others, urine specimens are screened with reagent strips for albumin and confirmed with a precipitation test such as the sulfosalicylic acid described in this book.

### Reagent Strip Tests for Protein

**Principle.** Reagent strip tests for urinary protein involve the use of pH indicators—

substances that have characteristic colors at specific pH values. At a fixed pH, certain pH indicators will show one color in the presence of protein and another color in its absence. This phenomenon is referred to as the "protein error of indicators." The pH of the urine is held constant by means of a buffer, so that any change of color of the indicator will indicate the presence of protein.

**Specificity.** The reagent strip tests for urinary protein are more sensitive to the presence of albumin than they are to other proteins such as globulin, hemoglobin, Bence Jones protein, and mucoprotein. If these proteins are present in the urine without albumin, false-negative results may be obtained. In other words, a negative reagent strip does not rule out the presence of protein. Therefore, depending on the patient population, it may be necessary for a given laboratory to test all urine specimens with both a reagent strip and a precipitation method for urinary protein so as not to miss certain abnormal proteins such as those seen in new, undiagnosed cases of multiple myeloma.

### Sensitivity (Minimum Detectable Level: Manufacturer's Values

| | |
|---|---|
| Multistix/Albustix | 15 to 30 mg/dL albumin |
| Micro-Bumintest | 4 to 8 mg/dL albumin |
| Chemstrip | 6 mg/dL albumin |
| | (in 90% tested) |

**Interferences.** If the urine is strongly pigmented, there may be interference with the color reaction. Bilirubin or drugs that give a vivid orange color, such as phenazopyridine (Pyridium) and other azo-containing compounds, may result in this interference.

#### False-Positive Results

- If the urine is exposed to the reagent strip for too long, the buffer may be washed out of the strip, resulting in the formation of a blue color whether protein is present or not.
- If a urine specimen is exceptionally alkaline or highly buffered, the reagent strip

*Bayer Corp, Diagnostics Division, Tarrytown, NY.

tests may give a positive result in the absence of protein.

- Contamination of the urine container with residues of disinfectants containing quaternary ammonium compounds or chlorhexidine may show a positive result because of increased alkalinity.
- Chemstrip products may give false-positive results during therapy with phenazopyridine and when infusions of polyvinylpyrrolidone (blood substitutes) are administered.

**False-Negative Results**

- When proteins other than albumin are present, the reagent strip will give a negative result in the presence of protein.

**Additional Comments.** The reagent strip tests for protein are not affected by turbidity, radiographic contrast media, most drugs and their metabolites, and urine preservatives, which occasionally affect other protein tests.

The color must be matched closely with the color chart when results are being read. The protein portion of the reagent strip is difficult to interpret, especially at the trace level. When results are in doubt, the slightly more sensitive SSA protein test or a test for microalbuminuria such as Micro-Bumintest (Bayer) might be helpful.

**Confirmatory Tests.** The sulfosalicylic acid (SSA) test or another protein precipitation method may be used to confirm the presence of

protein when reactions indicating a trace or more are obtained or when reagent strip results are in doubt. See Table 14-6 for comparison of urine protein test results with different methods.

### Sulfosalicylic Acid Test for Urine Protein

**Principle.** This test is based on the cold precipitation of protein with a strong acid, namely sulfosalicylic acid. Various concentrations of sulfosalicylic acid have been described for use in tests for urinary protein. In the procedure used at the Fairview-University Medical Center, University Campus, a 7 g/dL solution is employed so that 11 mL of cleared urine, resulting from the routine 12:1 concentration of the urinary sediment, can be used. See Procedure 14-3.

**Specificity.** The free sulfosalicylic acid in the working reagent serves to precipitate any protein in the specimen. It will detect albumin, globulins, glycoproteins, and light-chain immunoglobulins such as Bence Jones protein. Since the test does not rely on heat for precipitation, Bence Jones protein will precipitate like any other protein. To identify the actual type of protein present, further tests such as electrophoresis, immunoelectrophoresis, imunodiffusion, or ultracentrifugation may be necessary.

**Sensitivity (Minimum Detectable Level).** Five to 10 mg of protein per dL.

**Sulfosalicylic Acid Reagent (7 g/dL).** Dissolve 70.0 g of 5-sulfosalicylic acid

---

**TABLE 14-6**

Comparison of Urine Protein Test Results by Method

| Result/Grade | Sulfosalicylic Acid | Multistix/Albustix | Chemstrip |
|---|---|---|---|
| Negative | Negative | Negative | Negative |
| Trace | 5-20 mg/dL | Trace | Trace |
| 1+ | 30 mg/dL | 30 mg/dL | 30 mg/dL |
| 2+ | 100 mg/dL | 100 mg/dL | 200 mg/dL |
| 3+ | 300-500 mg/dL | 300 mg/dL | ≥500 mg/dL |
| 4+ | >500 mg/dL | >2000 mg/dL | No color block |

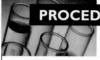

## PROCEDURE 14-3

### Sulfosalicylic Acid Test for Urine Protein

1. Centrifuge a 12-mL aliquot of urine.

2. Decant 11 mL of the supernatant urine into a 16 × 125 mm test tube. Note the clarity of the centrifuged urine.

3. Add 3 mL of 7 g/dL sulfosalicylic acid reagent.

4. Stopper the tube and mix by inverting twice.

5. Let stand exactly 10 minutes.

6. Invert tube twice.

7. Observe the degree of precipitation, and grade the results according to the descriptions in Table 14-7. To avoid making the test too sensitive, examine negative and trace reactions in ordinary room light, avoiding a Tyndall effect (scattering of light by colloidal particles), which might result from examination in too bright a light. If an agglutination viewer is available, use it to grade results higher than trace. To observe the degree of precipitation, tilt the test tube while simultaneously viewing the quality and quantity of precipitate in the mirror.

## TABLE 14-7

SSA Protein Test Results

| SSA Result | Description | Approximate Protein Concentration in mg/dL* |
|---|---|---|
| Negative | No turbidity, or no increase in turbidity. Clear ring is visible at bottom of tube when viewed from above (top to bottom) | <5 mg/dL |
| Trace | Barely perceptible turbidity in ordinary room light<br>Printed material distorted but readable through the tube<br>Cannot see a ring at bottom of tube when viewed from above | 5-20 mg/dL |
| 1+ | Distinct turbidity but no distinct granulation | 30 mg/dL |
| 2+ | Turbidity with granulation but no flocculation | 100 mg/dL |
| 3+ | Turbidity with granulation and flocculation | 300-500 mg/dL |
| 4+ | Clumps of precipitated protein or solid precipitate | >500 mg/dL |

*Based on a comparison of SSA values by reagent strip (Multistix) and Cobas protein results, UMHC, Jan 1993. Unpublished.

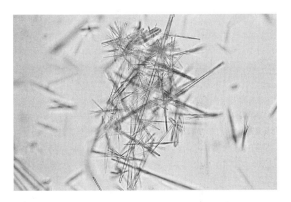

**FIG 14-5.** Microscopic appearance of the SSA precipitate due to radiographic media.

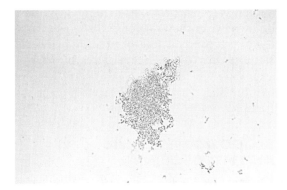

**FIG 14-6.** Microscopic appearance of the SSA precipitate due to protein.

($C_7H_6O_6S \cdot 2H_2O$) in deionized or distilled water and dilute to exactly 1 L.

### Interferences
#### False-Positive Results
- Turbidity (cloudiness) in the urine specimen. Urine must be clarified before testing—usually by centrifugation.
- The presence of organic iodides in radiographic contrast media, such as meglumine diatrizoate (Renografin, Hypaque), used for diagnostic procedures may precipitate in the acid test solution, giving a delayed positive reaction. When protein is present, precipitation begins immediately when the SSA reagent is added. Unusual crystals of the radiographic media may be found in the urinary sediment in such cases. This interference is suspected when very high specific gravity values (greater than 1.035 by refractometer) are obtained and the reagent strip test for protein is negative. It may be confirmed by checking the patient's history for the use of diagnostic radiographic procedures. The precipitated material in the SSA tube may also be observed microscopically for the presence of crystals. Such crystals are highly refractile needles that polarize light (Fig. 14-5). Precipitated protein shows an amorphous precipitate that does not polarize light (Fig. 14-6).

- Metabolites of drugs such as tolbutamide (an oral drug used to treat diabetes), massive doses of penicillin, sulfonamides, or cephalosporin, and the antiinflammatory drug tolmetin (Tolectin). These substances do not affect the reagent strip tests for protein; results would be negative or more than one grade lower than the SSA result. To confirm drug interference, check the patient history and/or observe the SSA precipitate microscopically for the presence of crystals.

#### False-Negative or Reduced Results
- The occurrence of a highly buffered alkaline urine if the buffer is sufficient to neutralize the acid in SSA. This is rare. Such specimens might also give a false-positive reaction with the reagent strip test. To resolve this discrepancy, acidify the urine specimen to pH 5 or 6 and retest with the reagent strip and SSA. Results should be similar on the acidified urine.

**Additional Comments.** With specimens showing a positive SSA test with a negative reagent strip, or a value more than one grade less than the SSA value, suspect the presence of a protein other than albumin. This might be a light-chain immunoglobulin (Bence Jones protein) seen in multiple myeloma. Confirm the identity of the problem by electrophoresis or immunoelectrophoresis.

Nonalbumin pancreatic fluid proteins may be excreted in the urine of patients who have received a pancreas transplant with anastomosis. Such urines will test negative by reagent strip and show a positive SSA reaction. Resolve by checking the patient history for pancreas transplant.

## BLOOD (HEMOGLOBIN AND MYOGLOBIN)

### Clinical Significance

Together with tests for protein, and the microscopic analysis of the urinary sediment, tests for blood in urine are used as indicators of the state of the kidney and urinary tract. Chemical tests for blood in urine react with red blood cells, hemoglobin, and myoglobin (which is muscle hemoglobin). Although the chemical tests are more sensitive to the presence of hemoglobin and myoglobin than to intact red cells, most positive reactions are actually caused by the presence of red cells (erythrocytes). Blood may represent bleeding at any point from the glomerulus to the urethra, and the actual location is important to the diagnosis and treatment of the patient. Although the chemical detection of blood in urine is a serious finding, the presence of a few red blood cells in urine is normal and hematuria may be associated with benign conditions.

It is clinically significant to differentiate between red cells and hemoglobin in the urine. Since tests for hemoglobin are positive in the presence of both free hemoglobin and red cells, it would seem that this differentiation is made mainly by the finding of red cells in the microscopic analysis of the urinary sediment. However, the presence of hemoglobin and the absence of red cells in the urine does not necessarily mean that the hemoglobin was originally free urinary hemoglobin. Red cells rapidly lyse in urine, especially when the specific gravity is low (<1.010) or the pH is alkaline. For this reason urine should be absolutely fresh when examined for the presence of red cells.

### Hematuria

**Hematuria** is the presence of red blood cells in the urine. It results from a great variety of conditions, including both lesions of the kidney itself and bleeding at any other point in the urinary tract. It may be an early sign of kidney or bladder tumor (benign or malignant) or result from stone formation in the kidney or bladder. Hematuria might be a sign of glomerular damage or interstitial nephritis (infection of the kidney), or it may be seen with a lower urinary tract infection such as cystitis (bladder infection). Generalized bleeding disorders or anticoagulant therapy may also result in hematuria.

Hematuria is a sensitive, early indicator of renal disease and should not be missed. Although blood will not be present in every voided specimen in every case of renal disease, **occult blood** (i.e., blood that is not grossly visible but is found by laboratory tests) may be present in almost every renal disorder. There may be little correlation between the amount of blood and the severity of the disorder, but its presence may be the only indication of renal disease. It is associated with glomerular damage and is typically seen in glomerulonephritis. Other laboratory findings besides hematuria indicate the presence of renal disease. Protein is usually present along with blood, and the presence of casts (especially red cell casts) and dysmorphic red cells in the urine sediment are particularly useful.

### Hemoglobinuria

**Hemoglobinuria,** or the presence of free hemoglobin in the urine, results from a variety of conditions and disease states. It may be the result of hemolysis in the bloodstream **(intravascular hemolysis),** in the kidney or lower urinary tract, or in the urine sample itself. The detection of intravascular hemolysis is important because the passage of free hemoglobin through the glomerulus and subsequent uptake by renal proximal convoluted epithelial cells are damaging to the nephron. Hemoglobin is carried in the bloodstream bound to a protein, **haptoglobin.** This hemoglobin-haptoglobin complex is a large molecule that is not filtered through the glomerulus. However, there is a limited amount of haptoglobin in the blood, and once it is saturated, the excess hemoglobin is filtered through the glomerulus into the renal tubules. Some of the excreted hemoglobin is absorbed into the renal tubular cells, converted to ferritin and **hemosiderin,** and subsequently excreted several days after an acute hemolytic episode. These hemosiderin-containing cells and granules may be observed in the urine sediment, especially when stained with Prussian blue.

Hematologic disease states resulting in hemoglobinuria include hemolytic anemias, hemolytic transfusion reactions, paroxysmal nocturnal hemoglobinuria, paroxysmal cold hemoglobinuria, and favism. Severe infectious diseases such as yellow fever, *Bartonella* infection, and malaria also result in hemoglobinuria, as do poisonings with strong acids or mushrooms, severe burns, and renal infarction. Finally, significant amounts of free hemoglobin occur whenever excessive numbers of red cells are present as a result of various renal disorders, infectious, or neoplastic diseases, or trauma in any part of the urinary tract.

### Myoglobinuria

Myoglobinuria is the presence of myoglobin in the urine. It is a rare finding. Chemical tests for occult blood are equally sensitive to the presence of hemoglobin and myoglobin. Myoglobin is released after **rhabdomyolysis**—acute destruction of muscle fibers. Myoglobinuria may result from traumatic muscle injury (such as from traffic accidents), excessive unaccustomed exercise, and beating or other crush injury. It is also seen in certain infections, after exposure to toxic substances and drugs, and in rare hereditary disorders.

The detection of myoglobinuria is important, as myoglobin is rapidly cleared from the blood and excreted into the urine as a red-brown pigment. Large amounts of myoglobin are damaging to the kidney and may result in anuria. It seems that myoglobin is more damaging than hemoglobin to the kidney.

### Differentiation of Hematuria, Hemoglobinuria, and Myoglobinuria

This may be difficult. It is done with a combination of gross observations of urine and serum (or plasma) and certain chemical tests. (See Table 14-8.) The occurrence of blood in urine will result in a coloration ranging from normal, to smoky, pink, amber, red to red-brown, brown, or frankly bloody. In general, with hemoglobin and myoglobin, the urine specimen is brown or red-brown. Although the presence of red blood cells would result in cloudiness, and hemoglobin or myoglobin by

---

**TABLE 14-8**

Differentiation of Red Blood Cells, Hemoglobin, and Myoglobin in Urine

| Finding | Red Cells | Hemoglobin | Myoglobin |
|---|---|---|---|
| Reagent strip for blood | Positive | Positive | Positive |
| Urine sediment for red cells | Present | Absent (few) | Absent (few) |
| Urine appearance | Cloudy red | Clear red | Clear red-brown |
| Plasma appearance | Normal | Pink to red (hemolysis) | Normal |
| Total serum creatinine kinase (CK) | Normal | Slight elevation (10 times normal upper limit) | Marked elevation (40 times normal upper limit) |
| Total serum lactate dehydrogenase (LD) | Normal | Elevated | Elevated |
| $LD_1$ and $LD_2$ | Normal | Elevated | Normal |
| $LD_4$ and $LD_5$ | Normal | Normal | Elevated |

Modified from Ringsrud KM, Linné JJ: *Urinalysis and Body Fluids: A ColorText and Atlas,* St Louis, Mosby, 1995, p 55.

itself would leave a clear specimen, other constituents often accompany all three entities, leading to cloudiness of the specimen. A gross observation of the serum or plasma accompanying these specimens is useful. If the urine contains only red blood cells, the serum would be normally colored. If intravascular hemolysis has occurred, the serum would appear to be hemolyzed (red). If rhabdomyolysis occurs, the myoglobin released into the blood is rapidly cleared into the urine, so that the serum appears normal in color.

In all cases, the reagent strip test for blood is positive. If red cells are present, they should be detectable in the microscopic examination of the urine sediment. With both hemoglobin and myoglobin, red cells would be absent, or very few would be present. In the case of rhabdomyolysis resulting in myoglobinemia and myoglobinuria, markedly elevated serum creatinine kinase (CK) is typical owing to the destruction of muscle. CK levels are not affected as markedly by hemolysis. Unfortunately, myoglobin-induced renal failure may not be seen clinically until a week or more after the clinical event, and by then myoglobin is no longer present in the urine. In some cases, it may be helpful to use serum lactate dehydrogenase (LD) isoenzyme values to differentiate hemolysis from rhabdomyolysis. The total LD is elevated in both cases, but the $LD_1$ and $LD_2$ isoenzymes predominate in hemolysis, and the $LD_4$ and $LD_5$ isoenzymes with rhabdomyolysis. In the future, immunochemical tests may prove to be useful.

## Principle and Specificity

Reagent strip tests for blood (hemoglobin, myoglobin) in urine make use of the peroxidase activity of the heme portion of the hemoglobin molecule. The reagent strips are impregnated with an organic peroxide, together with the reduced form of a chromogen. A positive reaction is seen when the peroxidase activity of the heme portion of the hemoglobin or myoglobin molecule catalyzes the release of oxygen from peroxide on the reagent strip. The released oxygen reacts with the reduced form of a chromogen, forming an oxidized chromogen, which is indicated by a color change. This reaction is summarized as follows:

| Peroxide | Heme | Water |
|---|---|---|
| + | → | + |
| Reduced chromogen | (Peroxidase activity) | Oxidized chromogen |

The reagent strips are equally sensitive to hemoglobin and myoglobin. Intact red blood cells are hemolyzed when they come into contact with the reagent strip, and the released hemoglobin reacts as described. It is essential that well-mixed urine be tested for the presence of blood. This is especially important when only a few intact red blood cells are present in the urine specimen. If intact red cells are allowed to settle and the supernatant urine is tested, false-negative results will be obtained.

## Sensitivity (Minimum Detectable Level): Manufacturer's Values

| | |
|---|---|
| Multistix/Hemastix | 0.015 to 0.062 mg/dL hemoglobin (equivalent to 5-20 intact RBC/µL) |
| Chemstrip | 5 RBC/µL or hemoglobin corresponding to 10 RBC/µL in 90% urines tested |

## Interferences
### False-Positive Results

■ Strong oxidizing cleaning agents, such as hypochlorite bleach, because of oxidation of the chromogen in the absence of peroxidase
■ Microbial peroxidase activity associated with urinary tract infection
■ The presence of blood as a contaminant from menstruation—no clinical significance

### False-Negative or Delayed Results

■ Ascorbic acid in urine specimens containing more than 25 mg/dL. This is seen after ingestion of large doses of vitamin C or when ascorbic acid is included as a reducing agent in certain parenteral antibiotics, such as tetracycline. Both Multistix and Chemstrip reagent strips claim no interference at reasonable or normally encountered levels. Chemstrip products include a blood-iodate scavenger to reduce false-negative results. Multistix products containing diisopropylbenzene dihydroperoxide as the organic peroxide are less subject to interference with ascorbic acid. (See also the section Ascorbic Acid).

- Testing the supernatant urine from centrifugation or settling when only a few intact red cells are present. Urine must be well mixed when tested.
- Elevated specific gravity (high salt concentration) or elevated protein may reduce the lysis or red blood cells necessary for a reaction to occur.
- When formalin is used as a urinary preservative
- Treatment with captopril (an antihypertensive)
- Extremely high nitrite levels (over 10 mg/dL), seen (rarely) in severe urinary tract infections

## Additional Comments

The presence of ascorbic acid in urine is a potential problem in the reagent strip tests for blood, as it is in any of the reagent strip tests that depend on the release of oxygen and subsequent oxidation of a chromogen. When present in sufficient quantity, the ascorbic acid (a strong reducing agent) reacts with the released hydrogen peroxide (rather than the chromogen), causing inhibited (negative) results or a delayed color reaction.

When the regent strip test for blood is negative, yet red blood cells are observed in the urine sediment, the presence of ascorbic acid should be suspected. This may be confirmed by testing the urine with a reagent strip for ascorbic acid or by the patient's clinical history.

## Confirmatory Tests

- Microscopic examination of the urinary sediment
- Reagent strip test for ascorbic acid if the test for blood is negative and red cells are seen in the urine sediment, or if blood is suspected

on the basis of the appearance of the urine specimen

# NITRITE

## Clinical Importance

Tests for the presence of **nitrite** in the urine have been included in the routine urinalysis as a rapid method of detecting urinary tract infection. Screening tests for nitrite are most useful when combined with tests for leukocyte esterase, another indicator of urinary tract infection. The presence of urinary nitrite indicates the existence of a urinary tract infection. It is especially useful in detecting asymptomatic infections. When certain, but not all, bacteria are present in the urinary tract, they will convert nitrate, a normal constituent of urine, to nitrite, an abnormal constituent. Nitrate converters are generally gram-negative bacteria, such as the common Enterobacteriaceae. Gram-positive organisms such as enterococci and yeast do not generally convert nitrate to nitrite. However, there must also be sufficient nitrate (primarily derived from vegetables in the diet) in the urine for conversion to nitrite to take place.

Urine must be retained (incubated) in the bladder for a sufficient period (generally 4 hours) for this reaction to take place. Thus, a first morning urine collection is the specimen of choice in testing for nitrite. A specimen collected at least 4 hours after previous voiding is also acceptable. Unfortunately, a common complaint with urinary tract infection is frequent urination, making collection of an adequate specimen difficult.

The early detection of urinary tract infection is important for the prevention of kidney damage. It is felt that most urinary tract infections begin in the lower urinary tract, as a result of fecal contamination. Most infections are due to organisms that are normally present in the feces, such as *Escherichia coli*. The infection is introduced into the normally sterile urinary tract via the urethra, and ascends to the bladder, ureters, and finally the kidney. The early detection and subsequent treatment of infection are important in preventing infection of the kidney and subsequent renal failure. From this discussion it should be apparent that because of anatomical differences, urinary tract infection is much more common in women than men. In fact, other than just after birth or with incontinence (often associated with aging or disability), urinary tract infection is typically a disease of women.

Traditionally, urinary tract infections are diagnosed through quantitative urine culture, in which the organism that causes the infection is cultured and identified (see Chapter 16). Nitrite tests are screening tests that aid quantitative urine cultures. The existence of urinary tract infections is also suggested by other findings in the routine urinalysis. Microscopic findings include the presence of white blood cells and bacteria in lower urinary tract infections; this plus the presence of casts, especially white cell or pus casts, indicates upper urinary tract infection (pyelonephritis). Chemical test results suggestive of urinary tract infection include the presence of leukocyte esterase and protein and a more alkaline urinary pH.

## Principle

Reagent strip tests for nitrite are based on the **Griess test.** This involves a **diazo reaction.** Nitrite will react with an aromatic amine (*p*-arsanilic or sulfanilic acid) in an acid medium to produce a diazonium salt. The diazonium salt is then coupled with another aromatic ring (quinolin) to give an azo dye, which is seen as a pink or red color.

## Specificity

The test is specific for nitrite.

## Results

Results are reported as positive or negative. Any overall pink coloration is a positive reaction. Pink spots or pink edges are a negative reaction. The intensity of color formation does not necessarily indicate the degree of bacterial infection. Any pink coloration suggests a significant infection.

## Sensitivity (Minimum Detectable Level)

| | |
|---|---|
| Multistix | 0.06 to 0.1 mg/dL nitrite ion |
| Chemstrip | As low as 0.05 mg/dL nitrite |

## Interferences
### False-Positive Results

- Medications such as phenazopyridine or other azo-containing compounds or dyes that color urine red or that turn red in an acidic medium
- In vitro conversion of nitrate to nitrite as a result of bacterial contamination of the specimen; prevented by testing fresh urine specimens

### False-Negative or Delayed Results

- Insufficient time in the bladder for the conversion of nitrate to nitrite—even with significant bacterial infection
- Insufficient dietary nitrate present for bacteria to reduce nitrate to nitrite, such as with starvation, fasting, or intravenous feeding
- Presence of bacteria that further reduce nitrite to nitrogen
- Sensitivity may be reduced in concentrated urine with low pH (less than 6). This is not typically seen with bacterial infection.
- Ascorbic acid in concentration of 25 mg/dL or greater in specimens with small amounts of nitrite, due to the reduction of the diazonium salt by ascorbic acid

## Additional Comments

The test is primarily useful if positive. If the nitrite test area shows a negative reaction, urinary infection cannot be ruled out. Organisms must contain the reductase enzyme necessary to reduce nitrate to nitrite. This is true of most of the gram-negative enteric pathogens that cause urinary tract infections. The gram-positive enterococci and yeast, however, do not. The urine must be retained in the bladder for 4 hours or more for adequate conversion of nitrate to detectable nitrite. Obtaining such specimens may be difficult because urgency and frequent urination are common in urinary tract infections.

Thus, lack of sufficient incubation time is a major obstacle to positive reagent strip results with significant infection.

### Confirmatory Tests

Microscopic examination of the urine sediment, Gram stain, and quantitative urine culture.

## LEUKOCYTE ESTERASE

### Clinical Importance

Chemical tests for leukocyte esterase have been included on the urine reagent strip tests as another means of detecting urinary tract infection. These tests are based on the measurement of leukocyte esterase, which is present in azurophilic or primary granules of granulocytic leukocytes. These granulocytes include polymorphonuclear neutrophils (PMNs or neutrophils), monocytes (histiocytes), eosinophils, and basophils. In practice, positive reactions occur with increased neutrophils. Conditions associated with sufficient quantities of other granulocytes to give positive reactions are extremely rare, if they ever occur. Lymphocytes and the various epithelial cells that make up the kidney and urinary tract do not contain leukocyte esterase and are not measured in this test.

The detection of leukocyte esterase as an indicator of infection is useful, since neutrophils are generally increased in response to bacterial infection. When bacteria infect the urinary tract, at any point from the urethra to the kidney, the presence of increased numbers of white cells, particularly neutrophils, is typical. Neutrophils are also seen in the urinary sediment. However, a frequent problem is the rapid lysis of neutrophils in urine, a result of their phagocytic activity. Once lysed, they are not detectable in the microscopic analysis of the sediment. However, the test for leukocyte esterase depends on its release from the azurophilic or primary granules of granulocytes. Thus the leukocyte esterase test is positive whether lysed or intact cells are present in the urine.

Urine normally contains a few (up to 5) white cells per high-power field in the microscopic analysis of the urinary sediment. This normal occurrence of white cells is not sufficient to cause a positive reaction with the leukocyte esterase test. The reaction requires 5 to 15 leukocytes per high-power field to give a positive reaction. Therefore, the absence of leukocyte esterase does not rule out a urinary tract infection. However, the presence of leukocyte esterase is helpful, especially when combined with an elevated (alkaline) urine pH and the chemical detection of nitrite in the urine together with the presence of bacteria and white cells in the urine sediment.

Increased leukocyte esterase may be seen in conditions in which bacteria are not seen in the urine sediment or cultured. These include inflammatory conditions that may occur without bacterial infection, bacterial infection after treatment with antibiotics, and infections by organisms such as trichomonads and chlamydia, which are not seen on standard culture media.

Negative or low results for leukocyte esterase may be seen in the urine of immunosuppressed patients who have significant bacterial infection, because of the inability to produce adequate granulocytes.

### Principle

Reagent strip tests for leukocyte esterase utilize a diazo reaction, much like the reagent strip tests for nitrite. In this case, the test area contains an ester that is hydrolyzed by leukocyte esterase to form its alcohol (which contains an aromatic ring) and acid. The aromatic ring is then coupled with a diazonium salt, present in the test area, to form an azo dye, which is seen as the formation of a purple color. Chemstrips use an indoxyl ester, and Multistix use a pyrrole amino acid ester.

### Specificity

The reaction is specific for esterase that is present in granulocytic leukocytes—primarily neutrophils in urine.

## Sensitivity (Minimum Detectable Level): Manufacturer's Values

| | |
|---|---|
| Multistix | 5 to 15 cells per high-power field in clinical urine |
| Chemstrip | 10 to 25 cells/µL |

## Interferences

The presence of substances that color urine, such as azo-containing compounds, nitrofurantoin, riboflavin, or bilirubin, may make color interpretation difficult.

### False-Positive Results

- Strong oxidizing agents like chlorine bleach and urinary preservatives such as formalin (formaldehyde). Preservatives should not be used.

### False-Negative or Reduced Results

- Drugs (antibiotics) such as cephalexin, cephalothin, tetracycline, and gentamicin
- Elevated glucose (over 3 g/dL)
- High specific gravity
- Oxalic acid—a metabolite of ascorbic acid
- High levels of albumin (over 500 mg/dL)

## Additional Comments

The presence of repeated trace and positive values are clinically significant and indicate the need for further testing to determine the cause of the presence of neutrophils (granulocytes) in the urine (pyuria). They may include microscopic analysis of the urinary sediment, Gram stain, and quantitative urine culture. The test is not affected by the presence of blood, bacteria, or epithelial cells. Results are especially useful when combined with reagent strip tests for nitrite.

## GLUCOSE (SUGAR)

### Clinical Importance

Chemical screening tests for glucose (**dextrose**) are generally included in every routine urinalysis. Unlike the parameters covered up to this point, they are used to diagnose and monitor a metabolic, rather than a renal or urinary tract, condition. The occurrence of glucose in the urine indicates that the metabolic disorder diabetes mellitus should be suspected, although several other conditions result in glucosuria.

Any condition in which glucose is found in the urine is termed **glycosuria (or glucosuria).** Tests for glucosuria were among the earliest laboratory tests. The "taste test" was used by the Babylonians and the Egyptians to detect diabetes by tasting for the presence of sugar (sweet) in what would normally be a salty solution, while Hindu physicians noticed that "honey urine" attracted ants.

The occurrence of measurable glucose in the urine is not normal. The blood glucose concentration normally varies between 60 and 110 mg/dL, depending on the method of analysis. After a meal it may increase to 120 to 160 mg/dL. Normally all the glucose in the blood is filtered by the glomerulus and reabsorbed into the blood. However, if the blood glucose concentration becomes too high (usually greater than 180 to 200 mg/dL), the excess glucose will not be reabsorbed into the blood and will be eliminated from the body in the urine. Other factors that might result in glucosuria are reduced glomerular blood flow, reduced tubular reabsorption, and reduced urine flow.

The lowest blood glucose concentration that will result in glycosuria is termed the renal threshold, and it varies somewhat from person to person. The most common condition in which the renal threshold for glucose is exceeded is diabetes mellitus. In simplified terms, diabetes mellitus is a deficiency in the production of, or an inhibition in the action of, the hormone insulin. Insulin has the effect of lowering the blood glucose concentration. As a result of the deficiency of insulin, the blood glucose concentration exceeds the renal threshold, and glucose is spilled over into the urine.

Tests for urine glucose have been used by diabetic patients to self-monitor the adequacy of insulin control. Although these urine tests have been replaced by home blood glucose testing for unstable diabetic patients, urine glucose testing is less expensive, is noninvasive, and remains useful for patients who do not have to make frequent insulin dose adjustments. Tests for diabetes mellitus include tests for blood glucose in addition to tests for urinary glucose. Additional tests, such as those for glycated hemoglobin, may also be used to monitor diabetes mellitus.

Although diabetes mellitus is suspected in cases of glycosuria, the occurrence of glycosuria is not diagnostic of the condition, since there are many other causes. For example, glycosuria may be observed after large amounts of sugar or foods containing sugar are eaten, in cases of acute emotional strain in which glucose is liberated by the liver for energy, and after exercise. It may also be associated with pregnancy, certain types of meningitis, hypothyroidism, certain tumors of the adrenal medulla, and some brain injuries.

In addition, certain abnormal conditions are characterized by the presence in the urine of sugars other than glucose. These are generally **reducing sugars,** which require detection by methods other than those employed in the reagent strip tests that are specific for glucose. **Galactosuria** is the presence of the sugar galactose in the urine. It results from a metabolic error whereby the enzyme galactose-1-phosphate uridyltransferase is lacking so that galactose is not metabolized, resulting in increased galactose in the blood (galactosemia) and urine. This condition results in permanent physical and mental deterioration, which may be controlled by early detection and dietary restriction of galactose. Therefore, urine from young pediatric patients should be screened with a nonspecific copper reduction test for reducing substances that will detect galactose and other reducing sugars in addition to glucose. State-required newborn metabolic screening tests for inherited disease often include a test for galactosemia.

Other reducing sugars, such as lactose, may be seen in the urine late in pregnancy or early lactation. Lactose intolerance in infancy and failure to gain weight may occur because of intestinal lactase deficiency, and lactosuria may be seen.

## Reagent Strip (Glucose Oxidase) Tests
### Principle and Specificity

The reagent strip tests for urinary sugar are specific for glucose because they are based on the use of the enzyme **glucose oxidase.** An enzyme may be described as a biological catalyst, a substance that must be present before a chemical reaction will occur. Glucose oxidase, like most enzymes, is absolutely specific. It will react only in the presence of glucose, and it will not react with any other substance.

Reagent strip tests for urine glucose are double sequential enzyme reactions. Glucose oxidase will oxidize glucose to gluconic acid and at the same time reduce atmospheric oxygen to hydrogen peroxide. The hydrogen peroxide formed will, in the presence of the enzyme peroxidase, oxidize the reduced form of a dye to the oxidized form, which is indicated by the color change of an oxidation-reduction indicator. This reaction is diagrammed below:

*Step 1:*

$$\underset{\text{(in urine)}}{\text{Glucose}} + \underset{\text{(from air)}}{O_2} \xrightarrow{\underset{\text{oxidase}}{\text{Glucose}}} \underset{\text{acid}}{\text{Gluconic}} + H_2O_2$$

*Step 2:*

$$H_2O_2 + \underset{\text{of dye}}{\text{Reduced form}} \xrightarrow{\text{Peroxidase}} \underset{\text{of dye}}{\text{Oxidized form}} + H_2O$$

The glucose oxidase, the peroxidase, and the reduced form of the oxidation-reduction indicator are all impregnated onto a dry reagent strip. Reagent strips differ in the chromogen used as the oxidation-reduction indicator. They all contain glucose oxidase and peroxidase.

It must be remembered that nonglucose reducing substances (NGRS) will not be detected by tests that are specific for glucose; therefore, specimens from infants and young pediatric patients and specimens in which NGRS are suspected should be subjected to nonspecific (usually copper reduction) tests for reducing substances in addition to the specific tests for glucose.

### Sensitivity (Minimum Detectable Level): Manufacturer's Values

| | |
|---|---|
| Multistix/Diastix | 75-125 mg/dL glucose (as low as 40 mg/dL in dilute urine containing less than 5 mg/dL ascorbic acid) |
| Chemstrip | 40 mg/dL in 90% of urines tested |

### Interferences

Since reagent strip tests are all specific for glucose, most interferences lead to reduced or false-negative results.

#### False-Positive Results

- Contamination by bleach or other strong oxidizing agents may oxidize the reduced form of the dye present on the reagent strip, causing a color change in the absence of glucose. This shows the importance of utilizing contamination-free urine containers and work surfaces.
- Trace values may be seen in very dilute urine specimens, because of increased sensitivity at low specific gravity.
- Reagent strips exposed to air by improper storage have been shown to give false positive results.[1]

#### False-Negative or Delayed Results

- Large urinary concentrations of ascorbic acid, from therapeutic doses of vitamin C or from drugs, such as tetracyclines, in which ascorbic acid is used as a reducing agent. Ascorbic acid blocks or delays the reaction by acting as a reducing agent reacting with the released hydrogen peroxide (rather than the chromogen in the reagent strip). Multistix products are inhibited by ascorbic acid concentrations of 50 mg/dL (500 mg/L) or greater in specimens containing small amounts (75 to 125 mg/dL) of glucose. Chemstrip is unaffected by ascorbic acid concentration less than 100 mg/dL (1000 mg/L). With questionable ascorbic acid interference, repeat tests on urine voided at least 10 hours after the last administration of vitamin C, or test for ascorbic acid.
- Ketone bodies at moderate levels (40 mg/dL or more) in specimens containing small amounts (75 to 125 mg/dL) of glucose. This combination of high ketone and low glucose is unlikely in a diabetic patient.
- Sodium fluoride is an enzyme inhibitor. Do not use as a preservative.
- Refrigerated specimens, because of decreased enzyme activity. Urine must be at room temperature when tested.

### Confirmatory and Follow-Up Tests

If semiquantitation beyond the color blocks on usual multiple-reagent strips is desired, urine may be tested with a test such as Chemstrip uG or uGK, or with the 2-drop Clinitest Tablet Test, which allows for semiquantitation to 5000 mg/dL (5 g/dL). The presence of ketones with glucose implies inadequate control of diabetes.

### Clinitest Copper Reduction Test for Reducing Sugars
#### Principle

The Clinitest Tablet Test (Bayer Diagnostics) is a nonspecific test for urinary sugar, which utilizes the ability of glucose (or any reducing substance) to reduce copper II (cupric) ions to copper I (cuprous) ions, in the presence of heat and alkali. A positive reaction is semiquantitated as a change in color ranging from blue to green, yellow, and orange, depending on the amount of sugar present. The reaction is:

$$2CuSO_4 + \text{Reducing substance} \xrightarrow[\text{heat}]{\text{alkali}}$$

(copper II)      (glucose et al)

$$Cu_2O + \text{Oxidized form of reducing substance}$$

(copper I)      (gluconic acid)

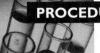

## PROCEDURE 14-4

### Clinitest Tablet Test for Reducing Sugars

**Five-Drop Method**

Follow the directions supplied with the Clinitest tablets.

1. Place five drops of urine in a $15 \times 85$ mm test tube and add ten drops of water.

2. Add one Clinitest tablet.

3. Watch while boiling takes place, but do not shake.

4. Wait 15 seconds after boiling stops, then shake the tube gently, and compare the color of the solution with the color scale supplied for the five-drop method.

5. Report results with the same units as used for reagent strip glucose results (mg/dL or g/dL).

6. Watch the solution carefully while it is boiling. If it passes through orange to a dark shade of greenish brown, the sugar concentration is more than 2.0 g/dL and the result should be recorded as greater than 2.0 g/dL without reference to the color scale. Urines showing this pass-through phenomenon should be retested with the two-drop method.

**Two-Drop Method**

Follow the directions supplied with the Clinitest tablets.

1. Place two drops of urine in a $15 \times 85$ mm test tube and add ten drops of water.

2. Add one Clinitest tablet.

3. Watch while boiling takes place, but do not shake.

4. Wait 15 seconds after boiling stops, then shake the tube gently, and compare the color of the solution with the color scale supplied for the two-drop method.

5. Watch the test throughout the entire reaction and waiting period, as the pass-through phenomenon may also occur with the two-drop test.

6. Report the results with the same units as used for other glucose methods.

The reaction is essentially **Benedict's qualitative test** for urine sugar in a solid form. The tablet combines copper sulfate, anhydrous sodium hydroxide, citric acid, and sodium carbonate in an effervescent tablet. The interaction of sodium hydroxide with citric acid and water results in moderate boiling, making an external boiling water bath unnecessary.

Results are semiquantitated at 15 seconds after boiling stops by comparison with a permanent color chart supplied with the tablets. Results must be read at this time, since the reaction continues and will result in falsely high values if observed at a later time.

Clinitest tests may be performed as either a five-drop or a two-drop method (see Procedure 14-4). The two-drop method was developed in response to a "pass-through" phenomenon, which may occur if more than 2 g/dL of sugar is present in the urine. Such concentrations of urinary glucose are possible in patients with diabetes mellitus. In the pass-through phenomenon, after the addition of the Clinitest tablet, the solution goes through the entire range of colors and back to a dark greenish brown because of caramelization of the large amount of sugar in the urine by heat. The final color does not compare with any section of the color chart; however, it corresponds most closely to a color indicating a significantly lower result. Thus it is extremely important to observe the entire Clinitest reaction, from the addition of the tablet to the end point. A pass-through reaction is indicated by a bright orange color before caramelization occurs.

### Specificity

Copper reduction tests such as Clinitest are nonspecific tests for reducing substances (sugars). The glucose is acting as a reducing agent, and any compound with a free aldehyde or ketone group will give the same reaction. Glucose is not the only reducing substance that may be found in urine. Nonglucose reducing substances (NGRS) include uric acid, creatinine, galactose, fructose, lactose, pentose, homogentisic acid, ascorbic acid, chloroform, and formaldehyde. Clinitest will give the same reaction with any reducing substance that may be present in the urine, either naturally or as a contaminant.

### Sensitivity

Clinitest reagent tablets will detect as little as 250 mg/dL sugar (0.25 g/dL). This is less sensitive than the reagent strip tests for glucose. Thus it is possible to see a positive reagent strip reaction for glucose with a negative Clinitest if only a small amount of glucose is present in the urine.

### Interferences

Clinitest tablets must be kept tightly closed at all times to prevent absorption of moisture and must be kept in a cool, dry place, away from direct heat and sunlight. The tablets normally have a spotted bluish white color. If not stored properly, they absorb moisture or deteriorate from heat, turning dark blue or blackish. In this condition they will not give reliable results. They are also available individually packaged in aluminum foil to help prevent absorption of moisture. Although they are more expensive in this form, it is useful when a limited number of tests are performed.

### False-Positive Results

- Since it is a reducing substance, the presence of **extremely** large amounts of ascorbic acid (over 200 mg/dL = 2000 mg/L) may cause low-level positive results—trace or 1+.
- Specimens that have a low specific gravity and contain glucose may give a slightly elevated result with Clinitest.
- Large quantities of nalidixic acid, cephalosporins, and probenecid.
- Radiographic contrast media may result in an unusual (black) color that might be interpreted as a positive result.

### False-Negative or Reduced Results

- Mixing the test tube before the 15-second wait after boiling stops; due to reoxidation of the cuprous ions to cupric ions by atmospheric oxygen.

### Additional Comments

The bottom of the test tube becomes very hot during the Clinitest reaction. Hold the test tube at the lip (not bottom) or place it in a test tube rack, to avoid burns.

Clinitest tablets will react with sufficient quantities of any reducing substance in the urine, including other reducing sugars such as lactose, fructose, galactose, maltose, and pentoses. Use reagent strips that are specific for glucose to confirm the presence or absence of glucose.

### Additional Tests

In cases when the presence of a reducing sugar other than glucose—such as galactose—is suspected in the urine, a nonspecific test such as Clinitest should be performed. Although specific reagent strip tests for glucose are commonly used as screening tests for the presence of glucose, all specimens obtained from young pediatric patients (less than 2 years of age) should be tested by a nonspecific method as well.

If a negative reagent strip test for glucose is obtained from a urine with a positive Clinitest, and the presence of another reducing sugar is suspected, it must eventually be identified. This is usually done by thin-layer chromatography (TLC). Note that common table sugar is sucrose. This is not a reducing sugar and will not react with copper reduction or glucose oxidase tests.

# KETONE BODIES

## Clinical Importance

Ketone bodies are a group of three related substances: acetone, acetoacetic (or diacetic) acid, and β-hydroxybutyric acid. Their structural similarity is illustrated in Fig. 14-7. They are normal products of fat metabolism and are not normally detectable in the blood or urine.

In fat **catabolism** (the phase of metabolism in which fats are broken down for energy), acetoacetic acid is produced first. It is converted either reversibly to β-hydroxybutyric acid or irreversibly to acetone. All three types of ketone

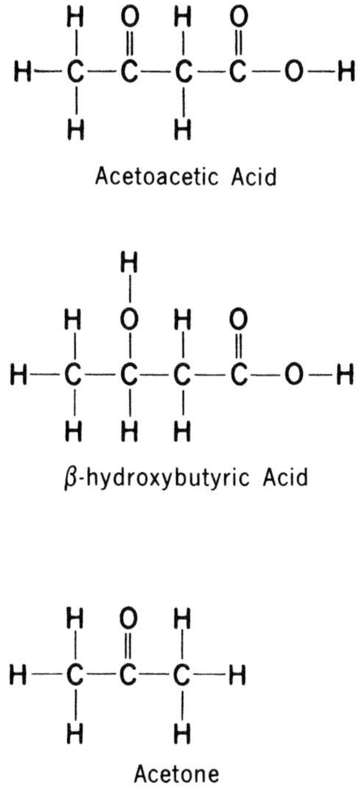

bodies are utilized as a source of energy and are eventually converted to carbon dioxide and water. When normal amounts of fat are utilized by the body, the tissues are able to use the entire ketone production as an energy source. However, if more fat than normal is metabolized, the body is unable to utilize all the ketone bodies. The clinical result is an increased concentration of ketones in the blood **(ketonemia)** and in the urine **(ketonuria). Ketosis** is the combination of increased ketones in both the blood and the urine.

Whenever fat (rather than carbohydrate) is used as the major source of energy, ketosis and ketonuria may result. The two outstanding causes of ketone accumulation are diabetes mellitus and starvation. In diabetes mellitus, the body is unable to use carbohydrate as an energy source and attempts to compensate by resorting to fat catabolism, which results in accumulation of the ketones. In starvation, the body is depleted of stored carbohydrate and must resort to fat as an energy source. In like manner, ketosis is seen in cases of dehydration, and conditions associated with fever, vomiting, and diarrhea. The same situation may occur in cases of severe liver damage. Most carbohydrate is stored as liver glycogen. In liver damage, there is no stored glycogen; hence the body must again resort to fat for energy. Finally, a **ketogenic diet** will result in ketone accumulation. A ketogenic diet is one that is high in fat and low in carbohydrates—specifically a diet containing more than 1.5 g of fat per 1.0 g of carbohydrate. Low-carbohydrate diets used for weight reduction may be ketogenic diets.

Since the presence of ketone bodies in urine is an early indication of lack of adequate insulin control, reagent strips that combine tests for glucose and ketones are often used by diabetics for home monitoring of their disease. The physiologic effect of ketone accumulation in the blood and urine (ketosis) is serious. Acetoacetic acid and β-hydroxybutyric acid contribute excess hydrogen ions to the blood, resulting in acidosis. Acidosis is an extremely serious condition and

**FIG 14-7.** The ketone bodies.

results in death if allowed to continue. Therefore, the body attempts to compensate for excess acid in the blood by eliminating acid through the urine. The kidney is capable of producing urine with a pH as low as 4.5. Thus, the occurrence of ketones in the urine is associated with a low urinary pH. Before insulin was used in the treatment of diabetes mellitus, acidosis was the cause of death in two thirds of all cases. In the treatment of diabetes mellitus, it is important to control the amount of insulin so that ketosis and acidosis do not occur. A typical urine specimen from an uncontrolled diabetic is pale and greenish, contains a large amount of sugar, has a high specific gravity by refractometer, has a low pH, and contains ketone bodies.

When ketones accumulate in the blood and urine, they do not occur in equal concentrations. Of the ketones, 78% are present as $\beta$-hydroxybutyric acid, 20% as acetoacetic acid, and only 2% as acetone. However, the reagent strip tests for ketones are most sensitive to the presence of acetoacetic acid. There are no simple laboratory tests for $\beta$-hydroxybutyric acid.

## Principle

The reagent strip tests for ketone bodies are based on Legal's (Rothera's) test, a color reaction with sodium nitroprusside (nitroferricyanide). Acetoacetic acid will react with sodium nitroprusside in an alkaline medium to form a purple color. If glycine is added, the test is slightly sensitive to acetone. Multistix and Ketostix have been formulated to react only with acetoacetic acid. They do not react with acetone. The Chemstrip products include glycine and detect both acetoacetic acid and larger amounts of acetone. None of the reagent strips detect $\beta$-hydroxybutyric acid.

## Acetest Tablet Test

The Acetest Tablet Test* is a tablet test for acetone and acetoacetic acid based on a color reaction with sodium nitroprusside. The principle is

---

*Bayer Diagnostics, Tarrytown, NY.

virtually identical to that of the reagent strip tests. In addition to urine, Acetest Tablets can be used to test whole blood, plasma, or serum. This test may be useful in testing urines containing interfering colors.

### Specificity and Sensitivity (Minimum Detectable Level): Manufacturer's Values

| Test | Specificity | Sensitivity |
| --- | --- | --- |
| Multistix/Ketostix | Acetoacetic acid | 5-10 mg/dL |
| Chemstrip | Acetoacetic acid | 9 mg/dL |
| | Acetone | 70 mg/dL |
| Acetest | Acetoacetic acid | 5-10 mg/dL |
| | Acetone | 20-25 mg/dL |

### Interferences

The presence of various pigments, drugs, or substances causing abnormal highly colored urine specimens presents problems in the reading of ketone results. False-positive reactions may occur as a result of the formation of a color that may be interpreted as positive, or true positive reactions may be masked in these urine specimens.

#### False-Positive Results

- Specimens containing phthaleins (Bromsulphalein, phenolsulfonphthalein), very large amounts of phenylketones, or the preservative 8-hydroxyquinoline
- Highly concentrated urine specimens (high specific gravity) or specimens containing large amounts of levodopa metabolites may give weak positive reactions
- 2-Mercaptoethanesulfonic acid (Mesna) or other compounds containing sulfhydryl groups. A positive reaction is seen initially, but the color fades to normal by the time specified for reading the color reaction. This interference is especially problematic when automatic reagent strip readers are employed, because these instruments are programmed to read the various chemical reactions in a shorter time frame than is done with visual readings. If such interference is suspected, reagent strips should be

checked visually, and the visual result reported. If the color persists and interference is still suspected, a drop of glacial acetic acid may be added to the test area on the reagent strip or the Acetest tablet. If the color is due to a sulfhydryl group, it will fade, whereas color due to diacetic acid will remain.

### False-Negative or Reduced Results

- Conversion of acetoacetic acid to acetone, with subsequent evaporation from the specimen, in improperly stored specimens. Urine specimens must be tested when freshly voided or immediately refrigerated.

### Additional Comments

When a patient is monitored with repeated determinations of acetone and acetoacetic acid in plasma or urine, the concentrations of these compounds may start at very high levels and fall, but still give results that correspond to "large" on the color chart. Repeated reports of "large" do not reflect the changes as they occur. In some instances it is desirable to dilute subsequent specimens to monitor and observe a decrease in ketone excretion. The urine specimen is diluted 1:2, 1:4, and so on, until a "large" value is no longer seen. The report in such cases should state at what dilution a "large" value is no longer obtained (e.g., large, 1:4 dilution moderate).

## BILIRUBIN AND UROBILINOGEN

As mentioned earlier, the routine urinalysis is used to provide information concerning the state of the kidney and urinary tract, or other metabolic or systemic disorders. Tests for urine bilirubin and urobilinogen are used as indicators of the latter, in particular as indicators of liver function. In order to better understand this, the following information on normal liver function and the formation and excretion of bilirubin and urobilinogen is included.

### Normal Liver Function

The liver is a large and complex organ, absolutely necessary for numerous body functions. The liver is responsible for many metabolic, storage, excretory, and detoxifying functions. More specifically, the liver is a major factor in the metabolism of carbohydrates, lipids, and proteins, in terms of both intermediary metabolism and the synthesis of many essential compounds. Many necessary enzymes and coenzymes for carbohydrate, lipid, and protein metabolism are present only in cells of the liver. Glycogen is formed, stored, and converted back to glucose in the liver. Energy derived from food is made available to the cells of the body through the process of glycolysis of the high-energy bonds in adenosine triphosphate (ATP), which were formed by oxidative phosphorylation in the cells of the liver. The liver is the site of detoxification of various substances. These toxic substances may be formed in normal body metabolism and converted or detoxified by the liver; an example is the formation of urea from the ammonia produced in protein metabolism. Toxic substances introduced into the blood from the intestine (such as dyes, heavy metals, and drugs) are excreted by the liver. The liver is essential in the formation and secretion of bile, bile pigments, and bile salts, which are necessary for digestion. These substances are derived from bilirubin, a major by-product of the destruction of red blood cells. In addition, the liver is the site of formation and synthesis of many of the factors involved in the clotting of blood.

These important functions of the liver may be altered when the liver is diseased or damaged. Numerous laboratory tests are available to determine both the existence of liver disease and the extent, location, and type of damage so that appropriate treatment can be initiated. No one test will give a complete clinical view of liver function; instead, a carefully selected group of tests may be necessary, depending on the process in question. These include tests for the presence and concentration of bilirubin in the blood and the urine.

## Normal Formation and Excretion of Bilirubin and Urobilinogen

Bilirubin is a normal product resulting from the breakdown of red blood cells. Individual red blood cells do not exist indefinitely in the body; they are degraded after approximately 120 days. As part of red blood cell degradation, the heme portion of the hemoglobin molecule is converted to the bile pigment bilirubin by the reticuloendothelial system (RES), primarily by RES cells in the liver, spleen, and bone marrow. A total of approximately 6 g of hemoglobin is released each day as red blood cells are eliminated from the body. The cells of the RES first phagocytose the red cells, and then convert the released hemoglobin through a complex series of reactions in which the heme portion of the molecule is finally converted to bilirubin. Bilirubin is a vivid yellow pigment. An increase in the concentration of bilirubin in the blood indicates the presence of **jaundice.** Although it is useful in the bile, bilirubin is a waste product that must eventually be eliminated from the body. When it is formed by the RES cells, bilirubin is not soluble in water. Therefore it is transported from the RES cells through the blood to the liver cells linked to albumin as a bilirubin-albumin complex. This insoluble form of bilirubin is referred to as **free bilirubin** or **unconjugated bilirubin.**

Bilirubin is normally excreted from the body by the liver by way of the intestine. It is excreted by the liver rather than the kidney because the bilirubin-albumin complex cannot pass through the glomerular capsule of the kidney. When free bilirubin reaches the liver, it is made water soluble by conjugation with glucuronic acid and other hydrophilic substances to form **bilirubin glucuronide.**

The water-soluble bilirubin glucuronide, referred to as **conjugated bilirubin,** can be eliminated from the body by way of the kidney or the intestine. Normally, conjugated bilirubin is excreted by the liver into the bile, and transported to the common bile duct and then to the gallbladder, where it is concentrated and emptied into the small intestine.

In the intestine, bilirubin is converted to **urobilinogen** by the action of certain bacteria that make up the intestinal flora. Urobilinogen is actually a group of colorless chromogens, all of which are referred to as urobilinogen. Part of the urobilinogen formed in the intestine is absorbed into the portal blood circulation and returned to the liver, where it is re-excreted into the bile and returned to the intestine. A very small amount of urobilinogen escapes this liver clearance and is therefore excreted from the body by way of the urine. This represents only about 1% of the urobilinogen produced in 1 day.

Part of the urobilinogen in the intestine is converted to **stercobilinogen** (colorless), which is oxidized to the colored **stercobilin.** This is the substance that gives the feces their normal color. The net effect is that, in normal circumstances, 99% of the urobilinogen formed from bilirubin is eliminated by way of the feces.

It is therefore apparent that the urine normally contains only a very small amount of urobilinogen and no bilirubin. Unconjugated (albumin-bound) bilirubin cannot be excreted by the kidney and is absent in urine. However, conjugated bilirubin can pass through the renal glomerulus, and if it is present in abnormal concentration in the blood, it will be excreted by the kidney.

### Clinical Importance

Tests for urinary bilirubin and urobilinogen should be performed when indicated by abnormal color of the urine or when liver disease or a hemolytic condition is suspected from the patient's history. Because these tests are part of most multiple-reagent strips, they are included in the routine urinalysis. The presence of bilirubin in the urine is an early sign of liver cell disease (hepatocellular disease) and of obstruction to the bile flow from the liver. It is especially useful in the early detection and monitoring of hepatitis, a highly infectious disease of particular importance to laboratory workers. The presence of urobilinogen in the urine is increased in any condition that causes an increase in the production of bilirubin glucuronide and any disease that prevents the liver from performing its normal function of returning urobilinogen to the intestine via the bile. Information about urinary bilirubin and urobilinogen, in addition to serum bilirubin levels, is useful in determining the cause of jaundice. The clinical significance of these substances and laboratory tests for them follow. (See also Bilirubin Metabolism and Liver Function, in Chapter 11.)

## Bilirubin
### Clinical Significance

Tests for urinary bilirubin (along with urobilinogen) are important in the detection of liver disease and the determination of the cause of the clinical condition known as jaundice. Normally, there is no detectable bilirubin in the urine with even the most sensitive methods. However, finding even very small amounts of bilirubin in urine is important, as it may be present in the earliest phases of liver disease. **Jaundice** is a condition that occurs when the serum bilirubin concentration becomes greater than normal and there is an abnormal accumulation of bilirubin in the body tissues. Since bilirubin is a vivid yellow pigment, its accumulation in the tissues results in yellow pigmentation of the skin, the sclera or white of the eyes, and the mucous membranes. The causes of jaundice are numerous and must be discovered as soon as possible so that treatment may be started. There are several classifications of the various types of jaundice; one of them describes three types: hemolytic (prehepatic), hepatic (hepatocellular), and obstructive (posthepatic). Laboratory findings in various types of jaundice are summarized in Table 14-9.

**Hemolytic (Prehepatic) Jaundice.** Hemolytic jaundice occurs in conditions in which there is increased destruction of red cells, such as hemolytic anemias and hemolytic disease of the newborn. The liver is basically normal, so there is an increased formation of conjugated bilirubin and subsequently of urobilinogen.

## TABLE 14-9

Laboratory Findings in Various Types of Jaundice

| Type of Jaundice | Clinical Examples | Blood Bilirubin (Unconjugated) | Urine Bilirubin (Conjugated) | Urine Urobilinogen | Color Feces |
|---|---|---|---|---|---|
| Normal | | 0-1.3 mg/dL | Negative | $\leq 1$ mg/dL | Normal, brown |
| Hemolytic (prehepatic) | Hemolytic anemia, Hemolytic disease of newborn | Increased | Negative | Increased | Increased (dark brown) |
| Hepatic (hepato-cellular) | Neonatal physiologic Hepatitis (viral, toxic) Cirrhosis | Increased (varies) | Increased (varies) | Increased or absent | Normal or pale |
| Obstructive (posthepatic) | Gallstones Tumor | Normal | Increased | None (decreased) | Pale chalky-white ("acholic") |

Modified from Ringsrud KM, Linné JJ: *Urinalysis and Body Fluids: A ColorText and Atlas*, St Louis, Mosby, 1995, p 65.

Increased formation of urobilinogen from bilirubin results in increased levels of urobilinogen in the blood. The liver is overwhelmed by the increased production of bilirubin and urobilinogen and unable to excrete the urobilinogen back into the intestine. Therefore, more urobilinogen is eliminated in the urine. However, all the bilirubin that is conjugated by the liver goes into the intestine, where it is converted to urobilinogen, and no bilirubin is found in the urine.

**Hepatic (Hepatocellular) Jaundice. Hepatic jaundice** results from conditions that involve the liver cells directly and prevent normal excretion of bilirubin. It is probably the most varied and difficult to understand; findings differ, depending on the disease or condition and the stage of disease. These include:

1. Failure to conjugate bilirubin, with increased concentration of free (albumin-bound) bilirubin in blood
2. Failure to transport conjugated bilirubin into the bile canaliculi, with increased conjugated bilirubin backing up (regurgitating) into the blood and urine
3. Failure of the liver to re-excrete the recirculated urobilinogen, with increased concentration of urobilinogen in the blood and the urine

**Neonatal physiologic jaundice** results when there is an enzyme deficiency in the immature liver, and thus failure to conjugate bilirubin, resulting in increased unconjugated (free) bilirubin in the blood with no bilirubin in the urine.

Disturbances of the transport mechanisms by which conjugated bilirubin is passed into the bile canaliculi are characteristic of **hepatocellular jaundice.** In conditions such as viral hepatitis, toxic hepatitis (caused by heavy metal or drug poisoning), and cirrhosis, there is a diffuse overall hepatic cell involvement. In these cases the bilirubin that is conjugated by the liver is not excreted into the bile; instead conjugated bilirubin backs up into the blood, and can now be

eliminated by the kidney. Of the conjugated bilirubin that reaches the gut, urobilinogen is formed, part of which is absorbed into the portal circulation and returned to the liver for excretion. However, the diseased liver cells may be unable to remove the urobilinogen from the blood, resulting in excretion of urobilinogen into the urine. As the disease progresses to later stages, the liver is unable to form and pass conjugated bilirubin into the bile, so that conjugated bilirubin regurgitates (backs up) into the blood and is eliminated from the body by way of the urine. Such cases would have little or no urobilinogen in the urine.

**Obstructive (Posthepatic) Jaundice. Posthepatic jaundice** is also known as **obstructive jaundice.** This occurs when the common bile duct is obstructed by stones, tumors, spasms, or stricture. As a result, the conjugated bilirubin is regurgitated back into the liver sinusoids and the blood. If the blockage is sufficiently extensive, liver cell function may be impaired so that both free and conjugated bilirubin are found in the blood. The conjugated bilirubin will be excreted by the kidney and therefore found in the urine. Since conjugated bilirubin is unable to reach the intestine, no urobilinogen is formed and it is absent in the blood and urine. Since urobilinogen is not formed, urobilin is absent and the stools have a characteristic chalky white to light brown color, also referred to as **acholic.**

### Reagent Strip Tests for Bilirubin

**Principle.** The reagent strip tests for bilirubin are based on a diazo reaction. Bilirubin is coupled with a diazonium salt in an acid medium to form azobilirubin. A positive reaction is seen as the formation of a colored compound. Tests differ in the diazonium salt used, and thus the color produced.

**Specificity.** Tests are specific for bilirubin. However, the presence of other highly colored pigments in the urine causes problems in interpreting results. This is especially true when metabolites of drugs such as phenazopyridine are present, which give the gross urine specimen a characteristic vivid red-orange color that might be mistaken for bilirubin and mask or give atypical color reactions on the reagent strip.

### Sensitivity (Minimum Detectable Level): Manufacturer's Values

| | |
|---|---|
| Multistix | 0.4-0.8 mg/dL |
| Chemstrip | 0.5 mg/dL in 90% of urines tested |
| Ictotest (Bayer) | 0.05-0.1 mg/dL |

**Interferences.** The reagent strip tests for bilirubin are difficult to read, and the color formed after reaction with urine must be carefully compared with the color chart supplied by the manufacturer. Proficiency in reading these results comes with experience and is essential for reliable results.

Atypical colors, which are unlike any of the color blocks, may indicate that other bile pigments derived from bilirubin are present in the urine and may be masking the bilirubin reaction. Testing the urine with a more sensitive test such as the Ictotest Tablet Test may be indicated. Large amounts of urobilinogen may affect the color reaction but not enough to give a positive result.

#### False-Positive or Atypical Results

- Substances that color the urine red or that turn red in an acid medium, such as phenothiazine, chlorpromazine, and metabolites of phenazopyridine (Pyridium) or ethoxazene (Serenium)
- Metabolites of etodolac (Lodine)
- A yellow-orange to red color with indican (indoxyl sulfate). Indoles are formed from bacterial overgrowth in the gut or in surgically constructed urinary bladders made from intestine.

#### False-Negative or Decreased Results

- Oxidation of bilirubin to biliverdin, especially when exposed to ultraviolet light
- In vitro hydrolyzation of bilirubin diglucuronide to free bilirubin. Tests are most sensitive to the conjugated form of bilirubin.

- Ascorbic acid in concentration of 25 mg/dL or more
- Elevated nitrite concentration, as seen in urinary tract infection, may decrease sensitivity.

**Additional Comments.** The presence of highly pigmented compounds may be mistaken for bilirubin in the gross urine specimen, and may mask the reaction of small amounts of bilirubin.

Urine specimens must be tested when absolutely fresh or bilirubin will oxidize to biliverdin. The test is specific for bilirubin—it will not react with biliverdin.

**Confirmatory and Related Tests.** The reagent strip tests for bilirubin are significantly less sensitive for bilirubin than the Ictotest Tablet Test. Because any detectable bilirubin in urine, even at a trace level, is a clinically significant finding, it may be necessary to test all urine specimens suspected of containing bilirubin (because of color, presence of a yellow foam when shaken, or clinical history) with a more sensitive method such as Ictotest. Since reagent strip colors are difficult to interpret and subject to masked or false-positive reaction, it has been recommended that all positive reactions be confirmed with another method, such as the Ictotest Tablet Test.

The presence of bilirubin and the presence of urobilinogen in urine are related, and the presence or absence of both constituents is useful in determining the cause of clinical jaundice. However, specific serum tests for liver function, such as serum bilirubin, aspartate transaminase (AST), alkaline phosphatase, and γ-glutamyl transpeptidase, are more useful than urine tests for bilirubin and urobilinogen.

#### Ictotest Tablet Test for Bilirubin

**Principle.** The Ictotest Tablet Test* is based on a diazo reaction, in which bilirubin is coupled

---

*Bayer Corp, Diagnostics Division, Tarrytown, NY.

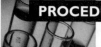

## PROCEDURE 14-5

### Ictotest Tablet Test for Bilirubin

Observe the precautions and follow the instructions supplied by the manufacturer.

1. Place 10 drops of urine on the center of either side of the special test mat supplied with the reagent tablets.

2. Place the Ictotest tablet in the center of the urine-moistened area. Do not touch the tablet with your hands.

3. Place 1 drop of water onto the tablet. Wait 5 seconds; then place a second drop of water onto the tablet so that the water runs off the tablet onto the mat.

4. Remove the tablet, and observe the mat for the appearance of a blue to purple color at 60 seconds.

5. Report the result as positive or negative according to the following criteria:

*Negative:* The mat shows no blue or purple within 60 seconds. Ignore any color that forms after 60 seconds, or a slight pink or red that may appear.

*Positive:* The mat around or under the tablet turns blue or purple within 60 seconds. Ignore any color change on the tablet itself.

with a diazonium salt in an acid medium. This is the same principle that is used in the reagent strip tests.

The tablets are supplied with a special absorbent mat. Urine is placed on the mat, the liquid portion is absorbed, and the bilirubin remains on the outer surface of the mat. The tablet contains the reactive ingredients. The tablet is placed over the urine on the mat, and water is added to the tablet. When bilirubin is present, it reacts with a solid diazonium salt present in the tablet to form azobilirubin. A positive reaction is seen as a blue or purple color on the mat. Other ingredients in the tablet provide the proper pH and ensure solution of the tablet when water is added, so that the reaction can take place. (See Procedure 14-5.)

**Specificity.** The test is specific for conjugated bilirubin. The absorbent mat concentrates bilirubin on the surface and minimizes interfering pigments.

**Sensitivity.** Ictotest will detect as little as 0.05 to 0.1 mg/dL bilirubin. This is more sensitive than any reagent strip test for bilirubin. For this reason, it is desirable to test any urine specimen suspected of containing bilirubin with Ictotest, even if the reagent strip test is negative.

**Interferences.** Interferences are generally the same as for the reagent strip tests for bilirubin. Suppression of results by large amounts of ascorbic acid and interferences by vivid pigments are especially troublesome.

**Additional Comments.** In order to minimize interferences and increase sensitivity (by concentration of bilirubin), the special absorbent mat provided must be used. Either side may be used. In order for the diazo reaction to occur, the reagent tablet must begin to dissolve, and water flow from the tablet onto the mat. When results are being read, it is desirable to move the tablet, as the color reaction is observed around and under the tablet. The reaction must be read at the time stated (60 seconds), since a confusing pink color may appear after this time.

Proper storage of tablets is essential. Tablets must be protected from exposure to light, heat, and ambient moisture. Deterioration is seen as a tan to brown discoloration of the tablet.

## Urobilinogen and Porphobilinogen
### Clinical Importance of Urobilinogen

Urobilinogens are normal by-products of red blood cell degradation; they are formed from bilirubin by bacterial action in the intestine and are excreted in the feces as stercobilin. Urobilinogens are closely related tetrapyrrols; they are colorless, labile, and oxidized to colored urobilins. Increased destruction of red cells may be accompanied by large amounts of urobilinogen in the urine. Therefore, urobilinogen will be seen in conditions such as various hemolytic anemias, pernicious anemia, and malaria. In the absence of increased red cell destruction, the tests may be considered liver function tests. One of the first effects of liver damage is impairment of the mechanism for removing urobilinogen from the blood circulation and re-excreting it through the intestine. This results in removal of urobilinogen by the kidney and its presence in the urine. Tests for urinary urobilinogen are thus useful for the early detection of liver damage. Urobilinogen is found in the urine in conditions such as infectious hepatitis, toxic hepatitis, portal cirrhosis, congestive heart failure, and infectious mononucleosis.

Normally, 1% of all the urobilinogen produced is excreted in the urine and 99% is excreted in the feces. However, under certain conditions urobilinogen is completely absent from the urine and the feces. When the normal intestinal bacterial flora is destroyed, as by antibiotic therapy, urobilinogen cannot be produced. Urobilinogen is also absent if the liver does not conjugate bilirubin, or if there is biliary tract obstruction, such as from gallstones, resulting in failure of conjugated bilirubin to reach the intestinal tract.

### Clinical Importance of Porphobilinogen

Another substance that is related to urobilinogen is porphobilinogen. **Porphobilinogen** is a normal, colorless, precursor of the porphyrins. The porphyrins are a group of compounds that are utilized in the synthesis of hemoglobin. The heme portion of hemoglobin is a type of porphyrin, namely ferroprotoporphyrin 9. In normal persons, porphyrins are eliminated from the body in the urine and feces, mainly as coproporphyrin I with a small amount of coproporphyrin III. However, certain errors of porphyrin metabolism lead to increased excretion of other porphyrins in the urine. These conditions are collectively called **porphyrias,** and in some of them porphobilinogen is present in the urine. Porphobilinogenuria is seen in acute attacks of acute intermittent porphyria, variegate porphyria, and hereditary coproporphyria. An acute attack may be precipitated by drugs affecting the liver, including barbiturates, sulfa drugs, heavy metals, hydantoins, and hormones, by infection, and by diet. The discovery of porphobilinogen in urine is a critical value that can eliminate or reduce adverse effects from drugs or anesthetics.

Tests for urobilinogen that use the Ehrlich aldehyde reaction will detect urobilinogen and porphobilinogen, in addition to other Ehrlich-reactive compounds.

### Reagent Strip Tests for Urobilinogen

**Principle.** The reagent strip tests for urobilinogen (unlike other reagent strip tests) differ in basic principle and specificity.

**Multistix** tests for urobilinogen are based on a modified **Ehrlich aldehyde reaction.** In this reaction, urobilinogen (also porphobilinogen and other Ehrlich-reactive compounds) reacts with $p$-dimethylaminobenzaldehyde in concentrated hydrochloric acid to form a colored (cherry-red) aldehyde. This is also the basis of the **Watson-Schwartz test,** which will be described in detail. An inverse Ehrlich's aldehyde reaction is the basis of the **Hoesch test,** which is used for the detection of porphobilinogen in urine.

**Chemstrip** reagent strips employ a diazo reaction in which a diazonium salt reacts with urobilinogen in an acid medium to form a red azo dye.

**Specificity.** The Multistix reagent strips react with substances known to react with Ehrlich reagent. These substances include porphobilinogen and various intermediate Ehrlich reactive substances, such as sulfonamides, p-aminosalicylic acid, procaine, and 5-hydroxyindoleacetic acid. Therefore, urine specimens that give a positive reaction with these reagent strips should be confirmed by using another method, such as Chemstrip, which is specific for urobilinogen, the Hoesch test for porphobilinogen, or the Watson-Schwartz test for urobilinogen, porphobilinogen, and intermediate Ehrlich-reactive compounds.

The Chemstrip reagent strips react with urobilinogen and stercobilinogen. However, differentiation between these two substances is not diagnostically important, as stercobilinogen is found in feces, not urine. Porphobilinogen and other Ehrlich-reactive substances are not detected with Chemstrips. This is helpful, as many interfering Ehrlich-reactive substances are commonly encountered in routine urinalysis. However, the existence of unsuspected or undiagnosed porphyria would be missed completely with this test.

### Sensitivity (Minimum Detectable Level): Manufacturer's Values

| | |
|---|---|
| Multistix | As low as 0.2 mg/dL |
| Chemstrip | Approximately 0.4 mg/dL |

The absence of urobilinogen cannot be determined. Results of 1 mg/dL or less should be reported as normal, rather than negative. There is normally up to 1 mg/dL urobilinogen present in urine.

**Interferences.** The presence of intermediate Ehrlich-reacting substances other than urobilinogen is a problem in any test based on the Ehrlich aldehyde reaction, such as Multistix. All strips are affected by highly colored pigments or their metabolites in the urine specimen. Strips based on the diazo reaction (Chemstrip) show interferences similar to reagent strip tests for bilirubin.

*False-Positive Results*

- Intermediate Ehrlich-reacting substances, such as sulfonamides, p-aminosalicylic acid (PAS) metabolites, procaine, and 5-hydroxyindolacetic acid, will react in tests based on the Ehrlich aldehyde reaction (Multistix).
- Methyldopa (Aldomet) will give a strong color reaction with Ehrlich's reagent.
- Highly colored pigments and their metabolites, including ethoxazene (Serenium), drugs containing azo dyes (phenazopyridine), nitrofurantoin, riboflavin, and p-aminobenzoic acid, may cause atypical or positive reactions with all reagent strips.
- Reactivity with Multistix increases with temperature and may give a false-positive reaction if the urine is tested at body temperature, because of a so-called "warm aldehyde reaction." Test urine at room temperature (22° to 26° C).

*False-Negative or Decreased Results*

- Oxidation of urobilinogen (colorless) to urobilin, an orange-red pigment. The urine specimen should be tested as soon as possible after collection.
- Formalin as a preservative with all reagent strips.
- Over 5 mg/dL nitrite with Chemstrip.
- Although porphobilinogen may be detected with tests based on the Ehrlich aldehyde reaction, Multistix is not a reliable test for the detection of porphobilinogen.
- Tests based on a diazo reaction (Chemstrip) will not detect porphobilinogen in the urine.

**Additional Comments.** The absence of urobilinogen is not detectable with any reagent strip.

It is extremely important that fresh urine specimens be tested, because urobilinogen is very unstable when exposed to room temperature or daylight. Urobilinogen, a colorless compound, is rapidly oxidized to urobilin, an orange-red pigment, which is not detected with either reagent strip test. This oxidation takes place so readily that most urine specimens that contain urobilinogen will show an abnormal color caused by partial oxidation to urobilin. The presence of urobilinogen and that of urobilin have the same clinical significance.

It is also extremely important that urine specimens be fresh and properly stored for testing for porphobilinogen. Porphobilinogen is a colorless compound that polymerizes (oxidizes) to a colored compound, namely porphobilin. Porphobilin gives a characteristic dark red or red-purple color, referred to as port-wine red. Fresh urine containing porphobilinogen is not usually colored, but some patients may have a dark red urine, or it may darken on standing as porphobilinogen polymerizes. To extend reactivity, the pH may be adjusted to 7 with sodium bicarbonate.

**Confirmatory and Additional Tests.** The normal urobilinogen concentration in urine is approximately 0.2 to 1.0 mg/dL. If the reagent strip result is 2 mg/dL, it may or may not be abnormal and requires further evaluation.

The presence of intermediate Ehrlich-reacting substances is a problem in any test that is based on the Ehrlich aldehyde reaction. It is therefore useful to use a second reagent strip, based on another methodology (the diazo reaction), with confirmation by the Hoesch test and the Watson-Schwartz test, to identify the reactant and establish the presence of abnormal concentrations of urobilinogen and porphobilinogen. The reactions of urobilinogen, porphobilinogen, and intermediate Ehrlich-reacting substances with these tests are outlined in Table 14-10.

The identity of the positive reaction with the Watson-Schwartz test is determined by extraction of the colored product of the reaction with chloroform and butanol, as shown in Table 14-11.

Generally, if Multistix and Chemstrip show a similar reaction, results may be reported for urobilinogen from the reagent strip. If the Multistix reaction is increased and the Chemstrip is normal, the presence of porphobilinogen or intermediate Ehrlich-reactive substances is suspected. If the Hoesch test (which is specific for porphobilinogen) is positive, the substance is porphobilinogen. If the Hoesch test is negative, the substance showing increased results with Multistix is probably an intermediate Ehrlich-reactive substance. This may be confirmed with the Watson-Schwartz test if results are uncertain.

---

**TABLE 14-10**

Reaction of Urobilinogen, Porphobilinogen, and Intermediate Ehrlich-Reacting Substances with Various Tests

| Method | Urobilinogen | Porphobilinogen | Intermediate |
|---|---|---|---|
| Multistix (Ehrlich reaction) | Positive | Positive (or negative) | Positive |
| Chemstrip (diazo reaction) | Positive | Negative | Negative |
| Hoesch test (inverse Ehrlich reaction) | Negative | Positive | Negative |
| Watson-Schwartz test (Ehrlich reaction) | Positive | Positive | Positive |

## TABLE 14-11

Results of Watson-Schwartz Test

| Result | Urine Ehrlich Reagent Sodium Acetate | Chloroform Extract | Butanol Extract |
|---|---|---|---|
| Negative | No pink color | Not done | Not done |
| Urobilinogen positive | Pink | Pink | Pink (if done) |
| Porphobilinogen positive | Pink | Colorless | Colorless |
| Intermediate Ehrlich-reactive compounds positive | Pink | Colorless | Pink |

### Watson-Schwartz Qualitative Test for Urobilinogen and Porphobilinogen

**Principle and Specificity.** The **Watson-Schwartz test** is a qualitative test that uses the Ehrlich aldehyde reaction for the detection and differentiation of urobilinogen, porphobilinogen, and intermediate Ehrlich-reactive compounds. The Ehrlich aldehyde reaction occurs with urobilinogen but not with urobilin. In the presence of Ehrlich's reagent, urobilinogen, porphobilinogen, and intermediate Ehrlich-reactive compounds give a characteristic cherry-red color. This color is the result of the reaction of *p*-dimethylaminobenzaldehyde in concentrated hydrochloric acid to form a colored aldehyde. The color is enhanced in the presence of saturated sodium acetate, which also inhibits color formation by skatoles and indoles, which might be present in the urine. It has been observed that if urobilinogen is present, the color development is characteristically delayed until the sodium acetate is added. If porphobilinogen is present, the aldehyde color characteristically develops as soon as the Ehrlich reagent is added.

To differentiate color formed by urobilinogen, porphobilinogen, and intermediate Ehrlich-reactive compounds, the test solution is extracted with the organic solvents chloroform and butanol. Color formed by urobilinogen is soluble in chloroform and butanol, porphobilinogen is not soluble in either organic solvent, and intermediate Ehrlich-reactive compounds are soluble in butanol but not in chloroform (see Table 14-11 and Fig. 14-8).

When the procedure is performed, it is not necessary to continue on to a butanol extraction if all of the color formed goes into the chloroform layer, as urobilinogen is the only compound soluble in chloroform. Extraction by butanol is necessary to differentiate porphobilinogen from the intermediate Ehrlich-reactive compounds. (See Procedure 14-6.)

**Sensitivity.** 2.0 to 10 mg/dL

According to Pietrach et al, the Watson-Schwartz test is somewhat more sensitive to porphobilinogen than the Hoesch test.[10]

**Reagents**

1. Ehrlich's reagent. Dissolve 0.7 g of *p*-dimethylaminobenzaldehyde in 100 mL distilled or deionized water.
2. Saturated sodium acetate. Add deionized or distilled water directly to bottle of reagent-grade sodium acetate. Shake daily for about 1 week. There should be a layer

COMMON REACTIONS:

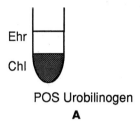

POS Urobilinogen

**A**

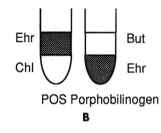

POS Porphobilinogen

**B**

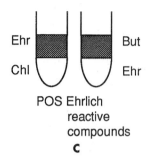

POS Ehrlich
reactive
compounds

**C**

RARE REACTIONS:

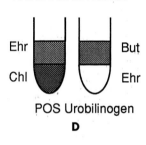

POS Urobilinogen

**D**

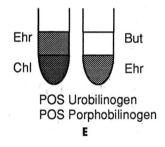

POS Urobilinogen
POS Porphobilinogen

**E**

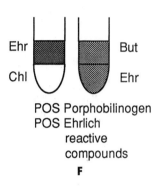

POS Porphobilinogen
POS Ehrlich
reactive
compounds

**F**

**FIG 14-8.** Watson-Schwartz test: interpretation of various results.

of undissolved crystals on the bottom of the stock and working reagent bottles.

3. Chloroform. Reagent grade.
4. Butanol. Reagent grade.

**Interferences.** Several compounds, such as methyldopa, methyl red, and azo dyes, give a confusing red color with Ehrlich reagent. Some will give a color reaction with acid alone, without the presence of Ehrlich reagent. To rule out such false-positive reactions, include a control reaction using 6 mol/L hydrochloric acid in place of the Ehrlich reagent.

***False-Positive Results***

■ The "warm aldehyde" reaction. This is seen when the urine is tested immediately after it is voided. It is a weak Ehrlich reac-

tion that takes place at body temperature with a chromogen (probably indoxyl) present in normal urine. To avoid this reaction, test urine that has cooled to room temperature.

■ Intermediate Ehrlich-reactive compounds: sulfonamides, procaine, 5-hydroxyindoleacetic acid, and others. Their presence makes interpretation of results difficult.

■ In patients receiving methyldopa (Aldomet), a strong color reaction is often observed. However, unlike the situation with porphobilinogen, there is an approximately equal distribution of the pink or red color between the aqueous and butanol layers in the second extraction.

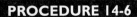

## PROCEDURE 14-6

### Watson-Schwartz Test For Urobilinogen and Porphobilinogen

1. Place 2.5 mL urine in a 15 × 125 mm test tube. Add 2.5 mL Ehrlich's reagent. Mix well by inversion.

2. Add 5.0 ml of saturated sodium acetate and mix. Observe for the development of a pink to deep cherry-red color. (Color development indicates the presence of urobilinogen, porphobilinogen, or intermediate Ehrlich-reactive compounds.)

3. If color develops, add 5 mL of chloroform to the test tube, stopper, and shake vigorously to extract the color.

   - If color is caused by urobilinogen, it will be extracted into the lower chloroform layer (Fig. 14-8, *A*). If all color is extracted into the chloroform layer, the test is positive for urobilinogen and further extraction is not necessary.

   - If color is caused by porphobilinogen or intermediate Ehrlich-reactive compounds, it will remain in the upper aqueous layer.

4. If color remains in the upper aqueous layer, remove one half of it to another test tube. Add 5 mL butanol. Stopper and shake vigorously to extract the color.

   - If the color is caused by porphobilinogen, it will remain in the lower aqueous layer. Porphobilinogen is not soluble in butanol (Fig. 14-8, *B*).

   - If the color is caused by intermediate Ehrlich-reactive compounds, it will be extracted into the upper butanol layer (Fig. 14-8, *C*).

   - If, in the first chloroform extraction, the color was caused by urobilinogen but was not completely extracted into chloroform, the color remaining in the aqueous layer will be extracted into butanol in the second extraction (Fig. 14-8, *D*) .

   - If both urobilinogen and porphobilinogen are present (an extremely rare situation), color caused by urobilinogen will be extracted into the chloroform layer. Color due to porphobilinogen will remain in the lower aqueous layer when extracted with butanol. The butanol layer will remain colorless in this extraction (Fig. 14-8, *E*).

   - It is possible to have situations in which the specimen contains intermediate Ehrlich-reactive compounds in addition to either urobilinogen or porphobilinogen. Interpretation is difficult and may require re-extraction with both chloroform and butanol (Fig. 14-8, *F*).

5. Report the results as:

   - Positive or negative for urobilinogen

   - Positive for porphobilinogen

   - Positive for both urobilinogen and porphobilinogen (very rare)

Do not report the finding of intermediate Ehrlich-reactive compounds. These are false-positive reactions of no clinical significance.

Modified from Ringsrud KM, Linné JJ: *Urinalysis and Body Fluids: A ColorText and Atlas*, St Louis, Mosby, 1995, p 71.

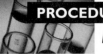

## PROCEDURE 14-7

### Hoesch Test For Porphobilinogen

1. Pour approximately 2 mL of Hoesch reagent into a 15 × 85 mm test tube.

2. Add two drops of well-mixed urine.

3. Observe for the appearance of an instantaneous cherry-red or bright-red color that appears on top of the solution. Agitate briefly, and look for a light to bright pink color throughout the test tube.

4. Report results as positive or negative for porphobilinogen.

■ An orange color in the chloroform layer is seen in the presence of indican. This should not be confused with urobilinogen.

■ Pale peach and light orange color should not be interpreted as positive reactions.

**False-Negative Results**

■ These are the result of inadequate specimen collection and processing. Specimens exposed to light or left at room temperature for more than 1 hour will show low or negative reactions because of conversion of urobilinogen to urobilin or porphobilinogen to porphobilin.

**Additional Comments.** The sodium acetate solution must be saturated for complete color enhancement. To ensure saturation, there should be a layer of undissolved crystals on the bottom of stock and working reagent bottles.

Chloroform is a known carcinogen, and exposure should be avoided. It should be used only if there is an adequate fume hood available. Exposure to chloroform can be avoided by limiting use of the Watson-Schwartz test. Screen specimens suspected of containing porphobilinogen with the Hoesch Test. If results are uncertain, confirm with the Watson-Schwartz test. In most cases, the presence of intermediate Ehrlich-reactive compounds can be established by comparing results with reagent strip tests based on the Ehrlich aldehyde reaction (Multistix) with diazo-based reactions (Chemstrip). (See also Table 14-10.)

### Hoesch Test for Porphobilinogen

**Principle.** This is a test for porphobilinogen based on an inverse Ehrlich's aldehyde reaction. In the Hoesch test, an acid solution is maintained by adding a small volume of urine to a relatively large volume of Ehrlich reagent. (See Procedure 14-7.)

**Reagents**

1. Hydrochloric acid, 6 mol/L. Dilute concentrated HCl (reagent grade) 1:2 with deionized or distilled water by slowly adding the acid to water.

2. Hoesch reagent. Dissolve 2.0 g $p$-dimethylaminobenzaldehyde in 6 mol/L HCl and dilute to 100 mL with HCl.

**Specificity.** The test is specific for porphobilinogen.

**Sensitivity.** 2.0 to 10.0 mg/dL porphobilinogen. This is similar to, but less sensitive than, the Watson-Schwartz test.

**Interferences.** These are similar to those seen with the Watson-Schwartz test.

**False-Positive Results**

■ Large doses of methyldopa, indoles in some patients with intestinal ileus, and phenazopyridine.

■ Urosein, a pigment related to indoleacetic acid, may produce a rose color in response to strong HCl, which may be confused with a positive porphobilinogen result. Such interference may be ruled out by separately testing the specimen in question with 6 mol/L HCl, along with the Hoesch reagent.

- Very large quantities of urobilinogen (over 20 mg/dL) will give a positive reaction. This is not a practical problem.

**Additional Comments.** A quantitative porphobilinogen test is necessary when either the Watson-Schwartz test or the Hoesch test is questionable.

# ASCORBIC ACID

## Clinical Importance

Unlike the analytes discussed to this point, tests for ascorbic acid are not part of the so-called routine urinalysis. Rather, specimens may be tested for ascorbic acid on the basis of findings in the routine urinalysis.

**Ascorbic acid (vitamin C)** is neither a normal nor a pathologic constituent of urine. Its presence in the urine is important because of the interfering effect it has on other chemical tests, especially the reagent strip tests for glucose and blood that depend on the release of hydrogen peroxide by peroxidase and subsequent oxidation of a chromogen to indicate a reaction. Ascorbic acid interferes by reducing the released hydrogen peroxide to water, preventing or delaying the desired oxidation of the chromogen indicator.

Ascorbic acid may also interfere with the various reagent strip tests that are based on the diazo reaction. In these tests, the ascorbic acid may react with the diazonium salt that is formed, causing a reduced or false-negative reaction.

Quantities of vitamin C in excess of those required by the body for normal function are quickly eliminated through the urine, which contains 2 to 10 mg/dL ascorbic acid when dietary intake is adequate. The urine of persons who have ingested large quantities of vitamin C

or who are receiving medications, such as intravenous antibiotics, that contain vitamin C may contain inhibiting quantities of ascorbic acid. With large amounts of ascorbic acid, generally more than 25 mg/dL (250 mg/L), inhibition is usually seen with low levels of the analyte in question in dilute urine. Ascorbic acid is metabolized to sulfate and oxalate. Oxalate stones may form in the kidneys of certain susceptible persons who ingest large amounts (1 gram or more per day) of vitamin C.

Neither Multistix nor Chemstrip contains a test area for ascorbic acid. The presence of ascorbic acid in the urine may be suspected when a reagent strip test for blood is negative even though the urinary sediment shows the presence of red cells. It may also be suspected when reagent strip tests for glucose on urine specimens from diabetic patients give inconsistent results, showing negative or reduced reactions even though the tests for ketones and the copper reduction tests for sugar are positive. In such cases, ascorbic acid may be confirmed by a reagent strip test specific for ascorbic acid. If this is not available, a clinical history of ingestion of large doses of ascorbic acid, or retesting a urine specimen that is voided at least 10 hours after the last administration of vitamin C, may suffice.

## Reagent Strip Test for Ascorbic Acid

At present, neither Multistix nor Chemstrip reagent strips contain a reagent pad for ascorbic acid. A reagent strip test was formerly available by the manufacturer of Multistix, but has been discontinued.

The Merckoquant ascorbic acid test* is intended for the semiquantitative determination of ascorbic acid in foodstuffs, such as fruit and vegetable juices, and in wine. However, it may be used to test urine for ascorbic acid by default, without reagent strips intended for urine.

---

*EM Science Div, EM Industries, Gibbstown, NJ, a division of E Merck, Darmstadt, Germany.

## Principle

The reaction is based on the reduction by ascorbic acid of phosphomolybdate, a yellow complex, to molybdenum blue.

## Specificity

The reaction is not specific for ascorbic acid but will react with other reducing substances with similar redox potential.

## Additional Comments

Results are read by comparison with a color chart in milligrams per liter (mg/L). Values for ascorbic acid throughout this chapter have been given in mg/dL. Therefore, values with the Merckoquant reagent strip should be converted to mg/dL.

## SUMMARY

A great deal of information is contained in this section on chemical tests in routine urinalysis. Much of this information is summarized in the following tables. False-positive and false-negative reactions in routine urinalysis tests are summarized in Table 14-12. Common confirmatory tests used in routine urinalysis are summarized in Table 14-13.

### TABLE 14-12

False-Positive and False-Negative Reactions in Routine Urinalysis Tests

| Test | False Positive or Masking of Results | False Negative or Decreased Results |
|---|---|---|
| Protein (reagent strip) | • Highly colored urine<br> Bilirubin or bile pigments<br> Azo-containing drugs or compounds—phenazopyridine (Pyridium)<br>• Loss of buffer on strip—overwetting<br>• Exceptionally alkaline or highly buffered specimen<br>• Residues of quaternary ammonium compounds or chlorhexidine (disinfectant contamination)<br>• Chemstrip: polyvinylpyrrolidone (blood substitutes) | • Presence of protein other than albumin |
| SSA protein | • Turbidity in specimen not cleared before testing<br>• Radiographic contrast media such as meglumine diatrizoate (Renografin, Hypaque)—delayed positive reaction<br>• Metabolites of tolbutamide<br>• Massive doses of:<br>  Penicillin<br>  Sulfonamides<br>  Cephalosporin<br>  Tolmetin (Tolectin) | • Highly buffered alkaline urine (acid in SSA is neutralized) |
| Blood | • Strong oxidizing cleaning agents like hypochlorite bleach (oxidation of chromogen) | • >2.5 mg/dL ascorbic acid<br>• Testing supernatant urine (settling of red cells) |

*Continued*

TABLE 14-12

False-Positive and False-Negative Reactions in Routine Urinalysis Tests—cont'd

| Test | False Positive or Masking of Results | False Negative or Decreased Results |
|---|---|---|
| Blood—cont'd | • Microbial peroxidase<br>• Menstrual contamination | • Elevated specific gravity or protein (reduces lysis of RBCs)<br>• Formalin as a preservative<br>• Captopril (antihypertensive)<br>• Nitrite level over 10 mg/dL (very rare) |
| Nitrite | • Phenazopyridine or other azo-containing compounds or dyes that color urine red or that turn red in an acidic medium<br>• In vitro conversion of nitrate to nitrite (bacterial contamination) | • Insufficient time in the bladder for the conversion of nitrate to nitrite<br>• Insufficient dietary nitrate for bacteria to reduce nitrate to nitrite<br>• Presence of bacteria that further reduce nitrite to nitrogen<br>• High specific gravity with low pH (less than 6)—not typical of bacterial infection<br>• ≥25 mg/dL ascorbic acid with small amounts of nitrite |
| Leukocyte esterase | • Strong oxidizing agents (chlorine bleach or formalin/formaldehyde) | • Drugs (antibiotics) such as cephalexin, cephalothin, tetracycline, and gentamicin<br>• Elevated glucose (>3 g/dL)<br>• High specific gravity<br>• Oxalic acid—metabolite of ascorbic acid<br>• High levels of albumin (>500 mg/dL) |
| Glucose (reagent strips) | • Contamination from strong oxidizing agents or bleach (oxidation of chromogen)<br>• Trace values in dilute urine (increased sensitivity)<br>• Improper storage of reagent strips | • Ascorbic acid (vitamin C)<br>  Multistix: ≥50 mg/dL (500 mg/L) in specimens containing small amounts (75-125 mg/dL) of glucose<br>  Chemstrip: >100 mg/dL (1,000 mg/L)<br>• Moderate ketone bodies (≥40 mg/dL) in specimens containing 75-125 mg/dL glucose—unlikely in a diabetic patient<br>• Sodium fluoride—enzyme inhibition<br>• Refrigerated specimens—decreased enzyme activity |
| Clinitest | • Extremely large amounts of ascorbic acid (over 200 mg/dL = 2,000 mg/L) may cause low-level positive results (equivalent to 500 mg/dL or less)<br>• Slightly elevated result with low specific gravity compared with reagent strip<br>• Large quantities of nalidixic acid, cephalosporins, and probenecid<br>• Radiographic contrast media—unusual (black) color | • Reoxidation of cuprous to cupric ions by atmospheric oxygen, due to mixing before the 15-second wait period |
| Ketones (reagent strip and Acetest) | • Phthaleins (Bromsulphalein, phenolsulfonphthalein) | • Conversion of acetoacetic acid to acetone with evaporation of acetone in improperly stored specimens |

**TABLE 14-12**

False-Positive and False-Negative Reactions in Routine Urinalysis Tests—cont'd

| Test | False Positive or Masking of Results | False Negative or Decreased Results |
|---|---|---|
| Ketones (reagent strip and Acetest)—cont'd | • Phenylketones—very large amounts<br>• 8-hydroxyquinoline—preservative<br>• Highly concentrated urine specimens (high specific gravity)<br>• Large amounts of levodopa metabolites<br>• 2-Mercaptoethanesulfonic acid (Mesna) or other compounds containing sulfhydryl groups | |
| Bilirubin (reagent strip and Icotest) | • Substances that color the urine red or turn red in an acid medium, including:<br>    Phenothiazine<br>    Chlorpromazine<br>    Phenazopyridine (Pyridium)<br>    Ethoxazene (Serenium).<br>• Metabolites of etodolac (Lodine)<br>• Indoles | • Oxidation of bilirubin to biliverdin<br>• In vitro hydrolyzation of bilirubin diglucuronide to free bilirubin<br>• ≥25 mg/dL ascorbic acid<br>• Elevated nitrite concentration (urinary tract infection) |
| Urobilinogen (reagent strips) | • Highly colored pigments and their metabolites, including:<br>    Ethoxazene (Serenium)<br>    Drugs containing azo dyes (phenazopyridine)<br>    Nitrofurantoin<br>    Riboflavin<br>    $p$-Aminobenzoic acid<br>• Multistix: intermediate Ehrlich-reacting substances, such as:<br>    Sulfonamides<br>    $p$-Aminosalicylic acid (PAS)<br>    Procaine<br>    5-Hydroxyindolacetic acid<br>• Multistix: Methyldopa (Aldomet)—strong color reaction<br>• Multistix: "warm aldehyde reaction" | • Oxidation of urobilinogen to urobilin<br>• Formalin (preservative)<br>• Chemstrip: >5 mg/dL nitrite<br>• Multistix: may or may not detect porphobilinogen<br>• Chemstrip: will not detect porphobilinogen |
| Watson-Schwartz test | • The "warm aldehyde" reaction<br>• Intermediate Ehrlich-reactive compounds<br>• Methyldopa (Aldomet)—strong color reaction<br>• Indican—orange color in the chloroform layer<br>• Pale peach and light orange color | • Conversion of urobilinogen to urobilin |
| Hoesch test | • Methyldopa, indoles, and phenazopyridine<br>• Urosein—rose color with strong HCl<br>• Very large quantities of urobilinogen (over 20 mg/dL)—not a practical problem | • Conversion of porphobilinogen to porphyrin |

**TABLE 14-13**

Confirmatory Urinalysis Tests

This is only a partial listing of confirmatory tests used in urinalysis. See a standard laboratory reference for additional tests and detailed information.

| Substance | Name of Test | Comments |
|---|---|---|
| Protein | Sulfosalicylic acid test | Based on the acid precipitation of protein with a strong acid—sulfosalicylic acid (SSA)<br>The reagent strip test is most sensitive to albumin<br>SSA reacts with any proteins; in addition to albumin: globulins, glucoproteins, and immunoglobulins<br>Delayed false positives with diagnostic radiographic media |
| Microalbuminuria | Micro-Bumintest (Bayer) | A tablet test for very small amounts of albumin; may be used to test for early, presymptomatic diabetic nephropathy; principle as for reagent strip test but will detect as little as 4-8 mg albumin/dL |
| | Nephelometer | Used to quantitate albumin by measuring the antibody-antigen complex in suspension |
| Blood | Microscopic examination | If microscopic analysis shows more than 2 RBC per high-power field and reagent strip is negative, test for the presence of ascorbic acid or otherwise account for the discrepancy |
| Hemoglobin and myoglobin | Centrifugation; then test supernatant with reagent strip test for blood | Separate hemoglobin from myoglobin by urine and plasma appearance, total serum creatine kinase (CK), total serum lactate (LD), and LD isoenzymes |
| Hemosiderin | Rous test | Based on a positive Prussian blue reaction of hemosiderin with potassium ferrocyanide |
| Glucose and other reducing substances (NGRS) | Clinitest (Bayer) | Tests for reducing substances in addition to glucose; based on the reduction of copper II to copper I in the presence of heat and alkali<br>Will detect glucose, galactose, lactose, fructose, and pentose (L-xylulose) but not sucrose |

## MICROSCOPIC ANALYSIS OF THE URINE SEDIMENT

Urinary sediment refers to all solid materials suspended in the urine specimen. Very few urine specimens are absolutely clear, and even those that appear clear to the naked eye have some solid material suspended in them. In addition, many urine specimens obviously contain solid material, as evidenced by their lack of clarity. Any amount of cloudiness that is visible to the naked eye must be accounted for in a microscopic analysis of the urine sediment. The solid material present in urine specimens can be identified only by microscopic examination. It may be the most important part of the urinalysis.

## TABLE 14-13

Confirmatory Urinalysis Tests—cont'd

| Substance | Name of Test | Comments |
|-----------|--------------|----------|
| Glucose and other reducing substances (NGRS)—cont'd | Clinitest (Bayer)—cont'd | False-positive results may be seen with large quantities of ascorbic acid, salicylates, and large amounts of some penicillins<br><br>Used routinely for pediatric specimens (less than 1 year old) to detect nonglucose reducing sugars |
| Carbohydrates | Thin-layer chromatography | Common tests are for fructose, sucrose, dextrose, lactose, xylose, galactose, and arabinose, as these are the sugars most often encountered in urine |
| Salicylates | Ferric chloride test | A rapid (spot) test for salicylate poisoning; also detects very large amounts of acetoacetic acid |
| Bilirubin | Ictotest (Bayer) | Used when very small amounts of bilirubin are suspected as more sensitive than the reagent strip tests; based on a diazo reaction |
| Urobilinogen and porphobilinogen | Watson-Schwartz test | This is the Ehrlich aldehyde reaction<br><br>Will differentiate urobilinogen, porphobilinogen, or intermediate Ehrlich-reacting substances if the Bayer reagent strip shows more than 1 EU |
| Porphobilinogen | Hoesch test | Test is specific for porphobilinogen<br>Based on the inverse Ehrlich reaction<br>Sensitivity similar to Watson-Schwartz test |
| Ascorbic acid | EM Quant (Merckoquant) | Use when interference of any of the reagent strip tests that depend on the presence of hydrogen peroxide is suspected<br><br>The reagent strip tests for blood are especially susceptible |

However, the examination of the urinary sediment is not a simple procedure, nor is it inexpensive. It requires well-trained, skilled, knowledgeable personnel, and it is time consuming. Personnel need to be skilled in the use of the microscope, and aware of the various microscopic techniques and other aids that are helpful in identifying the various components of the urinary sediment that may be encountered. This includes an understanding of the clinical correlation or significance of the various elements of the urinary sediment.

For all of these reasons, together with the need for cost containment in health care, it has been suggested that the microscopic analysis of the urinary sediment is not necessarily a part of every routine urinalysis. Rather, various protocols have been devised, which call for the microscopic analysis only when abnormal findings are seen in the physical and/or chemical analysis of the urine, or when determined by laboratory protocol (including the patient's condition or clinical history) or when requested by the physician. The NCCLS states: "The decision to perform microscopic examinations should be made by each individual laboratory based on its specific patient population."[7]

## SPECIMEN PREPARATION (CONCENTRATION)

When the urine sediment is to be examined, a concentrated portion of the urine is used. The sediment is concentrated before examination to ensure detection of less abundant constituents. To concentrate the sediment, a well-mixed, measured portion of urine is centrifuged. The clear supernatant is decanted, and the solid material, which settles to the bottom during centrifugation, is examined under the microscope (the supernatant may be further tested for chemical constituents, such as urine protein). The various parts of the sediment are identified and enumerated to give semiquantitative results. For these results to have any meaning, a constant amount of urine must be centrifuged and a constant volume of supernatant removed.

## STANDARDIZATION

Various aids to standardization of the preparation and examination of the urine sediment are available. Complete systems or portions of systems may be used by a given a laboratory. Complete systems include specially designed graduated centrifuge tubes with special devices or pipettes that allow for the easy decanting of the supernatant urine and retention of an exact volume of undisturbed concentrated urinary sediment. Systems differ in the final volume of urine sediment, although

they generally begin by centrifuging 12 mL of well-mixed urine. Standardized systems provide a capped centrifuge tube, transfer pipette, supravital stain, and choice of standardized slides. Various control solutions or preparations are also available. Systems include the KOVA system,* the UriSystem,[†] and the Count-10 system.[‡]

Traditionally, sediment was examined by placing a drop of concentrated sediment on a glass microscope slide and applying a coverglass. However, the size of the drop varied (it was generally not a measured drop), and results varied depending on the size of the coverglass used. Standardized systems employ specially designed slides of acrylic plastics with wells or applied cover glasses. They differ in the number of tests per slide, slide chamber volume (depth and surface area), availability of grided slides, and type of coverglass material (plastic or glass).

The NCCLS recommends the use of commercial standardized systems to ensure comparison between laboratories and consistency within laboratories.[8]

According to NCCLS guidelines, the following factors must be standardized, regardless of the system used, standardized or not.

1. Urine volume. 12 mL is used by standardized systems. Ten and 15 mL are also used. The final concentration of sediment should be reported with results.
2. Time of centrifugation. Five minutes is recommended.
3. Speed of centrifugation. The NCCLS recommends a relative centrifugal force (RCF) of 400 g. Others recommend 450 g or 400 to 450 g. Normograms can be used to relate the revolutions per minute (RPM) to RCF by measuring the radius of the centrifuge head in centimeters from the center

---

*ICL Scientific, Fountain Valley, Calif.
[†]Fisher Scientific, Pittsburgh, Pa.
[‡]V-Tech, Inc, Palm Desert, Calif.

pin to the bottom of a horizontal cup, using the following formula:

$$RCF (g) = 11.18 \times 10^{-6} \times Radius\ in\ cm \times RPM^2$$

4. Concentration factor of the sediment. This is based on the volume of urine centrifuged and the final volume of sediment remaining after the supernatant urine is removed. Standardized systems facilitate retention of a specific volume of urine sediment.
5. Volume of sediment examined. Standardized slides contain chambers that hold a specific volume of concentrated sediment. With traditional slide and coverglass: The volume of concentrated sediment placed on the glass slide should be measured; 20µL is common. The volume examined may be calculated based on the volume of sediment placed on the slide, size (area) of the coverglass, diameter of the microscope objective, and concentration of urine sediment used.
6. Reporting format. Every person in an institution who performs a microscopic examination of the urinary sediment should use the same terminology, reporting format, and reference ranges.

## SPECIMEN REQUIREMENTS

### Type of Specimen

Although any freely voided collection is acceptable, the ideal specimen for microscopic analysis of the urinary sediment is a fresh, voided, first morning specimen. A first morning specimen (an 8-hour concentration) is preferable because it is the most concentrated, and therefore small amounts of abnormal constituents are more likely to be detected. In addition, the formed elements (cells and casts) are less likely to disintegrate in more concentrated urine.

### Preservation

A fresh urine specimen is particularly important for reliable results. If the urine cannot be exam-

ined within 2 hours, it should be refrigerated as soon as possible after collection. Specimens left at room temperature for over 2 hours are not acceptable. However, a so-called "unacceptable" specimen should not be discarded until clinical personnel have been consulted and a mutually agreeable decision has been reached.

Although refrigeration retards decomposition of urine sediment constituents, amorphous deposits of urates and phosphates tend to precipitate out of solution as the urine cools. These findings are important in that they may obscure the presence of pathologic constituents that are present.

If the specimen must be kept in the refrigerator for more than a few hours, a chemical preservative might be considered. Formalin may be used as a preservative that will fix the various cellular elements and casts. However, it interferes with many chemical tests. Other preservatives, such as toluene or thymol, may be used to prevent bacterial contamination. None of the preservatives is completely satisfactory, and fresh collections are definitely preferred. If preservatives that may interfere with various chemical tests are added, it is advisable to split the well-mixed specimen so that the sediment constituents are preserved, yet the chemical constituents are not affected.

### Changes After Voiding

Changes that may occur as the urine stands include the following. Red blood cells become distorted because of the lack of an isotonic solution. They either swell or become crenated, which makes them difficult to recognize, and they finally disintegrate. White blood cells rapidly disintegrate in hypotonic solutions. Casts disintegrate, especially as the urine becomes alkaline, since they must have sufficient acidity and solute concentration to exist. Other components that are found only in acidic urine will disappear as the urine becomes alkaline. The increase in alkalinity results from the growth of bacteria and production of ammonia. Finally, bacteria multiply rapidly, obscuring various components.

## Protection From Contamination

In addition to being a fresh first morning collection, the urine specimen should be clean and free of external contamination. This is sometimes a problem, especially with female patients, since vaginal contamination will result in the presence of epithelial cells, red cells, and white cells. In such cases it may be necessary to use a clean voided midstream specimen, which is also required for quantitative urine culture. It may also be necessary to pack the vagina or use a tampon in some cases to avoid vaginal and menstrual contamination.

## NORMAL SEDIMENT

Normally urine contains little or no sediment, a reflection of the fact that normal urine is clear. However, a few constituents may be seen in any urine specimen. These generally consist of a very few red blood cells, white blood cells, hyaline casts, epithelial cells, and crystals. Each laboratory must establish its own reference values for normal urine on the basis of methodology and patient population. The reference values in Table 14-14 are those established for the Fairview-University Medical Center, University Campus, Minneapolis, Minn., and are included as an example of what might be encountered in so-called "normal" urine.

### TABLE 14-14

Reference Values For Urine Sediment*

| | |
|---|---|
| Red blood cells | 0-2/hpf |
| White blood cells | 0-5/hpf (female > male) |
| Casts | 0-2 hyaline casts/lpf |
| Squamous epithelial cells | few/lpf |
| Transitional epithelial cells | few/hpf |
| Renal tubular epithelial cells | few/hpf |
| Bacteria | Negative |
| Yeast | Negative |
| Abnormal crystals | Negative |

*These values are based on a 12:1 concentration viewed with low-power (10×) and high-power (40×) objectives with a 10× ocular. hpf = high-power field; lpf = low-power field.

## TECHNIQUES FOR EXAMINATION OF URINE SEDIMENT

The urinary sediment consists of a great variety of material. Some of the constituents are normal, while others are abnormal and represent serious conditions. It is important to learn to identify both the normal and the abnormal constituents. In general, the normal constituents are more easily seen under the microscope, and must be recognized so that they do not obscure the presence of the less obvious but more serious abnormal constituents. Recognition of the abnormal constituents is extremely important in the diagnosis and treatment of various renal diseases. They often give information about the state of the kidney and the urinary tract. In addition, the microscopic analysis of the sediment will help to confirm and account for findings in the chemical examination of the urine. For example, protein in the urine is often associated with the presence of casts and cellular elements in the sediment.

Traditionally, the urine sediment has been examined microscopically by placing a drop of urine on a microscope slide, applying a coverglass, and observing the preparation under the low-power (10×) and high-power (40×) objectives of a brightfield microscope. Since the preparation is a wet mount, oil immersion cannot be used in this examination. The brightfield examination of unstained sediment is difficult, and various microscopic techniques such as phase-contrast and polarizing microscopy have been developed to aid in the identification of the various entities that might be present in the urine sediment. Other useful techniques in the examination of the urine sediment include the use of stains and cytocentrifugation.

### Microscopic Techniques
(See also Chapter 5)
### Brightfield Microscopy

This is the traditional method of observation of the urinary sediment and the most difficult. When the sediment is examined with brightfield illumination, correct light adjustment is essential. The light must be sufficiently reduced, by correct positioning of the condenser and use of the iris diaphragm, to give contrast between the unstained structures and the background liquid. As described in Chapter 5, the condenser should be left in a generally uppermost position (at most only 1 or 2 mm below the specimen) and the desired contrast achieved by opening or closing the iris diaphragm. The condenser should not be "racked down." The correct light adjustment requires care and experience. Correct light adjustment is essential, and various translucent elements that may occur in the urine sediment are easily overlooked with this technique. Of particular difficulty are hyaline casts, mucous threads, and various cells, such as red cells, which have lost their hemoglobin content. If only a brightfield microscope is available, the use of a suitable stain is encouraged. Phase-contrast microscopy is helpful, and a combination of phase-contrast and brightfield microscopy is recommended. The hemoglobin pigment present in blood casts and red blood cell casts is more apparent with brightfield illumination, as are certain cellular details and the presence of highly refractile fat (free and in cells or casts). Most crystals are more easily visualized with brightfield or brightfield and polarizing microscopy.

### Phase-Contrast Microscopy

Phase-contrast microscopy is useful in the examination of unstained urine sediment, particularly for delineating translucent elements such as hyaline casts and mucous threads, which have a refractive index similar to that of the urine in which they are suspended. Some laboratories use a phase-contrast microscope for the routine examination of the urinary sediment. However, some elements are better visualized with brightfield, and the microscopist must be able to change from phase to brightfield with ease.

### Interference-Contrast Microscopy

This is also useful in the examination of unstained urinary sediment, but it is expensive and therefore not used routinely. Since it gives an apparently three-dimensional view of the object being observed, inclusions such as granules or vacuoles within a cell or cast can be better visualized. Besides increasing contrast, the geometric shape is observable.

### Polarizing Microscopy

**Polarized light,** with or without a full wave compensator, may be used to study substances that polarize light. Objects that **polarize** (bend or rotate) light are by definition **birefringent.** When viewed with crossed polarizing filters, they appear white against a black background. If a compensating filter is added, the birefringent body is seen against a magenta background, and certain crystals are identified by the pattern of their birefringence in relation to the direction of the slow wave of compensation. This is especially useful in the analysis of crystals in synovial fluid.

Objects found in the urine sediment that polarize light include most crystals, fat (as cholesterol esters), starch (which may be confused with fat), and fibers (which might be confused with some casts when viewed with brightfield or phase microscopy).

Both fat and starch show a characteristic Maltese cross pattern (a light cross against a black background) when polarized but appear different with brightfield illumination. Since protein material (e.g., casts, cells, bacteria) does not polarize light, polarizing microscopy may be used to differentiate amorphous urates or phosphates that polarize light from bacteria that do not, and an unusual ovoid form of calcium oxalate that is strongly birefringent from red blood cells that are not. It may also help distinguish certain fibers, such as diaper fibers, which polarize light, from waxy casts.

### Staining Techniques

Various staining techniques may be used to increase contrast and therefore visualize various components in the urinary sediment. They are especially useful in enhancing cellular detail, either free or within casts. They are also useful in accentuating many, although not all, casts.

Several stains are described, although the stain most often used for routine urinary sediment examination is a crystal violet and safranin stain, as described by Sternheimer and Malbin.

### Supravital Stains

**Crystal Violet and Safranin (Sternheimer-Malbin Stain).** This stain is useful in the identification of cellular elements. It is an all-purpose stain that is quick and easy to use. It is available as Sedi-Stain,* KOVA stain,[†] and Urisystem Stain,[‡] The staining reactions of the various cellular elements that may be encountered are supplied by the manufacturer and available on package inserts. Very alkaline urines may cause the dyes to precipitate, forming fine brown stellate crystals or purple granules that may obscure important pathologic constituents.

**Toluidine Blue.** A 0.5% solution of toluidine blue is an easy-to-use nuclear stain that can be prepared in the laboratory. It also has the disadvantage of precipitating and causing clumping in some specimens.

### Fat Stains

Fat stains such as Sudan dyes (Sudan III) or oil red O are used to stain neutral fat or triglycerides. These fats do not show as a Maltese cross with polarized light as cholesterol does, yet they have similar clinical significance. Both fat stains and polarizing microscopy should be used to help identify and confirm the presence of fat, either free, within renal epithelial cells or macrophages (oval fat bodies), or within casts (fatty casts).

### Gram Stain

This routine microbiological stain is used to differentiate gram-negative (red) and gram-positive (purple) bacteria. A dry preparation (smear or cytocentrifuged preparation) is necessary, which is heat fixed and then stained.

---

*Clay Adams, division of Becton Dickinson & Co, Parsippany, NJ.
[†]ICL Scientific, Fountain Valley, Calif.
[‡]Fisher Scientific, Pittsburgh, Pa.

### Acetic Acid

Although not a stain, acetic acid may be useful in differentiating white blood cells from red blood cells. A 2% solution of acetic acid may be added to a few drops of sediment in a test tube, or flowed under the coverglass of a mounted urine sediment. The acetic acid will accentuate the nucleus of leukocytes and epithelial cells and lyse red cells. Also, certain crystals that are sometimes present in urine will be dissolved or converted to other forms by acetic acid.

### Hansel's Stain

Hansel's stain* is a special eosinophil stain containing methylene blue and eosin-Y in methanol. It is usually used for the detection of eosinophils in nasal smears, to detect allergic rhinorrhea; however it is useful in the detection of eosinophils in the urine sediment, especially on slides that are prepared by cytocentrifugation.

## Cytocentrifugation

Although by no means a routine technique in urinalysis, cytocentrifugation is being increasingly recognized as a very useful adjunct in the examination of the urine sediment. Preparations may be stained with a Papanicolaou stain, the usual stain for cytologic studies in tumor detection. This stain is time consuming, and requires several solutions that are difficult to maintain, when not in use routinely. A Wright stain, either the traditional procedure used for blood films or a quick stain, may be sufficient.

Cytocentrifugation is useful in differentiating white blood cells from epithelial cells in addition to identifying the type of white blood cell present. Thus it is useful in the early detection of renal allograft rejection by the recognition of lymphocytes in the sediment or eosinophils in drug-induced interstitial nephritis. It is also useful in the detection of viral inclusion bodies, as with cytomegalovirus, fungi, and certain casts. Traditionally, it is used for cytologic studies of precancerous or malignant cells.

---

*Lide Labs, Florissant, Mo.

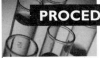

## PROCEDURE 14-8

### Microscopic Examination of the Urine Sediment

**General Procedure**

1. Pour exactly 12 mL of well-mixed urine into a labeled, graduated centrifuge (KOVA) tube.
   a. If less than 12 mL is available, use 3 mL.
   b. If less than 3 mL is available, examine the sediment without concentration. State this information on the report.

2. Centrifuge at a relative centrifugal force of 450 for 5 minutes. Let the centrifuge come to a stop without using the brake. Use of the brake will cause resuspension of the sediment and falsely low results.

3. Decant 11 mL of clear supernatant urine into a test tube, leaving 1 mL of sediment in the KOVA tube.
   a. Insert the KOVA Petter into the centrifuge tube. Push it to the bottom of the tube until it is firmly seated. Holding the Petter in place, decant the supernatant urine. This will leave exactly 1 mL of sediment in the bottom of the tube.
   b. If a 3-mL specimen is used, do not use a KOVA Petter. Decant all liquid quickly, retaining a small drop in which to resuspend the sediment. This is approximately equivalent to a 12:1 concentration.
   c. If the KOVA Petter is not available, pour off 11 mL of supernatant urine in one even motion so as not to resuspend the sediment. Use a disposable pipette to bring the volume of sediment to exactly 1 mL with the clear supernatant urine. Removal of more than 11 mL and readjustment to 1 mL are preferable to removal of less than 11 mL.

4. If using a brightfield microscope, use supravital staining. Add a drop or two of stain to the sediment and mix thoroughly. If the amount of original specimen is limited, or the urine is very alkaline, split the concentrated sediment and stain only one portion.

5. Thoroughly resuspend the sediment by gently squeezing the KOVA Petter.

6. Add the resuspended sediment to a standardized microscope slide, following the manufacturer's directions.

*Continued*

## LABORATORY PROCEDURE

Procedure 14-8 is based on the procedure used by the Fairview-University Medical Center, University Campus, Minneapolis, Minn. It uses a 12:1 concentration of the urine specimen and employs parts of the KOVA system. Well-mixed urine is measured and centrifuged in a special graduated centrifuge (KOVA) tube. It is decanted and exactly 1mL retained for microscopic examination by using a special disposable pipette with a built-in plastic disk (KOVA Petter). Results are reported according to the system in Table 14-15. Directions are included for both standardized slides and traditional glass microscope slides with coverglasses, using both unstained and stained sediment. If a phase-contrast microscope is used, staining is generally unnecessary. However, if only a brightfield microscope is used, staining is recommended.

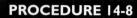

**PROCEDURE 14-8**

*Microscopic Examination of the Urine Sediment—cont'd*

- If traditional glass slides and coverglasses are used, place 20 µL (measured volume) of resuspended sediment on a glass microscope slide and cover with a 22 × 22 mm coverglass. The size of the drop and the size of the coverglass are important. The fluid should completely fill the area under the coverglass without overflowing the area or causing the coverglass to float. Take care that no bubbles appear when placing the coverglass over the sediment. If bubbles appear, a new preparation must be made on a clean slide. Bubbles are confusing and make enumeration impossible, since they prevent random distribution of the substances to be counted.

7. Place the preparation on the microscope stage, and focus. Adjust the light, using the low-power objective, by carefully positioning the condenser and iris diaphragm. The tendency is to have too much light, but the light must not be overly reduced. Be sure that the sediment itself is brought into focus, rather than the coverglass. It is easier to achieve focus with specimens that are stained. Finally, vary the fine adjustment continuously to maintain focus.

8. Be systematic in the examination. With standardized slides, scan the entire preparation. With traditional microscope slides and coverglasses, begin by looking around the four sides of the coverglass, then the center. First, look for the substances that are identified and graded under low power. Change to high power, refocus and readjust the light, and search for the substances that are graded and identified under high power. All gradings are based on the average number of structures seen in a minimum of ten microscopic fields. Describe separately the structures searched for under low and high power. Casts and cells are most important; look for these most carefully, observing the less important crystals and miscellaneous structures almost in retrospect.

9. Examine sediment preparations with the low-power (10×) and high-power (40×) objectives as outlined below. Report results as indicated in Table 14-15. All entities encountered must be reported using the appropriate objective and within the grading scale established for the individual laboratory.

**Low-Power Examination**

With the low-power (10 ×) objective, search for the following:

a. Casts. With standardized slides, scan the entire area for the presence of casts. With traditional slides, look for casts around all four edges of the preparation, and then in the center, since they tend to roll to the edges of the coverglass.
   - When a cast is discovered, change to high power to identify it.

## PROCEDURE 14-8

### Microscopic Examination of the Urine Sediment—cont'd

- Grade and report casts on the basis of the average number seen per low-power field, as shown in Table 14-15. If more than one type of cast is found in a single specimen, identify and grade each type separately.

b. Crystals and amorphous material. Look for these structures in the same way as for casts.
  - Normal crystals are reported as few, moderate, or many per high-power field, if present. However, they may be more apparent under low power.
  - Abnormal crystals are graded as the average number seen per low-power field, when present (see Table 14-15). Abnormal crystals must be confirmed by chemical test or clinical history before they are reported.
  - Crystals are generally identified by shape rather than size. Therefore, a combination of low- and high-power observation is necessary in the detection and identification.

c. Squamous epithelial cells. When they are present, report as few, moderate, or many per low-power field.

d. Mucus (mucous threads). These are reported as present when easily seen or prominent under low power. They are more apparent with phase-contrast microscopy.

**High-Power Examination**

With the high-power (40×) objective, search for the following:

a. Red blood cells. Grade and report on the basis of the average number seen per high-power field (see Table 14-15). Report the presence of unusual forms, such as dysmorphic red cells, if encountered.

b. White blood cells. Grade and report on the basis of the average number seen per high-power field (see Table 14-15). These are usually neutrophils (PMNs). If unusual cell types, such as lymphocytes or eosinophils, are morphologically identifiable, report this finding.

c. Normal crystals. Identify and report as few, moderate, or many per high-power field for each type of crystal encountered.

d. Casts. Identify with high power but grade under low power.

e. Epithelial cells. *Renal tubular, oval fat bodies (renal tubular cells with fat),* and *transitional.* When they are present, estimate and report as few, moderate, or many per high-power field.

f. Miscellaneous. This category includes various cell forms and other structures that may be encountered in the urine sediment, such as *yeast, bacteria, trichomonads, fat globules.* When they are present, identify the cell or structure and report as few, moderate, or many per high-power field. Report sperm as present in males only. It is considered a contaminant in routine urinalysis specimens from females and is not reported.

## TABLE 14-15

Reporting System for Urine Sediment*

| Average Number per Low-Power Field (×100) | | | | | | | |
|---|---|---|---|---|---|---|---|
| Casts (identify with high power) | Negative | 0-2 | 2-5 | 5-10 | 10-25 | 25-50 | >50 |
| Abnormal crystals | Negative | 0-2 | 2-5 | 5-10 | 10-25 | 25-50 | >50 |
| Squamous epithelial cells | Few | | Moderate | | Many | | |
| Mucus (if prominent) | Present | | | | | | |

| Average Number per High-Power Field (×400) | | | | | | | |
|---|---|---|---|---|---|---|---|
| Red blood cells | 0-2 | 2-5 | 5-10 | 10-25 | 25-50 | 50-100 | >100 |
| White blood cells | 0-2 | 2-5 | 5-10 | 10-25 | 25-50 | 50-100 | >100 |
| Normal crystals | Few | | Moderate | | Many | | |
| Epithelial cells (renal, oval fat bodies, transitional) | Few | | Moderate | | Many | | |
| Miscellaneous (bacteria, yeast, Trichomonas, free fat) | Few | | Moderate | | Many | | |
| Sperm (males only) | Present | | | | | | |

*Few = some are present; moderate = easily seen; many = prominent.

# CONSTITUENTS OF URINE SEDIMENT

In general, the constituents of the urinary sediment are either biological or chemical. The biological part, also called the **organized sediment,** includes red blood cells, white blood cells, epithelial cells, fat of biological origin, casts, bacteria, yeast, fungi, parasites, and spermatozoa. (Casts are long cylindrical structures that result from the solidification of material within the lumen of the kidney tubules.) The biological portion is the more important part of the sediment, the cells and casts being of primary importance; unfortunately, they are also the most difficult to detect.

The chemical portion, also called **unorganized sediment,** consists of crystals of chemicals and amorphous material. In general, it is less important than the biological portion. However, some abnormal crystals have pathologic significance. In addition, the constituents of the crystalline or chemical portion are sometimes so numerous that they tend to obscure the more important parts, which must be searched for with great care.

Constituents of the urinary sediment that may be encountered on microscopic examination will now be described. Unless otherwise specified, the staining reactions are those of the Sternheimer-Malbin crystal violet safranin stain (Sedi-Stain).

# CELLULAR CONSTITUENTS DERIVED FROM BLOOD

## Red Blood Cells (Erythrocytes)
### Clinical Importance

A few red cells are present in the urine of normal persons. The number varies, but generally five or fewer per high-power field in the concentrated sediment is considered "normal."[2] The condition in which red cells are found in the urine is termed **hematuria.** The degree of hematuria may vary from a frankly bloody specimen on gross examination to a specimen that shows no change in color. Hematuria may be the result of bleeding at any point along the urogenital tract and may be seen with almost any disease of the urinary tract, including renal disease or dysfunction, infection, tumor or lesions, stone formation, and generalized bleeding disorders, or it may result from anticoagulant usage. Hematuria is a sensitive early indicator of renal disease.

To determine the cause of hematuria, it is necessary to determine the site of bleeding. This involves various types of information, both laboratory and clinical. Part of this information will depend on other findings in the microscopic examination and other portions of the routine urinalysis. For example, bleeding through the glomerulus will often be accompanied by red cell casts, as seen in acute glomerulonephritis or disease of the glomerulus. This is an extremely serious situation, and red cell casts must be looked for carefully when red cells are found. There may be little correlation between the amount of blood and the severity of the disorder, yet the hematuria may be the only indication of renal disease. The occurrence of hematuria without accompanying protein and casts usually indicates that the bleeding is in the lower urogenital tract.

### Microscopic Appearance

Red cells are not easy to find under the microscope. Their detection requires careful examination. The high-power objective is used, and the light must be reduced by proper adjustment of the condenser and iris diaphragm or they will be missed. Their detection also requires continual refocusing with the fine adjustment of the microscope. The phase-contrast microscope is very useful in detecting red blood cells. Even after hemolysis has occurred, the red cell membrane is clearly visible with this technique.

In absolutely fresh urine, red cells will be unaltered or intact and appear much as they do in diluted whole blood. They are seen as pale yellowish orange, intact biconcave disks that are especially apparent as they roll over. Red cells

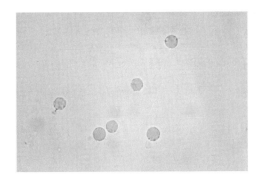

**FIG 14-9.** Red cells. Six intact red cells, unstained, ×400.

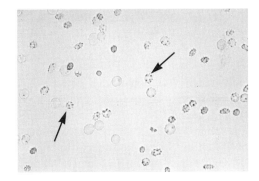

**FIG 14-10.** Crenated red cells *(arrows)*. Intact forms also present. Unstained, ×400.

have a generally smooth appearance, as opposed to the granular appearance of white cells, and are about 7 $\mu$m in diameter (Fig. 14-9). However, they rapidly undergo morphologic changes in urine specimens and are rarely observed as described. This is because urine is rarely an isotonic solution with red cells (the solute concentration within the red cell is rarely the same as the solute concentration of urine). The urine may be more or less concentrated than the blood, and the changes described below result.

When the urine is hypotonic or dilute, as evidenced by low specific gravity, the red cells appear *swollen* and *rounded* because of diffusion of fluid into them. If the urine is hypertonic or concentrated (high specific gravity), the red cells appear **crenated** and **shrunken** because they lose fluid to the urine (Fig. 14-10). When crenated,

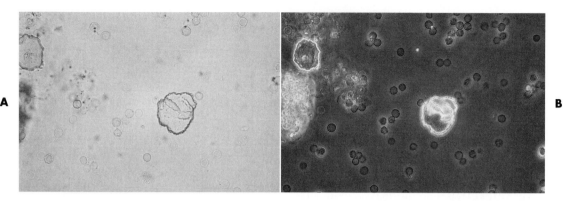

**FIG 14-11.** Red cells. Many ghost or shadow red cells, which are difficult to visualize with bright-field microscopy but are easily seen with phase contrast. Unusual uric acid crystals also present. Unstained, ×400. **A,** Brightfield. **B,** Phase contrast.

the red cells have little spicules, or projections, that cause them to be confused with white cells. However, a crenated red cell is significantly smaller than a white cell and has a generally smooth, rather than granular, appearance. Finally, when the urine is dilute and alkaline, the red cells will often appear as *shadow* or *ghost cells* (Fig. 14-11, A). In this situation the red cells have burst and released their hemoglobin; all that remains is the faint colorless cell membrane, a ghost or shadow of the original cell. This membrane is clearly visible with phase-contrast illumination, however (Fig. 14-11, *B*). Ghosts are often seen in old urine specimens. Eventually, even the ghosts will disappear as the cell completely disintegrates.

**Dysmorphic** red cells may also be seen (Fig. 14-12). These distorted or misshapen red cells may indicate the presence of glomerular disease. The distortion is best seen with phase-contrast illumination (Fig. 14-13). It is also possible to see nucleated red cells or sickle cells (in sickle cell disease) in urine (Fig. 14-14). However, this is extremely rare.

### Structures Confused With Red Cells

Red cells not only are difficult to detect in a urine specimen but also are often confused with

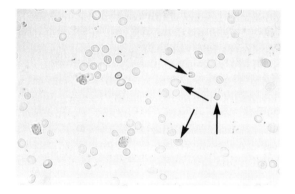

**FIG 14-12.** Dysmorphic red cells *(arrows)*, with many other red cells and three white cells. Sedi-Stain, ×400.

other structures that are found in the urinary sediment.

Red cells are often confused with *white cells (leukocytes);* however, the leukocyte is larger and has a generally granular appearance plus a nucleus. If morphologic differentiation is impossible, a drop of 2% acetic acid may be added to a new preparation or introduced under the coverglass. Acetic acid will lyse the red cells and at the same time stain (or accentuate) the nuclei of leukocytes. With a Sternheimer-Malbin stain, red cells in acidic urine may stain slightly purple or not at all. If the urine is alkaline, the alkaline

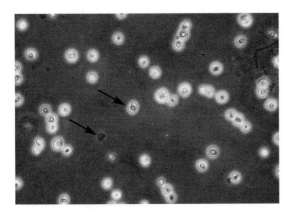

**FIG 14-13.** Dysmorphic red cells *(arrows)*. Phase contrast, ×400.

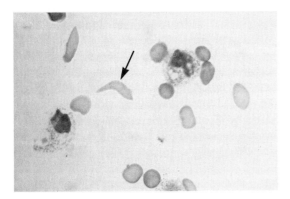

**FIG 14-14.** Sickle cell *(arrow)*, red cells, and two white cells from cytocentrifuged urine sediment of a patient with sickle cell anemia. Wright Stain, ×1000.

hematin that is formed stains dark purple. The reagent strip tests for blood and leukocyte esterase are also helpful.

*Yeast* may also be confused with red cells in urine. However, yeast cells are generally smaller than red cells, are spherical rather than flattened, and vary considerably in size within one specimen. In addition, since yeast reproduces by budding, the occurrence of buds or little outgrowths should identify yeast.

A very rare ovoid form of *calcium oxalate* may also be confused with red cells, especially when viewed with brightfield illumination. However, calcium oxalate crystals are more refractile and,

unlike red cells, polarize light. Thus they are easily differentiated with polarizing microscopy.

*Bubbles or oil droplets* are also confused with red cells, especially by the inexperienced. These vary considerably in size, are extremely refractive or reflective, and are obvious under the microscope.

### Other Considerations

The presence of red blood cells may be indicated by a tiny red button in the bottom of the centrifuge tube after centrifuging.

Red blood cells in the sediment should correlate with a positive reagent strip test for blood. However, since chemical tests are more sensitive to hemoglobin than to intact red cells, it is possible to have a negative reagent strip test when only a few intact red cells are present and no hemolysis has occurred. This is rare. Reagent strip sensitivity is reduced in urine with high specific gravity; the red cell must lyse in order to react. In this situation, red cells may be demonstrated by adding water to the sediment to lyse cells, and then retesting with the reagent test for blood.

When large amounts of vitamin C are present, reagent strip results may be negative or delayed even though red cells are seen in the sediment. In such cases, the sediment result can be confirmed by the use of a reagent strip test for ascorbic acid. Another clue would be the gross appearance of the urinary sediment, or a red button of cells in the bottom of the centrifuge tube.

If the reagent strip test for blood is positive, and red cells are absent in the urine sediment, the presence of hemoglobin or myoglobin in the urine should be considered.

### White Blood Cells (Leukocytes)
#### Clinical Importance

The presence of a few white blood cells or leukocytes in the concentrated urine sediment is normal. Again, reference values vary, but more than a few (as many as five per high-power field) is considered abnormal. The term *white blood cell* or *leukocyte* in urine usually refers to the presence of a neutrophil (polymorphonuclear neutrophil, or PMN). Unless otherwise specified, it is assumed that this is what is meant. However, any white cell type present in blood can also be found in the urinary sediment. The presence of lymphocytes and eosinophils is of particular diagnostic significance and is described later.

The presence of large numbers of white blood cells in the sediment indicates inflammation at some point along the urogenital tract. The inflammation may result from a bacterial infection or other causes. The presence of white blood cells is often associated with bacteria, but both bacteria and white cells can be present alone, without the other. In bacterial infections, ingested bacteria may be seen within the cell. These cells are extremely labile and rapidly disappear from the specimen. If the leukocytes originate in the kidney, rather than lower in the urinary tract (such as in the bladder), they may form cellular casts. Therefore, the presence of casts (usually cellular or granular) along with white blood cells and bacteria would help distinguish an upper (kidney) from a lower (bladder) urinary tract infection. Protein is usually present along with casts, and may or may not be present in a lower urinary tract infection. The condition in which increased numbers of leukocytes are found in urine is termed **pyuria**. Pyuria may cause clouding of the urine, and when this is severe enough the urine will have a characteristic milk-white appearance. Under the microscope the white cells may appear singly or in clumps. The presence of clumps is associated with acute infection.

### Microscopic Appearance

Leukocytes must be searched for with the high-power objective, reduced light, and continual refocusing with fine adjustment. Typically, they are about 10 to 14 $\mu$m in diameter (about twice the size of red cells); however, this size difference may not be obvious, as they often appear about the same size as a red cell. Leukocytes have thin cytoplasmic granulation and a nucleus. Even if the nucleus is not distinct, the center of the cell appears granular (Fig. 14-15). White cells are

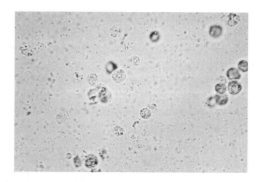

**FIG 14-15.** White cells and many bacteria. Unstained, ×400.

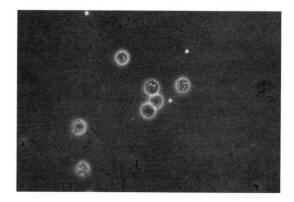

**FIG 14-16.** Several white cells with phase contrast illumination, ×400.

fragile and will disintegrate in old alkaline urine specimens. Various stages of disintegration may be observed in a single urine specimen. Neutrophil leukocytes are especially vulnerable in dilute alkaline urine specimens, and about 50% can be lost within 2 to 3 hours if the urine is kept at room temperature. In addition, the lobed nucleus tends to consolidate, and the neutrophil appears as a mononuclear cell as the cell begins to degenerate. If the urine is dilute, the cell cytoplasm may expand out in petals, without granules, before the neutrophil disintegrates.

Phase-contrast microscopy is especially useful in the detection and identification of white blood cells in the urinary sediment (Fig. 14-16), as is the use of a stain, such as the Sternheimer-Malbin stain (Fig. 14-17). However, precipitation of the stain in the highly alkaline urines associ-

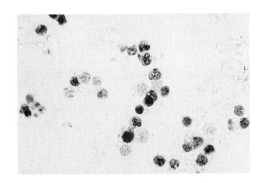

**FIG 14-17.** White cells and bacteria. Sedi-Stain, ×400.

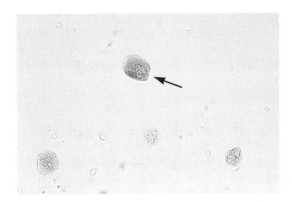

**FIG 14-19.** Renal tubular epithelial cell *(arrow)*. Sedi-Stain, ×400.

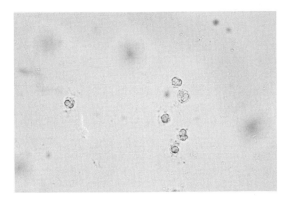

**FIG 14-18.** White cells treated with acetic acid to accentuate the nucleus and differentiate from red cells ×400.

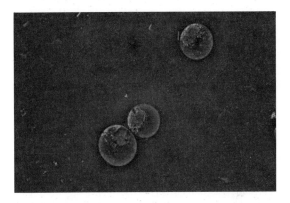

**FIG 14-20.** Glitter cells (swollen neutrophils showing Brownian motion in a wet preparation). Dark phase contrast, ×450.

ated with white cells and bacteria may pose a problem. When stained, neutrophilic leukocytes show a red-purple nucleus and violet or blue cytoplasm, although the same urine specimen may have a variety of staining reactions, and extremely fresh cells may fail to stain.

### Structures Confused With White Cells

Other structures may be mistaken for leukocytes. Most often this occurs with red cells and epithelial cells. White cells are generally larger than red cells, appear granular, and have a nucleus. A 2% acetic acid solution may aid in their identification (Fig. 14-18). There are several very different morphologic types of epithelial cells, but in general they are larger than white cells

and have smaller nuclei. Renal epithelial cells are most like white cells; however, the nucleus is generally round, more distinct, and surrounded by more cytoplasm (Fig. 14-19).

Other white blood cell types that may be seen in the urinary sediment include the following.

### Glitter Cells

These are larger, swollen neutrophilic leukocytes that appear in hypotonic urine with a specific gravity of about 1.010 or less. Their cytoplasmic granules are in constant random (brownian) movement, giving a glittering appearance. These cells are especially striking under phase-contrast illumination (Fig. 14-20). When stained, glitter cells have a light blue or almost colorless cytoplasm and the brownian motion of the granules may or may not be observed. Once thought to indicate chronic pyelonephritis, glitter cells are also seen in dilute urine specimens from patients with lower urinary tract infections.

### Eosinophils

Eosinophils may be present in the urine sediment. They are morphologically very similar to neutrophils and difficult to distinguish, especially with a wet preparation, under both brightfield and phase-contrast illumination. They are typically larger than neutrophils and oval or elongated. The cytoplasmic granules may not be prominent, but the presence of two or three distinct lobes of the nucleus with fresh specimens is helpful. Cytocentrifugation is useful in confirming the presence of eosinophils (Fig. 14-21). However, they do not stain as well with Wright stain as they do in blood smears. Use of special eosinophil stains, such as **Hansel's stain,** is helpful. Increased eosinophils are associated with drug-induced interstitial nephritis, as seen with treatment with penicillins. Detection is important because the treatment is fast and effective, namely discontinuation of the drug.

### Lymphocytes and Other Mononuclear Cells

A few small lymphocytes are normally present in urine, even though they are rarely recognized. They are very difficult to distinguish from red blood cells, especially with the normal

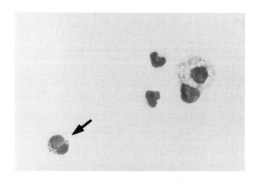

**FIG 14-21.** Eosinophil (arrow), neutrophils, and macrophage. Cytospin preparation, Wright stain, ×1,000.

wet preparation of the urinary sediment, under both brightfield and phase-contrast illumination. They are only slightly larger than red cells, with a single round nucleus and scant cytoplasm. The presence of many small lymphocytes is seen in the first few weeks after renal transplant rejection and is a useful early indicator of this rejection process. If their presence is suspected, identification is most easily confirmed by cytocentrifugation and staining with Wright stain. Since they are not granulocytes, lymphocytes will not react with the reagent strips for leukocyte esterase.

*Monocytes, histiocytes,* and *macrophages* may also be present in the urinary sediment. They are difficult to recognize on the standard wet preparation, but are generally larger than, and resemble, aging neutrophils. The cytoplasm is usually abundant, vacuolated, and granulated. These cells are granulocytes and capable of reacting with the reagent strips for leukocyte esterase. However, the sensitivity of the strips may not be sufficient to detect these cells, which, even when present, are seen in relatively small numbers. Monocytes and histiocytes are associated with chronic inflammation and radiation therapy.

Macrophages may be present with various inclusions within the cytoplasm. These include ingested fat, hemosiderin, red cells, or crystals. As with lymphocytes, identification of other mononuclear cells is most easily confirmed by cytocentrifugation and staining with Wright stain.

## EPITHELIAL CELLS

Except for the single layer of renal epithelial cells lining the tubules of the nephron, the structures that make up the urinary system are lined by several layers of epithelial cells. The layer of epithelial cells closest to the lumen of organs such as the urethra and bladder (besides contaminating cells of the male and female genital tracts) is continually sloughed off **(exfoliated)** into the urine and replaced by cells originating from deeper layers. Therefore, a few squamous epithelial cells are seen in most urine specimens.

The single-layered renal epithelial cells are also sloughed into the urine. The identification of the various epithelial cell types may be difficult yet clinically significant. They include squamous, transitional (urothelial), and renal epithelial cells.

## Squamous Epithelial Cells

Squamous epithelial cells line the urethra and bladder trigone in the female and the distal portion of the male urethra. They also line the vagina, and many of the squamous epithelial cells found in urine are the result of perineal or vaginal contamination in females or foreskin contamination in males. They are the most commonly encountered, and least significant, type of epithelial cell in urine specimens. Squamous epithelial cells can be divided into intermediate and superficial squamous cells. They form the most superficial layer of cells that line the mucosa and are continually sloughed off and replaced by newer, deeper cells.

Squamous epithelial cells are very large, flat cells made up of a thin layer of cytoplasm and a single distinct nucleus (Figs. 14-22 and 14-23). The nucleus is about the size of a red blood cell or lymphocyte, and the cell is about five to seven times the size of a red cell, about 30 to 50 μm. A thin flat cell, it may be rectangular or round. Epithelial cells are large enough to be seen easily under low power and sometimes roll into cigar shapes, which are mistaken for casts (Fig. 14-24). When stained, these cells show a purple nucleus and an abundant pink or violet cytoplasm. They are easily recognized until they begin to degenerate, when they may eventually appear as an amorphous mass. The presence of squamous epithelial cells is of little clinical significance unless they are in large numbers. When the urine is contaminated by vaginal secretions or exudates, sheets of squamous epithelial cells accompanied by many rod-shaped bacteria or yeasts, or both, may be seen.

### Clue Cells

Another type of squamous epithelial cell that might be encountered in the urine is of vaginal

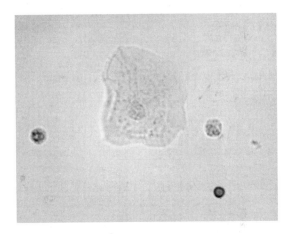

**FIG 14-23.** Squamous epithelial cell, two white cells, one red cell. Sedi-Stain, ×400.

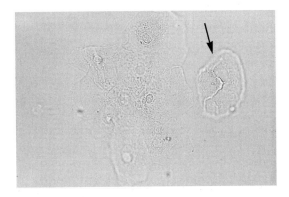

**FIG 14-24.** Several degenerating squamous epithelial cells with one folded cell (*arrow*) like a possible cast. Unstained, ×400.

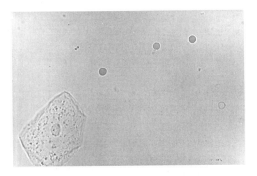

**FIG 14-22.** Squamous epithelial cell and three red cells. Unstained, ×400.

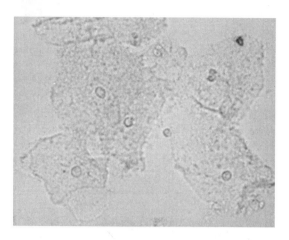

**FIG 14-25.** Several clue cells, vaginal squamous epithelial cells covered with *G. vaginalis*. Unstained, ×400.

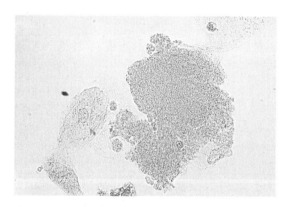

**FIG 14-26.** Clue cells. Sedi-Stain, ×400.

origin and is referred to as a clue cell. **Clue cells** are vaginal squamous epithelial cells that are covered, or encrusted, with a bacterium, *Gardnerella vaginalis.* They are usually searched for in wet mounts of vaginal swabs, and their presence indicates bacterial vaginitis caused by *Gardnerella.* They are coccobacilli and give the cytoplasm a characteristic refractile, stippled, or granular appearance with shaggy or bearded cell borders. Most, but not necessarily all, of the cell surface should be covered with bacteria, and the bacteria should extend beyond the cytoplas-

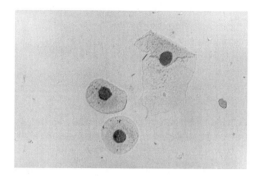

**FIG 14-27.** Two transitional epithelial cells, one folded squamous epithelial cell, and one dysmorphic red cell. Cytospin, Wright stain, ×400.

mic margins, in order for the cell to be called a clue cell (Figs. 14-25 and 14-26). The occasional keratohyaline granules in the cytoplasm of squamous epithelial cells should not be mistaken for clue cells.

### Transitional Epithelial (Urothelial) Cells

Transitional epithelial cells occur in multiple layers. They line the urinary tract, from the kidney pelvis in both females and males to the base of the bladder in the female and the proximal part of the urethra in the male. As the cell layers become deeper, the cells become thicker and rounded, looking more and more like renal epithelial cells or white blood cells. Their size varies with the depth and place of origin in the transitional epithelium. However, in general they are about four to six times the size of a red blood cell (20 to 30 $\mu$m), and appear smaller and plumper than squamous epithelial cells (Fig. 14-27). They are spherical or polyhedral in shape. Since they readily take on water, they are often spherical from swelling—like a balloon of water. They are generally larger than renal tubular cells and have a round nucleus (sometimes two nuclei) very similar in size and appearance to the nucleus seen in a squamous epithelial cell (Fig. 14-28). The more superficial bladder epithelial cells are large flat cells of a squamous na-

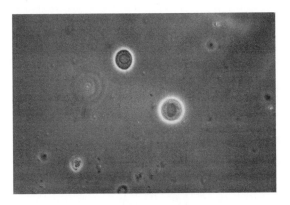

**FIG 14-28.** Two medium-sized transitional epithelial cells. Phase contrast, ×400.

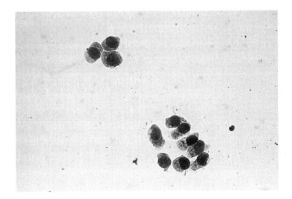

**FIG 14-29.** Many small transitional epithelial cells after catheterization of a 1-month-old infant. Sedi-Stain, ×400.

ture. Transitional epithelial cells stain with a dark blue nucleus and varying amounts of pale blue cytoplasm, which may have occasional inclusions. Some of these cells have tails and are indistinguishable from the caudate cells of the renal pelvis.

A few transitional epithelial cells are present in the urine of normal persons. Increased numbers are seen in the presence of infection. Clusters or sheets of these cells are seen after urethral or ureteral catheterization and with urinary tract lesions (Fig. 14-29). Urothelial cells may show malignant changes, and such cells should be referred for cytologic examination. Radiation therapy may result in large cells with multiple nuclei and vacuoles (Fig. 14-30).

### Renal Epithelial Cells

Renal epithelial cells are the single layer of cells that line the nephron from the proximal to the distal convoluted tubules, plus the cells lining the collecting ducts to the pelvis of the kidney. Their occurrence in urine is important, for it implies a serious pathologic condition and destruction of renal tubules, as does the presence of epithelial casts. Identification is difficult in wet preparations with both bright-field and phase contrast. Morphology varies, depending on the site of origin within the nephron, as shown in Fig. 14-31. Intact renal

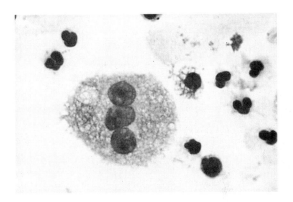

**FIG 14-30.** Multinucleated and vacuolated transitional epithelial cell as seen after radiation therapy. Cytospin, Wright Stain, ×1000.

epithelial cells are from three to five times the size of red cells—that is, slightly larger to twice as large as a neutrophil. Cells from the proximal convoluted tubules are relatively large and elongated or oval, with a granular cytoplasm. The granularity makes the proximal tubular cells, in particular, appear as small or fragmented granular casts (Fig. 14-32). The nucleus is extremely difficult to see in these renal epithelial cells in wet preparations. The use of cytocentrifugation and staining with Wright stain will help visualize the nucleus and show these structures to be cells rather

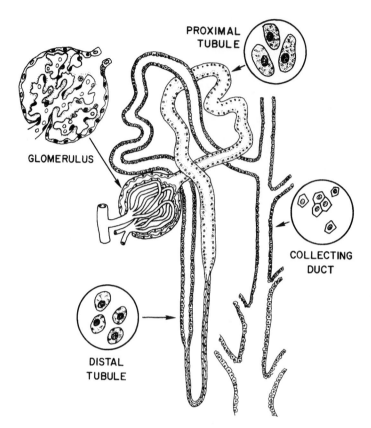

**FIG 14-31.** Diagram of nephron showing the locations of origin of the various types of renal epithelial cells seen in the urine sediment. (From Kaplan LA, Pesce AJ: *Clinical Chemistry,* ed 3, St Louis, Mosby, 1996, p 1131.)

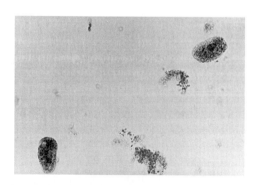

**FIG 14-32.** Two proximal renal tubular epithelial cells, appearing like small granular casts. Amorphous urates also present. Sedi-Stain, ×400.

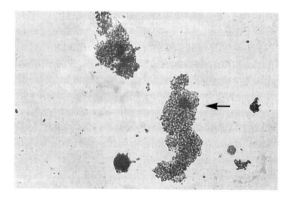

**FIG 14-33.** Cytocentrifuged preparation of proximal renal tubular epithelial cells appearing like granular casts (*arrow*). Cytospin, Wright stain, ×400.

than casts (Fig. 14-33). However, the traditional cytologic examination with the Papanicolaou stain is recommended (Fig. 14-34).

Renal epithelial cells are very difficult to identify in wet preparations. They resemble both white blood cells and smaller transitional epithelial cells. Morphologically, renal epithelial cells closely resemble leukocytes, especially degenerating ones, but they are typically larger and have a distinct single round nucleus (Figs. 14-35 and 14-36). Renal cells of the collecting tubules tend to be polyhedral or cuboid—one side tends to be flat, as opposed to the rounded cell more typical of transitional epithelial cells (Fig. 14-37). (Unlike transitional epithelial cells, renal cells do not absorb water and swell; therefore, they tend to retain their polyhedral shape.) When these cells are stained, the nucleus stains a dark shade of blue-purple and the cytoplasm a lighter shade of blue-purple. Again, cytocentrifugation and Pap stain are helpful, as seen in Figs. 14-38 and 14-39.

As is the case with all epithelial cells, renal epithelial cells will not react with the leukocyte

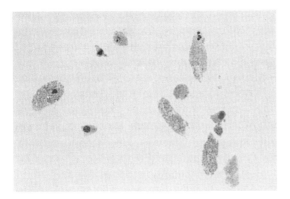

**FIG 14-34.** Cytocentrifuged preparation of proximal renal tubular epithelial cells appearing like granular casts. Cytospin, Papanicolaou stain, ×400.

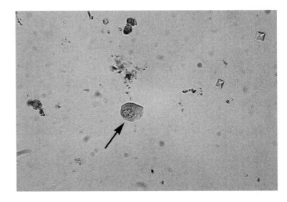

**FIG 14-36.** Renal epithelial cell (arrow). Sedi-Stain, ×400.

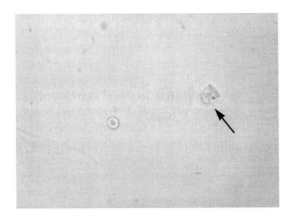

**FIG 14-35.** Renal epithelial cel (arrow) and one red cell. Unstained, ×400.

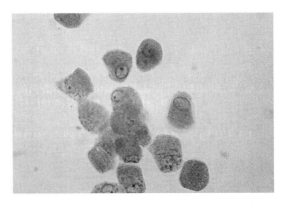

**FIG 14-37.** Cuboidial or polyhedral renal tubular epithelial cells, probably from the small collecting ducts; very difficult to differentiate from transitional epithelial cells. Sedi-Stain, ×400.

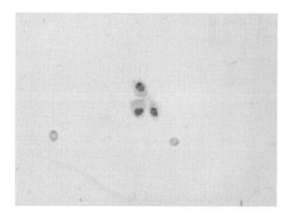

**FIG 14-38.** Three renal epithelial cells; two red cells also present. Cytospin, Papanicolaou stain, ×400.

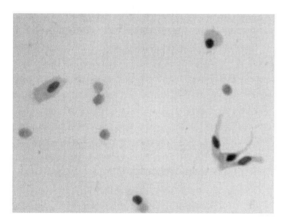

**FIG 14-39.** Renal epithelial cells, including three caudate forms. Red cells also present. Cytospin, Papanicolaou stain, ×400.

esterase reagent strips. This may be helpful in distinguishing them from neutrophils. Renal epithelial cells are associated with the presence of protein in the urine and are often found in association with casts. The presence of epithelial or granular casts will help confirm their identification, and when renal cells are suspected, casts should be searched for with great care. The phase-contrast microscope is particularly useful in such situations.

### Renal Epithelial Fragments

These are fragments or groups of three or more renal epithelial cells originating from the collect-

ing ducts. Their presence is more serious than the presence of individual renal epithelial cells, as they indicate renal tubular injury with disruption of the basement membrane.

### Oval Fat Bodies

These are a special type of renal epithelial cell that are filled with fat (lipid) droplets. **Oval fat bodies (OFB)** are sometimes referred to as **renal tubular fat (RTF)** or renal tubular fat bodies. They indicate serious pathology and must not be overlooked when present in the urinary sediment. The fat droplets are generally contained within degenerating or necrotic renal epithelial cells, although some oval fat bodies may be macrophages that have filled with fat. The fat droplets contained within these cells are highly refractive, coarse droplets that vary greatly in size (Figs. 14-40 and 14-41). They are more easily visualized with brightfield than phase-contrast microscopy. Although they are cells filled with fat, the cell nucleus is commonly invisible. Certain aids to the identification of oval fat bodies are available. When stained with Sternheimer-Malbin stain, fat globules do not become colored but appear highly refractive in a blue-purple background. When stained with fat stains such as Sudan III or oil red O, globules of triglyceride or neutral fat appear orange or red (Fig. 14-42). Polarized light is useful for indicating the presence of cholesterol esters in the fat. Cholesterol esters show a typical Maltese cross pattern when viewed with polarizing filters (Fig. 14-43). However, triglycerides or neutral fat do not show this pattern with polarized light. The appearance of a Maltese cross pattern is also seen with starch, a common urine contaminant. Fat should be confirmed by careful microscopic examination or specific staining. Oval fat bodies are often seen along with fat droplets and fatty casts in the urinary sediment, and the other two components should be searched for carefully when one is present. Oval fat bodies resulting from tubular epithelial degeneration of the nephron are associated with large amounts of protein in the urine, as in the nephrotic syndrome. The fatty material in the tubular cells

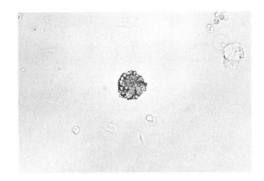

**FIG 14-40.** Oval fat body. Unstained, ×400.

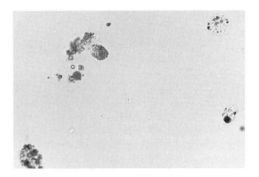

**FIG 14-42.** Several oval fat bodies and free fat stained with Sudan III stain, indicating the presence of neutral fat or triglycerides. (×400.)

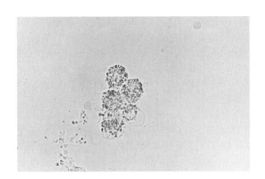

**FIG 14-41.** Clump of oval fat bodies. Unstained, ×400.

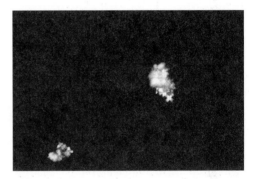

**FIG 14-43.** Oval fat bodies showing the typical Maltese cross of cholesterol esters when viewed with polarized light. (×400.)

may be the lipoprotein that passes through the damaged glomerulus in this syndrome. The lipoprotein may be ingested by the renal tubular cell, which metabolizes it into cholesterol. Clinically the presence of neutral fat (triglyceride) and the presence of cholesterol are equal.

### Fat Globules

Although not a cellular constituent, fat globules are discussed now because of their relationship to oval fat bodies. Fat globules may be found in the urinary sediment as highly refractive droplets of various sizes (Fig. 14-44). When their source is biological (rather than contamination), a serious pathologic condition implying severe renal dysfunction exists. Such lipiduria is also associated with the nephrotic

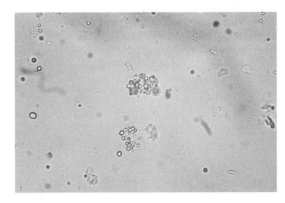

**FIG 14-44.** Free fat and oval fat bodies. Unstained, ×400.

syndrome and its various causes, diabetes mellitus, and conditions that result in severe damage to renal tubular epithelial cells, such as ethylene glycol or mercury poisoning. Fat globules are found in association with oval fat bodies and fatty casts. Fat stains orange or red with Sudan stains or oil red O. The identification may be aided by the use of polarized light, as cholesterol will show a Maltese cross pattern when so viewed. Fat in urine may also come from extraneous sources such as unclean collection utensils or oiled catheters (see Fig. 14-124). This is less common with the use of disposable urine collection containers.

### Hemosiderin

Occasionally, renal epithelial cells with granules of hemosiderin in the cytoplasm are seen in the urine sediment. This occurs several days after a hemolytic episode, when free hemoglobin has passed through the glomerulus into the nephron. The hemosiderin granules appear as yellow or colorless granules that are morphologically similar to amorphous urates. Unlike urates, they will stain blue with a Prussian blue stain for iron (the Rous test). Besides their presence in desquamated renal epithelial cells, granules of hemosiderin may be seen as free granules in the sediment, in macrophages, and in casts (Fig. 14-45).

### Viral Inclusion Bodies

Renal tubular epithelial cells may also be seen with viral inclusion bodies. This is especially characteristic of infection with cytomegalovirus. They are difficult to recognize on wet preparations. Cytocentrifugation and staining with the Papanicolaou stain are helpful in recognizing this condition (Fig. 14-46).

### Tumor Cells

Tumor cells and other cell forms with altered cytologic features may be found in the urine sediment. However, these cell forms cannot be diagnosed from the usual urinary sediment preparation but require special collection, cyto-

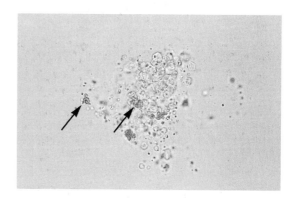

**FIG 14-45.** Hemosiderin, yellow-brown granules (arrows). Unstained, ×400.

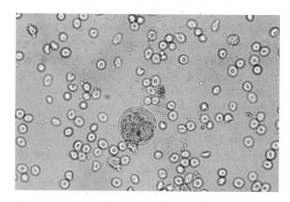

**FIG 14-46.** Inclusion bodies in macrophage or epithelial cell. Many red blood cells also present. Sedi-Stain, ×400.

centrifugation, and stains and examination by qualified personnel. If their presence is suspected from the examination of the sediment, the specimen should be referred accordingly. The presence of red cells in the chemical examination of the urine is an early diagnostic clue.

## OTHER CELLULAR CONSTITUENTS

### Spermatozoa

**Spermatozoa** may be present in the urine of both males and females. Laboratory protocol should be established and followed as to when the presence of sperm is to be reported. In fertility studies and cases of possible sexual abuse the presence of spermatozoa may be an important finding.

Spermatozoa are easily recognized by their oval body (head) and long delicate tail. The head is about 4 to 6 $\mu$m long (smaller and narrower than a red cell), and the tail is about 40 to 60 $\mu$m long. Spermatozoa may be motile in wet preparation (an aid to identification), or they may be stationary. Phase-contrast microscopy is especially helpful in identification (Fig. 14-47).

## Bacteria

Under normal conditions the urinary tract is free of bacteria. However, most urine specimens contain at least a few bacteria because of contamination when the urine is voided. Bacteria multiply rapidly when urine stands at room temperature. In specimens that are obtained in a manner suitable for urine culture and kept under sterile conditions, the presence of bacteria may indicate a urinary tract infection. In this case, they are likely to be associated with the presence of white blood cells, although this is not always true. Bacterial infection should be confirmed by quantitative urine culture.

Bacteria are recognizable morphologically in wet preparation under high power. They are extremely small, only a few micrometers long. They may be either rods or cocci and may occur singly, in pairs, in chains, or in tetrads. Rods are more easily recognized than cocci because of their larger size, although some rods are extremely short and difficult to tell from cocci. Bacteria are often motile, which helps in their identification. Occasionally, unusually long rod-shaped forms with central swelling are seen. These **protoplasts** are the result of damage to the cell wall by antibiotics (especially penicillins) used in therapy (Fig. 14-48).

Bacteria are most often seen in alkaline urine and may be confused with amorphous material at first, but this will not be a problem as experience in observation is gained. Phase-contrast microscopy is very useful in the visualization of bacteria, which are difficult to see with bright-field illumination. Although not normally part

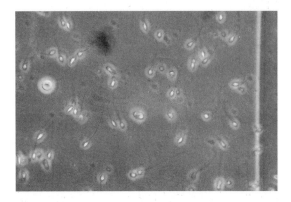

**FIG 14-47.** Sperm, many, in counting chamber. Phase contrast, ×400.

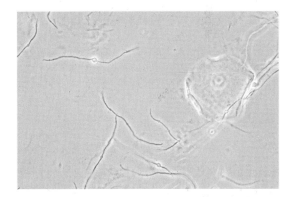

**FIG 14-48.** Many protoplasts (one at arrow), and a squamous epithelial cell. Phase contrast, ×400.

of urinalysis, Gram staining a drop of concentrated sediment is helpful in recognition of bacteria in difficult specimens. On Wright stained cytocentifuged preparations all bacteria will stain deep blue-purple (basophilic).

In lower urinary tract (bladder) infections, bacteria are generally, but not always, associated with the presence of white blood cells (leukocytes, PMNs). Mild proteinuria and a positive reagent strip test for nitrites or leukocyte esterase may also be seen. With upper urinary tract (kidney) infections, bacteria may be seen along with white cells and casts—leukocyte (white cell), cellular, or granular. There may be moderate proteinuria and a pos-

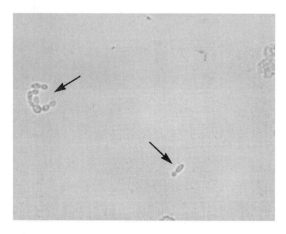

**FIG 14-49.** Yeast *(arrows)*. Unstained, ×400.

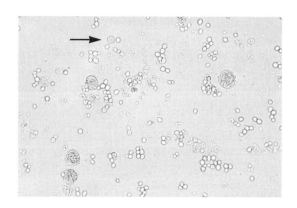

**FIG 14-51.** Many yeast, four white cells, and one red cell *(arrow)*. Sedi-Stain, ×400.

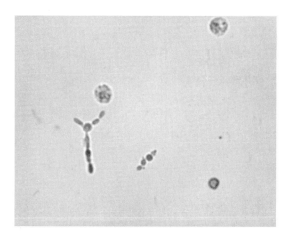

**FIG 14-50.** Yeast, two white cells, one red cell. Sedi-Stain, ×400.

itive reagent strip test for nitrites or leukocyte esterase.

## Yeast

Yeast cells are occasionally seen in urine, especially from females and diabetic patients. They are often present as the result of contamination of the urine from a vaginal yeast infection. They are associated with the presence of sugar in the urine. Sugar is the energy source for yeast cells, which grow and multiply rapidly when it is present. For this reason yeast cells are often discovered in the urine of diabetics, along with a

high sugar content, low pH, and ketones. Yeast cells are also common contaminants from skin and air, and infections are seen in debilitated and immunosupressed or immunocompromised patients.

Yeast cells are often mistaken for red blood cells. They are generally smaller than red cells and show considerable size variation, even within a specimen. They have a typically ovoid shape, lack color, and have a smooth and refractive appearance. The most distinguishing characteristic is the presence of little buds, or projections, because of their manner of reproduction (Figs. 14-49 to 14-51). Pseudomycelial forms of *Candida* sp. (the type of yeast usually present) may also be seen. These are elongated cells, which may be up to 50 μm long, and resemble mycelia of true fungi. These **pseudohyphae** may be branched and have terminal buds (Fig. 14-52). They are clinically significant in the urine of debilitated patients with severe *Candida* infection such as that seen in immunosuppressed patients. Other mycelial forms of yeast have been seen; these should not be mistaken for casts (Fig. 14-53).

## Trichomonas vaginalis

*Trichomonas vaginalis* is the parasite most frequently seen in urine specimens. This protozoan

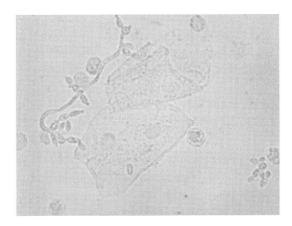

**FIG 14-52.** Yeast, several and with pseudohyphae. Two squamous epithelial and white cells. Unstained, ×400.

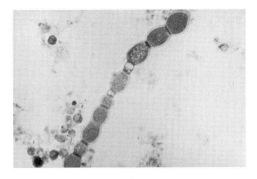

**FIG 14-53.** Large, unusual mycelia-like yeast, not to be mistaken for casts. Sedi-Stain, ×400.

is primarily responsible for vaginal infections; however, it also may infect the urethra, periurethral glands, bladder, and prostate. It generally resides in the vagina in women and prostate in men, where it feeds on the mucosal surface and ingests bacteria and leukocytes that may be present. The organism is motile, which is an aid to its identification. When an infection is suspected, direct swabs of the vagina or urethra are examined, although the organisms may be seen contaminating the urine sediment.

*Trichomonas* is a unicellular flagellated organism—a protozoan. It has a characteristic pear-shaped appearance, with a single nucleus, four anterior flagella, and an undulating membrane, and sharp protruding posterior axostyle (Fig. 14-54). The most distinguishing feature of trichomonas is its motility—a rapid, jerky, rotating, nondirectional motion that is easily recognized in wet preparations. The organisms are larger than typical leukocytes (up to 30 $\mu$m long) and may resemble transitional epithelial cells, especially when no longer motile. Phase-contrast microscopy is particularly useful in visualization, especially of the flagella (Fig. 14-55). When stained, the cells lose their characteristic motility as they round up and die, appearing very similar to degenerating transitional epithelial cell forms (Fig. 14-56). (See also under *Trichomonas vaginalis* in Chapter 16).

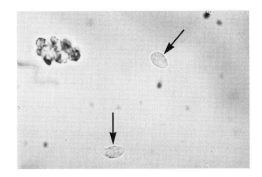

**FIG 14-54.** *Trichomonas,* pear shaped *(arrows).* Unstained, ×400.

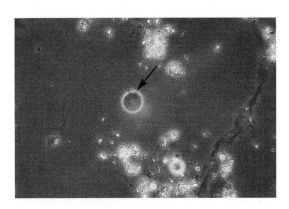

**FIG 14-55.** *Trichomonas,* rounded with flagella *(arrow).* Phase contrast, ×400.

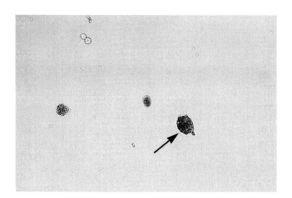

**FIG 14-56.** Presumed *Trichomonas (arrow)*, white cells, and yeast. Sedi-Stain, ×400.

## Other Parasites

Various other parasites may be seen in urine as the result of fecal or vaginal contamination and may be common to particular geographic areas and patient populations. All of these require special knowledge for identification; however, they may be noticed initially during urinalysis and then referred for identification.

Enterobius vermicularis, or pinworm, is a fairly common helminth infecting the intestinal tract, which may occasionally be seen in the urine in larval or egg (ova) form. (See also under *Enterobius vermicularis* in Chapter 16). Other parasites occasionally seen in urine include *Trichuris*, or whipworm, *Schistosoma, Strongyloides,* and *Giardia,* and various amebae. Various insects or "bugs" possibly seen in urine specimens include lice, fleas, bedbugs, mites, and ticks.

## CASTS

### Formation and Significance

Casts are at once the most difficult portion of the urinary sediment to discover and the most important. Their importance and their name derive from the manner in which they are produced. Casts are formed in the lumen of the tubules of the nephrons (the working units of the kidney) by solidification of material in the tubules. They are important because anything that is con-tained within the tubule is flushed out in the cast. Thus a cast represents a biopsy of an individual tubule and is a means of examining the contents of the nephron. It is believed that casts may be formed at any point along the nephron, either by precipitation of protein or by grouping together (conglutination) of material within the tubular lumen. In either case, the basic structure of the cast is a protein matrix. All casts have a matrix of Tamm-Horsfall mucoprotein; in addition, plasma proteins may be present. Before casts can form within the renal tubules, certain conditions must exist. Since the cast is made of protein, there must be a sufficient concentration of protein within the tubule. In addition, the pH must be low enough to favor precipitation and there must be a sufficient concentration of solutes. For the same reasons, casts are not likely to be found in dilute alkaline urine, since these conditions do not favor their formation. This also means that the urine must be examined when fresh, for as it becomes alkaline with aging the casts will disintegrate.

Since casts represent a biopsy of the kidney, they are extremely important clinically. They often contain red blood cells, white blood cells, epithelial cells, fat globules, or bacteria. These inclusions are not normally present within the renal tubule; they represent an abnormal situation. The formation of casts implies that there was at least a temporary blocking of the renal tubules. Although a few hyaline casts consisting only of precipitated Tamm-Horsfall mucoprotein may be seen in "normal" urine, increased numbers of casts indicate renal disease rather than lower urinary tract disease. The number of hyaline casts may increase in mild irritations of the kidney associated with dehydration or physical exercise. The presence of other types of casts represents a serious (pathologic) situation.

### Identification and Morphology of Casts

Casts are extremely difficult to see and must be searched for carefully with reduced light and the low-power objective. They are found and enumerated under low power, but must be

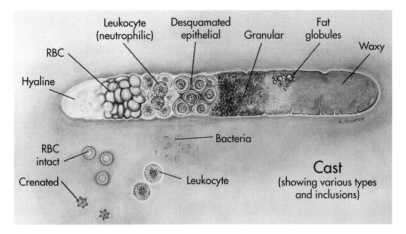

Leukocyte (neutrophilic) Desquamated epithelial Granular Fat globules Waxy

RBC

Hyaline

RBC intact

Crenated

Bacteria

Leukocyte

**Cast**
(showing various types and inclusions)

**FIG 14-57.** Archetypal cast (showing various types and inclusions).

identified as to type by means of the high-power objective. The refractive index of the cast is nearly the same as that of glass, which means that the image is very difficult to see under the microscope. It is for this reason that phase-contrast and interference-contrast microscopy are so useful in the examination of the urine sediment. Phase-contrast microscopy gives sufficient contrast that structures are not overlooked, while differential interference microscopy gives an appreciation of the shape and inclusions within these structures. Stains such as the Sternheimer-Malbin stain are also particularly useful for the discovery of casts in the urinary sediment. Casts that might otherwise be overlooked in brightfield examination, especially by the inexperienced observer, become obvious when so stained, although the presence of mucous strands in the sediment might be confusing, especially in searching for hyaline casts.

As might be imagined from the shape of the tubular lumen, casts are cylindrical bodies and have rounded ends. To be identified as a cast, a structure should have an even and definite outline, parallel sides, and two rounded ends. Although they vary somewhat in size, casts should have a uniform diameter (about seven or eight times the diameter of a red cell) and be several times longer than wide.

Although casts ideally have parallel sides and two rounded ends, this is not always the case. Casts take on the shape of the tubule in which they are formed. They may be serpentine or convoluted and are often folded. One end may taper off to a tail or point. Such structures have been referred to as **cylindroids,** but they should be considered to be, and enumerated along with, hyaline casts. Cylindroids are often confused with strands of mucus, and care must be taken to avoid this mistake. In addition, casts may be fragmented or broken, and waxy casts typically show blunt, rather than rounded, ends. Judgment is necessary in the enumeration of such structures. The whole urine sediment picture must be considered so that important pathologic findings are reported. Conversely, the occurrence of only one questionable cast, with no other pathologic indicators, should not be reported.

### Classification of Casts

Classification of casts is not always simple. In the laboratory it is done mainly on the basis of morphologic groupings: hyaline, cellular, granular, waxy, fatty, pigmented, or inclusion. However, a urine specimen may contain more than one morphologic type, and a particular cast may be of mixed morphology—for instance, one end may be hyaline and the other cellular. This is shown in the extreme in Fig. 14-57.

Casts are felt to arise either by precipitation of protein within the renal tubule or by conglutination (clumping) of material within the tubular lumen. Both types of casts may contain inclusions. Casts formed by protein precipitation may trap any other substance, such as leukocytes, fat, bacteria, red cells, desquamated renal tubular epithelium, or crystals, that may be present. Casts formed by either mechanism may appear coarsely or finely granular or waxy, as cells disintegrate when the cast is retained in the tubule before being flushed out of the kidney. Structures will also disintegrate if the urine specimen stands.

In any case, casts have a protein matrix, and the presence of casts in the urine is virtually always accompanied by proteinuria. Tamm-Horsfall protein is a specific mucoprotein that is secreted by the renal tubular cells. It has been identified immunologically and found to be present in all casts. Other immunoproteins have been identified in certain casts, although they are not found exclusively in any particular type of cast or disease state.

The following morphologic classification is based on appearance, physical properties, and existence of cellular components. The appearance of a cast when it is seen in the urine may not be the same as when it was originally formed in the renal tubule. If the cast is retained in the kidney (as happens in oliguric patients), cells present in it change in appearance. As the cells degenerate in the cast, their cytoplasm becomes granular. This is followed by loss of cell membranes, resulting in large or coarse granules. As these granules degenerate further, the cast shows smaller or fine granules. The final step in this degeneration is complete lack of structure, with the protein changed or coagulated into a thick, very refractive, opaque substance with a waxlike appearance, referred to as a **waxy cast.** These are the most serious casts pathologically, as the formation of the waxy material implies a greatly lengthened transit time, or shutdown of the portion of the kidney where the structure evolved. Such casts are sometimes referred to as renal failure casts.

The width or diameter of a cast is important clinically. Most casts have a fairly constant diameter, as do the tubules in which they are formed, although casts from small children are narrower than those from adults. **Narrow casts** probably result from swelling of the tubular epithelium, as in an inflammatory process, with narrowing of the tubular lumen. They are not particularly important and tend to be of a hyaline type. **Broad casts** are much more serious. Their diameter is several times greater than normal. This is felt to result from their formation in dilated renal tubules or in collecting tubules (several nephrons empty into a common collecting tubule, which has a greater diameter than the renal tubule). Severe chronic renal disease or obstruction (stasis) will often result in dilation and destruction of renal tubules. Cast formation in the collecting tubules must result from urinary stasis in the group of nephrons feeding a single collecting tubule. If not, the fluid pressure would be far too great for cast formation to occur. This represents serious stasis, and the presence of a significant number of broad casts in the urine sediment is considered to be a bad sign. Broad casts can be of almost any type, but because of the degree of stasis necessary for their formation, most tend to be waxy.

The types of casts that are encountered in the microscopic analysis of the urinary sediment will now be described in a morphologic classification. These are summarized in Table 14-16. Staining reactions that are described pertain to the Sternheimer-Malbin crystal violet safranin stain (Sedi-Stain).

### Hyaline Casts

Hyaline casts are colorless, homogeneous, nonrefractive, semitransparent structures (Fig. 14-58). They are the most difficult casts to discover under the microscope and the least important clinically. They require careful adjustment of light with the brightfield microscope; the light is adjusted to give contrast by lowering the condenser slightly and closing the iris diaphragm.

Phase-contrast and interference microscopy are especially valuable tools in the search for hyaline casts. Stain is also useful; hyaline casts stain a uniform pale pink or pale blue. However, they may take up a minimum of stain and remain difficult to visualize. Hyaline casts may be difficult to distinguish from mucous threads when they are present in the urine, both when stained and when observed by phase-contrast microscopy.

Hyaline casts result from solidification of Tamm-Horsfall protein, which is secreted by the renal tubular cells and may be seen without significant proteinuria. They will include any material that may be present in the tubular lumen at the time of formation, such as cells or cellular debris.

Although they are generally of the classic shape for identification as a cast (i.e., parallel sides, uniform diameter, definite borders, and rounded ends), very interesting modifications, representing molds of the tubular lumen where they are formed, may be observed. Some hyaline casts are broad, while others are thin and elongated; serpentine and folded forms are not unusual. **Cylindroids** are hyaline casts with one end that has not rounded off. They have the same significance, and should be enumerated and reported as hyaline casts (Fig. 14-59).

Hyaline casts are soluble in water and even more soluble in slightly alkaline solution. They are therefore more likely to be found in concentrated, acidic urine and may not form in advanced renal failure because of the inability to concentrate the urine or maintain the normal acid pH. In addition, hyaline casts dissolve if the urine stands and becomes alkaline. Hyaline casts may be further classified according to their

### TABLE 14-16

Morphologic Classification of Casts

Hyaline cast
Cellular cast
 White blood cell (leukocyte, neutrophil, pus) cast
 Red blood cell (blood, hemoglobin, hemoglobin pigment) cast
 Epithelial cell cast
 Bacterial cast
 Mixed cell cast
Granular cast
Waxy cast
Fatty cast
 Oval fat body cast
Pigmented casts
 Hemoglobin (blood) cast
 Myoglobin cast
 Bilirubin cast
 Drug pigment cast
Inclusion casts
 (Granular cast)
 (Fatty cast)
 Hemosiderin cast
 Crystal cast

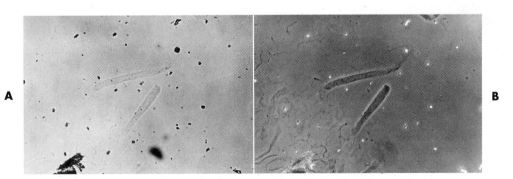

**A**                                                                 **B**

**FIG 14-58.** Two hyaline casts (cylindroids). Mucous threads also present. Note increased visibility with phase contrast. Unstained, ×100. **A,** Brightfield. **B,** Phase contrast.

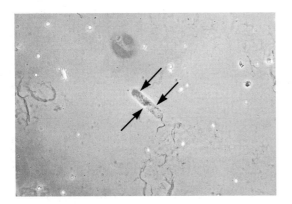

**FIG 14-59.** Cylindroid (hyaline cast with tail) at arrows. Mucus also present. Phase contrast, ×100.

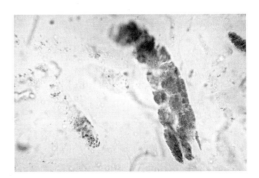

**FIG 14-60.** Cellular cast (probably epithelial cell in origin) Sedi-Stain, ×450.

inclusions, as hyaline cellular (red, white, or epithelial), hyaline granular, and hyaline fatty casts.

Simple hyaline casts are the least important clinically, and a few (less than two per low-power field) may be seen in urine from normal persons. They may be seen in increased numbers after strenuous exercise; however, the sediment returns to normal in 24 to 48 hours. They may be seen in large numbers (20 or 30 per low-power field) in moderate or severe renal disease.

### Cellular Casts

These casts contain intact white cells, red cells, or epithelial cells. They are called white cell (or pus) casts, red blood cell (or blood) casts, and epithelial casts. Bacterial casts have also been described. A truly cellular cast appears to result from clumping, or conglutination, of cells rather than simply precipitation of protein and entrapment of cells, although they are still incorporated in a protein matrix. Alternatively, smaller numbers of the same cell types may be embedded in a hyaline cast.

Cellular casts indicate the presence of cells in the renal tubules. Whenever this occurs, although there are a variety of causes and different degrees of severity, a serious situation exists.

It may be difficult, if not impossible, to distinguish the type of cell in a cast, especially

when cells begin to deteriorate. In such a situation, the best indicator is probably the nature of other constituents in the urine sediment. Leukocytes and bacteria in the sediment would be associated with leukocyte (white cell) casts, while epithelial casts are more likely to be accompanied by cells appearing to be renal epithelium (Fig. 14-60). Glitter cells are often seen when phagocytic neutrophils are present. When a morphologic distinction is impossible, the cast should be reported merely as a cellular cast, rather than misidentifying it (Fig. 14-61). The clinician will use other findings in the urine specimen, both chemical and microscopic, to infer the cell type or source.

Cellular casts are more easily detected under the microscope than hyaline casts, since the cells give them a definite structure as compared with homogeneous solidified protein of the hyaline cast. They must still be searched for with care, however, and proper illumination of the bright-field microscope is essential. Phase-contrast or interference microscopy and stains and cytocentrifugation are useful tools in the examination of the urinary sediment for cellular casts.

**White Blood Cell Casts.** These casts are also referred to as leukocyte casts, or pus casts, when neutrophilic leukocytes are present. When leukocytes are present in a cast, it is

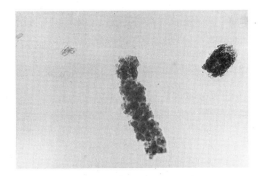

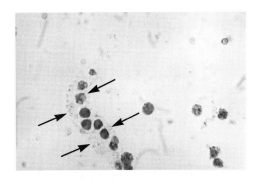

**FIG 14-61.** Cellular cast, probably red cell in origin. Sedi-Stain, ×400.

**FIG 14-62.** White cell cast (arrows) and white cells. Sedi-Stain, ×450.

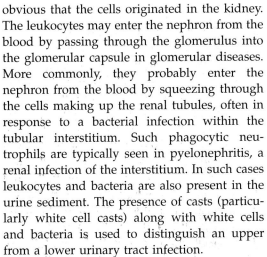

obvious that the cells originated in the kidney. The leukocytes may enter the nephron from the blood by passing through the glomerulus into the glomerular capsule in glomerular diseases. More commonly, they probably enter the nephron from the blood by squeezing through the cells making up the renal tubules, often in response to a bacterial infection within the tubular interstitium. Such phagocytic neutrophils are typically seen in pyelonephritis, a renal infection of the interstitium. In such cases leukocytes and bacteria are also present in the urine sediment. The presence of casts (particularly white cell casts) along with white cells and bacteria is used to distinguish an upper from a lower urinary tract infection.

White cell casts are seen fairly easily in the urinary sediment with the brightfield microscope (Fig. 14-62). The cells are fairly prominent, and the characteristic multilobular nucleus can usually be seen. Small leukocytes stain purple to violet, while large ones may be pale blue, in a pink matrix. As the cells disintegrate within the cast, their cytoplasm becomes granular, cell borders merge, and nuclei become indistinct, resulting in a granular cast when the cells are no longer distinguishable. The number of cells in a cast varies; some casts are packed with cells, while others show only a few cells in a hyaline matrix. White cell casts

packed with cells still have a protein matrix, and should have parallel sides and rounded ends. It is sometimes difficult to distinguish such a white cell cast from a clump of leukocytes **(pseudoleukocyte cast),** which may originate lower in the urinary tract. The presence of strands of mucus to which the white cells adhere is another complication. Yet it is important not to report such **pseudocasts** as casts, which imply renal involvement or disease.

**Epithelial Cell Casts.** At this point it should be obvious that to be called an epithelial cell cast, the epithelial cell must be renal tubular in origin. Epithelial casts represent a most serious situation, although they are infrequently seen in the urine. They may be seen in cases of exposure to nephrotoxic substances such as mercury or ethylene glycol (antifreeze), or in infections with viruses such as cytomegalovirus or hepatitis virus. They result from destruction or desquamation of the cells that line the renal tubules. These cells are responsible for the work done by the kidney. The damage may be irreversible, depending on the severity of the disease process. The time needed to replace renal epithelial cells, if the basement membrane is left intact, is unknown; however, cells do not show maximum concentrating ability for several months after severe loss of tubular epithelium.

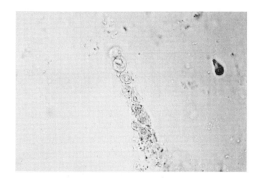

**FIG 14-63.** Epithelial cell cast. Unstained, ×400.

The epithelial cast often appears to consist of two rows of renal epithelial cells, implying tubular desquamation (Fig. 14-63). However, the cells may also vary in size, shape, and distribution, showing a varying amount of protein matrix (Fig. 14-64). When the cells are haphazardly arranged in the cast in varying stages of degeneration, cellular damage and desquamation from different and separate portions of the renal tubule are implied. The epithelial cast does not remain constant once formed, but undergoes a series of changes. These changes result from cellular disintegration as the cast remains within the kidney, as a result of decreased urine flow (stasis). Therefore, a range of epithelial casts from cellular to coarsely granular, finely granular, and finally waxy may be seen. The waxy type represents the most serious situation, as prolonged blockage of renal flow is required for them to form. All of these types of casts are often seen in the same specimen; such specimens are referred to as **"telescoped"** urinary sediments (Fig. 14-65). Epithelial casts may be difficult to distinguish from white cell casts, as previously discussed. When stained, the cells have a blue-purple nucleus and lighter blue-purple cytoplasm in a pink matrix. Phase-contrast and interference microscopy are also helpful in this examination, as is cytocentrifugation.

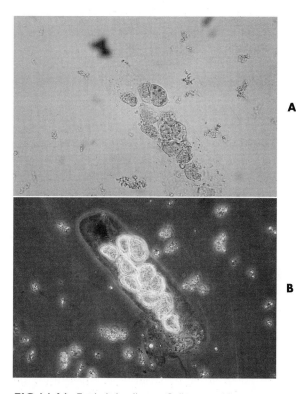

**FIG 14-64.** Epithelial cell cast. Cells stained by presence of bilirubin in the urine. (×400.) **A,** Brightfield. **B,** Phase contrast.

**Red Blood Cell (Blood and Hemoglobin) Casts.** The observation of red blood cell casts in the urinary sediment is a significant diagnostic finding and indicates a serious renal condition. Their presence must not be missed. The red cells enter the nephron by leakage through the glomerular capsule. It is possible that they bleed into the renal tubules at a point beyond the glomerular capsule; however, this would be a far less common path, as red cell casts are almost always associated with diseases that affect the glomerulus, such as acute glomerulonephritis and lupus nephritis. Once red cells are present in the lumen of the nephron, they clump together to form red cell casts. Red cell casts are probably the most fragile ones in the urinary sediment, which may be why they are rarely observed and

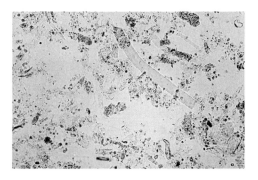

**FIG 14-65.** Telescoped urine specimen showing a mixture of casts, including; waxy, granular, cellular, and hyaline. Unstained, ×100.

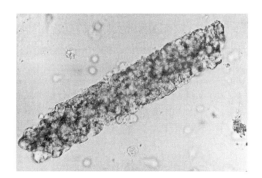

**FIG 14-67.** Blood cast. Unstained, ×400.

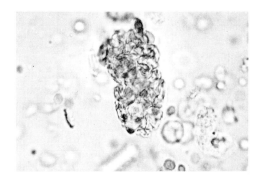

**FIG 14-66.** Red blood cell cast. Unstained, ×1,000.

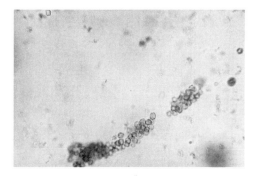

**FIG 14-68.** Red blood cell cast. Sedi-Stain, ×450.

why fragments are more often found. When physical conditions indicate that red cell casts may be present, it is imperative that the urine specimen be absolutely fresh and gently treated. The casts may be so fragile that they disintegrate under the microscope as the observer watches.

Red cell casts have a characteristic orange-yellow color caused by hemoglobin, which makes them unlike anything else seen in the urinary sediment (Figs. 14-66 and 14-67). Stain may or may not be useful in the identification of blood casts; however, the casts may have intact red cells, which stain colorless or lavender in a pink matrix (Fig. 14-68). Phase-contrast and interference microscopy are both very useful in detecting red cell casts. The characteristic color

is, however, best appreciated with brightfield observation of the unstained sediment.

The number of cells present in the red cell cast is variable. Often only a few intact cells are seen in a hyaline matrix. This may be referred to as a hyaline red cell cast. If many cells are clumped together to form the cast, the matrix is often not visible. These casts are more fragile and, unfortunately, more serious from the clinical standpoint.

Red cell casts or casts derived from red blood cells are often divided into **red blood cell casts, blood casts,** and **hemoglobin casts.** It is also possible to see **mixed cell casts,** which are a combination of all types. The red blood cell cast contains at least some recognizable red cells.

They may be present in a generally hyaline matrix, or appear as a solid mass of conglutinated red cells with little or no matrix between the packed cells. As the red cells degenerate, no longer showing a cell margin but remaining recognizable as probably being derived from blood, they are called blood casts. (This is analogous to the cellular or coarsely granular cast derived from white cells or epithelial cells.) The hemoglobin (pigment) cast shows a homogeneous matrix with no cell margins or recognizable red cells. Both blood and hemoglobin casts have a characteristic orange-yellow color. The hemoglobin pigment cast is then analogous to the waxy cast—representative of urinary stasis, and a more chronic than acute condition. The occurrence of red cells within a cast, regardless of the number of cells, represents a serious situation. When red blood cells are found in the urinary sediment, in conjunction with red cell casts of any sort, renal (usually glomerular) involvement is indicated.

**Bacterial Casts.** Casts made up of bacteria in a protein matrix have been described. They are an important finding and are diagnostic of acute pyelonephritis or intrinsic renal infections. They are probably mistaken for granular casts, which they resemble. The use of phase-contrast or interference-contrast microscopy and supravital stain is helpful. However, these casts are most easily recognized if a dry or cytocentrifuged preparation is stained with Gram stain. The bacteria in the cast may be packed closely together, sparsely distributed throughout, or concentrated in an area of a cast matrix. White cells may be present in addition to the bacteria within the cast.

### Granular Casts

The granules seen in granular casts may be the result of breakdown of cells within the cast or the renal tubule, or aggregates of plasma proteins including fibrinogen, immune complexes, and globulins in a Tamm-Horsfall matrix. Once all the cells have become granules, it is impossible to say for sure what sort of cell was originally present in the renal tubule. Such a distinction is useful, as red cell casts indicate glomerular injury, epithelial cell casts indicate renal tubular damage, and white cell casts indicate interstitial inflammation or infection. Often casts are seen that are basically granular but show some cells in transition to granules. When cells are present, they should be identified if possible. Once again, phase-contrast and interference microscopy are helpful in this distinction, as is cytocentrifugation. The end product of this disintegration is the waxy cast.

The size of the granules within the granular cast varies; they become progressively smaller as the cells disintegrate. The number of granules also varies, and casts range from those that are completely filled with granules to those that are basically hyaline and contain only a few granules. Such granules may have been present in the renal tubule and trapped in a protein matrix as the cast was formed. Although granular casts are sometimes reported as coarsely or finely granular, the term granular is sufficient (Figs. 14-69 and 14-70). The distinction between coarsely and finely granular is subjective, but relatively easily made. If the cast has a definite hyaline matrix with only a few granules, it is reported as hyaline. When large numbers of granules are present, it is described as granular. When many somewhat shortened granular casts

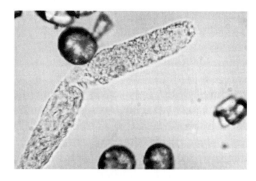

**FIG 14-69.** Granular cast; uric acid crystals also present. Unstained, ×400.

are seen, the possibility that they are actually proximal renal tubular epithelial cells should be considered (see also Renal Epithelial Cells.) They are more easily visualized with stained brightfield preparations, and cytocentrifugation and staining with Wright and Papanicolaou stain are especially helpful.

**Coarsely Granular Casts.** These casts contain large granules that appear to be degenerated cells (Fig. 14-71). They tend to be darker, shorter, and more irregular in outline than finely granular casts. They show a darker color and large granules that make them easier to find than either hyaline or finely granular casts. They stain with dark purple granules in a purple matrix.

**Finely Granular Casts.** These casts look much like hyaline casts; however, the presence of fine granules makes them more distinctive and easier to find (Fig. 14-72). When viewed with phase-contrast or interference microscopy, hyaline casts generally show a fine granulation. They are usually grayish or pale yellow in the unstained sediment and stain with fine dark purple granules in a pale pink or pale purple matrix.

### Waxy Casts

Waxy casts resemble hyaline casts and may be mistaken for them. They are much more significant clinically. The waxy cast is homogeneous, like the hyaline cast, but it is yellowish and more

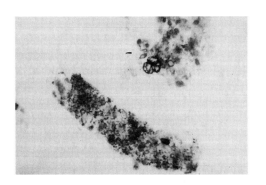

**FIG 14-70.** Granular cast. Sedi-Stain, ×400.

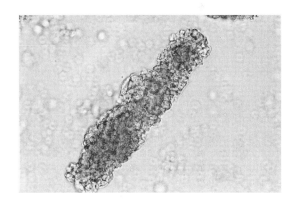

**FIG 14-71.** Granular cast with coarse granules (almost cells). Sedi-Stain, ×400.

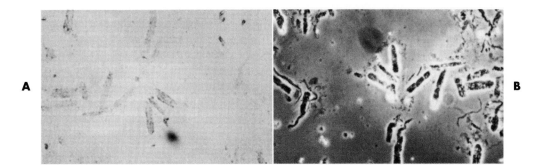

**FIG 14-72.** Several hyaline finely granular casts and mucous threads. Unstained, ×100. **A,** Brightfield. **B,** Phase contrast. Note improved visualization as compared with brightfield.

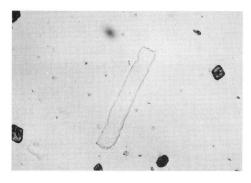

**FIG 14-73.** Waxy cast, resembling diaper fibers. Uric acid crystals also present. Unstained, ×160.

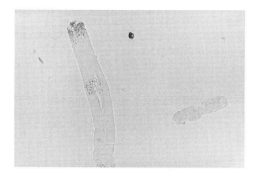

**FIG 14-74.** Waxy cast with fissure and granular end *(left)*, granular to waxy cast *(right)*. Unstained, ×160.

refractive, with sharper outlines. It appears hard, whereas the hyaline cast has a delicate appearance. Waxy casts tend to be wider than hyaline casts (they are described as broad casts or broad waxy casts) and usually have irregular broken ends and fissures or cracks in their sides (Figs. 14-73 and 14-74). Fairly long forms are also seen. Phase-contrast and interference microscopy and staining are useful in the examination of waxy casts. They generally stain with greater intensity than hyaline casts, making them easier to visualize (Fig. 14-75).

Waxy casts are felt to be the final step in the disintegration of cellular casts and are especially serious because they imply renal stasis. They are associated with severe chronic renal disease and renal amyloidosis, and are seen only rarely and in small numbers in acute renal diseases (Fig. 14-76).

### Fatty Casts

The importance and probable mechanism of formation of fatty casts have been discussed with oval fat bodies and fat globules. These three structures are often seen together in the same urine specimen, along with extremely large amounts of protein (greater than 2,000 mg/dL) and the pale foamy appearance of the specimen associated with the nephrotic syndrome. They are also seen in diabetes mellitus with renal degeneration and in toxic renal poisoning as from ethylene glycol or mercury.

Fatty casts, as the name implies, contain droplets of fat. These droplets are highly refractile under the microscope (Fig. 14-77). Although phase-contrast microscopy and interference microscopy are useful, the characteristic refractile appearance of fat droplets might be better appreciated with the brightfield microscope. If the droplets are neutral fat or triglyceride, they will stain bright orange or red with Sudan III or oil red O stains (Fig. 14-78). If cholesterol is present, they will show a Maltese cross pattern with polarized light (Fig. 14-79). With Sternheimer-Malbin stain, the cast matrix will stain, but the refractile fat globules will not.

Fatty casts may be seen as a protein matrix almost completely filled with fat globules, or as fat globules contained within a basically hyaline, cellular, or granular cast. In addition to free fat globules, intact oval fat bodies may be seen within the cast matrix; these are sometimes referred to as oval fat body casts.

### Other Casts

Various other structures that may be found in the urinary sediment may rarely be incorporated into the protein matrix of a cast. Pigmented casts may be seen including hemoglobin (already described), myoglobin, bilirubin, and drugs such as phenazopyridine. Hemosiderin casts contain granules of hemosiderin. Crystal casts, which contain urates,

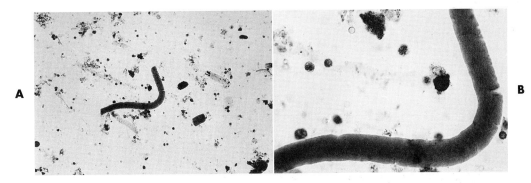

**FIG 14-75.** Mixture of casts from telescoped urine specimen, including waxy, granular, and hyaline. Stained with Sedi-Stain. Note affinity of waxy casts for stain. Brightfield. **A,** Low power, ×100. **B,** Enlarged view of the large cast in **A,** showing a broad cast in transition from granular to waxy, ×400.

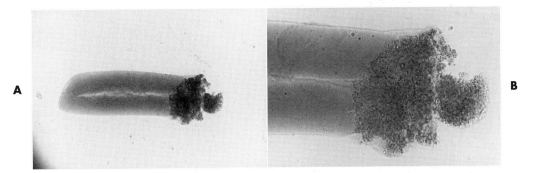

**FIG 14-76.** Broad waxy cast with central fissure and granular end. Sedi-stain. **A,** ×160. **B,** Higher magnification of same cast as A, showing granular end and fat inclusions, ×400.

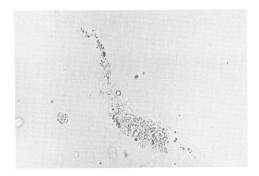

**FIG 14-77.** Fatty cast. Unstained, ×400.

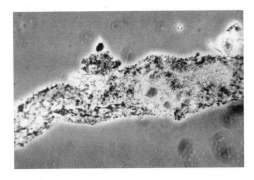

**FIG 14-78.** Large fatty cast with oval fat body inclusion, stained with Sudan III for neutral fat (triglyceride). Phase contrast, ×400.

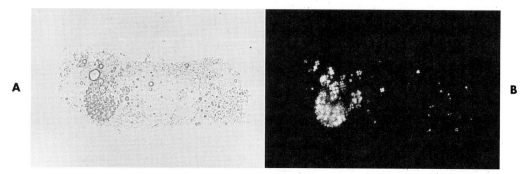

**FIG 14-79.** Large fatty cast, filled with fat and an oval fat body inclusion, showing the presence of cholesterol as a Maltese cross when viewed with polarized light. Unstained, ×400. **A,** Brightfield. **B,** Polarized light.

calcium oxalate, or sulfonamides, have also been seen. These must not be mistaken for crystals adhering to strands of mucus, however. Rather, the protein matrix must be visualized in a true crystal cast. Bacteria casts have also been described.

## Structures Confused With Casts
### Mucous Threads

The refractive index of mucous threads is similar to that of hyaline casts; however, the former are long ribbonlike strands with undefined edges and pointed or split ends. They also appear to have longitudinal striations. They are most apparent, and cause the most confusion, with phase-contrast or interference microscopy. They are often seen together with hyaline casts. Although difficult to distinguish, hyaline casts are generally more formed or structured.

### Rolled Squamous Epithelial Cells

These may be mistaken for casts when they have rolled into a cigar shape. However, they have pointed ends rather than rounded ones and are shorter, and a single round nucleus may be discovered with careful focusing.

### Disposable Diaper Fibers

These fibers are easily confused with waxy casts, appearing almost identically highly refractile

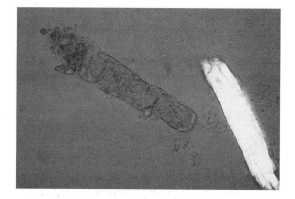

**FIG 14-80.** Waxy cast (left) and strongly birefringent fiber (right). Compensated polarized light, ×400.

with blunt ends. They may be seen in urine specimens from infants, or from geriatric patients or other adults who must use diapers. Unlike waxy casts, diaper fibers are rarely accompanied by other pathologic findings, especially proteinuria. The use of polarizing microscopy may be useful. Waxy casts do not polarize light; diaper fibers do (Fig. 14-80).

### Other Structures

Bits of hair or threads of material fibers are also mistaken for casts by the beginner. However, these are extremely refractive structures that have nothing in common with the appearance of protein microscopically. Likewise, scratches on the glass slide or coverglass may be mistaken for casts at first. Again, they are much too definite and obvious to be important. Finally, hyphae of molds are sometimes mistaken for hyaline casts. This is similar to mistaking yeast for red cells. Hyphae are much more refractive and are jointed and branching, as may be observed on closer examination.

## CRYSTALS AND AMORPHOUS MATERIAL

### Clinical Significance

Crystals and amorphous precipitates of certain chemicals make up what has been called the unorganized urinary sediment. These materials are generally obvious under the microscope. Because they are so striking, there is a natural tendency to pay considerable attention to them, but they are the most insignificant part of the urine sediment and deserve little attention. In the past, great emphasis was placed on the identification of these materials. However, it is generally preferable to search carefully for more pathologic constituents and note only briefly the occurrence of crystals.

The presence of crystals in the urine specimen is called **crystalluria.** As urine specimens stand, especially when refrigerated, many lose clarity and become cloudy because of the precipitation of amorphous material and crystals. However, crystalluria is generally important only when present in urine when voided (at body temperature). Yet it is necessary to identify crystals and amorphous materials that may be present, both normal and so-called abnormal forms, for the following reasons.

If crystals are abundant, they will obscure such important structures as red blood cells, white blood cells, and casts. The more important structures must be searched for with extreme care when crystals and amorphous materials are present. The use of a stain, such as the Sternheimer-Malbin stain, may be especially useful in this case.

The precipitation of certain crystals may accompany kidney stone formation **(lithiasis).**

When crystals are seen in the urine in cases of lithiasis, the chemical composition of the **calculi** (stones) may be implied. This is one reason for the attention that was formerly given to urinary crystals. However, stone formation may exist without the presence of crystals in the urine, and crystals are often present without stone formation.

Amino acids such as cystine, leucine, and tyrosine may crystallize in urine and indicate serious metabolic or inherited disorders. Administration of sulfonamide drugs may cause the formation of sulfonamide crystals, especially in acidic urine. The formation of sulfonamide crystals within the kidney may result in blockage of renal output and severe renal damage. This problem was greater when sulfonamide drugs were first introduced. Drugs that are currently used are more soluble, and thus less likely to precipitate. However, crystals are occasionally seen when high doses are given. More recently, crystals of the protease inhibitor indinavir sulfate have been associated with renal blockage and stone formation in HIV-positive individuals.

When the concentration of a salt in solution is greater than the solubility threshold for that salt, crystals will precipitate out of solution. Therefore, crystals are more likely to be seen in concentrated urine specimens with high specific gravity. This is often observed in the urine of persons with dehydration and fever.

### Classification of Urine Crystals

The various crystals that are encountered in urine specimens are usually classified as **normal** or **abnormal.** These are further subclassified as normal **acid** crystals (crystals seen in normal urine of an acidic pH), normal **alkaline** crystals (crystals seen in normal urine of an alkaline pH), abnormal crystals of metabolic origin, and abnormal crystals of **iatrogenic** origin. Iatrogenic refers to crystals that result from medication or treatment—that is, inadvertently caused by the physician. The various crystals found in the urine sediment are categorized and summarized in Table 14-17. The crystals in each category are arranged in approximately the order of importance or frequency in which they are encountered.

## Identification and Reporting of Urine Crystals

Identification of crystals is usually done on the basis of shape or morphology. This is aided by knowledge of the urine pH. Certain forms are seen in urine of an acid pH (generally 6.5 or less), while others are associated with urine of an alkaline pH (generally 7.0 or more). Although pH 7 is neutral, crystals present in urine of pH 7 are generally forms seen in a more alkaline pH.

The normal crystals are usually reported on the basis of morphology alone. They are observed with both low-power and high-power objectives, depending on size, and reported as few, moderate, or many per high-power field. Unlike the urine sediment constituents already described, crystals are characterized by shape rather than size. Although some crystals are typically large or small, crystals of chemicals such as uric acid may vary from extremely small crystals that can only be visualized with high power to extremely large forms that are easily seen with low power. The color of the crystals, both macroscopically on the basis of urine appearance and microscopically, is also helpful. In some instances, solubility with heat, acids, or alkalis is useful in the final identification.

The abnormal crystals generally require confirmation before they are reported to the clinician. They are observed under low and high power, depending on size, and reported on the basis of the average number per low-power field, as shown in Table 14-15. Confirmation may consist of a chemical test, such as a diazo reaction used for the sulfonamides, or a cyanide nitroprusside reaction for cystine. When chemical confirmatory tests are unavailable, confirmation may consist of the patient's drug history or history of various imaging procedures such as intravenous pyelograms or CAT scans.

Most crystals are birefringent when viewed with polarized light. The strength of birefringence depends both on the chemical composition of the crystal in question and on the thickness of the crystal. Thick crystals will show stronger birefringence than thin ones. As is the case with synovial fluid crystals, phosphates or phosphate-containing crystals generally show weaker birefringence than urates or uric acid.

## TABLE 14-17

Crystals Found in the Urine Sediment

**Normal Acid Crystals**
Amorphous urates
Uric acid
Acid urates
Monosodium urate or sodium urates
Calcium oxalate (also seen in neutral and
  alkaline urine)

**Normal Alkaline Crystals**
Amorphous phosphates
(Calcium oxalate)
Triple phosphates
Ammonium biurate
Calcium phosphate
Calcium carbonate

**Abnormal Crystals of Metabolic Origin**
Cystine
Tyrosine
Leucine
Cholesterol
Bilirubin
Hemosiderin

**Abnormal Crystals of Iatrogenic Origin (Drugs)**
Sulfonamides
Ampicillin
Radiographic contrast media
Acyclovir
Indinavir sulfate

The ability to polarize light is very helpful in the identification of crystalline structures as opposed to structures of biologic origin, such as cells, microoganisms, and casts, which do not polarize light.

## Normal Crystals
### Normal Acid Crystals

These are the crystals that are seen in normal urine of an acidic pH (pH 6.5 or less). In most cases, crystals seen at this pH are some form of uric acid or calcium oxalate. Uric acid is especially pleomorphic—when an unusual crystal is first encountered, it is often found to consist of uric acid or a salt of this acid. However, most of the abnormal crystals that have been encountered in urine are also associated with an acidic pH. Therefore, care must be taken to rule out the presence of pathologic crystals, before unusual forms are assumed to be a form of uric acid.

**Amorphous Urates.** This is the amorphous material found in urine of an acid pH. Chemically, amorphous urates are a sodium salt of uric acid (sodium, potassium, magnesium, or calcium). Amorphous means without shape or form. The urates show a characteristic yellowish red shapeless granulation (Fig. 14-81). They are strongly birefringent when viewed with polarized light. When present in sufficient numbers, they form a characteristic fluffy pink or orange precipitate referred to as brick dust.

Amorphous urates tend to precipitate out of urine that is highly concentrated, as in dehydration and fever. Such urine specimens are typically highly colored (dark amber) and show large amounts of fluffy pink or orange precipitate. Although of an alarming appearance to the patient, such specimens are of little concern clinically.

Amorphous urates will change to uric acid when acidified with glacial uric acid. They will dissolve when warmed to 60° C and when treated with 10% NaOH. Their solubility when heated is useful in differentiating them from amorphous phosphates, which are insoluble when heated. However, this differentiation is commonly made on the basis of urine pH—urates are seen in acidic urine, phosphates in alkaline urine. When treated with ammonium hydroxide, urates will change to ammonium biurate, the ammonium salt of uric acid.

**Uric Acid.** These crystals have a variety of shapes and colors. Typically they are yellow or reddish brown, much like the chemically related amorphous urates. The typical shape is the whetstone (Fig. 14-82). Other shapes include rhombic plates or prisms, somewhat oval forms

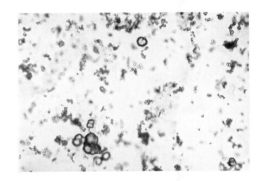

**FIG 14-81.** Amorphous urates. Acid urates also present. (×400.)

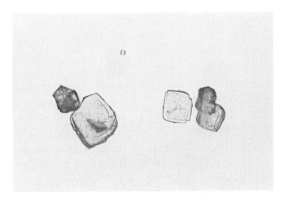

**FIG 14-82.** Uric acid, whetstone shape, ×160.

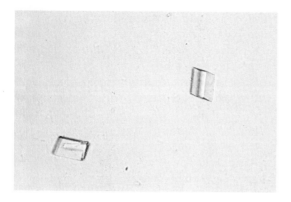

**FIG 14-83.** Uric acid, as rhombic prisms, ×400.

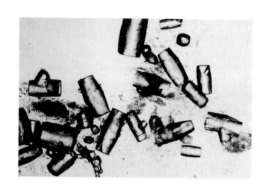

**FIG 14-85.** Uric acid, barrel shaped, ×100.

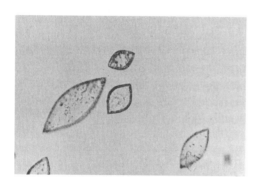

**FIG 14-84.** Uric acid, large lemon-shaped, ×400.

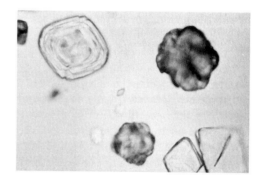

**FIG 14-86.** Uric acid, laminated forms, ×640.

with pointed ends ("lemon shaped"), and barrel-shaped forms (Figs. 14-83 to 14-85). Wedges, rosettes, irregular plates and laminated forms are also seen (Fig. 14-86). They are usually recognized by color, but some, especially the rhombic plates, may appear colorless. Unusual crystals, such as those seen in Fig. 14-87, in urine of an acid pH are generally forms of uric acid. A hexagonal form of uric acid may be mistaken for cystine crystals, which are abnormal and important to detect (Fig. 14-88). Several of the sulfonamides may mimic uric acid. When this situation is suspected, a drug history should be obtained and confirmatory test for sulfonamides performed.

Uric acid crystals are commonly seen in urine specimens, especially after the specimen has been standing. However, they are pathologic only when seen in fresh urine immediately after it is voided. Amorphous urates and uric acid, together with elevated serum uric acid, may be associated with gout or stone formation. The uric acid concentration in urine depends on dietary intake of purines and breakdown of nucleic acid. Therefore, large amounts of urates or uric acid are often seen in the urine of patients with leukemia or lymphoma who are receiving chemotherapy.

Uric acid is strongly birefringent and gives a beautiful play of colors when viewed with po-

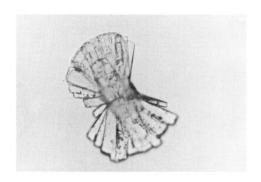

**FIG 14-87.** Uric acid, rare form, ×400.

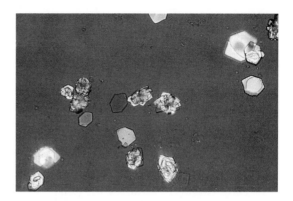

**FIG 14-89.** Uric acid showing strong birefringence when viewed with polarized light, ×160.

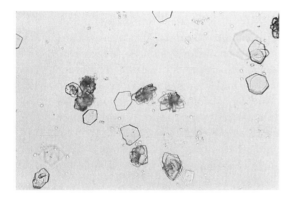

**FIG 14-88.** Uric acid, six-sided like cystine, ×160.

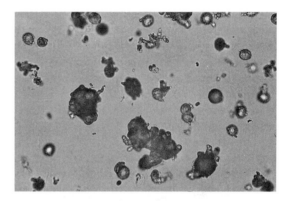

**FIG 14-90.** Acid urates, appearing like ammonium biurate or sulfonamide (sulfamethoxazole), ×400.

larized light (Fig. 14-89). Like amorphous urates, uric acid is soluble when heated to 60° C and when treated with 10% NaOH. However, uric acid crystals remain (are insoluble) when treated with glacial acetic acid.

**Acid Urates.** These rare forms of uric acid are seen in acidic or neutral pH. They may be sodium, potassium, or ammonium urates and are seen as brown spheres or clusters that resemble ammonium biurate. They are often seen in urine together with amorphous urates (see Fig. 14-81). They have the same significance as amorphous urates or uric acid. Acid urates resemble the alkaline counterpoint of uric acid,

namely ammonium biurate. They also resemble sulfamethoxazole, an abnormal crystal of pathologic significance, and are important to recognize for this reason (Fig. 14-90).

Like amorphous urates and uric acid, the acid urates are soluble at 60° C and in 10% sodium hydroxide and are changed to uric acid when treated with glacial acetic acid.

**Monosodium Urate or Sodium Urates.**

These are another rare form of uric acid that might be seen in urine. Monosodium urate is the form of uric acid seen in the synovial fluid of patients with gout. If present in urine, it appears as tiny, slender, colorless needles (Fig. 14-91).

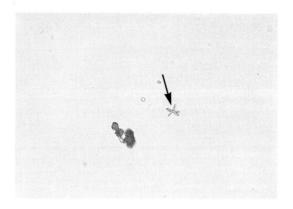

**FIG 14-91.** Monosodium urate, tiny needles or rod-shaped crystals *(arrow)*, ×400.

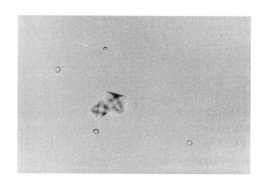

**FIG 14-94.** Calcium oxalate, typical octahedral and oval forms appearing like red blood cells, ×400.

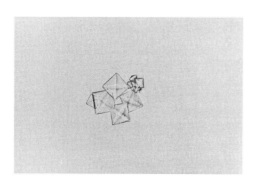

**FIG 14-92.** Calcium oxalate, typical envelope (octahedral) shape, ×400.

**Calcium Oxalate.** Calcium oxalate crystals have a characteristic shape, which has been referred to as an "envelope." These are octahedrons that vary somewhat in size but are typically small, colorless, and glistening (Fig. 14-92). Occasionally they are seen as rectangular forms with pyramidal ends (Fig. 14-93). Less frequently they may appear in a dumbbell shape or an ovoid shape that may resemble that of red blood cells (Fig. 14-94). Unlike red cells, calcium oxalate will polarize light (Fig. 14-95).

Although most common in acidic urine, calcium oxalate crystals may also be seen in neutral or alkaline urine specimens. They are of little clinical significance, although they may be present in association with stone formation, as calcium oxalate is the most common constituent found in kidney stones. There is a correlation between calcium stones and excess oxalate and uric acid in the urine. (Uric acid may be the nidus for stone formation.) Excess oxalate may result from ingestion of foodstuffs containing oxalic acid, such as spinach and rhubarb, and from ingestion of vitamin C, because oxalic acid is a breakdown product of ascorbic acid. Calcium oxalate crystals may also be seen in cases of ethylene glycol or methoxyfluran poisoning (Fig. 14-96).

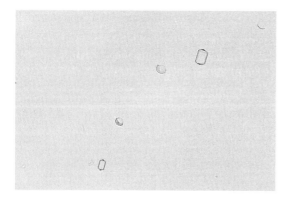

**FIG. 14-93.** Calcium oxalate, elongated with pyramidal end, plus two red blood cells, ×400.

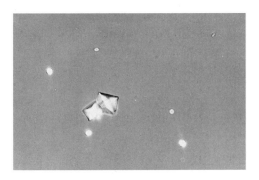

**FIG 14-95.** Calcium oxalate, typical octahedral and oval forms appearing like red cells, exhibiting strong birefringence with polarized light, ×400.

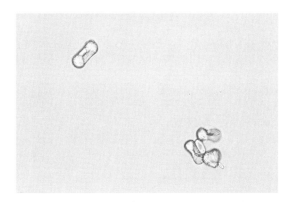

**FIG 14-96.** Calcium oxalate, rare large ovoid form of a type associated with ethylene glycol poisoning, ×400.

### Normal Alkaline Crystals

These are the "normal" crystals seen in urine of an alkaline pH (generally pH 7.0 and above). They are usually a phosphate- or calcium-containing crystal. However, the alkaline counterpoint of uric acid, ammonium biurate, is also seen. Phosphates have little clinical significance, although they are associated with an alkaline pH and infection.

**Amorphous Phosphates.** The amorphous material found in alkaline urine is amorphous phosphate. Generally, the phosphates give a finer or more lacy precipitate than the amorphous urates and are colorless (Fig. 14-97). Phosphates are the most common cause of turbidity in alkaline urine and are seen as a fine white precipitate microscopically. They do not dissolve when heated but are soluble in acetic acid and dilute hydrochloric acid. Phosphates appear like, and are often seen with, bacteria; care must be taken not to overlook bacteria when they are present. Use of phase contrast is helpful.

**Triple Phosphate.** Triple (ammonium magnesium) phosphates (also referred to as struvite) are colorless crystals and commonly show great variation in size, from tiny to relatively huge

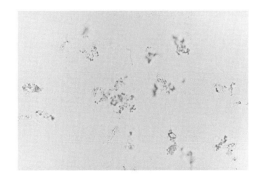

**FIG 14-97.** Amorphous phosphates, ×400.

crystals. They have a characteristic "coffin-lid" shape that is impossible to miss (Fig. 14-98). They may also be seen as large long prisms that are difficult to distinguish from calcium phosphate (Fig. 14-99). Both triple and calcium phosphates have similar clinical significance, and either may be reported as phosphates. Less commonly, triple phosphates occur in a fern-like form as they dissolve into solution (Fig. 14-100). They are soluble in dilute acetic acid.

**Ammonium Biurate.** This ammonium salt is the alkaline counterpart of uric acid and amorphous urates in urine. The crystals are spherical with radial or concentric striations and long prismatic spicules, resembling thorn apples

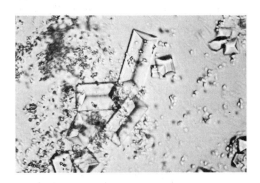

**FIG 14-98.** Triple phosphate, typical coffin-lid form. Amorphous phosphates also present. (×400.)

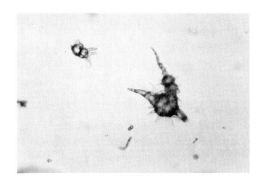

**FIG 14-101.** Ammonium biurate, large "thorn apples," ×400.

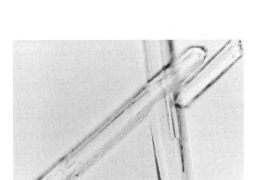

**FIG 14-99.** Triple phosphate or calcium phosphate (as brusite) seen as large long prisms, ×400.

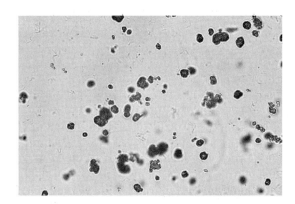

**FIG 14-102.** Ammonium biurates and bacteria, ×400.

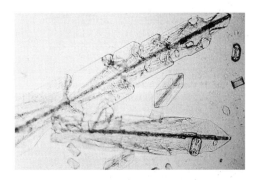

**FIG. 14-100.** Triple phosphate; unusual fern-leaf form of crystals dissolving into solution. Smaller, more typical forms also present. (×400.)

(Figs. 14-101 and 14-102). They are yellow and may be mistaken for some forms of the sulfonamide drugs that may precipitate out of urine. Sulfa crystals are usually seen in acidic urine, however. Ammonium biurates are often present in old alkaline urine specimens, especially those that contain unusual sediment constituents and have been retained for teaching purposes. They are much less frequently seen in fresh urine collections. They are soluble at 60° C with acetic acid and in strong alkali. They will convert to uric acid with concentrated hydrochloric acid or acetic acid.

**Calcium Phosphate.** Calcium phosphates are colorless crystals, occasionally seen in nor-

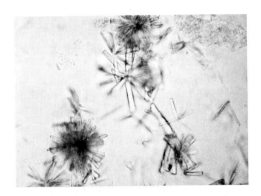

**FIG 14-103.** Calcium phosphate, most typical form of slender wedge-shaped crystals arranged in clusters or rosettes, ×400.

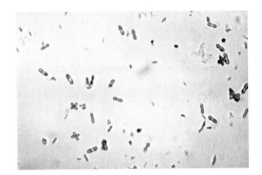

**FIG 14-105.** Calcium carbonate, tiny dumbbell form, ×400.

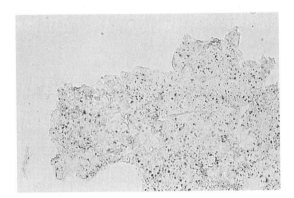

**FIG 14-104.** Calcium phosphate plate. Sedi-Stain ×400.

mal alkaline urine. Typically they appear as slender prisms with a wedge-like end occurring singly or arranged in rosettes (Fig. 14-103). They may appear like, and with, triple phosphate crystals as long prisms of calcium monohydrogen phosphate, also known as brusite. Calcium phosphate may also appear as flat plates, which might be mistaken for large degenerating squamous epithelial cells (Fig. 14-104).

Calcium phosphate is insoluble when heated to 60° C, slightly soluble in dilute acetic acid, and soluble in dilute hydrochloric acid.

**Calcium Carbonate.** Calcium carbonate crystals are tiny, colorless granules that typically

occur in pairs ("dumbbells") but may occcur also singly (Fig. 14-105). Because they are so small, calcium carbonate crystals represent part of the amorphous material seen in normal alkaline urine specimens. They are soluble in acetic acid with effervescence.

### Abnormal Crystals

With only a few, very rare exceptions, the abnormal urinary crystals are seen in urine specimens of an acid pH—6.5 or less. Normal crystals of urine may be reported on the basis of microscopic examination (morphology) and pH. However, the abnormal crystals require further confirmation. Whenever possible, this should be a chemical confirmation; however, a history of medications or treatment procedures may be the only possible confirmation. Unlike the normal crystals, which are reported as few, moderate, or many, the abnormal crystals are reported as the number seen per average low-power field.

Abnormal crystals may be further classified as metabolic (physiologic) or iatrogenic (see Table 14-15). The abnormal crystals of metabolic origin are the result of certain disease states or inherited conditions. These include cystine, tyrosine, leucine, cholesterol, bilirubin, and hemosiderin. **Iatrogenic** crystals are the result of medication or treatment and thus are inadvertently caused by the physician. Examples of iatrogenic crystals include the various sulfonamides, ampicillin, radiographic contrast media, acyclovir, and indinavir sulfate.

### Abnormal Crystals of Metabolic Origin

**Cystine.** Cystine crystals are colorless, refractile, hexagonal plates that are often laminated (Fig. 14-106). They may be seen in the urine of patients with the hereditary condition cystinuria. This is an amino acid transport disorder affecting cystine, ornithine, lysine, and arginine (COLA). Of these amino acids, only cystine crystallizes out in the urine. This crystallization of cystine is serious, as these patients are apt to form cystine stones, which may lead to kidney damage. Patients with this condition must always be well hydrated to prevent such stone formation. The crystals may be mistaken for a form of uric acid that is also hexagonal.

The presence of cystine should be confirmed with the **cyanide-nitroprusside reaction.** Cystine is reduced to cysteine by sodium cyanide. The free sulfhydryl groups that result react with nitroprusside to give a red-purple color. Cystine crystals are most insoluble in urine of an acid pH. However, they remain insoluble up to pH 7.4. They are soluble in alkali (especially ammonia) and dilute hydrochloric acid. They are destroyed by the presence of bacteria, because of the formation of ammonia. They are in-

soluble in boiling water, acetic acid, alcohol, and ether.

**Tyrosine.** Tyrosine crystals are rare, but may be present as the result of inherited amino acid disorders (hereditary tyrosinosis and oasthouse disease) and, together with leucine, in patients with massive liver failure.

They are colorless fine silky needles arranged in sheaves or clumps, which appear black as the microscope is focused (Fig. 14-107). They occur in urine of an acid pH. Tyrosine is soluble in alkali and dilute mineral acid. Tyrosine crystals are relatively soluble when heated, but insoluble in alcohol and ether. They are confirmed with a nitrosonaphthol test or by amino acid analysis by high-performance liquid chromatography (HPLC).

**Leucine.** Leucine crystals are yellow, oily-looking spheres with radial and concentric striations. They are of metabolic origin and extremely rare. Leucine and tyrosine crystals usually appear together and are associated with severe liver disease. Leucine is found in urine of an acid pH.

**Cholesterol.** Droplets of cholesterol that polarize as a Maltese cross are seen in the urine sediment as free fat, in oval fat bodies, and in

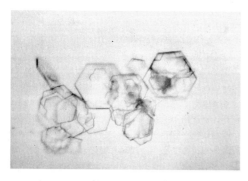

**FIG 14-106.** Cystine. Thin, colorless, laminated hexagon, ×640.

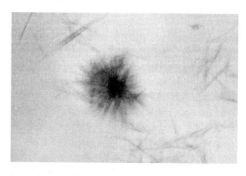

**FIG 14-107.** Tyrosine, fine silky needles, ×400.

fatty casts. However, cholesterol crystals or plates are extremely rare in freshly voided urine sediment; they have been seen rarely after the specimen has been refrigerated. When seen, they have the same clinical significance as the more common globules or droplets.

Like most abnormal crystals, cholesterol crystals are associated with urine of an acidic or neutral pH. Cholesterol crystals are large, flat, hexagonal plates with one or more corners notched out (Fig. 14-108).

When apparent cholesterol crystals are seen in large numbers, the presence of another drug or its crystals should be suspected. Crystals of radio-graphic media (such as meglumine diatrizoate) are found in urine collected immediately after intravenous radiographic studies. They are morphologically similar to cholesterol, but they are associated with a very high specific gravity (greater than 1.035 by refractometer) and a false-positive, delayed sulfosalicylic acid test for protein. They should not be mistaken for cholesterol (see Fig. 14-114).

If present, crystals of cholesterol should be associated with other findings, such as free fat, oval fat bodies, or fatty casts. They are more likely to be seen in urine specimens that have been retained and refrigerated.

Absolute, chemical confirmation of cholesterol may be difficult. However, cholesterol crystals are very soluble in chloroform, ether, and hot alcohol.

**Bilirubin.** The presence of crystals of precipitated bilirubin is occasionally seen in the urine sediment of patients with bilirubinuria. This finding has about the same clinical significance as the chemical detection of bilirubin in urine, and these crystals should not be reported in the absence of bilirubin. Bilirubin crystals are seen as reddish brown needles that cluster in clumps, or as spheres (Fig. 14-109).

**Hemosiderin.** The pathophysiology of hemosiderin was discussed in the section on renal epithelial cells. However, this abnormal crystal might be mistaken for amorphous urates, a common urine sediment finding.

Hemosiderin may be seen in acid or neutral urine a few days after a severe intravascular hemolytic episode. In unstained urine sediment, hemosiderin appears as coarse, yellow-brown granules. These may be seen as free granules, or they may be contained within renal epithelial cells, macrophages, or casts. Hemosiderin may be confirmed with the **Rous test,** a wet Prussian blue stain for iron (Fig. 14-110). Cytocentrifuged preparations of the urine sediment may also be stained with Prussian blue stain, as is done in hematologic stains for iron content.

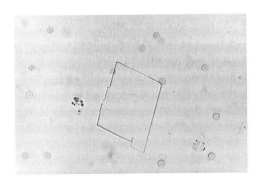

**FIG 14-108.** Cholesterol, large flat rectangle with notched corner. Fat and red cells also present. (×400.)

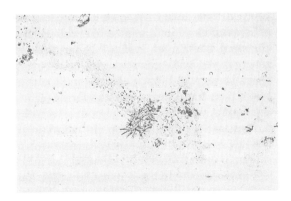

**FIG 14-109.** Bilirubin crystals. Cytospin, ×400.

**FIG 14-110.** Hemosiderin, stained with Prussian blue stain for iron (positive Rous test), ×400.

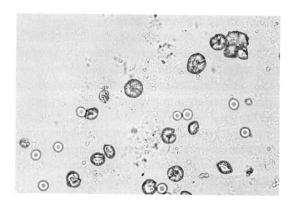

**FIG 14-111.** Sulfamethoxazole (Bactrim) and red blood cells, ×400.

### Abnormal Crystals of Iatrogenic Origin

**Sulfonamides.** The presence of these iatrogenic crystals in the urine sediment is an important pathologic finding. They are likely to cause renal damage, as the crystals precipitate in the nephron, causing bleeding (hematuria) and oliguria as a result of mechanical blockage of the renal tubules, which may lead to renal failure or shutdown. Precipitation or crystallization of the sulfonamides is prevented by adequate hydration of the patient and possibly alkalization of the urine with diet or medication. In the past much attention was given to the various forms of sulfonamides that might be encountered in the urine. However, current pharmacology uses more soluble forms of these drugs, and sulfonamide crystals are a fairly uncommon finding.

The sulfonamides are most likely to precipitate in urine with a low acid pH. The crystals are generally yellow to brown but may be colorless. Shape varies with the actual drug, and the various sulfonamides mimic various forms of uric aid, urates, and biurates. They have been described as colorless needles in sheaves or rosettes, arrowheads or whetstones; as brownish shocks of wheat with central binding; as colorless to greenish brown fan-shaped needles; and as dense brown or irregularly divided spheres.

All forms of sulfonamides may be confirmed by hydrolysis with heat and acid and application of a diazo reaction. Further confirmation may be made by requesting a list of medications administered to the patient.

A few of the more commonly encountered forms that crystallize in the urine follow.

*Sulfamethoxazole.* This is most commonly encountered sulfonamide crystal in the urine sediment. It is supplied as acetylsulfamethoxazole together with trimethoprim under the trade names Bactrim or Septra. Although this is a commonly used drug, occasionally it has been seen to crystallize in urine after unusually high dosage. When present, it is seen as a dense brown sphere or an irregularly divided sphere (Fig. 14-111).

*Acetylsulfadiazine.* This is a dangerous form of sulfonamide, because of its relative insolubility. It is now rarely used. It is seen as yellow-brown sheaves of wheat with eccentric binding (Fig. 14-112).

*Sulfadiazine.* This is another form of sulfonamide that is used only rarely. Sulfadiazine appears as dense brown globules like the crystals seen in Fig. 14-113. These crystals are morphologically similar to ammonium biurates and acid urates.

**Ampicillin.** Ampicillin crystals appear as long thin colorless needles in acidic urine. They are seen only rarely, as the result of large doses of the drug, which may be necessary for treatment of bacterial meningitis.

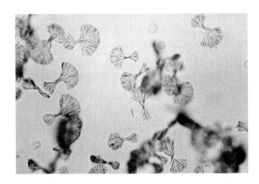

**FIG 14-112.** Acetylsulfadiazine, as sheaves of wheat with eccentric binding. Red blood cells also present. (×400.)

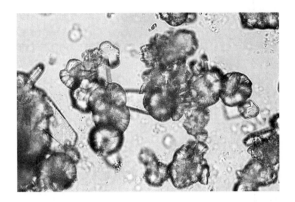

**FIG 14-113.** Sulfonamide crystals, possibly sulfadiazine, ×400.

**Radiographic Contrast Media.** Crystals of compounds, such as meglumine diatrizoate (Renografin, Hypaque), used for diagnostic radiographic procedures may be precipitated in the urine for a brief period after injection. They are primarily important because they might be misidentified as cholesterol crystals. Occasionally, their presence is of clinical importance, such as in dehydrated elderly patients, who may experience renal blockage from crystalline precipitation.

Crystals of meglumine diatrizoate may be seen in the urine sediment as flat, four-sided plates, often with a notched corner. They closely resemble cholesterol plates and should not be mistaken for them (Fig. 14-114). They may also occur as long, thin prisms or rectangles.

The presence of radiographic media should be suspected when many crystals resembling cholesterol plates are seen and the specific gravity by refractometer is extremely high (greater than 1.035). Since radiographic media do not ionize, the specific gravity by reagent strip is unaffected by their presence, however. When they are present, the urine may show a delayed false-positive sulfosalicylic acid precipitation test for protein. This should not be mistaken for true protein precipitation.

The presence of radiographic media may be confirmed by a clinical history of recent radiographic imaging procedures.

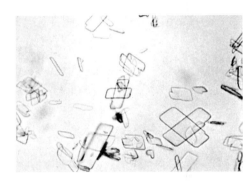

**FIG 14-114.** Radiographic contrast media (meglumine diatrizoate) appearing somewhat like cholesterol, ×400.

**Acyclovir.** This is another drug form that may be seen in the urine sediment in very rare cases of patients treated with high doses. Unlike most abnormal crystals, which are seen in acidic urine, acyclovir crystals have been seen in urine of pH 7.5. They appear as colorless slender needles that are strongly birefringent with polarized light (Fig. 14-115). They may be confirmed by obtaining a drug history.

**Indinavir Sulfate (Crixivan).** With the use of protease inhibitors in the treatment of HIV infection, the presence of crystals of indinavir sulfate (Crixivan) has been observed. According to product literature, 4% of patients treated with

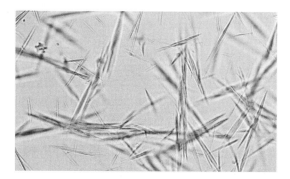

**FIG 14-115.** Acyclovir, tiny needle-shaped crystals, ×400.

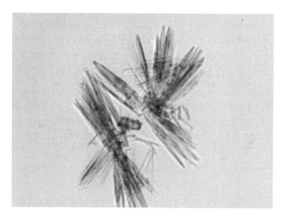

**FIG 14-116.** Indinavir sulfate (Crixivan). Slender rectangular plates arranges in fan or starburst. (×160.)

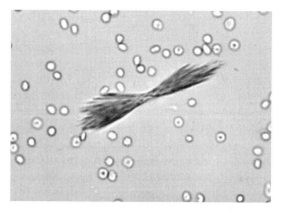

**FIG 14-117.** Indinavir sulfate (Crixivan). Slender needles in bundles or sheaves of wheat. Red blood cells also present. (×400.)

indinavir sulfate have renal stone formation.[13] As with other drugs that might precipitate in the urine, it is important that patients be well hydrated to avoid crystallization of the drug. The presence of these crystals in the urine might be an early sign of stone formation, especially when the patient has clinical evidence of stones such as pain and hematuria.

Crystals of indinavir sulfate are slender colorless needles or slender rectangular plates that tend to be arranged in fan-shaped or starburst forms, bundles or sheaves (Fig. 14-116 and 14-117). They resemble some forms of sulfonamides. Unlike most abnormal crystals, indinavir sulfate is most insoluble at an alkaline pH. The crystals are strongly birefringent with polarized light. Confirmation may depend primarily on the patient's drug history of indinavir use. Confirmation is possible by mass spectrometry or HPLC, but this is beyond the scope of the routine laboratory.

## CONTAMINANTS AND ARTIFACTS

Many objects and structures in the urinary sediment are contaminants or artifacts, and distract the attention of the observer from the important urinary constituents. These are the objects that beginning microscopists tend to see first when a microscopic examination of the urine sediment is attempted. It seems to be a general rule that if an object is easy to see, it is unimportant.

### Starch

Granules of starch are common contaminants in the urine sediment. They are the result of the use of barrier-protective gloves in all areas of the laboratory and medical care. Starch refers to cornstarch, a carbohydrate commonly used to line surgical or barrier-protective gloves. It is different from talc, or talcum, which is hydrated magnesium silicate, a chunky, irregular crystal.

Starch is a ubiquitous structure that is easily recognized, but must not be confused with globules or droplets of cholesterol. Both starch and cholesterol globules are birefringent and polarize as a Maltese cross (white cross on a black background) when viewed with polarized light. Starch is most easily recognized with brightfield microscopy (Fig. 14-118). It is seen as an irregular, generally round granule with a central dimple or slit. Even when viewed with polarized light, the Maltese cross formation produced by starch is more irregular and fussy than the very round, regular formation produced by droplets of cholesterol (Fig. 14-119).

## Fibers (Including Disposable Diaper Fibers)

Disposable diaper fibers are particularly troublesome in their resemblance to waxy casts (see Fig. 14-120). They may be seen in the urine of both infants and incontinent adults. They should be suspected when other findings associated with waxy casts, such as protein, are absent. As described earlier, diaper fibers will polarize light but waxy casts will not (Fig. 14-121).

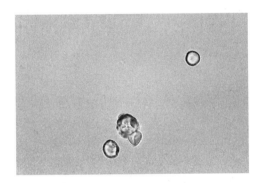

**FIG 14-118.** Starch granules, showing typical irregular, generally round, dimpled appearance with brightfield illumination, ×400.

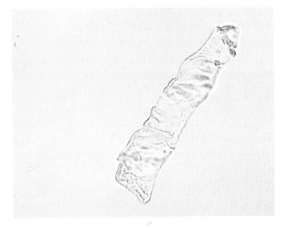

**FIG 14-120.** Diaper fiber resembling a waxy cast, ×400.

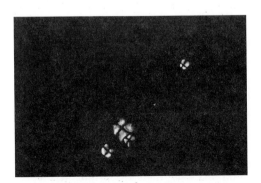

**FIG 14-119.** Starch granules showing Maltese cross formation with polarized light, ×400.

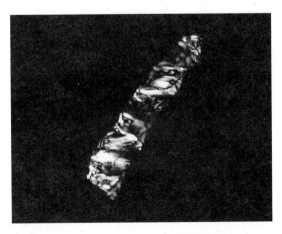

**FIG 14-121.** Diaper fiber, shown in Fig. 14-120, showing the presence of birefringence when viewed with polarized light, ×400. Waxy casts do not polarize light, as shown in Fig. 14-80.

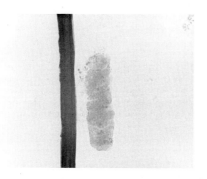

**FIG 14-122.** Fiber, probably hair *(left)*; waxy cast *(right)*. Sedi-Stain, ×400.

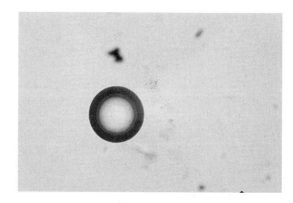

**FIG 14-123.** Air bubble (large), ×400.

Other contaminants may be introduced into the urine specimen at the time of collection, or by laboratory personnel at the time of specimen processing or examination. These include cotton threads, wood fibers, synthetic fibers, and hair. They are all highly refractile structures that should not be mistaken for casts (Fig. 14-122).

## Air Bubbles

These are highly refractile and structureless and easily recognized (Fig. 14-123). They may be introduced as the coverglass is applied to the urine sediment or as the sediment is introduced into the standardized slide.

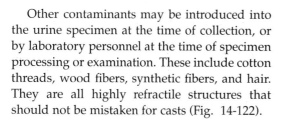

**FIG 14-124.** Oil droplets, extraneous oil (nonphysiologic), ×500.

## Oil Droplets

Oil droplets may be the result of contamination from lubricants such as vaginal creams, catheter lubricant, or mineral oil. They may be confused with red blood cells or fat globules of physiologic origin. Oil droplets are highly refractile and structureless (Fig. 14-124).

Contaminating oil should be distinguished from fat of physiologic origin. True lipiduria is usually associated with other findings, such as proteinuria, fatty casts, and oval fat bodies, as described previously.

## Glass Fragments

Colorless, highly refractile, pleomorphic fragments of glass (probably from very small pieces of coverglass) might appear like crystals (Fig. 14-125).

## Stains

The various supravital stains used in the examination of the urine sediment may precipitate, especially when added to urine of an alkaline pH. This may be seen as an amorphous purple granulation, or brown to purple needle-shaped crystals in clusters. Sudan III fat stain may also precipitate as clusters of needle-shaped crystals that are bright red or red-orange. When such precipitation occurs, identification of pathologic structures that might be present is difficult.

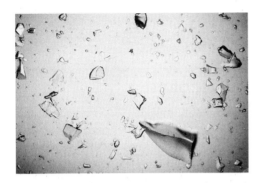

**FIG 14-125.** Glass fragments (from coverglass) appearing like crystals, ×100.

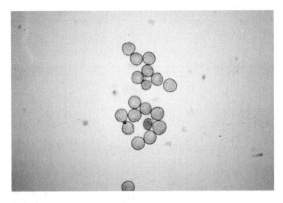

**FIG 14-126.** Pollen grains, seasonal contamination, ×100

## Pollen Grains

These may be seen as a urine contaminant, especially on a seasonal basis. They are fairly large and regularly shaped, with a thick cell wall. They may resemble the eggs of some parasitic worms (Fig. 14-126).

## Fecal Contamination

The presence of fecal elements in urine is usually the result of contamination during collection. However, if there is a **fistula** (an abnormal connection) between the colon and the urinary tract, fecal constituents may be seen in the urine. This is a serious pathologic condition, for it leads to recurrent infection of the urinary tract.

The presence of feces in the urine is usually observed as an overall yellow-brown color of the gross urine specimen. Microscopic findings include plant fibers, skeletal muscle fibers, and microorganisms (Fig. 14-127). Rarely, columnar epithelial cells from the gut mucosa or squamous epithelial cells from the anal mucosa are seen.

When detection of a fistula is clinically indicated, patients may be fed activated charcoal, which is carefully searched for in the urine. The presence of charcoal in the urine demonstrates an abnormal connection between the gut and the urinary tract (Fig. 14-128).

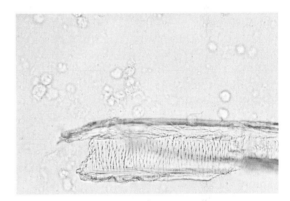

**FIG 14-127.** Fecal contamination, showing presence of large plant fiber, cells, and bacteria, ×400.

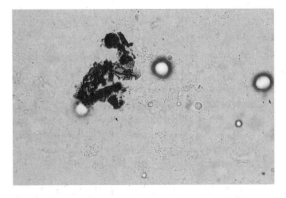

**FIG 14-128.** Charcoal in urine, indicating fecal contamination due to a fistula, ×400.

## QUALITY ASSURANCE

The urinalysis laboratory, like all departments of the clinical laboratory, requires a quality assurance program to ensure that results are meaningful for the physician and the patient. The use of multiple-reagent strips generally ensures rapid and reliable screening of all specimens for a greater range of abnormal constituents than was possible before they came into routine use. However, the principle of each test and its limitations and possible sources of interference and error must be understood. It is necessary to know which tests can be used only to screen for the presence or absence of a substance and which tests yield semiquantitative results. The necessity for and performance of confirmatory methods must be understood and employed. Tests must be performed in a technically correct manner, and the reagent strips and tablets must be stored properly so that they react as they are designed to. The latter is ensured by the use of control specimens.

The specifics of a given quality assurance program are beyond the scope of this book. However, it must meet CLIA '88 regulations. General principles follow. Details are contained within NCCLS urinalysis guidelines.[9] Quality assurance elements include record keeping, the procedure manual, materials and equipment, proficiency testing, and continuing education and training.

The quality assurance program begins with adequate and consistent record keeping. All procedures that are performed must be described in a procedure manual. This should include information regarding controls for the analyte in question, expected values, information regarding confirmatory testing, test principles for each procedure, and current product inserts. In addition, a record of lot number and expiration date for each container of reagent strips should be kept, along with control values. Information must also be recorded along with patient results. This includes time and date of collection, the lot number of the products used in testing the specimen, control solution results, and the identity of the person performing the test.

## CONTROL SOLUTIONS AND RECORDS

Control solutions must be used each day by each shift of workers. They are particularly necessary in the urinalysis laboratory because the least trained and most inexperienced personnel continue to be placed in this important department. Several quality control products are commercially available and suitable for use in the laboratory. Most are obtained in lyophilized form (freeze-dried human urine) and require reconstitution before use. Positive and negative controls are available, and both should be used in the routine testing program. The products are assayed for expected results with commonly used reagent strips and methods. The assayed values that are available for a product will be a factor in determining which product is used by a laboratory.

Urinalysis control solutions may be used both as a check on the urinalysis reagents and procedures and as a means of evaluating the ability of the laboratory personnel to correctly perform and interpret the tests. New bottles of reagent strips and tablets should be tested when they are first opened. All previously opened bottles of reagent strips and tablets should be tested at the beginning of each shift. Controls should be included whenever new reagents are used. Control solutions should be employed that check for both false-negative and false-positive results, the relative sensitivity at different concentrations, and the stability of the reagents. Results should be recorded or documented in such a way as to ensure that the laboratory remains in control and that problems are corrected when detected. The notation system used will vary from laboratory to laboratory; control results may be tabulated on daily and weekly graphs similar to those used for clinical chemistry analyses. One system describing when control specimens should be tested is the following:

1. Test all opened bottles of reagent strips or tablets each morning.
2. Test each new bottle on opening.
3. Record data on the record sheet daily.

All bottles should be covered tightly when not in use. Directions given by the manufacturer for storage should be carefully followed. If any discoloration appears on the reagent strips or tablets, discard the bottle immediately. Record the date on which a bottle is first opened. Note the expiration date, and do not use any product after that date.

Refractometers should also be checked daily for accuracy, and the data should be recorded in an acceptable manner. The method of checking urinometers and refractometers was described under Specific Gravity, earlier in this chapter.

## SPECIMEN COLLECTION AND HANDLING

Of course, the best quality control system will be useless if the urine specimen is not collected and handled in an acceptable manner, before and after reaching the urinalysis laboratory, or if it is mislabeled. Such mistakes remain the most frequent causes of error in routine urinalysis. One method of at least partial control of handling or specimen errors is to include blind controls or blind duplicates in the daily collection of urine specimens to be analyzed.

## INSPECTION OF RESULTS AND CORRELATION OF FINDINGS

Probably the oldest and still most useful tool in quality control of urinalysis is a final inspection of all the results that make up the urinalysis before they are reported to the physician or placed on the patient's laboratory record. Correlation of expected findings has been discussed throughout this section whenever applicable. To correctly inspect the laboratory record for correlated results, the worker must know the limitations of the tests and the reasons for their use. Physical properties, chemical test results, and constituents seen in the urinary sediment should be correlated, and if discrepancies are seen, they should be corrected or explained before results are reported.

## REFERENCES

1. Cohen HT, Spiegel DM: Air-exposed urine dipsticks give false-positive results for glucose and false-negative results for blood. *Am J Clin Pathol* 1991; 96:398-400.
2. College of American Pathologists 1996 Proficiency Testing Program: *Glossary of Terms.* Chapter 2: Clinical Microscopy. Northfield, Ill, College of American Pathologists, 1996, p 12.
3. Henry JB, Lauzon RL, Schumann GB: Basic examination of urine. In Henry JB (ed): *Clinical Diagnosis and Management by Laboratory Methods,* ed 19. Philadelphia, WB Saunders Co, 1996, p 416.
4. NCCLS: *Urinalysis and Collection, Transportation, and Preservation of Urine Specimens: Approved Guidelines.* Villanova, Pa, National Committee for Clinical Laboratory Standards, 1995, GP16-A (vol 12, no 15), p 1.
5. NCCLS: *Urinalysis and Collection, Transportation, and Preservation of Urine Specimens: Approved Guidelines.* Villanova, Pa, National Committee for Clinical Laboratory Standards, 1995, GP16-A (vol 12, no 15), p 4.
6. NCCLS: *Urinalysis and Collection, Transportation, and Preservation of Urine Specimens: Approved Guidelines.* Villanova, Pa, National Committee for Clinical Laboratory Standards, 1995, GP16-A (vol 12, no 15), pp 5-6.
7. NCCLS: *Urinalysis and Collection, Transportation, and Preservation of Urine Specimens: Approved Guidelines.* Villanova, Pa, National Committee for Clinical Laboratory Standards, 1995, GP16-A (vol 12, no 15), p 7.
8. NCCLS: *Urinalysis and Collection, Transportation, and Preservation of Urine Specimens: Approved Guidelines.* Villanova, Pa, National Committee for Clinical Laboratory Standards, 1995, GP16-A (vol 12, no 15), pp 8-9.

9. NCCLS: *Urinalysis and Collection, Transportation, and Preservation of Urine Specimens: Approved Guidelines.* Villanova, Pa, National Committee for Clinical Laboratory Standards, 1995, GP16-A (vol 12, no 15), pp 10-12.

10. Pietrach CA et al: Comparison of the Hoesch and Watson-Schwartz tests for urinary porphobilinogen. *Clin Chem* 1977; 23:166.

11. Ringsrud KM, Linné JJ: *Urinalysis and Body Fluids: A ColorText and Atlas.* St Louis, Mosby, 1995, pp 25-27. This section is reprinted with permission.

12. Schweitzer SS, Schumann JL, Schumann GB: Quality assurance guideline of the urinalysis laboratory. *J Med Technol* 1986; 3(11):569.

13. US package insert. West Point, Pa, Merck & Co, Inc, 1996.

## BIBLIOGRAPHY

College of American Pathologists 1996 Proficiency Testing Program: *Glossary of Terms.* Chapter 2: Clinical Microscopy. Northfield, Ill, College of American Pathologists, 1996.

Graff L: *A Handbook of Routine Urinalysis.* Philadelphia, JB Lippincott Co, 1983.

Haber MH: *A Primer of Microscopic Urinalysis,* ed 2. Garden Grove, Calif, Hycor Biomedical, 1991.

Haber MH: *Urinary Sediment: A Textbook Atlas.* Chicago, American Society of Clinical Pathologists, 1981.

Haber MH: *Urine Casts: Their Microscopy and Clinical Significance,* ed 2. Chicago, American Society of Clinical Pathologists, 1976.

Henry JB, Lauzon RL, Schumann GB: *Basic Examination of Urine.* In Henry JB (ed): *Clinical Diagnosis and Management by Laboratory Methods,* ed 19. Philadelphia, WB Saunders Co, 1996.

Kaplan LA and Pesce AJ: *Clinical Chemistry,* ed 3. St Louis, Mosby, 1996.

Mahon CR, Smith LA: Standardization of the urine microscopic examination. *Clin Lab Sci* 1990; 3:328.

NCCLS: *Continuous Quality Improvement: Essential Management Approaches and Their Use in Proficiency Testing, Proposed Guideline.* Villanova, Pa, National Committee for Clinical Laboratory Standards, 1997, GP 22-P.

NCCLS: *Physician's Office Laboratory Guidelines: Procedure Manual, Tentative Guidelines,* ed 3. Villanova, Pa, National Committee for Clinical Laboratory Standards, 1995, POL 1/2-T3 and POL 3-R.

NCCLS: *Urinalysis and Collection,Transportation, and Preservation of Urine Specimens: Approved Guidelines.* Villanova, Pa, National Committee for Clinical Laboratory Standards, 1995, GP16-A.

Ringsrud KM, Linné JJ: *Urinalysis and Body Fluids: A ColorText and Atlas,* St Louis, Mosby, 1995.

Schumann GB: *Urine Sediment Examination.* Baltimore, Williams & Wilkins Co, 1980.

Schumann GB, Schumann JL, Marcussen N: *Cytodiagnostic Urinalysis of Renal and Lower Urinary Tract Disorders,* New York, IGAKU-SHOIN Medical Publishers, Inc, 1995.

Schweitzer SS, Schumann JL, Schumann GB: Quality assurance guideline of the urinalysis laboratory. *J Med Technol* 1986; 3(11):569.

Ward PCJ: *The Urinary Sediment.* St Louis, Mosby, Image Premastering Services, 1992.

# STUDY QUESTIONS

1. Define urinalysis.

2. In general, urinalysis will provide information about what two disease systems or conditions?

   A.
   B.

3. List six considerations that must be kept in mind in performing a routine urinalysis.

   A.
   B.
   C.
   D.
   E.
   F.

4. Urine is primarily composed of what two dissolved substances?

   A.
   B.

5. What is the primary cause of decomposition of urine after it is voided?

6. What is the preferred method of preservation of the urine specimen if it cannot be examined immediately after it is voided?

7. Match the following descriptions of urine volume (1 to 5) with their definitions (A to E).

   1. Anuria
   2. Diuresis
   3. Nocturia
   4. Oliguria
   5. Polyuria

   _____ A. Any increase in urine volume, even temporary
   _____ B. Complete absence of urine formation
   _____ C. Consistent elimination of >2,000 mL urine per 24 hours
   _____ D. Excretion of <500 mL urine per 24 hours
   _____ E. Excretion of >400 mL urine at night

8. Complete the following sentence concerning normal urine color. The normal urine is some shade of _____.

9. Match the following abnormal urine colors (1 to 10) with their causes (A to J).

   1. Amber
   2. Black (or brown) on standing
   3. Bright orange
   4. Brown (yellow-brown or green-brown)
   5. Clear red
   6. Cloudy red
   7. Dark red or red-purple
   8. Dark red-brown
   9. Orange (orange-red or orange-brown)
   10. Pale

   _____ A. Bilirubin
   _____ B. Concentrated urine
   _____ C. Dilute urine
   _____ D. Hemoglobin
   _____ E. Melanin or homogentisic
   _____ F. Myoglobin
   _____ G. Phenazopyridine (Pyridium)
   _____ H. Porphyrins
   _____ I. Red blood cells (hematuria)
   _____ J. Urobilinogen

10. A urine specimen with a strong ammoniacal odor is *most often* the result of:

    A. Diabetes mellitus
    B. Improper handling and storage
    C. Ingestion of certain foodstuffs
    D. Urinary tract infection

11. Match each of the following causes of foam when a urine specimen is stoppered and shaken (1 to 3) with its appearance (A to C).

    1. Bilirubin
    2. Normal urine
    3. Protein

    _____ A. Yellow and abundant
    _____ B. White and abundant, persistent
    _____ C. White, small amount that dissipates

12. **Indicate whether the following statements concerning specific gravity are true (T) or false (F).**

_____ A. If the kidney is unable to concentrate or dilute urine, the specific gravity will be fixed at about 1.010.

_____ B. Reagent strips for specific gravity and the refractometer measure different things.

_____ C. Reagent strips measure any substances that is dissolved in the urine.

_____ D. Specific gravity is a measure of the amount of dissolved substances in solution.

_____ E. The refractometer measures only substances that ionize.

_____ F. The specific gravity of water is always the same.

_____ G. Within the error of the method, specific gravity by reagent strip is always equivalent to specific gravity by refractometer.

13. **Indicate whether the following statements concerning the measurement of urine pH are true (T) or false (F). Urine pH:**

_____ A. Is an indicator of proteinuria.

_____ B. Is helpful in the identification of crystals in the urine.

_____ C. Is unaffected by diet.

_____ D. Is useful in the assessment of specimen acceptability for examination.

_____ E. May be used as an indication of urinary tract infection.

14. **Detection of which of the following urine constituents is _most_ helpful in the detection and diagnosis of renal disease?**

A. Blood
B. Leukocyte esterase
C. Nitrite
D. Protein
E. Specific gravity

15. **Match the following protein types (1 to 5) with the following statements (A to E).**

1. Albumin
2. Globulin
3. Hemoglobin
4. Light-chain immunoglobulins (Bence Jones protein)
5. Tamm-Horsfall protein

_____ A. Associated with gammaglobulinopathies like multiple myeloma

_____ B. May be seen in urine as the result of intravascular hemolysis

_____ C. Molecule is generally too large to be filtered through the glomerulus

_____ D. Secreted by the distal convoluted tubules of the nephron

_____ E. The protein most associated with glomerular damage

16. **The reagent strip test for protein is most likely to show a positive reaction with which of the following?**

A. Albumin
B. Hemoglobin
C. Light-chain immunoglobulins
D. Tamm-Horsfall protein

17. **The sulfosalicylic acid test for protein is most likely to show a positive reaction with which of the following?**

A. Albumin
B. Globulin
C. Light-chain immunoglobulins
D. Tamm-Horsfall protein
E. All of the above

18. **Which of the following will give a false-positive sulfosalicylic acid test result for protein?**

A. Ascorbic acid
B. Azo-containing drugs or compounds
C. Highly buffered alkaline urine
D. Radiographic contrast media

19. **Which of the following is _not_ detected by the reagent strip test for blood?**

A. Hemoglobin
B. Hemosiderin
C. Myoglobin
D. Red blood cells

20. The presence of which of the following urine constituents might give a false-negative reaction if only supernatant urine is tested, rather than a well-mixed urine specimen?

A. Glucose
B. Hemoglobin
C. Nitrite
D. Protein
E. Red blood cells

21. Reagent strip tests that depend on the release of oxygen and subsequent oxidation of a chromogen, resulting in a color change, are subject to false-negative reactions because of the presence of:

A. Ascorbic acid
B. Azo-containing drugs or compounds
C. Chlorine bleach
D. Low specific gravity
E. Vitamin D

22. Indicate whether the following statements concerning the reagent strip test for nitrite in the urine are true (T) or false (F).

_____ A. Tests for nitrite tend to be positive when large numbers of gram-positive bacteria are present.
_____ B. Tests for nitrite tend to be positive when large numbers of gram-negative bacteria are present.
_____ C. Negative reactions for nitrite rule out the presence of urinary tract infection.
_____ D. Results are most useful if positive, as an indicator of urinary tract infection.
_____ E. A 4-hour incubation in the bladder is required for conversion of nitrate to nitrite.
_____ F. Results may be negative in the presence of severe urinary tract infection by gram-negative organisms in starving, fasting, or hospitalized patients being fed intravenously.

23. Reagent strip tests for urinary leukocyte esterase are most useful in the detection of:

A. Immunosuppression
B. Malignancy
C. Renal transplant rejection
D. Urinary tract infection

24. Reagent strip tests for urinary leukocyte esterase are most useful when results are evaluated together with the results for the reagent strip test for:

A. Blood
B. Nitrite
C. Protein
D. Specific gravity

25. A positive reagent strip test for glucose is most associated with which of the following conditions?

A. Anorexia nervosa
B. Diabetes insipidus
C. Diabetes mellitus
D. Starvation
E. Urinary tract infection

26. Match the tests for urine sugar (1 or 2) with the following statements (A to I).

1. Copper reduction test (Clinitest)
2. Reagent strip test

_____ A. May give false-negative reaction when sufficient ascorbic acid is present
_____ B. May give positive reaction when sufficient ascorbic acid is present
_____ C. Reacts with any reducing sugar or substance, including glucose
_____ D. Specific for glucose
_____ E. Test is based on a double sequential enzyme reaction
_____ F. Test is based on the conversion of copper II to copper I ions
_____ G. Test will be negative in the presence of galactose
_____ H. This test should be performed on patients less than 1 year of age
_____ I. Will detect a smaller quantity of glucose (more sensitive)

27. Name the three ketone bodies.

A.
B.
C.

28. Name two conditions that are associated with ketonuria.

A.

B.

29. Indicate whether the following statements concerning bilirubin and urobilinogen are true (T) or false (F).

_____ A. Bilirubin glucuronide is the conjugated form of bilirubin.

_____ B. Conjugated bilirubin is *not* soluble in water.

_____ C. Conjugation of bilirubin takes place in the intestine.

_____ D. Conversion of bilirubin to urobilinogen takes place in the intestine.

_____ E. Free bilirubin is also known as conjugated bilirubin.

_____ F. In cases of obstructive jaundice, urine bilirubin and urobilinogen are both increased.

_____ G. In order to be present in urine, bilirubin must be in a water-soluble form.

_____ H. Increased urine urobilinogen is associated with hemolytic jaundice and liver disease.

_____ I. Jaundice is the presence of an increased concentration of any form of bilirubin in the blood.

30. Match the following tests (1 to 4) with the statements concerning urinary urobilinogen and porphobilinogen (A to G). Tests may be used more than once.

1. Chemstrip reagent strip test
2. Hoesch test
3. Multistix reagent strip test
4. Watson-Schwartz test

_____ A. Test is based on a diazo reaction.

_____ B. Test is based on the inverse Ehrlich aldehyde reaction.

_____ C. Test is based on the Ehrlich aldehyde reaction.

_____ D. Test is specific for porphobilinogen.

_____ E. Test is specific for urobilinogen.

_____ F. Test may be positive with urobilinogen, porphobilinogen, and intermediate Ehrlich-reactive compounds.

_____ G. Test may react but is not a reliable means of detecting porphobilinogen.

31. Indicate which of the following tests (yes or no) may give a *false-negative* reaction in the presence of sufficient quantities of ascorbic acid.

_____ A. Bilirubin
_____ B. Blood
_____ C. Clinitest
_____ D. Glucose
_____ E. Nitrite
_____ F. Protein
_____ G. Sulfosalicylic acid test

32. Match the following urine constituents (1 to 11) with the test principles (A to I). Test principles may have more than one constituent.

1. Bilirubin
2. Blood
3. Glucose
4. Ketones
5. Leukocyte esterase
6. Nitrite
7. pH
8. Protein
9. Reducing sugars
10. Specific gravity
11. Urobilinogen

_____ A. Copper reduction test

_____ B. Diazo reaction

_____ C. Double pH indicator system

_____ D. Double sequential enzyme reaction based on glucose oxidase

_____ E. Ehrlich aldehyde reaction

_____ F. Peroxidase activity of heme

_____ G. $Pk_a$ change of polyelectrolytes (ionic concentration)

_____ H. Protein error of pH indicators

_____ I. Reaction with sodium nitroprusside

33. **List six factors that should be standardized in the microscopic examination of the urine sediment.**

    A.

    B.

    C.

    D.

    E.

    F.

34. **Phase-contrast microscopy is most useful in recognizing which of the following?**

    A. Crystals

    B. Hyaline casts

    C. Oval fat bodies

    D. Red blood cell casts

35. **The following elements seen in the urine sediment exhibit birefringence,** *except:*

    A. Diaper fibers

    B. Most crystals

    C. Oval fat bodies containing cholesterol

    D. Red blood cell casts

    E. Starch granules

36. **Complete the following. Birefringence is the ability of a crystal or substance to _____.**

37. **Match the following microscopic findings (1 to 4) with the statements concerning red cells (A to D).**

    1. Dysmorphic red cells

    2. Hematuria

    3. Ovoid calcium oxalate

    4. Shadow or swollen red cells

    _____ A. A sensitive early indicator of renal disease

    _____ B. Distorted or misshapen red cells that may indicate glomerular damage

    _____ C. May be differentiated from red cells with polarizing microscopy

    _____ D. Presence associated with dilute or hypotonic urine, difficult to see with brightfield microscopy

38. **Match the leukocytes or epithelial cells (1 to 9) with the following statements (A to I).**

    1. Clue cells

    2. Eosinophils

    3. Glitter cells

    4. Lymphocytes

    5. Neutrophils (PMNs)

    6. Oval fat bodies

    7. Renal epithelial cells

    8. Squamous epithelial cells

    9. Transitional epithelial cells

    _____ A. Indicate active kidney disease or tubular injury when 15 or more cells are seen in 10 high-power fields (1.5/hpf)

    _____ B. May be seen with infection and after urethral catheterization

    _____ C. Presence an early indicator of renal transplant rejection

    _____ D. Presence associated with drug-induced interstitial nephritis

    _____ E. Presence associated with the nephrotic syndrome

    _____ F. Presence usually indicates vaginal contamination

    _____ G. Squamous epithelial cells associated with vaginosis and *Gardnerella vaginalis* infection

    _____ H. Swollen neutrophils exhibiting Brownian motion; associated with hypotonic urine, specific gravity 1.010

    _____ I. The type of leukocyte most often seen in urine; indicates inflammation somewhere in the urogenital tract

39. **Match the following special microscopic or staining techniques (1 to 6) with the urine constituents (A to H). Techniques may be used more than once.**

    1. Gram stain

    2. Hansel's stain

    3. Phase-contrast microscopy

    4. Polarizing microscopy

    5. Rous test (Prussian blue stain)

    6. Sudan stain

    _____ A. Bacteria

    _____ B. Cholesterol esters

    _____ C. Eosinophils

    _____ D. Hemosiderin

    _____ E. Neutral fat/triglycerides

    _____ F. Oval fat bodies

    _____ G. *Trichomonas*

    _____ H. Yeast

40. **The presence of which of the following types of casts has the *least* clinical significance:**

    A. Fatty
    B. Granular
    C. Hyaline
    D. Red cell
    E. Waxy
    F. White cell

41. **Match the following types of cast (1 to 8) with the disease states or conditions (A to H).**

    1. Epithelial cell cast
    2. Fatty cast
    3. Hemosiderin cast
    4. Hyaline or granular cast
    5. Myoglobin cast
    6. Red blood cell cast
    7. Waxy cast
    8. White blood cell cast

    _____ A. Acute glomerulonephritis
    _____ B. Acute pyelonephritis
    _____ C. Chronic renal disease or renal failure
    _____ D. Heavy metal or nephrotoxic poisoning
    _____ E. Nephrotic syndrome or diabetic nephropathy
    _____ F. Severe crushing injury
    _____ G. Severe intravascular hemolysis
    _____ H. Strenuous exercise

42. **Indicate whether the following statements concerning crystals found in the urine sediment are true (T) or false (F).**

    _____ A. Ammonium biurate crystals are a common finding in freshly voided alkaline urine.
    _____ B. Cystine is an abnormal crystal associated with stone formation.
    _____ C. Hemosiderin may be seen as free granules, in cells or casts, several days after an acute hemolytic episode.
    _____ D. Most abnormal crystals are seen in urine of an alkaline pH.
    _____ E. Most crystals seen in urine exhibit birefringence.

    _____ F. Most kidney or bladder stones are made up of calcium oxalate or a calcium-containing compound.
    _____ G. The amorphous material seen in alkaline urine is amorphous urate.
    _____ H. The crystalline form of cholesterol (large, flat, hexagonal plate) is a common finding seen in most cases of the nephrotic syndrome.
    _____ I. The identification of normal crystals is based primarily on the urine pH and the morphology of the crystal.
    _____ J. The presence of abnormal crystals requires confirmation before they are reported.
    _____ K. The presence of crystals is most significant when they are seen in an absolutely fresh urine specimen.
    _____ L. The presence of crystals of the sulfonamides is a common finding in the urine and is of no clinical significance.
    _____ M. The use of phase-contrast microscopy is especially helpful in the identification of urine crystals.
    _____ N. The use of polarizing microscopy is not particularly helpful in the identification of urine crystals.
    _____ O. Uric acid crystals in the urine sediment indicate that the patient is probably suffering from gout.

43. **Finding which of the following chemical constituents is most helpful in differentiating waxy casts and disposable diaper fibers?**

    A. Bilirubin
    B. Blood
    C. Glucose
    D. Leukocyte esterase
    E. Protein

44. Which of the following urine sediment constituents is useful in detecting the presence of a fistula between the urinary tract and the gastrointestinal tract?

    A. Activated charcoal
    B. Ammonium biurate crystals
    C. Red blood cells
    D. Uric acid crystals
    E. Waxy casts

45. Twelve milliliters of urine is centrifuged and 1 mL retained for microscopic examination of the sediment. It is found to contain an average of 15 white blood cells, 3 hyaline casts, and no red blood cells. The presence of some squamous epithelial cells is noted. The results should be reported as:

    Concentration _____
    Hyaline casts _____
    Red cells _____
    White blood cells _____
    Squamous epithelial cells _____

## CASE HISTORIES

### ■ CASE I

A 20-year-old female college student with a sore throat is seen in the student health service. A throat swab is cultured and reported positive for group A beta-hemolytic streptococci. She is treated with an intramuscular injection of penicillin. Two weeks later, she wakes up in the morning and finds that she has decreased urine volume, and her urine is dark red. She also has a fever, and swelling in her feet. She returns to the student health service, where urine is collected for urinalysis. The following urinalysis results were obtained:

**Physical Appearance**

| | |
|---|---|
| Color | Red |
| Transparency | Cloudy |

**Chemical Screening**

| | |
|---|---|
| pH | 6 |
| Specific gravity | 1.025 |
| Protein (reagent strip) | 100 mg/dL |
| Protein (SSA) | 2+ |
| Blood | Large |
| Nitrite | Negative |
| Leukocyte esterase | Negative |
| Glucose | Negative |
| Ketones | Trace |
| Bilirubin | Negative |
| Urobilinogen | Normal |

**Microscopic Examination**

| | |
|---|---|
| Red blood cells | 10-25 per hpf |
| | Dysmorphic forms present |
| White blood cells | 0-2 per hpf |
| Casts | 2-5 red blood cell casts per lpf |
| Crystals | Moderate amorphous urates |

1. List the abnormal findings.
2. In this case, the proteinuria is probably due to which of the following?
    A. Glomerular damage
    B. Lower urinary tract disorders
    C. Prerenal disorders
    D. Tubular (or interstitial) damage
3. The presence of dysmorphic red cells and red cell casts indicates which of the following?
    A. Bleeding due to kidney stone formation
    B. Kidney disease located in the glomerulus
    C. Kidney infection
    D. Probable menstrual contamination
4. The trace reagent strip reaction for ketone and the presence of amorphous urates in the urine sediment of this patient are probably the result of:
    A. A false-positive ketone reaction due to sensitivity of the test
    B. Dehydration due to fever with concentration of urine
    C. The presence of dysmorphic red cells and red cell casts
    D. The presence of protein

5. Which of the following conditions is exhibited by this patient?
   A. Acute cystitis
   B. Acute drug-induced interstitial nephritis
   C. Acute glomerulonephritis
   D. Acute pyelonephritis
   E. Nephrotic syndrome

## ■ CASE 2

An 8-year-old girl complains of feeling like she needs to urinate all the time. Her urine burns when she does void and it is cloudy. She is seen by her pediatrician, where urine is collected for routine urinalysis and culture. The following urinalysis results were obtained:

**Physical Appearance**

| | |
|---|---|
| Color | Pale |
| Transparency | Cloudy |

**Chemical Screening**

| | |
|---|---|
| pH | 7.5 |
| Specific gravity | 1.010 |
| Protein (reagent strip) | Trace |
| Protein (SSA) | Trace |
| Blood | Negative |
| Nitrite | Positive |
| Leukocyte esterase | Positive |
| Glucose | Negative |
| Ketones | Negative |
| Bilirubin | Negative |
| Urobilinogen | Normal |

**Microscopic Examination**

| | |
|---|---|
| Red blood cells | 0-2 per hpf |
| White blood cells | 50-100 per hpf |
| | Clumps of white cells seen |
| Casts | None seen |
| Crystals | Moderate amorphous phosphates |
| Bacteria | Many rods |

1. List the abnormal results.
2. The positive reagent strip test for nitrite in this patient is probably due to which of the following?
   A. An infection due to gram-negative bacteria
   B. An infection due to gram-positive bacteria
   C. An infection due to yeast
   D. An old urine specimen, unsuitable for examination

3. The positive reagent strip test for leukocyte esterase in this case is due to the presence of which of the following?
   A. Amorphous phosphates
   B. Bacteria
   C. Nitrite
   D. Protein
   E. Red blood cells
   F. White blood cells
4. In this case, the alkaline pH is due to the presence of which of the following?
   A. Bacteria
   B. Leukocyte esterase
   C. Nitrite
   D. Protein
   E. White blood cells
5. In this case, the proteinuria is probably due to which of the following?
   A. Glomerular damage
   B. Lower urinary tract infection
   C. Prerenal disorders
   D. Upper urinary tract infection
6. Which of the following conditions is exhibited by this patient?
   A. Acute cystitis
   B. Acute drug-induced interstitial nephritis
   C. Acute glomerulonephritis
   D. Acute pyelonephritis
   E. Nephrotic syndrome

## ■ CASE 3

A 45-year-old man has been a paraplegic since being involved in a motorcycle accident 20 years ago. He has a history of recurrent urinary tract infections as a result of infection from an indwelling catheter. He now has severe back pain, with fever, chills, and vomiting. He has been exposed to "the flu" and seeks medical attention. A midstream urine specimen is collected for examination and culture. The following routine urinalysis results were obtained:

**Physical Appearance**

| | |
|---|---|
| Color | Yellow |
| Transparency | Cloudy |

## Chemical Screening

| | |
|---|---|
| pH | 6.5 |
| Specific gravity | 1.010 |
| Protein (reagent strip) | 100 mg/dL |
| Protein (SSA) | 2+ |
| Blood | Moderate |
| Nitrite | Negative |
| Leukocyte esterase | Positive |
| Glucose | Negative |
| Ketones | Negative |
| Bilirubin | Negative |
| Urobilinogen | Normal |

## Microscopic Examination

| | |
|---|---|
| Red blood cells | 2-5 per hpf |
| White blood cells | 10-25 per hpf |
| Casts | 5-10 cellular casts per lpf |
| Bacteria | Moderate rods |

1. List the abnormal findings.
2. In this case, the proteinuria is probably due to which of the following?
   A. Glomerular damage
   B. Lower urinary tract disorders
   C. Prerenal disorders
   D. Tubular (or interstitial) damage
3. Concerning the positive leukocyte esterase and the negative nitrite in this case, which of the following statements is correct?
   A. The leukocyte esterase test is probably a false-positive reaction.
   B. The negative nitrite reaction is probably due to insensitivity of the test or lack of sufficient incubation of urine in the bladder.
   C. The positive leukocyte esterase reaction indicates that an upper urinary tract infection is present.
   D. The presence of a bacterial infection is ruled out because of the negative nitrite reaction.
4. Concerning the positive reagent strip test for blood and the relatively low level of red blood cells seen in the urine sediment of this patient, which of the following statements is correct?
   A. The presence of hematuria is not consistent with the disease exhibited by this patient.
   B. The presence of protein is probably interfering with the chemical test for blood.

C. The reagent strip test is extremely sensitive and consistent with the microscopic findings.
   D. The reagent strip test is probably falsely positive because of the presence of ascorbic acid.
5. The presence of white blood cells, bacteria, and cellular casts in this urine specimen indicate which of the following?
   A. A urinary tract infection located within the kidney
   B. A urinary tract infection located in the bladder
   C. An inflammatory condition of the urinary tract
   D. The presence of a kidney stone
6. In this case, the cells present in the casts were probably derived from which of the following?
   A. Epithelial cells
   B. Lymphocytes
   C. Neutrophils
   D. Red blood cells
7. Which of the following conditions is exhibited by this patient?
   A. Acute cystitis
   B. Acute drug-induced interstitial nephritis
   C. Acute glomerulonephritis
   D. Acute pyelonephritis
   E. Nephrotic syndrome

## ■ CASE 4

A 12-year-old boy has a history of several infections in the past few months. He is now very lethargic and swollen, with generalized edema. He tells his mother that his urine is very foamy when he urinates and that he feels awful. He is seen by his pediatrician, and urinalysis is performed with the following results:

## Physical Appearance

| | |
|---|---|
| Color | Pale |
| Transparency | Cloudy |
| Foam | Abundant, white foam |

### Chemical Screening

| | |
|---|---|
| pH | 6.0 |
| Specific gravity | 1.010 |
| Protein (reagent strip) | >2000 mg/dL |
| Protein (SSA) | 4+ |
| Blood | Trace |
| Nitrite | Negative |
| Leukocyte esterase | Negative |
| Glucose | Negative |
| Ketones | Negative |
| Bilirubin | Negative |
| Urobilinogen | Negative |

### Microscopic Examination

| | |
|---|---|
| Red blood cells | 0-2 per hpf |
| White blood cells | 0-2 per hpf |
| Casts | 5-10 fatty casts per lpf |
| | 2-5 hyaline casts per lpf |
| Epithelial cells | Few renal epithelial cells |
| | Many oval fat |
| | bodies present |
| Other | Moderate free fat |
| | globules seen |

1. List the abnormal findings.
2. The abundant white foam in this urine specimen is due to the presence of which of the following?
   A. Blood
   B. Casts
   C. Fat
   D. Protein
3. The edema seen in this patient is due to the presence of which of the following?
   A. Blood
   B. Casts
   C. Oval fat bodies
   D. Protein
4. The presence of fatty casts, oval fat bodies, renal epithelial cells, and free fat in this case indicates which of the following?
   A. A lower urinary tract infection
   B. An allergic reaction
   C. An upper urinary tract infection
   D. Severe renal dysfunction, probably glomerular

5. Which of the following conditions is exhibited by this patient?
   A. Acute cystitis
   B. Acute drug-induced interstitial nephritis
   C. Acute glomerulonephritis
   D. Acute pyelonephritis
   E. Nephrotic syndrome

---

### ■ CASE 5

A 9-year old boy has a history of a recent viral infection. He now feels faint and is feverish, and is generally not well. He has to urinate frequently and is very thirsty. His breath smells fruity. He is seen in an urgent care clinic, where blood is drawn and urine collected for routine urinalysis. The following urinalysis results were obtained.

### Physical Appearance

| | |
|---|---|
| Color | Pale |
| Transparency | Clear |

### Chemical Screening

| | |
|---|---|
| pH | 5.0 |
| Specific gravity | 1.029 (refractometer) |
| | 1.005 (reagent strip) |
| Protein (reagent strip) | Negative |
| Blood | Negative |
| Nitrite | Negative |
| Leukocyte esterase | Negative |
| Glucose | >2000 mg/dL |
| Ketones | Large |
| Bilirubin | Negative |
| Urobilinogen | Negative |

### Microscopic Examination

| | |
|---|---|
| Red blood cells | 0-2 per hpf |
| White blood cells | 0-2 per hpf |

1. List the abnormal or discrepant findings.
2. The difference in the specific gravity values in this specimen is probably due to which of the following?
   A. Ability of the refractometer to measure only nonionizing substances
   B. Difference in the principles of the methods
   C. Failure to use proper quality control
   D. Instrument error
   E. Poor technique by the person performing the urinalysis

3. Calculate the concentration of glucose in this urine specimen, given the difference in specific gravity values.

4. The unusual fruity smell of the breath of this patient is due to the presence of:
   A. Acetone
   B. Beta-hydroxybutyric acid
   C. Diacetic acid
   D. Glucose

5. This patient is at risk of losing consciousness as a result of:
   A. Diabetic coma
   B. Diabetic shock
   C. Infection
   D. Kidney failure

6. Which of the following conditions is exhibited by this patient?
   A. Anorexia nervosa
   B. Diabetes insipidus
   C. Diabetes mellitus
   D. Galactosemia
   E. Nephrotic syndrome

## ■ CASE 6

A 60-year-old man who has a history of alcoholism is seen in an urgent care clinic; he complains of extreme pain in his upper abdomen. He has been experiencing pain on and off for the last ten days. Now he is yellow (jaundiced) and feels extremely ill. He also mentions that his stool specimens have lost their normal color, and look like clay. Blood is drawn for testing and urine collected for urinalysis. The following urinalysis results were obtained.

### Physical Appearance

| | |
|---|---|
| Color | Brown (yellow-brown) |
| Transparency | Clear |
| Foam | Abundant yellow foam |

### Chemical Screening

| | |
|---|---|
| pH | 6.5 |
| Specific gravity | 1.020 |
| Protein (reagent strip) | Negative |
| Blood | Negative |
| Nitrite | Negative |
| Leukocyte esterase | Negative |
| Glucose | Negative |
| Ketones | Negative |
| Bilirubin | Large |
| Urobilinogen | Normal |

### Microscopic Examination

| | |
|---|---|
| Red blood cells | 0-2 per hpf |
| White blood cells | 0-2 per hpf |

1. List the abnormal or discrepant findings.

2. The abnormal urine color is due to which of the following?
   A. Bilirubin glucuronide
   B. Free bilirubin
   C. Unconjugated bilirubin
   D. Urobilinogen
   E. More than one of the above

3. The lack of color in the feces is due to an absence of which of the following?
   A. Bilirubin glucuronide
   B. Free bilirubin
   C. Unconjugated bilirubin
   D. Urobilinogen

4. This patient's jaundice is the result of the presence of which of the following?
   A. Bilirubin glucuronide
   B. Free bilirubin
   C. Unconjugated bilirubin
   D. Urobilinogen
   E. More than one of the above

5. From the patient history and the urinalysis, this patient's jaundice is probably the result of:
   A. Acute alcoholism leading to a cirrhotic liver
   B. Hemolytic jaundice
   C. Infectious hepatitis
   D. Obstructive jaundice associated with gallstones

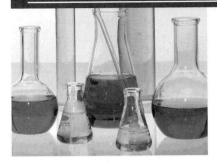

# CHAPTER 15

# Examination of Extravascular Fluids and Miscellaneous Specimens

## Learning Objectives

*From study of this chapter, the reader will be able to:*

➤ Define cerebrospinal fluid and describe the components of routine examination, including gross examination, cell counts, morphologic examination, and common chemical tests.

➤ Differentiate a traumatic tap from a hemorrhage on the basis of gross appearance of the spinal fluid.

➤ Define the serous fluids and describe the components of routine examination.

➤ Define effusion and differentiate a transudate from an exudate.

➤ Define synovial fluid and describe the components of routine examination.

➤ Describe the classification of synovial fluid seen in various joint diseases.

➤ Describe and perform the microscopic examination of synovial fluid for gout and pseudogout, using compensated polarizing microscopy for the identification of crystals.

➤ Describe the examination of nasal fluid for the presence of eosinophils, including collection, staining, and interpretation of results.

➤ Discuss the clinical significance of tests for fecal occult blood.

➤ Describe common interferences in tests for fecal occult blood and special dietary considerations necessary for specimen collection.

➤ Explain the chemical principle of the common slide tests for fecal occult blood.

➤ Describe the significance of testing for the presence of fecal leukocytes, and the procedure for slide preparation.

➤ Describe the cervical mucus test (Fern test) and the postcoital test (PCT).

➤ Describe the components of a qualitative sperm analysis.

# INTRODUCTION

**Extravascular fluids** (body cavity fluids other than blood or urine) are examined in various divisions of the clinical laboratory, depending on the nature of the test requested. Cell counts are routinely done on most body fluids, and for this reason the specimen is often sent directly to the hematology laboratory after collection (see Chapter 3). The extravascular fluids are termed **pleural** (around the lungs), **pericardial** (around the heart), **peritoneal** (around the abdominal and pelvic organs), **synovial** (around the joints), and **cerebrospinal** (around the brain and spinal cord). Each of these fluids is handled in special ways. Analyses of synovial fluid and cerebrospinal fluid are discussed separately. The examination of the other body fluids **(serous fluids)** is discussed in general terms.

Several general observations are made for all body fluids. Gross examination and cell counts are usual. Cytocentrifuged slides or smears are made and, after staining with Wright stain, are examined microscopically. Protein is measured, and clot formation is observed. For other tests ordered, the specimen is sent to a particular division, such as chemistry, microbiology, immunology, or cytology. (See Chapters 11, 16, and 17.)

Tests of miscellaneous other specimens are also included in this chapter. These include examination of nasal smears for eosinophils and examination of the feces for occult blood and leukocytes. In addition, a few tests used to assess reproduction by examination of semen and semen–cervical mucus interaction are included. These are all examples of either waived or provider-performed microscopic procedures according to CLIA '88.

# CEREBROSPINAL FLUID

The usual examination of the cerebrospinal fluid (CSF) specimen includes several observations. Abnormal color, the presence of turbidity, and clot formation are noted. The examination includes cell counts, morphologic examination, chemical analysis, Gram stain, and cultures. CSF is a clear, lymph-like, sterile, extravascular fluid that circulates in the ventricles of the brain, the subarachnoid spaces, and the spinal cord. The normal adult has from 90 to 150 mL of spinal fluid, and the newborn infant between 10 and 60 mL. Spinal fluid has four main functions: (1) it is a mechanical buffer that prevents trauma, (2) it regulates the volume of the intracranial contents, (3) it is a nutrient medium of the central nervous system, and (4) it is an excretory channel for metabolic products of the CNS.

Whenever a spinal tap (lumbar puncture) is performed, it is done for serious reasons, for it involves potential harm to the patient. The procedure is done by a physician. Indications for lumbar puncture include the following: the diagnosis of meningitis—bacterial, fungal, mycobacterial, and amebic; the diagnosis of hemorrhage—subarachnoid, intracerebral, and cerebral infarct; the diagnosis of neurologic disease, such as multiple sclerosis, demyelinating disorders, and the Guillain-Barré syndrome; the diagnosis and evaluation of suspected malignancy, such as leukemia, lymphoma, and metastatic carcinoma; and the introduction of drugs, radiographic contrast media, and anesthetics.

The greatest risk of lumbar puncture involves paralysis or death due to tonsillar herniation in patients with increased intracranial pressure. There is also a risk of infection from the procedure.

CSF, or spinal fluid, differs from serous and synovial fluids because of the selective permeability of the membranes and adjacent tissues containing it. This is referred to as the blood-brain barrier. As a result, the CSF is not an ultrafiltrate of plasma. Rather, there is active transport between the blood, CSF, and brain, in both directions, giving differing concentrations of substances in each.

Many drugs do not enter the cerebrospinal fluid from the blood. Electrolytes such as sodium, magnesium, and chloride are more concentrated in spinal fluid than in plasma or plasma ultrafiltrates, while bicarbonate, glucose, and urea are less concentrated in spinal fluid. Protein enters the spinal fluid in very small amounts. Very few cells are found in normal spinal fluid.

## Collection of Cerebrospinal Fluid

There is a certain risk to the patient in the procedure for obtaining a specimen of spinal fluid; hence such specimens must be handled with the utmost care. In practice, three sterile tubes containing about 5 mL each are collected during the spinal tap. These tubes are numbered in sequence of collection and immediately brought to the laboratory. The opening pressure is measured as the puncture is done. It is important that any cell count or glucose determinations be done as soon as possible after collection, to prevent deterioration of cells and glucose. Like other body fluids, spinal fluid is potentially infectious, and must always be collected and handled by using standard precautions. These specimens may be highly infectious and should be treated with extreme care.

The tubes that are sequentially collected and labeled in order of collection are generally dispersed and utilized for analysis (after gross examination of all tubes) as follows:

Tube 1. Chemical and immunologic tests
Tube 2. Microbiology
Tube 3. Total cell counts and differential cell count. This is least likely to contain cells introduced by the puncture procedure itself.

Excess fluid from any of these tubes should not be discarded until there is no further use for it.

## Routine Examination of Cerebrospinal Fluid
### Gross Appearance

All tubes collected by lumbar puncture are evaluated as to gross appearance. Normal spinal fluid is crystal clear. It looks like distilled water. Color and clarity are noted by holding the sample beside a tube of water against a clean white paper or a printed page.

**Turbidity.** Slight haziness in the specimen indicates a white cell count of 200 to $500/\mu L$, and turbidity indicates a white cell count of over $500/\mu L$.

Turbidity in spinal fluid may result from the presence of large numbers of leukocytes, as previously discussed, or from bacteria, increased protein, or lipid. If radiographic contrast media have been injected, the CSF will appear oily, and when mixed, turbid. This artifactual turbidity is not reported.

**Clots.** In addition to the gross observations of turbidity and color, the spinal fluid should be examined for clotting. Clotting may occur from increased fibrinogen resulting from a traumatic tap. Rarely, clotting may be associated with subarachnoid block, or meningitis.

**Color (traumatic tap versus hemorrhage).** Bloody fluid can result from a traumatic tap or from subarachnoid hemorrhage. If blood in a specimen results from a traumatic tap (inclusion of blood in the specimen from the puncture itself), the successive collection tubes will show less bloody fluid, eventually becoming clear. If blood in a specimen is caused by a subarachnoid hemorrhage, the color of the fluid will look the same in all the collection tubes. In addition, subarachnoid bleeding is indicated by the presence of xanthochromia.

*Xanthochromia.* This is the presence of a pale pink to orange or yellow color in the supernatant CSF. It is the result of the release of hemoglobin from hemolyzed red blood cells, which begins 1 to 4 hours after hemorrhage. Pale-pink or pale-orange xanthochromia due to oxyhemoglobin peaks in 24 to 36 hours and gradually disappears in 4 to 8 days. Because hemolysis of red cells will occur in vitro as well as in vivo, the examination for xanthochromia must be done within 1 hour of collection or false-positive results will be obtained.

When the hemorrhage is old, the supernatant fluid will show **yellow xanthochromia.** The yellow color is caused by bilirubin, formed from hemoglobin from the lysed red blood cells. This appears about 12 hours after a bleeding episode, peaks in 2 to 4 days, and gradually disappears in 2 to 4 weeks. When the CSF protein level is elevated over 150 mg/dL, a yellow color may also be seen, like the color of normal serum or plasma.

Finally, subarachnoid bleeding is associated with the microscopic observation of erythropha-

gia, which is the ingestion of red cells by macrophages in the CSF.

### Red and White Blood Cell Counts

Unlike cell counts on blood, cell counts on CSF (as is the case with all body fluids) are usually performed by manual methods (Procedures 15-1 and 15-2). Although electronic cell counts have been described, they are not generally used. The instruments are not standardized for the low cell counts generally seen in body fluids. Problems also occur owing to the viscosity of body (especially joint) fluids, the variation in cell size (especially when tumor cells are present), and background debris, which is generally higher than cell counts.

Since these fluids are often contaminated by pathogenic microorganisms, special procedures and equipment are employed to prevent contamination. Semiautomatic micropipettes or the Unopette system may be used to prepare dilutions, and disposable counting chambers may be employed. Traditional hemocytometers must be thoroughly disinfected after use.

If the spinal fluid appears clear, cell counts may be performed in a hemocytometer counting chamber without using diluting fluid. Cell counts should be done as soon as possible after the specimen is obtained, because cells lyse on prolonged standing and the counts become invalid. Therefore, counts should be done within 30 minutes of collection.

Normally there are no red cells in CSF. The normal white cell count in CSF is 0 to 8 per $\mu$L. More than 10 per $\mu$L is considered abnormal. A predominance of polynuclear cells usually indicates a bacterial infection, while the presence of many mononuclear cells indicates a viral infection.

### Morphologic Examination

When the cell count is over 30 white cells per microliter, a differential cell count is done. This may be done on a smear made from the centrifuged spinal fluid sediment, by recovery with a filtration or sedimentation method, or preferably on a cytocentrifuged preparation.

## PROCEDURE 15-1

### Cerebrospinal Fluid Red Cell Count

1. Insert a disposable Pasteur pipette directly into the well-mixed specimen. Carefully mount both sides of a clean counting chamber (hemocytometer).

2. With the low-power (10×) objective, quickly scan both ruled areas of the hemocytometer to determine whether red cells are present and to get a rough idea of their concentration.

3. With the high-power (40×) objective, count the red cells in 10 square millimeters. Count five squares on each side, using the four corner squares and the center square. (See Chapter 12, Fig. 12-10.)

4. Red cells will appear small, round, and yellowish. Their outline is usually smooth, although they may occasionally appear crenated.

5. If the number of red cells is fairly high (over 200 cells per ten squares), count fewer squares and adjust the calculations accordingly.

6. If the fluid is extremely bloody, it may be necessary to dilute it volumetrically with saline or some other isotonic diluent. It is preferable to count the undiluted fluid in fewer than ten squares, if possible. Adjust the calculations if dilution is necessary.

7. Calculate the number of cells per liter as follows:
   Total cells counted × Dilution factor × Volume factor = Cells/$\mu$L (mm$^3$)
   $$= \text{Cells} \times 10^6/\text{L}$$

   *Example:* If ten squares are counted, the volume counted is 1 $\mu$L (10 mm$^2$ × 0.1 mm), and if the fluid was not diluted, there is no dilution factor. Therefore, the number of cells counted in ten squares is equal to the number of cells per microliter, or × 10$^6$/L.

8. Decontaminate the hemocytometer by placing it in a Petri dish and flooding it with disinfectant solution. Allow the disinfectant to remain on the hemocytometer for at least five minutes; then rinse it well with 70% alcohol and wipe it dry.

**Cytocentrifugation.** This technique requires the use of a special cytocentrifuge, such as the Cytospin.*

It is a slow centrifugation method, which gives better cell yield and morphologic preservation than does ordinary centrifugation. It is relatively easy to learn and to perform and gives an excellent yield with a small amount of sample. The sample is slowly centrifuged from 200 to 1,000 rpm for 5 to 10 minutes. During centrifugation, the fluid portion of the specimen is absorbed into a filter paper and the cellular portion is concentrated in a circle 6 mm in diameter on a microscope slide. The cytocentrifuged preparation (often called a Cytospin) is stained with Wright stain or with a variety of stains for hematologic or cytologic studies.

**Smears From Centrifuged Spinal Fluid Sediment.** These may be used when a cytocentrifuge is not available. The spinal fluid is centrifuged for 5 minutes at 3,000 rpm. The supernatant is removed, and the sediment is used to prepare smears on glass slides. The smears are dried rapidly and stained with Wright stain. Recovery of cells is not as good as with other

*Shandon, Inc, Pittsburgh, Pa.

## PROCEDURE 15-2

### Cerebrospinal Fluid White Cell Count

1. Rinse a disposable Pasteur pipette with glacial acetic acid, drain it carefully, wipe the outside completely dry with gauze, and touch the tip of the pipette to the gauze to remove any excess acid. It is very important that no glacial acetic acid be left on the outside of the pipette, because it would contaminate the spinal fluid specimen when the pipette is placed in it.

2. Place the pipette in the well-mixed CSF sample, and allow the pipette to fill to about 1 inch of its length. Tilt the CSF tube slightly, if necessary, to allow filling by capillary action. Place a finger over the clean end of the pipette, and remove it from the sample.

3. Mix the spinal fluid with the acid coating the pipette by placing the pipette in a horizontal position and removing your finger from the end of the pipette. Rotate or twist the pipette to mix the CSF and acid together. Be careful not to allow any of the fluid to drip from the pipette.

4. Mount the acidified CSF on both sides of a clean hemocytometer. Wait for 3 to 5 minutes to allow time for red cell hemolysis.

5. With the low-power (10×) objective, quickly scan both ruled areas of the hemocytometer to determine whether white cells are present, and to get a rough idea of their concentration. The white cell nuclei will appear as dark, refractile structures surrounded by a halo of cytoplasm.

6. Using the low-power (10×) objective, count the white cells in 10 square millimeters, 5 on each side of the hemocytometer, using the four corner squares and the center square.

7. Do a chamber differential as the white cells are counted by classifying each white cell seen as polynuclear or mononuclear. This chamber differential is inaccurate, and a differential cell count on a stained cytocentrifuged preparation is preferred.

   a. To classify cells, change from the low-power (10×) to the high-power (40×) objective.

   b. Polynuclear white cells have a segmented or twisted, irregular nucleus, and a moderate amount of cytoplasm. They are usually neutrophils.

   c. Mononuclear white cells have a round grainy nucleus, and usually a smaller amount of cytoplasm. They may be lymphocytes, monocytes, or other nucleated cells.

8. If it appears that the number of white cells is over 200 cells per ten squares, count fewer squares and adjust your calculations accordingly.

9. Calculate the white cell count in cells per microliter as described in Procedure 15-1.

10. Decontaminate and clean the hemocytometer as described in Procedure 15-1.

techniques, and the cells tend to be distorted or damaged.

**Other Concentration Techniques.** These include special sedimentation methods and membrane filter techniques. These are more time consuming and expensive than cytocentrifugation and require more technical expertise.

**Differential Cell Count.** Exactly 100 white cells are counted and classified, and the percentage of each cell type is reported. Depending on the method of preparation, morphologic identification may be difficult. In some cases, cells can be identified only as polynuclear or mononuclear. With other preparation techniques (such as Cytospins), identification is more specific. Any of the cells found in blood may be seen in CSF, including neutrophils, lymphocytes, monocytes, eosinophils, and basophils. In addition, cells that originate in the CNS may be seen. These include ependymal, choroidal, and pia-arachnoid mesothelial (PAM) cells. If any tumor cells or unusual cells are encountered, the specimen should be referred for cytologic examination.

### Chemistry Tests

Several chemical determinations can be done on spinal fluid. The same chemical constituents are generally found in CSF and plasma, but because of the blood-brain barrier and selective filtration, normal CSF values are different from plasma values. Abnormal CSF values may result from alterations in the permeability of the blood-brain barrier, or from production or metabolism by neural cells in various pathologic conditions. There are relatively few important CSF chemical findings. Some of the more routine analyses will be described.

**Protein.** Protein tests and protein electrophoresis are common and of diagnostic significance for a variety of conditions and disease states. Protein fractions are generally the same as in plasma, but the ratios vary. The normal CSF protein varies with methodology and site of collection, with a reference range of 12 to 60 mg/dL. Increased CSF protein levels are the most common pathologic finding, and are seen with meningitis, hemorrhage, and multiple sclerosis. Low values are associated with leakage of fluid from the CNS. Electrophoresis has replaced the colloidal gold test for the evaluation of spinal fluid protein fractions.

**Glucose.** The glucose level in spinal fluid is about 60% to 80% of that in blood, but the amounts may vary. Both levels should be measured simultaneously, as it is the difference between these values that is clinically significant. Bacteria and cells utilize glucose. The glucose level in spinal fluid is especially reduced in bacterial meningitis, but not in viral meningitis, primary brain tumor, or vascular accidents. It is low in metastatic tumor and insulin shock, and elevated in diabetic coma.

**Lactate.** Determination of lactate levels in CSF is used in the diagnosis and management of meningitis, although usefulness is controversial and method dependent. Elevation over 25 mg/dL is seen in bacterial, fungal, and tubercular meningitis and is more consistent than a depression in glucose levels. The elevated serum lactate levels remain during initial treatment, but a fall indicates successful treatment. However, increased lactate levels occur in oxygen deprivation and are seen in any condition in which oxygen flow to the brain is decreased.

**Glutamine.** The presence of increased CSF glutamine is an indirect measure of the presence of excess ammonia in the CSF. Glutamine is produced by brain cells as a way of removing toxic ammonia from the CNS by combining ammonia and $\alpha$-ketoglutarate. Increased levels of blood and CSF ammonia are seen in some liver disorders. Measurement of glutamine is preferable to measurement of ammonia, as it is a more stable compound.

**Lactate Dehydrogenase.** The various isoenzymes of lactate dehydrogenase (LD) are used to help diagnose meningitis by helping to confirm the presence of neutrophils or lymphocytes, and by indicating destruction of brain tissue.

**Other Tests.** Tests for bilirubin and chloride are less commonly done. The chloride level in spinal fluid is normally higher than in blood, and determinations should be done simultaneously. Spinal fluid levels of other electrolytes are normally lower than blood levels but tend to rise during inflammation.

### Microbiological Examination

Gram stain and culture are done. Spinal fluid specimens are normally sterile. Gram stains are most useful in the diagnosis of acute bacterial meningitis, as the organisms can actually be seen in the Gram-stained specimen. Tuberculosis (acid-fast stain) and *Cryptococcus* infections (India ink preparations) may also be detected with microscopic examination of the CSF.

### Serology Tests

The VDRL test is a well-known serologic test for syphilis that is done on spinal fluid. However, it may be negative in 40% to 50% of cases. The fluorescent treponemal antibody absorption (FTA-ABS) test is more sensitive but less specific.

## SEROUS FLUIDS (PLEURAL, PERICARDIAL, AND PERITONEAL)

Serous fluids are the fluids contained within the closed cavities of the body. These cavities are lined by a contiguous membrane that forms a double layer of mesothelial cells, called the serous membrane. The cavities are the **pleural** (around the lungs), **pericardial** (around the heart), and **peritoneal** (around the abdominal and pelvic organs) cavities. A small amount of serous fluid fills the space between the two layers and serves to lubricate the surfaces of these membranes as they move against each other. The fluids are ultrafiltrates of plasma, which are continuously formed and reabsorbed, leaving only a very small volume within the cavities. An increased volume of any of these fluids is referred to as an effusion.

### Transudates and Exudates

Since normal serous fluids are formed as an ultrafiltrate of plasma as it filters through the capillary endothelium, they are **transudates.** Normally, serum protein exerts colloidal osmotic pressure and helps retard movement of

fluid into the serous cavity. If plasma protein levels decrease, the colloidal osmotic pressure falls and effusion results as movement of the transudate into the serous cavity increases. The formation is also affected by capillary pressure and permeability.

An increase in serous fluid volume **(effusion)** will occur in many conditions. In determining the cause of an effusion, it is helpful to determine whether the effusion is a **transudate** or an **exudate.** In general, the effusion is a transudate (which is an ultrafiltrate of plasma) as the result of a systemic disease. An example of a transudate includes ascites, an effusion into the peritoneal cavity, which might be caused by liver cirrhosis or congestive heart failure. Transudates may be thought of as the result of a mechanical disorder affecting movement of fluid across a membrane.

Exudates are usually effusions that result from an inflammatory response to conditions that directly affect the serous cavity. These inflammatory conditions include infections and malignancies.

Although it may be difficult to determine whether an effusion is a transudate or an exudate, the distinction is important from a practical standpoint. If the effusion is a transudate, further testing is generally unnecessary. However, if it is an exudate, further testing is required for diagnosis and treatment. If infection is suspected, Gram stain and culture are indicated, while suspected malignancies might require cytologic tests and biopsy.

Serous effusions have been classified as transudates or exudates on the basis of the amount of protein. Generally effusions with a total protein content under 3 g/dL are considered transudates, while those with a total protein over 3 g/dL are exudates. Unfortunately there is a good deal of overlap in separating the effusions. A more reliable method of separating transudates and exudates is the simultaneous measurement of the fluid and serum for protein and LD. Appearance of the fluid, cell counts, and spontaneous clotting are also useful in the differentiation. These findings are summarized in Table 15-1.

## Collection

Serous fluids are collected under strictly antiseptic conditions. The aspiration may be for diagnostic purposes or for mechanical reasons, to prevent an excess accumulation of fluid from inhibiting the actions of the lungs or heart. A pleural effusion may compress the lungs, a pericardial effusion may cause cardiac tamponade, and ascites (peritoneal effusion) may elevate the diaphragm, compressing the lungs. At least three anticoagulated tubes of fluid are generally collected and used as follows:

1. An EDTA tube for gross appearance, cell counts, morphology, and differential
2. A suitably anticoagulated tube for chemical analysis
3. A sterile heparinized tube for Gram stain and culture

Additional tubes, or the entire collection with a suitable preservative, are collected for cytologic examination for tumor cells. Sequentially collected tubes are observed for a possible traumatic tap.

## Description of Individual Serous Fluids
### Pleural Fluid

Normally, there is about 1 to 10 mL of pleural fluid moistening the pleural surfaces. It surrounds the lungs and lines the walls of the thoracic cavity. If inflammation occurs, the plasma protein level drops, congestive heart failure is present, or there is decreased lymphatic drainage, there can be an abnormal accumulation of pleural fluid.

### Pericardial Fluid

The pericardial space enclosing the heart normally contains about 25 to 50 mL of a clear, straw-colored ultrafiltrate of plasma, called pericardial fluid. This fluid forms continually and is reabsorbed by the nearby lymph vessels (lymphatics), leaving a small but constant volume. When an abnormal accumulation of pericardial fluid occurs, it fills up the space around the heart and can mechanically inhibit the normal action of the heart (cardiac tamponade). In this case, immediate aspiration of the excess fluid is indicated.

## TABLE 15-1

Differentiation of Serous Effusions: Transudate From Exudate*

| Observation or Test | Transudate | Exudate |
|---|---|---|
| Appearance | Watery, clear, pale yellow<br>Does not clot | Cloudy, turbid, purulent, or bloody<br>May clot (fibrinogen) |
| White cell count | Low, <1000/$\mu$L, with more than 50% mononuclear cells (lymphocytes and monocytes) | 500-1,000/$\mu$L or more, with increased PMNs<br>Increased lymphocytes with tuberculosis or rheumatoid arthritis |
| Red cell count | Low, unless from a traumatic tap | >100,000/$\mu$L, especially with a malignancy |
| Total protein | <3g/dL | >3g/dL (or greater than half the serum level) |
| Lactate dehydrogenase | Low | Increased (>60% of the serum level because of cellular debris) |
| Glucose | Varies with serum level | Lower than serum level with some infections and high cell counts |

Modified from Ringsrud KM, Linne JJ: *Urinalysis and Body Fluids: A ColorText and Atlas*, St Louis, Mosby, 1995.
*Note that some values are variable between the two effusions. Clinical considerations must always be used in combination with the laboratory findings.

### Peritoneal Fluid

Normally less than 100 mL of the clear, straw-colored fluid is present in the peritoneal cavity (the abdominal and pelvic cavities). An abnormal accumulation of the fluid is indicated by severe abdominal pain and may be caused by a ruptured abdominal organ, hemorrhage resulting from trauma, postoperative complications, or an unknown condition. The excess fluid is aspirated. The presence of such an accumulation must always be considered in the light of other findings.

## Routine Examination of Serous Fluids

The routine examination of serous fluids generally includes an observation of gross appearance, cell counts, morphology, and differential, Gram stain, and culture. Certain chemical analyses, and cytologic examination for tumor cells and tumor markers, are performed when indicated.

### Gross Appearance

Normal serous fluid is pale and straw colored. This is the color seen in a transudate. Turbidity increases as the number of cells and the amount of debris increase. An abnormally colored fluid may appear milky (chylous or pseudochylous), cloudy, or bloody on gross observation. A cloudy serous fluid is often associated with an inflammatory reaction, either bacterial or viral. Blood-tinged fluid can be seen as a result of a traumatic tap, and grossly bloody fluid can be seen when an organ such as the spleen or liver or a blood vessel has ruptured. Bloody fluids are also seen in malignant disease states, after myocardial infarction, in tuberculosis, in rheumatoid arthritis, and in systemic lupus erythematosus.

### Clotting

To observe the ability of the serous fluid to clot, the specimen must be collected in a plain tube with no anticoagulant. Ability of the fluid to clot indicates a substantial inflammatory reaction.

### Red and White Blood Cell Counts

Cell counts are done on well-mixed anticoagulated serous fluid in a hemocytometer. The fluid may be undiluted or diluted, as indicated by the cell count. The procedure is essentially the same as that described for CSF red and white cell counts. If significant protein is present, acetic acid cannot be used as a diluent for white cell counts, owing to the precipitation of protein. In this case, saline may be used as a diluent and the red and white cell counts are done simultaneously. The use of phase microscopy is helpful in performing these counts. As with CSF cell counts, 10 square millimeters are generally counted using the undiluted fluid. Results are reported as the number of cells per microliter (or liter).

Leukocyte counts over $500/\mu L$ are usually clinically significant. If there is a predominance of neutrophils (polynuclear cells), bacterial inflammation is suspected. A predominance of lymphocytes suggests viral infection, tuberculosis, lymphoma, or malignancy. Leukocyte counts over $1,000/\mu L$ are associated with exudates.

Red cell counts of more than $10,000/\mu L$ may be seen as effusion with malignancies, infarcts, and trauma.

### Morphologic Examination and White Cell Differential

Morphologic examination and white cell differential are essentially the same as described for CSF. Once again, slides prepared by cytocentrifugation are preferred to smears prepared after normal centrifugation. Slides are generally stained with Wright stain, and a differential cell count is done. The white cells generally resemble those seen in peripheral blood, with the addition of mesothelial lining cells. Generally 300 cells are counted and differentiated as to percentage of each cell type seen. If any malignant tumor cells are seen or appear to be present, the slide must be referred to a pathologist or qualified cytotechnologist.

### Microbiological Examination

Microbiological examination will include Gram stain and culture on all body effusions of unknown etiology (see Chapter 16).

### Chemical Analysis

**Protein.** Total protein is measured in the fluid and the plasma. The level and the ratio are helpful in distinguishing an exudate from a transudate. Protein electrophoresis is used in some cases.

**Lactate Dehydrogenase.** Lactate dehydrogenase is also measured in the fluid and the plasma. The level and the ratio, together with the total protein levels and ratios, are used to distinguish an exudate from a transudate. Increased levels are seen as a result of cellular debris from infection or malignancy.

**Glucose.** In bacterial infections, serous fluids have a lower concentration of glucose than does blood. Glucose determinations on serous fluids should be accompanied by a simultaneous blood glucose collection.

**Other Tests.** Determinations of amylase, lipase, other enzymes, ammonia, and lipids, among others, are also done in various conditions.

## SYNOVIAL FLUID

Synovial fluid is the fluid contained in joints. Synovial membranes line the joints, bursae, and tendon sheaths. Normal synovial fluid is an ultrafiltrate of plasma with the addition of a high-molecular-weight mucopolysaccharide called **hyaluronate** or **hyaluronic acid.** The presence of hyaluronate differentiates synovial fluid from other serous fluids and spinal fluid. It is responsible for the normal viscosity of synovial fluid, which serves to lubricate the joints so that they move freely. Hyaluronate is secreted by the synovial fluid cells (synoviocytes) that line the joint cavity. This normal viscosity is responsible for

some difficulties in the examination of synovial fluid, especially in performing cell counts.

### Normal Synovial Fluid

Normal synovial fluid is straw colored and viscous, resembling uncooked egg white. The word *synovial* comes from *syn*, with, and *ovi*, egg. About 1 mL of synovial fluid is present in each large joint, such as the knee, ankle, hip, elbow, wrist, and shoulder.

In normal synovial fluid the white cell count is low, less than $200/\mu L$, and the majority of the white cells are mononuclear, with less than 25% neutrophils. Red cells and crystals are normally absent, and the fluid is sterile. Since the fluid is an **ultrafiltrate of plasma,** normal synovial fluid has essentially the same chemical composition as plasma without the larger protein molecules. A small amount of protein is secreted by the synovial cells, resulting in less than 3 g/dL total protein.

### Aspiration and Analysis

The aspiration and analysis of synovial fluid may be done to determine the cause of joint disease, especially when accompanied by an abnormal accumulation of fluid in the joint (effusion). The joint disease (arthritis) might be crystal induced, degenerative, inflammatory, or infectious. Morphologic analysis for cells and crystals, together with Gram stain and culture, will help in the differentiation. Aspiration is also done with effusions of unknown etiology, and with pain or decreased joint mobility. Effusion of synovial fluid is usually present clinically before aspiration, and therefore it is often possible to aspirate 10 to 20 mL of the fluid for laboratory examination, although the volume (which is normally about 1 mL) may be extremely small, so that the laboratory receives only a drop of fluid contained in the aspiration syringe.

In the management of joint disorders, the differential diagnosis is essential so that the correct treatment can be instituted. The analysis of synovial fluid can be invaluable in this diagnosis. It can give an immediate diagnosis in some disorders, and provide valuable information concerning other diseases of the joints. If fluid volume or resources are limited, the most important aspects of analysis are microbiological study and an examination for crystals with compensated polarized light microscopy.

## Classification of Synovial Fluid in Joint Disease

The differential diagnosis of diseased synovial fluid usually classifies the fluid as noninflammatory, inflammatory, infectious, crystal-induced, or hemorrhagic. Although there is an overlap of disease states in this grouping, it is helpful.

### Noninflammatory

Noninflammatory synovial fluid is seen in degenerative joint disease, such as osteoarthritis, traumatic arthritis, and neurogenic joint disease. The fluid is usually clear and viscous; the white blood cell (WBC) count is less than 2,000/$\mu$L, less than 25% of which are neutrophils. The glucose and protein contents are approximately the same as in normal synovial fluid. Collagen fibrils or cartilage fragments may be seen, especially with phase microscopy.

### Inflammatory

Inflammatory effusions are associated with immunologic disease such as rheumatoid and lupus arthritis. The fluid is cloudy and yellow, has low viscosity, and has a moderately high white cell count (2,000 to 20,000/$\mu$L), with over 50% neutrophils. The glucose content is normal, and the protein content is high. The fluid may form spontaneous fibrin clots.

### Infectious

Infectious infusions suggest a bacterial infection. The fluid is generally cloudy and has low viscosity. The fluid may be yellow, green, or milky. The white cell count is very high, 500 to 200,000/$\mu$L, with over 90% neutrophils. The glucose content is characteristically very low. The protein content is high, and fibrin clot formation is common. Most infections are bacterial. *Staphylococcus aureus* and *Neisseria gonorrhoeae* are the most common infecting agents, although streptococci, *Haemophilus*, tuberculosis, fungi, or anaerobic bacteria are also seen. The most common type of organism found varies with the age of the patient.

### Crystal Induced

Crystal-induced effusions are seen in gout and pseudogout. The fluid is yellow or turbid and has a fairly high, but variable, white cell count (500 to 200,000/$\mu$L), with an increased percentage of neutrophils (up to 90%). Crystals of monosodium urate (MSU) are seen with gout, and calcium pyrophosphate dihydrate (CPPD) crystals with pseudogout. They are recognized by morphology and appearance when examined by polarized microscopy with the addition of a full-wave compensator.

### Hemorrhagic

Hemorrhagic effusions are characterized by the presence of red blood cells from bleeding or hemorrhage in the joint. This may be the result of traumatic injury, such as fracture, or tumor. Coagulation deficiencies, such as hemophilia, and treatment with anticoagulants may also result in hemorrhagic effusions.

## Collection of Synovial Fluid

Synovial fluid is collected by needle aspiration, which is called **arthrocentesis**. It is done by experienced persons under strictly sterile conditions. The fluid is collected with a disposable needle and plastic syringe, to avoid contamination with confusing birefringent material.

The fluid should be collected both anticoagulated and unanticoagulated. Ideally the fluid should be divided into three parts:

1. A sterile tube for microbiological examination

2. A tube with liquid EDTA (preferred) or sodium heparin for microscopic examination

3. A plain tube (without anticoagulant) for clot formation, gross appearance, and chemical and immunologic procedures. This should be a plain tube *without* a serum separator.

Oxalate, powdered EDTA, and lithium heparin anticoagulants should not be used, as they may appear as confusing crystals in the crystal analysis. This is especially true when only a small volume of fluid is aspirated, giving an excess of anticoagulant, which may crystallize.

Normal synovial fluid does not clot, and therefore an anticoagulant is unnecessary. However, infectious and crystal-induced fluids tend to form fibrin clots, making an anticoagulant necessary for adequate cell counts and an even distribution of cells and crystals for morphologic analysis. There is some disagreement as to whether anticoagulated or plain tubes should be used for analysis of crystals. A decision may be necessary on an individual basis. Ideally, both tubes would be made available so that if artifactual anticoagulant crystals are suspected, the plain clot tube could be examined.

Although an anticoagulant will prevent the formation of fibrin clots, it will not affect viscosity. Therefore, if the fluid is highly viscous, it can be incubated for several hours with a 0.5% solution of hyaluronidase in phosphate buffer to break down the hyaluronate. This reduces the viscosity, making the fluid easier to pipette and count.

## Routine Examination of Synovial Fluid

The routine examination of synovial fluid should include the following: (1) gross appearance (color, clarity, and viscosity); (2) microbiological studies; (3) WBC and differential cell counts; (4) polarizing microscopy for crystals; (5) other tests, as necessary. The most important tests are the microbiological studies, especially Gram stain, and crystal analysis. If the quantity of aspirated fluid is limited, these should be done first.

### Gross Appearance

The first step in the analysis of synovial fluid is to observe the specimen for color and clarity. The noninflammatory fluid is usually clear. To test for clarity, read newspaper print through a test tube containing the specimen. As the cell and protein content increases, or crystals precipitate, the turbidity increases, and the print becomes more difficult to read. In a traumatic tap of the joint, blood will be seen in the collection tubes in an uneven distribution, which diminishes as the aspiration continues. It may also be seen as an uneven distribution with streaks of blood in the aspiration syringe. A truly bloody fluid is uniform in color, and does not clot. Xanthochromia in the supernatant fluid indicates bleeding in the joint, but is difficult to evaluate because the fluid is normally yellow. A dark-red or dark-brown supernatant is evidence of joint bleeding rather than a traumatic tap.

### Viscosity

Viscosity is most easily evaluated at the time of arthrocentesis by allowing the synovial fluid to drop from the end of the needle. Normally, synovial fluid will form a string 4 to 6 cm in length. If it breaks before it reaches 3 cm in length, the viscosity is lower than normal. Inflammatory fluids contain enzymes that break down hyaluronic acid. Anything that decreases the hyaluronic acid content of synovial fluid lowers its viscosity.

Viscosity has been evaluated in the laboratory by means of the mucin clot test. However, this test is of questionable value, as results rarely change the diagnosis and are essentially the same as with the string test for viscosity. Therefore, it is no longer recommended as part of the routine synovial fluid analysis. The mucin clot test is based on the polymerization of hyaluronic acid. To perform the mucin clot test, synovial fluid is added drop by drop to dilute acetic acid. The resulting clot may fragment easily, indicating inflammatory fluid, or may remain firm, indicating noninflammatory fluid. Clots are graded as good, fair, poor, or very poor.

Viscosity can also be assessed by merely tipping the unanticoagulated collection tube and noting whether the fluid appears thick (viscous) or watery (thin).

### Red and White Blood Cell Counts

The appearance of a drop of synovial fluid under an ordinary light microscope can be helpful in estimating the cell counts initially and in demonstrating the presence of crystals. The presence of only a few white cells per high-power (40×) field suggests a noninflammatory disorder. A large number of white cells would indicate inflammatory or infected synovial fluid. The total WBC count and differential count are very important in diagnosis. When cells are counted in other fluids, such as blood, the usual diluting fluid is dilute acetic acid. This cannot be used with synovial fluid because it may cause mucin clotting. Instead, a solution of saline containing methylene blue is used. If it is necessary to lyse red blood cells, either hypotonic saline or saponinized saline can be used as a diluent. The undiluted synovial fluid, or, if necessary, suitably diluted fluid, is mounted in a hemocytometer and counted as described for CSF counts. Since acetic acid cannot be used as a diluent, both red and white cells are enumerated at the same time. This is most easily accomplished by using a phase-contrast rather than a brightfield microscope.

Cell counts below 200/$\mu$L with less than 25% polymorphonuclear cells and no red cells are normally observed in synovial fluid. Monocytes, lymphocytes, and macrophages are seen. A low white cell count (200 to 2,000/$\mu$L) with predominantly mononuclear cells suggests a noninflammatory joint fluid, while a high white cell count suggests inflammation and a very high white cell count with a high proportion of polymorphonuclear cells strongly suggests infection.

### Morphologic Examination

As with CSF, cytocentrifuged preparations of the synovial fluid are preferred for the morphologic examination and white cell differential. These preparations may also be used for crystal identification. The procedure is generally the same as that described for CSF. Slides should be prepared as soon as possible after collection, to prevent distortion and degeneration of cells. Digestion with hyaluronidase may be necessary with highly viscous fluids. If increased neutrophils are present, they are especially prone to disintegration, making them difficult to recognize.

If a cytocentrifuge is not available, smears are made, as for CSF, from normally centrifuged sediment. They should be thin, as hyaluronic acid will distort the cells. Smears are sometimes prepared from the fluid at the time of aspiration. The smears are air dried and stained with Wright stain.

Lupus erythematosus (LE) cells may be found in stained slides from patients with systemic lupus erythematosus and occasionally in fluid from patients with rheumatoid arthritis. The in vivo formation of LE cells in synovial fluid probably results from trauma to the white cells.

Eosinophilia may be seen in metastatic carcinoma to the synovium, acute rheumatic fever, and rheumatoid arthritis. It is also associated with parasitic infections and Lyme disease and has occurred after arthrography and radiation therapy.

### Microscopic Examination for Crystals

A drop of synovial fluid is placed on a slide and a coverglass applied, as is done for the examination of urinary sediment (see Chapter 14). To avoid confusion from extraneous particles that might polarize, it is recommended that slides and coverglasses be cleaned with alcohol and carefully dried with gauze or lens paper just prior to examination. It has also been recommended that the coverglass be immediately sealed with clear fingernail polish to reduce drying from evaporation. If nail polish is used, the slide should be allowed to dry for 15 minutes before microscopic examination, to prevent damage to the objective. An unsealed preparation can be examined during this waiting period if desired. Any crystals at the junction of the nail polish and synovial fluid should be ignored.

The unclotted synovial fluid is first examined with an ordinary brightfield or, preferably, phase-contrast microscope. Crystals are reported as being present or absent and, if they are present, as intracellular, extracellular, or both. The initial examination is followed by compensated polarized light microscopy. After examination of the wet preparation, a cytocentrifuged preparation may also be examined for the presence and identity of crystals.

**Brightfield or Phase-Contrast Microscopic Examination.** Needle-shaped, intracellular monosodium urate (MSU) crystals seen in a simple wet preparation of synovial fluid are characteristic of gouty arthritis (Fig. 15-1). Pseudogout, a crystal-deposition disease distinct from gout, is demonstrated by the presence of rhomboid calcium pyrophosphate dihydrate (CPPD) crystals (Fig. 15-2).

Cholesterol crystals are a rare finding in synovial fluid from persons with rheumatoid arthritis and are not seen in normal synovial fluid. They are flat, clear, rhombic crystals with one corner punched out, as shown in Chapter 14, Fig. 14-108.

Lipid crystals showing a Maltese cross for-

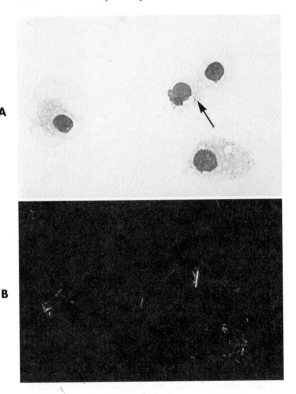

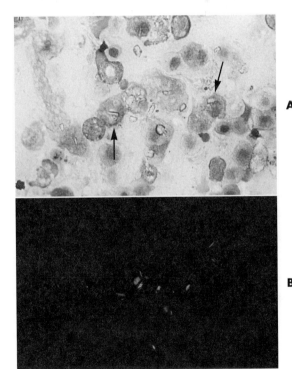

**FIG. 15-1.** Monosodium urate crystals in synovial fluid. Cells with needle-shaped intracellular crystals (*arrow and others*) morphologically resembling MSU. Cytospin, Wright stain, ×640. **A,** Brightfield. **B,** Polarized light, showing strongly birefringent needle-shaped crystals. Note that the number of crystals is more apparent with polarized light.

**FIG. 15-2.** Calcium pyrophosphate dihydrate crystals in synovial fluid. Degenerated neutrophils with chunky intracellular crystals (*arrows*) and some extracellular crystals, morphologically resembling CPPD, characteristic of pseudogout. Cytospin, Wright stain, ×640. **A,** Brightfield. **B,** Same field as A, with polarized light showing weak birefringence.

mation with polarized light have also been reported as causing acute arthritis. These should not be confused with starch (a common contaminant) (Fig. 15-3), or with a rare form of monosodium urate seen as a spherulite or "beachball."

Crystals of hydroxyapatite (HA) have been reported as causing apatite gout. They are too small to be seen with ordinary microscopy.

Clumps of these crystals may, however, be seen as spherical microaggregates.

Crystals of calcium oxalate may occur in oxalate gout, in patients receiving chronic renal dialysis, or in the very rare primary oxalosis.

Polyester fibers have been seen in the synovial fluid of patients who have had joint replacement, indicating deterioration of the artifi-

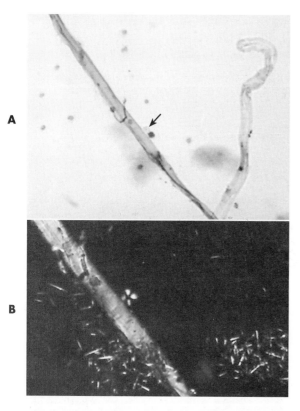

**FIG. 15-3.** Monosodium urates, starch, and filter paper fibers in synovial fluid. MSU crystals present in a mass of hyaluronate and extracellularly, a contaminating starch granule from gloves (arrow), and two contaminating filter paper fibers. Cytospin, Wright stain. **A,** Brightfield, ×100. **B,** Higher magnification, with polarized light showing strong birefringence of filter paper fiber, MSU crystals, and Maltese cross pattern of starch. (×400.)

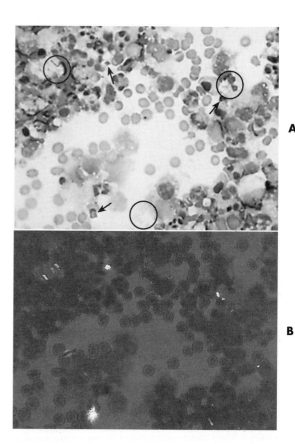

**FIG. 15-4.** Calcium pyrophosphate dihydrate and contaminating glove-lining powder in synovial fluid. The CPPD is more apparent morphologically with brightfield examination, in the Wright-stained preparation (as circled). The glove-lining powder (arrows) is more apparent with polarized microscopy, in which it is strongly birefringent as compared with the weakly birefringent CPPD. Cytospin, Wright stain, ×400. **A,** Brightfield. CPPD circled; glove-lining powder at arrows. **B,** Polarized light.

cial joint. These birefringent fibers are difficult to evaluate in the synovial fluid, especially on cytocentrifuged preparations that contain fibers derived from the filter paper (see Fig. 15-3).

Iatrogenic or extraneous crystals may be present in the synovial fluid. Starch might be introduced from gloves. These crystals show a Maltese cross pattern that might be confused with lipid droplets of cholesterol or spherulites of urates. Other substances lining gloves appear as tiny rectangles that might be mistaken for CPPD (Fig. 15-4).

If the joint has been treated with corticosteroids, crystals may be seen that resemble both monosodium urate and calcium pyrophosphate dihydrate. The crystals are generally extracellular and show numbers significantly greater than is typical of MSU or CPPD, but identification without the clinical history is very difficult (Figs. 15-5 and 15-6). Other substances that might be present and confusing are collagen fibrils, fibrin strands, and fragments of cartilage. The crystals seen in synovial fluid are summarized in Tables 15-2 and 15-3.

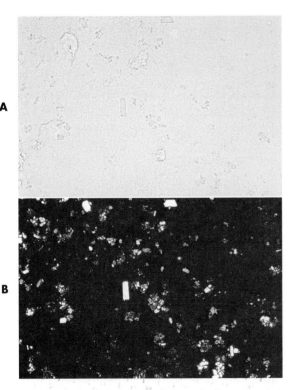

**FIG. 15-5.** Contaminating corticosteroid in synovial fluid. Crystals of triamcinolone diacetate (Aristocort), a corticosteroid used in treatment of arthritis. These appear like CPPD but polarize like MSU, causing confusion in crystal identification. Unlike CPPD, these crystals are soluble in alcohol. Wet preparation, unstained, ×400. **A,** Brightfield. **B,** Polarized light, showing strong birefringence.

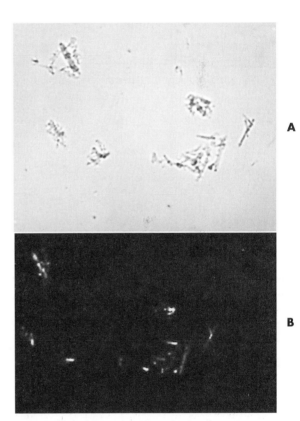

**FIG. 15-6.** Control suspension of betamethasone (CelestoneSoluspan), a corticosteroid suspension used for intraarticular injections. It is seen as jagged or needle-shaped crystals morphologically similar to MSU. These crystals will polarize in the same pattern as MSU and may be used as a control solution for compensated polarized light microscopy. Cytospin preparation, unstained, ×400. **A,** Brightfield. **B,** Polarized light.

**Polarized Light.** More definitive microscopic identification of crystals in synovial fluid can be made with the use of polarized light (see also Chapter 5). Both wet and cytocentrifuged preparations may be examined for the presence and identity of crystals. A polarizing microscope with a first-order red compensator (quartz compensator) is used. To set up the microscope, a polarizing filter (referred to as a polarizer) is placed between the light source (bulb) and the specimen. A second polarizing filter (referred to as an analyzer) is placed above the specimen, between the objective and the eye-piece. One of the polarizing filters (usually the polarizer) is rotated until the two are at right angles to each other. This is seen as the extinction of light through the microscope (one sees a black field, as all light waves are canceled when the filters are at right angles to each other). This is diagrammed in Chapter 5, Fig. 5-12.

Certain objects or crystals have the ability to rotate or polarize light so that they are visible when viewed through crossed polarizing filters. This property is called **birefringence,** and objects are termed weakly or strongly birefringent depending on how completely they polarize

## TABLE 15-2

Clinically Significant Crystals in Synovial Fluid

| Crystal | Morphology | Strength of Birefringence | Crystal Color When Parallel to Slow Wave | Crystal Size ($\mu$m) | Comments |
|---|---|---|---|---|---|
| MSU | Long slender needles | Strong | Yellow | 1-30 | Seen in gout |
| CPPD | Short chunky rectangles, or rhomboids | Weak | Blue | 1-20 (or more) | Seen in pseudogout |
| Hydroxy-apatite | Shiny clumps | Difficult to detect | N/A | 0.5-1 | Need electron microscope to visualize |
| Cholesterol plates | Large flat notched plates | Variable | Variable | 10-100 | Extremely rare, chronic effusion |
| Fat droplets (cholesterol) | Round spheres | Strong | Blue/yellow Maltese cross | 2-15 | Maltese cross appearance like starch |
| Cartilage fragments | Irregular | Strong | Variable | 10-50 | No definite crystal morphology |
| Polyethylene "wear" fragments | Long threads | Strong | Variable | Variable | Look like cytospin filter paper fibers Identification on wet prep only |
| Calcium oxalate | Bi-pyramidal (octahedrons) | Strong/variable | N/A | 2-10 | Seen in oxalate gout, especially with renal dialysis |
| Hematin | Vivid yellow-brown diamond shape | Weak | Might confuse with CPPD; use brightfield to avoid confusion | | Seen 2-4 weeks after hemorrhage |

light. Strongly birefringent crystals appear bright (white) against a dark background (see Fig. 15-1); weakly birefringent crystals appear less bright (see Fig. 15-2).

***Monosodium Urate.*** In synovial fluid, MSU crystals appear as strongly birefringent needle- or rod-shaped crystals from 1 to 30 $\mu$m in length (see Figs. 15-1 and 15-3). They may be intracellular or extracellular, and this distinction is recorded. The presence of intracellular crystals is characteristic of acute gout; extracellular crystals imply a more chronic condition. Crystals from a tophus may be quite large. MSU crystals are found in almost 100% of acute gouty arthritis, and in 75% of chronic gout.

***Calcium Pyrophosphate Dihydrate.*** CPPD crystals are also found in synovial fluid. These crystals are weakly birefringent, rod-shaped, rectangular, or rhomboid (see Fig. 15-2). Occasionally they are needle shaped. They may be very short and chunky, varying from 1 to 20 $\mu$m in length

and up to about 4 $\mu$m in width. These crystals are characteristic of pseudogout (also referred to as pyrophosphate gout or calcium pyrophosphate dihydrate crystal deposition disease). Pseudogout is seen in patients with degenerative arthritis, and in arthritides associated with hypothyroidism, hyperparathyroidism, hemochromatosis, and other conditions. Symptoms of pseudogout resemble those of gout, rheumatoid arthritis, and osteoarthritis.

**Compensated Polarized Light.** Crystals of monosodium urate and calcium pyrophosphate dihydrate that have been identified by polarized light are further identified by adding a full-wave compensator. This is also referred to as a first-order red plate (filter) or a full-wave retardation plate. Morphology and intensity of birefringence, although helpful, are not sufficient in separating these crystals.

Birefringent crystals have different properties

## TABLE 15-3

Artifacts and Contaminants in Synovial Fluid

| Crystal | Morphology | Strength of Birefringence | Crystal color When Parallel to Slow Wave | Crystal Size ($\mu$m) | Comments |
|---|---|---|---|---|---|
| Cortico-steroids | Variable Like MSU with blunt jagged edges Like CPPD, short, chunky | Strong | Yellow | 2-15 or more; variable | Common artifact from injection Soluble in alcohol Polarize like MSU Appear like MSU or CPPD |
| Starch | Variable Globule with irregular edges and central dimple Like tiny CPPD | Strong | Blue/yellow Maltese cross Yellow | 2-15 | Common contaminant Maltese cross like cholesterol Use BF to identify Like hydroxy-apatite or CPPD |
| Filter paper fibers | | Strong | Variable | 10-50 or more | Look like polyester fragments |
| Lipids from cells | | Strong | Blue/yellow Maltese cross | ~1-2 | Indicate degeneration of cells |
| Nail polish | | | | | Causes confusion; avoid edges of coverslip |

when viewed with polarized light with the addition of a compensator. When the compensator is in place, the background appears magenta, rather than black. The compensator may be inserted above either the analyzer or the polarizer. It is inserted in such a manner that the axis of slow vibration of the compensator (referred to as the slow wave) is at an angle of 45 degrees to the crossed polarizers. (See Chapter 5, Fig. 5-14.) In determining the type of crystal in question, the direction of the slow wave must be known. Crystals are identified by observation of the color of the long axis of the crystal in its relationship or orientation to the direction of the slow wave.

Crystals of MSU and CPPD have opposite characteristics when viewed with compensated polarized light. Crystals of MSU appear yellow when the long axis of the crystal lies parallel to the slow wave of the red compensator. These crystals appear blue when the long axis of the crystal lies perpendicular to the slow wave. This may be demonstrated by looking for crystals in the fluid that are so oriented, or by observing a crystal in a parallel orientation and then repositioning the slow wave at right angles to its original position. Alternatively, if the microscope has a rotating stage, the stage may be moved so that the crystal is rotated 90 degrees. In the case of MSU, the crystal will change from a yellow to a blue color. Crystals that appear yellow when parallel and blue when perpendicular to the slow wave exhibit **negative birefringence.** That is, the sign of birefringence is negative. The term *negative* should be avoided in reporting findings in synovial fluid so that the word is not taken to mean that the crystal in question is absent. Crystals are reported as being present or absent and are identified as to crystal type.

In the case of crystals of CPPD, the crystal appears blue when the long axis of the crystal is parallel to the direction of the slow wave. The same crystal will appear yellow when it lies perpendicular to the slow wave, which can be demonstrated as described above. The sign of birefringence in this case is positive **(positive birefringence),** which is by definition blue when the long axis is parallel to the slow wave. A determination of the type of birefringence with CPPD crystals may be troublesome, as it may be very difficult to determine their long axis, which may be very short, almost square.

An understanding of the polarizing microscope and the principle of birefringence is essential in examining synovial fluid for crystal identification. Although memorization of color patterns is discouraged, a useful mnemonic device is *yellow parallel equals gout.*

**Controls.** When crystals are analyzed with compensated polarized light for the type of birefringence, it is essential to use a control preparation to ensure the correct interpretation. Several control preparations are possible. A permanent cytocentrifuged preparation, or a prepared wet preparation of a specimen known to contain MSU crystals, may be used. Besides causing confusion when evaluating synovial fluid specimens, the birefringent properties of corticosteroids, which are commonly used to treat joint disease, may be utilized. A suspension of betamethasone acetate corticosteroid is very similar to MSU with compensated polarized light (see Fig. 15-6). Either a wet preparation or a more permanent cytocentrifuged preparation may be used. Other forms of corticosteroids are positively birefringent, showing the opposite pattern when viewed with compensated polarized light.

### Microbiological Examination

Pathogenic organisms can be identified by use of Gram stain and by culturing the synovial fluid. Cultures for suspected bacteria or mycobacterial or fungal infections are an essential part of the synovial fluid analysis. Immediate bedside inoculation of the sample onto chocolate agar and the use of special media for the propagation of gonococcal organisms are suggested. Gonococcal arthritis is a joint disease that is sometimes difficult to diagnose unless special techniques and care are used.

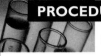

## PROCEDURE 15-3

### Nasal Smear for Eosinophils With Hansel's Stain

1. Flood the air-dried nasal smear with Hansel's stain* for 30 seconds. The staining time may be increased for thick mucous secretions.

2. Add distilled water to take up the stain, and allow the mixture to remain on the smear for another 30 seconds.

3. Tilt the slide to pour off the stain, and rinse with distilled water to remove excess stain.

4. Rinse the slide with 95% ethyl alcohol or 75% methyl alcohol to decolorize. Do not over-decolorize, or the cytoplasm of neutrophils will appear pink and confusing when you are looking for eosinophils.

5. Wipe the back and edges of the slide, and allow it to air dry.

6. Alternatively, Wright stain may be used for staining nasal smears; however, interpretation is more difficult.

———

*Lide Laboratories, Inc, Florissant, Mo.

### Chemistry Tests

**Glucose.** The determination of glucose in the synovial fluid is valuable when infectious diseases are suspected. For example, when the glucose level is significantly lower in synovial fluid than in serum or plasma, infection of the joint is suggested. Samples of the patient's synovial fluid and blood must be obtained at the same time for a comparison of the two values to be valid.

**Protein.** Total synovial protein is increased in several conditions. With inflammatory joint disease, such as rheumatoid arthritis, the total protein level approaches that of plasma. Normally it is about one third of the plasma value. Values are also increased in gout and infectious arthritis.

**Other Tests.** These include lactate dehydrogenase, uric acid, and lactate determinations.

### Immunologic Tests

The synovial fluid normally contains a lower immunoglobulin concentration than plasma. This is not the case in rheumatoid arthritis, in which the level of immunoglobulin is about equal to that in plasma, which suggests production of immunoglobulins in the affected joint.

Rheumatoid factor has been reported in the synovial fluid as well as in the serum of patients with rheumatoid arthritis. The presence of rheumatoid factor in the synovial fluid but not in the serum can be helpful in the diagnosis of this disease. Other immunologic tests include antinuclear antibodies, which are associated with systemic lupus erythematosus, and the demonstration of decreased complement levels. (See also Chapter 17.)

## NASAL SMEARS FOR EOSINOPHILS

Persons with an allergic reaction show a distinct increase in the number of eosinophilic cells in a differential count on a smear of the nasal discharge. Smears may be made directly from the nostril by using a swab, by aspiration with a soft rubber bulb, or from material blown into waxed paper by the patient. The nasal material is spread on a glass slide, as thinly as possible, and air dried. The slide is then stained with Wright stain, **Hansel's stain** (Procedure 15-3), or eosin and methylene blue. The eosinophils contain bright-red granules and are easily recognized under the high-power (40×) objective (Fig. 15-7). An increase in the number of eosinophils normally indicates that the patient may be in an allergic state rather than having an infection of some kind.

Examination of the nasal smear for eosinophils is simple and useful. It can indicate whether a patient's upper respiratory tract involvement or **rhinitis** (inflammation of the upper mucous membranes) is caused by an allergy (such as hay fever) or a nasal infection, which may be viral or bacterial. It may be necessary to prepare and examine several smears, especially if the specimen does not contain sufficient material, or if the picture is complicated by acute or chronic infection.

### Interpretation of the Nasal Smear

The stained smear is examined first under low power and then with the high-power (40×) objective. Eosinophils may be recognized by their red cytoplasm and large, deep red granules. The nucleus is stained blue (see Fig. 15-7).

Normally, the nasal smear contains mucus with scattered neutrophils, mononuclear cells, and occasional epithelial cells. If neutrophilia is pronounced, infection is probably present, especially if bacteria are present in large numbers.

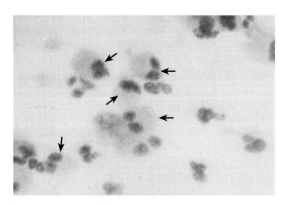

**FIG. 15-7.** Several eosinophils in nasal smear *(arrows).* Hansel's stain, brightfield, ×1,000.

Eosinophilia is positive evidence of nasal allergy. However, there can be a mixture of infection and allergy.

One method of evaluating the nasal smear is based on enumerating the eosinophils seen in four representative fields. If 10% or more eosinophils are seen in any of the four fields, nasal allergy is presumed to be present.

Hansel's stain can also be used to stain cytocentrifuged preparations of urinary sediment for the presence of eosinophils. In the case of urinary sediment, the presence of any eosinophils would be considered abnormal.

## FECAL (OCCULT) BLOOD

### Clinical Significance

Tests for hemoglobin in fecal specimens are often referred to as tests for occult blood. This is because hemoglobin may be present in the feces, as evidenced by positive chemical tests for blood, and yet not be detected by the naked eye. In other words, occult blood is hidden blood and requires a chemical test for its detection. Occasionally there will be enough blood in the feces to produce a tarry-black or even bloody specimen. However, even bloody specimens should be tested chemically for occult blood. In such cases the outer portion is avoided and the central portion of the formed stool is sampled. The detection of occult blood in the feces is important in determining the cause of hypochromic anemias resulting from chronic loss of blood and in detecting ulcerative or neoplastic diseases of the gastrointestinal system. Blood in the feces may result from bleeding anywhere along the gastrointestinal tract, from the mouth to the anus.

Tests for occult blood are especially useful for the early detection and treatment of colorectal cancer. Such tests are useful, for over half of all cancers (excluding skin) are from the gastrointestinal tract. Early detection results in good survival. Persons over age 50 years are commonly screened annually for occult blood. They sample their own stool specimens for three consecutive collections, apply a thin film to the test slides, and mail or bring them to the laboratory for testing. Dietary considerations are important to avoid false-positive results, and special instructions are generally included with the test slides. It is now rare for the laboratory to receive the actual fecal specimen to be tested for occult blood.

Bleeding at any point in the gastrointestinal system representing as little as 2 mL of blood lost daily may be detected by the tests for occult blood. However, false-negative results occur for unknown reasons, possibly because of inhibitors in the feces.

Implications of both false-positive and false-negative tests are important clinically. Early diagnosis and treatment of serious disease might be missed with false-negative results, resulting in poor prognosis and death. Positive results are serious, as any positive results require extensive further testing to determine the cause of bleeding, or to rule out false-positive reactions. Further testing is both unpleasant for the patient and expensive.

## Principle and Specificity

Numerous tests have been described for the detection of hemoglobin (or blood) in both urine and feces. Most of these tests are based on the same general principles and reaction. They all make use of peroxidase activity in the heme portion of the hemoglobin molecule.

Most tests for occult blood in feces use gum guaiac, a phenolic compound that produces a blue color when oxidized. The tests require the presence of hydrogen peroxide or a suitable precursor. The peroxidase activity of the hemoglobin molecule results in the liberation of oxygen from hydrogen peroxide ($H_2O_2$), and the released oxygen oxidizes gum guaiac to a blue oxidation product. The reaction is summarized below:

$$\text{Hemoglobin} + H_2O_2 \rightarrow \text{Oxygen}$$
(peroxidase activity)

$$\text{Oxygen} + \text{Reduced gum guaiac} \rightarrow$$
(colorless)

$$\text{Oxidized gum guaiac} + H_2O$$
(blue)

## Interfering Substances and Dietary Considerations

Several interfering substances may give false-positive results for occult blood. These include those of dietary origin with peroxidase activity, especially myoglobin and hemoglobin in red meat. Vegetable peroxidase, as found in horseradish, can also cause positive results. Several foods have been identified as causing erroneous reactions. These include turnips, broccoli, bananas, black grapes, pears, plums, and melons. Cooking generally destroys these peroxidases, and therefore patients are generally instructed to eat only cooked foods. White cells and bacteria also have peroxidase activity, which might result in false-positive reactions. Various drugs, including aspirin and aspirin-containing preparations and iron compounds, are known to increase gastrointestinal bleeding, causing positive results. Vitamin C and other oxidants may give false-negative results.

Patients are generally instructed to eat no beef or lamb (including processed meats and liver) for 3 days before collecting the first specimen and to remain on this diet through the collection of three successive samples. They may eat well-cooked pork, poultry, and fish. They are also instructed to avoid raw fruits and vegetables, especially melons, radishes, turnips, and horseradish. Cooked fruits and vegetables are acceptable. Ingestion of high-fiber foods, such as whole wheat bread, bran cereal, and popcorn, is encouraged. The ingestion of over 250 mg/day of vitamin C is to be avoided, as it may cause false-negative results. The mechanism of this interference is the same as for reagent strips used in urinalysis. Aspirin and other non-steroidal anti-inflammatory drugs should be avoided for 7 days prior to and during the test period.

## Guaiac Slide Test for Occult Blood

Various commercial tests have been developed to test for the presence of hemoglobin in the feces. At least eight guaiac-based tests for occult blood are available commercially. The

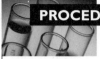

## PROCEDURE 15-4

*Testing for Occult Blood With Hemoccult II*

### Application of Specimen to Hemoccult II Slide *(Often done by patient)*

1. Collect a small amount of fecal specimen on one end of the applicator stick provided. Open the cover flap and apply a thin smear inside box A on the front side of the slide.

2. Collect a second sample from a different part of the stool, using the same applicator. Apply a thin smear inside box B.

3. Close the cover flap, and allow the slide to air dry.

### Color Development *(Performed in laboratory)*

1. Open the perforated window on the back of the slide.

2. Apply two drops of the peroxide solution (developer) to guaiac paper directly over each smear.

3. Read the results within 60 seconds. Any trace of blue on or at the edge of the fecal smear is positive.

4. Develop on slide performance monitor areas (controls): Apply one drop only of the peroxide solution between the positive and negative performance areas. Always test the specimen, and read and interpret the results, before developing the controls. A blue color from the positive control might spread into the specimen and cause confusion or a false-positive reaction. Read the results within 10 seconds. A blue color will appear in the positive, and no color in the negative, performance monitor area if the slides and developer are reacting according to product specifications.

### Interpretation

Any trace of blue color is positive, whether the intensity of color development is weak or strong. Reagent paper that has turned blue or blue-green before use should be discarded. If discolored test paper has been used by the patient, the test should be repeated if there is any question in interpretation.

---

Hemoccult II,* which seems to have the lowest rate of false-positive results, is described here (Procedure 15-4). Other tests are similar. In all cases, the manufacturer's directions should be followed.

Hemoccult II is available as a slide test that contains filter paper uniformly impregnated with gum guaiac. The specimen is applied in a thin film in each of two boxes on the front side of the slide. This may be done by the patient or the laboratory. The specimen is applied with a

wooden applicator, which is supplied with the test kit. The kit includes dietary information for the patient and instructions for collecting the specimen.

The American Cancer Society recommends that two samples from three consecutive specimens be collected for colorectal screening. Therefore, test kits are usually supplied to patients in groups of three slides. The patient is instructed to allow the test slides to dry overnight, and then to return them to the physician or laboratory. If the slides are to be mailed, they must be placed in an approved U.S. Postal Service

---

*SmithKline Diagnostics, Sunnyvale, Calif.

mailing pouch. They may not be mailed in a standard paper envelope.

When the slides are received in the laboratory, the specimen is tested on the back (opposite side) of the test slide. When the perforated window on the back of the slide is opened, two specimen windows plus positive and negative performance monitor areas (controls) are revealed. If the specimen is applied in the laboratory, it must air dry before the developer solution is applied so as to increase the sensitivity of the test.

The developer solution is a stabilized mixture of hydrogen peroxide and denatured alcohol, which is supplied with the test. Only reagent supplied with the test slides can be used for color development. When the fecal specimen containing occult blood is applied to the guaiac-impregnated test paper, peroxidase in the specimen comes in contact with the guaiac. When the developing solution is then applied to the test paper, a reaction between the guaiac and peroxidase results in formation of a blue color.

The reaction requires that blood cells be hemolyzed for proper release of peroxidase. This usually takes place within the gastrointestinal tract. If whole, undiluted blood is applied to the test paper, the red cells may not hemolyze and the reaction may be weak or atypical. The test is significantly more sensitive to the presence of occult blood if the specimen is allowed to dry on the slide before the developing solution is applied. The American Cancer Society recommends that slides be tested within 6 days of preparation, and that the slides not be rehydrated. They also recommend that a single positive smear be considered a positive test result, even in the absence of dietary restriction.

## FECAL LEUKOCYTES

It is occasionally useful to examine the feces for the presence of neutrophils as an indication of the presence of certain enteric pathogens. About 70% of cases of dysentery due to *Shigella* have neutrophils present in the feces. However,

dysentery due to *Salmonella* or *Campylobacter* shows neutrophils in only 30% to 50% of the cases. Dysentery resulting from noninvasive organisms like *Rotavirus* and toxigenic *E. Coli* shows neutrophils in only 5% of cases.

To test for the presence of neutrophils in a fecal (stool) specimen, smears are prepared by selecting flecks of mucus from the fecal material with a cotton swab. This is then rolled across a glass slide, and the slide is allowed to air dry. It is then stained with Wright stain, and observed microscopically for the presence of neutrophils.

Although neutrophils are usually easily recognized, in fecal smears artifacts, cellular distortion, and degeneration are common. The nuclear lobes may appear eccentric, and the cytoplasm may show toxic changes. Morphologic changes due to autolysis, such as nuclear pyknosis and fragmentation, may make identification of the cell type difficult.

## CERVICAL MUCUS TEST (FERN TEST)

The evaluation of the cervical mucus and sperm and their interaction is useful in the area of fertility evaluation, in which the desired outcome is pregnancy, or for the purpose of contraception. Specimens must be obtained and handled and tests performed according to specific laboratory protocol and procedure. A general description follows.

The secretion of cervical mucus is regulated by ovarian hormones. The estrogens stimulate the production of copious amounts of watery mucus, and progesterones inhibit the secretory activity of the cervical epithelial cells. Thus, there is a cyclic variation in the amount of cervical mucus secreted. The largest volume is at mid-cycle in normal premenopausal women. The consistency of the cervical mucus also varies during the menstrual cycle. It is highly viscous and often cellular premenstrually, and watery at mid-cycle, just before ovulation, because of the effect of estrogen. Viscosity begins to increase again by the time ovulation is completed, because of the effect of progesterone. Viscosity, and therefore the stage of the menstrual cycle, is sometimes evaluated microscopically by the fern test. It is used to predict the day of ovulation and to determine whether ovulation occurs.

For the **fern test,** mucus aspirated from the cervix is spread on a glass slide and allowed to dry for a few minutes. The slide is examined microscopically for a characteristic "ferning" pattern. During a normal ovulatory cycle, at mid-cycle from about the seventh to about the eighteenth day, a characteristic fern-like pattern of the dried cervical mucus, also described as a "palm leaf pattern," is normally seen microscopically.

This is the period of watery mucus production, during which sperm are able to penetrate the cervical mucus, beginning at approximately the ninth day of a normal cycle and with a peak penetration just before ovulation. The ability of sperm to penetrate the cervical mucus begins to diminish even before large changes in mucus properties are clinically apparent, and individual variations in time and degree of sperm penetration are common.

Although the fern test is prone to false-positive results, it has been used for many years and is still used in clinics and physicians' offices because it is easy to do and quick to perform.

## POSTCOITAL TEST

The evaluation of cervical mucus includes assessment of spinnbarkeit (fibrosity, threadability, or elasticity), ferning (crystallization), consistency, and pH. These properties are scored according to a scale of 1 to 15 (15 is best) in the **postcoital test (PCT).** Spinnbarkeit is assessed by touching cervical mucus on a glass slide with a coverslip or a second slide held crosswise, which is lifted gently. The length of the cervical mucus thread stretched in between is estimated in centimeters and scored. The overall score is based on volume, consistency, ferning, spinnbarkeit, and cellularity. The pH is recorded but not scored.

The postcoital test should be performed as closely as possible to the time of ovulation. This is determined by clinical criteria, which include usual cycle length, basal body temperature, cervical mucus changes, vaginal cytology plus plasma or urine estrogen assays, and ovarian ultrasound examination when available.

In general, in the postcoital test, the couple is instructed to abstain from sexual intercourse for two days prior to the day on which the test is performed. The cervical mucus is then examined by the laboratory at a standard time after coitus—from 9 to 24 hours.

A sample of the fluid pool in the posterior vaginal fornix is aspirated and examined to ensure that semen has been deposited in the vagina. A sample of mucus is then aspirated from the endocervical canal. This cervical mucus is placed on a glass microscope slide, coverslipped, and examined with a phase-contrast microscope for the number of sperm present and sperm motility.

The purpose of the postcoital test is to determine the number of active spermatozoa in the cervical mucus and to evaluate sperm survival many hours after coitus. The optimum time for this evaluation of longevity is 9 to 24 hours after coitus. Cervical factors as possible causes of infertility can be excluded if there is an adequate number of motile spermatozoa at this stage. If the initial result is negative or abnormal, the postcoital test should be repeated, as it may be due to incorrect timing—too early or too late in the menstrual cycle in an otherwise fertile woman.

## SEMEN ANALYSIS (QUALITATIVE)

Semen analysis is done for several reasons. These include assessment of fertility or infertility, forensic purposes, determination of the effectiveness of vasectomy, and determination of the suitability of semen for artificial insemination procedures.

Semen (seminal fluid) consists of a combination of products of various male reproductive organs (testes, epididymis, seminal vesicles, prostate, and bulbourethral and urethral glands). During ejaculation, the products are mixed, producing the normal viscous semen specimen or ejaculate. This ejaculated human semen is a viscous, yellow-gray fluid, which forms a fairly firm gel-like clot immediately after ejaculation. At room temperature, this clot liquefies spontaneously and completely within 5 to 60 minutes. If this liquefaction process requires more than 1 hour, the specimen is considered abnormal. Liquefaction must be complete before any laboratory analysis can be done.

## Macroscopic Examination

Macroscopic examination includes time for complete liquefaction, appearance, volume, viscosity (consistency), and pH.

## Wet Mount Analysis

Wet mount analysis is used to determine the approximate sperm count and motility. A drop of the thoroughly mixed, liquefied, semen specimen is placed on a clean glass slide and coverslipped. The volume of semen delivered onto the slide and the dimensions of the coverslip must be standardized. A standardized volume of 10 $\mu$L covered with a 22 × 22 mm coverglass will result in a fixed depth of about 20 $\mu$m and allow for a qualitative estimate of sperm number, morphology, motility, and velocity. The freshly made preparation is allowed to stabilize for about 1 minute before microscopic analysis. This is done by observing 10 to 20 microscope fields, using a 40× or 60× (high-power) objective.

Normally, mature sperm cells make up the majority of cells seen. Other cells typically seen are epithelial cells from the male genital tract, immature germ cells, and white blood cells. Percentages of the various types of cells are determined and reported. The approximate sperm count is reported as few, several, many, or numerous. Although subjective, this estimate should correlate with the actual chamber sperm count. The relative percentage of motile sperm is

determined while the sperm count is estimated. Because mobility and velocity are temperature dependent, a microscope with a warm stage should be used. At least 200 motile and non-motile sperm are counted in at least five different microscope fields, and the percentage of motile sperm is calculated as follows:

$$\% \text{ motility} = \frac{\text{Total sperm} - \text{Nonmotile sperm}}{\text{Total sperm}} \times 100$$

Normally, 50% or more sperm are motile.

## Other Tests

Qualitative semen analysis is subjective and generally requires further testing, including tests or observations of agglutination, viability, and morphology, counting chamber sperm counts, and sperm antibody assays.

## BIBLIOGRAPHY

College of American Pathologists 1996 Proficiency Testing Program: *Hematology, Clinical Microscopy and Body Fluids Glossaries.* Northfield, Ill, College of American Pathologists, 1996.

Huicho L, Sanchez D, Contreras M, et al: Occult blood and fecal leukocytes as screening tests in childhood infection diarrhea. *Pediatr Infect Dis J* 1993; 12:474.

Kao YS, Liu FJ: Laboratory diagnosis of gastrointestinal tract and exocrine pancreatic disorders. In Henry JB (ed): *Clinical Diagnosis and Management by Laboratory Methods,* ed 19. Philadelphia, WB Saunders Co, 1996, pp 537-541.

Keel BA, Webster DW, eds: *CRC Handbook of the Laboratory Diagnosis and Treatment of Infertility,* Boston, CRC Press, 1990.

Kjeldsberg CR, Knight JA: *Body Fluids: Laboratory Examination of Amniotic, Cerebrospinal, Seminal, Serous and Synovial Fluids,* ed 3. Chicago, American Society of Clinical Pathologists Press, 1993.

Litt M: Eosinophils and antigen-antibody reactions. *Ann NY Acad Sci* 1964; 116:964.

McCarty DJ (ed): *Arthritis and Allied Conditions: A Textbook of Rheumatology,* ed 12. Baltimore, Williams & Wilkins, 1992.

Ringsrud KM, Linne JJ: *Urinalysis and Body Fluids: A ColorText and Atlas.* St Louis, Mosby, 1995.

Schumacher RH Jr, Reginato AJ: *Atlas of Synovial Fluid Analysis and Crystal Identification.* Philadelphia, Lea & Febiger, 1991.

Smith GP, Kjeldsberg CR: Cerebrospinal, Synovial, and Serous Body Fluids. In Henry JB (ed): *Clinical Diagnosis and Management by Laboratory Methods,* ed 19. Philadelphia, WB Saunders Co, 1996, pp 457-506.

World Health Organization: *WHO Laboratory Manual for the Examination of Human Semen and Sperm–Cervical Mucus Interactions,* ed 3. New York, Cambridge University Press, 1992.

## STUDY QUESTIONS

1. **Which of the following fluids is *not* an ultrafiltrate of plasma?**

   A. Cerebrospinal fluid
   B. Pericardial fluid
   C. Peritoneal fluid
   D. Pleural fluid
   E. Synovial fluid

2. **Regarding gross appearance, normal spinal fluid is:**

   A. Crystal clear
   B. Pale yellow
   C. Slightly cloudy
   D. Slightly pink
   E. Xanthochromatic

3. **Match the following causes (1 to 6) with the gross appearances of cerebrospinal fluid (A to F).**

   1. Bilirubin from old hemorrhage
   2. Infection
   3. Normal appearance
   4. Recent hemorrhage
   5. Subarachnoid hemorrhage
   6. Traumatic tap
      _____ A. Cloudy fluid in all tubes
      _____ B. Crystal clear fluid in all tubes
      _____ C. Pale-pink or pale-orange xanthochromasia in supernate
      _____ D. Three sequentially collected tubes are equally bloody.
      _____ E. Three sequentially collected tubes are progressively less bloody; the third is clear, or almost clear.
      _____ F. Yellow xanthochromasia in supernate

4. **An increased spinal fluid white cell count with a preponderance of neutrophils is most characteristic of which of the following?**

   A. Bacterial meningitis
   B. Tuberculosis
   C. Viral meningitis
   D. Yeast infection

5. **A lower than normal spinal fluid glucose in relation to blood glucose is most characteristic of which of the following?**

   A. Bacterial meningitis
   B. Brain tumor
   C. Diabetic coma
   D. Viral meningitis

6. **Match the following fluids (1 to 9) with the definitions (A to I).**

   1. Cerebrospinal fluid
   2. Effusion
   3. Exudate
   4. Pericardial fluid
   5. Peritoneal fluid
   6. Pleural fluid
   7. Serous fluids
   8. Synovial fluid
   9. Transudate
      _____ A. An effusion that is usually the result of a systemic disease
      _____ B. An effusion that is usually the result of an inflammatory process
      _____ C. An increase in fluid volume
      _____ D. Around the abdominal and pelvic organs
      _____ E. Around the brain and spinal cord

_____ F. Around the heart
_____ G. Around the joints
_____ H. Around the lungs
_____ I. Fluids contained with the closed cavities of the body

7. **The presence of which of the following distinguishes synovial fluid from other extravascular fluids?**

A. Glucose
B. Hyaluronic acid
C. Lactate dehydrogenase
D. Protein
E. Xanthochromasia

8. **Match the following types of synovial fluid seen in joint disease (1 to 5) with the disease states or causes (A to H). Types of fluids may be used more than once.**

1. Crystal-induced fluid
2. Hemorrhagic fluid
3. Infectious fluid
4. Inflammatory fluid
5. Noninflammatory fluid
_____ A. Degenerative joint disease
_____ B. Fracture
_____ C. Gonorrhea
_____ D. Gout
_____ E. Hemophilia
_____ F. Immunologic disease
_____ G. Lupus arthritis
_____ H. Osteoarthritis
_____ I. Pseudogout
_____ J. Staph infection

9. **Which of the following anticoagulants is preferred for microscopic examination of the synovial fluid?**

A. Liquid EDTA
B. Lithium heparin
C. Oxalate
D. Plain serum separator tube
E. Powdered EDTA

10. **The viscosity of synovial fluid may be assessed by which of the following?**

A. Mucin clot test
B. String test

C. Tipping and observing the unanticoagulated tube
D. More than one of the above
E. All of the above

11. **The presence of monosodium urate (MSU) crystals in the synovial fluid is characteristic of:**

A. Gout
B. Osteoarthritis
C. Pseudogout
D. Rheumatoid arthritis

12. **The presence of calcium pyrophosphate dihydrate (CPPD) crystals in the synovial fluid is characteristic of:**

A. Gout
B. Osteoarthritis
C. Pseudogout
D. Rheumatoid arthritis

13. **The final identification of crystals in crystal-induced arthritis is best accomplished with which of the following?**

A. Brightfield microscopy
B. Compensated polarized light microscopy
C. Phase-contrast microscopy
D. Polarized light microscopy

14. **Match the following crystals seen in crystal-induced arthritis (1 and 2) with the following statements (A to H).**

1. Calcium pyrophosphate crystals (CPPD)
2. Monosodium urate crystals (MSU)
_____ A. Appear blue when parallel and yellow when perpendicular to the slow wave of vibration of compensated polarized light
_____ B. Appear yellow when parallel and blue when perpendicular to the slow wave of vibration of compensated polarized light
_____ C. Exhibit weak birefringence
_____ D. Exhibit strong birefringence
_____ E. "Sign" of birefringence is negative
_____ F. "Sign" of birefringence is positive
_____ G. Typically seen as chunky rectangles
_____ H. Typically seen as long slender needles

15. **Nasal smears are examined for the presence of eosinophils to diagnose the presence of:**

    A. Acute bacterial sinusitis
    B. Allergic rhinitis
    C. Bacterial rhinitis
    D. Viral rhinitis

16. **Tests for fecal occult blood are in general use as a screening test for which of the following?**

    A. Breast cancer
    B. Colorectal cancer
    C. Enteric infection of the colon
    D. Malabsorption syndrome
    E. Prostate cancer

17. **Indicate whether the following statements concerning tests for fecal occult blood are true (T) or false (F).**

    _____ A. Aspirin and nonsteroidal antiinflammatory drugs should be avoided to prevent gastrointestinal bleeding.

    _____ B. False-positive reactions are commonly due to peroxidase activity.

    _____ C. Most tests are slide tests that involve the reduction of gum guaiac from a colorless to a colored compound.

    _____ D. Tests are based on the peroxidase activity of heme.

    _____ E. The presence of large amounts of ascorbic acid may cause false-positive results.

    _____ F. To minimize false-positive reactions, patients should be instructed to eat only raw fruits and vegetables.

    _____ G. To minimize false-positive reactions, patients need to be on a special diet for three days before specimen collection begins, and for the duration.

18. **Indicate whether the following statements concerning tests of cervical mucus and sperm are true (T) or false (F).**

    _____ A. A positive fern test is seen when estrogen levels are high.

    _____ B. A positive fern test is seen when progesterone levels are high.

    _____ C. In normal semen, spermatozoa are the minority of cells seen.

    _____ D. Qualitative semen analysis is subjective, and further testing is generally required.

    _____ E. Qualitative semen analysis must take place before liquefaction of the specimen.

    _____ F. Sperm are more easily able to penetrate the cervical mucus when the fern test is negative

    _____ G. The fern test may be used to predict the day of ovulation.

    _____ H. The postcoital test is used to determine the number of active spermatozoa in the cervical mucus and to evaluate sperm survival after coitus.

    _____ I. The secretion of cervical mucus in regulated by ovarian hormones.

## CASE HISTORIES

### ■ CASE 1

A 15-year-old high school student with fever, chills, and severe headache is seen in an urgent care clinic. He felt nauseated and vomited before reporting to the clinic. At the clinic his temperature is 104° F; he has neck rigidity and complains of back pain. Some small petechial spots are noted on his chest and back and in the mouth. Blood is drawn for CBC and blood glucose, and a lumbar puncture is performed. Cerebrospinal fluid is collected sequentially in three sterile tubes and examined.

#### Blood Results

| | |
|---|---|
| White cell count | $25 \times 10^9$/L |
| Differential | 80% neutrophils |
| | 10% lymphocytes |
| | 10% monocytes |
| Glucose | 95 mg/dL |

#### Cerebrospinal Fluid Results

| | |
|---|---|
| CSF pressure | Increased |
| Gross appearance | All tubes equally cloudy, not bloody |
| Glucose | 15 mg/dL |
| CSF white count | 12,000/$\mu$L; 90% neutrophils |
| Gram stain | Many gram-negative cocci in pairs, some intracellular |

1. Does the white cell count and differential on venous blood indicate a bacterial or a viral infection?
2. What is the significance of the gross appearance of the spinal fluid in this case?
3. What is the significance of the blood and spinal fluid glucose in this patient?
4. Based on the Gram stain, what is the likely cause of infection in this patient?

### ■ CASE 2

A 75-year-old woman has had a long history of joint pain in the large joints. She now has shoulder pain and a swollen, red knee joint. She has a slight fever, and bilateral muscle weakness in the lower limbs. Blood is drawn for hematology, her knee is x-rayed, and arthrocentesis is performed on her knee.

#### Hematology Results

| | |
|---|---|
| Hemoglobin | 11.9 g/dL |
| White cell count | $12 \times 10^9$/L |

#### X-ray Findings

Calcification in the cartilage and meniscus (chondrocalcinosis).

#### Synovial Fluid Findings

| | |
|---|---|
| Appearance | Cloudy and watery |
| Microscopic exam | Many neutrophils. Intracellular and extracellular crystals present, appearing as small chunky rectangles that show weak birefringence and appear blue when parallel and yellow when perpendicular to the slow wave of vibration of compensated polarized light. |

1. The pattern of birefringence in this case is consistent with:
   A. Calcium pyrophosphate dihydrate (CPPD)
   B. Cholesterol
   C. Hydroxyapatite
   D. Monosodium urate (MSU)
2. The sign of birefringence in this case is:
   A. Negative
   B. Positive
3. The disease exhibited by this patient is referred to as:
   A. Gout
   B. Osteoarthritis
   C. Pseudogout
   D. Rheumatoid arthritis
4. What is the significance of the hemoglobin and the white cell count in this patient?

# CHAPTER 16

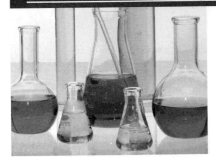

# Microbiology

## Learning Objectives

*From study of this chapter, the reader will be able to:*

➤ Appreciate the importance of collection requirements for the various specimens used in microbiological studies.

➤ Describe the various Gram stain reactions for common bacteria.

➤ Prepare and examine a Gram stained smear for common bacteria.

➤ Select and inoculate the appropriate media for commonly collected specimens—urine, throat swabs, genitourinary exudates, blood.

➤ Collect an appropriate specimen for a urine culture, quantitatively plate it, and interpret results.

➤ Collect a throat swab for a throat culture on sheep blood agar, plate it, and interpret results.

➤ Collect blood for culture and describe how to process and interpret the result of the culturing.

➤ Discuss the major sexually transmitted diseases and the laboratory tests used in their diagnosis.

➤ Collect genitourinary specimens for culture.

➤ Discuss the purpose and process of testing for antimicrobial susceptibility or sensitivity.

➤ Discuss the factors that are considered in the selection of an antimicrobial agent.

➤ Discuss the characteristics of fungi and the common methods used to detect fungi in the laboratory.

➤ Discuss the specimen collection and identification process for common intestinal parasites.

# INTRODUCTION TO MICROBIOLOGY

The field of clinical or medical microbiology involves the isolation and identification of organisms so small that they cannot be seen with the naked eye. They can be observed only with a microscope and are therefore known as microorganisms or microbes. Microorganisms are distributed throughout nature and interact in the human life cycle and in the life cycles of other species. Some microorganisms inhabit the human body normally and do not cause disease; these are called **normal flora.** Other microorganisms can cause disease; these are called **pathogens.**

Several different groups of microorganisms are studied in the microbiology laboratory, including bacteria, viruses, rickettsiae, fungi, protozoa and other parasites, and algae. Organisms in each of these groups can cause disease. Medical microbiology is concerned with identifying pathogens and developing effective ways to eliminate or control them.

The field of clinical microbiology is generally divided into areas of specialization, according to the type of microorganism being studied. For example, the study of bacteria is **bacteriology,** the study of viruses is **virology,** the study of fungi is **mycology,** the study of rickettsiae is **rickettsiology,** and the study of parasites is **parasitology.** In this chapter, the discussion centers more on bacteriology than on any other area of microbiology. It is possible, however, to apply the general skills covered when discussing bacteriology to the other areas. As with other divisions of the clinical laboratory, if the basic skills are understood and learned well, other specific tests and procedures may more easily be done.

The routine procedures, such as the specimen collection itself, the initial media inoculation, handling of media, staining of slides, and microscopic examination of the slides, are extremely important for the final identification process. Techniques involved in these routine procedures—the growth (culture) and identification of various common pathogenic microorganisms—are discussed in this chapter. Monoclonal antibodies have been employed in many tests involving antigen-antibody reactions. Some are described in this chapter and in other chapters where applicable.

Molecular diagnostic techniques have added a new dimension to the microbiology laboratory. Genetic probes are also being used, these being known, labeled sequences of DNA or RNA used to detect complementary sequences in target specimens. Currently, in the microbiology laboratory, application of DNA probes includes the detection of bacterial, fungal, and mycobacterial pathogens.

**599**

## Normal Flora

Microorganisms are present under normal conditions in certain sites of the body. Examples of these normal flora are the normal constituents of the human intestinal tract, especially the large intestine and colon. These microorganisms benefit from this association, for they derive essential food materials from the host. The host also benefits, for the microorganisms synthesize and aid in the digestion of vitamins that are essential for human life. Normal flora also may be found in the mouth and oral cavity, in the nose, and on the surface of the skin. Sites of the body that normally are **sterile,** or that contain no normal flora, are the blood, the cerebrospinal fluid, and the urinary bladder.

## Pathogenic Microorganisms

Although microorganisms are generally beneficial and essential for life, some are harmful to their hosts. These are the disease-producing, or pathogenic, microorganisms. It is important that the laboratorian be able to distinguish normal flora from pathogens in the specimens being cultured from specific sites. The discussion in this chapter is primarily concerned with pathogenic microorganisms.

An **opportunistic pathogen** is an organism that does not usually cause disease in a person with an intact immune system but can cause disease when the host's immune system has been compromised by disease or other condition that has damaged or changed the immune status of the host. Infectious microorganisms can reside in the health care facility itself and can become a large problem if they start infecting the patients. **Nosocomial infections** are those acquired in the hospital or health care facility—the organism is not present in the patient, nor is it incubating in the patient before he or she is admitted into the health care facility. Infection control is critical to prevent this from occurring, and health care facilities of all types have active infection control departments for this purpose. Common nosocomial microorganisms include the *Staphylococcus* bacterium and the fungus *Candida albicans*. In contrast, a **community-acquired infection** results from organisms residing in or incubating in the patient before admission into the health care facility.

The pathogenic microorganisms include living organisms of both the plant and animal kingdoms. The only true microbes of the animal kingdom are the protozoa, which are single-celled animals, classified as parasites in this chapter. Most of the protozoa are harmless, but some may be pathogenic. The protozoa are subdivided into amebas, ciliates, flagellates, and sporozoa. An example of a disease resulting from protozoa is amebic dysentery, which is caused by a specific protozoan ameba.

Certain pathogenic worms are often included in the field of microbiology, although they are not microorganisms (see under Tests for Parasites). Examples of worms that cause disease are the tapeworm *Taenia solium*, the fluke *Fasciolopsis buski,* and the roundworm *Strongyloides stercoralis*. An even higher class of parasitic animals, the arthropods, are included in microbiology assays in some instances. These organisms themselves rarely cause disease; however, they serve as vectors in certain microbial infections. Some insects are essential in one stage of the life cycle of true microorganisms that cause malaria. Also, some ticks are bloodsucking parasites themselves. A relatively well known tick-borne disease is Lyme disease, the etiologic agent being the bacterium *Borrelia burgdorferi*. Transmission occurs by inoculation by a bite of a tick of the genus *Ixodes;* diagnosis of Lyme disease depends on finding antibodies in the serum or spinal fluid.

Microorganisms that are bacteria, fungi, protozoa, or algae are neither plant nor animal, but belong to a separate kingdom called Prokaryotae. Bacteria make up the most numerous group in the Prokaryotae. The systematic classification of the microorganisms is complex. Fungi are simple colorless plants that are further subdivided into the molds, yeasts, and bacteria. Microorganisms more simple than bacteria include pleuro-pneumonia and pleuropneumonia-like organisms, rickettsiae, and viruses.

## CLASSIFICATION OF MICROORGANISMS: TAXONOMY

In discussing microorganisms, it is necessary to refer to the method by which living things are classified or named. By using biological classification methods, it is possible for the laboratory microbiologist to systematically identify microbes. The scientific study of the classification process is known as **taxonomy.** The traditional classification system provides a relatively simple, orderly method for placing microbes into categories according to their similar morphologic and biochemical properties. *Bergey's Manual of Systematic Bacteriology* is a definitive source for the naming and classifying of bacteria.[11]

### Genus and Species

In the terminology of biological classification, the word **species** is frequently used; it is the basic unit of the biological world. The species category is based on reproduction: members of the same species are able to mate successfully and produce others of their kind. The **genus** is the next larger classification—members of the same genus sharing common biological likenesses.

The microbes studied in the medical microbiology laboratory will have two Latin names, the genus name (often abbreviated with the first initial only) and the species name. These Latin names are printed in italics. A genus can include several species, all of which differ somewhat from one another. For example, the genus *Haemophilus* includes several species. Depending on the species, the organisms can cause different diseases in humans. *Haemophilus influenzae* type b is a pathogen that causes acute respiratory tract infections and can lead to meningitis, while *Haemophilus parainfluenzae* and *Haemophilus aphrophilus* are both a cause of subacute endo-

carditis. Other species of this genus can cause different human diseases.

Continuing up the classification system, microbes that have common characteristics are grouped into successively larger categories: similar genera are grouped into families, related families are classified as an order, related orders make up a class, and classes with common characteristics constitute a phylum (Fig. 16-1). Traditionally, bacterial species are placed into three categories: a family, a genus, and a species. An example is the family Enterobacteriaceae. In this single family are many different genera and species categorized by their key features, some of these being their biochemical reactions. In this family, the genus *Escherichia* contains several species, including *coli*, written *Escherichia coli* or *E. coli*, a common causative pathogen of urinary tract infections.

### Classification by Morphology and Biochemical Properties

Organisms have traditionally been classified and placed into groups on the basis of the similarity

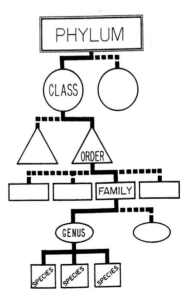

**FIG 16-1.** Biological classification system.

of their phenotypical or observable characteristics for all members of a particular group. This includes observation of their morphology on culture and Gram stain and on their biochemical reactions when they are tested for metabolic characteristics.

## Classification by Cell Type and Function: Prokaryotes and Eukaryotes

Another system of classification of organisms is by cell structure and function. Three groups have been identified: prokaryotes, eukaryotes, and archaeobacteria, all belonging to the kingdom, Prokaryotae. Prokaryotes and eukaryotes are most relevant to medical microbiology and will be briefly discussed. Bacteria are prokaryotic, while fungi, algae, protozoa animals cells and plant cells are eukaryotic in function and cell structure.

**Prokaryotes** (bacteria) are the smaller and often less complex organisms containing DNA in a single, circular chromosome. Structures also unique to prokaryotes are their cell membranes and cell walls. The cell membrane is a lipoprotein that surrounds the cytoplasm. The cell wall is a rigid structure that protects the organism and is extremely complex, being made up of peptidoglycan layers, proteins, and lipids, depending on the specific organism. The cell wall maintains the shape of the organism, and its components contribute to the gram-negative or gram-positive staining reaction of the organism. Features of the cell wall also contribute to the acid-fast staining attribute of mycobacteria. Many bacteria are enclosed with a polysaccharide capsule.

**Eukaryotes** (fungi, algae, protozoa) are more structurally complex than prokaryotes and contain a variety of membrane-enclosed organelles such as mitochondria, lysosomes, and endoplasmic reticulum; they have a true membrane-enclosed nucleus. Their cell walls, when present, are composed of polysaccharides such as cellulose, unlike the complex components in the cell walls of prokaryotes. Eukaryotes do not have capsules. The DNA in the nucleus is organized into multiple chromosomes covered with histones (protein).

# PROTECTION OF LABORATORY PERSONNEL AND DECONTAMINATION AND STERILIZATION OF MATERIALS

All clinical laboratories have procedures in place that must be followed for the general safety and protection of the workers (see Chapter 2). Since the material to be examined in the microbiology laboratory is likely to contain infectious pathogens, it is necessary to also protect the microbiologist from any potentially infectious specimens.

Microbiology laboratories pose a hazard in addition to the hazards of blood and body fluid specimens themselves (involving the standard precautions policies). Potentially hazardous infectious cultures of pathogenic agents are necessarily prevalent in these laboratories and require extra precautionary measures. Laboratorians who engage in microbiology work and who routinely handle these agents must pay special attention to all measures employed by the laboratory for their protection and safety. Protection from infection from pathogenic microbiological agents requires specific additional safety practices for laboratorians working in a microbiology laboratory setting.

## Classification of Biological Agents Based on Their Hazard to Persons Handling Them

The Centers for Disease Control and Prevention (CDC) has published a list that classifies biological agents, or etiological agents, on the basis of the assessment of the relative risk of working with them.[5] The more common of these agents are listed below, but in general, patient specimens pose a greater hazard to laboratory workers than do cultures of microorganisms, because the nature of the etiological agent in patient specimens is usually not known.

### Biosafety Level I

These are agents that pose no known pathologic potential for persons with normal immune systems. Good standard working practices should be used in handling agents of this level. Examples of Level I agents include *Bacillus subtilis* and *Mycobacterium gordonae*.

### Biosafety Level 2

These agents are the ones most commonly being identified in patient specimens. They include all of the common agents of infectious diseases, including HIV. Biosafety Level 2 agents also include the causes of laboratory-acquired infection, such as hepatitis B virus, and other less common organisms, such as *Mycobacterium tuberculosis* and *Salmonella* and *Shigella* species. The general principles of safety and infection control discussed must be used for handling these agents, including the use of barrier protection, limited access to the laboratory, and use of a biological safety cabinet when necessary when aerosolization of the agent is possible.

### Biosafety Level 3

Agents in this category are not usually ones encountered in a routine microbiology laboratory. Agents in Biosafety Level 3 include certain arboviruses, arenoviruses, and cultures of *M. tuberculosis* and certain mold stages of systemic fungi. Laboratories where these agents are in use must have special engineering features for careful control of air movement and a requirement for personnel to wear protective clothing and other special barrier devices.

### Biosafety Level 4

These agents are not found in routine microbiology laboratories in the United States, unless they are in special maximum containment facilities or research laboratories.

## General Safety Practices in the Microbiology Laboratory

Access to the microbiology laboratory should be limited to those persons who understand the potential risk involved in simply being in this area. Specific high-risk work can be done in an area separate from the main microbiology laboratory, where access is strictly limited.

The air-handling system of the microbiology laboratory should operate to move air from low-risk areas to high-risk areas and not the reverse. Air should ideally not be recirculated after it has been in this area. If special procedures are done that generate aerosols that are infectious, a biological safety cabinet should be in place. Several diseases may be contracted by inhalation of the infectious particles—tularemia, tuberculosis, brucellosis, histoplasmosis, and Legionnaires' disease, to name a few. These infectious particles are known as **aerosols;** several processes carried out in microbiological studies can create aerosols. Techniques like mincing, vortexing, and preparation of direct smears have been known to produce aerosol droplets. These selected procedures should be carried out in a biological safety cabinet (see under Protection From Aerosols, in Chapter 2).

It is essential that strict adherence to the policies of standard precautions be maintained (see Standard Precautions, in Chapter 2). One important aspect of this is the conscientious use of barrier precautions, the most common barrier being the use of gloves for handling patient specimens and for any work done in the microbiology laboratory. Gloves must be worn at all times during laboratory procedures dealing with all specimens and microbiological work. Protective laboratory clothing, such as laboratory coats, should also always be worn in the laboratory. These coats should be removed before leaving the laboratory (see under Barrier Precautions, in Chapter 2).

Other general safety practices include keeping the laboratory free of dust, which can be the cause of infection by dangerous pathogens. An important consideration also is the transportation and handling of laboratory specimens. Specimen containers must always be transported to the laboratory in plastic, leak-proof, sealed bags, and the outside surface of the container should not be contaminated with any of the specimen contents.

The hands should be washed thoroughly before a laboratorian leaves the microbiology laboratory, according to the laboratory's established protocol; they must also be washed in case of contamination. The microbiologist should not work with uncovered open cuts or broken skin; these should be covered with a bandage or some suitable material before gloves are put on.

Each health care facility will have its own policies for safety protocol specifically pertaining to the microbiology laboratory, and these must be followed explicitly by the laboratorians working in that area.

### Disposal of Waste and Process of Decontamination

Any material that has become contaminated with an infectious agent must be decontaminated before final disposal. All such materials must first be placed into biohazard containers, clearly marked as such. These materials include media that have been inoculated, along with any remaining patient specimens. The biohazard bags or containers are then disposed of in the way established by the health care facility. Any sharp objects, needles, blades, and so forth, must be placed in special puncture-resistant sharps containers for disposal prior to decontamination. The actual decontamination can take place by several means—by steam sterilization as in an autoclave or by incineration or burning.

The work area should be cleaned with a phenolic compound or bleach before and after use each day. A mild disinfectant or diluted solution of bleach is commonly used for cleaning. Diluted bleach is a very effective decontaminant against viral agents and is the antiseptic of choice for laboratories where viral studies are done. There are commercially available decontaminants, which are used in some laboratories. The longer the surface is allowed to remain wet with the cleaning agent, the more effective the decontamination—a minimum of ten minutes is recommended. Decontamination is an ongoing process in the microbiology laboratory.

### Use of Flame Burners: Adherence to Protection from Fire Hazards

If open flame burners are used in the laboratory to sterilize the inoculating loops and needles, special caution must be taken. Fire hazards may be minimized by turning off burners whenever they are not in use. In addition, burners should be kept away from material that is flammable. When inoculating loops or needles are flamed in a flame burner, care must be taken to prevent splattering of material during the process (Fig 16-2). These burners should be housed in a protective container to prevent accidental burns. An alternative to the open flame burner is the incinerator burner.

## Disinfection and Sterilization Techniques

It is essential that sterile media be used to grow pure cultures of bacteria and that contamination by any of the microorganisms normally so widely distributed in nature be avoided (organisms in the air, on the hands, on laboratory equipment and supplies, and so forth). In general, all equipment and glassware and all media used in the microbiology laboratory must be absolutely sterile to ensure the preparation of pure cultures of microorganisms. Media in which microorganisms have been cultured or anything contaminated by infected material must be disinfected or sterilized. Media must also be decontaminated or sterilized or placed in special biohazard discard bags before being discarded, in order to prevent infection of those responsible for its removal.

Disinfection is the process of removing pathogenic organisms but not necessarily bacterial or other spores. Physical or chemical means may be used, but most disinfection is done by use of a chemical agent such as a bleach solution applied to an inanimate object such as a desktop or work area.

**Sterilization** refers to the killing or destruction of all microorganisms, including bacterial spores. There are various ways in which sterilization may be achieved. In general, physical means such as heat or filtration and chemical means such as oxidation are involved.

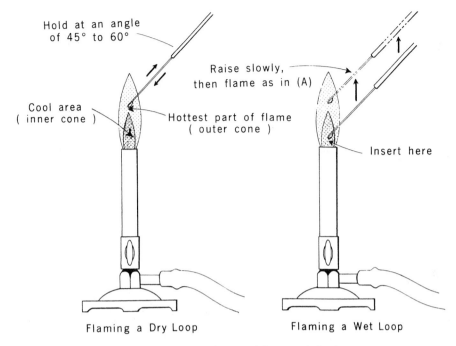

Hold at an angle
of 45° to 60°

Raise slowly,
then flame as in (A)

Cool area
( inner cone )

Hottest part of flame
( outer cone )

Insert here

Flaming a Dry Loop

Flaming a Wet Loop

**FIG 16-2.** Flaming of wet and dry inoculating loops.

### Use of Bleach or Antiseptic Agents

If the work area is actually contaminated, a strong disinfectant such as 5% phenol or 5% household bleach (sodium hypochlorite) solution must be used. For example, if a culture is dropped or spilled, a bleach solution should be poured over the contaminated area, covered with paper towels, and let stand wet for at least 10 minutes. Then the contaminated material is removed and placed in an appropriate container for discarding of biohazardous materials.

### Use of Heat or Burning

The effect of heat on organisms is generally known, and heat is a widely used and efficient physical means of sterilization. Heat may be employed in the form of dry heat or moist heat. Dry heat destroys bacteria by oxidation, while moist heat works through the coagulation of protein. Except for burning or incineration, sterilization by moist heat is generally more rapid. However,

the type of sterilization method that is used will depend on the nature of the material being treated, since many materials are destroyed by burning and many are harmed by the application of moist heat. Sterilization by dry heat includes burning and the use of hot air. Sterilization by moist heat includes the use of boiling water, "live" steam (steam at atmospheric pressure), and steam under pressure—the autoclave.

**Sterilization of the Inoculating Loop or Wire.** Burning is a useful means of sterilization in various steps in the culture and identification of microorganisms. Infected material from the original specimen, material from isolated colonies, and material from liquid cultures are usually manipulated by means of a transfer needle or inoculating loop. These needles and loops are made of inert metals such as platinum or suitable alloys such as Nichrome. They are unharmed when held in an open flame burner or an incinerator burner and are decontaminated or sterilized in this manner (Fig. 16-2). Therefore, when material is to be transferred, the inoculating loop or wire is flamed until it glows, cooled to room temperature by waiting approximately 30 seconds, and then reflamed after use to sterilize it. The open flame burner (Bunsen burner) and the incinerator burner are commonly used pieces of equipment in the microbiology laboratory (see also Use of Inoculating Loop or Needle and Culture Plates or Tube Cultures).

**Use of Dry Air.** Sterilization by dry heat is achieved by use of a dry-air chamber that is similar to an oven. The material must be kept at a temperature between 150° and 160° C for at least 1 hour. To be sterilized in this time, the material must be a good heat conductor; this method is most useful for materials that are destroyed by moist heat. Sterilization by dry heat is used for glassware in the microbiology laboratory when it must be reused.

**Use of Moist Heat.** Moist-heat sterilization by boiling water is convenient because it requires little special equipment. Boiling in water for 5 minutes is sufficient to kill all vegetative forms of bacteria, but the spores remain. Certain species of bacteria of the genus *Bacillus* have the ability to form spores under unfavorable conditions, but return to normal when favorable conditions return. Since spores are highly resistant forms of bacteria, they pose a problem in decontamination or sterilization. To kill spores by boiling in water generally requires 1 to 2 hours, although certain spores have been known to survive 16 hours of boiling. For this reason, certain chemicals may be added to the water to achieve more rapid sterilization by boiling. For example, 1 g/dL sodium carbonate makes the destruction of spores more rapid and also prevents rusting of certain metals sterilized in this manner. Moist heat is used to sterilize heat-stable objects.

**Use of Steam Under Pressure (the Autoclave).** The most effective means of sterilization with moist heat involves the use of steam under pressure, and a special device called an **autoclave.** It is the method of choice for any material that can fit in the apparatus and is not injured by moisture, high temperature, or high pressure. Some equipment is sterilized in this manner, as are some infected materials that are to be discarded.

Several types of autoclaves are available. Basically, the device is a heavy metal chamber with a door or lid that can be fastened to withstand the internal steam pressure, a pressure gauge, a safety valve, and a temperature gauge. The steam may be supplied by boiling water in the chamber or from heating pipes. Whatever type of autoclave is used, it is essential that all the air be displaced from the chamber by steam before the system is sealed. If this is not done, the chamber will contain unsaturated steam, which is a mixture of dry heat and moist heat and is significantly less efficient in achieving complete sterilization.

The exact details of operation of the autoclave may be found in the operating instructions provided with the autoclave. The material is exposed to pure steam in the autoclave at 121° C for 15 to 20 minutes. This temperature is achieved by applying pressure. Generally, 15 lb above atmospheric pressure is required to reach 121° C. This time and temperature will kill all forms of bacterial life, including spores. The temperature of steam in an autoclave at 15-lb gauge pressure at sea level is 121.3° C.

Temperature chart recorders must be used for documentation of autoclave maintenance, and quality assurance programs require that the maintenance of the autoclave be checked and documented regularly. This may be done by one of several methods, using biological or chemical indicators. To monitor sterilization, chemically impregnated tape is available that, when exposed to 121° C for 15 minutes, changes color to show the word "autoclaved."

### Use of Filtration

In the preparation of certain media that are used in microbiology, none of the preceding methods of sterilization is applicable, since they result in deterioration of the media. In these cases, some other means, such as filtration through thin membrane filters composed of plastic polymers or cellulose esters, may be used. Heat-sensitive solutions such as vaccines or antibiotic solutions can be sterilized by filtration.

# SPECIMENS FOR MICROBIOLOGICAL EXAMINATION

When a patient has particular disease symptoms and a microbiological infection is suspected, the causative agent must often be identified. The laboratory should be alerted to possible suspected organisms or tentative diagnoses, and sufficient clinical information should be included to assist the laboratorian in the selection of proper media and the use of appropriate laboratory testing procedures. Positive identification of the causative agent is important in selecting the best treatment for the patient. It is important, therefore, that only appropriate specimens be sent to the laboratory. Information accompanying the specimen must include its site of origin ("wound" culture, sputum, etc.). In the case of a possible kidney or urinary tract infection, a urine specimen will be collected for bacterial analysis. If the patient has a sore throat, the throat will be swabbed, and this specimen will be submitted for testing. Possible dysentery will require the examination of stool specimens, while the examination of infected wounds will require swabs or appropriate material from the area of infection. Other sites of infection from which swabs or material is submitted to the laboratory for culture and identification include the blood, various body fluids (from the cervix, urethra, vagina, ear, endometrium), eye, cerebrospinal, ventricular, or subdural fluid, bronchi or trachea (sputum material), and various tissues (see also Chapter 3).

## Specimen Collection Requirements for Culture

The microbiologist must be aware of the types of infective agents that may be responsible for a disease and test for these accordingly. Likewise, for each source of infected material, there is a certain set of tests that must be performed to discover the cause of infection. It is the responsibility of the laboratory to inform the hospital staff of correct procedures for collecting microbiological specimens and to provide or suggest suitable containers for this purpose.

The treatment of a disease or infection often involves the use of antibiotics or other agents that destroy various pathogens. The antibiotics are often administered before the causative agent is identified, since such identification takes 1 day or more and the patient requires immediate treatment. However, culture of the causative agent will often be impossible once antibiotics have been administered. Therefore, the appropriate specimen should be obtained before antibiotics are administered.

It is important to remember that material should be collected for culture from the location where the suspected organism is most likely to be found. An example is the culture of specimens from draining lesions containing coagulase-positive staphylococci. This type of specimen should also be collected with as little external contamination as possible from areas around the lesion—the actual wound must be cultured, not the surrounding area, where there may be only normal skin flora. Another example is the collection of sputum to assist in the diagnosis of a lower respiratory tract infection. Sputum is needed for this culture and not saliva from the oral cavity, which may yield only normal mouth flora.

Another factor that contributes to the successful isolation of the causative agent is the stage of the disease during which the specimen is collected. Enteric pathogens are found in much greater numbers in the acute stage of certain diarrheal intestinal infections and are therefore more likely to be isolated from specimens obtained at this stage. Viruses causing meningitis are isolated from cerebrospinal fluid with greater frequency when the fluid is obtained at the onset of the disease. It is important that the necessity of collecting microbiological specimens at the correct time, as well as in the proper manner, be understood.

The laboratory should be informed of the source of the material to be examined and of the tentative diagnosis. This information will help to ensure that the correct medium is inoculated with the specimen, aiding in the correct identification of the pathogen.

### Specimen Containers

Correct identification of a causative agent requires isolation and growth of a pure culture of that organism in the laboratory. To do this, the original specimen must be collected in a sterile container and not be contaminated at any stage in its subsequent transfer to or isolation in the laboratory. The microbiology laboratory should provide appropriate sterile containers to the patient care unit or physician, with specific information about the type of container to be used for various types of specimens and about the manner of collection. It is also important, for the protection of the laboratory personnel and anyone else handling the specimen, that the specimen be placed entirely within the appropriate container and not allowed to contaminate the outside. Proper transport procedure must be followed. Microbiology specimens often contain infectious pathogens that could infect anyone coming in contact with the infected material.

The container holding the specimen should neither contribute its own microbial flora nor increase or decrease the original flora contained in the specimen. A variety of containers have been manufactured for collecting microbiology specimens. Most are disposable. One of the most useful pieces of collecting equipment is a wooden applicator stick tipped with cotton, calcium alginate, or polyester. Applicator sticks tipped with the appropriate fiber, packaged in a capped sterile container, are available commercially. These sticks may be used for the collection of material from the throat, nose, eye, or ear; from wounds and surgical sites; from urogenital orifices; and from the rectum. In many instances, another container with sterile broth media is included with these units, and when the specimen has been collected on the swab it is immediately placed in the broth media to prevent it from drying out. Many innovations have been made in sterile, disposable culture units of various types. To prolong the survival of microorganisms that have been collected, transport media can be used. This is especially desirable when a significant delay occurs between collection and culturing. Swabs of infectious material can be prevented from drying out by immersion in broth or another holding medium until culture is done. The whole culture unit must be properly labeled and promptly sent to the laboratory.

If the suspected organism is an anaerobe, conventional transport tubes should not be used. The crucial factor in the successful final culturing of anaerobic (oxygen-sensitive) organisms is the transport of the original specimen. Atmospheric oxygen, which kills such organisms, must be kept out until the specimen has been processed anaerobically by the laboratory. Special double-stoppered collection tubes containing oxygen-free carbon dioxide or nitrogen can be used. The specimen is injected through the rubber stopper, avoiding the introduction of air. If only a swab can be obtained, the swab should be one that has been prepared in a special "gassed-out" tube and then transported to the laboratory in a rubber-stoppered tube partially filled with an anaerobic medium (see under Requirements for Culture Media, Oxygen, Aerobes, and Anaerobes).

### Transport to the Laboratory

Once the specimen has been placed in the appropriate container, it should be delivered to the laboratory immediately and not allowed to stand at the patient care unit or clinic. Although many organisms remain alive for long periods after collection, some are extremely **fastidious** (sensitive to change) outside the host, requiring protected conditions for culture, including rapid inoculation into a suitable culture medium, in order to be detected. In fact, some organisms are so fragile that arrangements must be made to take a special culture medium to the patient so that the material can be placed directly on it. Some pathogens will be obscured by the rapid and overwhelming growth of other organisms that are normally present in the material to be cultured. For example, fecal samples normally contain several types of bacteria—normal flora—that will obscure the detection of such pathogens as *Shigella* if the specimen is not delivered to the laboratory and plated onto a suitable medium soon after collection.

### Handling and Storing the Specimens in the Laboratory

Immediate culture of freshly collected specimens is always best but is not always practical. If culture must be delayed, refrigeration at 4° to 6° C provides a safe method for temporary storage of most pathogenic organisms or specimens until they can be tested. Exceptions are those samples that must be immediately cultured (specimens that may contain gonococcal organisms) or certain bacteria causing meningitis, such as meningococci *(Neisseria meningitidis)*, in cerebrospinal fluid that are susceptible to low temperatures and also require immediate culturing. Most pathogenic organisms are not greatly affected by small changes in temperature, but they are generally susceptible to drying out. Although most specimens can be temporarily refrigerated, some specimens require freezing to preserve the organism. It is the responsibility of the laboratory personnel to know which organisms require immediate inoculation and which can be safely stored until culturing can be done.

Refrigeration will prevent overgrowth of other organisms that are present, which could make the isolation of the significant microbe more difficult. Refrigeration is particularly effective for specimens of urine, feces, sputum, and material on swabs from a variety of sources. It is not effective for anaerobic organisms from wound cultures; these specimens should be kept at room temperature until cultured. Specimen collection and handling requirements should be consulted in testing for specific microorganisms or in using unique biologic samples. Only when the specimens are properly collected and han-

dled by the laboratory will the final results of the culturing be valid.

### Types of Microbiology Specimens Collected
#### Blood

A blood sample for culture is extremely useful—normal blood is sterile and should not contain any microorganisms. Special blood-collecting equipment is used. Sterile collecting bottles containing the proper nutrient broth media, blood-collecting sets with needles and tubing that allow the blood to flow into the collecting bottle, and the proper skin-cleaning supplies are necessary to ensure a properly collected blood specimen for culture.

Special care must be taken to clean the venipuncture site carefully before puncture to avoid possible contamination of the blood sample with skin contaminants. One method uses an initial cleaning with a 70% to 95% solution of alcohol to remove dirt, lipids, and fatty acids. A circular motion moving from the venipuncture site out is used. A 2% iodine or iodophor scrub solution is used, followed by an alcohol rinse (see Venous Blood Collection by Venipuncture in Chapter 3 and Blood Cultures in this chapter). The protocol is determined by the facility.

#### Cerebrospinal Fluid (CSF)

Cerebrospinal fluid is collected only by a physician by means of a lumbar puncture. Rapid handling of spinal fluid samples in the laboratory is extremely important, since some of the organisms associated with meningitis quickly "self-destruct" after collection—they are prone to damage from chilling or drying. Spinal fluid is collected by lumbar puncture, usually into three sterile tubes. Because the first tubes may contain contaminants, it is recommended that any microbiologic culture be done using the third tube. The tubes are sent to the laboratory immediately for testing, including culture.

#### Feces

Feces normally contain large numbers of bacteria (normal flora), and a specimen of feces is usually cultured only to isolate certain types of pathogenic organisms, such as parasites or enteric organisms. Feces are usually collected early in the day and should be cultured immediately. Swabs of the rectal area are also commonly used.

### Sputum

When a specimen of sputum is collected, the patient must cooperate fully to ensure that a proper specimen is obtained. Sputum is usually collected in the morning, and it should be sent to the laboratory and processed immediately. Deep coughing will usually bring up a good sputum specimen. It is necessary to avoid collecting nasal or salivary fluids. A wide-mouthed sterile container is best used for collecting this type of specimen.

An acceptable or suitable sputum specimen that is free from contamination with saliva can be gram-stained and checked microscopically for the presence of squamous epithelial cells. Finding more than 10 squamous epithelial cells per low-power field indicates the specimen is saliva and is therefore not an acceptable specimen to culture.

When sputum is being collected from a suspected or confirmed patient with tuberculosis, extra biohazard precautions must be taken by the person collecting the sample. The use of a special barrier device—a respirator—is necessary (see Respirators or Masks for Tuberculosis Control, in Chapter 2). Because of the possible aerosolization of these organisms, it is important to handle the specimens carefully, preferably using a biological safety cabinet or biohazard hood.

### Swabs of Various Fluids

Swabs are used to collect cultures from various openings of the body, such as the nose, throat, mouth, vagina, anus, and wounds. These swabs must be collected carefully and placed in the proper transport media before they are taken to the laboratory for processing. If swabs are not properly handled, the microorganisms may dry out and/or not be in sufficient numbers to be cultured. It has been found that some organisms survive longer when polyester rather than cotton swabs are used.

### Urine

The collection of urine for microbiological studies also requires the cooperation of the patient. A midstream sample "clean catch," usually the first morning specimen, is suitable for culture, provided care has been taken to clean the urethral area before the collection (see also Collection of Urine for Culture, in Chapter 3). Urine in the bladder is normally sterile. A sterile container must be used for the collection of urine for culture. When a patient is too ill or cannot void properly, a specimen is obtained by catheterization. This is not done unless necessary, because of the risk of introducing an infection into a previously sterile bladder via the catheter. After collection, specimens should be sent to the laboratory for immediate processing.

## SPECIAL TECHNIQUES AND EQUIPMENT USED IN MICROBIOLOGY

Microbiologists use special techniques and methods to grow and isolate pure cultures of microorganisms free of contamination by other microorganisms that are present everywhere. Most work in the microbiology laboratory involves efforts to culture, identify, and characterize the various microbes being studied. With the information gained through these studies, knowledge about three important areas is gained: (1) culture of organisms present in the patient specimens, (2) classification and identification of the organisms when isolated, and (3) interpretation for the use of an appropriate antimicrobial agent. Such efforts require the use of specific techniques and equipment, which includes the inoculating needle or loop, tube cultures, Petri dish cultures, and stained slides for microscopic examination. (See also Smear Preparation and Stains Used in Microbiology.)

### Inoculating Needle or Loop

Probably one of the most important tools of the microbiologist is the **inoculating transfer needle** or **loop**. Disposable and reusable types are used. Disposable inoculating loops are made of plastic

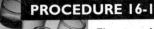

## PROCEDURE 16-1

### Flaming the Inoculating Loop or Needle

1. Hold the inoculating loop between the thumb and index finger. This leaves the three outer fingers free to remove tops from test tubes or culture plates.

2. Push the loop into the upper flame of the Bunsen burner at an angle of about 45 to 60 degrees. (Observe the special technique described below if the loop is wet.) Continue heating until the entire loop is red hot. Then briefly flame the hub of the loop holder. An incinerator burner can also be used for this step (and is preferable).

3. Allow the loop to cool to room temperature before using. If used hot, it will kill the organism under study.

and are meant to be discarded after use. The classic reusable type may be either a straight wire or a wire with a loop at one end inserted into a suitable holder. The wire is usually platinum or an alloy, such as Nichrome, that can be sterilized by being heated to glowing without being harmed and returned to room temperature fairly rapidly (Procedure 16-1 and Fig. 16-2). An object that can be safely heated until it is red is sterilized almost instantaneously. The needle or loop is used to transfer microorganisms from one medium to another or from a culture to a microscope slide. Because it can be sterilized quickly, it can be used repeatedly for this purpose. When a transfer is to be made, the needle or loop is sterilized in a flame, used to perform the transfer, and then resterilized before it is set aside. The process for sterilizing the inoculating loop by flaming with a Bunsen burner is described in Procedure 16-1.

### Flaming the Loop or Needle (Sterilization)

A flame normally has two parts: the outer part is the outer cone, and within this part, extending down to the base or origin of the flame, is the inner cone. The hottest part of the flame is the upper portion, above the top of the inner cone. The inner cone at the base of the flame is cool. If an inoculating needle or loop filled with bacteria is inserted into the hottest part of the flame, a small amount of steam will form. This will result in explosive sputtering of the material to the desk top, hands, and clothing of the worker. This is extremely dangerous, as the bacteria are often still viable when this occurs and can produce infection. To prevent this, an alternative method of flaming must be followed. If the needle or loop is wet, it must be first inserted into the cool inner cone at the base of the flame. It is then slowly raised through the inner cone and finally flamed in the hottest part of the flame (Fig. 16-2). The needle or loop must always be flamed before it is set aside.

An improvement to the use of Bunsen burners is the use of an electronic incinerator burner which does not have an open flame. The insulation in these burners must be checked regularly, as use of the equipment can be an electrical hazard if the insulation has worn thin.

### Transfer From Tube Culture Using an Inoculating Needle

Microorganisms are commonly grown and maintained in presterilized test tubes that contain a liquid or liquefiable solid medium and have been covered with loose-fitting metal caps or screw caps. In general, the cap is removed with and held in the hand holding the inoculating needle. The lip of the tube is flamed before and after entry to prevent contamination of the culture. The transfer is performed with a sterilized inoculating needle.

## Tube Cultures

If the medium is to be used as a **test tube culture,** it is usually dispensed and autoclaved directly in the tubes. If liquefiable solid medium is to be used in slant tubes, it is dispensed in the liquid state into test tubes, autoclaved, and then allowed to harden while set at an angle (Fig. 16-3).

## Petri Plate Cultures

The **Petri dish** or **plate** is often used for culture. It is a shallow glass or plastic plate with a loose-fitting cover of the same material, shape, and depth as the dish but slightly larger in diameter. The deep cover prevents contamination of the dish. Petri dishes are used for liquefiable solid media. The medium is poured into the dish, allowed to harden, covered, and stored in an inverted position in order to prevent condensation on its surface. The plates are also stored in an inverted position after inoculation; they are labeled on the back of the portion of the plate in which the medium is contained. Plates of liquefiable solid media may be used as streak plates or as pour plates.

### Streak Plates

**Streak plates** are prepared by streaking material across the surface of the hardened medium contained in a Petri dish. Streaking is especially useful for isolating individual colonies originating from a single bacterial cell (Fig 16-4). These isolated colonies may then be transferred to another medium. Thus, pure cultures may be prepared from mixtures of bacteria. Characteristics of isolated colonies may also be observed on streak plates.

The technique of streaking a plate will vary from laboratory to laboratory and even within a particular laboratory, depending on the source of material and the characteristics of the microorganism under investigation. It should be remembered that the streak plate is used primarily as a means of obtaining isolated colonies of microorganisms (see Throat Cultures and Genitourinary Cultures). The aim is therefore to inoculate successively smaller quantities of material onto the medium, so that at one point the organisms are plated thinly enough to allow the growth of individual isolated colonies.

If a swab is submitted for culture, it may be used to make the inoculation onto the medium, instead of an inoculating loop (see under Throat Cultures).

There are certain important things to remember when using the plate culture method. Plates should be perfectly dry before use, or the organism will tend to spread; this will hinder the for-

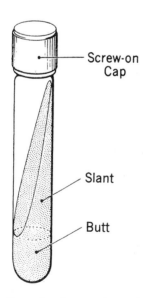

**FIG 16-3.** Slant tube, showing slant and butt.

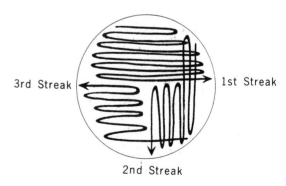

**FIG 16-4.** Preparation of a streak plate.

mation of individual colonies. When a loop is used to inoculate the plate, it should be held lightly and not be allowed to dig into the medium.

In general, a small and sometimes measured amount of material is streaked onto the periphery at one side of the plate (see Fig. 16-4). Streaking is achieved by drawing the inoculating loop across the surface of the medium in a zigzag motion. The first streak is continued across approximately half the plate. The plate is then turned 90 degrees and streaked again, beginning at the periphery, overlapping the previously inoculated area once or twice. The second streak is continued across half the plate. Finally, the plate is turned 90 degrees once again and streaked a third time, beginning at the periphery, drawing the loop through the second streak once, and continuing across the remaining quarter of the plate. The **isolated colonies** will generally be found in the third area of streaking.

Sometimes the needle must be flamed between each streak as well as before and after inoculation. Sheep blood agar plates are often cut one or more times with the inoculating loop at the conclusion of streaking in order to observe hemolysis reactions of certain bacteria.

### Pour Plates

Pour plates represent another manner of inoculating culture media in Petri dishes. They are less commonly used than streak plates. **Pour plates** are generally used to determine the number of viable organisms in a liquid—particularly in testing such liquids as milk and water for bacterial contamination.

In using the pour plate, one generally first dilutes the specimen serially to achieve isolation of colonies. The diluted specimen is then inoculated into a liquefiable solid medium that is in the liquid state. The medium and inoculum may be mixed in a test tube and poured onto the plate or mixed in the plate itself, depending on the technique being used. Thorough mixing must be achieved in any case. When the medium has been inoculated and incubated at the appropriate temperature for the desired length of time, it is al-

lowed to harden. Plates are then observed for growth, and the colonies are counted to obtain an estimate of the concentration of microorganisms in the original specimen. The use of pour plates rather than streak plates provides at least partially anaerobic conditions in the deeper layers of the plate, facilitating the culture of anaerobic microorganisms. As with streak plates, colonies may be observed on the pour plate itself or introduced into additional media in order to obtain pure cultures or observe growth on different media.

## USING MICROBIOLOGY TO DIAGNOSE DISEASE

For the microbiologist to correctly identify the etiologic or causative agent of an infection, several steps must be carried out. The steps used involve a general knowledge of microorganisms and their modes of action. The field of microbiology is too extensive to be covered in this textbook; this chapter therefore deals only with the routine laboratory aspects of the subject. The study of the routine specimen collection and identification processes for common bacteria, fungi, and parasites found in clinical specimens will be briefly discussed.

### TESTS FOR BACTERIA (BACTERIOLOGY)

One of the principal roles of a laboratorian working in a microbiology laboratory is to isolate, identify, and present interpretive information about bacteria that cause disease in humans—the subspecialty of bacteriology. The identification of most bacteria involves microscopic observations, culture studies, and biochemical tests.

In the laboratory, bacteria are generally classified into groups based on two major microscopic observations: (1) the Gram staining reaction of the bacteria and (2) the shape or morphology of the bacteria—round **(cocci)**, rod-shaped **(bacilli)**, or spiral (spirilla). Culture studies, including morphologic characteristics and the oxygen requirements of the bacteria (whether they require oxygen for growth [aerobes] or grow without oxygen [anaerobes]), are done and patterns of biochemical reactions are noted.

## Smear Preparation and Stains Used in Microbiology

One necessary step in the identification of a particular species of bacteria involves morphologic examination under the microscope. If unstained bacteria are placed on a glass slide and observed under the microscope, they appear as transparent, colorless structures and may be homogeneous or granular. Bacterial motility may also be observed by studying unstained wet preparations of bacteria. Most bacteria can be seen unstained with the ordinary brightfield microscope, but bacteria have a refractive index close to that of glass and therefore should be stained to be made more visible. If they are unstained, the use of phase-contrast microscopy is helpful in visualization. Various staining procedures may be used, depending on the information desired.

### Smear Preparation

To stain bacteria, the material to be examined is spread thinly on a glass microscope slide and allowed to dry. The film should be thin enough so that individual bacteria can be seen. If the material to be examined is a liquid, such as a broth culture, it may be transferred by means of a sterile, cooled inoculating loop and spread directly on the dry slide. If it is taken from an isolated colony on a Petri plate or other dry material, a drop of sterile water must first be placed on the slide and the material added and mixed by using the sterile, cooled inoculating loop or needle.

If the specimen to be stained is on a single swab obtained directly from the patient, culture media must be inoculated first and then the swab rolled onto the surface of the dry, clean glass slide. Slides are not sterile and thus are prepared last, after all other culture media are inoculated.

When a smear is prepared, it is essential to use only clean slides. The material is spread thinly but evenly over the appropriate area of the slide, using an inoculating loop. This material may be

from a suspension of bacteria in a liquid medium, a colony on a solid medium, or a patient specimen directly. All slides prepared must be labeled with sufficient patient identification information. It is sometimes helpful to draw a circle on the back (underside) of the slide, directly under the area where the specimen has been placed on the slide, using a wax pencil, so that the examination area may more easily be identified after staining.

After the material has air dried completely, it must be heat fixed to the slide—that is, hardened and preserved for microbiological study. The fixing process prevents many of the bacterial cells from washing off the slide in subsequent staining operations. Fixation is achieved by simply passing the back of the microscope slide through the burner flame two or three times. The film side of the slide must not be exposed to heat, and the bottom of the slide must not be so hot that it cannot be held against the back of the hand. This heating coagulates the bacterial protein, causing cells to adhere to the slide. The air-drying and fixation do not necessarily kill all the bacterial cells on the slide, and to prevent accidental infection, the slides must be handled carefully and placed in biohazard containers for glass and discarded appropriately.

Several staining procedures are used in the microbiology laboratory, but a **gram-stained smear** is used routinely and is most likely to yield valuable information; it should be done in all cases when a staining procedure is indicated. Gram stains are also used for the examination of cultures to determine purity and for preliminary identification of bacterial microorganisms. Properly prepared and stained preparations of specimens may give excellent clues to the media for inoculation or further tests to be done. Preliminary reports on the results of Gram staining of spinal fluid, urethral smears, and sputum, for example, can be of great value regarding early treatment of the patient.

### Types of Stains

To observe gross morphologic features, a simple stain such as crystal violet, fuchsin, methylene blue, or safranin may be used. However, the most widely used stain in the bacteriology laboratory is a differential stain, Gram stain, which differentiates bacteria as gram positive or gram negative, in addition to showing gross morphologic features. Other stains include acid-fast stains, capsule stains, flagella stains, stains for metachromatic granules, spore stains, relief stains, and stains for spirochetes, rickettsiae, yeast, and fungi. (See also Staining Techniques.)

### Morphology of Bacteria

Each species of bacteria has a characteristic shape, which is one of three basic shapes. Spherical or round bacteria are **cocci,** straight rod-shaped ones are **bacilli,** and spiral rod-shaped ones are **spirilla.** Most bacteria are either cocci or bacilli, the bacilli being the most numerous.

There are certain variations of the three basic shapes, such as club-shaped bacilli and bacilli with square ends. The particular species may be further classified according to whether the cells normally occur singly, in diploids or pairs, in chains, or in clusters. The prefix *diplo-* describes bacteria that occur as pairs of cells, *strepto-* describes bacteria occurring as chains of cells, and *staphylo-* refers to irregular clumps or clusters of bacterial cells.

Although bacteria can be seen under the ordinary brightfield microscope, they are extremely small structures. They are normally observed under oil immersion with a 100× objective, giving a total magnification of 1,000 times when the 10× ocular is used. Bacteria are measured in micrometers (1 $\mu$m = 1/1,000 millimeter or about 1/25,000 in.). There is a good deal of variation in size among bacteria. Cocci may range from 0.15 to 2.0 $\mu$m in diameter, although most pathogens measure 0.8 to 1.2 $\mu$m. This is near the limit of resolution of the common light microscope, namely 0.25 $\mu$m. The bacilli show an even greater size variation. *Hemophilus influenzae* is a very small rod, about 0.5 $\mu$m long by 0.2 $\mu$m wide. *Bacillus anthracis* is a relatively large rod, 5 to 10 $\mu$m long and 1 to 3 $\mu$m wide. For comparison, a red blood cell is approximately 7 $\mu$m in diameter.

Each bacterium has four distinct morphologic parts: protoplasm, cytoplasmic membrane, cell wall, and capsule. Different stains may be used to accentuate these parts. Other morphologic structures have been discovered by means of the electron microscope.

The morphologic character of a bacterium is useful for identifying it. One should determine its general shape (sphere, straight rod, or spiral rod), its Gram staining reaction, and its association with other bacterial cells (single, in chains, or in clusters). However, these and other morphologic characteristics only rarely lead to the final identification of the bacterium. For the final identification, it is necessary to know the cultural characteristics of the bacterium. This is discussed later in this section.

Each bacterium is a single cell, and, like most cells, it possesses cytoplasm surrounded by a cell membrane, which in turn is surrounded by a cell wall. Some bacteria also have other external structures, such as flagella or capsules. Some typical organelles found within a single bacterium are the nucleus, ribosomes, vacuoles, and granules. The cytoplasm of bacteria can contain a variety of granules, many of which can be identified by special staining procedures.

An important organelle contained within the cytoplasm is the spore. **Spores** are an inert stage of a microorganism that the organism reverts to when its environment becomes hostile. Spores are resistant to heat, cold, drying conditions, and chemicals. Some bacteria have spores, or endospores, in their cytoplasm. Spores are able to survive under extremely unfavorable conditions, even when the active or vegetative bacterial cell dies. Thus, spore-forming bacteria can survive conditions that would kill non-spore-forming bacteria.

Bacteria can manufacture a slimy gelatinous layer around the cell wall, and this layer of slime often becomes an integral part of the bacterial cell structure called a capsule. If special staining techniques are used, the capsule may be seen more easily. The presence or absence of a capsule is used clinically to help identify the microorganism.

**PROCEDURE 16-2**

*Staining With Methylene Blue*

1. Spread a thin film of material on the clean microscope slide; air dry and heat fix. Place the slide on the staining rack.

2. Flood the surface of the slide with methylene blue staining solution. Allow the stain to remain on the slide for 2 minutes.

3. Wash the slide gently with running water to remove excess stain.

4. Blot the slide to air dry with paper towels.

5. Examine the smear with the oil-immersion microscope lens, noting the size, shape, and uniformity of staining of the microorganisms present.

The most significant external structures of bacteria are flagella—long, threadlike structures anchored within the cell wall and cell membrane. The whiplike motion of the flagella enables the bacterial cell to move. Flagella vary in their number and position on the bacteria, and this pattern is also helpful in identifying the species.

### Staining Techniques

Biological staining is the microscopic procedure most commonly used in microbiology to identify a particular bacterial species. Stains are chemical substances that contain colored dyes. Certain bacterial structures have affinities for particular dyes. It is common to use commercially prepared stains. These are usually purchased in a ready-to-use state. Actual methods will vary from manufacturer to manufacturer, so the directions included with the stains must be followed carefully. Special stains are useful for showing the morphology of bacteria and specific structures such as capsules, flagella, spores, and granules. Simple stains such as methylene blue or more complex differential stains are used to show special cellular details. One commonly used differential stain is Gram stain. The way bacteria react to this stain depends on the chemical composition of the cell wall.

**Simple Stains.** Simple staining procedures employing crystal violet, fuchsin, methylene blue, or safranin have only limited use in the microbiology laboratory. These are termed **simple stains** because only one stain is used and all structures present are stained the same color. They accentuate the otherwise colorless bacterial cell, but that is about all. When a simple stain is used, organisms should be observed for size, shape, and uniformity of staining.

*Methylene Blue Stain.* The procedure for using one simple stain in microbiology, the methylene blue stain, appears in Procedure 16-2.

**Differential Stains.** Differential stains are used to show specific cellular details not shown by a simple stain. The most commonly used differential stain is Gram stain.

*Gram Stain.* **Gram stain** is used to differentiate various types of bacteria that have similar morphologic features. The cell wall of the particular bacterium contributes to the gram staining reaction of the organism. There are several modifications of the Gram stain method, but most conventional stains involve the primary stain crystal violet, the addition of iodine, which serves as a mordant, decolorization with an alcohol-acetone solution, and counterstaining with a secondary stain such as safranin. (A mordant is a substance that combines with a particular dye, forms an insoluble complex, or "lake," and fixes the color in the substance dyed.)

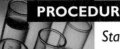

## PROCEDURE 16-3

### Staining With Rapid Gram Stain (Conventional Method)

1. Flood the heat-fixed slide with crystal violet stain and wait 10 seconds.

2. Pour off the stain and rinse with the iodine solution.

3. Cover with the iodine solution and wait for 10 seconds.

4. Rinse with running water, shaking off the excess.

5. Decolorize quickly with the alcohol-acetone solution, or with 95% alcohol if the alcohol-acetone decolorization proves to be too rapid. Continue until no more color is extracted by the solvent. This usually takes 10 to 20 seconds, but take care not to decolorize the film too much.

6. Flood with safranin for 10 seconds.

7. Rinse with water; blot dry with paper towels.

The Gram stain method divides bacteria into two broad groups. Bacteria that stain purple (dark blue/black) as a result of retention of the crystal violet–iodine complex are termed **gram positive.** Bacteria that stain red from the counterstain are termed **gram negative.** When bacteria are exposed to a solution of crystal violet stain, a purple-blue color, in combination with an iodine dye complex, and then washed with alcohol (or acetone-alcohol), some organisms retain the purple color and others are decolorized. The organisms that retain the purple color are called gram positive, and those that lose this purple color when washed with alcohol are called gram negative. Another dye of a contrasting color is used as a counterstain. Safranin, a red dye, is used in Gram stain as a counterstain; it colors the gram-negative organisms red, making them visible. A conventional method of Gram staining (Hucker modification) is described in Procedure 16-3. Another modification (rapid Kopeloff modification), uses sodium bicarbonate added to the crystal violet to decrease the reaction time needed.

In the first step of the procedure for the Gram stain, all organisms present are stained violet by the primary stain, crystal violet. The iodine added in the second and third steps forms a crystal violet–iodine complex, which is fixed or re-

tained in gram-positive but not in gram-negative organisms. The mechanism involved in the retention of this complex in gram-positive but not gram-negative organisms is not completely understood, but it reflects significant differences between the two groups.

The fifth step of the procedure, decolorization with a mixture of acetone and alcohol, removes all color from gram-negative organisms but does not affect gram-positive ones, which remain purple. Since the gram-negative organisms are colorless after the fifth step, they are counterstained in the sixth step with the red secondary stain safranin so that they can be visualized under the microscope.

If a slide were observed under the microscope after each step of the Gram staining process, the following results would be noted. After steps 1, 2, and 3, all organisms would be colored purple. After step 5, gram-positive organisms would appear purple, and gram-negative organisms would be colorless. After step 6, all gram-positive organisms would appear purple and all gram-negative organisms red.

Differentiation into these Gram staining categories is particularly helpful in determining the subsequent tests and means of culture for eventual identification of the bacteria. It is also a

---

**PROCEDURE 16-4**

*Staining for Acid-Fast Organisms Using the Kinyoun Carbolfuchsin Method*

1. Flood the heat-fixed smear with Kinyoun's carbolfuchsin stain containing Tergitol 7 for 1 minute.

2. Wash with water.

3. Decolorize by adding acid-alcohol reagent drop by drop with continuous agitation until carbolfuchsin no longer washes off. This requires approximately 2 minutes for smears of average thickness.

4. Wash with water.

5. Counterstain with methylene blue for 20 to 30 seconds.

6. Wash with water; blot dry with paper towels.

---

guide to treatment of the patient, for certain antibiotics are generally effective against gram-positive bacteria, while gram-negative bacteria are not as susceptible to their action, and vice versa.

*Acid-Fast Stain.* Acid-fast stain is used mainly to detect organisms that cause tuberculosis and leprosy. Because of the possible aerosolization of these organisms, it is important to handle the specimens carefully, preferably using a biological safety cabinet or biohazard hood. These organisms are extremely difficult to stain by ordinary methods because of their highly resistant fatty (or lipid) cell membranes. Once stained, they retain the dye color and decolorization is difficult, even with an acid-alcohol solution—hence the term **acid-fast bacteria (AFB).** Other bacteria are easily decolorized by the acid-alcohol reagent.

The traditional Ziehl-Neelsen acid-fast method uses carbolfuchsin as the primary stain, heat as the mordant, a mixture of hydrochloric acid and alcohol as the decolorizer, and methylene blue as the counterstain. The Kinyoun acid-fast modification (Procedure 16-4) uses a slightly different carbolfuchsin preparation and Tergitol 7 as the mordant. After the first step of the acid-fast staining procedure, all bacteria present on the slide appear red. Following decolorization with acid-alcohol reagent, the acid-fast bacteria appear red and all other bacteria are colorless.

After counterstaining with methylene blue, the acid-fast bacteria appear red and all other cells appear blue.

### Microscopy Techniques Used

Although brightfield microscopy is used for most routine microscopic examinations in the microbiology laboratory, the use of varying microscopy techniques is important in some microbiological assays.

**Brightfield Microscopy.** For most routine microscopy needs, the brightfield microscope is used. With this type of illumination, the organism appears dark against a bright background. Gram stains are usually examined with an ordinary brightfield microscope using the oil-immersion objective (100×).

**Fluorescence Microscopy.** Fluorescent antibody (FA) techniques are used in many laboratories and are replacing some of the older serologic methods for the identification of certain microorganisms. It is possible to pretreat certain antibodies with fluorescent dye and then react them with bacteria specific for the complementary antigen. The antibody-antigen complex is fluorescent and can be observed by using the fluorescence microscope.

In fluorescence microscopy, the specimen is self-illuminating and a light image is observed against a dark background. A special darkfield fluorescence microscope is used (see under Other Types of Microscopes [Illumination Systems], in Chapter 5). Group A $\beta$-hemolytic streptococci may be identified on pure cultures isolated from throat swabs from patients with acute pharyngitis (strep throat), although FA techniques for this have been mostly replaced by tests utilizing the rapid detection of the streptotoccal antigen. There is a rapid FA method for detecting human influenza virus infection by utilizing nasal smears. In some cases, FA techniques completely replace time-consuming culture methods. In others, preliminary identification of microorganisms by FA methods may be followed by culture confirmation.

## Culture Studies

Culture studies used in the identification of microorganisms require growing and isolating the suspected organism. A pure culture of the organism grown from that in the patient specimen must be obtained.

### Growth of a Pure Culture

Specimens for microbiological analysis must be collected in sterile containers because the identification of microorganisms generally requires isolation and growth of a pure culture of bacteria. A bacterium placed on a suitable culture medium will multiply until an **isolated colony** of bacteria is formed. It is assumed that each colony of bacteria originates from a single cell. In culturing bacteria in the laboratory, the infected material is treated in such a way that single bacterial cells are separated on the primary or initial culture medium and allowed to grow into isolated colonies. Material from a single isolated colony is then further inoculated onto additional media, so that several colonies will appear, all arising from a single bacterium. The growth of several colonies originating from a single colony, and hence a single cell, is what is meant by a **pure culture.**

### Isolating Colonies on the Primary Culture Plate

Bacteria from patient specimens are almost always isolated by first streaking on the surface of a primary culture medium in a culture plate or Petri dish. A suitable medium will allow a single bacterial cell to grow into a colony. Various culturing methods enable the microbiologist to separate individual cells on the primary culture media and eventually allow them to grow into separate colonies.

In doing the initial culture, or **primary culture,** it is important that the streaking be done properly to provide the best opportunity for isolation of the bacterial colonies. When isolated colonies are grown, a portion of the pure culture may be picked up for identification by using the inoculating needle. There are several ways in which a plate may be streaked to ensure the appearance of isolated colonies on incubation. One method is illustrated in Fig. 16-4. Special streaking methods are used for certain types of specimens (see Petri Plate Cultures, Streak Plates).

### Types of Culture Media

Bacteria are grown in or on specially prepared culture media, although future trends in clinical microbiology are pointing toward more use of non-growth-dependent methods. The isolation and identification of viable pathogenic organisms on culture media are still the gold standard for diagnosis of infectious disease processes. Specimens are plated and inoculated on several different growth media, depending on the etiologic agent that is suspected. Choosing appropriate culture media is essential for the isolation, growth, and final identification of pathogenic organisms. By studying the cultural characteristics of a particular bacterium, certain growth patterns may be seen and the presumptive species identification may be made.

The types of culture media vary greatly. They may be prepared in liquid or solid form. Most are in a solid medium form and may be prepared in a flat, circular culture dish called a Petri dish or culture plate. When the specimen is placed on the medium in the plate, it is said to be **inoculated.** A tube of solid medium can be prepared as a stab or a slant. In a **slant culture,** the surface of the medium is inclined at an angle (Fig. 16-5) and an inoculating loop or needle is used to place the specimen on the surface of the medium. A tube of medium can also be inoculated by stabbing or passing through the medium with an inoculating needle, thus leaving the specimen behind in the medium. A tube prepared in this way is referred to as a **stab tube.** In a stab culture the surface of the medium is perpendicular to the sides of the test tube (see Fig. 16-5). Tubes containing liquid broth media can also be inoculated with bacteria by using an inoculating loop or needle (see Fig. 16-5). Liquid media are well suited to studying the production of a gas, odor, or change in pH. Media in a semisolid or solid form are most useful for the observation of colony size, shape, and color.

The media used in clinical microbiology are generally prepared from precisely measured quantities of known substances that are formulated to give highly repeatable culture results.

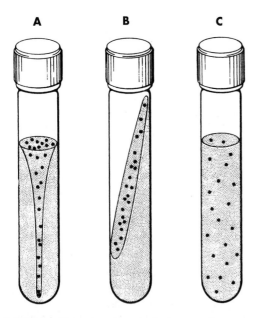

**FIG 16-5.** Examples of types of culture media in tubes. **A,** Stab culture tube. **B,** Slant culture tube. **C,** Liquid broth culture tube.

Media of this type are produced synthetically and consist of the specific amino acids, sugars, salts, vitamins, and minerals needed to ensure the proper growth of certain bacterial species. They are usually produced commercially and used for diagnostic purposes. Commercially prepared media in disposable culture plates or tubes have generally replaced media prepared in the individual laboratory. The National Committee for Clinical Laboratory Standards (NCCLS) has published recommendations to be followed by manufacturers of commercial media.[10] (See also under Quality Control of Media.) Broths are also sometimes used as culture media. They are less well chemically defined and are used mainly to maintain bacterial growth. They are generally not used for identification of bacterial species. Broths are meat extracts of protein materials—either peptone, an intermediate product of protein digestion, or digested protein.

**Agar** is used extensively in the preparation of solid media; it is a seaweed extract that is liquid when heated and solid when cooled. It does not affect bacterial growth and is an excellent base for nutrient media. Agar can be melted and poured into tubes or plates, where it will solidify when cool. The more agar used, the more solid the final medium will become. Plates, slant tubes, and stab tubes are all prepared with agar as the base.

In addition to the use of culture plates or Petri dishes to observe growth characteristics of the microorganisms, culture studies include the use of **agar slants** for maintenance of cultures or for certain biochemical studies, semisolid media for motility or biochemical studies, and **broth media** for maintenance or biochemical studies. Many (but not all) microorganisms may be grown in the laboratory away from their natural habitat. To grow microorganisms artificially, it is necessary to provide the proper nutrients and growth conditions. The growth of microorganisms on artificial material is referred to as **culture** of the microorganism, and the mixture of nutrients on which the microorganism is grown is the **culture medium.**

## Colony Characteristics (Appearance) of Bacterial Cultures

When inoculated onto suitable semisolid or solid nutrient media with the proper temperature and moisture, bacteria rapidly multiply and form macroscopic colonies. Under ideal conditions, the growth of a microbial cell is a geometric progression with time. For example, a single bacterium such as *Escherichia coli*, having a generation time of 20 minutes, would produce $2.2 \times 10^{43}$ cells in 48 hours. Certain limiting factors come into play that ultimately terminate growth, however. A culture that is a closed system will eventually stop growing as a result of exhaustion of essential nutrients, accumulation of toxic products, or development of an unfavorable pH.

The type of culture medium used—liquid or solid—can affect the appearance or growth of the colonies. In liquid media, bacterial growth does not have a characteristic appearance, and organisms cannot be separated from "mixed cultures." By contrast, on solid media the appearance of a culture is extremely useful in initially differentiating the colony type, and pure cultures can be isolated.

Bacteria multiply by binary fission, or division into two equal parts. Macroscopic bacterial colonies form in 24 to 48 hours. The colonies originate from individual cells, although each colony is a mass of individual cells, each of which functions independently. Different species of bacteria form colonies that differ in appearance; therefore, colony appearance is useful in identifying the species of bacteria. Colony characteristics that are observed for the purpose of identification include the following:

1. Bacteria without slime capsules produce colonies that appear dry and rough.
2. Bacteria with slime capsules produce colonies that appear smooth and shiny.
3. Bacteria may possess a pigment that gives a characteristic color (e.g., white, red, yellow, or orange) to the colony.
4. Bacteria may spread from the original colony, which indicates that they are motile. Nonmotile bacteria remain in discrete colonies.

Bacterial colonies should be observed for their relative size, shape, elevation, texture, marginal appearance, and color. This information, in addition to morphologic appearance under the microscope, various staining reactions, such as with Gram stain, and results of biochemical tests performed, helps in the eventual identification of a particular species of bacteria.

**Temperature of Incubation for Routine Cultures.** Human pathogens generally multiply best at temperatures close to those of the host. Most often, therefore, only two incubators are necessary for a routine microbiology laboratory—one set at 35° C, close to the normal human internal body temperature, and one set at 30° C, the temperature of the surface of the body. Most incubations are carried out at 35° C. The temperature of the incubators must be periodically monitored as part of the maintenance documentation required by quality assurance programs.

**Time for Incubation of Routine Cultures.** A certain amount of time is needed for any final identification using the routine plate culture media and testing procedures—usually about 2 days. Most bacteria will be seen growing on culture media within 24 hours (Fig. 16-6).

### Requirements for Culture Media

Bacteria, like all living things, have specific requirements to sustain life and to reproduce. The culture requirements for bacteria include a source of nutrients, the proper temperature, an adequate supply of oxygen (or in some cases the absence of oxygen), and the correct pH.

**Oxygen Requirements: Aerobes and Anaerobes.** An important factor that must be considered in culturing microorganisms is the presence or absence of oxygen. Pathogenic organisms are either **aerobes,** utilizing oxygen for their growth; **anaerobes,** intolerant to oxygen;

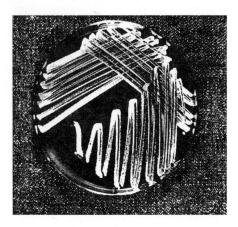

**FIG 16-6.** Culture plate with bacterial growth after 24 hours. (From Becan-McBride K, Ross DL: *Essentials for the Small Laboratory and Physician's Office.* St Louis, Mosby, 1988, p 344.)

or microaerophilic, growing best in an atmosphere of reduced oxygen tension. Aerobes can be incubated in room air. Most clinically significant aerobes are really facultative anaerobes, which can grow under either aerobic or anaerobic conditions. Most of the common pathogenic bacteria are aerobic and grow well in the presence of oxygen. Aerobes require an atmosphere containing oxygen for growth.

Some pathogenic organisms are incapable of growth in oxygen and are classified as anaerobic organisms. All specimens for anaerobic studies must be cultured as soon as possible after collection to avoid loss of viability. Special methods are required for the isolation and study of anaerobic bacteria. Anaerobes are able to derive oxygen from their food sources and are actually inhibited by atmospheric oxygen; to culture these anaerobes or anaerobic organisms, atmospheric oxygen must be excluded.

There are also organisms with oxygen requirements between those of the obligate aerobes and those of the obligate anaerobes—**facultative** microorganisms, able to grow under either aerobic or anaerobic conditions. Microaerophilic organisms grow best under conditions of low oxygen tension and are inhibited by high oxygen tension.

Specimens originating from sites where an anaerobic agent is suspected are cultured on both aerobic and anaerobic media. Enriched media as well as differential and selective media are inoculated. The enriched and selective media are needed because anaerobes are fastidious and because most anaerobic infections are mixed with aerobic and other anaerobic organisms present also. Inoculated plates are immediately placed in an anaerobic environment for incubation. Jars, chambers, or commercially produced pouches and bags can be used. Cultures are incubated for 48 hours at 35° C. Usually these cultures should not be exposed to any oxygen until after 48 hours of incubation. Colony morphology can change dramatically between 24 and 48 hours. If plates are in a chamber or an anaerobic bag, they can be observed after 24 hours without oxygen exposure. Anaerobic conditions may be produced in the laboratory in a number of ways, including displacement of air by carbon dioxide, use of special media such as thioglycolate broth, or inoculation into the deeper layers of solid media. The techniques for culturing anaerobic organisms are essentially of three types, involving the use of (1) media containing reducing substances that eliminate oxygen, (2) media and methods by which oxygen can be excluded, and (3) anaerobic jars, plates, and incubators from which oxygen can be removed and replaced by hydrogen or nitrogen.

One of the most useful media for growing anaerobic organisms is thioglycolate broth. It contains sodium thioglycolate, which absorbs oxygen from the medium (see under Commonly Used Types of Media). It can be used to study and identify anaerobes, but is generally not very satisfactory for the isolation of microbes. For isolation, it is desirable to streak plates of blood agar, infusion agar, or thioglycolate agar. When the plates have been streaked, they are placed in an anaerobic jar or other special container and the oxygen is removed (Fig. 16-7). Prereduced media are commercially available and appear to be very practical and reliable for the isolation of anaerobic bacteria.

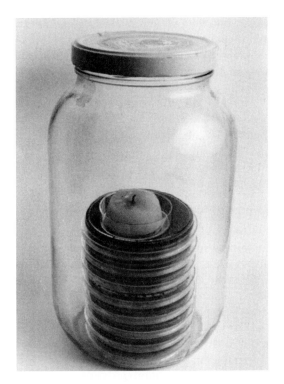

**FIG 16-7.** Anaerobic candle jar for culture of anaerobic organisms. (From Baron EJ, Finegold SM: *Bailey and Scott's Diagnostic Microbiology*, ed 8. St Louis, Mosby, 1990, p 53.)

**Nutrients.** The proper nutrient elements must be available, as microorganisms differ in their food requirements. Some grow on media containing simple mixtures of inorganic salts, since they are able to synthesize their own organic compounds. Others, especially many pathogens, are very particular and may require complex mixtures of nutrients, including many of the B vitamins and certain amino acids. In general, the culture medium must be able to supply carbon, nitrogen, and inorganic salts. Peptone is used in a variety of culture media, as it contains nitrogen in a form (amino acids and simple nitrogen compounds) that can be used by most microorganisms. Certain bacteria require media to which serum, blood, or ascitic fluid has been added. In some media it is ad-

vantageous to add carbohydrates, and in some instances, salts of calcium, manganese, magnesium, sodium, and potassium are required by the microorganism for growth.

In addition to nutrient sources, dyes or indicators may be added to culture media as a means of detecting metabolic activity by the microorganism or of promoting the growth of some microorganisms by inhibiting the growth of others. Finally, certain microorganisms either require or are enhanced by the presence of growth-promoting vitamin-like substances in the media.

**Temperature.** All organisms have a minimum temperature below which development ceases, an optimum temperature at which growth is maximum or luxuriant, and a maximum temperature above which death occurs. The majority of bacteria grow within the temperature range of 15° to 43° C. However, the pathogens generally have a narrow temperature range, with optimum growth at 35° C, and for this reason most cultures are incubated at 35° C. Since the heat of an incubator would promote drying, the incubator should always be equipped with containers of water or some other suitable source of humidity. In addition, most microorganisms grow best in the absence of light, and sunlight should be avoided.

**pH.** Another factor affecting the growth or culture of microorganisms is the pH of the medium. Not only must a culture medium contain the proper nutrients in the correct concentrations; it also must have the correct degree of acidity or alkalinity. Most microorganisms prefer culture media that are approximately neutral, although some require a medium that is acid. Most microorganisms grow within a pH range of 3 to 9. Although changes in pH may not actually prevent the growth of a particular organism, its metabolic activities may not be normal if the pH is not optimum.

The pH of media is controlled by use of buffers, or substances that resist changes in hydrogen ion concentration. Buffers are especially useful for microorganisms that produce acid as part of their metabolism. These microorganisms would kill themselves by their own acid production if a suitable buffer were not present. Conversely, some bacteria produce alkaline products such as ammonia, which must also be buffered or the culture would destroy itself. Blood, milk, and seawater are all solutions that are naturally buffered and are therefore useful as culture media. Synthetic media often contain phosphate buffer systems.

**Sterile Conditions.** To obtain a pure culture of a microorganism, the culture medium must be sterile. Not only is sterilization necessary for separation of the inoculated organism, but contamination by other microbe forms may influence or prevent the growth of the desired microorganism. Most culture media are sterilized by use of the autoclave. Commercially prepared media are sterilized and packaged ready for use. Media prepared by the laboratory must be sterilized prior to use. Quantities of media up to 1 L should be autoclaved for 15 minutes at 121° C, and larger volumes may require a longer period. The culture media should be prepared according to directions and then placed in test tubes or Erlenmeyer flasks. These are loosely capped and placed in the autoclave. The test tubes should be autoclaved in racks or baskets, and the flasks should not be more than two-thirds full. Over-sterilization or prolonged heating must be avoided, as it can change the composition of the medium; it may cause precipitation in agar media or an increase in acidity. Some culture media may be harmed by autoclaving and may have to be sterilized by filtration.

**Moisture.** All microorganisms require some moisture for growth. Bacteria in general require a high concentration of water in their environment for growth and multiplication. Formation of highly resistant spores by bacteria that are spore formers is stimulated by drying or lack of water. Water is required for the metabolic reactions that take place in the bacterial cell and is the means of supplying nutrients to and removing waste products from the cell. Water is an integral part of the organism's protoplasm and accounts for much of the weight of the bacterial cell.

The amount of moisture in culture media varies. A medium may be used as a liquid, solid, liquefiable solid, or semisolid. Liquid media, or broths, may be converted to solid media by adding whole egg, egg white, or blood serum and heating until the mixture coagulates.

### Storage of Media

Culture media must be protected from external contamination. Media and cultures in Petri dishes are protected from external contamination by the design of the dish. Test tubes and flasks may be covered with screw caps or loosely fitting metal or autoclavable plastic covers. The cover must not be too tight or too loose, and it must protect the lip of the container from contamination by dust. Screw caps must be used with care, for their improper use may result in production of anaerobic or partially anaerobic conditions.

Media are generally stored under refrigeration (4° C) to prevent deterioration and dehydration. Certain media require special storage, but such information will be provided with the media. In general, a medium should be allowed to warm up to room temperature before it is inoculated, or microorganisms may be destroyed.

### Classification of Media

Although culture as well as morphologic characteristics are essential in the identification of bacteria, additional determinations are often necessary. Culture media may be simply supportive, or they may be employed to give additional information; in this context, media are classified as selective, differential, or enrichment media.

**Supportive Media.** Supportive media contain nutrients that allow most nonfastidious organisms to grow at their normal rate. These media do not give one organism any growth advantage over another. The organism's own metabolism affects the progress of its growth.

**Selective Media.** Selective media are semisolid plating media prepared by adding dyes, antibiotics, or other chemical compounds to certain media. In **selective media,** these substances selectively inhibit the growth of certain microorganisms and permit the growth of others. Selective media are used for fecal and sputum specimens, in which many normally occurring bacteria could obscure the presence of the pathogenic material. The normally occurring bacteria are selectively inhibited so that the pathogens can be seen if they are present.

**Enrichment Media. Enrichment media** permit one organism to grow rapidly while inhibiting the growth of other organisms. Enrichment media are especially useful in the isolation of *Salmonella* or *Shigella* species from stool cultures, which contain several bacteria—the normal intestinal flora—that are so numerous that they would obscure the growth of the pathogens, if present. Therefore, cultures of stool specimens for pathogens normally include an enrichment medium that inhibits the normal intestinal flora and promotes the growth of the pathogens that must be identified. Subculture to a solid plating medium from the enrichment broth must be made to obtain isolated colonies for final identification.

**Differential Media. Differential media** contain dyes, indicators, or other constituents that give colonies of particular organisms distinctive and easily recognizable characteristics. The final identification of an organism often involves isolation on a suitable culture medium and then the characteristic reaction or growth being noted on a differential medium. Such a characteristic reaction constitutes a confirmatory test for the microorganism.

## Commonly Used Types of Media

The eventual identification of a particular microorganism requires its culture on various media (selective, enrichment, or differential). No one system is universally employed in the identification of pathogens (see also Biochemical and Enzymatic Tests).

Most microbiologists can now purchase the majority of materials needed for culture, identification, and susceptibility testing of pathogenic microorganisms. In the past, much of the media was prepared by the laboratory. The commercial production of testing materials for microbiologic use has simplified much of what used to be a time-consuming effort by the laboratory personnel.

Most culture media are purchased already in Petri plate form, but some are in the form of a dehydrated powder that must be reconstituted. If media must be prepared, they must be prepared by following the manufacturer's directions carefully. If the media are to be sterilized in an autoclave, the container is capped. Safety precautions should be taken when the autoclave is used for this purpose.

Many hundreds of types of media are available for culture purposes. Some are used as part of routine culture protocol and others are used only rarely. Descriptions of available media can be found in the *Difco Manual: Dehydrated Culture Media and Reagents for Microbiology,* tenth edition (Difco Laboratories, Inc., Detroit, 1985).

**Bordet-Gengou Agar (BG).** This is a selective, enrichment media used for the isolation of *Bordetella pertussis* in the diagnosis of whooping cough. Colonies of the organism have a special diagnostic appearance on this medium. Penicillin may also be added to the medium to inhibit growth of the normal bacterial flora. However, certain strains of *B. pertussis* are also inhibited by penicillin, so two BG plates should be inoculated, one with and one without penicillin.

**Chocolate Agar (Choc).** Choc is an enrichment medium that especially promotes the growth of *Haemophilus* species. Choc is prepared by adding blood to a nutrient base medium at 75° to 80° C. The heat denatures proteins in the blood, causing the blood to coagulate and turn brown. This gives a richer medium than ordinary blood agar, providing a higher moisture content required by some fastidious organisms. Choc is also used in the cultivation of the pathogenic *Neisseria* species. These organisms cause gonorrhea and meningitis and are difficult to grow. They require an atmosphere of 10% carbon dioxide in addition to the special medium.

**Eosin-Methylene Blue Agar (EMB).** EMB is both a selective and a differential medium used in the primary plating of routine urine cultures. It promotes the growth of gram-negative organisms and inhibits that of gram-positive organisms. In addition, many gram-negative organisms have a characteristic appearance on EMB. In culturing urine, EMB plates as well as sheep blood agar plates are inoculated, since many urinary tract infections are caused by gram-negative rods. Lactose fermenters produce acid, which precipitates the two dyes present in the EMB medium (eosin, giving a metallic sheen to *E. coli,* and methylene blue, inhibiting gram-positive organisms) and gives colonies of the lactose-positive organisms a purple center. MacConkey agar can be used in place of EMB in urine cultures.

**Löwenstein-Jensen Medium (LJ).** This medium is used to cultivate and isolate *Mycobacterium* species. It is an egg-based medium containing whole eggs, potato flour, and glycerol to support the growth of mycobacteria, the genus causing tuberculosis and leprosy. The presence of malachite green in the medium inhibits the growth of other bacteria that may be present in the specimen. Malachite green is light sensitive, so the medium must be kept out of direct light. Specimens are inoculated onto the LJ medium and incubated anaerobically for 6 to 10 weeks. Alternate media used to cultivate *Mycobacterium* species are Middlebrook 7H10 and 7H11. Isoniazid-resistant strains grow better on these media than on egg-based media.

**MacConkey Agar (Mac).** Mac is both a selective and a differential medium for Enterobac-

tericeae and other gram-negative rods and is used in the primary plating of routine urine cultures in particular. It differentiates between lactose-fermenting and non-lactose-fermenting gram-negative rods. Crystal violet is included to inhibit the growth of gram-positive organisms, and bile salts are present to inhibit nonpathogenic gram-negative organisms. The medium is also used in the diagnosis of dysentery, typhoid, and paratyphoid bacteria, which do not ferment lactose. Colonies of organisms that do ferment lactose are red in this medium because the lactic acid that results from fermentation reacts with the bile salts, with subsequent absorption of neutral red. Neutral red is an acid-base indicator (red indicates an acid reaction, yellow an alkaline reaction). Therefore, the pathogens that do not ferment lactose are seen as yellow or colorless colonies on this medium.

Mac medium is sometimes used in place of EMB, since it tends to inhibit the spread of *Proteus* species more than EMB does.

**Methyl Red–Voges-Proskauer Broth.** This medium is important as the culture medium for two differential tests, the methyl red test and the Voges-Proskauer test, used in the identification of gram-negative rods.

**Phenylethyl Alcohol Agar (PEA).** This is essentially sheep blood agar with phenylethyl alcohol added. The medium permits the growth of gram-positive cocci and inhibits the growth of gram-negative organisms except *Pseudomonas aeruginosa.* It permits growth of the gram-positive cocci and allows their identification and separation, even when they are mixed with gram-negative organisms. If *P. aeruginosa* is present in a mixed culture and isolation of gram-positive organisms is desired, the culture is mixed with ether and then streaked onto the PEA plate, since ether destroys *Pseudomonas.* Hemolysis cannot be observed on the PEA plate.

**Sabouraud Dextrose Agar With Antibiotics (SAB).** This medium promotes the growth of fungi while inhibiting bacterial growth. It has a low pH and high osmotic pressure. It should always be incubated at room temperature. Chloramphenicol is included to inhibit bacterial growth. Cycloheximide may be included to inhibit nonpathogenic fungi.

**Salmonella-Shigella Agar (SS).** SS is a highly selective medium that is very inhibitory to **coliform bacilli** (gram-negative organisms that are part of the normal intestinal flora) and gram-positive organisms. Brilliant green is present to inhibit the gram-positive organisms. It is used along with Mac in routine stool cultures. The medium should be heavily inoculated. It is designed to isolate the *Salmonella* species and some *Shigella* species in the presence of other gram-negative organisms. It can also differentiate lactose-fermenting from non-lactose-fermenting strains. Colonies of lactose fermenters are red, and those of nonfermenters are yellowish or colorless. Neutral red is an acid-base indicator. Organisms that produce hydrogen sulfide show black centers on this medium.

**Selenite Broth.** This is an enrichment medium used for stool cultures. The medium inhibits the growth of gram-positive organisms and coliform bacilli, while favoring and therefore isolating *Shigella* and *Salmonella,* the causative agents of dysentery and typhoid fever, respectively. The medium suppresses growth of organisms other than *Shigella* and *Salmonella* for 12 to 18 hours. After this time, coliform bacilli and streptococci (enterococci) grow rapidly; overgrowth occurs. Therefore, after 18 hours of incubation, cultures grown in selenite broth must be subcultured onto a MacConkey plate or other suitable differential medium. Selenite broth is most effective at a neutral pH and under reduced oxygen tension. Therefore, it is dispensed into tubes to a depth of 2 in. The broth should be inoculated heavily with fecal material—an amount about the size of a pea.

**Sheep Blood Agar (SBA or BA).** This medium supports the growth of most ordinary bacteria. It is therefore used for primary plating and for subculturing. It is a good general medium for the growth of pathogens, since the blood adds many of the accessory substances that pathogens require. Most pathogens can be recognized on sheep blood. The medium is also useful in distinguishing different types of organisms, such as streptococci, by their ability to hemolyze the red blood cells present in the medium. They are differentiated as producing alpha hemolysis—green (or partial) hemolysis; beta hemolysis—clear (or complete) hemolysis; or gamma hemolysis—no hemolysis.

**Simmons Citrate Agar.** Simmons citrate agar is used to differentiate gram-negative enteric bacilli. It is an agar slant and is not a nutrient agar, but contains simple inorganic salts. It is used to test the ability of the organism to utilize sodium citrate as its sole source of carbon and to utilize the medium's ammonium salt (monoammonium phosphate) as its sole source of nitrogen. The breakdown of the ammonium salt results in a pH change to the alkaline range; the pH indicator, bromthymol blue, changes color from green to blue. Bromthymol blue is green (the color of the uninoculated medium) when gram-negative enteric bacilli are not growing but turns blue when they are—growth of gram-negative enteric bacilli utilizes the ammonium salt and changes the pH. Therefore, a positive reaction is observed as a change of the color of the medium from green to blue.

**Thayer-Martin Agar (Modified Thayer-Martin Agar).** This is a selective, enrichment medium for *Neisseria gonorrhoeae* and *Neisseria meningitidis.* It is a modification of chocolate agar, containing hemoglobin along with the various nutrients from the lysed red cells. Several antibiotics are present in the medium to inhibit the growth of normal flora and most other types of bacteria and fungi. When these plates are used, the cultures should be incubated anaerobically.

**Thioglycolate Broth (Thio Broth).** Thio broth is an all-purpose medium that can be used to isolate a wide range of bacteria, but it is used particularly for the cultivation of anaerobic organisms. It contains thioglycolic acid (sodium thioglycolate) and agar to encourage anaerobic growth. The medium is in a reduced state and contains the indicator resazurin, which turns pink if the medium is oxidized. If more than one third of the medium is pink, it contains too much oxygen for anaerobic growth. The oxygen can be driven off by heating the tube of medium. All cultures in which an anaerobic organism is suspected are inoculated into thio broth.

**Triple Sugar Iron Agar (TSIA) Slants.** TSIA slants are slant tubes having a lump, or butt, of medium at the bottom and a slant above (see Fig. 16-3). TSIA contains glucose, sucrose, and lactose (fermentable sugars), phenol red pH indicator, peptone (nutrient source), and iron salt, plus sodium thiosulfate (sulfur source and hydrogen sulfide indicator). It is essential that the slants be inoculated with a pure culture. Therefore, a single, well-isolated colony should be used for the inoculum. The medium is inoculated by streaking the slant and then stabbing the butt with a straight inoculating needle.

The medium is especially useful as a first step in the identification of gram-negative rods. It is used to test the ability of gram-negative rods to ferment dextrose, sucrose, and lactose, and to produce hydrogen sulfide ($H_2S$). Fermentation of sugars is accompanied by acid production, which is indicated by a change in the color of the phenol red indicator from red to yellow (yellow in acid pH and red in alkaline pH). Ferrous ammonium sulfate is present; this is black in the presence of hydrogen sulfide. Production of hydrogen sulfide is therefore indicated by the formation of a black color, as hydrogen sulfide combines with ferrous ammonium sulfate. Splitting of the agar in the butt indicates gas production.

There are other media that are similar to TSIA. One such medium is Kligler's iron agar (KIA). This medium differs in that it tests fermentation of only dextrose and lactose; sucrose is not included. (See also under Biochemical or Enzymatic Tests.)

**Trypticase Soy Broth (TSB).** TSB is a very good general-purpose medium. Almost everything grows well in it. All TSB contains dextrose, some type of peptone, inorganic salts, and water. Most cultures are inoculated into TSB to maintain the growth of all organisms in the specimen. A small amount of agar is added to the medium to make it thicker, but not enough to solidify it. This permits the growth of some anaerobic organisms, since oxygen does not diffuse to the bottom of the medium if agar is added.

**Tryptophan Broth and Peptone Water (Indole Medium).** This is a culture medium that can be used for the indole test. The broth contains trypticase, a peptone rich in the amino acid, tryptophan. The ability of bacteria to split indole from the tryptophan molecule is highly diagnostic. If a microorganism growing in peptone water with tryptophan has produced indole, the addition of Kovac's reagent to the culture results in a red color. Therefore, a positive test for indole production is the production of a red color after addition of Kovac's reagent. The indole test is useful in the identification of gram-negative rods.

**Urea Agar.** This is an enrichment agar slant that is used to test the ability of a microorganism to utilize urea as its only source of nitrogen. To do this, the organism must produce the enzyme urease. Breakdown of urea by the action of urease results in the production of ammonia, which raises the pH of the medium, as indicated by a color change of the phenol red indicator to red. The organism is streaked onto the slant only. The butt is not stabbed. Some organisms give a red color in only the slant; others color both the butt and the slant.

Tests for urease production may also be done on urea broth, which contains a buffered urea solution and phenol red indicator.

### Quality Control of Media

The NCCLS has developed recommendations for use of abbreviated quality control testing for media that have been commercially prepared when, in the process of preparation, the manufacturer has followed these recommendations. If a manufacturer has followed the NCCLS recommendations, it has been found that the performance of its media is consistent and adequate and that these media do not require further testing in the local laboratory as to quality.

There are some commercially prepared media that must be tested in the local laboratory before use. The NCCLS has identified the media that need quality control testing on a local basis. For this purpose, there are quality control organisms that can be purchased, along with their expected results. The relevant NCCLS publication, *Quality Assurance for Commercially Prepared Microbiological Culture Media: Approved Standard,* second edition, should be consulted for this information.[10] All media prepared in the laboratory must be tested before being used for routine culture. Clones of stock organisms for which the media are intended are used for testing the media for quality and must be maintained by the laboratory for CLIA-mandated participation in quality assurance programs.

## Biochemical or Enzymatic Tests

Many bacteria cannot be identified on the basis of microscopic or cultural characteristics alone. The biochemical properties and reactions of bacteria form the basis for an important series of identification procedures. Biochemical identification has been used increasingly and is an important function of the microbiology laboratory. Biochemical tests rely on bacterial physiology and the end products produced in reactions of bacterial cells themselves. Important biochemical reactions involve oxidation and fermentation, starch hydrolysis, hydrogen sulfide production, urea hydrolysis, and tryptophan hydrolysis.

In each biochemical procedure, the unknown bacterium causes a change of some type in the medium, to which a specific test substance has been added. The change may be indicated by the formation of gas or by the formation of color. In some media a pH indicator is used—for instance, to show when an acid is produced during fermentation. Some bacteria can break down starch in the medium, and iodine is used to test for the presence or absence of starch. Metabolism of the amino acid tryptophan can produce indole, which can be detected by a color change in another indicator. Biochemical tests may be done individually, or they may be incorporated into culture media.

Some biochemical tests can be performed directly on colonies seen growing on primary culture plates. Some of these are rapid tests taking only minutes, and others take a few hours of incubation for results to be seen. Use of information gained from the results of biochemical tests can place an organism into a further category, together with colony characteristics and morphologic and microscopic information. In this way, a tentative or preliminary identification can be made, which is often valuable diagnostic information needed in cases of serious infections.

Modifications of the traditional biochemical tests have been made to facilitate inoculation of media, shorten the incubation time, automate procedures, or in some way make the identification of species based on reaction patterns easier to do. In some modifications, a heavy suspension of organism being tested is inoculated on a small volume of media. Some commercial suppliers prepare reagent-impregnated paper disks or filter paper strips that are used along with small volumes of water (elution process) or saline to produce the desired test substrate. Tablets are also available that can be added to water to produce the substrate needed. This type of substrate is useful for differentiating two similar species that differ in only one characteristic.

There are also multitest systems in which conventional biochemicals are prepared in microdilution trays. Some of these substrate products are shipped in a frozen state and stored frozen until needed. They must be thawed prior to inoculation and require overnight incubation, as conventional biochemicals also need. Some substrate products are provided in a dried state in a tray.

These products are rehydrated with a suspension of the organism during inoculation.

There have been many innovations devised commercially to include the traditional biochemical tests. Biochemicals have been placed in trays, tubes, and other holding devices. Many different substrates are included in wells in a single test tray. The suspension of the organism being tested is inoculated into the plastic wells, the tray incubated, and the organism allowed to mix with the various substrates. In many instances, results are available after 4 hours of incubation. These multitest systems can often be used in conjunction with a computer-generated database that will identify the biochemical patterns generated by the organism being tested. By use of automation, more precision is attainable than with use of the conventional biochemical tests.

Some of the more traditional biochemical tests are described below.

### Bile Solubility Test

Some organisms contain an active autocatalytic enzyme that will lyse the organism's own cell wall during cell division. Upon the addition of a bile salt, such as sodium deoxycholate, these organisms rapidly autolyze. When a drop of bile salt detergent reagent is added to isolated colonies of *Streptococcus pneumoniae* on a blood agar or chocolate agar plate, there will be visible dissolution (autolysis) of the colony within 30 minutes after exposure to the test reagent. Species of *S. pneumoniae* give a positive reaction, which is the disappearance of the suspected colony, leaving a flat area. Other streptococcal species will not be affected by the addition of the bile salt reagent.

### Catalase Test

In this test, the enzyme catalase breaks down hydrogen peroxide into oxygen and water. The test is usually performed on a glass slide. If a small amount of an organism that produces catalase is added to hydrogen peroxide, bubbles of oxygen are seen immediately. The oxygen bubbles represent the gaseous product of the enzyme's activity occurring in this reaction. This test is commonly used to differentiate streptococci from staphylococci. All staphylococci are catalase-positive and will produce copious bubbles. The genus *Streptococcus* does not produce catalase and consequently is catalase negative, producing no visible bubbling of the hydrogen peroxide reagent.

### Coagulase Test

The clumping factor test (coagulase test) is cell associated and binds plasma fibrinogen, causing agglutination of the organisms by binding them together by means of aggregated fibrinogen. Detection of a positive test is seen by observation of clumping of cells. The coagulase test is used primarily to identify isolates of *Staphylococcus aureus*, an important human pathogen. *S. aureus* is almost always coagulase positive. Immediate visible aggregation will be seen when coagulase plasma reagent is mixed with coagulase-positive organisms, usually resulting in the complete clearing of the suspension background. Coagulase-negative organisms will retain the smooth, milky appearance of the original suspension. A control is always included with this test. A specific immunologic particle agglutination test for *S. aureus* has replaced the clumping factor coagulase test in many laboratories.

### Rapid Carbohydrate Fermentation Reaction Test

Various bacteria ferment different carbohydrates (sugars), producing lactic acid. The ability of microorganisms to ferment certain carbohydrates often serves to identify them. Tubes for these tests contain peptone broth in addition to a solution of the sugar in question. The medium also contains a pH indicator, phenol red, which is red in alkaline solutions and yellow in acid solutions.

In the carbohydrate fermentation tests, carbohydrates are metabolized by certain organisms, with subsequent changes in pH. The pH indicator in the peptone broth tubes is phenol red, which changes from red to yellow in the presence of positive organisms. One portion of the broth should be retained without carbohydrate to serve as a control. This control tube should remain red after the incubation period. The presence of buffers controls the pH change, and the use of a heavy amount of inoculum allows rapid detection of the positive reaction. The broth tubes are incubated for up to 4 hours and should be observed periodically for any color change.

If a microorganism ferments the sugar into which it has been inoculated, it produces lactic acid from the sugar and therefore lowers the pH of the medium. This change of pH is indicated by a color change of the phenol red indicator from red to yellow. Hence, the formation of a yellow color indicates fermentation of the sugar, or a positive reaction. Growth may occur in sugar tubes without the production of lactic acid (i.e., without fermentation). There will be no color change in this case. The sugars used most in the identification of bacteria are glucose, maltose, fructose, and sucrose.

### Rapid Urease Test

Organisms that produce the enzyme urease are able to hydrolyze urea-releasing ammonia as an end product. The production of ammonia changes the alkalinity, thus causing the pH indicator phenol red to change from yellow to red. This test can be used to screen lactose-negative colonies on differential media that have been plated with a stool specimen, thereby assisting in the differentiation of the pathogenic *Salmonella* and *Shigella* species, which are urease negative, from the urease-positive nonpathogens. Commercial urease testing supplies are available with reagent-impregnated swabs that are rubbed across the colony to be tested—this being done directly on the culture plate. Reagent tablets are also available. Another method uses a urea broth that is inoculated with a heavy suspension of the organism to be tested. The observance of a color change from a pale straw or yellow to a red identifies the presence of a urease-positive organism, such as *Proteus* or *Klebsiella* species.

### Spot Indole Test

Organisms that produce the enzyme tryptophanase can degrade the amino acid tryptophan to yield indole as one end product. Indole can be detected by its ability to combine with certain aldehydes to form a colored compound. Indole reagent, containing the indicator aldehyde, is added to filter paper in the bottom of a Petri dish. The reagent should saturate the filter paper. A portion of the isolated colony to be tested is rubbed onto the filter paper. Indole-positive organisms will result in the rapid development of a blue color on the filter paper if the indicator aldehyde is paradimethylaminocinnamaldehyde. This test can be used to differentiate swarming *Proteus* species from one another and as a presumptive identification of *Escherichia coli*. Positive organisms such as *E. coli* will give a blue-green color on the filter paper, and negative organisms remain colorless.

### Spot Oxidase Test

Organisms that produce the enzyme cytochrome oxidase are able to oxidize the test reagent tetramethyl-*p*-phenylenediamine dihydrochloride (Kovac's reagent), forming a colored end product. A dark-purple end product will be visible when an organism producing the enzyme is added to filter paper that has been impregnated with the reagent substrate. The test is primarily done to presumptively identify *Neisseria* species and to initially characterize gram-negative bacilli. *Neisseria* species, oxidase-positive organisms, will turn the filter paper a dark purple within 10 seconds. Oxidase-negative organisms will remain colorless or keep the color of the original colony within 10 seconds.

### Triple Sugar Iron Agar (TSIA) and Kligler's Iron Agar (KIA)

By use of TSIA or KIA, initial presumptive identification of gram-negative bacilli may be made, especially members of the Enterobacteriaceae family—the common enteric intestinal pathogens screened. Use of these media can determine three primary characteristics of these organisms: ability to ferment gas from sugars, production of large amounts of hydrogen sulfide gas (visualized by appearance of black iron-containing precipitate), and ability to ferment lactose in KIA and lactose and sucrose in TSIA. The medium is inoculated with an inoculating needle, using a small amount of growth from a pure colony of the organism being tested, by streaking the surface of the medium and by stabbing the butt of the medium all the way down to the bottom of the tube. (See also under Commonly Used Types of Media.)

After incubation, reactions are noted and the organism presumptively identified on the basis of fermentation reactions, hydrogen sulfide production, and gas formation. Since there is such a variety of reactions occurring in the TSIA slants, there must be a scheme for observing and recording these reactions. Reactions in the slant and butt are recorded as acid (A) or alkaline (Alk), and the production of hydrogen sulfide ($H_2S$) and gas (G) is noted. An acid reaction is indicated by the presence of a yellow color and an alkaline reaction by a red color. No reaction would be recorded as NR. Various observations and interpretations are shown in Table 16-1.

Failure of the organism to ferment any of the three sugars results in an Alk/Alk reaction (or no reaction), indicated by a red slant and butt. An Alk/A reaction (red slant and yellow butt) results when only dextrose is fermented. Organisms fermenting only dextrose will initially give an A/A reaction, or yellow slant and butt; the small amount of dextrose present is used up as the incubation continues. The slant is under aerobic conditions and reverts to alkaline (or red) in 18 to 24 hours. In the butt, however, anaerobic conditions exist, there is no reversion to alkaline pH, and the acid (or yellow) reaction remains.

An A/A reaction (yellow slant and butt) results when dextrose and lactose or sucrose or both are fermented. The medium contains ten times more lactose and sucrose than dextrose. Therefore, organisms fermenting lactose or sucrose or both do not use up the sugars except after very prolonged incubation. Fermentation of sucrose or lactose is indicated by acid (yellow) conditions in both the slant and the butt. However, with prolonged incubation (48 to 72 hours), lactose and sucrose may also be used up and formerly acid reactions may revert to alkaline. Therefore, the time of incubation is critical. The time recommended to obtain typical reactions is 18 hours.

## URINE CULTURES

Cultures are done on urine to diagnose bacterial infections of the urinary tract (bladder, ureter, kidney, and urethra). Urinary tract infections (UTI) are of two main types: (1) lower urinary tract infection, such as cystitis, an infection of the bladder, and (2) upper urinary tract or kidney infection, such as pyelonephritis, an infection of the renal parenchyma (kidney). Routine urine cultures are usually done by using one selective culture medium and one nonselective, or general or supportive, medium.

### Collecting the Specimen

The urine specimen for culture must be collected in a clinically reliable manner; proper cleaning of the collection site, especially for females, is very

---

**TABLE 16-1**

Observations of Triple Sugar Iron Agar (TSIA)

| Notation | Color Change | Metabolic Change |
|---|---|---|
| A/A | Yellow slant, yellow butt | Dextrose fermented, lactose or sucrose or both fermented |
| Alk/A | Red slant, yellow butt | Dextrose fermented, lactose and sucrose not fermented |
| Alk/Alk or NR | Red slant, red butt | None of the three sugars fermented, or no reaction |
| $H_2S$ | Black in butt | $H_2S$ production |
| G | Splitting of agar in butt | Gas production |

important. A voided clean-catch, midstream urine sample collection is the one utilizing the least invasive technique and, consequently, the one most commonly used (see also Specimens for Microbiological Examination, in this chapter, and Collection of Urine for Culture, under Collecting Urine Specimens in Chapter 3).

The specimen must be collected into a sterile container and, if not cultured immediately in the laboratory, must be refrigerated to prevent bacterial growth. Urine is normally sterile within the bladder but is easily contaminated during the collection process if caution is not used in cleaning the collection site.

Quantitative urine culture methods are needed to differentiate true **bacteriuria** (bacteria in the urine) from contamination. The presence of bacteria in the urine does not necessarily indicate a urinary tract infection unless the number of organisms is significant. The classic criterion of infection is the presence of greater than 100,000 ($10^5$) **colony-forming units (CFU)** of bacteria per milliliter of urine. If a quantitative culture results in a colony count between 10,000 and 100,000 CFU/mL urine, a repeat culture is done on a fresh urine specimen to confirm the result. An increased number of white cells present as polymorphonuclear neutrophils (PMNs) in the urine specimen, in conjunction with the results of the urine culture, increases the diagnostic value of both tests.

## Methods for Detection of Bacteriuria
### Rapid Screening Test Strips

Rapid screening test strips have been developed to test for bacteriuria. Nitrite tests have been incorporated into reagent strips used in many laboratories for routine urine analysis (see Chapter 14). Common organisms that cause urinary tract infections, such as species of *Enterobacter, Escherichia, Proteus, Klebsiella, and Pseudomonas*, contain enzymes that reduce nitrate in the urine to nitrite (see Nitrite in Chapter 14.) Organisms must contain the reductase enzyme necessary to carry out this process.

The rapid screening test strips for bacteriuria are most useful when the test for nitrite is com-

bined with that for leukocyte esterase. Chemical test strips are available that combine nitrite and leukocyte esterase tests. Multiple-reagent test strips contain test pads for these constituents. Test strips for leukocyte esterase utilize a diazo reaction that is specific for esterase. Leukocyte esterase is an enzyme present in the primary or azurophilic granules of granulocytes such as neutrophils. Since neutrophils are generally increased in a urinary tract infection, the presence of leukocyte esterase in the urine is an indicator of infection (see Leukocyte Esterase in Chapter 14). The absence of leukocyte esterase does not rule out a urinary tract infection, however. The finding of nitrite-positive and leukocyte esterase–positive urine using chemical screening tests is helpful in detecting bacteriuria, especially in combination with the presence of bacteria and white cells in the urine sediment. To identify the organism causing the infection, a Gram stain and a quantitative urine culture are done.

### Quantitative Culture Methods

To determine true bacteriuria, quantitative methods are used to determine the number of colony-forming units of organism per milliliter of urine specimen and cultures are done to identify the pathogenic organism present. The traditional streak plate culture method is done in many laboratories, but automated screening methods are also available.

**Streak Plate for Quantitative Urine Culture.** A streak plate method for quantitating the growth of microorganisms in the urine is the classic culture method commonly used in many clinical laboratories (Procedure 16-5). A calibrated standardized inoculating loop, containing 0.001 or 0.01 mL of urine, is used to transfer the well-mixed specimen to the culture plates and to streak the plates. The larger volume (0.01 mL) gives a greater amount of inoculum and can be used to gain more accurate quantitation. Care must be taken in obtaining the specimen with the calibrated loop (see Fig. 16-8).

**PROCEDURE 16-5**

*Quantitative Urine Streak Plate*

1. Ensure that the urine specimen is well-mixed

2. Flame the calibrated inoculating loop, allow it to cool, and insert it into the bubble-free surface of the specimen (see Fig. 16-8.)

3. Streak the loopful of undiluted urine over the surface of the SB plate. Repeat the process and streak the EMB or Mac plates (see Figs. 16-9 and 16-10). After streaking the SB plate, make three or four small cuts in the agar to more readily observe hemolysis after incubation.

4. Incubate the culture plates at 35 to 37° C in an inverted position for 18 to 24 hours.

5. Interpret the results.

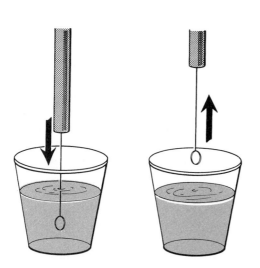

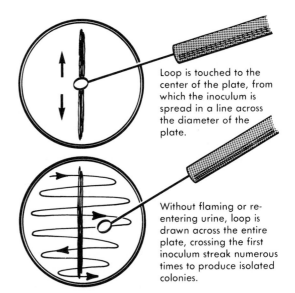

Loop is touched to the center of the plate, from which the inoculum is spread in a line across the diameter of the plate.

Without flaming or re-entering urine, loop is drawn across the entire plate, crossing the first inoculum streak numerous times to produce isolated colonies.

**FIG 16-8.** Method for inserting a calibrated loop into urine to ensure that the proper amount of specimen will adhere to the loop. (From Baron EJ, Finegold SM: *Bailey and Scott's Diagnostic Microbiology*, ed 8. St Louis, Mosby, 1990, p 260.)

**FIG 16-9.** Method for streaking a loopful of urine with a calibrated inoculating loop to produce isolated colonies and countable colony-forming units of organisms. (From Baron EJ, Finegold SM: *Bailey and Scott's Diagnostic Microbiology*, ed 8. St Louis, Mosby, 1990, p 260.)

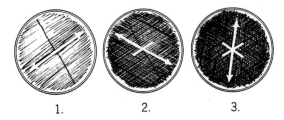

**FIG 16-10.** Streak plate for quantitative urine culture.

In common practice, a general or supportive medium such as sheep blood (SB) agar and a selective or differential medium such as Mac or EMB are streaked with the urine specimen. This is done in such a way that the drop of urine is spread as uniformly as possible on the plate (Figs. 16-9 and 16-10). After streaking and incubation, the number of colonies seen is multiplied by 1,000 (for the 0.001 mL loop) or 100 (for the 0.01 mL loop) to give the number of colonies in 1 mL of urine. The blood agar plate gives a total colony count, as most common organisms grow on it. The selective medium indicates whether gram-negative rods (and some inhibited gram-positive organisms) are present. The EMB and Mac media also indicate whether the organisms are lactose positive or lactose negative. The most common cause of UTIs is *E. coli,* associated with approximately 90% of all UTIs in ambulatory patients and in a large percentage of hospitalized patients also. *E. coli, Klebsiella* species, and *Enterobacter* species are lactose fermenters that show pink colonies (lactose positive), whereas *Proteus* species and *Pseudomonas* species are lactose negative (do not ferment lactose) and show yellowish colonies. *Proteus* species may also be recognized on blood agar by their spreading growth. Gram-positive organisms such as staphylococci and streptococci (enterococcus) grow well on blood agar but are inhibited on EMB or Mac medium.

**Interpreting Results of Quantitative Urine Cultures.** Normal urine is sterile. Plates that show no growth may be discarded and reported as no growth. Bacteriuria is considered clinically significant when laboratory findings show the presence of 100,000 ($10^5$) or more bacteria colonies per milliliter of urine specimen. After the incubation period, the number of colonies growing on the plates is counted and multiplied by 1,000 (if 0.001 mL urine has been plated) to determine the number of microorganisms per milliliter of original urine specimen. A count of 100,000 CFU/mL urine indicates a UTI in asymptomatic patients. A count of 1,000 CFU/mL urine may be significant for a UTI in a symptomatic patient. Therefore, it is always important to combine the results of colony counts with the clinical information available.

The growth characteristics of the colonies on the plates are also observed. As discussed previously, the EMB or Mac plates are observed for presumptive identification of gram-negative organisms, and growth on the blood agar plates is noted. Any cultural observations should agree with the results of the Gram stain. Further biochemical tests can be done to identify the suspected organism.

### Automated Screening Systems

Automated methods have been developed to screen urines rapidly for bacteriuria. One such device is the Bac-T-Screen system,* which employs a filter paper detection method screening out negative urine specimens in about 2 minutes. With this colorimetric filtration system, a measured amount of the urine sample is drawn by suction through a paper filter. Bacteria and other particles such as white blood cells adhere to the filter paper. A stain is passed through the filter paper, giving a color, the depth of which depends on the number and type of stainable particles. The intensity of color on the filter paper is read by a spectrophotometric device in the instrument, which compares the unknown filter paper color with that of a standard. The filter paper can also be examined visually, and if the color is less than that of the control, the testing can be stopped at this point, as it is considered to

---

*bioMerieux Vitek Systems, Hazelwood, Mo.

be negative. The Bac-T-Screen system has shown excellent correlation with the clinical diagnoses of urinary tract infections.[2]

The AutoMicrobic System* is another automated method to detect UTI pathogens. This system measures bacterial growth photometrically. The urine sample is introduced by vacuum into the tiny wells of the system's plastic cartridge card, and the card is placed into the instrument. The card is incubated and measured photometrically at periodic intervals to determine the amount of light that passes through the wells. The wells contain substrates that can be utilized only by certain organisms causing urinary tract infections—etiologic agents of UTI. After 6 to 8 hours, microorganisms grow in the appropriate wells and are detected by their increased turbidity as determined photometrically. The internal computer of the instrument issues a colony count and preliminary identification of the organism. Low counts are considered negative urine cultures.

### Nonculture Method: Gram Stain

If a screening test is positive for leukocyte esterase or nitrite using multiple-reagent strips, a Gram stain should be done on the well-mixed urine sample. One drop of uncentrifuged urine is placed on a glass slide, allowed to air dry, and then stained with Gram stain. The stained smear is examined microscopically by using the oil-immersion objective. If at least one organism per field (after examining at least 20 fields) is seen, this correlates with a significant bacteriuria of greater than 100,000 CFU/mL urine.[12] If three or more morphologic types of bacteria are detected, the urine is contaminated with distal urethral or perianal bacteria and another specimen must be collected.

## THROAT CULTURES

Throat cultures are done primarily to differentiate the Lancefield group A β-hemolytic streptococcal (*Streptococcus pyogenes*) sore throat

*bioMerieux Vitek Systems, Hazelwood, Mo.

(pharyngitis) from the more common viral throat infections. Sore throats caused by the group A streptococcal organism, the major throat pathogen, must be identified and treated because, if untreated, in some instances, sequelae can occur, leading to acute rheumatic fever followed by chronic rheumatic heart disease and valvular cardiac disease. Acute glomerulonephritis can also follow an untreated group A streptococcal throat infection in some patients.

### Collecting the Specimen

The proper collection of the sample is important. A sterile swab is used to collect the specimen. Throat cultures are done by swabbing the rear pharyngeal wall and the tonsillar area (see also Throat Culture Collection, in Chapter 3). The swab used to collect the specimen must be transported quickly to the laboratory for plating; transport media can be used to sustain the swab if transport to the laboratory must be delayed. These media will allow survival of suspected streptococcal organisms for 24 to 48 hours at 4° C. Culture of the throat swab specimen is traditionally done by using sheep blood agar plates.

### Methods of Detection of Group A β-Hemolytic Streptococci

The traditional culture using sheep blood agar plates continues to be used by many laboratories. Several nonculture methods—direct antigen tests—are also used, their advantage being that results are obtained more rapidly.

### Culture on Blood Agar

Culture on sheep blood agar will isolate bacterial pathogens from the pharyngeal area, if they are present (Procedure 16-6).

**Interpreting Results of Throat Culture Plates.** After suitable incubation has taken place, the colony morphology and the appearance of hemolysis on the blood agar plates are used in the identification of streptococci. Streptococci typically appear as translucent to milky, circular, small colonies.

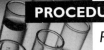

## PROCEDURE 16-6

### Plating Throat Cultures

1. Using the throat swab obtained from the patient, roll the swab onto one edge of an SB plate, being certain to get as much of the specimen off and onto the plate as possible.

2. Flame the inoculating loop and use it to streak the plate out from the inoculated area, as shown in Fig. 16-11. The streaking is done so as to isolate the bacterial colonies as much as possible. Make three or four cuts into the agar to more readily observe hemolysis after incubation.

3. Incubate for 18 to 24 hours at 35 to 37° C; then examine the culture plates for pathogens. If pathogens are present, do appropriate subculturing for final identification.

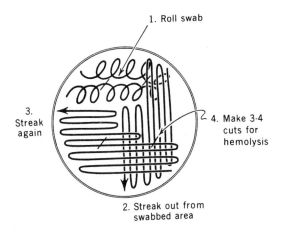

**FIG 16-11.** Streak plate for throat culture.

**Appearance of Hemolysis.** After incubation, hemolysis on the sheep blood agar can be observed. Hemolysis is determined by holding the culture plate directly in front of a light source. This phenomenon is useful in distinguishing different types of streptococci by their ability to hemolyze the red cells present in the medium. Hemolysis is of three types, depending on the type of streptococci: (1) **alpha** (green) or incomplete (partial) **hemolysis,** produced by *Streptococcus viridans* (part of the normal flora of the throat) and, less commonly, by *Streptococcus pneumoniae* (which can also be a cause of meningitis and pneumonia), in which hemolysis is seen macroscopically as a green discoloration of the medium surrounding the colony—hemolysis is incomplete; (2) gamma hemolysis, which macroscopically shows "no hemolysis" (gamma streptococci do not hemolyze the red cells in the media); and (3) **beta** (clear) or complete **hemolysis.** Most *Streptococcus pyogenes* organisms (the common throat pathogens) are beta-hemolytic, and the hemolysis will appear macroscopically as a clear zone surrounding the surface colonies or in the stabs in the blood agar—representing complete hemolysis of the red blood cells in the media.

Since throat cultures are done primarily to detect the presence of the Lancefield group A beta-hemolytic streptococci, plates are read with this organism in mind. Other pathogens may sometimes be clinically significant. Normal throat cultures show a predominance of alpha-hemolytic streptococci *(Streptococcus viridans)* and commensal Neisseria species. Other organisms can also constitute normal flora. If pathogens are not present, the result should be reported as normal flora.

**Subculturing and Use of Bacitracin Test.** To identify the group A β-hemolytic streptococci from other β-hemolytic streptococci, the bacitracin test can be used. With a sterile inoculating loop, a single presumptive colony of group A β-hemolytic streptococci is picked from the primary culture plate and streaked completely onto a segment of a new blood agar plate.

A bacitracin disk (with 0.04 unit bacitracin) is placed in the center of the inoculated area aseptically, and the plate is incubated overnight. A zone of inhibition of growth around the disk is indicative of bacitracin susceptibility and should be reported as "group A streptococci by bacitracin."

A bacitracin filter paper disk can also be placed directly on the area of initial inoculation on the primary plate, and after an overnight incubation period, presumptive identification of *Streptococcus pyogenes* can be made. All group A and a small percentage of group B streptococci are susceptible to the bacitracin. Since the bacitracin test is recommended to be used with a pure culture, it should be used for presumptive identification only when used on the primary culture plate. Final identification requires use of a pure culture of the organism isolated from the specimen. Identification of group A streptococci is shown by a zone of growth inhibition around the disk after the plate has been incubated for 18 to 24 hours.

**Use of Bile Solubility or Optochin Susceptibility Tests.** To ensure that the appearance of any green hemolysis seen on the primary culture plate is from the normal throat flora, *Streptococcus viridans*, and not *Streptococcus pneumoniae*, a bile solubility test or test for susceptibility to optochin can be done (see also under Biochemical or Enzymatic Tests). *Streptococcus pneumoniae* organisms will be lysed by the addition of a bile salt (a detergent reagent), or their growth will be inhibited by the anti-bacterial agent ethylhydrocupreine hydrochloride (optochin) impregnated onto a filter paper disk.

If the bile salt detergent reagent is used, a drop of the reagent is added to isolated colonies on a blood agar plate, and visible dissolution of the *Streptococcus pneumoniae* colonies is noted within 30 minutes if they are present. The optochin disk, when used, is placed on a subculture of the suspected colonies on a blood agar plate, and the plate is incubated overnight. Zones of inhibition are seen around the optochin disk

as presumptive identification for *Streptococcus pneumoniae* .

### Direct Visual Identification Using Fluorescence Antibody Techniques

Smears using direct fluorescent antibody techniques have been used in the identification of group A β-hemolytic streptococci in throat specimens. Use of one of the many commercially available rapid testing products to directly detect the streptococcal antigen in throat specimens has mostly replaced the use of fluorescent antibody smear examination (see Rapid Detection Methods: Nonculture Techniques).

### Rapid Detection Methods: Nonculture Techniques

Numerous commercial products are available for the rapid detection of group A β-hemolytic streptococcal pathogens. Instead of waiting for an overnight incubation period for culture plate methods, these results are available within a much shorter time—15 to 30 minutes—and antibiotic therapy can be started immediately. These rapid streptococcal antigen detection systems use enzyme immunoassays or latex or coagglutination techniques or gene probe technologies.

Specific procedures will vary with the product, and the manufacturer's directions must always be followed carefully for optimal results. Controls should be used with all methods.

Most laboratory comparisons of conventional culture methods and rapid testing methods have shown good sensitivity (>90%) and excellent specificity (>97%). If results are positive using rapid testing methods, it is sufficient reason to begin antibiotic therapy, as the rapid test is very specific for the group A β-hemolytic streptococcal antigen. Because of the lower test sensitivity, a negative test result does not mean the absence of disease. In some facilities, protocol recommends that two throat swabs be taken. If the first swab gives a positive rapid strep test result, the second swab can be discarded. If the rapid strep test is negative, the second swab can be inoculated onto a blood agar plate, incubated, and read in the traditional way. In this way, a negative rapid test result is confirmed with a culture plate method, which then accounts for a possible false-negative result, which can occur with some rapid strep testing methods.

Most rapid strep tests commonly first require extraction of any group A–specific antigen from the specimen on the throat swab. The group A–specific carbohydrate antigen is present in the cell wall of the streptococcal organisms. The swab is incubated with an acid solution or an enzyme—commonly nitrous acid is used—to extract the group A–specific carbohydrate antigen.

**Latex Slide Agglutination Tests.** Many rapid strep test products are latex slide agglutination tests for the direct detection of the group A streptococcal antigen extracted. For the latex agglutination tests, any extracted group A–specific antigen is mixed on a slide with specific antibody-coated latex beads, resulting in a visible agglutination, which occurs within a few minutes, indicating the presence or absence of the bacterial infection, depending on the product being used.

**Membrane-Bound Enzyme Immunoassay (EIA) or Enzyme-Linked Immunosorbent Assay (ELISA).** Another commonly used rapid strep testing methodology is the membrane-bound enzyme immunoassay (EIA) or the enzyme-linked immunosorbent assay (ELISA). In these immunoassays, the extracted antigen from the throat swab is added to a disposable plastic cassette chamber whose bottom portion contains an antibody-coated membrane (usually made from nitrocellulose or nylon) and an underlying absorbent bed of material (usually a cellulose acetate). When the extraction sample is added to the chamber, the absorbent material below it pulls the fluid through the antibody-coated membrane by a wicking action. This serves to present a relatively large amount of antigen (if present) to the antibody and to bind it. Bound antigen is detected by a second enzyme-labeled antibody using a variety of means,

depending on the product being used. With the TestPack Strep A kit,* a positive result is indicated by a plus sign appearing in the detection area; for a negative result, a minus sign appears. Positive and negative controls are also built into the product. These products have become known as "flow-through" tests, and they have become very popular because the results are easily read and they have excellent specificity and good sensitivity (>90%).

**Optical Immunoassay.** Antigen-antibody interactions that occur on an inert surface can be detected by changes in light reflectance due to an alteration in the thickness of the reactants on the surface. This technology is used in a product, Strep A OIA† optical immunoassay for group A streptococcus, using a reflective surface for enhanced detection of antigen-antibody reactions. With this technology, antigen can be detected, or the presence of an antigen-antibody complex, by allowing the sample containing antigen to react with an appropriate reflective surface to which a specific antibody is attached. Light reflecting off the surface film containing bound antibody only is viewed as one color, while group A–specific antigen binding increases the thickness of the film, causing the surface to appear a different color.

In a series of studies, the Strep A OIA product demonstrated a sensitivity of 98.9% and a specificity of 98.6%.[6] The manufacturer believes that with this excellent sensitivity, use of its Strep A OIA product eliminates the need for subsequent cultures of a specimen giving negative Strep A OIA results, as is recommended for other rapid antigen tests.

## GENITOURINARY CULTURES

Microbiological examination of genitourinary tract specimens is done primarily to determine the cause for urethritis, vaginitis, and cervicitis.

---

*Abbott Laboratories, Diagnostics Division, Abbott Park, Ill.
†Biostar, Inc, Boulder, Colo.

The organisms commonly detected are *Neisseria gonorrhoeae,* the etiologic agent of gonorrhea, and *Chlamydia trachomatis,* a common cause of a nongonococcal chlamydial infection in the urethra and cervix. These can all be sexually transmitted diseases. Chlamydial infections have surpassed the number of gonorrheal infections as the most prevalent sexually transmitted bacterial disease in the United States; in males they cause 30% to 50% of nongonococcal urethritis. Other microorganisms that can cause vaginitis in females include *Gardnerella vaginalis* and *Trichomonas vaginalis. T. vaginalis* is a parasite and is a commonly recognized sexually transmitted organism, which can be identified in a wet mount of vaginal secretions. *G. vaginalis* is one cause of bacterial vaginosis, a condition resulting from the disruption of the normal flora in the vagina. Vaginosis is not necessarily a sexually transmitted disease. *G. vaginalis* organisms are gram-negative coccobacilli and are associated with the presence of "clue cells." When the exfoliated vaginal epithelial cells are covered with tiny gram-variable rods and coccobacilli, they are known as clue cells. (See also Tests for Parasites, in this chapter, and Clue Cells in Chapter 14, Figs. 14-25 and 14-26.) Genitourinary fungal infections are common also and can often be the cause of vaginitis in women, especially women who are receiving antibiotic therapy that inhibits the growth of the normal vaginal bacterial flora. A common fungal infection is caused by *Candida albicans.* (See also Tests for Fungi.) Herpes simplex virus is another frequent cause of genitourinary infections.

## Collecting the Specimen

It is essential that genitourinary tract specimens, usually from the vaginal cervix or inflamed perineal areas in women and the anterior urethra in men, be appropriately collected in order that the organisms may be detected. Specimens must be handled carefully to avoid any contamination with other viable infectious material.

For detecting chlamydial organisms, it is important that columnar epithelial cells are collected along with the vaginal or urethral secre-

tions, as the organism resides in the cells. A separate sample must be taken for detection of gonococcal organisms (see under Gonorrheal Infections), in which case the specimen is inoculated directly onto the appropriate culture medium and a smear made for Gram stain. Genitourinary specimens must be transported immediately to the laboratory and culturing done without delay or appropriate storage precautions followed. There are commercially available transport systems for transit and storage of genitourinary tract specimens, which enhance the survival of the organisms, if present. Kits are available that include collection swabs and transport tubes containing specially formulated stabilizing media.

### Vaginal Smears

Vaginal smears or cultures must be collected with the swab inserted well into the vagina. The outer lips of the labia must be held apart so that the swab does not touch them. An endocervical specimen is necessary for suspected gonorrheal infections and requires the use of a speculum. Lubricants should not be used, as some of these are toxic to the microorganisms.

### Urethral Smears

Urethral samples are taken with a urogenital swab designed for this purpose. The swab must be inserted approximately 2 cm into the urethra and rotated gently before withdrawing. Special loop swabs are available for collection from the distal urethra if the discharge is minimal. Urethral smears from men are done by collecting the urethral discharge from the penis using a swab and rolling the collected specimen onto a microscope slide. Gram stained smears are examined for the presence of gram-negative intracellular diplococci indicative of gonococci in males.

## Methods of Detection for Common Genitourinary Tract Infections

The physician must alert the laboratory to the probable organisms causing the infection so that the identification process can be initiated using the appropriate culture media and assay protocol.

## Gonorrheal Infections

When *N. gonorrhoeae* is suspected, a special agar medium and a carbon dioxide atmosphere for incubation are required for optimal recovery from the clinical specimen being tested. Various supplemental media can also be inoculated. Thayer-Martin agar is a selective medium for *N. gonorrhoeae*. It contains various antibiotics to inhibit the growth of other types of bacteria and fungi. Chocolate agar is also a support medium for *N. gonorrhoeae*, but it does not inhibit the growth of normal flora because it does not contain the antibiotics. Special media kits are available that contain Thayer-Martin agar on one side and chocolate on the other. Some systems have self-generating carbon dioxide that will provide the anaerobic atmosphere necessary for growth of the gonococcal organisms. Otherwise, classic candle jars or other anaerobic incubation is used. Appropriate inoculation of the medium is important. The swab should be rolled over the surface of the medium in a W or Z pattern (Fig. 16-12) and incubated as quickly as possible.

After 24 to 48 hours of incubation on Thayer-Martin and chocolate agar, colonies of N. gonorrhoeae appear small, gray, translucent, and shiny. A Gram stain should be made of one of these colonies, and if the organism is *N. gonorrhoeae*, the characteristic gram-negative diplococci ("coffee-bean" appearance) will be observed. In addition, the biochemical oxidase test should be performed for presumptive identification purposes (see under Biochemical Tests). Only when the Gram stain results, the appearance of the colony on Thayer-Martin and chocolate agar, and an oxidase-positive biochemical reaction all support *N. gonorrhoeae* can the laboratory report indicate "presumptive *N. gonorrhoeae*." Other testing can be done on the isolates to detect penicillin-resistant strains of the organism. The culture plates should be maintained for at least 72 hours before a negative result is sent out. There are latex agglutination, coagglutination, or carbohydrate utilization tests that can be used as additional confirmatory tests for this organism. Several manufacturers have developed kits for this purpose.

## Chlamydial Infections

Infection with *Chlamydia trachomatis* is a prevalent sexually transmitted disease in the United States. It is important that the specimen be collected properly from the appropriate site by using a scraping technique or by vigorously rubbing against the involved site to dislodge the necessary epithelial cells where the chlamydial organism re-

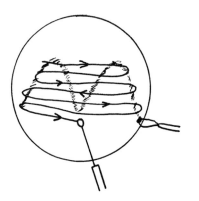
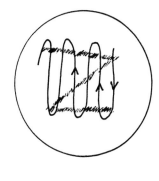

**FIG 16-12.** Method for streaking genital specimens. Two appropriate inoculation methods for *Neisseria gonorrhoeae*. The swab should be rolled over the plate in a W or Z pattern, followed by cross-streaking with a sterile inoculating loop. (From Becan-McBride K, Ross DL: *Essentials for the Small Laboratory and Physician's Office.* St Louis, Mosby, 1988, p 370.)

sides and not to collect only an exudate. The organism resides in columnar epithelial cells and not in squamous epithelial cells or other inflammatory cells. The specimen must be transported to the laboratory immediately. *C. trachomatis* is a fastidious organism—one that requires complex or extensive nutritional requirements—that must be grown in protected conditions.

The gold standard for identification of the chlamydial organism is cell culture and staining for the typical intracytoplasmic inclusion bodies present in the cells. Nonculture methods include direct fluorescent antibody studies using monoclonal antisera and an ELISA test. These are direct tests that give relatively rapid results and are very sensitive. A negative nonculture test result does not rule out the presence of chlamydial infection.

Tests employing a direct fluorescent antibody stain for the inclusion elementary bodies of the chlamydial organism present in the cells collected in the sample are quite sensitive and specific. The characteristic "green apple" elementary body is visualized under the fluorescence microscope when chlamydial organisms are present. A fluorescent monoclonal antibody stain is considered the most sensitive test for chlamydia. PCR and gene probes are also used to detect chlamydia. Complete collection and test systems are available commercially for these tests.

### Trichomonal and Yeast Infections

*Trichomonas vaginalis* can be observed on a direct wet mount of the vaginal fluid. This is the simplest and most rapid means of detection of this parasitic organism (see also under Tests for Parasites, in this chapter, and Figs. 14-54 to 14-56). Fungal elements can also be visualized at the same time. By addition of a 10% KOH reagent to the preparation, host cell protein is dissolved, allowing the pseudohyphae of the yeast to be seen more easily (see also under Tests for Fungi, in this chapter, and Figs. 14-49 to 14-53). KOH also makes the discharge alkaline, causing it to emit a fishy, aminelike odor that is characteristically associated with bacterial vaginosis.

### Bacterial Vaginosis

Bacterial vaginosis is produced by a mixed infection with anaerobic and facultative organisms. These are organisms that live on or in a host but that may also survive independently. Bacterial vaginosis is characterized by a foul-smelling vaginal discharge, and a Gram stain will show a mixed flora. The vaginal discharge can be observed microscopically for diagnosis of the condition; in a wet preparation, sloughed epithelial cells, many of which are covered with tiny, gram-variable rods and coccobacilli, will be seen. When epithelial cells have this appearance, the coating by the tiny bacteria, they are called "clue cells"; *Gardnerella vaginalis* organisms are often associated with this condition and are often the organisms coating the epithelial cells (see Fig. 14-25).

## BLOOD CULTURES

Blood is normally sterile, and no microorganisms should be present. The careful and expeditious detection of blood-borne pathogens is a very important function of the microbiology laboratory.

Bacteremia (bacteria in the blood) can be a serious consequence of an infectious disease. Positive blood cultures can help provide a clinical diagnosis. Bacteria can be detected in the blood in the absence of disease, especially after dental extractions or any incident in which there has been a loss of integrity of the capillary endothelial cells; this would be called a transient bacteremia. **Septicemia** or **sepsis** indicates a situation in which the bacteria in the blood or a toxin produced by the bacteria is causing harm to the host (patient). **Fungemia,** the presence of fungi in the blood, can be found frequently in immunosuppressed hosts.

Symptoms of septicemia include increased pulse, fever, chills, and respiratory alkalosis. Some gram-negative organisms produce endotoxins when they break down, which can activate complement and the clotting factors and decrease the circulating granulocytes. Effects of certain bacterial products include disseminated intravascular coagulation, which may lead to septic shock accompanied by lowered blood pressure (hypotension), metabolic acidosis, intravascular coagulation, congestive heart failure, hyperventilation, oliguria, toxicity, and respiratory failure.

## Organisms Commonly Isolated from Blood

Portals of entry for organisms that can cause bacteremia or septicemia are the genitourinary tract (25%), the respiratory tract (20%), abscesses (10%), surgical wound infections (5%), and miscellaneous uncertain sites (25%).[1] Organisms most commonly cultured from blood are the gram-positive cocci, including *Staphylococcus aureus*, coagulase-negative *Staphylococcus*, the viridans *Streptococcus*, *Streptococcus pneumoniae*, and *Enterococcus* species. Organisms also found in blood are *Escherichia coli*, *Klebsiella*, *Pseudomonas*, *Enterobacter*, *Proteus*, *Salmonella*, and *Haemophilus*. Many of these organisms are likely to be found in the health care facility's environment and as normal flora; they are likely to colonize the skin, oropharyngeal area, and gastrointestinal tract of hospitalized patients.

The incidence of bacteremia or septicemia has increased over the past 25 years, most likely as a result of several factors—the decreased immunocompetency status of several patient populations, the increased use of invasive procedures such as intravenous catheters and vascular prostheses, the prolonged survival of debilitated and seriously ill patients, the increase in the aging population in general, and the increased use of therapeutic drugs such as broad-spectrum antibiotics, suppressing normal flora and allowing emergence of resistant strains of bacteria. These factors have made the interpretation of significant growth of microorganisms in the blood more difficult.

*Candida albicans* is the most common cause of fungemia. The incidence of fungemia is increased in immunocompromised patients. Standard blood culture systems are usually sufficient to isolate most fungi.

## Collecting the Specimen

Collection of blood for culture requires more exacting protocol than blood for most other laboratory tests. It is critical that additional care be taken to clean the skin at the venipuncture site in a special way to prevent any contamination from normal skin organisms present. The NCCLS has published recommendations for the collection of blood for culture, along with its information on venipuncture for routine laboratory testing.[9] Timing of the collection is also critical. After dental, colonoscopic, or cystoscopic procedures, bacteria may be present in the blood only for a brief period following the procedure. For intermittent bacteremias, bacteria are in the highest concentration before a fever spike. Intermittent bacteremia can occur as a result of wound abscesses or other infections. For continuous bacteremia, in which the organisms are from an intravascular source and are present in the blood consistently, the timing is not as critical. Ideally, blood should be collected before any antimicrobial agents are administered, as previous antimicrobial therapy may delay the growth of some organisms. A single culture is usually not sufficient to diagnose bacteremia.

Ideally, three cultures are drawn from separate sites, spaced at least 1 hour apart during a febrile episode. If two specimens must be drawn simultaneously, they should be drawn from two separate sites (e.g., the left arm and the right arm); one hour later the third culture should be drawn. Collecting more than three sets in a single day is discouraged, as additional cultures do not add to the recovery of significant organisms.

Since the volume of blood being tested is a major factor in detecting bacteria in blood cultures, for adults 8 to 10 mL of blood should be collected for each of the culture bottles—or approximately 30 mL total when three cultures are done. Into each of the three culture bottles, approximately 10 mL blood is inoculated. Smaller amounts are collected from children. Protocol for specific blood culture collection is established by each health care facility.

### Cleansing the Collection Site

Since it is necessary to avoid any normal skin flora contaminating the collection, it is critical that extra precautions be taken to cleanse the venipuncture site when blood is collected for culture. Proper disinfection of the skin is essential (see also under Blood Collection for Culture, in Chapter 3). The skin is cleaned by using a triple scrub with a povidone-iodine solution. Three times the skin is cleaned by using a concentric outward-moving circle beginning with the chosen venipuncture site and using a separate scrub applicator for each cleansing. An alternative disinfectant scrub is chlorhexidine gluconate, which can be used if a patient is allergic to the povidone-iodine solution most commonly used.

### Culture Media for Blood

The medium into which the blood is drawn is of an enrichment type, which encourages the growth and multiplication of all organisms present, even stray bacterial contaminants found as part of the normal skin flora. Blood can be collected by using a syringe and needle or, ideally, directly into culture bottles or tubes by using an evacuated (vacuum) system, which helps to prevent accidental needle sticks.

The basic culture medium for blood is a liquid that contains both a nutrient broth and an anticoagulant. Most commercially available blood culture media contain trypticase soy broth, brain-heart infusion agar, peptone supplement, or thioglycolate broth. In addition, an anticoagulant, 0.025% to 0.05% sodium polyanethol sulfonate (SPS), is commonly used in blood culture bottles because it does not harm the bacteria. A ratio of 1:5 or 1:10 blood to medium is found to be adequate for most laboratories.

For optimal recovery of blood-borne pathogens, the use of two different types or systems of blood culture media is recommended. One system can be vented, permitting oxygen from the air to enter the system for growth of aerobic organisms. The other can be incubated anaerobically, allowing growth of most facultative and anaerobic organisms.

If the blood to be cultured is not drawn directly into the culture medium, it must be collected into a collection tube with an anticoagulant. The best anticoagulant is sodium polyanethol sulfonate; SPS does not inhibit the growth of microorganisms, as other anticoagulants have been found to do. These tubes are then sent to the laboratory for inoculation into the culture media.

## Blood Culture Methods
### Incubating the Blood Cultures: Traditional Method

The protocol for blood culture followed by most clinical laboratories includes one culture bottle designated for recovery of aerobic organisms and one for recovery of anaerobic organisms.

After 6 to 18 hours of incubation at 35° to 37° C, most bacteria will be present in large enough numbers to detect. Detection includes doing blind subcultures on the aerobic bottle and direct smears on both anaerobic and aerobic bottles. The blind subcultures are made after the first 6 to 18 hours of incubation, and the bottles are reincubated for 7 days. A "blind" subculture means that culture bottles are subcultured to an appropriate medium (such as a chocolate blood agar plate, sheep blood agar, MacConkey agar) even if visible growth of organisms is not noted. In addition to the blind subculture, a routine direct smear is made, Gram stained, and examined for all culture bottles. This is done because some organisms do not produce turbidity, hemolysis, or gas in the growth medium—evidence of "growth." When there is macroscopic evidence of growth, use of a Gram stain of the medium is rewarding and a rapid identification procedure should be used (see under Biochemical or Enzymatic Tests, in this chapter). A number of rapid tests can be done using the broth blood culture. The use of phase microscopy may reveal morphologic details that will aid the physician in diagnosis and early treatment.

The blood culture bottles are examined visually at least once a day for 7 days. Growth of organisms is indicated by hemolysis of red blood cells, gas bubbles in the medium, turbidity, or the appearance of small colonies in the broth, on the surface of the red cell layer, or sometimes along the walls of the bottle. After 7 days, if no evidence of growth is noted, a report is made: "no aerobic and/or anaerobic growth after 7 days of incubation." If specific infections are suspected (bacterial endocarditis, fungemia, brucellosis, or anaerobic bacteremia), the bottles should be held for 2 weeks.

Subcultures of positive blood cultures are done to a variety of media types so that the growth of most organisms, anaerobes included, can be supported. All isolates from blood cultures should be stored for an indefinite period, preferably by freezing at $-70°$ C in 10% skim milk. An alternative is to store an agar slant of the isolate under sterile mineral oil at room temperature.

Any presumptive positive finding must be reported to the physician as soon as possible. The presumptive result must be verified by using conventional procedures and a pure culture of the organism isolated. The physician will use the report concerning any isolated organism to determine its significance for his or her patient.

### Automated Blood Culture Systems

Many laboratories now use an automated system to culture blood. The advantages of use of an automated system are a more rapid detection time for many pathogens, monitoring of growth without visual inspection or subculture of the culture bottles, and the ability to use the report in conjunction with a computerized laboratory management information system.

One automated system, Bactec,* allows a faster detection time for many pathogens, monitors growth without visual inspection or subcultures, and can automatically handle large numbers of blood culture bottles. Blood is inoculated into bottles that contain the necessary substrates, and at predetermined intervals the bottles are

---

*Becton Dickinson Diagnostic Instrument Systems, Towson, Md.

monitored by passage by a detector. The detector inserts two needles into each bottle through a rubber separator seal at the top of the bottle; the needles draw out the carbon dioxide gas that has accumulated above the liquid in the bottle—called headspace gas—and replace it with fresh gas. This system measures the production of carbon dioxide by the metabolizing organisms by using either radiometry or spectrophotometry. A level of carbon dioxide above a preset baseline value is considered suspicious of microbial growth in the specimen. The medium is automatically agitated during the incubation process, which encourages growth of aerobic and facultative organisms.

Newer technology has introduced blood culture systems that automatically and continuously monitor the carbon dioxide produced by using noninvasive means. Gas-permeable sensors use fluorescence to detect carbon dioxide. In some of these systems, the bottles are not punctured again once the initial sample has been inoculated. These systems improve the time to detection and show a reduced frequency of false positives.

## ANTIBIOTIC SUSCEPTIBILITY TESTS

One of the important functions of the medical microbiology laboratory is to test the isolated organisms for susceptibility to antimicrobial agents or antibiotics. To a large extent, the laboratory report showing susceptibility or resistance to a particular antibiotic determines whether the agent is used or withdrawn. In choosing an appropriate antimicrobial agent, the one with the most activity against the pathogen, the least toxicity to the host, the least impact on the normal flora, and the appropriate pharmacologic considerations, in addition to being the least expensive, should be selected to attain a more certain outcome for the treatment of the patient's infectious process.

In doing tests for antibiotic susceptibility (sensitivity), the laboratory must maintain a high level of accuracy in the testing procedures, there must be a high degree of reproducibility of results, and there must be a good correlation between the results and the clinical response of the patient.

## Sensitivity (Susceptibility) Versus Resistance

**Sensitivity** or **susceptibility** of an organism to an antibiotic is the ability of an antibiotic to inhibit the growth of the microorganism. Since the pattern of resistance and susceptibility is unpredictable, it is necessary to test isolated pathogenic organisms against the appropriate antimicrobial agents. Patterns of sensitivity and resistance are constantly changing. The organism is said to be **resistant** to an antibiotic if the antibiotic does not inhibit the growth of the organism. Many microorganisms, including bacteria and some fungi, have developed resistance even to the newest antibiotics.

## Minimal Inhibitory Concentration Versus Minimal Bactericidal Concentration

The lowest concentration of an antimicrobial agent that will inhibit the growth of the organism being tested is known as the **minimal inhibitory concentration (MIC).** This is detected by the lack of visual turbidity, matching that of a negative control included with the test. Many factors must be considered in choosing the specific antimicrobial agent, the MIC being one important consideration. MIC is determined by use of dilution antimicrobial susceptibility test methods.

The ability of an antimicrobial agent to inhibit the multiplication of an organism is measured by the MIC. Since MIC is a measure of organism inhibitory status, it is possible that when the antimicrobial agent is removed, the organism could begin once again to grow. In this case, the antimicrobial agent is called bacteriostatic or inhibitory. Sometimes, for certain infections, it is necessary to determine the ability of the agent to actually kill the organism. To determine the ability of the antimicrobial agent to kill the organism, a bactericidal activity test can be performed by

using a modification of the broth dilution susceptibility testing method; a **minimal bactericidal concentration (MBC)** is thus determined.

## Methods Used to Determine Antimicrobial Susceptibility

Susceptibility (or sensitivity) and resistance are functions of the site of the infection, the microorganism itself, and the antimicrobial agent being considered. By using a standard method, the microbiology laboratory can produce consistent results to aid the physician in his or her therapeutic choice. Two principal methods are employed to determine antimicrobial susceptibility: **agar disk diffusion tests,** employing antibiotic-impregnated disks, and **dilution tests,** such as broth tube dilution or agar plate dilution. Disk diffusion methods are not used as commonly now as in the past; they have been replaced by either broth microdilution or automated instrument methods in many laboratories.

Approved groupings of antimicrobial agents that should be considered for routine testing have been devised by the U.S. Food and Drug Administration for combinations of various groups of organisms.[7,8] Each laboratory must determine which of the many antimicrobial agents are appropriate for testing against the various organisms in its particular setting. The number of antimicrobials being tested against a single isolated organism is limited usually by the particular method being used. Disk diffusion plates (with 150 mm of agar) can usually accommodate no more than 12 disks, whereas some of the commercially available panels can test slightly more drugs on the same panel.

It is important to remember that any in vitro test for antibiotic sensitivity is an artificial measurement and will give only an estimate of the effectiveness of an agent against a microorganism in vivo. The only absolute test of antibiotic sensitivity is the clinical response of the patient to the dosage of the antibiotic.

The classic method for testing the susceptibility of microorganisms is the broth dilution method, yielding a quantitative result for the amount of antimicrobial agent needed to inhibit the growth of a specific microorganism, or the MIC. The NCCLS has published the complete protocol for this method.[7,8] The adaptation of the broth dilution methods to a microbroth method, either automated or done manually, is used by many laboratories because it saves time for the laboratorian doing the test, is cost effective, and gains efficiency from replicate inoculation of the prepared systems being used.

The preparation of the **inoculum** is the most important step in doing the susceptibility test.

The isolated organism being tested is first inoculated into a broth medium, whether a diffusion method or a macrodilution or microdilution method is used.

### Preparation of Inoculum

The number of organisms in an inoculum can be determined in different ways. One practical method is to compare the turbidity of the test liquid medium with that of a standard that represents a known number of bacteria in suspension. Chemical solutions of standard turbidity have been prepared using barium sulfate. Tubes with varying concentrations of this chemical were developed by McFarland to approximate numbers of bacteria in solutions of equal turbidity, as determined by doing colony counts in a counting chamber.[8] (See more about preparation of inoculum under Disk Diffusion Method [Kirby-Bauer Test] in this chapter.)

**McFarland Standards.** The standard used most frequently is the McFarland 0.5 standard, which contains 99.5 mL of 1% sulfuric acid and 0.5 mL of 1.175% barium chloride to obtain a barium sulfate solution with a very specific optical density. This provides a turbidity comparable to that of a bacterial suspension containing approximately $1.5 \times 10^8$ CFU/mL.

### Microdilution Method

The microdilution method utilizes plastic microdilution trays or panels and is used in many laboratories to give MIC results as part of the rou-

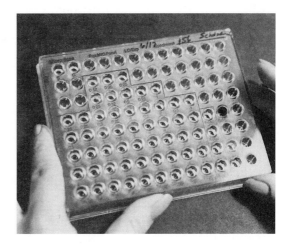

**FIG 16-13.** Plastic microdilution tray used for microbroth dilution antibiotic susceptibility testing. Antimicrobial agents are arranged in linear arrays of serial twofold dilutions. (From Baron EJ, Finegold SM: *Bailey and Scott's Diagnostic Microbiology*, ed 8. St Louis, Mosby, 1990, p 180.)

tine protocol for microbiology laboratory tests. This method permits a quantitative result to be reported (the MIC), indicating the amount of a drug needed to inhibit (or kill) the microorganism being tested. Most laboratories purchase the microdilution panels commercially. These have been prepared with the wells each holding a microamount of the varying concentrations of the various antimicrobial agents being tested, along with the necessary controls for growth and sterility tests (Fig. 16-13). They have been prepared under strict quality control standards, which assure the laboratory of consistent performance when they are used according to the manufacturer's directions. Usually a variety of panels containing different drug combinations are available for testing various groups of organisms.

Some microdilution systems are prepared and shipped in a frozen state. These are stored frozen until needed by the laboratory and must be thawed before use. These systems are easy to inoculate and usually include a disposable inoculating device, which allows a single inoculation of all the wells on the plate simultaneously. An-

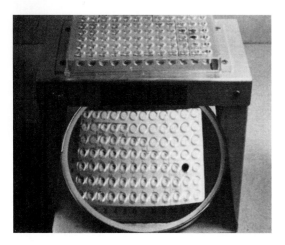

**FIG 16-14.** Reading microbroth dilution results using a magnifying mirror reader. (From Baron EJ, Finegold SM: *Bailey and Scott's Diagnostic Microbiology*, ed 8. St Louis, Mosby, 1990, p 180.)

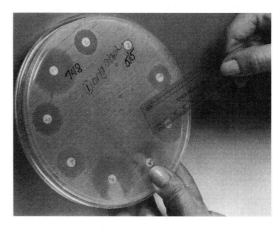

**FIG 16-15.** Measuring zones of inhibition on a disk diffusion susceptibility test plate. (From Baron EJ, Finegold SM: *Bailey and Scott's Diagnostic Microbiology*, ed 8. St Louis, Mosby, 1990, p 181.)

other type of system consists of dried or lyophilized antimicrobial agents, requiring reconstitution before use.

The standardized inoculum used to set up the microtiter panels is prepared and, by use of an intermediate dilution of this inoculum as determined by the manufacturer, the wells of the chosen panel are inoculated. Some manufacturers have special devices to facilitate inoculation of the panel, and most have prepared their systems to be read automatically or semiautomatically by being viewed with one of several panel-reading devices—a light box or from the bottom with a mirror reader (Fig. 16-14).

One completely automated system is the Vitek System,* in which the antimicrobial agents are contained in wells in a plastic card. The system includes a filler/sealer module, a reader incubator, a computer module, a data terminal, and a printer. The cards are incubated, and the wells are monitored for optical density. Results can be obtained in as early as 4 hours; however, the mean time is 7 hours for antimicrobial sus-

ceptibility testing. Other automated systems read the end point photometrically. One such system is the Baxter MicroScan AutoScan Walkaway.*

### Disk Diffusion Method (Kirby-Bauer Test)

Methods utilizing disks impregnated with various antimicrobial agents placed on an agar culture plate inoculated with the organism to be tested were used extensively before the advent of microdilution methodology.

For this test, the standardized inoculum is prepared as described and is swabbed over the surface of the agar plate, paper disks containing a single concentration of the chosen antimicrobial agent are placed onto the inoculated surface, and the plate is incubated overnight. The antimicrobial agent on the disk diffuses into the medium in a circle around the disk, inhibiting the growth of the organism wherever the concentration of the agent is sufficient. Large zones of inhibition are an indication of more antimicrobial activity or greater diffusibility of the drug, or both (Fig. 16-15). An area in which there

---

*bioMerieux Vitek, Hazelwood, Mo.

*Baxter Healthcare Corp, West Sacramento, Calif.

is no zone indicates complete resistance to the drug. This method is also commonly known as the Kirby-Bauer test.

By use of this method, several drug agents can be tested against one organism isolate at the same time. This method was first described by Bondi et al in 1947.[4] In 1966, Bauer et al standardized the method and correlated it with MICs.[3] They introduced standardized filter paper disks and enabled this method to be one that yielded qualitative results that correlated well with results obtained by MIC tests. This agar disk diffusion method continues to be used by many laboratories, as it is less expensive than the commercial microdilution method and standardization is not difficult. The results can be correlated directly with MIC values, but clinical interpretation of this method depends on performing the test with the established protocol.

Disks are commercially available for this method, and a special disk dispenser is used to distribute the appropriate disks on the inoculated plate. The plate is incubated overnight and observed the following morning. There will be a zone of growth inhibition around the disk containing the agent to which the organism is susceptible, whereas the organism will grow up to and under the periphery of the disks containing agents to which it is resistant. Much work has been done to standardize the disk procedure, and one modification used in many laboratories is that of Bauer et al.[3]

The disk diffusion test is more flexible than the commercially prepared microdilution panels, which are available only in standard panels of antimicrobials. The disk diffusion method allows a laboratory to choose any number of appropriate antimicrobial agents on the agar plate used for the test (usually 10 to 12 will fit on one plate). Because of this flexibility, it is also a cost-effective test.

The disk diffusion method is subject to Food and Drug Administration requirements, which cover standardization of media, formula, pH, agar depth, inoculum density, temperature, zone sizes, interpretative tables, and reference strains of bacteria for controls.

**Selection of Media for Plating.** For antibiotic sensitivity testing, the Mueller-Hinton (MH) agar plate is used. MH agar can be purchased commercially. The plates should be stored in the refrigerator until used and checked periodically for signs of water loss by evaporation. Plates can be saved longer by wrapping them in polystyrene and keeping them refrigerated.

**Handling and Storage of Antibiotic Disks.** Disks for antibiotic susceptibility testing are usually supplied in separate containers with a suitable desiccant to prevent deterioration. Most antibiotic disks should be refrigerated until used, but some require freezing to maintain their potency. The manufacturer's instructions for storage and handling should be followed. All disks must be discarded on their expiration dates.

**Preparation of Inoculum.** A tube of trypticase soy broth (5 mL) is inoculated with a pure culture of the organism to be tested, using four to five isolated colonies of similar morphology, and is incubated at 35° C for 4 hours or until the culture is visibly cloudy. For organisms that grow unpredictably in broth, fresh colonies (16- to 24-hour) grown overnight on an agar plate are inoculated directly into broth or saline and not incubated.

The turbidity of the test organism is compared with that of a McFarland barium sulfate standard. The standard must be vigorously mixed before use. The turbidity of the broth culture may be adjusted, if necessary, by being diluted with uninoculated broth in another tube. If the 4-hour broth tube does not have enough growth, it can be reincubated until adequate growth is observed. MH plates should be inoculated within 15 minutes of standardizing the broth.

**Inoculation of the Mueller-Hinton Agar Plate.** A sterile swab is dipped into the standardized, well-mixed broth culture inoculum, and any excess fluid is removed from the swab by squeezing it on the side of the tube. The swab is streaked across the plate in much the same way as for the quantitative urine culture plate (see Fig. 16-10). While the MH plate is being streaked, the same swab is used to inoculate an SB plate to check for purity. All organisms being tested should be inoculated onto their respective plates before any disks are applied. Plates should be labeled with the patient's name, type of specimen, organism, and date. They should be allowed to dry for at least 3 minutes before the disks are applied.

**Application of Disks.** The appropriate disks are applied to all the plates, using a disk dispenser if one is available. Special disk dispensers are available with different combinations of antibiotic-impregnated disks. Each disk should be firmly pressed down onto the surface of the agar with flamed and cooled forceps to ensure complete contact with the agar. The disks should be distributed so that they are no closer than 15 mm to the edge of the Petri dish and so that no two disks are closer than 24 mm from center to center. Once a disk has been placed, it should not be moved, as some diffusion of the antibiotic occurs almost immediately. The plates are incubated at 35° C for 18 hours.

**Reading of Results.** After incubation, the diameters of the zones of inhibition are measured with calipers or a zone reader and recorded to the nearest whole millimeter (see Fig. 16-15). Susceptibility of the organism to the antibiotic is demonstrated by a clear zone of growth inhibition around the disk. Within the limitations of the test, the diameter of the inhibition zone is a measure of the relative susceptibility to a particular antibiotic. The diameters are compared with a sensitivity table for each antibiotic to see whether the organism is sensitive, intermediate, or resistant to that particular antibiotic. These results are reported to the physician. The term susceptible or sensitive implies that an infection caused by the strain tested may be expected to respond favorably to the particular antibiotic. Resistant strains, on the other hand, are not inhibited completely by the usual therapeutic concentration of the antibiotic.

## QUALITY CONTROL IN THE MICROBIOLOGY LABORATORY

Quality control is necessary in microbiology as in the other areas of the laboratory. Established quality control procedures must be performed and results recorded.

### Control of Equipment

Equipment used in the microbiology laboratory can be easily controlled—for example, by monitoring the temperatures, daily or weekly, of incubators, refrigerators, water baths, freezers, and autoclaves. All monitoring data must be recorded as part of the laboratory's ongoing quality assurance program. Every laboratory handling biological material must have a biohazard safety hood and a biological safety cabinet for handling hazardous specimens and organisms.

### Control of Media

Most media are purchased ready-made from media companies. They are generally of high quality and provide good batch-to-batch consistency of results. Commercially prepared media must be stored and used in accord with manufacturers' directions and must be used within the specified expiration dates. Quality control measures are used during manufacture of commercial media to follow NCCLS recommendations (see Quality Control of Media, under Classification of Media).[10] If media are prepared by the laboratory, strict controls must be employed in the preparation. The best way to control the quality of media is by performance testing—checking the media with cultures of known stock microorganisms. Control strains of bacteria are available commercially.

### Control of Reagents and Antisera

Reagents should be tested daily, with few exceptions, using both positive and negative controls. New batches of reagents must also be tested in the same manner. Reagents should be dated when they are prepared, as are reagents in other areas of the laboratory. New reagents should be tested with known control cultures.

Gram-staining reagents are best checked by staining and examining slides prepared with known suspensions of gram-negative and gram-positive organisms.

## Control of Antimicrobial Tests

Laboratories must periodically monitor their performance of methods used for antimicrobial testing, following NCCLS recommendations.[8] Control organisms are specific strains of common organisms available for this purpose. The commercially available microdilution broth plates contain their own controls—some for sterility of the plate itself and others for growth. It is always important to carefully follow directions supplied with commercial products used.

## Maintenance of Stock Cultures

Each microbiology laboratory must maintain known stock cultures of organisms to participate in a quality control program. They are available from several sources—commercially, from proficiency testing isolates, from patient isolates, and so forth. In participating in a quality control program, when the testing appears to have failed, it is, more often than not, the stock culture that has failed rather than the test itself.

## Control of Specimens and Specimen Collection

If proper protocols and procedures are not in place regarding the collection of patient specimens and the procedures for handling these specimens in the laboratory, the identification of pathogens is not very meaningful and quality assurance is not being practiced. Strict adherence to proper procedures for sample collection must be enforced and repeat collections made if the circumstances demand it.

## TESTS FOR FUNGI (MYCOLOGY)

In the clinical laboratory, identification of yeasts and molds is an important service. Fungi are well recognized as a common cause of infection, and to provide a sufficient mycology service (the study of fungi), the microbiology labora-tory should include the direct examination of clinical specimens and information about the proper collection, culturing, and transportation of these specimens to a reference laboratory, if needed.

With the advent of chemotherapy, radiation treatment, and diseases such as acquired immunodeficiency syndrome (AIDS)—factors altering the human immune system—fungi existing in the environment that were not previously considered pathogenic are now causing disease in certain patient populations. When an organism is isolated in an immunocompromised patient, it must be considered a significant finding and used in the course of treatment of that patient, even if the finding of that organism had formerly been considered insignificant for an immune-intact individual.

## Characteristics of Fungi

Fungi include both yeasts and molds and differ significantly from bacteria. Fungi are eukaryotes, possessing a true nucleus with a nuclear membrane and mitochrondria, while bacteria are prokaryotes, lacking these structures. The fungi that are seen in the clinical laboratory—yeasts and molds—can be separated into the two groups on the basis of the macroscopic appearance of the colonies formed.

Yeasts are one-celled organisms that reproduce by budding. Yeasts produce moist, opaque, creamy, or pasty colonies on culture media, whereas molds produce fluffy, cottony, woolly, or powdery colonies. All yeasts look similar microscopically and therefore need to be differentiated on the basis of results of biochemical tests.

Molds have a basic structure that is made up of tube-like projections called **hyphae** or **mycelium.** As hyphae grow, they intertwine to form a loose network called a mycelium, which can be aerial or vegetative. Most molds have mycelia; yeasts do not, although some have pseudomyelia, or pseudohyphae (see also under Characteristics of Fungi). Pseudohyphae project from the edges of the colony as filamentous extensions with constrictions. The walls of true hyphae are parallel and do not have constrictions.

Molds are filamentous fungi. Types of mycelium can be recognized microscopically, which can assist in the early identification of certain molds. Molds have their characteristic "fuzzy" or woolly appearance because of their mycelia.

## Fungi as a Source of Infection

Fungi normally live a nonpathogenic existence in nature, enriched by decaying nitrogenous material. Humans become infected with fungi through accidental exposure by inhalation of spores or by their introduction into tissue through trauma. Any alteration in the immunologic status of the host can result in infection by fungi that are normally nonpathogenic; most yeast infections are opportunistic. The most frequently isolated yeast is *Candida albicans*, part of the normal flora of the gastrointestinal tract in persons with intact immunity.

Fungal infections (or mycoses) can be superficial, cutaneous, subcutaneous, or systemic. A superficial mycosis is one confined to the outermost skin and hair layer, with symptoms of discoloration, scaling, or depigmentation of the skin. Cutaneous infections affect the keratinized layer of the skin, hair, or nails. Symptoms of these infections include itching, scaling, or ring-like patches of the skin; brittle or broken hairs; and thick, discolored nails. Subcutaneous infections affect the deeper layers of the skin, including muscle and connective tissue; these infections do not usually disseminate through the blood to other organs. Symptoms include ulcers that progress and do not heal and the presence of draining sinus tracts. Systemic mycoses affect internal organs or the deep tissues of the body. Commonly the original site of these systemic infections is the lung, from which the organisms usually disseminate via the bloodstream (hematogenous spread) to other sites in the body. Infiltrates may be seen in the pulmonary system on x-ray. Symptoms can be very general, such as fever and fatigue; other symptoms include a chronic cough and chest pain.

Fungal infections can occur in persons with diabetes mellitus or other chronic, debilitating diseases, or in persons with impaired immuno-logic function resulting from drug therapies with corticosteroids or antimetabolites. In recent years, there have been more fungal infections in immunocompromised patients. Fungi are not communicable in the usual person-to-person or animal-to-person transmittance.

## Collection of Specimens for Fungal Studies

Any tissue or body fluid can be cultured for fungi, but the most common specimens are respiratory secretions (sputum, bronchial washings); *C. albicans* can be found in the sputum of immunocompromised individuals, for example (Fig. 16-16). Other specimens cultured for fungi include hair, skin, nails and nail scrapings, urine, blood or bone marrow, tissue, other ordinarily sterile body fluids, and cerebrospinal fluid. **Fungemia,** or fungi in the bloodstream, is most commonly caused by *C. albicans*. Many of the specimens collected for fungal identification will be contaminated with bacteria and/or rapidly growing fungi. For this reason, the media used should contain antibiotics to inhibit these organisms and allow the pathogens to grow; an example of such a medium is Sabouraud dextrose agar with antibiotics (SAB). The selection of specimen

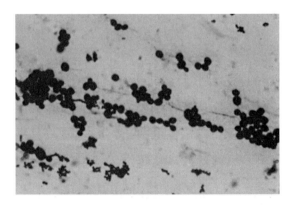

**FIG 16-16.** Gram stain of sputum with *Candida albicans* showing purple, blue/black oval yeast cells with some budding. (From Delost MD: *Introduction to Diagnostic Microbiology: A Text and Workbook*, St Louis, Mosby, 1997, p 379.)

to be tested, along with collection techniques for specimens to be used for fungal studies, is directly related to the diagnosis of fungal infections. It is extremely important that specimens be appropriately collected from the proper site in order that the fungi be recovered.

It is also important that a specimen for fungal studies be transported to the laboratory as quickly as possible. Because many pathogenic fungi grow slowly, any delay in transporting or processing a specimen can compromise the quality of the specimen and the eventual prospects of isolating the causative organism. Overgrowth with contaminating bacteria is common when slow-growing fungi are being tested.

## Methods for Detection of Fungi

Because there has been an increase in the number of fungal infections—specifically yeast infections, primarily in immunocompromised patients—there is an increased need for the detection of these infecting organisms so that treatment may be started.

To begin the identification process in the laboratory, specimens for fungal studies should be microscopically examined directly and cultured immediately to ensure the recovery of the suspected fungal organism from the specimen.

### Direct Microscopic Examination of Fungi

Examination of the specimen microscopically is an important part of the microbiology laboratory's fungal identification process. It provides a rapid method, which in some cases leads to a tentative immediate diagnosis; this, in turn may result in the early initiation of treatment. Direct microscopic examination can often provide the first microbiological evidence of fungal etiology in patients with suspected fungal infections; several stains can be used for this purpose. Direct examination can also show specific morphologic characteristics and present a rationale for choice of special media to be inoculated immediately. The initial stain used is generally Gram stain, but other direct stains or procedures can give more specific information regarding the identity of the infecting organism.

**Gram Stain.** This is the stain commonly used for most clinical microbiological specimens. It also will detect most fungi, if present in the specimen (see also Smear Preparation and Stains Used in Microbiology). Yeast will appear gram positive (purple, blue/black) and will often show its budding tendencies when examined microscopically using the oil-immersion objective (see Fig. 16-16).

**Potassium Hydroxide Preparation.** This has been the traditionally recommended preparation for detecting fungal elements in the skin, hair, nails, and tissue. Addition of a 10% solution of potassium hydroxide (KOH) reagent clears the specimen, making the fungi more easily visible. On a glass slide, a drop of the specimen is mixed with a drop of 10% KOH, a coverglass is applied, and the slide is scanned for fungal elements using the low-power objective. Any fungi present will be seen, because the KOH reagent has dissolved the keratin and cellular material in the specimen. If the specimen is extremely viscous, an overnight incubation of the wet-mounted slide in a humidified chamber may be necessary. If the slide appears cloudy, warming may help to clear it for viewing the fungi.

**KOH with Calcofluor White.** Calcofluor white, a fluorescent dye, can be mixed with potassium hydroxide, a drop mixed with the specimen on the glass slide, coverslipped, and observed using a fluorescence microscope. Use of this preparation detects the presence of fungi rapidly (in 1 minute) by visualization of a bright apple green or blue-white fluorescencee, depending on the filters used in the microscope. The calcofluor white binds to polysaccharides present in the fungus or to cellulose; any element with a polysaccharide skeleton fluoresces. This method does require a fluorescence microscope, but fungi exhibit an intense, easily recognizable fluorescence with this type of microscopy.

**India Ink.** A drop of India ink may be added to a drop of cerebrospinal fluid sediment from the centrifuged specimen and the specimen examined under high-power magnification. The presence of the encapsulated yeast *Cryptococcus neoformans* can be seen by using this preparation. This is a negative staining method, whereby the budding yeast will be seen surrounded by a large clear area against a black background, and is presumptive evidence of an infection with *C. neoformans*. India ink preparations have, for the most part, been replaced with direct antigen detection tests for cryptococcus.

**Acid-Fast Stain.** This stain is used to detect mycobacteria but can also detect *Nocardia* (see also Smear Preparation and Stains Used in Microbiology). Acid-fast stain is primarily used to differentiate *Nocardia* species from other actinomycetes.

### Culture of Fungi

Specimens to be cultured for fungi should be inoculated on a general-purpose medium with and without cycloheximide (see Culture Media below). Mold cultures should be handled in a class II biological safety cabinet to prevent aerosol dissemination of fungal elements—mold can be highly mobile. Yeast cultures can be handled on a regular bench top with no extra protection other than the usual universal precautions for safety. Numerous species of *Candida* and other yeasts have been identified. Relatively few types of media are needed to culture fungi. Laboratories will differ in their protocols for media chosen for fungal culture.

**Culture Media.** Sabouraud dextrose agar with antibiotics (SAB) medium favors growth of fungi over bacteria and is recommended for primary isolation of dermatophytes. The addition of the antimicrobial agents cycloheximide and chloramphenicol inhibits bacterial growth. Media with a combination of equal parts of Sabouraud dextrose agar and brain-heart infusion (BHI) agar have proved to be useful for isolation of clinically significant fungi, particularly from specimens also containing bacteria,

such as sputum specimens. Most specimens for fungal identification are also contaminated with bacteria and other rapidly growing fungi, and it is important that antibacterial and antifungal agents be included in the culture medium. Some fungi require the presence of blood in the medium (sheep blood agar).

Culture dishes or screw-capped culture tubes are used for satisfactory recovery of fungi.

### Examination of the Culture

Fungal cultures are incubated at room temperature (at 25° to 30° C) for 4 to 6 weeks and examined weekly or twice a week for growth before being reported as negative. One of the first decisions is whether the microorganism is a yeast or a mold. Characteristic gross culture growth and microscopic features are observed to make this determination. Gross features, such as colony color, texture, and growth rate are necessary initial observations.

**Microscopic Examination of the Isolated Microorganism.** Once the organism has been isolated, a direct mount is commonly done and examined microscopically. Identification of yeasts requires that certain microscopic features be present, as well as the use of biochemical tests to confirm the species identification. Identification of molds also requires that certain microscopic morphologic features be present (see also under Characteristics of Fungi).

Yeasts are usually unicellular microorganisms that reproduce asexually by budding; the appearance of the colony is a collection of distinct individual organisms that resemble the appearance of bacterial colonies on the agar surface. On culture media, *Candida albicans* colonies appear heaped and dull and may resemble those of staphylococci. Some yeasts may have pseudohyphae, which project from the edges of the colony as filamentous extensions; these are not the true hyphae of molds. The walls of true hyphae are parallel and do not have the constrictions seen in the pseudohyphae. In contrast, molds are filamentous fungi with tube-like projections or hyphae, and as the hyphae grow, they intertwine to form a loose network called the mycelium. Identification of different types of hyphae can be done to identify the various types of molds. With practice, laboratorians are able to identify the fungi commonly found in clinical specimens. A practical working schema has been suggested by Winn and Westenfeld, which can assist the laboratorian in this identification.[13]

**Germ-Tube Test.** Another test done to specifically identify *Candida albicans* is the germ-tube test. This test depends on *C. albicans* being able to produce germ tubes from their yeast cells when placed in a liquid nutrient environment and incubated at 35° C for 3 hours. It is important that the incubation time be limited to 3 hours, as other species will begin to form structures resembling germ tubes with prolonged incubation. This allows an early identification of the most common and important yeast pathogens; 75% of yeasts recovered in the laboratory can be identified by using the germ-tube test. A **germ tube** is defined as an appendage that is one-half the width and three to four times the length of the yeast cell from which it arises; germ tubes are the beginnings of true hyphae (Fig. 16-17).

### Biochemical Screening Methods

Biochemical tests are necessary for yeast identification, but microscopic confirmation is also im-

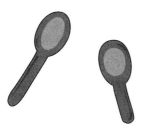

**FIG 16-17.** *Candida albicans* germ tube. (From Delost MD: *Introduction to Diagnostic Microbiology: A Text and Workbook,* St Louis, Mosby, 1997, p 380.)

portant. Rapid manual biochemical screening tests are used by some laboratories, and commercially available yeast identification systems have provided others with standardized identification procedures. Biochemical tests include a rapid urease test, used to screen urease-producing yeasts, and a rapid nitrate reductase test (see also Biochemical or Enzymatic Tests). An alternative to this rapid test is the use of urea agar, which requires incubation (see also Urea Agar, under Commonly Used Types of Media).

Commercially available yeast identification systems are also in common use by many laboratories. These methods are, for the most part, rapid, and the results are available within 72 hours. These systems utilize a large database of information based on thousands of yeast biotypes and consider a number of variations and reaction patterns when presenting the result. One method utilizes a number of biochemical tests whose reactions are monitored by various indicator systems after addition of a reagent to certain substrates. This system is designed to give an identification within 4 hours. Some systems take longer for the final identification process. In general, these commercial identification systems are easy to use, easy to interpret, and relatively inexpensive when compared with the conventional testing methods.

## TESTS FOR PARASITES (PARASITOLOGY)

Human parasitic infections occur worldwide, although more of these problems arise in tropical areas. Parasites affect their hosts by their actions; parasites and hosts represent symbiotic relationships in which two or more organisms live together. An **obligate parasite** cannot survive without its designated host. A **facultative parasite** can exist in a free-living state as a commensal or as a parasite. In the **commensal state,** the parasite and the host exist together with no harm coming to the host; the relationship is beneficial to both. **Parasitism** results when the parasite injures its host by its actions.

## Parasites as a Source of Infection

Because many persons have lived or traveled in tropical areas and because there has been a great influx of refugee populations into the United States, many organisms endemic elsewhere are being seen in people now living in this country. Still another consideration is the number of immunocompromised patients, who are very much at risk for certain parasitic infections.

Human parasites belong to five main groups. These are the Protozoa (amebae, flagellates, ciliates, sporozoans, etc.); the Platyhelminthes or flatworms; the Acanthocephala or thorny-headed worms; the Nematoda or roundworms; and the Arthropoda (insects, spiders, mites, and ticks). Parasitic infections are usually diagnosed by detecting and identifying the **ova** (parasite eggs), **larvae** (immature form), or adults of some types of parasites, usually the helminths, and the **cysts** (inactive stage) or **trophozoites** (motile forms) of others, usually the protozoa. Most protozoa have two developmental stages, the ova, usually found in the formed feces, and the trophozoite, usually found in loose or watery stools. Finding protozoan ova usually indicates that the infection is in an inactive or carrier state, while finding trophozoites—the active feeding stage—usually indicates an active infectious disease.

The identification of the various types of parasitic organisms depends on morphologic criteria. There are also various immunologic tests now available to detect parasitic infections. It is important that the infecting parasitic organism be identified specifically, because treatment is dependent on the type of parasite found and its site of infestation. Any identification process first depends on correct specimen collection and adequate fixation. Specimens for parasitic identification include feces, urine, blood, sputum, and tissue biopsies.

The patient's symptoms and clinical history, including travel, are significant pieces of information to be collected and shared with the clinical laboratory. Good lines of communication between the laboratorian and the physician will ensure that the appropriate specimen is collected and handled properly during the clinical workup

of the patient. Since the field of medical parasitology is vast and the knowledge base of practitioners variable, medical parasitology textbooks should be consulted for in-depth studies. There are excellent resource textbooks and other references, which contain the specific morphologic criteria needed to correctly identify the more common parasites. One recommended reference for medical parasitology is Garcia and Bruckner's *Diagnostic Medical Parasitology*, second edition (American Society for Microbiology, Washington, D.C., 1993).

## Collection of Specimens for Parasite Identification

Specimens for parasite identification come primarily from the intestinal tract as fecal specimens, from the urogenital tract as a vaginal or urethral discharge or as a prostatic secretion, from sputum, from cerebrospinal fluid, or from biopsy material from other body tissues. Blood can also be examined for malarial parasites such as *Plasmodium*. Each specimen has unique morphologic criteria for the particular parasites inhabiting the area. Inadequate or improper specimen collection may result in misidentification or failure to identify the infecting organism.

### Fecal Specimens

Identification of intestinal parasites, particularly protozoa, requires that specific collection protocol be followed; the quality of the specimen being analyzed is directly related to the ability to detect and identify intestinal parasites. Specimen requirements for the identification processes should be consulted. A single fecal specimen may not be sufficient to isolate an intestinal parasite, for example, as many intestinal parasitic organisms shed eggs or cysts on a variable schedule. It has been recommended that the collection of three fecal samples spaced a day or two apart, but all collected within a 10-day period, be done to provide optimal detection of intestinal parasites.

Collection of fecal samples for parasites should always be done before radiological studies involving barium sulfate are done; the use of barium will affect the sample for at least a week. Certain medications can also affect the detection of parasites in fecal samples.

A clean, dry, waterproof container with a tight-fitting lid is an appropriate collection container for a fecal sample for parasite studies. Contaminating the specimen with water or urine should be avoided. The sample should be sent to the laboratory as soon as possible. Commercially available transport systems are available that will preserve the fecal sample. Any fecal sample should be handled carefully, as it is a potential source of infection.

### Blood Specimens

Thick and thin blood smears are made, to allow for better detection of malarial parasites. The thick smear is used to screen a larger volume of blood; the thin smear to identify the parasite specifically when the screen is positive. Giemsa hematologic stain can be used to detect the blood parasites. (See under Blood and Tissue Microorganisms.)

## Methods for Detection of Parasites

Methods for parasite detection vary with the specimen and its source. Since many parasitic infections are diagnosed through identification of eggs or larvae in a fecal sample, methods of detection in feces are discussed more completely than detection using other specimens. Examination of a direct wet mount of a fecal specimen is used to detect the presence of motile protozoan trophozoites and flagellates. A fecal concentration method—flotation or sedimentation—can be done to enhance the detection of smaller numbers of parasites. Commercial products are available for the specimen collection and detection of some parasites. Permanent stained smears are made to confirm identification. Quality assurance of detection and identification results begins with the use of properly collected specimens. (See more under Common Parasites Identified.)

### Wet Mount, Direct Smear

A smear is prepared by mixing a small amount of the sample (usually feces) with a drop of phys-iologic saline on a glass slide, adding a coverslip, and examining the slide for trophozoites. The smear is also examined for helminth ova (eggs), larvae, and protozoan cysts. Motility is also observed.

## Common Parasites Identified
### Trichomonas vaginalis

*Trichomonas vaginalis* is an intestinal flagellate, a parasite that can inhabit the urogenital system of both males and females. It is considered a pathogenic parasite; it is the cause of vaginitis, urethritis, and prostatitis, usually considered sexually transmitted diseases. The motile trophozoite stage is found in freshly voided urine of both sexes, in prostatic secretions, and in vaginal wet preparations. The diagnosis is usually made by observation of the motile trophozoite—a pear-shaped, elongated form—in fresh urine and urogenital specimens. The parasites are observed to move with a jerky and undulating motion; they are approximately the size of a neutrophil. As movement slows down, the undulating membrane may usually be seen (Fig. 16-18).

Motile trophozoites of *T. vaginalis* can be identified only in very fresh urine specimens and fresh genital secretions; they cannot be identified in old urine specimens or dry vaginal or prostatic secretions because they are no longer motile or viable and their morphology generally has

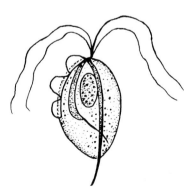

**FIG 16-18.** *Trichomonas vaginalis* trophozoite. (Illustration by Nobuko Kitamura. From Baron EJ, Peterson LR, Finegold SM: *Bailey and Scott's Diagnostic Microbiology*, ed 9. St Louis, Mosby, 1994, p 796.)

changed, becoming rounded up and resembling a white blood cell or a transitional epithelial cell. For this reason, proper specimen collection and immediate transportation to the laboratory for analysis are very important in the identification process (see also Chapter 14).

The most sensitive identification method for *T. vaginalis* is culture, and commercial products are available for this purpose. One product is a self-contained system, the InPouch TV System,* used for detection of the organism by both culture and direct microscopic examination. The transport and culture vessel is a flexible, clear plastic pouch with water-vapor and oxygen barrier qualities. Use of this product results in a reduced-oxygen environment, which enhances and maintains the desired selective growth characteristics of the media. The system consists of two pouches; one can be used for immediate microscopic examination and the other for culture. An open plastic viewing frame comes with the system, which allows for correct positioning and viewing of the pouch under the microscope. With this viewing system, when no trichomonads are seen under low power—confirmed by high-power examination—the inoculum has fewer than 100 organisms.

### Intestinal Ova and Parasites

Many parasitic infections are diagnosed through identification of their eggs (ova) or larvae in a fecal sample; the parasites are residing in the intestinal tract. Fecal specimens for ova and parasite studies must be preserved or fixed immediately. A pH indicator is also added to attain an approximate pH of 7. Most commercial collection kits for these tests contain the appropriate preservative and pH indicator. The preservative-fixative for specimens to be tested for ova and parasites is formalin or polyvinyl alcohol (PVA). It is important to be aware of possible collection problems, such as that any collection of ova and parasite fecal specimens should be done prior to radiologic studies using barium sulfate, since an excess of the

barium crystalline materials interferes with the detection of the parasites for up to a week after the use of barium. Other interfering substances are mineral oil, bismuth, some antidiarrheal preparations, antimalarials, and some antibiotics. Contamination with urine should also be avoided.

For a routine examination for intestinal parasites—prior to any treatment—a minimum of three specimens should be collected. Many parasitic organisms do not appear in fecal specimens in consistent numbers on a daily basis; thus many procedures call for the collection of specimens on alternate days. A series of three specimens should be collected within no more than 10 days, and a series of six within no more than 14 days. If amebiasis is suspected, a series of six specimens should be collected.

**Macroscopic Examination.** Macroscopic examination includes observation of the consistency of the specimen. A fecal specimen of normal consistency—in which the moisture content is decreased—will more likely yield cyst stages because the protozoan parasite has encysted to survive. In a soft or liquid sample, the trophozoite stages are more likely to be found. Occasionally, adult helminths can be seen on the surface of the feces. The presence of blood should be noted; dark feces may indicate bleeding high in the gastrointestinal tract, whereas bright red feces indicates bleeding at a lower level.

**Microscopic Examination.** Direct wet mounts of the specimen are observed to detect helminth eggs and motile trophozoite stages of the protozoa. It is not sufficient to identify the protozoa by using only the direct wet mount preparation. Permanent stained smears should also be examined to confirm the identification of the parasitic organism.

The microscopic identification of intestinal protozoa and helminth ova is based on recognition of specific morphologic characteristics by a laboratorian experienced in parasitology. In these studies, it is imperative that a good microscope, with a good light source, be used. The micro-

---

*BioMed Diagnostics, San Jose, Calif.

scope should be equipped with a calibrated ocular micrometer to measure the size of the ova and parasites seen. Quality control requirements demand that each calibrated microscope be recalibrated once a year.

To observe the sample microscopically, a small amount of the sample is mixed with a drop of physiologic saline on a glass slide and the mixture is coverslipped. Correct light adjustment, as for unstained urine sediment, is needed to see the motile trophozoite stages of the protozoa, as they are very pale and transparent.

After examination of the wet preparation is complete, a drop of weak iodine solution can be placed at the edge of the coverslip. This stained preparation will assist in the identification of protozoan cysts that stain with iodine. These will be seen as cysts with yellow-gold cytoplasm, brown glycogen material, and paler refractile nuclei. Other stains are used to reveal nuclear detail in the trophozoite stages of the protozoa. A permanent stained smear is used to confirm the identification of intestinal protozoa.

**Concentration Procedures.** Concentration of fecal material should be included in a complete parasite examination. Concentration procedures allow the visualization of small numbers of parasite organisms that may be missed if only a direct mount is observed. Various concentration procedures are used; sedimentation or flotation techniques are generally employed.

Flotation procedures allow the separation of protozoan cysts and certain helminth eggs. In this procedure, a reagent with a high specific gravity is used, such as zinc sulfate. The parasitic elements will be in the surface layer of the mixture, and the debris will be in the bottom layer. Some helminth or protozoan eggs do not concentrate well with the flotation method.

Sedimentation procedures use gravity or centrifugation and allow recovery of all protozoa, eggs, and larvae present in the specimen.

**Permanent Stained Smears.** The confirmation of identification of intestinal protozoa requires the preparation of a permanent stained smear. Permanent smears also provide a permanent record of the examination. To prepare slides for staining, fixation/preservation is first necessary. Fresh feces fixed in Schaudinn fixative or a PVA-preserved sample can be stained. PVA-preserved samples are made by mixing polyvinyl alcohol reagent with one or two drops of fecal material directly on a slide and allowing the slide to dry for several hours (at 35° C) or overnight (at room temperature). Permanent stains used include iron hematoxylin and trichrome. Trichrome stains are most commonly used.

### Enterobius vermicularis (*Pinworm*)

*Enterobius vermicularis,* or pinworm (also known as seatworm), is a common parasite in children worldwide. It is a roundworm whose adult female migrates from the anus during the night, depositing her eggs in the perianal region—making a fecal sample not an optimal specimen, as the eggs may not be observed in the feces. Most laboratories use the clear cellophane tape method to collect and prepare the specimen for examination.

**Cellophane Tape Collection Method.** The cellophane tape method is commonly used to collect the specimen. A piece of clear cellophane tape (not Magic transparent tape), with the sticky side toward the patient, is pressed against the skin across the anal opening to collect any eggs, using even, thorough pressure. The sticky side of the tape is then placed down against the surface of a clean glass slide with a glass coverslip. The slide should be labeled with the patient's name and any other identifying data. Commercial collection kits are available, simplifying the collection process. These specimens must be collected first thing in the morning, before bathing, defecating, or urinating. Negative findings must be confirmed with more tests done on subsequent days.

The microscopic examination is performed by adding a small drop of toluene or xylene under the tape and coverslip on the slide. This will clear the tape so that the ova of the pinworm may be observed. The slide is scanned for the characteristically shaped eggs of the organism, using low- and high-power magnification. They are ellipsoid (football shaped) with one slightly flattened side (Fig. 16-19). A known control slide of pinworm ova should be used for comparison purposes.

### Blood and Tissue Microorganisms

Malaria is the most common infectious disease worldwide, and its rapid laboratory diagnosis is important. Diagnosis is dependent on clinical symptoms (headache, low-grade fever, chills, sweats, nausea) and identification of the *Plasmodium* malarial parasites in the red blood cells. The malarial parasite enters the human through a bite from an infected mosquito.

Tick-borne infectious agents can cause disease; some agents are parasites, others are not. A sample of these infectious processes includes babesiosis, Lyme disease, and ehrlichiosis. Babesiosis is a disease that clinically resembles malaria. *Babesia* organisms are tick-borne sporozoan parasites. Diagnosis of babesiosis is made through identification of *Babesia* parasites in the red blood cells. Another tick-borne disease is Lyme disease, the etiologic agent being the bacterium *B. burgdorferi.* Transmission occurs by inoculation by a bite of a tick of the genus *Ixodes.* Diagnosis of Lyme disease depends on finding antibodies in the serum or spinal fluid. Ehrlichiosis is another infectious process that is tick borne. The organism, *Ehrlichia chaffeenis,* is a gram-negative, obligate intracellular rickettsia-like organism that multiplies in the white cells. Diagnosis is made by direct visualization of clusters of the organisms in the phagosomes of white cells, using Giemsa stain or by indirect immunofluorescence for detection of antibodies.

Lung tissue or secretions can be infected with *Pneumocystis carinii,* usually only symptomatic in immunosuppressed individuals. *P. carinii* pneumonia is seen in patients with AIDS and is a leading cause of death for these patients.

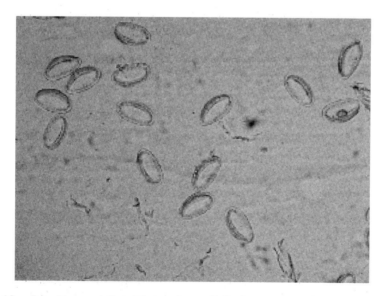

**FIG 16-19.** *Enterobius vermicularis* (pinworm) eggs. Cellophane tape preparation used for collection. (From Baron EJ, Peterson LR, Finegold SM: *Bailey and Scott's Diagnostic Microbiology,* ed 9. St Louis, Mosby, 1994, p 852.)

**Malarial Parasites.** The malarial parasites enter the bloodstream and invade the red blood cells. Blood should be drawn for this test immediately before a fever spike is expected, as this is when the greatest number of organisms is likely to be present. Smears made from fresh capillary blood, at the bedside of the patient, are preferred. Thin and thick smears are prepared, stained with Wright or Giemsa stain, and examined for presence of the blood parasites. The thick smears are more difficult to interpret but increase the sensitivity by concentrating the cells and the organisms. The thin smears are used to better identify the species of the malarial parasite. Correct therapy is dependent on identification of the specific variety of malarial organism present in the blood.

# REFERENCES

1. Baron EJ, Peterson LR, Finegold SM: *Bailey and Scott's Diagnostic Microbiology*, ed 9. St Louis, Mosby, 1994, p 197.
2. Baron EJ, Tyburski M, Almon R, et al: Visual and clinical analysis of Bac-T-Screen urine screen results. *J Clin Microbiol* 1988; 26:2382.
3. Bauer AW, Kirby WWM, Sherris JC, et al: Antibiotic susceptibility testing by a standardized single disc method. *Am J Clin Pathol* 1966; 45:493-496.
4. Bondi A, Spaulding EH, Smith ED, et al: A routine method for the rapid determination of susceptibility to penicillin and other antibiotics. *Am J Med Sci* 1947; 214:221-225.
5. Centers for Disease Control and National Institutes of Health: *Biosafety in Microbiological and Biomedical Laboratories*, ed 2. Washington, DC, US Department of Health and Human Services, Public Health Service, 1988, HHS publication no (NIH) 88-8395.
6. Harbeck RJ, Teague J, et al: Novel, rapid optical immunoassay technique for detection of group A streptococci from pharyngeal specimens: comparison with standard culture methods. *J Clini Microbiol* 1993; April:839-844.
7. NCCLS: *Methods for Dilution Antimicrobial Susceptibility Tests for Bacteria That Grow Aerobically: Approved Standard*, ed 4. Villanova, Pa, National Committee for Clinical Laboratory Standards, 1997, document no M7-A4.
8. NCCLS: *Performance Standards for Antimicrobial Disk Susceptibility Test: Approved Standard*, ed 6. Villanova, Pa, National Committee for Clinical Laboratory Standards, 1990, document no M2-A6.
9. NCCLS: *Procedures for the Collection of Diagnostic Blood Specimens by Venipuncture: Approved Standard*, ed 3. Villanova, Pa, National Committee for Clinical Laboratory Standards, 1991, document no H3-A3.
10. NCCLS: *Quality Assurance for Commercially Prepared Microbiological Culture Media: Approved Standard*, ed 2. Villanova, Pa, National Committee for Clinical Laboratory Standards, 1996, document no M22-A2.
11. Sneath PHA, Mair NS, et al (eds): *Bergey's Manual of Systematic Bacteriology*, vol 2. Baltimore, Williams & Wilkins, 1986.
12. Washington JA II, White CM, Laganiere M, et al: Detection of significant bacteriuria by microscopic examination of urine. *Lab Med* 1981; 12:294.
13. Winn WC, Westenfeld FW: Mycotic diseases. In Henry JB (ed): *Clinical Diagnosis and Management by Laboratory Methods*, ed 19. Philadelphia, WB Saunders Co, 1996, p 1219.

# BIBLIOGRAPHY

Baron EJ, Peterson, LR, Finegold SM: *Bailey and Scott's Diagnostic Microbiology*, ed 9. St Louis, Mosby, 1994.

Becan-McBride K, Ross DL: *Essentials for the Small Laboratory and Physician's Office*. St Louis, Mosby, 1988.

Delost MD: *Introduction to Diagnostic Microbiology: A Text and Workbook*. St Louis, Mosby, 1997.

Garcia LS, Bruckner DA: *Diagnostic Medical Parasitology*, ed 2. Washington, DC, American Society for Microbiology, 1993.

Henry JB (ed): *Clinical Diagnosis and Management by Laboratory Methods*, ed 19. Philadelphia, WB Saunders Co, 1996.

Jacobs DS, DeMott WR, Grady HJ, et al (eds): *Laboratory Test Handbook*, Hudson, Ohio, Lexi-Comp, Inc, 1996.

Koneman EW, Roberts GD: *Practical Mycology*, ed 3. Baltimore, Williams & Wilkins, 1985.

Mahon CR, Manuselis G Jr: *Textbook of Diagnostic Microbiology*. Philadelphia, WB Saunders Co, 1995.

Murray PR, Drew WL, Kobauashi GS, et al: *Medical Microbiology*. St Louis, Mosby, 1990.

NCCLS: *Development of In Vitro Susceptibility Testing Criteria and Quality Control Parameters: Tentative Standard,* ed 2. Villanova, Pa, National Committee for Clinical Laboratory Standards, 1992, document no M23-T2.

NCCLS: *Physician's Office Laboratory Guidelines, Procedure Manual, Tentative Guideline,* ed 3. Villanova, Pa, National Committee for Clinical Laboratory Standards, 1995, document no POL2-T3.

Prescott LM, Harley JP, Klein DA: *Microbiology.* Dubuque, Iowa, William C Brown, 1990.

## STUDY QUESTIONS

1. Microbiology laboratory-acquired infections from an aerosol:

   A. Largely occur in persons who are new to the job.
   B. Can occur from an accidental needle puncture wound.
   C. Can cause disease with an organism of usually low infectivity.
   D. Are associated with improper venting of air in the laboratory setting.

2. Prevention of aerosolization can best be accomplished by:

   A. Disinfecting the work areas with a bleach solution.
   B. Using puncture-proof sharps discard containers.
   C. Using a biological safety cabinet when working with aerosols.
   D. Discarding all specimen-contaminated materials in a biohazard bag.

3. Media that are used to selectively inhibit the growth of certain organisms while permitting the growth of other organisms are called:

   A. Enrichment media
   B. Differential media
   C. Supportive media
   D. Selective media

4. Media that are used to permit the rapid growth of one organism while inhibiting the growth of other organisms are called:

   A. Enrichment media
   B. Differential media
   C. Supportive media
   D. Selective media

5. Media that are used to permit the normal rate of growth of most nonfastidious organisms are called:

   A. Enrichment media
   B. Differential media
   C. Supportive media
   D. Selective media

6. Which of the following media is *not* a general purpose medium?

   A. Trypticase soy broth
   B. Thayer-Martin agar
   C. Sheep blood agar
   D. Thioglycolate broth

7. Which of the following media are used to promote the growth of gram-negative organisms while inhibiting the growth of gram-positive organisms?

   A. MacConkey agar
   B. Sheep blood agar
   C. Thayer-Martin agar
   D. Chocolate agar

8. Which of the following media is used to promote the growth of *Neisseria gonorrhoeae* and *Neisseria meningitidis?*

   A. MacConkey agar
   B. Sheep blood agar
   C. Thayer-Martin agar
   D. Phenylethyl alcohol agar

9. Automated microbiology systems have generally been designed to replace:

   A. Manual antibiotic susceptibility procedures.
   B. Manual procedures that are repetitive and that are performed daily on a large number of specimens.
   C. Manual procedures that are done infrequently but are labor intensive.
   D. All manual procedures done in the microbiology laboratory.

10. The lowest concentration of antimicrobial agent that will inhibit the growth of the organism being tested is known as the:

    A. Minimal inhibitory concentration (MIC).
    B. Minimal bactericidal concentration (MBC)
    C. Agar disk diffusion test
    D. Dilution test

11. Use of triple sugar iron agar or Kligler's iron agar can identify *all but which one* of the following characteristics of members of the Enterobacteriaceae family (common enteric intestinal pathogens)?

    A. Ability to ferment gas from sugars
    B. Ability to produce hydrogen sulfide gas
    C. Ability to produce ammonia
    D. Ability to ferment lactose

12. Pathogenic *Shigella* species organisms characteristically are:

    A. Urease negative
    B. Urease positive
    C. Coagulase positive
    D. Producers of indole

13. MacConkey agar is quantitatively inoculated with a urine specimen and incubated appropriately. Results are: >100,000 col/mL urine of gram-negative lactose-fermenting organisms. Which of the following would be statistically the most likely organism to cause a urinary tract infection?

    A. *Escherichia coli*
    B. *Proteus* species
    C. *Staphylococcus aureus*
    D. *Klebsiella* species

14. Which of the following quantitative urine culture results would be considered clinically significant for bacteriuria in an asymptomatic patient?

    A. $10^3$ col/mL urine
    B. $10^4$ col/mL urine
    C. $10^5$ col/mL urine
    D. $10^6$ col/mL urine

15. Which of the following organisms can be recognized by its spreading growth appearance on sheep blood agar?

    A. *Escherichia coli*
    B. *Proteus* species
    C. *Staphylococcus aureus*
    D. *Klebsiella* species

16. Urogenital swabs to be cultured for gonococci should be plated onto culture media:

    A. Immediately; at the bedside preferably
    B. Within 2 hours of collection
    C. Within 4 hours of collection
    D. Within 24 hours of collection

17. In culturing a throat swab for group A $\beta$-hemolytic streptococci testing, which of the following media is preferred?

    A. Sheep blood agar
    B. Horse blood agar
    C. MacConkey agar
    D. Chocolate agar

18. What is the purpose of making cuts in the sheep blood agar when a throat culture is plated?

    A. To count the colonies growing after incubation
    B. To observe the appearance of any hemolysis present
    C. To determine whether the organism is lactose positive or negative
    D. To note the morphologic appearance of the colony growth

19. In some people, untreated pharyngitis infections with group A $\beta$-hemolytic streptococci can eventually result in :

    A. Nephrotic syndrome
    B. Acute pyelonephritis
    C. Chronic glomerulonephritis
    D. Acute glomerulonephritis

20. In observing a sheep blood plate inoculated with a throat swab and showing the presence of alpha or green hemolysis after incubation, what test can be done to determine whether the organism is *Streptococcus viridans*, part of the normal throat flora, or *Streptococcus pneumoniae*?

   A. Bile solubility test, in which most *Streptococcus pneumoniae* colonies would be dissolved by the reagent used (or inhibited by optochin disk)
   B. Bile solubility test, in which most *Streptococcus viridans* colonies would be dissolved by the reagent used (or inhibited by optochin disk)
   C. Bacitracin susceptibility test, in which most *Streptococcus pneumoniae* colonies would be inhibited by the bacitracin disk
   D. Bacitracin susceptibility test, in which most *Streptococcus viridans* colonies would be inhibited by the bacitracin disk

21. In identifying the presence of most group A β-hemolytic streptococci, as opposed to those that are non-group A, which of the following tests can be done?

   A. Bile solubility test, in which most group A β-hemolytic streptococci colonies would be inhibited by an optochin disk
   B. Bile solubility test, in which most non-group A β-hemolytic streptococci colonies would be inhibited by an optochin disk
   C. Bacitracin susceptibility test, in which most group A β-hemolytic streptococci colonies would be inhibited by the bacitracin disk
   D. Bacitracin susceptibility test, in which most non-group A β-hemolytic streptococci colonies would be inhibited by the bacitracin disk

22. Which of the following antibiotics is used to inhibit nonpathogenic fungi from growing in media that have been designed to promote growth of pathogenic fungi (such as Sabouraud dextrose agar)?

   A. Penicillin
   B. Streptomycin
   C. Chloramphenicol
   D. Cycloheximide

23. A gram-stained sputum smear shows 40 to 50 squamous epithelial cells per low-power (10×) field, along with gram-positive cocci, many gram-negative rods, and many gram-positive cocci in pairs, using the oil-immersion objective. How should the laboratorian report the result for this smear?

   A. Call physician directly to report life-threatening situation.
   B. Report: gram-positive cocci, many gram-negative rods, and many gram-positive cocci in pairs and many squamous epithelial cells.
   C. Subculture must be done to confirm, report pending.
   D. No report; request another specimen, as this one is contaminated with mouth flora (is probably saliva, not sputum), as evidenced by the large numbers of squamous epithelial cells.

24. "Clue cells" are best seen in which of the following specimens?

   A. Wet preparation of vaginal discharge
   B. Gram stain of vaginal discharge
   C. KOH-wet preparation of vaginal discharge
   D. KOH-Gram stain of vaginal discharge

25. When antibiotic therapy is needed, specimens for culture and organism identification should be collected:

   A. At any time; administration of antibiotics does not affect the tests.
   B. While the antibiotics are being administrated.
   C. Before the antibiotics have been administered.
   D. After the antibiotics have been administered.

26. If the antibiotic does *not* inhibit the growth of an organism, the organism is said to be which of the following?

   A. Susceptible
   B. Sensitive
   C. Resistant
   D. Intermediate

27. The specimen of choice for finding pinworm organisms in children is:

   A. Feces
   B. Rectal swab
   C. Skin area around the anus
   D. Blood

28. **What are the requirements for collection of an appropriate specimen for the detection of chlamydia?**

    A. Examine the collected specimen while it is still fresh, when the organisms are still motile.
    B. Vigorously rub the cervical or urethral canal with a swab to dislodge the necessary columnar epithelial cells where the chlamydial organism resides.
    C. Use the cellophane tape collection procedure on the skin area around the anal opening.
    D. Culture at the bedside is preferred, using chocolate agar and sheep blood agar.

29. **What are the requirements for collection of an appropriate specimen for the optimal detection of *T. vaginalis*?**

    A. Examine the collected specimen while it is still fresh, when the organisms are still motile.

    B. Vigorously rub the cervical or urethral canal with a swab to dislodge the necessary columnar epithelial cells where the organism resides.
    C. Cleanse the site carefully before any collection is done.
    D. Culture at the bedside is preferred, using chocolate agar and sheep blood agar.

30. **Collection of fecal samples for identification of intestinal parasites should be done:**

    A. After radiological studies using barium sulfate have been completed.
    B. Before radiological studies using barium sulfate have been done.
    C. First thing in the morning, before the patient has bathed, defecated, or urinated.
    D. Before the onset of an acute phase of the intestinal disease.

## CASE HISTORIES

### ■ CASE I

A mother brings her 10-year-old daughter to a clinic complaining of a sore throat and a low-grade fever (99.6° F.). The mother states that the child has had a runny nose and a cough for the last few days. Upon examination, the physician notes that her pharynx appears red and that her tonsils are slightly swollen; no exudate is noted. Her temperature is 99° F. Blood is drawn for a CBC, and a rapid strep test is done. Results are as follows:

CBC:
| | |
|---|---|
| Hemoglobin | Normal |
| WBC | High normal |
| Rapid strep test | Negative |

What is the most likely diagnosis for this patient's condition?
  A. Viral infection, the cause of most cases of pharyngitis
  B. Strep throat infection; treat with antibiotics for 10 days
On what information in the case history and other findings is this diagnosis based? (List findings.)

### ■ CASE 2

A 50-year-old male comes to the emergency room complaining of right-sided chest pain each time he breathes and a cough that has produced a rust-colored sputum. He also states that his symptoms began abruptly with chills just the day before this visit to the ER; he had previously been healthy. Examination by the physician shows a fever of 102° F and coarse breathing sounds in the right anterior chest. A chest x-ray shows a right upper lobe infiltrate. Blood is drawn for a CBC, and a sputum sample is collected, Gram stained, and cultured. Results of laboratory tests are as follows:

CBC:
| | |
|---|---|
| Hemoglobin | 14.5 g/dL (normal) |
| WBC | Elevated |
| Differential | 90% neutrophils |

Sputum:
| | |
|---|---|
| Gram stain | Gram-positive diplococci (cocci in pairs) |
| Culture | Grew *Streptococcus pneumoniae* |

The diagnosis is pneumonia caused by *Streptococcus pneumoniae*.

What findings (history, physical exam, laboratory results) support the diagnosis? (List findings.)

The observation of which cells on the Gram-stained smear will assure the laboratorian that a sputum specimen has been collected and tested?

A. >10 squamous epithelial cells per low-power field (10×)

B. <10 squamous epithelial cells per low-power field (10×)

## ■ CASE 3

A 20-year-old female presents to her family practice physician for a routine pelvic examination. It has been several years since her last visit to this clinic, when she was diagnosed and treated for a nongonococcal sexually transmitted disease (STD). She is now sexually active only with her fiancé, but has also had sexual encounters with others in the past. She now desires to become pregnant. There are no apparent physical abnormalities, but the physician decides to culture the cervical discharge for gonorrhea and to perform a direct immunofluorescence test for chlamydia. A serum sample is also collected for HIV testing. All laboratory tests are normal, with the exception of the test for chlamydia, which is positive.

Note: Symptoms of chlamydial infections include dysuria and vaginal/urethral discharge—symptoms similar to those of gonorrhea. Twenty-five percent of infected patients exhibit no symptoms of a chlamydial infection. Laboratory diagnosis of chlamydial infection relies on the quality of the sample collected; samples must contain columnar epithelial cells taken from the infected sites, particularly if direct microscopic exam or culture is done. The specimen must be collected from the anterior urethra or endocervical canal by vigorous swabbing or scraping; simply swabbing the purulent discharge is inadequate sampling.

What are some of the findings in the history, physical exam, and laboratory test results that would lead to the diagnosis of a sexually transmitted disease? (List findings.)

What is still the "gold standard" for the laboratory diagnosis of chlamydial infections?

A. Culture

B. Immunofluorescence antibody test

C. Enzyme immunoassay (EIA)

D. DNA probe

## ■ CASE 4

A disoriented, 58-year-old male patient with a history of poorly controlled diabetes mellitus and chronic obstructive pulmonary disease comes to the emergency room. The patient has been smoking cigarettes for many years. He has been taking steroid medications for his pulmonary disease. Physical examination shows that he is slightly febrile, lethargic, and in respiratory failure. A diagnosis of meningitis is being considered. A lumbar puncture is done and cerebrospinal fluid collected for a smear and culture.

Laboratory results: A cytocentrifuged preparation of the CSF is done and stained with a Gram stain and with calcofluor reagent to specifically stain for yeast present by staining the yeast cell walls. The smear shows encapsulated budding yeasts. A cryptococcal antigen test is done and is positive. The culture of CSF identifies *Cryptococcus neoformans*.

What observations in the history, physical exam, and laboratory findings support the diagnosis of meningitis caused by this type of infectious organism? (List findings.)

Fungi are widespread in the environment, but only rarely cause CNS infection. *Cryptococcus neoformans* is the most common cause of fungal meningitis. It is especially common among patients that are immunocompromised. This type of infection is known as a (an):

A. Nosocomial infection

B. Opportunistic infection

C. Community-acquired infection

D. Hospital-acquired infection

## ■ CASE 5

An 18-year-old female college student complains of fever and chills and that her head hurts and she has been vomiting. She goes to the college health service emergency department, where she is examined. She appears lethargic, and her temperature is 102° F. Blood is drawn for a CBC and culture, urine is collected for analysis, and a serum chemistry profile is ordered. A lumbar puncture is performed, and cloudy cerebrospinal fluid is collected. Laboratory results are as follows:

CBC:

| | |
|---|---|
| WBC | $20.0 \times 10^9$/L (increased) |
| WBC differential | Shows marked neutrophilia with a shift to the immature forms (shift to the left) |

CSF results:

| | |
|---|---|
| WBC | 1200 cells/$\mu$L with 95% neutrophils (normal = 0-5 lymphocytes) |
| Glucose | 25 mg/dL (decreased, compared with normal blood glucose value) |
| Protein | 150 mg/dL (increased) |
| Gram stain | Many neutrophils, gram-negative cocci in pairs |
| Urinalysis | Increased protein, few RBC, few granular casts |
| Serum chemistries | Within normal reference values |

Note: *Haemophilus influenzae* (gram-negative coccobacillus) type b is the most common cause of men-ingitis in children 1 to 6 years of age. *Streptococcus pneumoniae* (gram-positive diplococcus) is a causative agent of meningitis in adults. *Neisseria meningitidis* (gram-negative cocci) is most frequently identified as the causative organism for meningococcal infections in adolescents and young adults and has occurred in epidemics in the United States.

From the history and laboratory results, *all but which one* of the following findings in the blood and cerebrospinal fluid substantiate a bacterial rather than a viral meningeal infection?

A. Decreased CSF glucose
B. Increased WBC in CSF, with neutrophils predominating
C. Gram stain showing gram-negative coccal organisms
D. Increased protein, few RBC, few granular casts in urine

# CHAPTER 17

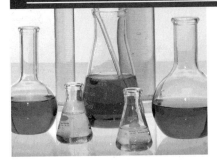

# Immunology and Serology

## Learning Objectives

*From study of this chapter, the reader will be able to:*

➤ Explain the function of the immune system and its lymphoid tissue components, chiefly the B and T lymphocytes.

➤ Define the terms antigen and antibody.

➤ List and discuss characteristics of the five major classes of immunoglobulins.

➤ Define monoclonal and polyclonal antibodies.

➤ Discuss principles of commonly used detection systems of antigen-antibody reactions, such as precipitation, flocculation, agglutination, fluorescent microscopy techniques, lysis, complement fixation, enzyme immunoassays, and Western blot technology.

➤ Define titer and know how to dilute a serum specimen serially.

➤ Understand the basis for immunologic tests for pregnancy.

➤ Understand immunologic tests for heterophil antibodies seen in infectious mononucleosis.

➤ Understand screening tests for antinuclear antibody (ANA) in systemic lupus erythematosus.

➤ Understand tests for rheumatoid factor (RF) in the serum of some patients with rheumatoid arthritis.

➤ Explain routine tests for syphilis.

# INTRODUCTION TO IMMUNOLOGY AND SEROLOGY

Humans are equipped with two strong lines of defense against the invasion of foreign substances. One is a nonspecific resistance to certain diseases that comes about through physiologic and anatomic mechanisms such as the inflammatory response, skin and mucous membranes as barriers, and phagocytic cells. The other is the **immune response,** a major body defense system, having the ability to distinguish "self" from "nonself." Together, these mechanisms or systems normally work effectively to protect humans throughout life.

The immune response is the human body's unique defense system against foreign substances; it is extremely complex and plays a variety of roles in maintaining health. The immune response serves as a defense against invasion by infectious agents as well as against certain abnormal cells in the body itself that have developed through various conditions or mutations. Study of the immune system also includes the autoimmune antibodies that can be produced in response to certain of the body's own cells. The primary function of the immune system is to recognize self from nonself and to protect the body against nonself.

**Clinical immunology** involves the study of antigen-antibody reactions in vitro. In clinical immunology tests, there must be a reaction between an antibody and an antigen that results in a recordable event. **Serology** is a division of immunology that specializes in detecting and measuring specific antibodies that develop in the blood during a response to exposure to a disease-producing antigen. Several techniques and detection systems are utilized in clinical immunologic and serologic assays. These include precipitation, immunoelectrophoresis, agglutination, complement fixation, cytolysis, neutralization, flocculation, immunodiffusion, enzyme immunoassays, enzyme-linked immunosorbent assays (ELISA or EIA), and fluorescent antibody (FA) methods. Immunohematology, or blood banking, also utilizes serologic methods to determine blood groups and unexpected antibodies for persons donating or receiving blood (see Chapter 18).

## The Immune Response

The response to an antigenic or "foreign" stimulus is referred to as an immune response. It involves the recognition and elimination of foreign substances by the immune system, a complex interrelated system of tissues and organs that are generally derived from lymphoid tissue. In the human, the bone marrow and the thymus are classified as primary or central lymphoid organs. Secondary lymphoid tissue includes the spleen and lymph nodes.

### Lymphoid Tissue and Lymphocytes

Lymphoid cells (lymphocytes) are derived from a common stem cell in the bone marrow. The lymphocytes are further classified as T and B cells. **T lymphocytes** are lymphocytes that are derived from the thymus or are influenced by thymic hormones. **B lymphocytes** are derived from the bone marrow and secrete antibodies. (See also Chapter 12.) About 70% to 80% of the lymphocytes circulating in the blood are T lymphocytes. They are responsible for defenses against viruses, fungi, and incompatible cells seen in cases of rejection of foreign tissues and in tumors. About 20% of the circulating lymphocytes are B lymphocytes. They are responsible for defenses against extracellular bacteria. T and B lymphocytes as seen in a stained blood film cannot be distinguished one from the other. Subsets of the various lymphocytes are identified and enumerated by evaluating their various surface membrane markers by means of monoclonal antibody tests. An immune response may be cellular or humoral, and there is much interaction between the two responses.

**Humoral Response and B Lymphocytes.** The **humoral response** involves antibodies produced by B lymphocytes and the complement system. The B cells originate in the bone marrow, being processed there to develop receptors for their specific antigens. B cells are processed in the thymus gland to respond to specific antigens. When the B cells encounter their specific antigens, they undergo antigenic stimulation, forming immunoblasts, with the subsequent development of two forms of cells—effector B cells, which produce plasma cells, and memory B cells. **Plasma cells** produce antibodies, the immunoglobulins, which enter the bloodstream. The antibodies produced by the B cells make their way through the blood and lymphatic system to all parts of the body to form a complex with the antigens for which they are specific.

**Cell-Mediated Response and T Lymphocytes.** The **cellular** or **cell-mediated response** involves actions of T lymphocytes (especially subsets of T lymphocytes) together with plasma cells and macrophages. The subsets of T cells that develop are: (1) killer T cells, which produce cytokines to destroy the antigen; (2) T helper cells, which assist B cells to destroy the antigen; (3) T suppressor cells, which turn off the immune response when its activity is no longer needed; and (4) T memory cells, which react to protect at a later time when a subsequent antigenic encounter takes place. Mature T lymphocytes survive for several months or years, while the B lymphocytes survive for only a few days. Taken all together, the immune response is a finely tuned regulatory mechanism that involves B lymphocytes together with T lymphocytes and mononuclear phagocytic cells.

## ANTIGENS AND ANTIBODIES

An **antigen** is a foreign substance; if it is introduced into the body of a person who does not already have the antigen, an antisubstance called an **antibody** will be produced. The antibody produced in response to the foreign antigen is found in the plasma and in other body fluids and reacts with the foreign antigen in some observable way. It is specific for the antigen against which it is formed; that is, it reacts with only its corresponding antigen and no other antigen.

The significance of antigens and antibodies is basic to the study of immunity and immunology. Various microorganisms have antigenic properties. Therefore, when introduced into a host, they elicit antibody formation. The antibody formed in response to the foreign antigen (in this case, the microorganism) protects the person from subsequent infections by that particular organism.

Foreign antigenic substances are recognized by lymphoid and plasma cells. Each specific type of antigen stimulates the production of equally specific antibodies by various body tissues. If an antibody has been formed against a foreign antigenic substance, one good way to identify the infecting organism is to identify the antibody produced in response to it. This is the basis for immunologic and serologic determinations. Many years ago researchers in the field of immunology showed that if a known antigen, such as a certain bacterium, is exposed in a test tube to a patient's serum containing antibodies against that antigen, a **serologic** or **immunologic reaction** will be observed. If the specific antibody is not present in the patient's serum, no reaction will be observed.

Antibodies that have been produced in response to a specific antigenic stimulus can be identified in the serum. This serologic reaction produces an observable change in the mixture in one of several ways, such as precipitation or agglutination reactions. The reaction takes different forms because of variations in the technique being used and the type of antigen being assayed.

### Nature of Antigens

An antigen is generally described as a substance that, when injected into an animal, is recognized as foreign and—provided immunologically active cells are present—provokes an immune reaction or response. As stated previously, this immune response is the production of antibodies—substances that usually protect the body against the foreign antigen. There are times, however, when antibodies are not protective, as in the case of antibody-antigen reactions that cause hay fever, rash, or anaphylactic shock. Antigenicity is not confined to proteins. Certain nonantigenic, nonprotein substances known as **haptens** may bind themselves to protein, and the resulting hapten-protein complex is antigenic.

Chemically, antigens are usually proteins, although polysaccharides, polypeptides, or polynucleotides may also be antigenic; they are usually large molecules with a molecular weight of 10,000 or more. The specificity of an antigen is related to its chemical composition together with the spatial configuration or arrangement of the amino acids, simple sugars, and fatty acids that make up the chemical composition of the molecule. However, not all antigens are equally antigenic. Some are extremely effective in their ability to cause antibody production, while others are relatively weak and not as likely to result in antibodies. Antigenicity is influenced by several things. These include the molecular size and electrical charge, the solubility, the shape of the molecule, and the biological and chemical composition.

## Production of Antibodies

Antibodies are proteins and are produced in response to foreign antigenic stimuli. It is believed that they are synthesized from gamma globulin by B lymphocytes or plasma cells. For example, a person who has had chickenpox is immune to the disease in the future—that is, has protection from getting the disease again. The immunity is a function of antibody production by the host.

Some antibodies occur in humans naturally as a result of exposure throughout life to bacteria and plant material, in the form of food, and through inhalation and ingestion. Antibodies can also be produced in response to natural infections, as with pneumonia and typhoid fever organisms, and their production can be artificially stimulated by the injection of antigens in vaccine form. Natural and artificial infections stimulate the production of immune, or protective, antibodies.

### Natural and Immune Antibodies

**Natural antibodies** appear to exist without antigenic stimulus, whereas **immune antibodies** are the result of stimulation by specific foreign antigens. An example of natural antibodies in blood are the anti-A and anti-B antibodies found in the ABO blood group system (see Chapter 18). Immune antibodies are also referred to as unexpected antibodies and are usually the result of specific antigenic stimulation. They can also result from immunization from pregnancy, transfusion, or injection of transfused red cells. Once immunization exists, it is permanent. Immune antibodies include the IgG, IgA, and IgM types.

### Antibody Response

Immunity is not immediate, as can be seen from the fact that on first infection the person is ill or incapacitated by the disease. Antibodies require about 2 weeks to develop sufficiently, after which subsequent exposure to the antigen will elicit an effective antigen-antibody reaction and therefore **protective immunity.** Another example of antibody response is in the ABO blood group system; persons whose red cells contain group A antigen are unable to form anti-A antibody but do form naturally occurring anti-B antibodies (see Chapter 18).

**Primary Response.** When a foreign antigen is first introduced, the antibody cannot be detected immediately in the serum or plasma. It is observed about 10 to 14 days after antigenic stimulation, and the **antibody titer,** or the concentration of antibody, is greatest at about 20 days, after which it gradually decreases. (See also under Testing for Antibody Levels.) This is known as the **primary response** or first response.

**Secondary Response.** A second exposure to the same antigen, however, rapidly results in detectable amounts of antibody in the plasma or serum, which is known as the **secondary response.** There appears to be a memory phenomenon elicited by the lymphocytes that results in an immediate antibody response on the second exposure or subsequent exposures. This secondary antibody response also produces a higher and longer-lasting titer of antibody. In addition, the antibody is more effective in its reaction with antigen or has better combining properties.

**Factors Influencing the Immune Response.** Several factors influence the amount of antibody that will be formed after foreign antigen stimulation. Generally, the stronger the antigen, the greater the antibody response. The number of foreign antigens that are introduced at a particular time also influences the amount of antibody production. In general, exposure to only one antigen elicits a stronger antibody response than simultaneous exposure to more than one antigen. The number of exposures to foreign antigen also plays a role in antibody response. Repeated exposures result in greater antibody formation. The interval between exposures to a foreign antigen also has a role in antibody formation. A number of exposures repeated rapidly are less likely to result in antibody formation than the same number of exposures spaced over a longer period of time. The quantity of antigen introduced has some effect, but the number of exposures and the interval between them are more important in terms of antibody production.

There is apparently a threshold amount of antigen related to antibody production. If more than this threshold amount of antigen is introduced, the amount of antibody produced is relatively small in proportion to the quantity of antigen. In addition, a large excess of antigen may completely inhibit an antibody response. This is especially important in blood banking, for a relatively small amount of incompatible blood produces as much antibody as a relatively large amount—the transfusion of any incompatible blood may result in serious sensitization of the patient.

There are individual and age differences in antibody formation. Some persons are more prone to form antibodies than others. Newborn infants do not form antibodies but may have received them passively from the mother across the placenta. They begin forming gamma globulin and therefore antibody at about 3 months and usually have a normal gamma globulin level by 6 months. This is important when serum from newborn infants is tested for antibodies (as in testing for ABO groups in immunohematology laboratories; see Chapter 18).

## Types of Antibodies

Antibodies are mainly proteins of the gamma globulin type of serum protein; they are therefore also referred to as **immunoglobulins (Ig).** When antibodies result from exposure to antigenic material from another species, they are referred to as **xenoantibodies** or **heteroantibodies.** When antibodies result from antigenic stimulation within the same species, they are referred to as **alloantibodies** or **isoantibodies.** Blood group antibodies are isoantibodies (alloantibodies); these are the antibodies that cause transfusion-related problems. In blood banking, antibody formation does not result in protective immunity. The blood antigens are present on the red cells, and the antibody is found in the plasma or serum. The antigen-antibody reaction results in the destruction of the antigen-carrying red cell by antibody in the serum of the person receiving the red cells—clinically known as a transfusion reaction.

## Classes of Immunoglobulins (Antibodies)

Five classes of gamma globulin antibodies occur in human body fluids. These are IgA, IgD, IgE, IgG, and IgM. These immunoglobulins differ in molecular size, carbohydrate content (all are glucoproteins), biological activity, and plasma half-life. The sizes and relative amounts present in serum are shown on Table 17-1.

IgG is the predominant immunoglobulin of serum and makes up about 80% of the total immunoglobulin present. It is the smallest of the immunoglobulins in size. IgM is the largest of the immunoglobulins and makes up about 6% of the total. IgM and IgG can activate complement. IgM is the type of antibody that results from primary exposure to foreign antigen. Secondary exposure results in IgG formation. Repeated stimulation results in IgG antibody formation. IgA is the immunoglobulin component of external secretions such as saliva and tears; it is the primary

## TABLE 17-1

Immunoglobulins in Serum or Plasma

| Immunoglobulin Type | Molecular Weight (in daltons) | Proportion of Total Immunoglobulin |
| --- | --- | --- |
| IgA | 160,000-500,000 | 13% |
| IgD | 180,000 | 1% |
| IgE | 196,000 | Trace |
| IgG | 150,000 | 80% |
| IgM | 900,000 | 6% |

defense against ingested or inhaled antigens. The serum levels of IgA, IgG, and IgM are influenced by a number of factors, including age and race. IgM is the first type of antibody that the newborn infant is able to form, and it is effectively synthesized at about 9 months. IgG is effectively synthesized at about 3 to 4 years, whereas IgA is not produced until adolescence. Because of its small molecular size, IgG is the only type of antibody that is able to cross the placenta.

### Antibody Structure

All of the immunoglobulins have a similar chemical structural configuration, as shown in Fig. 17-1. The common configuration consists of a monomer composed of two identical heavy chains and two identical light chains connected by disulfide bonds or bridges in the hinge region. The chains are polypeptides; the light chains have a molecular weight of approximately 22,500 daltons, and the heavy chains range from 50,000 to 75,000 daltons. As shown in Fig. 17-1, IgG is a simple monomer while IgM is a pentamer (made up of five monomers). Each monomer has reactive sites capable of combining with corresponding antigens.

The chemical structure of the heavy chains is responsible for the differences in the various classes of antibodies. However, the light chains are of only two types (kappa and lambda) and are common to all classes of immunoglobulins.

### Monoclonal and Polyclonal Antibodies

**Polyclonal antibodies** are derived from multiple ancestral clones of antibody-producing cells.

Although of a particular specificity, polyclonal antibodies contain a mixture of about two-thirds kappa light chains and only one-third lambda light chains. Most antibodies found in serum are of the polyclonal type. Polyclonal antibodies recognize a broader range of antigenic determinants than do monoclonal antibodies directed against the same antigen. Polyclonal antibodies are characteristically produced in infectious diseases.

**Monoclonal antibodies** are of a more homogeneous, restricted nature. They are more precise in recognition of the corresponding antigen than the polyclonal antibody directed to the same antigen. They are derived entirely from a single **clone** or a single ancestral antibody-forming parent cell. Unlike polyclonal antibodies, monoclonal antibodies of a given specificity are entirely either kappa or lambda light chains, but not both. Monoclonal antibodies are secreted into the serum in large quantities when associated with malignant proliferations of plasma cells or their precursors, as in multiple myeloma. Monoclonal antisera used as testing reagents, produced by hybridization, are utilized in diagnostic testing because of their greater diagnostic precision.

## PRINCIPLES OF IMMUNOLOGIC AND SEROLOGIC METHODS

Antibodies can be detected by several different techniques or reactions. In some cases, antibodies to an agent may be detected by more than one method, but the different methods may not detect the same antibody.

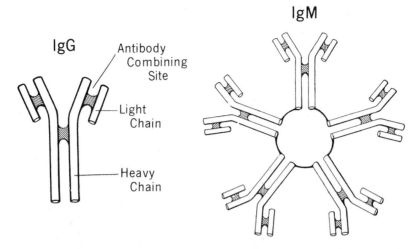

**FIG 17-1.** Examples of antibody molecular structure. Two antibody molecules shown are IgG and IgM. IgG *(left)* is a simple monomer composed of two heavy chains and two light chains connected by disulfide bonds or bridges. IgM *(right)* is in the form of a pentamer. Each has reactive sites capable of combining with corresponding antigens.

## Agglutination

**Agglutination** means clumping. In this type of observable reaction, the combination of specific antigens and antibodies results in the formation of visible clumps, which settle out of the solution. Antibodies that form clumps are called **agglutinins,** and the associated antigens are called **agglutinogens.** Agglutination occurs only if the antigen is in the form of particles, such as bacteria, red blood cells, latex particles, white blood cells, or any substance that appears cloudy when suspended in saline.

**Slide agglutination** tests are the easiest to perform and are generally quite sensitive. Reagents for many of these tests are available commercially. Artificial carriers, such as latex particles or treated red blood cells, or biological carriers, such as bacterial cells, can carry antigen on their surface that will bind with antibody that has been produced in response to the specific antigen when it was introduced into the host. Agglutination tests have a wide range of application in the clinical diagnosis of both infectious diseases and noninfectious immune disorders. There are many commercial agglutination procedures available for use in large and small laboratories and in physicians' office laboratories. These tests can determine many constituents of importance to clinicians, and the techniques utilizing agglutination are ideally suited for use in a variety of settings to facilitate diagnosis and expedite the overall treatment of the patient. Agglutination tests are also utilized in immunohematologic typing procedures (see Chapter 18).

### Mechanisms of Agglutination

Agglutination reactions are influenced by several factors. The first phase of the agglutination reaction is **sensitization.** This is the physical attachment of the antibody molecule to the antigen; it is a reversible reaction subject to certain conditions being present. Physical conditions such as pH, temperature, and length of time of incubation will affect the reaction. The **antigen-antibody ratio,** or the number of antibody molecules in relation to the number of antigen sites per cell, is another factor influencing antigen-antibody association reactions.

If the amount of antigen is gradually decreased while the antibody concentration remains constant, a point is reached where large amounts of agglutinate or precipitate appear rapidly. Conversely, when increasing amounts of antigen are added, a point is reached where no agglutinate or precipitate is observed. An excess of antibody is known as the **prozone phenomenon.** This excess of antibody concentration can result in false-negative reactions.

The second phase of the agglutination process is **lattice formation.** Lattice formation results in the visible aggregation or clumping reaction, necessary for the agglutination technique. To produce this lattice formation, a cross-linking between sensitized particles and antibodies, it is necessary that the cell with the antibody attached to its surface come close enough to another cell to permit the antibody molecules to combine with the antigen receptor sites on the second cell. This bridging action, necessary to lattice formation, takes place slowly.

### Direct Bacterial Agglutination

Antibodies produced by the host in response to infection by some bacterial agents can be measured by agglutination tests. In these tests for bacterial antibody, the specific antibodies produced in the infectious process bind to the surface antigens of the bacterial agent and cause the bacteria to clump together in visible aggregates. A thick suspension of the bacteria is needed for this test. The reaction is called direct bacterial agglutination. This type of agglutination reaction can be performed on the surfaces of glass slides or in test tubes (Fig. 17-2). Incubation periods can be included when test tubes are used, allowing more antigen and antibody to interact, often making these methods more sensitive. Direct bacterial agglutination tests are used to diagnose diseases in which it is difficult to culture the pathogenic agent in the laboratory. Diseases that are commonly diagnosed by using this immunologic assay include tetanus, brucellosis, and tularemia.

### Latex Agglutination

Antibody molecules can be artificially bound to the surfaces of latex beads for **latex agglutination** procedures. The surface of each latex particle can contain many antibody molecules, in-

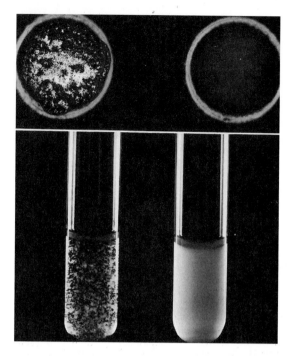

**FIG 17-2.** Agglutination patterns. *Top,* Slide agglutination of bacteria with known antisera or known bacteria. A positive reaction is demonstrated by the specimen on the left, a negative reaction by the specimen on the right. *Bottom,* Tube agglutination. A positive reaction is demonstrated by the specimen on the left, a negative reaction by the specimen on the right. (From Barrett JT: *Textbook of Immunology,* ed 5. St Louis, Mosby, 1988.)

creasing the potential number of exposed antigen-binding sites. If antigen is present in the specimen being tested, such as the C-reactive protein antigen, the antigen will bind to the combining sites of the exposed antibody on the latex bead surface, forming visible cross-linked aggregates of antigen and latex beads (Fig. 17-3). In other testing systems, such as that for rubella antibody, the latex particles can be coated with antigen. These specific antigen-coated latex particles and any rubella antibody present in the patient's serum will result in visible clumping of the latex particles. These are called **direct agglutination** tests. **Indirect agglutination** tests show agglutination when no positive constituent (antibody)

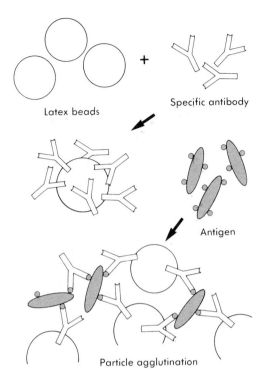

Latex beads    Specific antibody

Antigen

Particle agglutination

**FIG 17-3.** Alignment of antibody molecules bound to the surface of a latex particle and latex agglutination reaction. (From Baron EJ, Finegold SM: *Bailey and Scott's Diagnostic Microbiology*, ed. 8. St Louis, Mosby, 1990, p 128.)

is present to react and therefore produce no agglutination reaction when the constituent is present (see also Latex Particle Agglutination Inhibition, under Types of Pregnancy Tests.)

Procedures utilizing latex agglutination must be performed under strict standardized conditions. Complete systems employing the use of latex or other particle agglutination technology are commercially available for detection of some pathogenic agents. The amount of antigen-antibody binding is influenced by pH, osmolarity, and the ionic concentration of the solution. Other important factors include the time of incubation of the coated particles with the patient's serum (or other source of antibody) and the amount and avidity of the antigen attached to the carrier. It is important that the manufacturer's directions be followed carefully. Immunologic assays em-

ploying latex agglutination can be used for the human gonadotropin hormone of pregnancy testing, C-reactive protein, IgG and IgM rheumatoid factors, cytomegalovirus (CMV), and rubella antibody.

### Coagglutination

To enhance the visibility of the agglutination reaction, antibodies are sometimes bound to a particle; this technique involves **coagglutination**. It is highly specific but may not be as sensitive as the latex agglutination system.

### Hemagglutination

Animal red blood cells have been treated for use as carriers of antigen for some agglutination tests. These are called indirect or passive agglutination tests because it is not the antigens of the blood cells themselves, but the passively attached antigens, that are bound by the antibody. **Hemagglutination (HA)** is the agglutination of red blood cells. One test commonly performed that utilizes hemagglutination is the microhemagglutination test for antibody to *Treponema pallidum* (MHA-TP). This test is performed on a microtiter plate. Other tests include the hemagglutination treponemal test for syphilis (HATTS), the passive hemagglutination tests for antibody to extracellular antigens of streptococci, and the rubella indirect hemagglutination tests. All of these tests are commercially available in kits.

## Precipitation and Flocculation

**Precipitation** may be defined as the visible result of an antigen-antibody reaction between a soluble antigen and its antiserum (serum containing antibodies). Electrolytes are also needed to bring the process to its desired conclusion, along with the proper pH and temperature of the mixture. Antibodies that react to form precipitates are called **precipitins**. The interaction of a soluble antigen with antibody thus results in the formation of a **precipitate**, a concentration of fine particles. **Flocculation** is the clumping together of fine particles to form a visible mass. A visible flocculation or precipitation reaction results because the precipitated product is forced to remain in a particular space within a matrix. The precipitin end product clumps that are formed are visible either macroscopically or microscopically.

Two variations of flocculation tests are used in serologic tests for syphilis (see also under Syphilis). These are the Venereal Disease Research Laboratory (VDRL) and the Rapid Plasma Reagin (RPR) tests. The RPR test is used by many laboratories and is available commercially as a complete testing system, containing positive and negative controls. The RPR test appears to be a more specific screening test for syphilis than the VDRL test.

Precipitin tests have been used historically in the identification of bacteria, specifically in the classification of streptococci into groups A through K using the grouping methods originated by Lancefield. Serologic typing of the streptococcal cell wall components by means of the Lancefield precipitin method has classically been used to group these bacteria.

Abnormal globulins produced as a result of certain inflammatory diseases can also be identified by precipitin techniques. Certain diseases alter the quantities of some proteins found in the serum, such as immunoglobulin, haptoglobulin, and complement. These increases or decreases are valuable diagnostic tools. Modifications of the precipitin test include the use of counterimmunoelectrophoresis (CIE) or gel diffusion detection of antigen-antibody reactions.

## Fluorescent Antibody Techniques

Antigen-antibody complexes formed can also be demonstrated by means of **fluorescent antibody (FA)** techniques. In this method, antibody against insoluble or particulate antigen, such as bacteria or cellular materials, may be detected. In the FA technique, antibody is labeled with fluorescein isothiocyanate (FITC), a fluorescent compound that has an affinity for proteins. A conjugate is formed when the fluorescein compound forms a complex with the protein in the bacteria or tissue, and this conjugate is

then able to react with antibody-specific antigen. Fluorescent techniques are very specific and sensitive. Antibodies may be conjugated to other markers, in addition to the fluorescent dye. An example is the use of enzyme-substrate marker systems. Systems are available commercially to measure antibodies developed against a number of infectious agents as well as against some self-antigens, as in detecting the presence of autoimmune antibodies. Monoclonal antibodies have been conjugated to fluorescein in detection systems used for chlamydia and other pathogenic microorganisms in specimens that are used for direct staining techniques.

### Indirect Fluorescent Antibody Tests

Serologic tests used for the detection of many types of antibodies apply the concept of indirect fluorescent antibody (IFA) techniques. When the IFA technique is used, the antigen against which the patient makes antibody is fixed to the surface of a clean glass microscope slide. Serum from the patient is added to the slide, covering the area in which the antigen was placed. If the specific antibody in question is present in the serum, the antibody will bind to the specific antigen. To remove any unbound antibody, the slide is washed. In the second part of this process, antihuman globulin that has been conjugated to the fluorescent dye is placed on the slide. The conjugated marker will bind to any antibody already bound to the antigen on the slide. This will serve as a marker for the antibody when the slide is viewed under a fluorescence microscope. The dye marker fluoresces apple green. If antibody is absent, the antihuman globulin dye marker will be removed during the washing procedure and no fluorescence will be seen. The fluorescence does not fade appreciably for a few days if the stained slides are coverslipped using a drop of buffered glycerol and if the slides are kept refrigerated in the dark. It is best to examine the prepared slides immediately after staining, however.

Commercially available systems utilizing fluorescence techniques are used in many laboratories. These IFA systems include slides with the antigens, positive and negative control sera, diluent for the patient's sera, and the properly diluted conjugated marker. These IFA techniques, if performed properly, will give extremely specific and sensitive results. **Immunofluorescence** is used in the detection of autoantibodies and antibodies to tissue and cellular antigens. **Antinuclear antibodies (ANAs),** a group of circulating immunoglobulins that react with the whole nucleus or nuclear components, are frequently assayed by using an IFA technique. Indirect fluorescent studies are commonly done to test for antibodies to *Legionella* species, *Borrelia burgdorferi*, varicella-zoster virus, cytomegalovirus, Epstein-Barr virus, herpes simplex viruses types 1 and 2, rubella virus, *Mycoplasma pneumoniae, T. pallidum,* and several rickettsiae.

## Lysis

Some serologic reactions cause the destruction of red blood cells containing antigens. Such reactions are used in blood bank procedures. **Lysis,** or **hemolysis,** of the red cells is a positive indication that a specific antigen-antibody reaction has taken place. For lysis to occur, complement must be present. The lysing antibody that causes the reaction is known as a **lysin.** One form of *Streptococcus* produces streptolysin, an antigen that can destroy human or rabbit red blood cells.

## Complement Fixation

A valuable but time-consuming means to detect and quantitate soluble antibody is by **complement fixation** tests. These tests detect soluble antigen by virtue of the availability of complement. **Complement** is a group of serum proteins that, when present or combined with antigen-antibody complexes, lyse antigen if it consists of bacteria or other cellular material. The antigen-antibody complex binds the complement present, and thus it is no longer available to promote additional antigen-antibody reactions. In the hemolysis of red cells, for example, and in the destruction of bacteria (called bacteriolysis), three elements must be present for the reaction to be observed: antigen, antibody, and complement.

Complement fixation tests involve two stages of reactions (Fig. 17-4). The first is a serologic reaction between a test serum and antigen, in which complement is adsorbed or bound by the

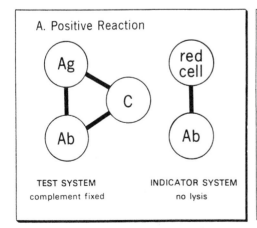
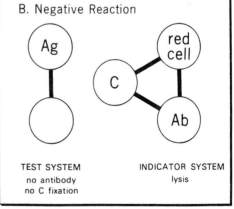

**FIG 17-4.** Complement fixation test. Antigen *(Ag)* and antibody *(Ab)* are incubated with complement *(C)*. The indicator system, consisting of red cells coated with antibody, is added. **A,** Positive reaction. When antigen and antibody are present in the test system, they fix or bind the available complement and none remains to lyse the added indicator cells. **B,** Negative reaction. When antigen or antibody is lacking in the test system, complement is available to lyse the sensitized indicator cells.

antigen-antibody complex, but no visible lysis occurs. The second occurs when red cells coated with anti-red cell serum are added to the suspension. The absence of hemolysis is caused by the fixation of complement in the first step of the reaction. It is primarily the availability of complement in the system that determines whether lysis occurs, and the test thus indicates indirectly the presence or absence of specific antibody.

Complement fixation tests have been used to identify some infectious disorders. A well-known historical example is the Wassermann complement fixation test for syphilis.

## Enzyme Immunoassays

Enzyme immunoassays employ the use of enzymes as immunochemical labels in the detection of antigen-antibody reactions. Other names for these tests include **enzyme-linked immunosorbent assay (ELISA), enzyme immunoassay (EIA),** and enzyme-multiplied immunoassay (EMIT*). Enzyme immunoassays can detect extremely small quantities of antigen-antibody reactants. Either an antibody or an antigen conjugate can be labeled with the appropriate enzyme and used in a number of immunologic assays for a variety of antigens or antibodies, respectively. The enzyme with its substrate can detect the presence and quantity of antigen or antibody in the patient specimen. In this technique, the conversion of a colorless substrate to a colored product allows for either visual or colorimetric detection.

A variety of enzymes can be used in enzyme immunoassays. The most commonly used enzymes are peroxidase and alkaline phosphatase. In a classic enzyme immunoassay, plastic plates, paddles, or beads are coated with the antigen. When the patient's serum is added to the antigen, specific antibody present in the serum will react with it to form an **antigen-antibody complex.** The plate or bead is next incubated with an enzyme-labeled antibody conjugate. If antibody is present, the conjugate reacts with the antigen-antibody complex present. After the addition of a

specific chromogenic substrate, the enzyme activity is measured spectrophotometrically or visually by a change in color.

### Enzyme-Linked Immunosorbent Assay

This system consists of antibodies that are bound to enzymes that remain able to catalyze a reaction that yields a visually observed end product while still being attached to the antibody. Furthermore, antibody-binding sites remain free to react with their specific antigens. There are several variations of this method; the enzyme tag can be conjugated to either antigen or antibody. These enzyme-conjugated substrates are quite stable and can be stored for relatively long periods of time. The formation of a colored end product can be observed visually or read with a simple photoelectric instrument. The use of monoclonal antibodies has increased the specificity of these testing systems.

**Monoclonal Antibodies Used in Assays.** Monoclonal antibodies are highly specific and purified antibodies that have been produced from the daughter cells (clones) of a single hybrid cell. They are engineered to bind to a single specific antigen. Since all of the cells are derived from a single cell producing one antibody molecule type, these are called monoclonal antibodies. Monoclonal antibodies have been used successfully in many commercial systems for the detection of infectious agents. In one test used for the rapid detection of a chlamydial infection, a monoclonal antibody to a protein of *Chlamydia trachomatis* is conjugated to a fluorescent dye. When viewed with a fluorescence microscope, the elementary bodies and inclusions present in specimens from patients infected with chlamydiae can be seen.

**ELISA "Sandwich" Technology.** One type of ELISA method involves the use of a sandwich technique. It is utilized in several commercially available testing products. In the sandwich ELISA technology, the specific antigen is conjugated or fixed to a solid support medium. The pa-

---

*Syva Corp, Palo Alto, Calif.

tient's serum containing the antibodies is added. A complex is formed with the antibody and its specific antigen in the testing system. Unbound materials are washed away as part of the test procedure. An anti-IgG antibody that has been labeled with an enzyme is added and, after an incubation period, the anti-IgG complexes with the specific antibody if it is present. The enzyme tags commonly used are alkaline phosphatase, glucose oxidase, and peroxidase. After rinsing, a chromogenic substrate is added. The product that is formed by the catalytic action of the enzyme is measured by an observed reaction. The amount of product formed is directly proportional to the amount of antibody in the patient's specimen.

**Solid-Phase Immunosorbent Assay.** If the antibody directed toward the agent being assayed is fixed firmly to a solid matrix, either to the inside of the wells of a microdilution tray or to the outside of a spherical plastic or metal bead or some other solid matrix, the system is called a solid-phase immunosorbent assay (SPIA).

## Western Blot Technology

With **Western Blot technology,** the antigenic proteins or nucleic acids of an organism are separated by gel electrophoresis and transferred or blotted onto membrane filter paper. Antiserum from the patient is allowed to react with the filter paper and, by use of labeled anti-antibody detectors, the specific antibody bound to its homologous antigen is detected. That is, if present, the antibodies being sought will bind to the protein or nucleic acid against which they were created. Detection is by use of enzyme-labeled probes or fluorescent markers. Specific assays using the Western Blot technology are utilized to detect antibodies to human immunodeficiency virus (HIV), the causative agent of acquired immunodeficiency syndrome (AIDS). Before an HIV result using a screening enzyme immunoassay is considered positive, the result should be confirmed by the use of at least one additional test. A current standard test for confirming positive HIV-1 tests uses Western blot technology.

# SPECIMENS FOR SEROLOGY AND IMMUNOLOGY

Immunologic testing is done in many areas of the clinical laboratory—microbiology, chemistry, toxicology, immunology, hematology, surgical pathology, cytopathology, and immunohematology (blood banking), to list a few—and a great variety of specimens are tested. With the advent of procedures devised to give rapid, accurate results—especially those based on the use of monoclonal antibodies and enzyme immunoassay technology—many clinical constituents can be determined immunologically. Many types of body fluids can be evaluated by using immunologic technology. It is always important to determine the specimen of choice for each procedure being considered. The many commercial kits available for the various assays will state specific specimen requirements and acceptable criteria for collection.

## Testing for Antibody Levels

In obtaining specimens for serologic testing, it is important to consider the phase of the disease and the condition of the patient at the time of the specimen collection. This is especially important in assays for diagnosis of infectious diseases. If serum is being tested for antibody levels for a specific infectious organism, generally the blood should be drawn during the **acute phase** of the illness—when the disease is first discovered or suspected—and another sample drawn during the **convalescent phase,** usually about 2 weeks later. Accordingly, these samples are called acute and convalescent serum. A difference in the amount of antibody present, or the antibody titer, may be noted when the two different samples are tested concurrently. An important concept in any serologic testing is the manifestation of a rise in titer.

### Antibody Titer

The antibody titer is defined as the reciprocal of the highest dilution of the patient's serum in which the antibody is still detectable. That is, the titer is read at the highest dilution of serum that give a positive reaction with the antigen. If a serum sample has been diluted 1:64 and it reacts positively with the antigen suspension used in the testing process and the next highest dilution of 1:128 does not give a positive reaction, the titer is read as 64. A high titer indicates that there is a relatively high concentration of the antibody present in the serum. For some infections, the titer of antibody rises slowly—months after the acute infection for Legionnaires' disease, for example. For most pathogenic infections, an increase in the patient's titer of two doubling dilutions, or from a positive result of 1:8 to a positive result of 1:32 over several weeks, is an indication of a current infection. This is known as a fourfold rise in the antibody titer. To serially dilute a serum specimen, progressive, regular increments of serum are diluted (Table 17-2). Most commonly, serial dilutions are "twofold." This means that each dilution is half as concentrated as the preceding one. The total volume is the same in each tube. As previously stated, titers are usually reported as the reciprocal of the last dilution showing the desired reaction, such as agglutination, lysis, or a change in color.

## Types of Specimens Tested

The majority of immunology tests are done on serum. Blood is collected in a plain tube and allowed to clot completely before being centrifuged. Serum should be removed from the clot as soon as possible after processing. Lipemia, hemolysis, or any bacterial contamination can make the specimen unacceptable. Icteric or turbid serum may give valid results for some tests but may interfere with others. Blood specimens should be collected before a meal to avoid the presence of chyle, an emulsion of fat globules that often appears in serum after eating, during digestion. Contamination with alkali or acid must be avoided, as these substances have a denaturing effect on serum proteins and make the specimens useless for serologic testing. Excessive heat and bacterial contamination are also to be avoided. Heat coagulates the proteins, and bacterial growth alters protein molecules. If the test cannot be performed immediately, the serum should be refrigerated. If the testing cannot be done within 72 hours, the serum specimen must be frozen.

For some testing, the serum complement must first be inactivated. To inactivate complement, the tubes of serum are placed in a hot-water bath at 56° C for 30 minutes. If the protein complement is not inactivated, it will promote lysis of the red cells and other types of cells and can produce invalid results. Complement is also known to interfere with certain tests for syphilis.

Other specimens include urine for pregnancy tests and for tests for urinary tract infections. It is important that the urine specimen be collected after thorough cleaning of the external genitalia to prevent contamination for any microbiological assays. Urine for the human chorionic gonadotropin (hCG) assay (pregnancy test) must be collected at a suitable time interval after fertilization, to allow the concentration of the hCG hormone to rise to a significant detectable level. Any specimen must be collected into a suitable container to prevent in vitro changes that could affect the assay results. Proper handling and storage of the specimen until testing is done are essential. Immunologic assays are also done on

---

**TABLE 17-2**

Preparation of a Serial Dilution

|  | Tube 1 | Tube 2 | Tube 3 | Tube 4 | Tube 5 | Tube 6 | Tube 7 |
|---|---|---|---|---|---|---|---|
| Saline, mL | 1 | 1 | 1 | 1 | 1 | 1 | 1 |
| Serum, mL, or mL of diluted serum | 1 | 1 of 1:2 | 1 of 1:4 | 1 of 1:8 | 1 of 1:16 | 1 of 1:32 | 1 of 1:64 |
| Final dilution | 1:2 | 1:4 | 1:8 | 1:16 | 1:32 | 1:64 | 1:128 |

cerebrospinal fluid, on other body fluids, and on swabs of various types of body exudates and discharges. The established protocol for each specific assay must be followed in terms of specimen collection requirements and conditions for the assay itself.

# COMMON IMMUNOLOGIC AND SEROLOGIC TESTS

As previously discussed, the advent of monoclonal antibody technology has given rise to the development of many new, highly specific and sensitive immunoassays. Classical serologic testing has been an important part of some diagnostic tests in the clinical laboratory for many years; traditional serologic tests have been done for viral and bacterial diseases. The use of monoclonal antibodies has allowed the identification of specific bacterial and viral proteins and the isolation and characterization of cell surface histocompatibility markers. Monoclonal antibodies continue to play a significant role in advancing the knowledge of malignant processes, as more tumor antigens and hormone receptors are identified. In addition, immunologic processes are involved in transplantation technology, including allograft rejection of normal organs. Immunologic testing is employed in tissue typing procedures for organ transplantation. The immune mechanism is currently recognized as a very important factor in diseases across all medical disciplines, as immunologic deficiencies or abnormal immune responses are seen in many types of diseases and disorders.

Among some of the common serologic and immunologic tests that are important in clinical laboratory diagnoses are tests for syphilis; infectious mononucleosis (heterophil antibodies); C-reactive protein; streptococcal infections (antistreptolysin O antibodies); cold agglutinins; human gonadotropin hormone (hCG) in tests for pregnancy; rheumatoid arthritis (RA) factors; hepatitis, rubella, herpes simplex, and human immunodeficiency viruses; autoantibodies such as antinuclear antibodies (ANAs); thyroid disorder antibodies; and febrile disease antibodies. Some of these tests are discussed in the following sections of this chapter.

## Pregnancy Tests (Measurement of hCG Hormone)

Immunologic tests are done frequently in the laboratory to detect pregnancy in the early stages. Laboratory tests for pregnancy are based on the fact that during pregnancy, the placenta produces a hormone called **human chorionic gonadotropin (hCG).** This hormone rapidly disappears after delivery. In pregnancy, hCG is produced by trophoblast cells of the developing placenta. HCG is a glycoprotein consisting of two subunits, alpha and beta, with a combined molecular weight of about 35,000. The alpha-subunit is also a part of the pituitary hormones, but the beta-subunit is distinctive to hCG and is what gives immunologic and biologic specificity. Both free $\beta$-subunit and the intact $\beta$-subunit hCG are measured as hCG in most current testing methodologies. In the nonpregnant state, there is normally no detectable hCG present in the serum.

Human chorionic gonadotropin is also produced in other conditions, as in gestational trophoblastic neoplasms, in which the tumors can produce large amounts of hCG. Examples of these tumors are hydatidiform mole and choriocarcinoma, both of which arise from the fetal placenta. Abnormal amounts of hCG can also be produced by malignant teratomas of the ovaries and testes.

In a normal pregnancy, detectable amounts of about 25 mIU/mL hCG are secreted 2 to 3 days (48 to 72 hours) after implantation or approximately 8 to 10 days after conception or fertilization. Current tests are sensitive to the low levels first produced. At between the eighth and tenth weeks of gestation (60 to 80 days), a peak production of hCG in the serum (and urine) of approximately 30,000 mIU/mL is attained. After the tenth week of gestation, during the last part of the first trimester, hCG production sharply declines and then plateaus at 15 to 16 weeks to a level of about 10,000 mIU/mL, which is maintained throughout the remainder of the pregnancy.[5]

Concentration of hCG in serum is paralleled by its concentration in the urine, with some variations. Serum levels of hCG are higher than urine levels for generally the first 2 weeks after conception. Urine levels are about the same as serum levels during the third week and, after this period, the urine levels are generally higher than serum. The rate of excretion of hCG into the urine of a pregnant woman parallels its production and increases rapidly between the 30th and 60th days of pregnancy doubling every 2 days during the first 6 weeks of gestation, with peak levels between the 60th and 80th days of gestation (8 to 10 weeks). After delivery, the urinary hCG level drops rapidly over a 2- to 3-day period, and it is undetectable 2 weeks after delivery.

The international reference unit for human gonadotropin activity is determined by using a dried gonadotropin World Health Organization (WHO) standard. Manufacturers use the WHO standard against which to prepare their products.

The presence of hCG is routinely measured in the urine because a urine sample is easy to obtain. Urinary hCG parallels the rise and fall of the hCG levels in serum. Laboratory tests for pregnancy are routinely used to detect hCG no earlier than 10 days after the last missed menstrual period and are used through the first trimester, or to about the twelfth week of pregnancy. After the first trimester, the levels of hCG may be undetectable by many routine laboratory methods.

Most of the kits currently can be used for both serum and urine hCG but show better sensitivity with serum than with urine, because the concentration of hCG in serum is not subject to the wide variation found in urine hCG as a result of changes in urine concentration. Urine for hCG testing should be a first morning collection, which would be more concentrated, have a higher specific gravity, and thus contain a higher concentration of hCG.

The stage of pregnancy has a marked influence on the test results, especially on the incidence of false-negative results. Between the seventh or eighth and twelfth weeks of gestation, even a relatively insensitive assay will be almost 100% positive. Since the levels of hCG fall after the first trimester, false-negative results may be obtained in an obviously pregnant woman.

The most common reason for a positive test is pregnancy, but greatly increased levels of hCG may be seen in other instances, as previously described. An increase in the level of hCG after the removal of a hydatidiform mole, for example, would indicate either that the mole was not completely removed, or that it was malignant and is redeveloping. The test for hCG is therefore a valuable tool for purposes other than the confirmation of pregnancy.

A minimum quality control program for hCG assays requires that known negative and positive samples be assayed to check the system, and that tests be done regularly with samples of different, known hCG levels to check the low and high sensitivity of the system.

Early methods for the determination of pregnancy were biological and involved the use of animals. These tests were costly and very time-consuming. Test results were not available for several days, and often the animals had to be sacrificed to carry out the determination. Early biological tests employing animals, usually frogs, toads, rabbits, or rats, were the Aschheim-Zondek test and the Friedman test. The accuracy, economy, and convenience of immunologic tests for pregnancy have made animal tests a thing of the past.

Immunologic pregnancy tests are done in one of several ways. They differ in the carrier for the external source of hCG, which is commonly monoclonal antibodies, and less commonly, latex particles or red blood cells. Rapid slide agglutination or test tube agglutination methods or enzyme immunoassays are used. A variety of commercial kits are available for these methods. The kits also include positive and negative controls, sensitized particles, and antiserum.

## Interpretation of Measurement of hCG

Two to three days after implantation, hCG concentration is generally greater than 25 mIU/mL (25 IU/L). Serum hCG levels of about 500 mIU/mL are reported at 14 to 18 days after conception, or about 28 to 32 days after the beginning of the last menstrual period. These values generally confirm pregnancy. Therefore, test kits with sensitivities of 25 mIU/mL are currently best used to test for pregnancy. Test kit methodology sensitivity must always be considered in interpreting the outcome of the test result, as results vary according to the sensitivity of the test. Serum tests with a sensitivity of 25 mIU/mL or better have a false-negative rate of 1% to 2%.[5] False-negative results are obtained in up to 40% of home pregnancy tests because of failure to comply with kit instructions.[2] Kits using EIA methodologies are very accurate when directions are followed. A false-negative test result with home pregnancy testing should be repeated within one week, using a fresh specimen, to avoid any delay in seeking needed prenatal care.

## Specimens for Pregnancy Tests

Many pregnancy tests are routinely performed on urine specimens. A first morning urine specimen is required, and it should have a specific gravity of at least 1.015. It should be tested immediately or refrigerated until the test can be performed. Specimens that contain blood and those with heavy proteinuria are likely to cause interference and give false-positive results. Drugs can also contribute to false-positive tests. False-negative results may be obtained if the urine is too dilute (low specific gravity) or it is too early in the pregnancy. Most pregnancy tests give reliable results about 42 days after the onset of the last normal menstrual period and are not reliable after the first trimester of the pregnancy. ELISA tests give a positive reaction with a much lower concentration of hCG and consequently will give positive hCG results earlier in the pregnancy. Urinary hCG levels

generally parallel the rise and fall of the serum levels.

## Types of Pregnancy Tests

Most pregnancy tests, both for home and laboratory use, employ EIA (ELISA) methodologies and have almost completely replaced older, less sensitive methods. The accuracy of the commercial immunologic pregnancy tests depends on several factors. The manufacturer's directions must be followed carefully, the reagents must be properly shipped and stored, and the specimens be properly collected and delivered promptly to the laboratory for testing. Other important factors are the stage of pregnancy, whether the pregnancy is normal or abnormal, the presence of interfering substances in the urine (including drugs, proteins, and red cells), the sensitivity and specificity of the assay procedure, and the use of quality control programs.

Types of tests include enzyme immunoassay, hemagglutination inhibition, latex particle inhibition, direct latex particle agglutination, sol particle immunoassay, and radioimmunoassay. For the most part, these tests are easy to perform with both serum and urine, and some of them have been incorporated into home test kits for pregnancy.

**Hemagglutination Inhibition.** This test involves a two-stage testing process and can be carried out in a test tube. The hCG in the patient's urine or serum will neutralize anti-hCG antiserum that is added to the sample (an antigen-antibody reaction occurs if hCG is present in the specimen). Red cells coated with hCG are next added to the tube, and the tube is observed for agglutination. If the hCG in the patient's specimen has reacted with the anti-hCG in the first stage, no agglutination will be observed in the second stage when the coated red cells are added, and the unagglutinated red cells settle in a ring in the bottom of the tube. Agglutinated red cells settle in a button. A positive test for pregnancy is therefore reported when no agglutination is observed in the second stage of the test. A negative test is reported when agglutination occurs in the second stage. This test may be used with both urine and serum samples.

**Latex Particle Agglutination Inhibition.** This type of test is based on the interference of hCG in a specimen when it is added to a system of latex particles that have been coated with hCG. As part of the first stage of the test, an anti-hCG serum reagent is mixed with the patient's urine on a slide. For stage 2 of the test, the hCG-coated latex particles are added. If hCG is present in the specimen, it has been neutralized by the anti-hCG reagent and no agglutination is observed. If the patient's urine contains hCG in sufficient quantities (because of pregnancy or another condition previously described), an antigen-antibody reaction occurs between the patient's hCG and the anti-hCG in the reagent serum, leaving no anti-hCG to react with the coated latex particles added during the second stage of the test. Therefore, a negative agglutination reaction is interpreted as a positive pregnancy test. Conversely, the absence of hCG in the specimen allows agglutination of the latex particles by the anti-hCG reagent within approximately 2 minutes, the specific reaction time depending on the test kit being used.

The anti-hCG for the reagent is manufactured by injecting purified hCG into animals (usually rabbits) and allowing the animal to produce the specific antibodies to the hCG in its serum.

**Latex Particle Agglutination Test.** In this test, latex particles are coated with anti-hCG antiserum. These are agglutinated when the urine specimen being tested contains hCG. A positive pregnancy test is indicated by the presence of agglutination. This is in contrast to the latex particle inhibition test described above.

**Enzyme Immunoassays.** There are several ELISA tests available as a result of monoclonal antibody technology. In these tests, two types of monoclonal antibodies are used.

One is an hCG-specific antibody bound to a membrane or other solid support medium. This can be a membrane in a tube or on a disk. The characteristics of nitrocellulose, nylon, or other membrane material can be used to enhance the speed and the sensitivity of ELISA reactions. When there is an absorbent material below the membrane, it can help to pull the liquid reactants through the membrane and help separate components that have not reacted from those that have formed antigen-antibody complexes and have bound to the membrane during the testing process. The washing steps are simplified in this way. When a specimen containing hCG is added (urine, plasma, serum, or whole blood can be used), the hCG molecules present are bound to the antibodies on the solid support membrane.

The second monoclonal antibody is an hCG antibody that has been linked to a specific enzyme (alkaline phosphatase). This enzyme-linked antibody is added to the testing system and will bind to a different site on the hCG molecule, creating a sandwich of bound antibody–hCG–enzyme-labeled antibody. After an incubation period, any unbound enzyme-labeled antibody is washed free. A chromogenic substrate reagent is next added, which undergoes a specific color change in the presence of the alkaline phosphatase enzyme, indicating the presence of hCG. The color change is often blue. Variations in these tests include the use of impregnated membranes and strips.

Test results should be reported as "hCG positive" or "hCG negative," not as "pregnancy positive" or "pregnancy negative," owing to the possibility of a false-positive pregnancy test reaction. False-positive results are less common with the ELISA tests. ELISA tests are very sensitive, giving positive reactions as early as 10 days after conception (well before the first missed menses). Most pregnancy tests use these methodologies.

**Abbott TestPack hCG Combo.** By use of the commercial ELISA test kit, TestPack Plus hCG Combo, hCG in serum and urine can be measured (Procedure 17-1). By using a combination of both monoclonal anti-hCG antibodies and polyclonal antibodies, hCG in both serum and

## PROCEDURE 17-1

### hCG in Urine or Serum, Using Abbott TestPack Plus Combo*

1. Remove the reaction disc from the protective pouch and place on a flat, dry surface.

2. Using the transfer pipette supplied with the kit, dispense three drops of specimen into the sample well on the reaction disc. For urine, the first morning urine specimen usually contains the highest concentration of hCG and therefore is the specimen of choice; any urine specimen may be tested, however.

3. The test results should be read immediately after the appearance of a red color in the end of assay window. Test results are observed in the result window. Positive results can be observed in as little as 3 minutes, but the appearance of a red color in the end of the assay window is required for maximum sensitivity or to confirm negative results.

4. Interpret results as follows: A positive (+) sign indicates that the specimen contains elevated levels of hCG; the manufacturer's instructions must be followed in regard to specific interpretation details. A negative (−) sign indicates the absence of detectable hCG. This test will detect serum and urine hCG concentrations of 25 mU/mL or greater. Occasionally, specimens containing less than 25 mU/mL may also give a positive result.

5. If neither a positive (+) or a negative (−) sign appears in the Result Window, or if no color appears in the End of Assay Window, the specimen should be retested.

*Abbott Diagnostics, Abbott Park, Ill.

urine can be identified selectively with a high degree of sensitivity. The specimen is allowed to migrate through the membrane in the reaction disc. As it passes through the membrane, it first mobilizes the anti-alpha hCG antibody-coated complex. The specimen and antibody-colloid complex move through the immobilized anti-beta hCG antibody capture region and then on to the end of the membrane. The plus (+) and minus (−) sign format gives a clear-cut readout for positive or negative specimens. The appearance of the negative (−) sign with a negative specimen gives an added assurance of quality control by demonstrating antibody recognition, assuring that the procedure was performed correctly and that the reagents were chemically active. This becomes a procedural control. If neither a plus nor a minus sign appears, the test must be repeated.

With this test, if hCG is present at serum or urine levels of 25 mU/mL or greater, a positive (+) sign will be seen in the result window. If hCG is absent, a negative (−) sign will appear in the result window. The appearance of a red color in the end of assay window assures the user that the test is complete. Quality control samples should be used daily to ensure proper kit performance, and samples should be tested according to the established protocol of the laboratory. It is always essential to follow the manufacturer's instructions carefully. Package inserts will also indicate causes for false-positive or false-negative reactions. This information should always be considered in performing the test.

### Heterophil Antibodies in Infectious Mononucleosis

Infectious mononucleosis is an acute infectious disease, viral in origin, that is characterized by clinical symptoms of extreme fatigue, malaise, sore throat, fever, enlarged lymph nodes in the neck, and enlarged spleen. A significant number of cases do not show these classic signs and symptoms. The Epstein-Barr virus (EBV) was first identified in 1964 as the cause of infectious mononucleosis. EBV is a human herpes DNA virus, and there are a variety of antigens encoded by this virus. An infection with EBV results in the expression of viral capsid antigen, early antigen, and nuclear antigen, each with their corresponding antibody responses. There are also specific assays for IgM and IgG antibodies to the EBV antigens; these tests are usually performed in virology laboratories or reference laboratories. Antibodies to EBV virus are produced early in the disease and can also be detected by complement fixation tests and immunofluorescence techniques.

Heterophil antibodies are commonly produced in high titer in infectious mononucleosis and are quite easily detected in the laboratory. For this reason, routine immunologic tests for the presence of heterophil antibodies are used for the diagnosis of infectious mononucleosis, along with characteristic clinical and hematologic findings. Common characteristic laboratory findings for infectious mononucleosis include peripheral blood with abnormal, enlarged lymphocytes with atypical nuclei (see Examination of the Blood Film, in Chapter 12) and serum that contains a high titer of heterophil antibodies.

### Heterophil Antibodies

**Heterophil antibodies** are antibodies that appear in cells and fluids of apparently unrelated animals and microorganisms; they are stimulated by one antigen and react with an entirely unrelated surface antigen present on cells from different mammalian species. Heterophil antibodies react with an antigen entirely different from and phylogenetically unrelated to the antigen responsible for their production.

Heterophil antibodies are made up of a group of antibodies that cross-react with antibodies against any one member of the particular heterophil group. Heterophil antibodies are present in low titer in the serum of normal persons. Included in the heterophil antibody group are Forssman, infectious mononucleosis, and serum sickness antibodies.

An example of one of the earliest heterophil antibodies identified is that discovered by Forssman in 1911, known as the **Forssman antibody.** The Forssman antibody was formed when an emulsion of guinea pig organs was injected into rabbits. The production of this Forssman antibody in the rabbit was shown to lyse sheep red cells in the presence of complement. Forssman antibodies resemble the antibodies found in infectious mononucleosis in that they agglutinate sheep red cells, but differ from them in that they are absorbed by an emulsion of guinea pig kidney, which is rich in Forssman antigen, and are not absorbed by beef cells, which are poor in Forssman antigen. In cases of serum sickness, or sensitization to animal (usually horse) serum, a further type of sheep red cell agglutination antibody is found and may be present in high titer. However, this is again distinguished from the antibody of infectious mononucleosis by being absorbed by guinea pig kidney, and from Forssman antibodies by being absorbed by beef red cells. This is summarized in Table 17-3. This comparison was devised by Davidsohn in 1937 and is used today as the basis for presumptive and differential tests.

### Tests for Infectious Mononucleosis Heterophil Antibody

The sheep cell agglutinins of infectious mononucleosis can be distinguished from those of serum sickness and other conditions by means of a differ-

**TABLE 17-3**

Comparison of Forssman, Serum Sickness, and Infectious Mononucleosis Antibodies[1]

| Antibody | Absorbed by | |
| --- | --- | --- |
| | Guinea Pig Kidney | Beef Red Blood Cells |
| Forssman | Yes | No |
| Serum sickness | Yes | Yes |
| Infectious mononucleosis | No | Yes |

ential test, using absorption with guinea pig kidney and beef red cell antigens. The antibody that can be removed by absorption with guinea pig kidney is known as the Forssman antibody, and with the guinea pig kidney as the Forssman antigen. The classic sheep red cell agglutination test is carried out in two steps: the presumptive test of Paul and Bunnell and the differential test of Paul, Bunnell, and Davidsohn. These are the reference tests from which the rapid testing procedures have evolved. Modifications of these classic procedures utilize horse red cells instead of sheep red cells.

Under normal circumstances, rapid screening tests for EBV infectious mononucleosis (IM) are done for the presence of IgM heterophil antibodies. Horse red cells are usually used rather than sheep red cells, as they are more sensitive to heterophil antibodies. Persons suffering from infectious mononucleosis begin developing heterophil antibodies shortly after the appearance of the clinical symptoms, usually during the first 2 weeks. Highest titers are found during the second and third weeks of the illness. The titer bears no relationship, however, to the severity of the illness. As a rule, heterophil sheep cell agglutinins appear in only 50% to 80% of cases of infectious mononucleosis, so negative results can be obtained when the disease is present. This is especially true in young children with EBV infection, in whom the heterophil test is usually negative. Negative tests therefore do not rule out the possibility of the disease.

The immunologic test for heterophil antibodies is of confirmatory diagnostic importance in cases of infectious mononucleosis with typical clinical and hematologic findings. It is of a deciding diagnostic importance early in the disease when there are unusual clinical findings and hematologic signs, some of which may be caused by complicating factors.

Faster and easier screening tests have been introduced commercially and most laboratories employ them, replacing the laborious presumptive and differential tests done in the past.

The heterophil antibody produced in infectious mononucleosis is IgM and usually appears during the acute phase of the disease or as early as the fourth day and usually by the 21st day of illness. Detectable levels of the IM heterophil antibody may persist for months and for years, in rare instances. These heterophil antibodies have the following characteristics: they react with horse, ox, and sheep red blood cells; they are absorbed by beef red blood cells; they are not absorbed by guinea pig kidney cells; and they do not react with any of the EBV-specific antigens. These characteristics have enabled the development of several immunologic and serologic tests that are commonly used in the diagnosis of infectious mononucleosis.

**Paul-Bunnell Test.** Paul and Bunnell developed their test in 1932, when they first observed that heterophil antibodies developed in persons with infectious mononucleosis.[4] This test is presumptive, as it indicates only the presence or absence of heterophil antibodies. It does not distinguish between antibodies associated with infectious mononucleosis, serum sickness, or the Forssman antigen. That is, the Paul-Bunnell test is not specific. If the test is negative, however, it does eliminate the need for further testing. In this test, patient serum is mixed with antigen-bearing sheep red blood cells. Sheep cells carry antigens associated with infectious mononucleosis and serum sickness and also the Forssman antigen. Dilutions of the patient serum are mixed with the sheep cells, incubated, centrifuged, and examined macroscopically for agglutination. A positive agglutination reaction is primarily associated with infectious mononucleosis, but as previously stated, the test is not specific.

**Davidsohn Modification of the Paul-Bunnell Test.** In 1937, Davidsohn modified the classic Paul-Bunnell test to distinguish the infectious mononucleosis heterophil antibodies from the heterophil antibodies of the Forssman antigen and serum sickness.[1] This is the classic test for infectious mononucleosis heterophil antibodies and has been used as a basis for the rapid testing systems that are currently used in many laboratories.

The Davidsohn differential test is dependent on the fact that sheep red blood cells and beef (ox) red blood cells bear some common antigens that are not present on the guinea pig kidney cells. When the patient's serum is exposed to both the guinea pig kidney cells (rich in the Forssman antigen) and beef red blood cells (poor in the Forssman antigen), differential absorption takes place. The guinea pig kidney will absorb or remove any Forssman antibodies present, and the beef red cells will absorb or remove any infectious mononucleosis heterophil antibody present. Any absorbed antibodies are removed by centrifugation, and the supernatant fluid is tested with the sheep red blood cells. The agglutination patterns are shown in Table 17-3. Positive reactions are recorded only if the differential absorption pattern is typical for the disease. A baseline titer of 1:56 is needed using the preliminary Paul-Bunnell test before this test is performed. In patients with the clinical signs and hematologic features of infectious mononucleosis, a positive Davidsohn differential test establishes the diagnosis.

The sensitivity of this test depends in part on the time after onset of the disease when the specimen is collected and when the test is performed. Peak titers of the heterophil antibody are found during the second and third weeks of the illness. Tests for heterophil antibodies should not be used to follow the clinical course of the disease, as there is a poor correlation between the titer of the infectious mononucleosis antibody and either the stage and severity of the illness or the numbers of atypical lymphocytes seen in the peripheral blood.

In 1968, Lee and Davidsohn found that by using horse red blood cells instead of sheep cells, there was a greater sensitivity in the detection of infectious mononucleosis heterophil antibodies. This adaptation of the classic Davidsohn-Paul-Bunnell test is specific for the disease and has increased the sensitivity. It has also simplified the criterion for a positive test, and baseline titers are not needed. The Lee modification has been utilized in the commercially manufactured rapid slide tests for infectious mononucleosis het-

erophil antibody.[3]

Use of a rapid slide screening test for infectious mononucleosis heterophil antibody is indicated in a patient with the clinical or laboratory evidence of the disease. A positive slide test in a patient with the appropriate clinical signs and symptoms is strong evidence of acute infectious mononucleosis. The slide test is not indicated for screening purposes in an asymptomatic patient.

**Rapid Slide Tests.** Rapid slide tests (also called spot tests) have been developed by several manufacturers. Most of these screening tests utilize fine suspensions of guinea pig kidney for the rapid differential absorption and horse red cells for the sensitive detection of infectious mononucleosis (IM) heterophil antibodies. These rapid screening tests are based on the following general principles: (1) the use of horse red cells instead of sheep red cells makes the test more sensitive and thus is especially valuable for low-titer serum found in the early stages of the disease; (2) the unwashed preserved horse red cell reagent remains in a usable condition for at least 3 months and gives stronger and quicker agglutination with infectious mononucleosis serum than do horse red cells preserved with formalin; (3) some noninfectious mononucleosis serum also has a high horse agglutinin titer, and therefore serologic tests cannot depend on titers alone; and (4) fine suspensions of guinea pig kidney give satisfactory instant absorption of antibodies and a clear-cut differentiation between infectious and noninfectious mononucleosis serum. Before any reagents are used for the test, the reagent test cells should be shaken well to provide a homogeneous mixture. The reagents should be used at room temperature.

For many of these rapid tests, serum, plasma, or whole blood (capillary or anticoagulated venous blood) from the patient can be used and, as part of the test, is mixed thoroughly with guinea pig kidney on one section of the slide to absorb or neutralize any Forssman antibodies present, since both IM antibodies and Forssman antibod-

---

**PROCEDURE 17-2**

*MonoSlide\* Test for Infectious Mononucleosis*

1. Place the slide on a flat surface.

2. Resuspend the guinea pig antigen (Reagent A) to mix thoroughly. Add one drop of Reagent A to the left side of the test circles being used.

3. Invert the horse red cells (Reagent B) to mix thoroughly. Add one drop of Reagent B to the right side of the test circles being used.

4. Using the pipette provided, add one drop of the patient's serum or plasma to the guinea pig antigen (Reagent A, which has previously been added to the left side of the circle). Thoroughly mix the serum with the antigen, using the paddle end of the pipette. When the guinea pig antigen is mixed with the patient's serum, absorption of any Forssman antibodies will take place if any are present in the specimen.

5. Gradually mix the antigen-serum solution into the horse red cells (Reagent B), which have previously been added to the right side of the test circles, covering the entire circle with the mixture.

6. Rock the card by hand slowly and gently for one minute.

7. Immediately observe the mixture macroscopically for the presence or absence of agglutination or clumping.

8. Interpretation of results: *Positive test for infectious mononucleosis:* observation of agglutination or dark clumps against a blue-green background, distributed evenly throughout the test circle. *Negative test for infectious mononucleosis:* no agglutination or clumping observed. A negative test may show a fine granularity against a brown/tan background. Peripheral color development associated with fine granularity should be interpreted as negative. (*Note:* Some persons with infectious mononucleosis do not develop detectable heterophil antibody. Specific EBV antibodies can be identified in these cases.)

---

\*Becton Dickinson Microbiology Systems, Cockeysville, Md.

---

ies will agglutinate the horse red cells in the test reagent (both are heterophil antibodies). The IM antibodies, if present, will remain reactive and will agglutinate the test horse red cells when they are added to the absorbed serum mixture. The test reagents are available commercially as part of the specific test kit being used. Directions must always be followed carefully for each specific product. Agglutination is observed at a specific time after the final mixing, generally after one minute of mixing. If agglutination is observed, the test is positive. If no agglutination is observed, the test is negative. Specific instructions about interpretation of a test are included with the product information. One commercially available test kit utilizing this principle is Mono-Slide, described in Procedure 17-2. This product utilizes specially treated horse red cells that provide color enhancement to increase the specificity, sensitivity, and readability of the test.

When serum is used for the rapid IM screening tests, the presence of hemolysis in the specimen makes it unsuitable for testing. If testing cannot be done immediately, serum or plasma may be stored at 2° to 8° C for several days after being collected.

Most of the widely used rapid immunologic assays for infectious mononucleosis are highly sensitive. It is still necessary, however, to use adequate and proper control programs as the only dependable method of detecting sources of technical errors. Control sera should be tested, using both a positive and a negative control specimen, once during each shift of use to ensure proper kit performance. When the results are not clear-cut, it is always important to repeat the test and to conduct additional serologic tests if needed.

False-negative slide tests may be obtained in patients with a low heterophil titer. This can occur early, in the first 1 or 2 weeks after onset of symptoms. False-negative tests can also be seen in the patient who does not mount a heterophil antibody response to the infection. This can be true especially in young children. The slide test can be repeated at a later date, or an EBV titer for IgM can be performed to help establish the diagnosis for these persons.

False-positive tests for heterophil antibody have been reported in cases of CMV infections, rubella infections, leukemia, Hodgkin's disease, Burkitt's lymphoma, rheumatoid arthritis, viral hepatitis, and multiple myeloma.

## Antinuclear Antibody Tests for Systemic Lupus Erythematosus

Antinuclear antibody (ANA) procedures are used as a screening test for systemic lupus erythematosus (SLE), an autoimmune disease of the connective tissue. SLE is a generalized disorder that affects more women than men and expresses itself as an inflammatory condition of the vessels. It usually involves many organ systems—skin, kidney, blood vessels, blood cells, heart, joints, and central nervous system. The primary cause of death in severe cases of SLE is a pathologic decrease in kidney function. There is no cure for SLE, although steroids and immunosuppressive drugs can help control the course of the disease.

Severe immunologic findings are associated with SLE. A striking laboratory finding is the appearance in the serum of numerous globulins with the properties of antibodies that are directed against various self cell nuclei. These are known as **antinuclear antibodies (ANAs)** or **LE (lupus erythematosus) factor.** ANAs are usually IgG, but they may also be IgM or IgA.

The ANA tests have virtually replaced the LE cell test, formerly the classic diagnostic test for SLE. The LE cell is a neutrophil that has ingested a homogeneous globular mass of altered nuclear material. The LE factor present in the blood of persons with SLE has the ability to cause depolymerization of the nuclear chromatin of polymorphonuclear (PMN) leukocytes. The depolymerized material is subsequently phagocytosed, or ingested, by an intact PMN leukocyte, giving rise to the LE cell.

The transformed nuclear material in the white cell attracts phagocytes, usually segmented PMNs and occasionally monocytes. The phagocytes with the ingested nuclear material are the LE cells. Formation of LE cells requires the presence of the LE factor, damaged leukocytes, and normal active leukocytes. In patients with SLE, LE cells are found in the bone marrow and the peripheral blood when the smears are prepared according to specific procedures. The classic method to observe the LE cells is to mash the blood clot, centrifuge the clot fragments, and make buffy coat smears from the resulting cell suspension. This test has been replaced, for the most part, by immunologic assays for antinuclear antibodies.

### *Antinuclear Antibodies*

Antinuclear antibodies are immunoglobulins that react with the whole cell nucleus or nuclear components such as nuclear proteins, DNA, or histones in the tissue of the host. They are **autoantibodies,** or antibodies directed against self antigens. The presence of ANAs is the serologic hallmark of SLE. ANAs are found in other diseases, such as scleroderma, polymyositis, and rheumatoid arthritis, are associated with the use of certain drugs, and are found in aging persons without disease. Thus the assays for ANAs are not specific for SLE. ANAs are, however, present in more than 95% of persons with SLE. Since the detection of ANAs is not diagnostic of only SLE, their presence cannot confirm the disease. However, the absence of ANAs can be used to help rule out SLE. The significance of the presence of ANAs in a patient's serum must be considered in relation to the patient's age, sex, clinical signs and symptoms, and other laboratory findings. **Fluorescent antinuclear antibody (FANA)** techniques are commonly used in screening tests for SLE. An indirect fluorescent technique is usually used.

### Indirect Immunofluorescent Tests for ANA.

The use of indirect immunofluorescent tests for ANA is based on the utilization of fluorescein-conjugated antiglobulin. These methods are extremely sensitive. In one assay, the serum specimen is delivered into a well on a microscope slide that contains a mouse liver substrate. Substrates of rat or mouse liver or kidney, or cell-cultured fibroblasts, can also be used as the antigen and are fixed to the slides. If antibody is present in the serum of the patient, the unlabeled antibody will attach to the nuclei of the cells in the substrate. After the substrate is washed in buffer, the slide is incubated with fluorescein-labeled goat antihuman immunoglobulin. If the patient antibodies have attached themselves to the nuclear antigens in the substrate, the fluorescein-tagged goat antihuman immunoglobulin will attach to these antibodies. Fluorescence will be seen microscopically using ultraviolet light. The slides should be examined as soon as possible. If immediate examination is not possible, the slides can be stored in the dark at 4° C for up to 48 hours prior to being read.

Several different patterns of fluorescence reactivity are seen, depending on whether the ANAs have reacted with the whole nucleus or with nuclear components such as the nuclear proteins, DNA, or histone (a simple protein). This difference in nuclear fluorescence pattern reflects specificity for various diseases. Patterns are described as being diffuse or homogeneous, peripheral, speckled, or nucleolar fluorescence. Nuclear rim (peripheral) patterns correlate with antibody to native DNA and deoxynucleoprotein and bear correlation with SLE, SLE activity, and lupus nephritis. Homogeneous (diffuse) patterns suggest SLE or another connective tissue disorder. Speckled patterns are found in many diseases, including SLE. Nucleolar patterns are seen in patients with progressive systemic sclerosis and Sjögren's syndrome. After ensuring that the results for positive and negative control specimens are giving the expected reactions, the results for the patient are reported. Results from the screening tests are reported as positive or negative. The normal person is expected to give a negative reaction: no green or gold fluorescence is observed. The degree of positive fluorescence may be semiquantitated on a scale of 1+ to 4+. Positive samples give a green-gold fluorescence of a characteristic pattern (homogeneous, peripheral, speckled, or nucleolar).

## Rheumatoid Factor

The identification of rheumatoid factor (RF) in the serum or synovial fluid of patients with clinical features of rheumatoid arthritis (RA) assists in confirming the diagnosis. Rheumatoid arthritis is a chronic inflammatory disease, primarily affecting the joints and joint tissues. It is generally accepted that immunologic reactions contribute significantly to the pathogenesis of the disease. Rheumatoid factors are autoantibodies that are directed against the Fc fragment of IgG—usually an IgM antibody to the altered IgG antibody, an antibody to an antibody. The sera of most patients with RA have detectable abnormal protein immune complexes. These protein complexes circulate and are known collectively as **rheumatoid factor.** RF is now generally accepted to be actually a group of immunoglobulins that interact specifically with antigenic determinants on the IgG molecule. RF is associated with either IgG or IgM, more commonly with IgM. RF is present in many persons with RA, but not all. RF can also be present in other diseases, but the highest titers are found in persons with RA.

Patients with tuberculosis, bacterial endocarditis, hepatitis, or collagen diseases may also have RF in their serum. RF that appears in chronic diseases virtually disappears when the infectious process is treated with the appropriate therapy; RF that is present in RA persists indefinitely. RF is not found in degenerative joint diseases like osteoarthritis or in gout or infectious joint diseases. The determination of the presence of RF is important in the prognosis and management of RA. High titers of RF are indications of greater amounts of joint destruction, possible increased systemic involvement, and generally more severe disease. RF can also be detected in synovial fluid, but its significance is little more than that of RF in serum.

### Tests for Rheumatoid Factor

The tests for RF are based on the reaction between antibodies in the patient's serum (RF) and an antigen derived from gamma globulin. Generally, all tests are designed to detect antibodies to immunoglobulins. A latex-coated suspension coated with albumin and chemically bonded with denatured human gamma globulin serves as the antigen in one commonly used test for RF. If RF is present in the serum, macroscopic agglutination will be visible when the latex reagent is mixed with serum. Latex agglutination procedures have a 95% correlation with a clinical diagnosis of probable or definite RA. False-positive tests are possible with other rheumatic diseases, such as lupus erythematosus, in chronic infectious diseases such as hepatitis, tuberculosis, and syphilis, and in other diseases, such as liver cirrhosis and sarcoidosis. Other RF tests utilize sensitized sheep cells in hemagglutination procedures. The latex agglutination and sheep cell agglutination tests are the most popular of the routine tests used for RF. There are several commercial kits available for assay of RF; some use test tubes and some are rapid slide tests.

**Rapid Latex Agglutination Test for RF.** Serum is usually the specimen used for this test. If the test cannot be performed immediately, the specimen should be refrigerated. If the test cannot be performed within 72 hours, the specimen should be frozen. Frozen serum should be thawed rapidly at 37° C prior to testing. Before the test is done, the specimen should be at room temperature. All reagents used for the rapid slide RF tests must be at room temperature. It is always important to carefully follow all instructions provided with the testing product.

### Syphilis

Serologic tests are among the most important diagnostic procedures for syphilis. The laboratory results, together with clinical signs and the patient's history, aid the physician in making the diagnosis. Syphilis tests were some of the first serologic determinations done. The first diagnostic blood test for syphilis was introduced by Wassermann in 1906, when syphilis was a great threat to humans and many researchers had devoted years to the problem of finding a laboratory diagnosis for the disease. To many, the terms syphilis and serology have become synonymous.

Syphilis is a sexually transmitted disease that continues to be a medical problem. In the United States more than 80,000 cases of syphilis are reported annually. The number of reported cases has continued to rise over the last several years. Early detection and treatment of syphilis are of critical importance to prevent the infection from spreading and doing further harm to the patient.

Adequate diagnosis and treatment are important in all three stages of syphilis. The first stage extends from the initial inoculation with a spirochete type of bacterium, *Treponema pallidum*, by direct contact (usually sexual) with an infectious lesion, to the formation of the chancre at the initial port of entry. The chancre is a primary lesion that appears 3 to 4 weeks after the initial inoculation. In this first stage, both the blood and the local lesion are infective. The sores often heal by themselves. In the second stage, there is a generalized illness that suggests a viral infection, along with appearance of a rash of the skin and mucous membranes. Exudates from the lesions contain large numbers of the syphilitic spirochetes. The patient is still highly contagious. Specific antibodies to the spirochete begin to appear about 4 to 6 weeks after the initial inoculation or 1 to 3 weeks after the appearance of the primary sore or chancre. In the third, or latent, stage of the disease, no clinical signs or symptoms are seen; it is recognized only by serologic tests. If the disease is untreated, severe systemic complications can occur. Complications include cardiovascular and central nervous system problems (strokes and seizures), personality changes, and dementia.

Direct microscopic examination of the treponemes is best done by use of darkfield microscopy. Microscopically, these organisms appear as fine, spiral organisms. The treponemes cannot be cultured in artificial laboratory media, so immunologic testing is usually done to diagnose the presence of syphilis. In addition to formation of specific antibodies to *T. pallidum*, patients with a syphilitic infection respond immunologically by producing a nonspecific reagin antibody-like substance. Serologic tests for syphilis are therefore divided into two categories based on the two types of antibodies present in persons with syphilitic infections: tests for treponemal antibodies and tests for nontreponemal antibodies.

### Treponemal Antibody Tests

Treponemal antibodies are produced against the antigen of the *T. pallidum* organism itself. Serologic tests for the treponemal antibody include the fluorescent treponemal antibody absorption test (FTA-ABS) and the MHA-TP (microhemagglutination *Treponema pallidum*) test. These procedures are used to confirm that a positive nontreponemal test result has been caused by syphilis rather than one of the other biological conditions that can also produce a positive nontreponemal test result. In the FTA-ABS test, the patient's serum is first absorbed with non-*T. pallidum* treponemal antigens to reduce any nonspecific cross-reactivity. Then a fluorescein-conjugated antihuman antibody reagent is applied as a marker for specific antitreponemal antibodies in the patient's serum. The test slide is examined with a fluorescence microscope and the intensity of fluorescence noted.

### Nontreponemal Antibody Tests

Nontreponemal antibodies are also called **reagin antibodies.** These antibodies are produced by the infected person against components of their own or other mammalian bodies. Reagin antibodies are almost always produced by persons with syphilis, but can also be produced in other infectious diseases, such as leprosy, tuberculosis, malaria, measles, chickenpox, infectious mononucleosis, and hepatitis. The reagin antibodies can also be seen in noninfectious disorders such as autoimmune conditions and rheumatoid disease and in nondiseases such as pregnancy and old age. The two most widely used tests for nontreponemal antibody are the VDRL (Venereal Disease Research Laboratory) test and the RPR (Rapid Plasma Reagin) test. Both of these tests are based on an agglutination or flocculation reaction in which soluble antigen particles are coalesced to form larger particles that are visible as clumps when aggregated by the antibody. These nontreponemal screening tests can be confirmed by another testing method, usually the FTA-ABS test or the MHA-TP test, tests for the presence of specific treponemal antibody.

**VDRL Flocculation Test.** This test is performed using cardiolipin-lecithin-cholesterol antigen and heat-inactivated serum from the patient, or with cerebrospinal fluid. It is commonly a slide test. Technique must be strictly adhered to and standardized reagents must be used to ensure good results. Quality control measures must be employed to ensure reproducible and reliable results from laboratory to laboratory. Positive and negative control sera of predetermined reactivity indicate when corrective action should be taken. Since this procedure tests for nonspecific reagin, antibodies other than those of syphilis may react with the antigen. The test is therefore not 100% specific for syphilis, but it is practical, inexpensive, and reproducible. A positive VDRL test should be confirmed with the FTA-ABS or TP-MHA test.

**Rapid Plasma Reagin (RPR) Card Test.** In this test, the patient's serum is mixed with an antigen suspension of a carbon particle cardiolipin antigen on the special disposable card provided with the test kit. If the suspension contains reagin, the antibody-like substance present in the serum of persons with syphilis, flocculation occurs with a coagglutination of the carbon particles of antigen. This flocculation appears as black clumps against the white background of the plastic-coated RPR card. This reaction is observed and graded macroscopically. A diagnosis of syphilis cannot be made solely on the basis of a positive RPR card test, without clinical signs and symptoms or supportive history. Positive reactions are occasionally seen with other infectious conditions or inflammatory states, thus necessitating confirmation of all positive results with the qualitative RPR test. Various manufacturers produce RPR kits, and the instructions included with the kits must be followed carefully. Positive and negative control sera should be tested daily to ensure the accuracy of the test antigen reagent.

## REFERENCES

1. Davidsohn I: Serologic diagnosis of infectious mononucleosis. *JAMA* 1937; 108:289.

2. Lee C, Hart LL: Accuracy of home pregnancy tests: DICP. *Ann Pharmacother* 1990;24:712.

3. Lee CL, Davidsohn I, Panczyszyn O: Horse agglutinins in infectious mononucleosis. II. The spot test. *Am J Clin Pathol* 1968; 49:12.

4. Paul JR, Bunnell WW: The presence of heterophile antibodies to infectious mononucleosis. *Am J Med Sci* 1932; 183:90-104.5.

5. Ravel R: *Clinical Laboratory Medicine,* ed 6. St Louis, Mosby, 1995, pp 543-545.

## BIBLIOGRAPHY

Baron EJ, Peterson, LR, Finegold SM: *Bailey and Scott's Diagnostic Microbiology,* ed 9. St Louis, Mosby, 1994.

Henry JB (ed): *Clinical Diagnosis and Management by Laboratory Methods,* ed 19. Philadelphia, WB Saunders Co, 1996.

NCCLS: *Glossary and Guidelines for Immunodiagnostic Procedures, Reagents, and Reference Materials: Approved Guideline.* Villanova, Pa, National Committee for Clinical Laboratory Standards, 1992, Document DI1-A2.

NCCLS: *Physician's Office Laboratory Manual: Tentative Guideline.* Villanova, Pa, National Committee for Clinical Laboratory Standards, 1995, POL 1/2-T3.

Turgeon ML: *Immunology and Serology in Laboratory Medicine,* ed 2. St Louis, Mosby, 1996.

## STUDY QUESTIONS

1. Which immunoglobulin is typically found in external secretions such as saliva and tears?

   A. IgA
   B. IgE
   C. IgG
   D. IgM

2. Substances that gain antigenicity only when coupled to a protein carrrier are:

   A. Agglutinins
   B. Agglutinogens
   C. Haptens
   D. Opsonins

3. Antibodies that result from exposure to antigenic material from another species are referred to as:

   A. Heteroantibodies
   B. Alloantibodies
   C. Isoantibodies
   D. More than one of the above

4. Which of the following is the visible result of an antigen-antibody reaction between a soluble antigen and its specific antibody?

   A. Sensitization
   B. Precipitation
   C. Agglutination
   D. Complement fixation

5. Which of the following is true about immunoglobulins?

   A. Produced by T lymphocytes
   B. Produced by B lymphocytes
   C. Purified (cloned) from a single ancestral cell
   D. Derived from the thymus and influenced by thymic hormones

6. Which of the following is used to confirm a positive screening test in testing a patient for HIV antibody?

   A. ELISA
   B. Immunofluorescence assay
   C. Western blot
   D. Complement fixation test

7. Which of the following immunoglobulins can cross the placenta and therefore provides passive immunity to the infant for the first few months of life?

   A. IgA
   B. IgD
   C. IgG
   D. IgM

8. Which of the following immunoglobulins is found in the greatest amounts in the serum, yet is the smallest in size?

   A. IgA
   B. IgD
   C. IgG
   D. IgM

9. Agglutination occurs only if the antigen is in which of the following forms when the antigen-antibody complex occurs?

   A. Is a particle such as a bacterium or blood cell
   B. Is soluble
   C. Both of the above
   D. Neither of the above

10. Most commonly, the rheumatoid factor in rheumatoid arthritis is associated with which immunoglobulin?

    A. IgA
    B. IgD
    C. IgG
    D. IgM

11. The most specific assays for human chorionic gonadotropin (hCG) utilize antibody reagents against which subunit of hCG?

    A. Alpha
    B. Beta
    C. Gamma
    D. Chorionic

12. The concentration of hCG is generally at a particular level in serum about two to three days after implantation. This is the concentration at which most sensitive laboratory assays can give a positive serum hCG result. What is the lowest level of hormone for which most current serum hCG tests can give a positive result?

    A. 25 mIU/mL
    B. 50 mIU/mL
    C. 100 mIU/mL
    D. 100,000 mIU/mL

13. The heterophil antibody produced in infectious mononucleosis is of which class of immunoglobulins?

    A. IgA
    B. IgD
    C. IgG
    D. IgM

14. Heterophil antibodies produced in infectious mononucleosis have *all but which one* of the following characteristics?

    A. They are absorbed by guinea pig kidney cells.
    B. They are not absorbed by guinea pig kidney cells.
    C. They are absorbed by beef red cells.
    D. They react with horse, ox, and sheep red cells.

15. **T lymphocyte function is characterized by *all but which one* of the following?**

    A. Produce and secrete immunoglobulins
    B. A subset develops killer cells that produce cytokines
    C. A subset suppresses the immune response
    D. A subset develops helper cells

16. **The primary requirement for a substance to be an antigen in a particular individual is that it:**

    A. Have a large molecular weight.
    B. Be composed of protein and polysaccharide.
    C. Be different from "self."
    D. Have several different combining sites.

17. **Of the circulating lymphocytes in the peripheral blood, which are in the greatest percentages, B or T lymphocytes?**

18. **In certain disease states, antibodies are made to self antigens; this is known as:**

    A. Autoimmune disease
    B. Infection
    C. Inflammatory response
    D. Phagocytosis

## CASE HISTORIES

### ■ CASE 1

A 25-year-old woman comes to the clinic for pregnancy testing. She reports that her last menstrual period began 30 days ago. The clinic uses a rapid indirect latex slide agglutination pregnancy test. A random urine specimen is collected for testing. The result for this test is reported as negative. The physical examination indicates that the woman is pregnant.

1. What is a possible reason for the negative test result? (More than one answer may be correct.)
    A. The specific gravity was greater than 1.015.
    B. The lack of agglutination seen on the test slide was interpreted as a negative test result.
    C. The test lacks the sensitivity to detect the concentration of hCG present in the specimen.
    D. The urine specimen is not concentrated enough, specific gravity below 1.015.

2. If conception is estimated to have taken place 16 days prior to the visit to the clinic, and if this is an average pregnancy, what would be the normal average serum hCG concentration at the time of her visit?
    A. 25 mIU/mL
    B. 50 mIU/mL
    C. 500 mIU/mL
    D. 30,000 mIU/mL

3. What should be the next step(s) to follow up this clinic visit?

### ■ CASE 2

A 45-year-old woman comes to a clinic with complaints of morning stiffness in her ankle joints, worse on rising in the morning and improving during the day. Her discomfort is responsive to aspirin. She has also been fatigued and weak. During the last week she has noticed that her wrist and ankle joints on both sides of her body are also painful and swollen. Blood is drawn to test for rheumatoid factor (RF) and antinuclear antibodies (ANA), and synovial fluid is aspirated and analyzed. Results from analysis of the synovial fluid rule out crystal deposition diseases, such as gout and pseudogout, and no infectious microorganisms are seen. Results of immunologic blood tests for RF and ANA are as follows:

RF        Positive
ANA      Negative

1. On the basis of the above findings (history and the test results), the patient is likely to have:
    A. Degenerative arthritis
    B. Rheumatoid arthritis
    C. Systemic lupus erythematosus with joint involvement
    D. Joint disease from a gonococcal infection
2. Which immunoglobulin serves as the antigen in this disease?

## ■ CASE 3

A male college freshman is seen at the college health service complaining of general fatigue, a sore throat, and swollen lymph nodes in his neck. A throat culture is done, and blood is drawn for hematology studies and a heterophil antibody test.

Hematology results show a normal hemoglobin and a slight increase in the white cell count, with many large reactive lymphocytes being seen in the differential. A rapid strep test is negative, but a second swab is cultured on sheep blood and incubated, the result to be read in 18 hours. The result from the heterophil antibody test is positive.

1. From the above findings, what is the probable diagnosis for this patient?
   A. Systemic lupus erythematosus
   B. Infectious mononucleosis
   C. Strep throat, infection with $\beta$-hemolytic streptococcus, group A
   D. Viral infection
2. Knowing the above, what would you expect the result from the 18-hour incubated throat culture to be?
   A. Normal throat flora, no $\beta$-hemolytic streptococcus seen on sheep blood
   B. Group A $\beta$-hemolytic streptococcus seen on sheep blood

# CHAPTER 18

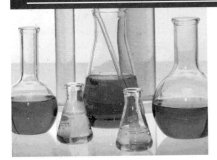

# *Immunohematology*

## Learning Objectives

*From study of this chapter, the reader will be able to:*

- ➤ Define immunohematology, blood banking, and blood transfusion.
- ➤ Appreciate the complexity of the field of immunohematology and transfusion medicine and the need for strictly enforced procedures and regulations.
- ➤ Explain the role of antigens and antibodies in immunohematology.
- ➤ Define natural and immune antibodies and their roles in blood banking.
- ➤ Describe the means of detecting antigen-antibody reactions in blood banking, including the role of complement.
- ➤ Define antisera and discuss preparation and requirements.
- ➤ Define genotype and phenotype as used in immunohematology.
- ➤ Describe ABO cell and serum typing procedures.
- ➤ Explain Landsteiner's rule and how it applies to blood banking procedures.
- ➤ Explain the concept of universal donors and recipients.
- ➤ Explain what is meant by Rh negative and Rh positive.
- ➤ Discuss CDE and Rh-Hr terminology and inheritance.
- ➤ Explain and describe the direct and indirect antihuman globulin reaction (Coombs' test).
- ➤ Discuss hemolytic disease of the newborn, including detection and prevention.

# INTRODUCTION

The field of immunohematology has advanced rapidly, and all indications point to further advancement as techniques in transfusion medicine continue to change. Since 1951, new discoveries have been made at a rapid pace and the nature of the immunologic response to different antigens has been shown to be vastly more complicated than was at first supposed. Before 1951, nine independent blood group systems had been discovered. These important systems and their approximate dates of discovery are ABO (1900), MN (1927), P (1927), Rh (from rhesus) (1939), Lutheran (1945), Kell (1946), Lewis (1946), Duffy (1950), and Kidd (1951). As of 1993, over 600 antigens had been organized into twenty-two blood group systems. The complexity of the red cell and its antigenic polymorphism seems almost endless, and it is expected that as methodology for studying red cell antigen-antibody reactions improves, the boundaries of knowledge will continue to expand.

The risk of transfusion-transmitted infections such as viral hepatitis and human immunodeficiency virus (HIV) infection has significantly changed the practice of transfusion medicine. Changes have occurred in the manner in which blood is tested before transfusion, the way in which donors are selected, and the nature of the blood component or derivative used for transfusion.

A study of the immunologic reactions of blood cells is critical when therapeutic replacement of blood is necessary. The many possible antigen-antibody reactions that can occur must be anticipated and tested for by using the laboratory procedures available in the immunohematology laboratory. In many diseases and health problems, therapeutic administration of blood and blood products is indicated. Severe illness and death are closely associated with loss of blood, which impairs the ability of the circulatory system to deliver adequate amounts of oxygen to the body cells and critically upsets the delicate homeostatic water and acid-base balance of body fluids. Blood loss may be caused by hemorrhage, excessive destruction of red cells, or the body's inability to replenish its own blood supply. In specific instances, administration of blood or its components is indicated. The technique of replacing whole blood or its components is known as **blood transfusion.** The procedures involved in collecting, storing, processing, and distributing blood are called **blood banking.** The techniques and procedures involving the study of the immunologic responses of blood cells are called **immunohematology.**

Immunohematology and blood banking are unlike other fields of clinical laboratory investigation. Although accuracy is always important in the laboratory, it is absolutely essential in blood banking. Even the smallest error can directly result in the death of a patient from a hemolytic transfusion reaction. As R.R. Race said, "Blood group tests are different from most laboratory tests used in medicine in a vital way—the reported result must be correct, for the wisest physician cannot protect his patient from the consequences of a blood grouping error."[1]

This chapter is meant only as a very general introduction to the subject of blood banking and immunohematology. It is definitely not sufficient in itself as preparation for work in blood banking laboratories. Specific blood banking procedures are not presented; only principles are discussed. Several excellent texts are available in the field of blood banking; however, most of them seem complex (even unintelligible) to the person who has no background in this area. Probably the best single reference, in a practical sense, is the *American Association of Blood Banks (AABB) Technical Manual.* This indispensable reference will be found in any licensed blood bank and should be consulted by the regular blood bank staff.

To carry out blood banking procedures, a thorough knowledge of the principles involved, recognition of the many difficulties that may be encountered, and exactness of technique are essential. Shortcuts must never be taken. Everyone working in a particular blood bank must use exactly the same technique. Also, an elaborate system of safeguards must be established and thoroughly understood by all personnel. These are the standard operating procedures, which must be established and followed for each blood bank laboratory. These safeguards and checks may seem repetitive but are essential. When an incompatible transfusion reaction occurs, it is usually caused by a breakdown of, or failure to observe, the established system.

Complete, permanent, legible records must be kept of every sequence of the many steps involved in administering a unit of blood. Manual or computerized record keeping systems may be employed. Manual results and observations are always entered directly on the permanent record, in ink, and never recopied, as recopying will invariably result in error at some time. If changes are made to computerized results, they must be appropriately documented in the computer.

## Blood

Whole human blood consists of two major portions: solid and liquid. The solid portion consists primarily of the formed elements—red blood cells, white blood cells, and platelets—and makes up about 45% of the total blood volume. The liquid portion consists of the **plasma,** which makes up about 55% of the total volume. The blood volume of normal adults is approximately 5 to 6 L. In blood banking, reference is often made to a unit of blood. For practical purposes, a unit may be considered about 500 mL of whole blood.

Infused blood, or blood that is administered by transfusion, must be anticoagulated. However, the portion of blood that is used for blood bank testing procedures such as typing and crossmatching is generally clotted blood. Although **serum** (from clotted blood) is preferred, plasma may be used. If plasma from anticoagulated blood is used, there is a chance that small fibrin clots may be present in the plasma and may be incorrectly interpreted as a positive result. Therefore, laboratory blood bank tests generally employ red cells and serum (the liquid remaining after blood has been allowed to clot), not red cells and plasma. Another important reason for using serum rather than plasma in labo-

ratory testing is that complement activation is usually prevented by an anticoagulant. Most anticoagulants bind calcium, which is necessary for complement integrity. Persons doing blood banking procedures are repeatedly reminded that complement activity occurs in laboratory tests only when serum is used. In the body, plasma does not have the added anticoagulant, and therefore the complement integrity is not lost. Therefore, complement activation occurs as readily in serum in the laboratory as it does in plasma in the body. This is important in the laboratory, as several blood group antibodies require complement activation in order for an observable reaction to be seen.

## Historical Interest in Transfusions

The importance of blood must have been realized from the earliest times. Early humans must have observed that loss of blood could lead to death. In addition, some primitive groups had rituals in which the blood of one person was given to another; it was thought that in this way various characteristics of the donor could be given to the recipient. The discovery of the circulation of blood by Harvey in 1616 did much to advance interest in blood transfusion. In one early transfusion, attempted by Denis in 1667, lamb's blood was transfused into a man. At first this seemed to benefit the man, who was given a total of three such transfusions. However, after the third transfusion of lamb's blood the man suffered a reaction and died. It was found that it is impossible to successfully transfuse the blood of one species of animal into another species (isogenic), whether from animal to human, human to animal, or animal of one species to animal of another species. Transfusions were also attempted within the same species of animal, such as from human to human, or from one animal to another of the same species. These species-specific transfusions seemed to work about half the time, but far too often the result was death.

## Blood Groups

It is now known that the incompatibility of many transfusions was caused by the presence of certain factors that we now know are antigens on red cells. Each species of animal, humans included, has certain antigens that are unique to that species and are present on the red cells of all members of that species. If the red cells of sheep, for example, are transfused into a human, an anti-sheep substance **(antibody)** will be produced in the blood of the human. The anti-sheep substance will destroy any sheep red cells that are subsequently introduced. This cell destruction is what is meant by an incompatible hemolytic transfusion reaction, and it results in the death of the recipient.

It is also known that certain antigens are common to some, but not all, members of a particular species. If blood containing such antigens is transfused into a recipient whose red cells do not contain that antigen, the recipient will form an antibody that may result in an incompatible transfusion reaction. These antibodies from different members of the same species are referred to as **alloantibodies.**

So far, this seems rather simple. Why all the difficulty in blood banking? All that is necessary is to find the antigen present on the red cell and transfuse only blood containing that antigen. The principle is correct, but over 600 red cell antigens have been described and organized into units referred to as blood group systems. Twenty-two blood group systems have been described. A partial list includes:

| ABO | Kidd | Lutheran | Kell |
|-----|------|----------|------|
| Rh | P | I | Xg |
| Lewis | Diego | MNSs | Duffy |

The antigens that exist on a person's red cells within a particular blood group system represent that person's type for that system. The number of possible types within one system varies. In the ABO system there are six main types, plus additional types determined by less frequent subgroups. The more complex Rh-Hr system alone has over 100 possible types. Taking all systems and type combinations into account, over 500 billion different types of blood

are possible. In essence, each person has a unique blood type.

At this point it would seem that blood transfusion is impossible, since no two persons should have exactly the same type of blood. Fortunately, only certain antigens are likely to give problems in transfusion (i.e., incompatible transfusion reactions), although there is always the possibility that an unknown or untested-for antigen may occur that will result in such a reaction. The antigens most likely to cause reactions are located within the ABO and Rh-Hr systems and must be tested for whenever blood is administered. Other antigens are routinely tested for indirectly through crossmatching and antibody screening techniques. Persons who are given an antigen not present on their red cells may produce an alloantibody in their plasma that will react with the foreign antigen. This is evidenced by the destruction of the red cell containing the foreign antigen.

## Inheritance of Blood Groups
### Genes

All the factors or antigens present on a person's red cells are inherited. Each antigen is controlled by a gene, which is the unit of inheritance. In other words, antigens are inherited as genes. If the gene for a particular antigen is present, that antigen will be found on all the red cells.

### Chromosomes

Each cell (except for mature red cells) consists of cytoplasm and a nucleus. If the nucleus is observed under the microscope at approximately the time of cell division, several long, threadlike structures will be visible. These structures are referred to as chromosomes. Each species has a specific number of chromosomes, and the chromosomes occur in pairs. Humans have 46 chromosomes (23 chromosome pairs). The paired chromosomes are similar in size and shape and have their own distinct functions. A complete set of 23 chromosomes is inherited from each parent. Chromosomes occur in pairs in all cells of the body, except the sex cells (sperm and ovum), which contain 23 single chromosomes.

### Gene Location (Linkage)

Since the gene is the unit of inheritance, it must also be located within the nucleus. Genes are exceedingly small particles that, when associated in linear form, make up the chromosome. They are too small to see under the normal brightfield microscope but together are visible as the chromosome. Genes are made up of deoxyribonucleic acid (DNA). Each trait that is inherited is controlled by the presence of a specific gene. The genes responsible for a particular trait always occur at exactly the same point or position on a particular chromosome; this position is referred to as the locus of the gene. Research in the field of genetics is continually revealing new information about the location or sequence of genes on the chromosome and about diseases that are genetically inherited or environmentally induced. If genes for different inherited traits are known to be carried on the same chromosome, they are said to be syntenic. This term is useful in referring to genes on a single chromosome that are too far apart to display absolute linkage in inheritance. Genes that are located on the same chromosome and are normally inherited together are known as **linked genes.** The closer the loci of the genes, the closer the **linkage** is said to be.

### Alleles

Inherited traits are somewhat variable within a species. For example, eye color varies, and it is known to be inherited. Therefore, each possible eye color must be the result of a gene for that color. Variants of a gene for a particular trait are referred to as **alleles** for that trait. Since we have only two genes (one pair) for any given trait, our cells will have only two alleles. However, the number of possible alleles for a trait varies. A person who has identical alleles for a trait is said to be **homozygous** for that trait. For example, a person with blue eyes carries two blue-eye genes and is homozygous for blue eyes.

A person who has two different alleles for a trait is **heterozygous** for that trait—for example, having a blue-eye gene in addition to a brown-eye gene.

In general, certain alleles may be stronger than, or may mask the presence of, other alleles. In the case of eye color, brown-eye genes mask the presence of blue-eye genes, and are said to be dominant over blue-eye genes. Persons who have one brown-eye and one blue-eye gene have eyes that appear brown. Blue-eye genes are then said to be recessive in relation to brown-eye genes. One must have two blue-eye genes in order to have blue eyes. However, in blood banking, the various alleles for a particular blood group system are equally dominant, or codominant. If the gene is present (and there is a suitable testing solution available), it will be detected.

### Phenotypes and Genotypes

Two other genetic terms that are often used in blood banking are phenotype and genotype. The **phenotype** is the blood type determined by tests made directly on the blood, even though other antigens may be present. The **genotype** refers to the actual total genetic pattern for any system. It is usually impossible to determine the complete genotype in the laboratory; this usually requires additional studies, especially family studies.

## ANTIGENS AND ANTIBODIES IN IMMUNOHEMATOLOGY

All blood banking is based on a knowledge of antigens and antibodies. Unfortunately, they cannot be defined simply. In general, an antigen may be thought of as a foreign substance—foreign in the sense that if it is introduced into the body of a person who does not already have the antigen, an antisubstance called an antibody will be produced. The antibody is found in the plasma and other body fluids. It reacts with the foreign antigen in some observable way, and it is specific for the antigen against which it is formed—that is, it reacts with only its corresponding antigen and no other antigen. The significance of antigens and antibodies is not limited to blood banking. See the information on antigens and antibodies in Chapter 17.

## Transfusion Reactions

In blood banking, antibody formation does not result in protective immunity. The blood group antigens are present on the red cells, and the antibody is found in the plasma or serum. The antigen-antibody reaction results in the destruction of the antigen-carrying red cell by antibody in the serum of the person receiving the red cells. Clinically the result of this red cell destruction is the transfusion reaction. It may be a hemolytic reaction or decreased red cell survival as a result of antibodies coating the red cells being removed by the reticuloendothelial system (RES). The reaction varies from patient to patient, but generally the immediate reaction is characterized by chills, high temperature, pain in the lower back, nausea, vomiting, and shock as indicated by decreased blood pressure and rapid pulse. These first effects of the reaction are rarely fatal; however, the by-products of red cell destruction pose many problems, primarily severe renal involvement. The patient may eventually die from kidney failure. The same blood group antigens are found not only on the red cells but also in the other body fluids, such as urine, saliva, plasma, and gastric juice.

## Natural and Immune Antibodies

A different antibody classification in immunohematology includes natural and immune antibodies. The **natural antibody** appears to exist without antigenic stimulus, whereas the **immune antibody** is the result of stimulation by specific blood group antigens. Examples of natural antibodies in blood are the anti-A and anti-B antibodies found in the ABO blood group system. In this system, if the red cell lacks the A antigen, anti-A antibody will be found in the serum. If the red cell lacks the B antigen, anti-B antibody will be found in the serum. Hence the name natural antibody. Substances very similar to blood group antigens A and B are so widely distributed in nature that the antibody will develop in anyone if the antigen is not present. Certain bacteria and foods may have A-like or B-like antigens. The natural anti-A and anti-B antibodies are routinely used in testing for the ABO blood group. (They are saline solution-active and of the IgM type.) There are several other natural IgM blood group antibodies.

Immune antibodies are also referred to as **unexpected antibodies.** They are usually the result of specific antigenic stimulation, and they result from immunization by way of pregnancy, transfusion, or injection of red cells. Once immunization exists, it is permanent. Immune antibodies are of the IgG, IgA, or IgM type.

## Means of Detecting Antigen-Antibody Reactions in Blood Banking

Two terms that are used in discussing biological reactions are in vivo and in vitro. **In vivo** means in the living body, and **in vitro** means in glass (or in a laboratory setting). A biological reaction that normally occurs in the body (in vivo) may be demonstrated in vitro, or under laboratory conditions. Blood banking reactions that are used in determining blood groups and compatibility are in vitro reactions.

### Antisera

To determine a person's blood type, some sort of substance must be available to show what antigens are present on the red cell. The substance used for this purpose is referred to as an antiserum or antisera. An **antiserum** is a prepared and highly purified solution of antibody. It is named on the basis of the antibody it contains. For example, a solution of anti-A antibodies is called anti-A antiserum.

**Preparation of Antisera.** Most of the antisera that are used in blood banking are prepared commercially and purchased by the blood bank. In general, antiserum is prepared as follows:

1. Animals are deliberately inoculated with antigen, and the resulting serum, which contains antibody, is purified and standardized for use as an antiserum.
2. Serum is collected from humans who have been sensitized to an antigen through

transfusion, pregnancy, or intramuscular injection.

3. Monoclonal antisera are produced by hybridization, a fusion of a single clone of human neoplastic antibody-producing cells with sensitized splenic lymphocytes obtained from a rodent species.

**Antisera Requirements.** Antiserum must meet certain requirements to be acceptable for use. It must be specific for the antigen to be detected—that is, specific under the manufacturer's recommended test conditions. It must have a sufficient titer to detect antigen. It must have a certain avidity for, or strength of reaction with, corresponding red cells. It must also be sterile, clear, provided in a good container with a dropper, and stable. It should be marked with an expiration date and must never be used after this date. In addition, it must be stored at 4° C when not in use.

Exact requirements for antisera are defined by the Food and Drug Administration (FDA) Center for Biologics Evaluation and Research. When commercial antisera are used, the manufacturer's directions must be followed carefully and quality assurance procedures established and documented. For antisera that are produced locally, and unlicensed, there must be records of reactivity and specificity as described in the AABB manual.

**Reaction of Antisera With Red Cells.** When antiserum is mixed with red cells, an antigen-antibody reaction may or may not occur. If a reaction does occur, the corresponding antigen must be present on the red cell, and the result is a positive reaction. If a reaction does not occur, the antigen is absent, and the result is negative. A positive reaction with anti-A antiserum demonstrates the presence of A antigen on the red cell, and so on.

In the original definition of antibody, it was stated that antibody resulting from antigenic stimulation will react with the antigen in an observable manner. In blood banking, two types of observable reactions may occur: *agglutination* and *hemolysis.*

## Agglutination

**Agglutination** is clumping, or close association, of red cells caused by a specific antibody or antigen present on the cells. A positive antigen-antibody reaction results in an immediate combination of antibody and antigen on the red cell, followed by the visible agglutination, which takes longer to form. The IgG antibody, for example, is thought to be a somewhat Y-shaped structure with a reactive site at the end of each arm of the Y (see Fig. 17-1). Each reactive site is capable of combining with corresponding antigen. Agglutination is thought to be the result of bridging of the red cells by antibody reacting with antigen sites on adjacent red cells. This bridging causes the red cells to stick together. Several such bridges result in visible clumping. The degree of agglutination varies. Very strong agglutination forms a large mass of cells that can be easily seen macroscopically. Less strong agglutination results in correspondingly smaller clumps of cells that can also be seen macroscopically, and finally in clumps of cells that can be seen only microscopically. The ability to observe all degrees of agglutination requires great care and experience. It is not a simple task, yet it is imperative that the degree of agglutination be detected.

## Hemolysis

**Hemolysis** is the result of lysis, or destruction, of the red cell by a specific antibody. It is probably the third stage in an antigen-antibody reaction and does not occur in all cases. The antibody causes rupture of the cell membrane with release of hemoglobin. The result is a crystal-clear red solution, with no cloudiness since no cells are present. Whenever hemolysis occurs, it is a positive antigen-antibody reaction. However, it may be overlooked and reported as negative, since agglutination is much more common and hemolysis looks much like a negative reaction with no agglutination. In the case of a negative reaction, however, the cells remain in a smooth, cloudy suspension.

It is also possible to have partial hemolysis, when some cells are hemolyzed and others agglutinate. This is particularly difficult to interpret. Misinterpretation of hemolysis is a cause of false-negative results in the blood bank and may end in disaster for the patient.

### Role of Complement in Hemolysis

For hemolysis to occur, a substance called complement must be present in the serum being tested. Complement is a complex substance with at least nine components. It is important in blood banking because some antigen-antibody reactions require the presence of complement to be demonstrated in vitro, and although almost all normal sera contain complement when fresh, complement is destroyed by heat. Therefore, to have complement activity, the serum must be either fresh or stored correctly. Complement will remain active if stored for 24 to 48 hours at 4° C or for 2 months at −50° C. If an antibody is to be detected that utilizes complement, it must be provided in the test medium.

### Blood Banking Techniques

In summary, the detection of antigen on red cells requires the demonstration of a positive reaction of the cells with a specific solution of antibodies (antiserum). The technique by which the red cell and antiserum are brought together varies widely, depending on a number of factors. The most important factor is the manner of action of the particular antigen-antibody system being tested for; in other words, knowledge of the antibodies of the blood group system involved is necessary.

In general, blood group tests are performed either on a microscope slide or in test tubes. When test tubes are used, they are $10 \times 75$ or $12 \times 75$ mm. Results are seen as agglutination or hemolysis, as described above. Other methods of detecting antigen-antibody reactions include inhibition of agglutination, immunofluorescence, radioimmunoassay, enzyme-linked immunosorbent assay (ELISA), and solid-phase red cell adherence tests using indicator red cells. Each of these is described in the AABB manual and in Chapter 17 of this book.

Many factors affect red cell agglutination, which is thought to occur in two stages. The first stage involves the physical attachment of antibody to red cells, and is referred to as sensitization. Sensitization is affected by temperature, pH, incubation time, ionic strength, and the antigen-antibody ratio. These factors are influenced by the testing medium that is employed: isotonic saline solution, low-ionic-strength saline, or albumin solution.

The second stage of agglutination involves the formation of bridges between sensitized red cells to form the lattice that is seen as agglutination. Factors that influence this stage include the distance between the cells, the effect of enzymes, and the effect of positively charged molecules such as hexadimethrine (Polybrene).

In all, many factors affect the reactions that are used to detect an antibody-antigen reaction. These include the use of adequate serum and red cells, the concentration of cell suspensions, the testing medium, the temperature and duration of incubation, the use of centrifugation, the use of reagents and glassware, and the reading and interpretation of agglutination reactions. The correct conditions are essential for reliable tests. Development of correct techniques requires thorough knowledge of all these considerations as well as of the blood groups. The technique will also depend on the brand of antiserum that is used and the manufacturer's directions, which must be followed for accurate results.

## THE ABO BLOOD GROUP SYSTEM

The ABO blood group system was first discovered and described in 1900 and 1901 by Karl Landsteiner. By taking the blood of six of his colleagues, separating serum and cells, and mixing each cell suspension with each serum, Landsteiner was able to divide the blood into three groups: A, B, and O. In 1902 the fourth group, AB, was discovered by von Decastello and Struli, two of Landsteiner's pupils.

### ABO Phenotypes

The ABO system consists of the blood groups, or phenotypes, A, B, AB, and O. These four groups may be explained by the presence of two antigens (or factors) on the red cell surface, the A antigen and the B antigen. If a person belongs to group A, the A antigen is present on the red cell. Group B persons have B antigen on their cells. Group AB individuals have both A and B, while group O people have neither A nor B.

## ABO Genotypes

The antigen present on the red cell is determined by genes on the chromosomes. Three allelic genes can be inherited in the ABO system: the A, B, and O genes. Since each person has two genes for any trait, one from each parent, the following combinations of alleles are possible: AA, AO, AB, BB, BO, and OO. These combinations represent the possible genotypes in the ABO system.

If the A gene is present on the chromosome, A antigen will be present on the red cell. The presence of B gene results in B antigen on the red cell. The presence of O gene results in neither antigen on the red cell.

However, group O individuals have significant H antigen on their red cells, since H is the precursor of A and B antigen.

## ABO Typing Procedures
### Red Cell Typing for Antigen

In testing blood for the ABO group, a suspension of red cells in saline solution is prepared. This suspension is tested by mixing one portion with a solution of known anti-A antiserum (anti-A antibodies). A second portion is mixed with known anti-B antiserum (anti-B antibodies). The mixtures are then observed for a reaction. A positive reaction is the occurrence of agglutination or hemolysis. A negative reaction is the absence of agglutination or hemolysis. Results may be grouped as follows:

Group A blood— positive reaction of cells with anti-A antiserum
Group B blood—positive reaction of cells with anti-B antiserum
Group O blood—negative reaction of cells with both anti-A and anti-B antiserum
Group AB blood—positive reaction of cells with both anti-A and anti-B antiserum

In these typing reactions, the blood is merely tested for the presence or absence of A and B antigens. No direct test is made for the presence or absence of the O gene. This is phenotyping, or typing by means of tests made directly on the blood. Since blood is tested only for the A and B antigens, genotypes AA and AO will both type as blood group A. Genotypes BB and BO both contain B antigen and will type as blood group B. Genotype AB will type as group AB, since both antigens are present to react with the appropriate antisera. All blood that types as group O must belong to the genotype OO, since the blood will not react with either anti-A or anti-B antiserum.

### Landsteiner's Rule

As is the case with any blood group system, corresponding antigens and antibodies cannot normally coexist in the same person's blood. In other words, persons who are blood group A cannot form anti-A antibodies and will not have anti-A antibodies in their serum. However, in the ABO system, unlike other blood group systems, if the A or B antigen is lacking on the red cell, the corresponding antibody will be found in the serum. These are the so-called natural antibodies discussed previously. Adults lacking group A antigen will be found to have anti-A antibody in their sera. The sera of adults with red cells lacking B antigen have anti-B antibody. This occurrence of natural anti-A or anti-B antibody when the corresponding antigen is lacking from the red cell is known as **Landsteiner's rule.** It exists only in the ABO system.

### Serum Typing for Antibody

Naturally occurring anti-A and anti-B antibodies are important for several reasons, especially for ABO blood grouping in the laboratory. It is essential to avoid giving a blood transfusion to a person whose serum contains an antibody for an antigen present on the transfused red cells. If this occurred, there would be an immediate and severe hemolytic transfusion reaction. It is absolutely essential that the correct ABO blood type be transfused, or a severe reaction and death might result. For these reasons, the occurrence of

## TABLE 18-1

ABO Typing Reactions

| Blood Group | Antigen on Red Cells | Antibody in Serum | Antigen, Front, or Direct Typing | | Antibody, Back, or Indirect Typing | | Possible Genotype |
|---|---|---|---|---|---|---|---|
| | | | Reaction of Undetermined Cells With Anti-A Antiserum | Reaction of Undetermined Cells With Anti-B Antiserum | Reaction of Undetermined Serum With $A_1$ Cells | Reaction of Undetermined Serum With B Cells | |
| A | A | Anti-B | + | − | − | + | AA, AO |
| B | B | Anti-A | − | + | + | − | BB, BO |
| AB | A and B | Neither | + | + | − | − | AB |
| O | Neither | Anti-A and anti-B | − | − | + | + | OO |

natural anti-A and anti-B antibodies is made use of in the ABO typing procedure. In addition to testing red cells with known antibody, as described, the serum is tested with known group $A_1$* and group B red cells to determine what antibodies are present. In these tests, serum from the undetermined blood group is separated from the cells. One portion of the serum is mixed with red cells known to contain group $A_1$ antigen. A second portion of serum is mixed with cells known to contain group B antigen. The mixtures are then observed for a positive or negative reaction as evidenced by agglutination or hemolysis. If there is a positive reaction with known group $A_1$ cells, the serum contains anti-A antibodies. If there is a positive reaction with known group B cells, the serum contains anti-B antibodies. If the serum reacts with both $A_1$ and B cells, both anti-A and anti-B antibodies are present. If no reaction occurs with either cell type, both antibodies are lacking. Remembering that in the ABO system the serum contains the corresponding antibody for the A or B antigen lacking from the red cell, the results may be grouped as follows:

Group A blood—positive reaction of serum with group B cells

Group B blood—positive reaction of serum with group $A_1$ cells

Group O blood—positive reaction of serum with both $A_1$ and B cells

Group AB blood—no reaction with either $A_1$ or B cells

### Summary

**Typing** reactions that employ undetermined red cells and known antibody or antiserum are referred to as antigen, cell, direct, or front typing reactions. Typing reactions that employ undetermined serum and known red cells are referred to as antibody, serum, indirect, or back typing reactions. These reactions are summarized in Table 18-1.

When the ABO group is to be determined, both the cells and the serum should be typed as described. The antigen and antibody typing results should then be compared to be sure that mistakes have not occurred and that the results are consistent. This is an excellent way to guard against mistakes in ABO grouping. However, in certain instances the antigen and antibody typing results show discrepancies.

### Natural Antibodies of the ABO System

One cause of cell and serum discrepancies in ABO typing procedures involves the natural antibodies, which are expected to occur in most adults. They cannot be expected to exist in newborn infants, since infants do not normally begin to produce antibodies until they are 3 to 6

---

*$A_1$ is a subgroup of A antigen that will be defined later. For the present it may be considered synonymous with A antigen.

months of age. The titer of natural antibodies normally increases gradually through adolescence and then decreases gradually. For this reason, serum-grouping results may also show discrepancies in very elderly patients.

### Variation in Titer

It should also be mentioned that there is a variation of the antibody titer in the population. In general, the anti-A titer seems to be higher than the anti-B titer. In the laboratory the antibody titer of serum will only rarely approach the antibody titer of commercially prepared antiserum. For this reason, reactions with cell grouping tests are generally stronger and easier to read than serum grouping reactions.

### Subgroups

The occurrence of subgroups of group A or group B antigen might also result in discrepancies between cell and serum grouping reactions. The classification of blood in the ABO system into groups A, B, AB, and O is an oversimplification. Both group A and group B may be further classified into subgroups. The most important subdivision is that of group A into $A_1$ and $A_2$. Both $A_1$ and $A_2$ cells react with anti-A antisera. However, anti-$A_1$ reagent can be prepared from group B human serum or with the lectin of *Dolichos biflores* seeds. This anti-$A_1$ antibody will react with $A_1$ cells only. Practically, the subgroups should be kept in mind when there is difficulty in ABO grouping or compatibility testing.

### H Substance

H substance is a precursor of A and B blood group antigens. Thus, the ABO system is concerned with substances A, B, and H.

Genetically, the ABO system is controlled by at least three sets of genes. We have described one set, the A, $A_1$, B, and O gene set, which occupies a specific locus or position on corresponding chromosomes.

Another set is described as H and h, which are alleles for another locus or position. The H gene is extremely common; over 99.9% of the population inherits the H gene. Very few people carry an h allele, and the hh genotype, called Bombay or Oh, is extremely rare. It is a cause of unexpected blood typing reactions, as the cells type as group O. However, the serum of these Bombay individuals reacts strongly with group O red cells, owing to the presence of a potent anti-H antibody. Anti-H antisera are also prepared from the anti-H lectin of *Ulex europeaus*. Anti-H antisera will not agglutinate red cells from Bombay individuals, but will give a strong reaction with group O red cells.

Finally, the Se and se alleles occupy a third locus. The Se and se genes regulate the presence of A, B, and H antigenic material in the body secretions. About 78% of the population has inherited the Se gene (SeSe or Sese). These persons are secretors who have H, A, or B substance produced by their secretory cells. Thus, corresponding H, A, or B substance will be found in the saliva of these persons.

### Summary

It is because of the existence of subgroups that $A_1$ test cells must be used in ABO serum grouping. Subgrouping tests will involve the use, for example, of anti-AB serum, absorbed anti-A serum, and lectins.

It must be stressed that if discrepancies between the results of cell and serum grouping occur, they must be resolved. These problems should be referred to a person with sufficient training and experience in the area of blood banking.

### Immune Antibodies of the ABO System

Thus far, only natural anti-A and anti-B antibodies have been discussed. However, anti-A and anti-B antibodies may also be of the immune type. Serum may contain immune antibodies in addition to the natural ones. Natural antibodies are normally found in the serum of adults if the red cell lacks the corresponding antigen, and they probably arise from the inevitable stimulation by ABH substances widely distributed in nature. Immune anti-A or anti-B antibodies result from specific antigenic stimulation. This stimulation may occur through incompatible transfusion, pregnancy, or injection of ABH substances or substances having ABH activity.

### Physical and Chemical Properties

Immune and natural antibodies differ in physical and chemical properties and in their serologic behavior. In addition, natural ABO antibodies react best if the red cells are suspended in saline solution and the test is carried out at room temperature or 4° C. Immune antibodies differ in that they react better if cells are suspended in albumin or serum and incubated at 37° C. There are other differences in mode of reaction in the laboratory, and they must be taken into account when the occurrence of an immune-type anti-A or anti-B antibody is suspected or possible—for example, in cases of hemolytic disease of the newborn (HDN) with ABO incompatibility and in screening blood for low titers of anti-A and anti-B.

### Size

The natural antibody is a large molecule with a molecular weight of about 900,000, whereas the immune antibody has a molecular weight of about 150,000. Probably because of this size difference, natural antibodies are unable to cross the placental barrier, whereas immune antibodies may cross it. This is important in HDN. Natural antibodies are of the IgM type, whereas immune antibodies are of the IgG type.

## Universal Donors and Recipients

One concept that must be discussed in conjunction with the ABO system is that of the "universal donor" and the "universal recipient." These are terms familiar to most people, yet to the blood banker the concept is considered oversimplified and is therefore avoided. The concept is made use of only in cases of extreme emergency.

When blood is to be transfused, two questions must be kept in mind:

1. Does the patient's serum contain an antibody against an antigen on the transfused red cell?

2. Does the serum to be transfused contain an antibody against an antigen on the patient's red cells?

The first situation is the more serious one. It can result in a major reaction and in the death of the patient. This is because all the transfused blood will be destroyed by antibody in the patient's circulatory system, resulting in accumulation of toxic waste products and probably in severe renal failure and death.

The second situation, in which the donor serum contains antibody against the patient's red cells, is not as serious. A minor reaction would occur, because only a small amount of blood compared with the patient's total blood volume is infused. As a result, only a small proportion of the patient's red cells are actually destroyed by donor serum, and this is offset by the benefits of the donor red cells that remain intact and viable.

These transfusion situations are made use of in the concepts of universal donor and recipient. Universal donor blood is group O blood. It is felt that group O red cells can be safely transfused into a person with any ABO blood type, because the patient's serum cannot contain an antibody to group O cells. In other words, a major reaction cannot occur. However, group O blood does contain anti-A and anti-B antibodies. Therefore, if it is given to group A persons, a minor reaction can occur with anti-A antibodies. In the case of group B persons, there can be a minor reaction with anti-B antibodies, while the AB person can have a minor reaction with both anti-A and anti-B.

Because these minor reactions can occur, it is preferable that group O blood that is to be used as universal donor blood have most of the plasma removed. This is common practice, as whole blood is very rarely transfused. In virtually all cases, the transfusion of red cells, without plasma, is preferable. If this is not possible, the donor blood must be screened with certain additional tests. There is no universally accepted method of screening for "safe" blood for such use. An additional problem is the possible presence of immune anti-A or anti-B antibodies in addition to the natural forms.

In the case of the group AB patient, it is even more dangerous to transfuse group O blood, since both anti-A and anti-B antibodies are present to react with the patient's red cells. For this reason, if group AB blood cannot be secured for transfusion it is preferable to use either group A or group B red cells, rather than group O. The so-called universal recipients are those with group AB blood, since they may be infused with group A, B, or O red cells in emergency situations.

In summary, it should be stressed that ABO type-specific blood should be used whenever possible. Whenever group O blood is used for the A, B, or AB patient and A or B blood for the AB patient, a certain risk does exist. Although screening methods are available to test the titer of anti-A and anti-B, these methods are not perfect, and a severe transfusion reaction may still take place. Transfusion of non-type-specific blood includes situations in which group-specific blood is not available and blood must be transfused, or there may not be enough time to type the patient's blood and test for compatibility, or the patient's blood group cannot be accurately determined. In cases of ABO HDN, group O red cells are generally used. Finally, there may be such unusual circumstances as disasters or military situations in which blood cannot be typed for use before it is transfused.

## THE Rh BLOOD GROUP SYSTEM

### Definition of Rh Factors and Inheritance

#### Rh Antigens

The Rh blood group system is considerably more complex than the ABO system. Basically, it consists of six related blood group factors, or antigens, C, D, E, c, d, and e, and the corresponding antibodies anti-C, anti-D, anti-E, anti-c, and anti-e (anti-d antibody does not exist). Because of the lack of an anti-d antibody, the existence of d as an antigen is disputed. For this reason, the so-called presence of d should be thought of as the absence of D antigen.

The six antigens that have been defined are not the only antigens in the Rh system, for over 40 variants have been described. To date, there are at least 35 related factors in the system. However, C, D, E, c, and e are the most important factors. The weak expression of D antigen, referred to as $D^u$, is also important in blood banking procedures.

### Nomenclature

More than one system of nomenclature is used to define the antigens of the Rh-Hr system. There is the Rh system of Wiener, the CDE system of Fisher and Race, and the numerical system of Rosenfield et al. These systems are compared in Table 18-2. The CDE nomenclature is commonly used.

### CDE Terminology and Inheritance (Fisher-Race)

The Rh factors that have been discovered on red cells are inherited traits, as are the antigens of the ABO system. However, in the ABO system only three allelic genes could be inherited. In the Rh system, D, C, E, d, c, and e are not all alleles for the same position. Rather, C and c are alleles for the same trait, while D and d are alleles for another chromosome position, as are E and e. The factors are inherited in groups of three, so that a particular chromosome will have one position for the Dd alleles, a second position for the Cc alleles, and a third position for the Ee alleles. In other words, each chromosome carrying the Rh determinants has three closely linked loci for the three related Rh alleles. Everyone has loci for six Rh genes.

### TABLE 18-2

Comparative Nomenclature of the Rh Antigens

| CDE System (Fisher-Race) | | Rh System (Wiener) | | Numerical System (Rosenfield et al.) | |
|---|---|---|---|---|---|
| D | d | $Rh_o$ | $Hr_o$ | Rh1 | |
| C | c | rh' | hr' | Rh2 | Rh4 |
| E | e | rh" | hr" | Rh3 | Rh5 |

Thus, there are three pairs of Rh-Hr factors that are genetically related. Everyone must have at least one of or both of the paired alleles Cc, Dd, and Ee. Since D and d are alleles for the same trait, if D is absent, d must be present, and if d is absent, D must be present. This means that there are three possible combinations of genes for the Dd alleles. A person may possess two D genes, DD, and be homozygous for D. Or a person may possess a D gene and a d gene, Dd, and be heterozygous for D. Finally, the person may possess two d genes, dd, and be homozygous for d. This is also true of the Cc and the Ee alleles: persons may be homozygous or heterozygous for Ee and Cc.

Since the Rh alleles are inherited in groups of three paired factors, and each person has two chromosomes for the Rh factors, each person has a total of six Rh factors. This means that there are eight possible combinations of three factors that can be carried on a particular chromosome. These possible combinations of factors in CDE notation and the corresponding Rh notation, and their approximate frequency, are given in Table 18-3. These frequencies are for the white population and differ for other races. They are included to give a general idea of the relative frequencies that might be seen in blood banking. For more defini-

tive frequencies, consult the AABB manual or one of the standard immunohematology textbooks in the Bibliography at the end of this chapter.

One of the eight possible Rh-Hr gene combinations is inherited from each parent, so that the total Rh-Hr genotype for a person would be denoted as CDE/cde or CDe/cDe, and so on. In Wiener's Rh-Hr notation corresponding to the CDE system, the capital letter R refers to the presence of D ($Rh_0$) antigen, while r refers to the presence of d ($Hr_0$). The superscript in Wiener's notation refers to the antigens C, c, E, and e.

Thus far, only one theory of Rh-Hr inheritance has been presented here—the theory of Fisher and Race. In this theory the three genes on each chromosome carrying the Rh-Hr determinants are felt to be so closely linked that, in effect, they are inherited as a unit. In other words, the unit of inheritance is considered to be the chromosome rather than the gene in this case. This theory recognizes the existence of six genes, each gene controlling the identical factor in the blood. There is no difference between the gene and the factor.

### Rh-Hr Terminology and Inheritance (Wiener)

Another theory of Rh-Hr inheritance is that proposed by Wiener. Wiener differentiated between the genes and the factors that are found in the blood. Wiener felt that there is a single gene on each Rh-Hr chromosome that determines the presence of three factors in the blood. Since there are eight possible combinations of Rh-Hr factors, this theory recognizes eight possible genes. In other words, inheritance of the $R^1$ gene will result in the presence of C (rh'), D ($Rh_0$), and e (hr") antigens on the red cells. A person inheriting an $R^1$ gene from one parent and an $R^z$ gene from the other would be of genotype $R^1/R^z$ (or CDe/CDE), and that person's red cells will contain C (rh'), D ($Rh_0$), E (rh"), and e (hr") antigens. Wiener supported his theory of inheritance with the fact that examples of crossovers (mutations resulting from paired chromosomes breaking and recombining) have not been found.

| **TABLE 18-3** | | |
|---|---|---|

**Rh Chromosomes and Approximate Frequency**

| CDE Notation (Fisher-Race) | Rh-Hr Notation (Wiener) | Approximate Frequency in White Population* |
|---|---|---|
| CDe | $R^1$ | Common |
| cDE | $R^2$ | Common |
| CDE | $R^z$ | Rare |
| cDe | $R^o$ | 2% |
| Cde | r' | 1% |
| cdE | r" | 1% |
| CdE | $r^y$ | Very Rare |
| cde | r | Common |

*Data from Stratton F, Renton PH: *Practical Blood Grouping.* Springfield, Ill, Charles C Thomas, Publisher, 1958, p 154.

In virtually every other case of closely linked inherited traits, crossovers have been found.

In any case, the net effect is the same. People will always have six Rh-Hr factors in their blood. The only real difficulty is that the two theories of inheritance have resulted in more than one system of nomenclature that must be learned by the student.

### Rh Inheritance From Molecular Genetics Research

New information from molecular genetics research shows that the Rh system antigens are controlled by a set of two closely linked genes that are located on chromosome 1. In D-positive people, the D gene produces a membrane protein containing the D antigen. A second CE gene produces two separate highly related proteins containing the Cc and Ee antigens. In D-negative persons, one of the Rh system genes is completely lacking. It appears that the two genes may have developed from a common ancestor gene by duplication.

### Historical Background

The discovery of the Rh system was based on work by Landsteiner and Wiener in 1940 and by Levine and Stetson in 1939. A woman who delivered a stillborn fetus was studied by Levine and Stetson. The woman had never received a blood transfusion; however, after delivery she was transfused with her husband's blood. Both the woman and her husband were blood group O. Following transfusion, the woman experienced a severe hemolytic reaction.

Similar transfusion reactions had previously been known to occur following the first transfusion after childbirth, and they did not seem to be associated with the ABO system. Levine and Stetson developed an explanation of their patient's transfusion reaction that has been proved to be correct. They explained the reaction by proposing that the woman's red cells did not contain a "new" antigen. However, the child inherited this new antigen from the father, and the fetal cells containing it found their way into the mother's circulatory system. This resulted in the formation of antibody to the new antigen. Therefore, when the woman was transfused with her husband's blood, her serum contained an antibody to the new antigen contained on her husband's red cells. It was also found that the woman's serum agglutinated not only her husband's red cells but the red cells of 80 of 104 ABO-compatible bloods. Levine and Stetson did not name this new antigen.

The naming of this new factor eventually resulted from studies by Landsteiner and Wiener in 1940. They inoculated rabbits and guinea pigs with the red cells of rhesus monkeys, and found that the resulting rabbit antibody agglutinated the red cells of all rhesus monkeys and, more important, the red cells of about 85% of samples of the white population of New York City. The 85% of the cells that were agglutinated by the anti-rhesus serum were called **Rh-positive,** and the remaining 15% not agglutinated were called **Rh-negative.** Later it was shown that an antibody found in the serum of certain patients who had hemolytic reactions after transfusion of ABO-compatible blood was apparently the same as the antibody in the anti-rhesus serum. It was also found that the antibody contained within the serum of the women studied by Levine and Stetson in 1939 was similar to the antibody in the anti-rhesus serum.

### Rh-Positive and Rh-Negative

It is now known that the new antigen described by Levine and Stetson is the D (or $Rh_o$) antigen. Persons whose red cells contain D antigen either as D/D or D/d are now termed Rh-positive. They represent approximately 85% of the population. In other words, the antibody responsible for several transfusion reactions is the anti-D (anti-$Rh_o$) antibody. Persons whose red cells lack the D ($Rh_o$) antigen are termed Rh-negative. Rh-negative persons are then d/d. They represent about 15% of the population. (The great majority of Rh-negative persons are cde/cde. This genotype is what is meant by a truly Rh-negative person. Other very rare genotypes that are d/d must be considered Rh-negative as blood recipients.)

## Characteristics of the Rh Antigens

The factors C, D, E, c, and e are all antigenic. This means that they are capable of stimulating the production of antibodies if introduced into the body of a person whose red cells completely lack them. The Rh antigens are permanent inherited characteristics that remain constant throughout life. However, not all the Rh antigens are equally antigenic. The D ($Rh_o$) antigen is the strongest and will generally result in immunization if introduced into a foreign host. For this reason the term Rh-positive merely refers to the presence of D antigen without respect to the other Rh factors. The antigenic strength of D also makes it imperative that blood be tested for Rh type before transfusion. Rh-negative persons should not be transfused with Rh-positive (D-positive) blood, for they will certainly develop anti-D antibodies over 80% of the time according to the AABB manual. This would not be lethal at the time of the first transfusion; however, subsequent transfusion with D-positive blood would result in a transfusion reaction. In the case of the woman who was sensitized by an Rh-positive fetus, transfusion with D-positive blood resulted in a hemolytic reaction with the first transfusion.

While D is the most antigenic of the Rh antigens, the other factors (except d) are also antigenic. If strength is considered in terms of antibody frequency, anti-c is most common, followed by anti-E, anti-C, and finally anti-e. Combinations of antibodies in the same blood are also seen.

### Weak Expression of D Antigen ($D^u$)

Not all red cells that contain D antigen react equally well with anti-D blood grouping reagent. Some of these cells may even appear to be D-negative, depending on methodology. This weak reactivity with anti-D sera is referred to as $D^u$. An explanation is not simple, nor is $D^u$ a single entity. It can be the result of several different genetic circumstances, or result from a position effect on the chromosome. The degree of reactivity

results in the terms high-grade and low-grade $D^u$. Although typing of red cells for transfusion only tests for the presence of D antigen, donor blood must be tested with techniques that demonstrate $D^u$. These cells require antiglobulin testing to show agglutination.

## Characteristics of the Rh Antibodies

Like all antibodies, the Rh antibodies are made from the gamma globulin portion of the blood plasma. They are specific for the antigen against which they were formed. Unlike the ABO antibodies, all Rh antibodies are immune or unexpected antibodies. There are no naturally occurring Rh antibodies. They all result from specific antigenic stimulation, whether by transfusion, pregnancy, or injection of antigen. The lack of natural antibodies in the Rh system is important for several reasons. Practically, it means that antibody typing is impossible in the Rh system. All typing methods in this system depend upon antigen-typing or cell-typing procedures involving unknown antigen and known antiserum.

## Rh Typing Procedures

Commercial antiserum is available for the C, D, E, c, and e factors. There is no way of testing for the d factor, since no anti-d antibody has been found. However, routine testing for Rh antigens other than D is not recommended. Antisera other than anti-D may be scarce, and the time and cost involved are unnecessary unless specifically indicated.

### Types of Rh Typing Reagents (Antisera)

Two types of Rh antibodies are available commercially. High-protein antisera are used for routine D and $D^u$ testing. The sera may be used for slide, rapid tube, or microplate methods. The sera contain 20% to 24% concentrations of protein, and other macromolecular additives that accelerate the antigen-antibody reaction. An Rh control supplied by the manufacturer must be used along with high-protein antisera, and the manufacturer's directions must be followed.

Saline-reactive Rh antisera are also commercially available. These are low-protein, saline-reactive antisera that require a test tube method. Saline-reactive antisera are designed to determine the Rh status of red cells that are known or suspected to be giving false or unreliable reactions with reagents containing a high concentration of protein.

### High-Protein Antisera

It was found that some of the Rh antibodies, although not detectable in saline suspensions of red cells, could be demonstrated if a slightly different technique was used. Rather than saline solution, the cells were suspended in serum or a medium containing sufficient protein. The antibodies that were detectable only when suspended in protein were termed incomplete, or albumin-active, antibodies, as opposed to the complete, or saline solution–active, antibodies. Later, another class of antibody was found to be demonstrable only by means of antihuman globulin, or Coombs' reagent. This type of antibody was termed incomplete univalent. It is now known that all antibodies have more than one valence (i.e., reactive site), although some are detectable in saline suspension, others require sufficient protein, and still others are demonstrable only by means of the antihuman globulin test.

Commercial antisera of the albumin-active, high-protein variety contain IgG-type antibodies. In general, the albumin-active antisera are more avid preparations, and for this reason many of them may be used with either a slide or the test tube technique. In addition, the reaction takes place in less time than with saline solution–active antibody, and the incubation time is shortened. The tube methods with albumin-active antiserum may not even require incubation at 37° C but may produce a reaction at room temperature. In general, Rh antibodies will not react unless the preparation is warmed to (or incubated at) 37° C. Antisera of the incomplete, or albumin-active, variety are labeled "for slide or rapid tube test (or modified tube test)." Again, it is essential to follow the manufacturer's directions.

### High-Protein Antiserum Control.

There are several causes of false-positive results when high-protein antisera are used. For this reason, a high-protein control must always be included. There may be spontaneous agglutination of IgG-coated red cells, or there may be factors in the patient's own serum that affect the test, which often uses unwashed red cells suspended in the patient's own serum or plasma. Other causes of false-positive results include strong autoagglutinins, abnormal serum protein that causes rouleaux formation, or antibodies against an additive in the reagent itself.

The best control consists of an immunologically inert control reagent, generally the diluent used for manufacturing the particular antiserum. Thus, it is desirable to use the high-protein control provided by the same manufacturer as the maker of the antiserum in use.

### Low-Protein (Saline-Active) Antisera

Antibody of the saline solution-active type is labeled "for saline tube tests." When this preparation is used, reactions must be carried out on saline suspensions of red cells, and the test must be performed in a test tube. Slide tests cannot be performed. The first Rh antibodies discovered were active in saline solution.

Anti-C and anti-E antisera (in addition to anti-D) are normally available in a saline solution-active form. Antisera of this type will be labeled "for saline tube tests," and the tests must be performed in test tubes. In general, equal amounts of antiserum and 2% to 4% suspensions of red cells (one or two drops of each) are mixed in $10 \times 75$ or $12 \times 75$ mm test tubes and incubated at 37° C for about 1 hour. After incubation, the tubes may be centrifuged. Most blood banking laboratories use a special high-speed centrifuge. This centrifuge is set to run at a constant speed and is used to spin serum-cell mixtures before reading. By using this high-speed centrifuge, time can be saved and the results of typing tests determined quickly. The results are very carefully read macroscopically by resuspending the cells and tipping the tubes. Negative results are often confirmed by observation under the microscope. The exact technique will vary with different brands of antiserum, and the manufacturer's directions must be followed.

### Nature of the Rh Antibody Molecule

The differences in reactivity of antibodies have been found to depend on the length of the antibody molecule. The molecules that are reactive in saline suspensions of cells are of the larger IgM type. Their length is sufficient to cause bridging of adjacent cells in suspension (agglutination). However, red cells in suspension are known to carry an electrical charge, the zeta potential, which causes them to repel each other. The IgM-type antibody molecules are so long that they extend beyond the range of the zeta potential and can react with antigenic sites on adjacent cells. Molecules of the smaller IgG type are so short that they do not extend beyond the zeta potential and cannot react with adjacent cells. To demonstrate the existence of IgG molecules by means of agglutination, the repulsion caused by the zeta potential must be overcome or reduced. It can be reduced by suspending the cells in a sufficiently high protein medium (either their own serum or a commercial protein preparation, or both). Other techniques for the demonstration of IgG include high-speed centrifugation and enzyme methods.

### Typing Blood for Transfusion

When blood is to be transfused, the patient must be tested for the presence or absence of the D (Rh$_o$) antigen. This is because the D factor is so antigenic that most persons who are D-negative (Rh$_o$-negative) or d/d may produce an anti-D antibody if transfused with D-positive blood. All persons who are D-negative (d/d) must be transfused with Rh-negative or d/d blood. Conversely, since d (Hr$_o$) has never been shown to be antigenic, Rh-positive persons may be safely transfused with Rh-negative (d/d) blood.

Since the D (Rh$_o$) factor is the most antigenic of the Rh factors, laboratories test only for the presence or absence of this factor and transfuse Rh-

positive or Rh-negative blood accordingly. In most cases this is sufficient, since other Rh antibodies are comparatively rare and are tested for indirectly by compatibility testing or antibody screening techniques. If only the D factor is to be tested for, the incomplete, albumin-active, anti-Rh$_o$ (anti-D) antiserum is usually used. Weaker forms of the D antigen (D$^u$) are not detectable with saline solution-active anti-D antiserum. If only one test is to be performed, the incomplete, albumin-active form of anti-D must be used. Blood that is negative with this test should be further tested for the presence of the D$^u$ variant by means of the anti-human globulin (Coombs') reaction.

Blood is routinely tested for D antigen with both these antisera as a means of checking the accuracy of the test for D antigen. Since all Rh antibodies are immune ones and it is impossible to antibody-type, it is useful to have a means of checking results for the D antigen. The saline and albumin forms of anti-D antiserum should give the same result. The use of albumin-active anti-D allows for the detection of D antigen in a shorter period of time than with saline anti-D. In the case of the D$^u$ variants of the D antigen, only the incomplete form of anti-D antiserum will give positive results. For a more complete explanation of D$^u$ testing, the AABB manual should be consulted.

### Typing for Additional Rh Antigens

By performing additional Rh tests, either the complete Rh genotype may be determined positively, or the most probable genotype may be determined by consulting the frequency charts that are available from these typing reactions. This may be useful in determining the probability of occurrence of HDN in mothers negative for a factor that the father is positive for. In this case, both the mother and the father are typed and the most probable genotypes are determined, to predict the possibility of HDN in their children. The results of tests with these other Rh-typing sera may be used to check the laboratory results by consulting frequency charts. The occurrence of a very infrequent typing reaction will often point to an error in the typing procedure itself.

## Conclusion

The Rh system is considerably more complex than the ABO system. Everyone has six Rh blood group factors but only two ABO blood group factors. One may be either homozygous or heterozygous for the three paired Rh factors, as for the A, B, and O factors. The ABO system has both natural and immune antibodies, while the Rh system has only immune antibodies. In transfusions, ABO type-specific blood should always be given. With the Rh system, blood is routinely tested for only the presence or absence of D antigen and transfused accordingly. However, blood is screened for the presence of unexpected antibodies before transfusion, by means of the antihuman globulin test.

Commercial Rh antiserum may be of either the saline solution–active or the albumin-active type. The procedure used depends on the form of antiserum employed. Techniques vary with different brands of antiserum.

Experience is invaluable in testing for the Rh factors. Techniques must be mastered and performed with great care. Shortcuts must never be taken, and the testing methods and reasons for them must be thoroughly understood.

## THE ANTIHUMAN GLOBULIN REACTION (COOMBS' TEST)

The antihuman globulin reaction or test is also referred to as the antiglobulin test (AGT) or the Coombs' test (named for Robin R.A. Coombs, who described the use of antihuman globulin for the detection of weak and incomplete Rh antibodies in serum in 1945, along with Mourant and Race).

Different types of antibodies and their laboratory reactions were discussed under Rh Typing Procedures. Antibodies were classified as complete or incomplete, depending on their ability to react in saline suspensions of red cells or the requirement for additional techniques, such as the addition of protein to the test medium. This was related to the size of the antibody molecule and its ability to overcome electrical charges on red cells in suspension (the zeta potential). In general, IgM antibodies are large enough to extend beyond the zeta potential and agglutinate red cells in saline suspensions. However, many IgG antibodies are unable to bring about agglutination unless the zeta potential is reduced by such means as adding protein to the red cell suspension. Even after the addition of protein, some IgG antibody molecules will not bring about agglutination. Antibodies that are unable to cause agglutination in any of the laboratory techniques mentioned thus far are detectable by means of the antiglobulin technique. They have been described in the past as incomplete univalent antibodies; however, they are now known to be bivalent in action, although this can only be demonstrated by the antiglobulin technique.

## Principle of the Antihuman Globulin Test

The antibodies that are detectable by the antiglobulin technique react with red cells. However, the reaction is not observable in terms of agglutination. The antibodies coat the red cells by reacting with antigenic sites on the cell surfaces. The other arm of the antibody molecule is not able to react with antigen on a second red cell, with resultant bridging and agglutination. To demonstrate the coating of red cells by this incomplete antibody, some sort of reagent must be available to show that the cells have reacted with antibody, as seen in the example in Fig. 18-1. It must be remembered that these incomplete antibodies are capable of reacting in the body and, if present, may result in severe transfusion reactions.

In developing a reagent to demonstrate the coating of incomplete antibody on red cells, use is made of the fact that all antibodies are some form of human globulin. The reagent need only be an antibody to human globulin. This is the basis of the antiglobulin, or Coombs', test. The reagent is an antibody to human globulin, or anti–human globulin antibody. This antiglobulin antibody will react with any antibody coating a red cell. Since it is sufficiently long (it is actually an IgM-type antibody), it will react with antibody coating adjacent red cells, and bridging or agglutination of the red cells results.

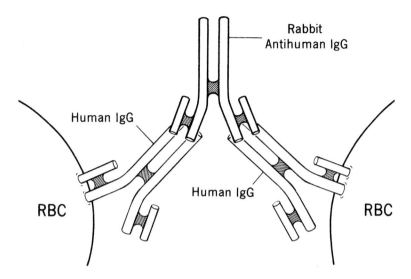

**FIG 18-1.** Antiglobulin (Coombs') reaction. Rabbit IgG with antihuman IgG specificity is shown combining or reacting with human IgG on human red blood cells.

## Preparation and Nature of Antihuman Globulin Reagent

Antihuman globulin reagent is produced commercially by the companies that produce blood group antisera. The antihuman globulin reagent may be prepared by inoculating laboratory animals (usually rabbits) with human serum or a purified globulin fraction of human serum. The laboratory animals produce an antibody to the human globulin, or antihuman globulin antibody. The animal is bled and the serum collected. This serum is purified by various techniques until it is specific for human globulin. The antihuman serum is often prepared in such a way that it reacts with both gamma globulin and complement. The antiglobulin portion of the serum is anti-IgG globulin. However, antibodies other than those of the IgG type must be detected by the antiglobulin test, and it has been found that some of these other antibodies utilize complement in their reaction—they are said to fix complement. Antihuman globulin reagent that contains both anti-IgG and anticomplement antibodies is called polyspecific antihuman globulin reagent. Current requirements for polyspecific antihuman globulin

reagent require antibody to human IgG and the C3d component of human complement. Current polyspecific reagents are a blend of polyclonal IgG antibodies against all human subclasses of IgG and monoclonal antibodies against C3b and C3d complement components.

The nature of the anticomplement and its inclusion in the antihuman globulin reagent is debatable, and varies. A variety of reagents are available, and different types have different uses in the laboratory. These may be polyspecific reagents, or monospecific reagents. Examples of monospecific reagents include anti-IgG with no anticomplement activity or anti-C3d and other complement components with no anti-immunoglobulin activity. These monospecific reagents may be produced as the result of injection of purified fractions of human serum into rabbits, or by the production of murine (mouse) monoclonal antibodies. Monospecific antibodies may be pooled to form polyspecific reagents.

## Antihuman Globulin Test Procedures

There are two ways in which the antiglobulin test is performed. These are the direct and the indirect methods. Both tests are essentially the same; only the starting points differ. With the direct test, the starting point is red cells suspected of being coated with antibody. With the indirect test, the starting point is a serum that may contain antibody. With the indirect test, the serum must first be reacted with a suitable red cell indicator, and then the test is carried out as for the direct procedure.

### The Direct Antihuman Globulin Test

The direct antihuman globulin test or direct antiglobulin test (DAT) is performed on red cells that are suspected of being coated with antibody. It demonstrates an in vivo antigen-antibody reaction; antibody has coated red cells in the body.

The direct test is used to investigate transfusion reactions, and to diagnose autoimmune hemolytic anemia, HDN, and drug-induced hemolytic anemia.

In performing the test, the cells are first washed meticulously with saline solution to remove all traces of serum (human globulin) from the test medium. Any serum remaining will react with the antihuman globulin reagent, causing false-negative results.

The test is performed in test tubes measuring $10 \times 75$ or $12 \times 75$ mm. The cells are washed by completely filling the test tube with a forceful stream of saline solution, resulting in a homogeneous suspension of cells in saline solution. The tube is then centrifuged, and the cells are packed at the bottom of the tube. After centrifuging, the tube is inverted and all the saline solution is decanted in one motion, with the tube being shaken to remove all saline solution. The tube is then turned upright and shaken to resuspend the cells. The tube must never be covered with the finger or palm of the hand at any stage of mixing, for protein from the skin can inactivate or neutralize the antiglobulin reagent.

The cells are washed with saline solution in this manner at least three times. More washing may be necessary if periodic evaluation of the washing technique shows that three times is not adequate. An alternative way to wash and centrifuge the cells is to use one of the cell-washing centrifuges that are available. These centrifuges can be preset to the desired number of washes and are extremely useful for antiglobulin tests. After the final washing, the saline solution is decanted as completely as possible. The cells are shaken to facilitate resuspension, and the antiglobulin reagent is added. The test tube is then incubated and centrifuged as the manufacturer's directions specify, and the results are read macroscopically and microscopically for the presence or absence of agglutination.

### The Indirect Antihuman Globulin Test

The indirect antihuman globulin test or indirect antiglobulin test (IAT) is an in vitro test of unknown serum for an antigen-antibody reaction. It tests for antibodies that are freely circulating in the plasma and react with specific antigens on red cells in a test tube. Antibodies may be present in serum when sensitized by transfusion or pregnancy. Patients with autoimmune hemolytic anemia may have free circulating antibody in addition to antibodies coating their red cells. In any case, the indirect test begins a step before the direct method, although it eventually requires the same washing technique and reaction with antihuman globulin reagent.

The indirect antihuman globulin test is the final stage of many antibody detection procedures and has several uses. It is a step in compatibility testing (crossmatching) for transfusion. It is used to detect and identify antibodies in the serum of potential blood donors and transfusion recipients. The demonstration of certain red cell antigens with known antisera, such as Kell typing and $D^u$ testing, requires the indirect test. It is also used in the titration of incomplete antibodies.

The indirect test begins with a serum suspected of containing antibodies. The serum is mixed with red cells that contain antigen for the suspected antibody in the serum. The test cells are suspended in saline solution, albumin, or serum (depending on the antibody), mixed with the suspected serum, and incubated for a sufficient period of time for a reaction to occur. Incubation is usually for 15 to 30 minutes at 37° C, but this varies with the antigen-antibody system involved. If the serum contains an antibody for an antigen on the test cells, there will be a reaction—a coating of antibody on the test cells. To demonstrate the reaction, the cells must be washed with saline solution and treated in the same way as in the direct test.

### Antibody-Coated Control Cells

One major source of false-negative reactions with the antihuman globulin test is inactive antihuman globulin reagent. The whole vial of antisera may be inactive because of poor storage or contamination by serum globulins. In a given test, the antihuman globulin reagent may be inactive because it has reacted with globulins remaining after inadequate washing of cells. A control that consists of red cells that have been coated with human IgG antibody is used to detect such false-negative reactions. Thus, all tubes that appear to be negative, in both the direct and indirect tests, are reacted with coated control red cells after the final microscopic reading. If the antisera are reactive, agglutination should be seen with the coated control cells. No agglutination after addition of coated control cells indicates inactivation of the antihuman globulin reagent, and the total test procedure must be repeated.

### Conclusion

Neither the indirect nor the direct antihuman globulin test is specific for any one antibody. They give the same reaction with any antibody contained in human serum. To determine the identity of the antibody responsible for a positive reaction, the antigens present on the red cells must be known. This is done by a process of elimination, using various commercial red cell preparations containing known antigens.

The test is not simple. The reagent is a particularly unstable preparation and must be stored with great care. It is inactivated in several different ways. There are many causes of false-negative and of false-positive results, which must be understood before the antihuman globulin test can be performed with reliability. Because of these numerous sources of error, quality assurance procedures must be followed and controls included when the test is performed.

## HEMOLYTIC DISEASE OF THE NEWBORN

### Pathophysiology

Hemolytic disease of the newborn (HDN), also called erythroblastosis fetalis, occurs when a child inherits an antigen for which his or her mother is negative. The disease most commonly involves factors of the Rh and ABO blood group systems, although it may result from incompatibilities in virtually any blood group system. For this disease to occur, however, the child must be positive for an antigen for which the mother is negative.

This condition develops while the fetus is in the uterus. The mechanism involves sensitization or immunization of the mother to foreign antigen present on her child's red cells. Although the circulatory systems of a mother and her child are separate, and only small molecules such as nutrients can cross the placenta, there can be some seepage of fetal red cells into the mother's circulatory system. This is most likely to occur very late in pregnancy or at the time of birth. If any incompatible fetal red cells do find their way into the mother's circulatory system, she may well develop an antibody to the antigen on them. Once such immunization occurs, it is permanent. The antibody formed by the mother is of the IgG type, and it can cross the placenta into the circulatory system of the fetus, where it reacts with corresponding antigen on the red cells of the fetus, with resultant destruction of the cells. HDN is the condition that exists when maternal antibody crosses the placenta and reacts with antigen on fetal red cells. This was the cause of death of the child delivered by the woman studied by Levine and Stetson in 1939, which led to the discovery of the Rh blood group system.

### Rh Factors in Hemolytic Disease of the Newborn

HDN most commonly involves the Rh blood group system. It most often involves the D antigen, the mother being negative for D (d/d) and the father positive for D. The child inherits this factor from the father and is D positive (D/d). If any of the D positive red cells of the fetus cross into the mother's circulatory system, she may develop an immune anti-D antibody. This antibody, of the IgG type, crosses the placenta and reacts with the red cells of the fetus. Fortunately, sensitization usually occurs only very late in pregnancy or at the time of delivery, so the first child is rarely affected by HDN. Furthermore, any child who is D negative cannot be affected by anti-D antibody in the mother's circulatory system. For this reason, genotyping parents in possible cases of HDN is very useful in predicting the chance of occurrence of the disease. For example, if the husband is heterozygous for the D antigen (D/d) and the mother is D negative (d/d), chances are that only half the children will inherit the D antigen (Fig. 18-2). On the other hand, if the father is homozygous for D (D/D), all the children will inherit the D antigen and there is a 100% chance of HDN (see Fig. 18-2). (Only children who are D-positive can be affected by the disease, since only they are positive for a factor that the mother is negative for.)

It has been mentioned that the first child is rarely affected by HDN. In fact, fewer than 20% of Rh-negative women actually become immunized during pregnancy. Although a woman can usually have one or two children who are both Rh-positive and encounter no difficulties, her immunization is permanent. Furthermore, once the disease develops in one child, subsequent children positive for the antigen are likely to be af-

fected at least as severely. More important, if a woman has been sensitized before pregnancy as a result of transfusion of incompatible blood or injection of antigenic material, even the first child can be severely affected.

It has been mentioned that the anti-D antibody is the most common cause of HDN. Other antibodies causing this disease include anti-c, anti-K (Kell), anti-E, and even incompatibilities in the ABO system.

## Prevention of Rh Immunization (Use of Rh Immune Globulin)

In the 1960s a dramatic decrease in the incidence of HDN was seen following the introduction of **Rh immune globulin (RhIG)**, which could prevent immunization to the D antigen during pregnancy. This was an extremely important advance, and the incidence of immunization by pregnancy to the Rh antigen D is very different now. It was found that if RhIG is injected into Rh-negative women who deliver Rh-positive babies within 72 hours of delivery, they are well protected against Rh problems in subsequent pregnancies. The use of RhIG is based on immunosuppression of an Rh-negative mother to prevent immunization (sensitization) by her child's red blood cells. The mother is passively immunized by the administration of RhIG when sensitization by fetal red cells is most likely. This generally occurs at the time of delivery.

About 1 in 10 pregnancies involve an Rh-negative woman and an Rh-positive father. Ac-

|   | D | d |
|---|---|---|
| d | D/d | d/d |
| d | D/d | d/d |

|   | D | D |
|---|---|---|
| d | D/d | D/d |
| d | D/d | D/d |

**FIG 18-2.** Chance of development of hemolytic disease of the newborn. Chance is based on genotypes for the D factor.

cording to the AABB manual, an Rh-negative woman with an Rh-positive infant who is not protected by passive immunization has a 7% to 8% chance of developing anti-D antibodies. When given RhIG postpartum, this risk drops to about 1%. This risk is further reduced to 0.1% when RhIG is administered antepartum at 28 to 30 weeks' gestation. It has been found that infants whose mothers have received up to two antepartum doses of RhIG show no adverse effects.

RhIG is injected intramuscularly within 72 hours of delivery in mothers (1) who are D-negative, (2) who have no detectable anti-D antibody, and (3) whose newborn infants are D-positive. Antepartum treatment at 28 weeks' gestation has also been advocated by the American College of Obstetricians and Gynecologists. If so done, a sample of blood obtained immediately prior to treatment should be tested for ABO group, Rh type, antibody screen, and identification of antibody if present.

RhIG is supplied as a sterile, clear 1-mL solution to be injected intramuscularly. It is a concentrated solution (300 $\mu$g/mL) of IgG anti-D derived from human plasma. It does not transmit hepatitis or HIV infection.

The anti-D antibody can be detected 12 to 60 hours after the administration of RhIG and is sometimes found for as long as 5 months thereafter. If it is detected 6 months after delivery, active immunization and failure of the RhIG can be assumed. Such failures are infrequent, but they can occur if RhIG is given too late or in too small a dose, or if Rh immunization has already occurred during the pregnancy. Most of the D-positive fetal cells enter the maternal circulation at the time of delivery. The amount of fetal blood present in the maternal circulation is important for the RhIG dosage.

If the amount of Rh-positive fetal red cells entering the mother's circulation is greater than 30 mL of whole blood, the standard dose of RhIG is not enough to prevent anti-D antibody formation. Thus, it is important to determine the presence and amount of fetomaternal hemorrhage. This may be done by use of the rosette test and

acid elution or an enzyme-linked antiglobulin test.

### The Rosette Test

This is used as a screening test for the detection of large fetomaternal hemorrhage. The test will detect fetomaternal hemorrhage of approximately 10 mL. It uses D-positive indicator red cells to form rosettes around individual D-positive fetal cells that may be present in the maternal circulation. The test gives only qualitative results. For quantitative results, an acid elution test (Kleihauer-Betke) or an enzyme-linked antiglobulin test is necessary to determine the amount of the hemorrhage.

### Acid Elution Stain (Modified Kleihauer-Betke Method)

This stain is based on the fact that fetal hemoglobin is resistant to acid elution (separation of a substance by extraction), whereas adult hemoglobin is not. That is, when a thin blood smear is exposed to an acid buffer, the adult red cell loses its hemoglobin into the buffer, leaving only the red cell stroma, whereas the fetal red cell is unaffected and retains its hemoglobin. The smears are examined under the microscope after staining, and the percentage of fetal cells in the maternal blood is used to calculate the approximate volume of fetal hemorrhage into the maternal circulation. Either clotted blood or anticoagulated blood may be used for this test.

## ABO Factors

HDN can also occur as a result of factors in the ABO system. In this case, the mother is usually blood group O and the child inherits the A or B antigen from the father. If this occurs and any fetal cells find their way into the mother's circulation, she develops an immune IgG antibody in addition to her natural IgM anti-A or anti-B antibody. If an immune IgG antibody is produced, it crosses the placenta and reacts with corresponding antigen on the red cells of the fetus. Fortunately, although ABO sensitization may occur fairly often, hemolytic disease caused by ABO incompatibility is less severe, and the child may be only mildly affected and require little or no treatment.

## Treatment of Hemolytic Disease of the Newborn

When HDN does occur, it varies considerably in severity. In its most severe form, the child is still-born or aborts early in pregnancy. If the child is alive when born, it may be affected so mildly as to require little treatment, or it may be severely affected by the products of destruction of the red cells and by anemia. The cell destruction results in hemolytic anemia accompanied by abnormal levels of serum bilirubin with the clinical appearance of jaundice. The bilirubin will result in irreversible brain damage if present in sufficient concentration. If the child survives and is not treated adequately, the brain damage will result in severe mental retardation.

Treatment in severe cases of HDN includes blood transfusion. This is referred to as an exchange transfusion, for most of the child's blood is replaced with the transfused blood. The exchange transfusion will serve to correct the anemia and remove the abnormal levels of serum bilirubin, thus preventing brain damage.

The type of blood used for transfusion depends on the antibody responsible for the disease. The outstanding consideration is that the blood be negative for the factor against which the antibody has been formed. In other words, the child is given blood that is compatible with the mother. In the case of HDN caused by the formation of anti-D antibody in the mother's serum, the child is transfused with red cells that are specific for its own ABO type but negative for the D antigen. This is because not all of the child's blood is replaced at the time of exchange, and some maternal antibody is left. Therefore, red cells are given that will not react with the remaining antibody yet will not harm the child. In cases of ABO incompatibility that require exchange, the mother is usually group O and the child group A or B. In such cases the child is transfused with group O red cells of the child's Rh type.

In cases of severe HDN, it is sometimes necessary to attempt to treat the fetus before birth. This intrauterine transfusion may be necessary to correct severe anemia and prevent death in utero when the risk of early delivery is too great. In such cases, based on maternal antibody titer, obstetric history, and ultrasound, amniocentesis is performed. The amniotic fluid is tested for bilirubin level and fetal maturity. If the fetus appears to be severely affected, an intrauterine transfusion may be indicated. In an intrauterine transfusion, packed red cells are infused through the fetal abdominal wall into the peritoneum. Direct transfusion into the umbilical vein may also be attempted.

## Laboratory Tests in Hemolytic Disease of the Newborn

Many laboratory tests are performed in cases of HDN, on the parents' (primarily the mother's) blood prior to birth and on the child's blood after birth. The first step is to type the mother and father for ABO and Rh early in pregnancy to see if HDN can occur. In other words, is the father positive for any factor that the mother is negative for? Depending on the results of genotyping the mother and father, with reference to frequency charts and family studies, the probability of occurrence of the disease can be predicted. The mother's serum is usually screened by means of the indirect antihuman globulin test to see if an antibody exists. If an antibody is found, it is identified and the titer is determined. This titer is rechecked throughout pregnancy as an indication of the possible severity of the disease.

After birth, several tests may be performed on the child's blood, in addition to further tests on the maternal serum. Initially, a sample of umbilical cord blood is tested for ABO group and Rh type, and a direct antihuman globulin test is performed. Some other laboratory tests include hemoglobin determinations, blood smear examination and differential, reticulocyte count, and serum bilirubin determinations on the child's blood.

The decision to perform exchange transfusion will depend on a combination of laboratory results and on the clinical condition of the child. Preparation can and should be made before birth, so that the exchange can be done as soon as possible if necessary.

## COMPATIBILITY TESTING AND CROSSMATCHING

### Compatibility Testing: Definition and General Considerations

Whenever blood is to be transfused, two considerations must be kept in mind. First, blood must be selected that will not be harmful to the patient or result in a transfusion reaction. Second, blood must be selected that will be of maximum benefit to the patient. For these reasons, whenever blood is to be transfused it must be tested for compatibility between the donor and the recipient (patient). Compatibility testing is much more than crossmatching, which is just one part of the testing procedures. Compatibility testing involves a series of tests that must include the following:

1. Correct identification of donor and recipient
2. A review of the patient's past history and blood bank records for type and the presence of unexpected antibodies
3. ABO and Rh typing of both donor and recipient
4. Testing of serum (or plasma) of the donor and recipient for the presence of unexpected antibodies (unexpected antibody screen)
5. Crossmatching of the donor red cells with the patient's serum

In general, compatibility testing is used to help detect:

1. Unexpected antibodies in the patient's serum
2. Some ABO incompatibilities
3. Some errors in labeling, recording, or identifying patients or donors

Unfortunately, compatibility testing is not a perfect or foolproof method that guards against all problems that may arise. The most frequent causes of transfusion of incompatible blood are errors of an organizational, clerical, or technical nature. Although these errors may be detected by means of compatibility testing and the crossmatch, this is not always the case. The laboratory must always work with great care to avoid mistakes of this nature. In addition, although ABO incompatibility may be detected in the crossmatch, not all such errors are found by this method. Correct typing and unexpected antibody screening are also necessary.

Incompatibility in the crossmatching procedure will be discovered only if the patient's serum contains an unexpected antibody to the donor's red cells. Compatibility testing will not prevent immunization if the patient is transfused with foreign antigen. For example, an Rh-negative person who has never been exposed to Rh-positive antigenic material will not show incompatibility if crossmatched with Rh-positive blood, but the person may develop an anti-D antibody. Errors of Rh typing will be detected only if the recipient's serum contains an Rh antibody.

No single crossmatching procedure or antibody screening procedure will detect all unexpected antibodies that may be present in the patient's serum. Even if the blood is found to be compatible, testing procedures will not ensure the normal survival of donor red cells. The blood must be processed and stored correctly.

### ABO and Rh Typing of Donor and Recipient

When blood is selected for transfusion, the patient and the donor are tested for ABO type and for the presence or absence of the D ($Rh_0$) antigen. The ABO group is matched and the Rh type is selected with respect to the D factor. Patients whose cells contain the D antigen are given blood positive for the D factor (Rh-positive blood), while patients who are negative for the D antigen are always given blood that is negative for the D antigen (Rh-negative blood). The other antigens that collectively make up a person's complete blood type are not matched when blood is to be transfused.

## Unexpected Antibody Screening

When blood is to be transfused, the patient's serum must be tested for unexpected antibodies. This is done by testing the patient's serum with a panel (or series) of group O reagent red cells that are known to contain antigens to the most important clinically significant unexpected antibodies. Antibody screening with reagent red cells allows for testing of the patient's serum in advance of the actual transfusion, allowing for selection of rare donor blood, when necessary. This prior testing for antibodies will often make it unnecessary to perform an antiglobulin crossmatch, as the serum will already have been tested for unexpected antibodies with the antiglobulin procedure.

The group O red cells for antibody screening are available as commercially prepared products. They are supplied in sets of two or three vials, suspended in a preservative solution, and must be refrigerated when not in use. There are federal requirements for antigens that must be present on reagent red cells for antibody screening, and additional antigens are used by various investigators. However, it should be remembered that all antibodies of potential clinical significance cannot be detected by antibody screening.

## Crossmatching

As mentioned previously, crossmatching is just part of compatibility testing. There are several different ways to perform the crossmatch. **Crossmatches** have historically been divided into major and minor crossmatches. This concept is presently outdated, as the screening of patient and donor serum for unexpected antibodies has generally replaced the minor crossmatch procedure.

The **major** crossmatch involves testing the patient's serum with the donor's red cells. It is used to detect any unexpected antibodies in the patient's serum that will react with antigens on the donor's red cells. In transfusion, the primary consideration must be what the patient's serum will do to the infused red cells, as destruction of infused red cells will result in a severe transfusion reaction.

The **minor** crossmatch is just the opposite; it tests the donor's serum with the patient's red cells. It is used only rarely to detect the presence of an unexpected antibody in the donor's serum that has reacted with an antigen on the patient's red cells in investigation of transfusion reactions.

The division into major and minor crossmatches is related to the principles involved in considering group O persons as universal donors and group AB persons as universal recipients. The major crossmatch involves testing the donor's red cells with the patient's serum to detect any antibody in the patient's serum that will react with the donor's red cells. The presence of such antibody in the patient's serum would certainly result in a major transfusion reaction, for all the infused donor cells would be destroyed by the patient's antibodies. Of course, even if the patient's serum did contain an unexpected antibody, it would be detected only if the donor's cells contained the corresponding antigen. For this reason, the patients' serum is screened with a panel of group O reagent red cells to detect a greater variety of unexpected antibodies than may be detected by means of a major crossmatch of prospective donors.

### Crossmatch Procedure

The crossmatch involves mixing serum and a 2% to 4% suspension of cells in saline solution in a test tube. The test tube is first incubated at room temperature, centrifuged, and observed for the presence of agglutination or hemolysis. At this stage ABO incompatibility will be observable, as will incompatibility caused by antibodies of the P, MNSs, Lewis, Lutheran, or Wright systems.

If the test is negative at this point, the test tube is further incubated at 37° C for a sufficient period of time and observed once again. Saline solution-reacting antibodies of the Rh-Hr and Lewis systems will be detected, and antibodies of the P, MNSs, and Kell systems may sometimes react at this stage. If the crossmatch is still negative, it may be further tested by means of the antihuman globulin crossmatch.

### Antihuman Globulin Crossmatch

The antihuman globulin crossmatch is an extension of the crossmatch. After incubation at 37° C, the cells are thoroughly washed with saline solution, as described for the direct and indirect antihuman globulin tests. The antihuman globulin serum is added and the test carried out as recommended by the manufacturer. This is an indirect test between the patient and the prospective donor. The crossmatch will detect almost all Rh antibodies. In addition, it may be the only means of detecting some antibodies, especially in the Duffy, Kidd, and Kell blood group systems. It is no longer necessary when the patient's serum has been screened for unexpected antibodies with reagent cells.

### Abbreviated Crossmatch

The major crossmatch as described was required until 1984, when the AABB eliminated the incubation at 37° C and conversion to an antiglobulin test requirement as long as the antibody screen on the patient is completely negative and there is no known history of previous clinically significant antibodies. Instead only a crossmatch procedure designed to detect ABO incompatibility is required. This consists of testing the donor cells and patient serum (major crossmatch) at room temperature by immediate spin or by centrifugation after incubation for 5 minutes at room temperature.

### Other Crossmatching Techniques

As in typing procedures, several other techniques may be applied to crossmatching and antibody screening. Low-ionic-strength (LIS) salt solution may be used to ensure the formation of antigen-antibody complexes. Hexadimethrine has been used as a rapid and sensitive crossmatch method. It is useful in detecting ABO incompatibility when the patient has demonstrated a negative antibody screen. Microplate methods for antibody detection using low-ionic-strength salt solution are also used to screen large numbers of sera for unexpected antibodies. A technique that uses polyethylene glycol (PEG) is also used for antibody detection and identification. This may be used as a supplement to more conventional methods when weak reactions are encountered.

### Computer Crossmatching

Computer crossmatching may be used in blood bank services where it is permissible to omit the AHG phase of the crossmatch and perform only a procedure to detect ABO compatibility. The computerized selection of blood may be used if the requirements described in the AABB technical manual are met. Use of a computerized crossmatch requires FDA approval of a request for variance to regulations on compatibility testing.

### Summary

A well-defined compatibility testing regimen is required whenever blood is to be transfused. Unfortunately, there is no one ideal method to guarantee that all mistakes or incompatibilities have been discovered. If an incompatibility is discovered at any point, its cause must be determined. This determination is far beyond the scope of this brief outline of compatibility testing. Numerous technical problems may be encountered that have not been described. Yet, if compatibility testing has been performed with care, with strict adherence to the procedures established by the particular blood bank, transfusion of blood can be a relatively safe procedure of tremendous benefit to the patient.

## BLOOD TRANSFUSION

The therapeutic replacement of blood or its components is indicated in many instances. However, appropriate **blood transfusion** is not a simple matter and requires several considerations. The reason for the transfusion must be carefully evaluated, and the potential benefit should outweigh any potential harm to the patient. Potential harm includes such considerations as the risk of transfusion-transmitted disease, and other possible transfusion reactions. The practice of blood banking is regulated by several different agencies in the United States. These include the National Center for Drugs and Biologics of the FDA, the Health Care Financing Administration (HCFA), the Occupational Safety and Health Administration (OSHA), and the state departments of health, which perform inspections to ensure regulatory compliance. The American Association of Blood Banks (AABB) is a professional association that provides the scientific leadership and mechanisms to deal with progress and change by providing the AABB Standards. In addition, the AABB, the College of American Pathologists (CAP), and the Joint Commission on Accreditation of Healthcare Organizations (JCAHO) all have their own written standards and make available voluntary inspections by peers.

### Transfusion Reactions

Transfusion reactions can generally be characterized as hemolytic, febrile, allergic, or circulatory overload. Although the most life-threatening transfusion reaction is the hemolytic reaction that occurs with the destruction of incompatible red cells by antibodies in the patient's serum (usually ABO incompatibility), several other forms of transfusion reaction, with varying severity to the patient, also exist. These include immediate and delayed effects, both immunologic and nonimmunologic.

Immediate immunologic effects include febrile nonhemolytic reactions, usually to the donor's granulocytes. Anaphylaxis from antibody to IgA, urticaria (hives) from antibody to plasma proteins, and noncardiac pulmonary edema from antibody to leukocytes or complement activation are other immediate immunologic causes of transfusion reactions. Nonimmunologic immediate transfusion effects include marked fever with shock from bacterial contamination, congestive heart failure from increased blood volume, and hemolysis of infused red cells from the physical destruction of blood, such as from freezing or overheating or mixing nonisotonic solutions with red blood cells.

In addition to the immediate causes of transfusion reactions, there are delayed adverse effects of transfusion. Delayed hemolysis may occur from prior sensitization to red cell antigens by antibodies that are not present or detectable in the blood immediately prior to transfusion. Graft-versus-host disease may result from engraftment of transfused functional lymphocytes. Purpura (the presence of purple patches in the skin and mucous membranes) from bleeding as a result of the development of antiplatelet antibodies may occur. Or the patient may be sensitized and form antibodies to donor antigens on red cells, white cells, platelets, or plasma protein. Other delayed nonimmunologic adverse effects include iron overload from multiple (over 100) transfusions and the transmission of disease as a result of transfusion. Such diseases include hepatitis, acquired immunodeficiency syndrome (AIDS), and protozoan infections.

### Benefits and Reasons for Transfusion

There are many indications for the transfusion of blood components or derivatives. In general, these may be divided into four major categories, and the component to be transfused will depend on which of these categories applies.

First, transfusion may be used to restore or maintain oxygen-carrying capacity or hemoglobin. This is best done by the transfusion of red blood cells with plasma removed. The transfusion of whole blood is both unnecessary and contraindicated, as the inclusion of plasma will increase blood volume with possible circulatory overload.

The second basic indication for transfusion is to restore or maintain blood volume. This is necessary in cases of acute blood loss, as seen with massive bleeding, to prevent shock. Although whole blood may sometimes be indicated, as in actively bleeding patients who have lost over 25% to 30% of their blood volume, it is usually preferable to replace lost blood volume with crystalloid (electrolyte) solutions such as 0.9% sodium chloride (isotonic saline) or plasma substitutes. Lost hemoglobin can be replaced later with packed red cells, although in most patients, about 20% of blood volume can be replaced with crystalloid solutions alone.

A third indication for transfusion is to replace coagulation factors in order to maintain hemostasis. This is done with a variety of blood components and derivatives, which vary with the particular situation in question. These include platelet concentrates, fresh frozen plasma, cryoprecipitate, and factor VIII and factor IX concentrates.

Finally, transfusion may be indicated in order to restore or maintain leukocyte function. This is quite rare but may be necessary for severely granulocytopenic patients with infections that do not respond to antibiotics.

## Donor Selection and Identification

The selection and proper identification of the potential blood donor are essential in ensuring that the blood that is collected for transfusion is safe and will be of benefit to the recipient. Previously much of the blood used for transfusion was obtained from donors who were paid for their blood donations. This practice has been almost completely replaced by voluntary donations, which have significantly decreased the risk of hepatitis, as it has been demonstrated that paid donors are less likely to give a reliable history.

The selection of the blood donor involves a medical history and a mini physical examination. Two considerations must be kept in mind when the donor is to be selected: whether the procedure might be harmful to the donor and whether the donor's blood might be harmful to the recipient. The actual selection process involves a series of questions to ensure safety to both the donor and the recipient. Medical guidelines and requirements for the selection of donors have been developed by the FDA, the AABB, the American Red Cross, and the College of American Pathologists (CAP). It is essential that guidelines and requirements be established for each blood bank and be codified in its own standard operating procedures manual.

## Collection of Blood

Blood for transfusion must be collected and handled under strictly sterile conditions to prevent contamination. According to the AABB, it is col-

lected only by trained personnel working under the direction of a qualified, licensed physician. The collection must be aseptic, must use a sterile closed collection system, and must use a single venipuncture. If more than one venipuncture is done, a new container and donor set must be used for each skin puncture. The AABB also requires that the phlebotomist sign or initial the donor record, whether or not a full unit is collected. The usual amount of blood drawn for 1 unit of whole blood is 450 mL. This is added to 63 mL of citrate phosphate dextrose (CPD) or CPD adenine (CPDA-1) anticoagulant solution, which brings the total volume of a unit of blood to about 500 mL. When the proper amount of blood has been collected, extra tubes and segments must be filled with up to 30 mL of blood for the various testing procedures that are required before the blood can be used.

### Anticoagulants and Preservatives

Blood collected for transfusion must be treated with an anticoagulant. It must be collected into an FDA-approved container. These are usually plastic blood collection bags. They must be pyrogen free, sterile, and contain anticoagulant sufficient for the amount of blood to be collected. The anticoagulant and preservative solution is generally a combination of citrate and dextrose. Citrate is used as an anticoagulant, which binds calcium, thus preventing activation of the coagulation cascade. Dextrose is used to provide an energy source for the red blood cells. Inorganic phosphate buffer is added to increase adenosine triphosphate (ATP) production, which increases red cell viability. Adenine is another additive which is used to improve red cell survival and extend the storage period of blood. As mentioned, two commonly used anticoagulants are CPD and CPDA-1. CPD is approved by the FDA for 21-day storage of red cells at 1° to 6° C. CPDA-1 is approved for storage for up to 35 days at 1° to 6° C.

### Labeling

Proper labeling of the collecting container is of the utmost importance. According to the AABB, each unit of blood or blood component must include the following information at a minimum: the name of the product (i.e., whole blood, red cells), the kind and amount of anticoagulant, the volume of the unit, the required storage temperature, the name and address of the collecting facility, the expiration date, and the unique donor identification number, together with an indication of whether the donor is a volunteer, autologous, or paid. The ABO blood group and Rh type are also shown on the label, once these tests are completed. The pilot tubes and segments for testing must also be properly labeled, and a stoppered or sealed sample of donor blood must be retained and properly stored by the transfusion service for at least 7 days after transfusion.

## Storage of Blood

Blood bank blood must be stored in a refrigerator with a constant temperature of 1° to 6° C. Some sort of alarm must be available that will go off whenever the temperature is not within these limits. A thermometer for recording the temperature should also be installed. Whole blood collected with CPD can be stored for only 21 days; whole blood with CPDA-1 for 35 days. After 21 or 35 days, this blood is outdated and must be removed from the blood supply or treated with a rejuvenation solution and the time extended as described below.

Stored whole blood is inspected daily for color, turbidity, appearance of clots, and presence of hemolysis. Blood is removed when it does not meet the appearance criteria established by the laboratory.

## Blood Processing Tests

The testing of each unit of donated blood is neither simple nor inexpensive. A series of tests must be performed to ensure that the blood will be as safe as possible so that it will truly benefit the patient. These tests include methods that ensure compatibility between donor and recipient (described previously) and tests to screen for transfusion-transmitted diseases. Tests to ensure compatibility include ABO and Rh typing and antibody screening. Screening for transfusion-transmitted disease includes tests for syphilis, hepatitis, and AIDS. Since one unit of blood is normally separated into several components, which are transfused into several different recipients, the presence of viruses such as those causing hepatitis or AIDS would be truly disastrous.

### Screening for Transfusion-Transmitted Disease

The most important factor in ensuring that blood is free of transmittable disease is the careful selection of the blood donor. The virtual elimination of commercial blood donation has significantly decreased the risk of hepatitis. This, together with procedures to allow for self-deferral of donors who have risk factors for human immunodeficiency virus (HIV), the causative agent of AIDS, has done much to ensure the safety of the blood supply. Nevertheless, blood is routinely screened for transmissible disease. The number of routine screening tests has increased dramatically in the past few years, from a single screening test for syphilis to a battery of tests for hepatitis and HIV.

**Tests for Syphilis.** A serologic test for syphilis continues to be required, although it has been questioned for years. It is now used as a surrogate marker for detecting donors who might be high risk for transmitting transfusion-related disease.

**Tests for Hepatitis.** Transmission of hepatitis remains a risk in transfusion. Eighty to ninety percent of post-transfusion hepatitis is caused by hepatitis C (formerly non-A, non-B). Hepatitis B virus is responsible for about 10%, and a small percentage is caused by cytomegalovirus (CMV), Epstein-Barr virus, and hepatitis A virus. For this reason, donated blood is screened with several tests for hepatitis virus. At present these include a test for hepatitis B surface antigen (HBsAg), and antibody tests for hepatitis C (HCV) and hepatitis B core antibody (HBc). In addition, a test for alanine aminotransferase (ALT) is used by some blood centers to detect liver damage of many kinds.

**Tests for AIDS.** Because of the long incubation period of HIV, donor selection methods and self-deferral of donors are essential in the screening of blood for HIV. All donated blood must be tested for HIV-1 and HIV-2 antibodies. A combination test may be used. At present, all donated blood is also tested for HIV-1-antigen.

**Tests for HTLV.** All units of blood must also be tested for human T-cell lymphotropic virus type 1 (HTLV-1) antibody. The test should be sensitive enough to detect most examples of anti-HTLV-II.

## Autologous Transfusions

A relatively new and now common practice in transfusion medicine is the use of autologous transfusions. This is based on the knowledge that the safest blood a recipient can receive is his or her own blood. Not only does this prevent transfusion-transmitted infectious diseases, but it eliminates the formation of antibodies to antigens in the transfused blood and the possibility of graft-versus-host disease and stimulates erythropoiesis by repeated preoperative phlebotomy. For these reasons, patients who meet certain criteria are encouraged to donate blood for themselves before anticipated surgery if they are likely to need blood transfusion.

## Directed Transfusions

These are transfusions in which the patient directly solicits blood for transfusion from family or friends. Directed transfusion is the public's response to concern about AIDS. However, it is based on a false assumption that blood donated by family or friends is safer than that from the regular volunteer donor population. This has not been found to be true, as the directed donor is under significantly more pressure to donate than an anonymous donor. It is also felt that the extra paperwork and other logistics increase the probability of clerical errors.

## Blood Components and Derivatives for Transfusion

From the preceding, it should be evident that whole blood is rarely used when transfusion is indicated. Rather, a variety of preparations, including red cells, plasma, albumin, platelet concentrates, leukocytes, and other preparations and derivatives, are used. These are summarized in Table 18-4 and in the material that follows. Materials prepared from blood by mechanical methods, especially by centrifugation, are called **components,** whereas those separated by more complex processes are called blood **derivatives** or **fractions.** Modern equipment, such as refrigerated centrifuges and plastic bags, has made blood component preparation within reach of almost every blood bank laboratory. Blood fractionation is still a complex process and is done by the pharmaceutical industry from plasma pools of thousands of donor units.

The use of plastic bags for blood containers has been the most important advance for component blood therapy. By using plastic instead of glass, several containers can be interconnected in a sterile system. Blood drawn into the primary container bag can be easily separated into components, which are then transferred aseptically into one or more of the satellite container bags. In this way, plasma and cells can be prepared, stored, and administered individually, without the potential for contamination that is always present when the blood container is "entered" for transfusion into the recipient or patient.

### Whole Blood

Whole blood is made up of plasma and the formed elements (red cells, white cells, platelets). It is collected aseptically and must be free from transmissible diseases such as hepatitis and AIDS. Clotting is prevented by use of an anticoagulant solution such as CPD or CPDA-1. Whole

## TABLE 18-4

Some Blood Components and Derivatives and Their Uses

| Blood Component or Derivative | Use |
| --- | --- |
| Whole blood | Acute blood loss where both red cells and volume are desired; rarely indicated |
| Red blood cells | To increase red cell mass (e.g., therapy for anemia); use with colloids or crystalloids in active bleeding or massive transfusion |
| Red blood cells | |
|   Additive solution added | Like red cells or whole blood |
|   Leukocytes removed by centrifugation, washing, or filtration | To increase red cell mass and avoid febrile and allergic reactions from leukocytes or plasma proteins and to prevent anaphylactic reactions |
|   Deglycerolized | To extend storage of red cells with rare blood types and autologous transfusion or to prevent HLA sensitization |
| Platelets (platelet concentrates, platelet-rich plasma, random or single donor by apheresis | Functional or quantitative platelet defects |
| Granulocytes, apheresis | Rare; for septic, severely granulocytopenic patients who do not respond to antibiotic therapy after 48 hrs of treatment |
| Fresh frozen plasma | In bleeding patients with multiple coagulation defects; also for treatment of factor V or XI deficiency |
| Cryoprecipitate | For treatment of von Willebrand's disease, factor XIII deficiency, or hypofibrinogenemia |
| Factor VIII concentrate | For hemophilia A (Factor VIII deficiency) |
| Factor IX concentrate | For hereditary deficiency of factors II, VII, IX (hemophilia B), or X |
| Albumin/plasma protein fraction (plasma substitutes) | For volume expansion and colloid replacement without risk of hepatitis or AIDS |
| Immune serum globulin | For treatment or prophylaxis of hypogammaglobulinemia and to prevent or modify hepatitis A and non-A, non-B hepatitis |
| Rh immune globulin | To prevent hemolytic disease of the newborn in Rh-negative women exposed to Rh-positive red cells |

blood can be stored for up to 21 days with CPD solution or 35 days with CPDA-1 if refrigerated at 1° to 6° C.

In cases of severe hemorrhage, whole blood may be used to replace red cells and plasma. However, whole blood is rarely transfused. It is generally separated into various components and derivatives both to ensure economic use of a valuable resource and for clinical appropriateness.

### Packed Red Blood Cells (PRBC)

Blood component preparation begins with the separation of plasma from whole blood, leaving the red cells. Red cells for transfusion can be pre-

pared by sedimentation or centrifugation. The technique used must maintain the sterility of both the plasma and the red cells. If the container is not entered when the red cells are prepared, the expiration date for the red cells remains the same as for the original whole blood. If the container is entered, the red cells are considered usable for only 24 hours. Packed red cells are used when oxygen-carrying capacity is diminished or lost, such as in treating certain anemic conditions.

Packed red cells have essentially replaced whole blood in transfusion except in the case of massive bleeding when over 25% to 30% of blood volume is lost. In most cases, even in massive bleeding, red cells, together with isotonic saline or plasma substitutes, are preferred.

Red cells may be further treated by removing leukocytes by centrifugation, washing, or filtration. Red cells may also be treated with additive solutions consisting of saline, adenine, glucose, or mannitol. In this case, maximum amounts of plasma are removed shortly after phlebotomy, and additive solutions are used to maintain red cell function. This process extends the shelf life of red cells to 42 days. Rejuvenation solutions have also been licensed to extend the life of stored blood for immediate use, or it can be frozen for transfusion later. This is especially useful for rejuvenating outdated units of autologous donor blood.

### Plasma

When the red cells are removed from whole blood, plasma remains. It is the liquid portion of blood that has been anticoagulated. Slightly more than half the volume of whole blood is plasma. Plasma should not be used to replace lost blood volume or protein, as much safer products exist. These include plasma substitutes such as albumin or plasma protein fractions, synthetic colloids, and balanced salt solutions. These have the advantage of not transmitting disease or causing allergic reactions. Plasma is appropriately used to replace coagulation factors.

**Fresh Frozen Plasma.** When plasma is used, it is often in the form of fresh frozen plasma. Fresh frozen plasma is a good source of labile clotting factors and can be used to replace all coagulation factors. It is especially useful in treating multiple coagulation deficiencies, as seen with liver failure, disseminated intravascular coagulation (DIC), vitamin K deficiency, warfarin toxicity, or massive transfusions.

**Cryoprecipitate.** Plasma is used to make other blood derivatives. One of these is cryoprecipitated antihemophilic factor (AHF). It is prepared by slowly thawing a unit of fresh frozen plasma at 1° to 6° C overnight. A small amount of white precipitate is formed. This is cryoprecipitate. The

unit is centrifuged, and all but 10 to 15 mL of the supernatant plasma is removed. The preparation contains AHF, also called factor VIII; fibrinogen; von Willebrand's factor; and factor XIII. Cryoprecipitate used to be the product of choice for severe hemophilic patients who were bleeding, but newer methods that inactivate viruses make pooled concentrates of factor VIII the product of choice. Cryoprecipitate is presently used in the treatment of severe von Willebrand's disease.

**Plasma Substitutes.** These include albumin and plasma protein fractions, which are prepared by the chemical fractionation of pooled plasma. The products are heat treated to eliminate the risk of infectious disease such as hepatitis and AIDS. They are used to treat patients who need replacement of blood volume. Alternatively, crystalloid (either saline or electrolyte) solutions are used. The preferred product is debatable.

### Platelets

Platelet concentrates are prepared from random donor whole blood units by differential centrifugation shortly after donation. They are used for patients who are bleeding as a result of low platelet counts or, occasionally, abnormally functioning platelets. Massive transfusions may also result in thrombocytopenia and require platelet concentrates. Occasionally, patients develop HLA antibodies that make transfused platelet concentrates ineffective. In such cases it may be necessary to select HLA-matched donors and prepare platelets by apheresis.

## CONCLUSION

This chapter has been only a brief introduction to the complex field of immunohematology and blood banking, also known as transfusion medicine. Specific blood-grouping and crossmatching methods have been omitted. The current edition of the *Technical Manual of the American Association of Blood Banks* is useful for these procedures. Also, it is extremely important to always follow the manufacturer's instructions in using any specific blood-grouping or blood-typing antisera. Complete instructions are always included with the reputable commercial products. Other topics that have not been discussed completely in this chapter but must be understood before the student can work in the blood bank include causes of error, cleaning of glassware, organization of the blood bank, selection of blood donors, labeling of blood, and record-keeping protocols. Excellent discussions of these subjects have been published in standard blood bank texts. In addition, knowledge may be gained from firsthand experience in a licensed blood bank. Areas that have not been covered in this discussion include bone marrow transplants, organ transplants, and HLA typing and matching.

In the field of blood banking there are numerous situations that may result in error. In general, these may be organizational, clerical, or technical errors. Organizational and clerical errors may be made by the blood bank staff or by personnel in other services involved in the transfusion of blood. These errors often involve incorrect identification of the patient or of the blood removed from the patient and sent to the laboratory for testing.

Transfusion involves a series of tests that are performed by several persons. Included are clerical manipulations in which even a mistake on the part of a typist in transcribing a laboratory report could result in fatal errors if adequate checks did not exist. Because of the number of persons and tests involved in blood transfusion, a blood bank has elaborate organizational procedures that must be followed exactly to ensure that the correct blood is transfused into the correct patient. The AABB and the FDA have definite requirements and recommendations. Organizational systems involve such items and procedures as request forms, methods of label-

ing tubes of blood from the patient, manner of recording results in the laboratory, labeling and numbering of donor blood, selection of blood donors, and storage of blood.

Technical errors are the direct responsibility of the blood banking laboratory and its staff. They may be personal errors, for which the laboratorian is directly responsible, or nonpersonal errors resulting from various factors that enter into the laboratory technique. In any blood-grouping or compatibility testing method, nonpersonal technical factors can produce false-positive or false-negative results. Some may happen in all tests, and some are peculiar to a specific method. These sources of error are beyond the scope of this discussion, but they must be understood by blood bank personnel if the results are to be reliable and accurate.

It is hoped that this brief outline of blood banking will serve as a useful introduction to the student. Work in this area will require much additional knowledge and study.

## REFERENCES

1. Dunsford I, Bowley CC (eds): Techniques in Blood Grouping. Edinburgh, Oliver & Boyd, Ltd, 1955, Preface.

## BIBLIOGRAPHY

Bryant NJ: *An Introduction to Immunohematology,* ed 3. Philadelphia, WB Saunders Co, 1994.

Harmening D: *Modern Blood Banking and Transfusion Practices,* ed 3. Philadelphia, FA Davis Co, 1994.

Henry JB: *Clinical Diagnosis and Management by Laboratory Methods,* ed 19. Philadelphia, WB Saunders Co, 1996.

Issitt PD: *Applied Blood Group Serology,* ed 3. Miami, Montgomery Scientific Publications, 1985.

Judd WJ: *Methods in Immunohematology*, ed 2. Durham, NC, Montgomery Scientific Publications, 1994.

Malloy D (ed): *Immunohematology Methods*, ed 1. Rockville, Md, American National Red Cross, 1993.

McCullough J: *Transfusion Medicine*, New York, McGraw-Hill, 1998.

Rudmann SV: *Textbook of Blood Banking and Transfusion Medicine*, Philadelphia, WB Saunders Co, 1995.

Standards Committee of the American Association of Blood Banks: *Standards for Blood Banks and Transfusion Services*, ed 17. Bethesda, Md, American Association of Blood Banks, 1996.

Vengelen-Tyler V (ed): *Technical Manual of the American Association of Blood Banks*, ed 12. Bethesda, Md, American Association of Blood Banks, 1996.

## STUDY QUESTIONS

1. **Match each of the following terms (1 to 8) with its definition (A to H).**

   1. Allele
   2. Blood banking
   3. Blood transfusion
   4. Genotype
   5. Immune antibody
   6. Immunohematology
   7. Natural antibody
   8. Phenotype

   _____ A. Actual genetic makeup; may not be evident by direct tests

   _____ B. Antibodies that appear to exist without antigenic stimulus, such as the anti-A and anti-B antibodies in the ABO system

   _____ C. Blood type as determined direct tests

   _____ D. The procedures involved in collecting, storing, processing, and distributing blood and its components

   _____ E. The technique of replacing whole blood and its components

   _____ F. The techniques and procedures involving the study of the immunologic responses of blood cells

   _____ G. Unexpected antibodies that result from specific antigenic stimulation

   _____ H. Variants of a gene for a particular trait

2. **Tell if the following statements are true (T) or false (F).**

   _____ A. A positive reaction in blood banking procedures is seen as hemolysis or agglutination.

   _____ B. Agglutination is clumping caused by the presence of any antigen present on red cells.

   _____ C. An antiserum is a solution of antigens.

   _____ D. Blood group tests in general may be performed either on a microscope slide or in a test tube.

   _____ E. In order for hemolysis to be seen as a positive reaction in blood banking procedures, complement must be present in the serum.

3. **List the six common genotypes in the ABO blood group system, and indicate the corresponding phenotypes.**

4. **Complete the following table by placing a plus sign or a minus sign in each of the boxes.**

| Blood group | Reaction of patient red cells with anti-A antisera | Reaction of patient red cells with anti-B antisera | Reaction of patient serum with group A red cells | Reaction of patient serum with group B red cells |
|---|---|---|---|---|
| A | | | | |
| B | | | | |
| AB | | | | |
| O | | | | |

5. **When blood is to be transfused, the most important consideration is:**

   A. Do the donor's red cells contain an antibody against the patient's red cells?
   B. Do the patient's red cells contain an antibody against the donor's red cells?
   C. Does the donor's serum contain an antibody against the patient's red cells?
   D. Does the patient's serum contain an antibody against the donor's red cells?

6. **Patients are generally described as Rh positive or Rh negative on the basis of the presence of which of the following antigens on the red cells?**

   A. C
   B. c
   C. D
   D. E
   E. e

7. **Match the type of antiglobulin test (1 or 2) with the statement concerning antihuman globulin testing (A to E).**

   1. Direct antiglobulin test (DAT)
   2. Indirect antiglobulin test (IAT)
   _____ A. Part of the major crossmatch
   _____ B. Part of screening for unsuspected antibodies with group O red cell panels
   _____ C. Test performed on red cells suspected of being coated with antibody
   _____ D. Test performed on serum suspected of containing antibodies
   _____ E. Used to detect antibody coating donor red cells in cases of incompatible transfusion reactions
   _____ F. Used to detect unsuspected antibodies in the patient's serum

8. **The most important reason for the decrease in the number of cases of hemolytic disease of the newborn is the:**

   A. Acid elution stain
   B. Rosette test
   C. Use of improved typing procedures
   D. Use of Rh immune globulin

9. **Which of the following is *not* part of usual compatibility testing?**

   A. ABO and Rh typing of donor and recipient
   B. Correct identification of donor and recipient
   C. Crossmatching of the donor red cells with the patient serum
   D. Crossmatching of the patient red cells with the donor serum
   E. Testing of the patient's serum with a panel of group O cells for unexpected antibodies

10. **Compatibility testing is used to help detect:**

    A. Some ABO incompatibilities
    B. Some errors in labeling, recording, or identification
    C. Unexpected antibodies in the patient's serum
    D. More than one of the above
    E. All of the above

11. **What is the primary consideration in transfusion of red cells?**

12. **Which of the following are generally character-ized as a transfusion reaction?**

    A. Hemolytic
    B. Febrile
    C. Allergic
    D. Circulatory overload
    E. All of the above

13. **Which of the following tests is *not* required in the screening of potential blood donors for trans-fusion-transmitted disease?**

    A. Alanine aminotransferase (ALT)
    B. Hepatitis B surface antigen (HBsAg)
    C. Hepatitis C antibody (HCV)
    D. Hepatitis B core antibody (HBc)
    E. HIV antigen
    F. HIV-1 and HIV-2 antibodies
    G. Human T-cell lymphotropic virus (HTLV-1) antibody
    H. Serology for syphilis

14. **Match each of the following blood components or derivatives (1 to 6) with the use or statement (A to F).**

    1. Cryoprecipitate
    2. Crystalloid solutions or plasma substitutes
    3. Fresh frozen plasma
    4. Packed red blood cells
    5. Platelet concentrates
    6. Whole blood
       _____  A. Bleeding due to low or dysfunc-tional platelets
       _____  B. Rarely, if ever used in transfusion
       _____  C. Restore or maintain blood volume
       _____  D. Restore or maintain oxygen-carrying capacity
       _____  E. Source of labile clotting factors
       _____  F. Treatment of severe von Willebrand's disease

# APPENDIX A

## Prefixes, Suffixes, and Stem Words

Every specialty has a vocabulary of its own. The clinical laboratory is no different. Progress in learning the vocabulary of the laboratory and of medicine in general will come with experience, but some introductory information is important for anyone coming into the laboratory for the first time.

Most modern medical words are made up of parts derived from Greek or Latin, some with changes that have gradually been made over the years as the ancient words were adopted into English. All but the simplest medical terms are made up of two or three parts. For example, *pathology* is the study of disease. The root word is *pathos-*, from the Greek, meaning disease. The suffix *-logy* is from the Greek word *-logia,* from *logos,* meaning the study of. By examining the root or stem word along with the prefix or suffix, the meaning of most medical words can be understood.

Many of the common prefixes, suffixes, and stem words are listed below.

| Prefix/Stem Word | Meaning |
| --- | --- |
| a-, an- | lack, not |
| ab-, a- | away from, outside of |
| ad- | to, toward |
| ambi-, ambo- | both |
| amyl-, amylo- | starch |
| angi-, angio- | vessel, vascular |
| ante- | before, preceding, in front of |
| arteri-, arterio- | artery, arterial |
| arthr-, arthro- | joint |
| aur-, auri-, auro- | ear |

| Prefix/Stem Word | Meaning |
| --- | --- |
| bi- | two, twice, double |
| bi-, bio- | life |
| brachi-, brachio- | arm, brachial |
| brady- | slow |
| bronch-, broncho- | bronchus, bronchial |
| cardi-, cardia-, cardio- | heart, cardiac |
| cephal-, cephalo- | head |
| cerebr-, cerebri, cerebro- | cerebrum, cerebral, brain |
| cervic-, cervico- | neck, cervix, cervical |
| chol-, chole-, cholo- | bile, gall |
| circum- | around, about |
| co-, com-, con-, cor- | with, together |
| col-, coli-, colo- | colon |
| contra-, counter- | against, opposite |
| crani-, cranio- | cranium, cranial |
| cyan-, cyano- | dark blue, presence of the cyanogen group |
| cyst-, cysti-, cysto- | gallbladder, urinary bladder, pouch, cyst |
| de- | undoing, reversal |
| dec-, deca- | ten, multiplied by ten |
| deci- | tenth, one tenth of |
| derm-, derma-, dermo- | dermis, dermal, skin |
| dextr-, dextro- | toward, of, or pertaining to the right |
| di-, dis- | two, twice, double |
| dipl-, diplo- | twofold, double, twin |
| dis-, di- | separation, reversal, apart from |
| dys- | abnormal, diseased, difficult, painful, unlike |
| en-, em- | in, inside, into |
| end-, endo- | within, inner, internal |
| enter-, entero- | intestine, intestinal |
| ep-, epi- | upon, beside, among, above |
| erythr-, erythro- | red |
| eu- | good, well, normal, true |

| Prefix/Stem Word | Meaning | Prefix/Stem Word | Meaning |
|---|---|---|---|
| ex-, e-, ef- | out, away, without | | small, minute, one millionth |
| extra- | outside of, beyond the scope of | micr-, micro- | single, one, alone |
| ferri- | ferric, containing iron III | mon-, mono- | form, structure |
| ferro- | ferrous, containing iron II | morph-, morpho- | many, much, affecting many parts |
| fibr-, fibro- | fiber, fibrous | multi- | muscle |
| gastr-, gastro- | stomach, gastric | my-, myo- | marrow |
| gluc-, gluco- | glucose | myel-, myelo- | nose, nasal |
| glyc-, glyco- | sweet, sugar, glucose, glycine | nas-, naso- | new, recent |
| | | ne-, neo- | death |
| gyne- | female, woman | necr-, necro- | kidney |
| hem-, hema-, hemo- | blood | nephr-, nephro- | neural, nervous, nerve |
| hemi- | half, partial | neur-, neuro- | nitrogen |
| hepat-, hepato- | liver, hepatic | nitr-, nitro- | not, ninth, nine |
| heter-, hetero- | other, another, different | non- | normal |
| hex-, hexa- | six | normo- | nucleus, nuclear |
| hom-, homo- | common, like, same | nucle-, nucleo- | egg, ovum |
| hydr-, hydro- | water, hydrogen | oo- | straight, direct, normal |
| hyp-, hypo- | deficiency, lack, below | orth-, ortho- | bone |
| hyper- | excessive, above normal | ost-, oste-, osteo- | ear |
| hyster-, hystero- | uterus, uterine, hysteria | ot-, oto- | oxygen |
| icter-, ictero- | icterus, jaundice | oxy- | near, beside, adjacent to |
| immuno- | immune, immunity | par-, para- | pathologic |
| in-, im- | not, in, into | path-, patho- | about, beyond, around |
| inter- | between, among | peri- | eating, feeding |
| intra- | within, inside | phag-, phago- | pharynx, pharyngeal |
| is, iso- | equality, similarity, uniformity | pharyng-, pharyngo- | vein, venous |
| | | phleb-, phlebo- | sound, speech, voice |
| juxta- | near, next to | phon-, phono- | light |
| kerat-, kerato- | horn, horny, cornea | phot-, photo- | natural, physical, physiologic |
| ket-, keto- | presence of the ketone group | physi-, physio- | plant, vegetable |
| kilo- | thousand | phyt-, phyto- | plasma, protoplasm, cytoplasm |
| lact-, lacti-, lacto- | milk, lactic | plasm-, plasmo- | air, gas, lung, respiratory |
| lapar-, laparo- | flank, abdomen | | multiple, compound, complex |
| laryng-, laryngo- | larynx, laryngeal | pneum-, pneumo- | |
| latero- | lateral, to the side | poly- | after, behind |
| leuk-, leuc-, leuko-, leuco- | white, colorless, leukocyte | post- | before |
| levo- | left, on the left | pre- | front, forward, before |
| lith-, litho- | stone | pro- | rectum, anus |
| lymph-, lympho- | lymph, lymphatic | proct-, procto- | first, primitive, early |
| macr-, macro- | large, great, long | prot-, proto- | false, deceptively resembling |
| mal- | wrong, abnormal, bad | pseud-, pseudo- | psyche, psychic, psychology |
| mamm-, mammo- | breast | psych-, psycho- | lung, pulmonary |
| medi-, medio- | middle, medial, median | pulmo- | pus |
| meg-, mega-, megal- | large, extended, enlarged, one million times as large as | py-, pyo- | |

| Prefix/Stem Word | Meaning |
|---|---|
| pyel-, pyelo- | renal, pelvic |
| pykn-, pykno-, pycn- pycno- | compact, dense |
| pyr-, pyro- | fire, heat |
| radio- | radiation, radioactivity |
| re- | again, back |
| ren-, reni-, reno- | kidney, renal |
| retro- | back, backward, behind |
| rhin-, rhino- | nose, nasal |
| rubr-, rubri-, rubro- | red |
| sarc-, sarco- | flesh, fleshlike, muscle |
| semi- | half |
| ser-, seri,- sero- | serum, serous |
| sub- | under, less than |
| super- | above, upon, extreme |
| supra- | upon, above, beyond, exceeding |
| syn-, sym- | together, with |
| tachy- | rapid, quick, accelerated |
| thorac-, thoraci-, thoracio-, thoraco-, thorax, thoracic | thorax, thoracic |
| thromb-, thrombo- | clotting, coagulation, blood platelets |
| thyr-, thyreo-, thyro- | thyroid |
| tox-, toxi-, toxo- | toxic, poisonous |
| trache-, tracheo- | trachea, tracheal |
| trans- | through, across |
| trich-, tricho- | hair, filament |
| un- | not, without |
| uni- | one |
| ur-, uro- | urine, urinary |
| uter-, utero- | uterus, uterine |
| vas-, vasi-, vaso- | vessel, vascular |
| ven-, vene-, veni-, veno- | vein, venous |

| Suffix/Stem Word | Meaning |
|---|---|
| -algia | a painful condition |
| -ase | enzyme |
| -ation | action, process |
| -blast | sprout, shoot, germ, formative cell |
| -cele | tumor, hernia, pathologic swelling |
| -cyte | cell |
| -desis | binding, fusing |
| -ectomy | surgical removal |
| -emia | blood |
| -ethesia | feeling, sensation |
| -gram | drawing, record |
| -graph | something written, recorded |
| -itis | inflammation |
| -logy | field of study |
| -lysis | dissolving, loosening, dissolution |
| -megaly | abnormal enlargement |
| -oma | tumor, neoplasm |
| -opia, -opy | defect of the eye |
| -osis | process, state, diseased condition |
| -pathy | disease, therapy |
| -penia | deficiency |
| -phil, -phile | having an affinity for |
| -plasty | plastic surgery |
| -rrhage, -rrhagia | abnormal or excessive discharge |
| -scope | viewing instrument |
| -scopy | inspection, examination |
| -stoma | mouth, opening |
| -stomy | operation establishing an opening into a part |
| -tomy | cutting, incision, section |
| -uria | of or in the urine |

# Abbreviations

| | | | | |
|---|---|---|---|---|
| ADH | antidiuretic hormone | | DIC | disseminated intravascular coagulation |
| AGN | acute glomerulonephritis | | DNA | deoxyribonucleic acid |
| AGT | antiglobulin test or reaction | | EA | early antigen |
| AHG | antihuman globulin | | EBV | Epstein-Barr virus |
| AIDS | acquired immune deficiency syndrome | | EDTA | ethylenediaminetetraacetic acid |
| AIN | acute interstitial nephritis | | EIA | enzyme immunoassay |
| ANA | antinuclear antibody | | ELISA | enzyme-linked immunosorbent assay; enzyme-labeled immunosorbent assay |
| APTT | activated partial thromboplastin time | | | |
| ASCLS | American Society for Clinical Laboratory Science | | EMB | eosin methylene blue agar |
| ASCP | American Society of Clinical Pathologists | | ESR | erythrocyte sedimentation rate |
| | | | FIA | fluorescence immunoassay |
| ASO | antistreptolysin O | | Hb | hemoglobin |
| BAP | blood agar (plate) | | HBV | hepatitis B virus |
| BT | bleeding time | | HCFA | Health Care Financing Administration |
| CAP | College of American Pathologists | | Hct (or Ht) | hematocrit |
| CBC | complete blood count | | HCV | hepatitis C virus; formerly called non-A, non-B hepatitis virus |
| CDC | Centers for Disease Control and Prevention | | | |
| | | | HDN | hemolytic disease of newborn |
| CFU | colony-forming unit | | Hgb | hemoglobin |
| CFU-C | colony-forming unit, culture | | HHS | Department of Health and Human Services |
| CFU-L | colony-forming unit, lymphoid | | | |
| CFU-S | colony-forming unit, spleen | | HIS | hospital information system |
| CLA | clinical laboratory assistant | | HIV | human immunodeficiency virus |
| CLIA '88 | Clinical Laboratory Improvement Amendments of 1988 | | HLA | human leukocyte antigen |
| | | | HMWK | high-molecular-weight kininogen |
| CLT | clinical laboratory technician | | IAT | indirect antiglobulin test |
| COLA | Commission on Office Laboratory Accreditation | | IDDM | insulin-dependent (type 1) diabetes mellitus |
| CPD | citrate phosphate dextrose | | IF | intrinsic factor |
| CPDA-1 | citrate phosphate dextrose with adenine | | Ig | immunoglobulin |
| | | | IL | interleukins |
| CPU | central processing unit | | IM | infectious mononucleosis |
| CQI | Continuous Quality Improvement | | IU | international unit |
| CRT | cathode ray tube | | IV | intravenous |
| CSF | colony stimulating factor; cerebrospinal fluid | | JCAHO | Joint Commission on Accreditation of Healthcare Organizations |
| DAT | direct antiglobulin test | | L | liter |

| | |
|---|---|
| **LAP** | leukocyte alkaline phosphatase |
| **LIS** | laboratory information system |
| **LISS** | low-ionic-strength saline solution |
| **M** | meter |
| **Mac** | MacConkey (agar) |
| **MBC** | minimal bactericidal concentration |
| **MCH** | mean cell hemoglobin |
| **MCHC** | mean cell hemoglobin concentration |
| **MCV** | mean cell volume |
| **MIC** | minimal inhibitory concentration |
| **MKC** | megakaryocyte |
| **MLA** | medical laboratory assistant |
| **MLT** | medical laboratory technician |
| **mol** | mole |
| **MPV** | mean platelet volume |
| **MSDS** | material safety data sheets |
| **MT** | medical technologist |
| **NA** | numerical aperture |
| **NAD+** | nicotinamide adenine dinucleotide, oxidized form |
| **NADH** | nicotinamide adenine dinucleotide, reduced form |
| **NBS** | National Bureau of Standards |
| **NCA** | National Certification Agency for Medical Laboratory Personnel |
| **NCCLS** | National Committee for Clinical Laboratory Standards |
| **NCEP** | National Cholesterol Education Program |
| **NIDDM** | non-insulin-dependent (type 2) diabetes mellitus |
| **OFB** | oval fat body |
| **OGTT** | oral glucose tolerance test |
| **OSHA** | Occupational Safety and Health Administration |
| **PCT** | postcoital test |
| **PCV** | packed cell volume |
| **PEP** | post-exposure prophylaxis |
| **PKK** | plasma prekallikrein |
| **PMN** | polymorphonuclear neutrophil |
| **PPM** | provider-performed microscopies |
| **PRP** | platelet-rich plasma |
| **PT** | prothrombin time |
| **PTT** | partial thromboplastin time |
| **PV** | predictive value |
| **QA** | quality assurance |
| **QC** | quality control |
| **RAM** | random access memory |
| **RBC** | red blood cell |
| **RCF** | relative centrifugal force |
| **RDW** | red cell distribution width |
| **RES** | reticuloendothelial system |
| **RF** | rheumatoid factor |
| **RhIG** | Rh immune globulin |
| **RIA** | radioimmunoassay |
| **RTF** | renal tubular fat |
| **SB** | sheep blood (agar) |
| **SEM** | scanning electron microscope |
| **SI** | International System of Units (le Système International d'Unités) |
| **SLE** | systemic lupus erythematosus |
| **SPIA** | solid-phase immunosorbent assay |
| **TEM** | transmission electron microscope |
| **TLC** | thin-layer chromatography |
| **TQI** | Total Quality Improvement |
| **TT** | thrombin time |
| **VAD** | vascular access device |
| **VDRL** | Venereal Disease Research Laboratory (test for syphilis) |
| **vWD** | von Willebrand's disease |
| **vWF** | von Willebrand's factor |
| **WBC** | white blood cell |

# APPENDIX C

# *Reference Values*

Selected reference values for common clinical laboratory tests follow. Values will differ slightly with individual laboratories and methodology. Reference values must be established for each laboratory.

## HEMATOLOGY*

Values are for adults (unless indicated otherwise).

| | | |
|---|---|---|
| Hemoglobin | M | 14.0-17.5 g/dL |
| | F | 12.3-15.3 g/dL |
| Hematocrit[†] | M | 40%-54% |
| | F | 37%- 47% |
| RBC | M | $4.5\text{-}5.9 \times 10^{12}$/L |
| | F | $4.1\text{-}5.1 \times 10^{12}$/L |
| MCV | M/F | 80-96.1 fL |
| MCH | M/F | 27.5-33.2 pg |
| MCHC | M/F | 33.4-35.5 g/dL (%) |
| RDW | M/F | 11.5%-14.5% |
| WBC | M/F | $4.4\text{-}11.3 \times 10^9$/L (over 21 years) |
| | | $6.0\text{-}17.5 \times 10^9$/L (12 months) |
| Platelets | M/F | $172\text{-}450 \times 10^9$/L |

---

*Hematology reference values are taken from Beutler E et al: *Williams Hematology,* ed 5. New York, McGraw-Hill, Inc, 1995, unless indicated otherwise.

†Hematocrit values are from NCCLS: *Procedure for Determining Packed Cell Volume by the Microhematocrit Method: Approved Standard, ed* 2. Villanova, Pa, National Committee for Clinical Laboratory Standards, August, 1993, H7-A2.

Reticulocyte count*

| | | |
|---|---|---|
| Relative count | M | 1.1%-2.1% |
| | F | 0.9%-1.9% |
| Absolute count | M/F | $50 \times 10^9$/L |

Leukocyte differential cell count (M/F, age 21 and above)

| | Mean % (relative count) | Mean absolute count $\times$ $10^9$/L |
|---|---|---|
| Neutrophils | 59 | 4.4 |
| Band | 3.0 | 0.22 |
| Segmented | 56 | 4.2 |
| Lymphocytes | 34 | 2.5 |
| Monocytes | 4.0 | 0.3 |
| Eosinophils | 2.7 | 0.20 |
| Basophils | 0.5 | 0.04 |

Erythrocyte sedimentation rate (ESR)[†]

| | Less than 50 years | Over 50 years | Over 85 years |
|---|---|---|---|
| Male | 0-15 mm/hr | 0-20 | 0-30 |
| Female | 0-20 mm/hr | 0-30 | 0-42 |

## URINALYSIS‡

Specific gravity

| | |
|---|---|
| Random urine | 1.001-1.035 |
| Normal diet and fluid | 1.016-1.022 |

---

*Reticulocyte count reference values are from Williams WJ et al: *Hematology,* ed 4. New York, McGraw-Hill Book Co, 1990.

†ESR reference values are from Henry JB (ed): *Clinical Diagnosis and Management by Laboratory Methods,* ed 19. Philadelphia, WB Saunders Co, 1996.

‡Urinalysis reference values are those established for the Fairview-University Medical Center, University Campus, Minneapolis, Minn.

Chemical screen

| | |
|---|---|
| pH | 5-7 |
| Protein | Negative |
| Blood | Negative |
| Glucose | Negative |
| Ketones | Negative |
| Nitrite | Negative |
| Leukocyte esterase | Negative |
| Urobilinogens | To 1 EU/dL |
| Bilirubin (conjugated) | Negative |

Sediment examination (12:1 concentration)

| | |
|---|---|
| RBC | 0-2/hpf |
| WBC | 0-5/hpf (female > male) |
| Casts | 0-2 hyaline/lpf |
| Squamous epithelial cells | Few/lpf |
| Transitional epithelial cells | Few/hpf |
| Renal tubular epithelial cells | Few/hpf |
| Bacteria | Negative |
| Yeast | Negative |
| Abnormal crystals | Negative |

## CHEMISTRIES, SERUM (ADULT)*

| | |
|---|---|
| Alanine aminotransferase (ALT) | 10-35 U/L |
| Alkaline phosphatase | |
| Male | 30-90 U/L |
| Female | 20-80 U/L |
| Aspartate aminotransferase (AST) | 10-40 U/L |
| Bicarbonate | 22-29 mmol/L |
| Bilirubin | |
| Total | 0.3-1.2 mg/dL |
| Direct, conjugated | 0.0-0.2 mg/dL |
| Calcium, total | 8.5-10.2 mg/dL |
| Chloride | 98-107 mmol/L |

| | |
|---|---|
| Cholesterol | |
| Desirable | <200 mg/dL |
| Borderline/moderate risk | 200-239 mg/dL |
| High risk | >240 mg/dL |
| Creatinine | |
| Male | 0.7-1.3 mg/dL |
| Female | 0.6-1.1 mg/dL |
| Creatinine clearance | |
| Male (under 40 yr) | 90-139 mL/min/1.73 m² |
| Female (under 40 yr) | 80-125 mL/min/1.73 m² |
| Creatine kinase (CK) | |
| Male | 15-105 U/L |
| Female | 10-80 U/L |
| Glucose (fasting) | 70-105 mg/dL |
| Iron | |
| Male | 65-170 μg/dL |
| Female | 50-170 μg/dL |
| Total iron binding capacity (TIBC) | 250-450 μg/dL |
| % saturation of iron | |
| Male | 20%-55% |
| Female | 15%-50% |
| pH (arterial blood) | 7.35-7.45 |
| Potassium | 3.5-5.1 mmol/L |
| Protein, total | 6.4-8.3 g/dL |
| Protein, albumin | 3.9-5.1 g/dL |
| Sodium | 136-145 mmol/L |
| Triglyceride (10-12 hr fast required) | |
| Male | 40-160 mg/dL |
| Female | 35-135 mg/dL |
| Urea | 5-39 mg/dL |
| Urea nitrogen | 7-18 mg/dL |
| Uric acid | |
| Male | 4.4-7.6 mg/dL |
| Female | 2.3-6.6 mg/dL |

---

*Reference values are from Burtis CA, Ashwood ER (eds): Tietz Fundamentals of Clinical Chemistry, ed 4, Philadelphia, WB Saunders Co, 1996, pp 773-821.

# GLOSSARY

## A

**absolute cell count (absolute numbers)** Concentration of a cell type expressed as a number per volume of whole blood, usually per liter; obtained by multiplying the relative percentage value by the total leukocyte count per liter.

**absorbance** Amount of light that is absorbed or retained and therefore not able to pass through or be transmitted through a solution.

**absorbance spectrophotometry** Methodology that utilizes Beer's law, whereby the amount of light absorbed by a solution is directly proportional to the concentration of the solution; this measurement can be made only by mathematical calculation from the transmission data obtained by use of a quantitative analytical method, such as spectrophotometry.

**absorbance units** Units of measure for light that is absorbed by a colored solution.

**absorbed light** Light that is not transmitted.

**acceptable control range** Statistically determined range of values within which a test result must fall to be considered acceptable; it is a means of quality control or assurance.

**accuracy** Correctness of a result, freedom from error, or how close the answer is to the "true" value.

**accurate and precise technology (APT)** "Easy" or automated quantitative tests or easy qualitative tests for which the manufacturer of the automated instrument has been granted special standing under CLIA '88 definitions of laboratory tests.

**acholic stool** Absence of bile; results in formation of colorless, chalky-appearing fecal specimens.

**acid crystals** Crystals seen in urine of an acidic pH, less than pH 7.0.

**acid-base balance** Maintenance of a constant balance between acids and bases; maintenance of constant pH.

**acid-fast bacteria (AFB)** Bacteria that retain staining dye and make the decolorization step difficult.

**acid-fast stain** Used to detect organisms that are difficult to decolorize, even with acid-alcohol solutions; typical organisms are those that cause tuberculosis or leprosy.

**acidophilic** Acid loving; on blood films, the cell components that stain with the acidic portion of Wright or Wright-Giemsa stain, such as hemoglobin and eosinophilic granules, which stain orange to pink.

**acidosis** Decrease in blood pH.

**activated partial thromboplastin time (APTT)** A test sensitive to heparin; useful in detecting deficiencies in intrinsic and common pathway factors.

**active reabsorption** A form of reabsorption that requires the expenditure of energy. This is usually against a concentration gradient, from a region of lower to one of higher concentration.

**acute glomerulonephritis (AGN)** Also postinfectious glomerulonephritis. A disease of the kidney glomerulus that is an immunologic sequela of a bacterial infection. Characteristics include, oliguria, edema, proteinuria, with red blood cell or granular casts, and hematuria.

**acute interstitial nephritis (AIN)** An inflammation of the interstitial tissue of the kidney that is an immunologic, adverse reaction to certain drugs, such as sulfonamide or methicillin. The condition is characterized by fever, rash, proteinuria, and the presence of eosinophils in urine.

**acute phase** Early in the course of a disease, when the disease is first suspected; blood is drawn (acute phase serum) when little or no antibody has had time to develop and is compared with antibody level in convalescent serum.

**acute-phase reactants** Group of glycoproteins associated with nonspecific inflammatory conditions.

**acute pyelonephritis** An infection of the pelvis and parenchyma of the kidney; usually the result of an ascending infection from the lower urinary tract.

**additives, anticoagulants** Additives usually are anticoagulants that prevent coagulation of the blood specimen. Several different anticoagulants are available for different testing purposes. Some laboratory tests require the use of plasma or whole blood for the assay, and these must be anticoagulated during the collection process.

**aerobes** Microbes that require oxygen for growth.

**aerosols** Infectious particles that are airborne; fine mist in which particles are dispersed.

**agar** A seaweed extract that is liquid when heated and solid when cooled; used as base medium for preparation of culture plates, slant tubes, and stab tubes.

**agar disk diffusion tests** Tests that employ antibiotic-impregnated disks placed on an agar culture plate inoculated with the organism to be tested.

**agar slant** Tubes of agar media that are solidified on a slant (the surface of the medium is on an incline); useful for particular cultures.

**agglutination** Visible clumping or aggregation of red cells or any particles; used as an indication of a specific antigen-antibody reaction.

**agglutinins** Antibodies that form visible clumps, or agglutinate, with their specific antigens.

**agglutinogens** Antigens that form visible clumps, or agglutinate, with their specific antibodies.

**aggregometer** Instrument that measures platelet aggregation in platelet dysfunction studies.

**albuminemia** Decreased blood albumin.

**albuminuria** Presence of albumin in urine.

**aldosterone** Hormone that controls the sodium-potassium pump, the primary mechanism for sodium reabsorption in the kidney; regulator of blood sodium and potassium levels.

**alignment** Microscope adjustment that ensures that the light path from the light source throughout the microscope and ocular is physically correct.

**aliquot** One of a number of equal parts.

**alkaline crystals** Crystals seen in urine of an alkaline pH; generally pH 7.0 and above.

**alkalosis** Increase in blood pH.

**alleles** Variants of a gene for a particular trait.

**alloantibodies** Antibodies resulting from antigenic stimulation within the same species.

**alpha hemolysis** Incomplete or partial hemolysis (appears green).

**ambulatory patient** A patient not confined to bed; example, an outpatient or clinic patient.

**American Standard Code for Information Interchange (ASCII)** Standardized codes allowing the keyboard of the computer to be used to enter alphanumeric as well as numerical data into the computer.

**Americans with Disabilities Act (ADA)** Mandates that specific plans be developed for any person with a disability employed by a clinical laboratory, to ensure that the person is working in a safe atmosphere.

**amorphous material** Crystalline material seen in the urine sediment as granules without shape or form.

**anaerobes** Microbes that cannot grow in an atmosphere of oxygen; special steps must be taken to provide an oxygen-free atmosphere for incubation and growth of these organisms.

**analog computation** Measurement derived directly from an instrument signal.

**analytical balance** Instrument used to weigh substances to a high degree of accuracy (e.g., chemicals used in the preparation of standard solutions).

**analytical functions** Process whereby analytical analyses are carried out; includes generating work lists, doing the analyses, entering the results, quality control measures, and results verification.

**analyzer** In polarizing microscopy, a polarizing filter located above the specimen, between the objective and the eyepiece.

**anemia** A condition in which there is a decrease in hemoglobin in the blood and therefore in the amount of oxygen reaching the tissues and organs. May be the result of a decrease in the number of erythrocytes (decreased red cell mass), decreased hemoglobin concentration, or abnormal hemoglobin.

**anion gap** Concentration of unmeasured anions; calculated as the difference between measured cations and measured anions.

**anisocytosis** A general term indicating increased variation in the size of red cells in the blood film.

**antibiotic resistance** Exists if the growth of a microorganism is not inhibited by the presence of an antibiotic; the organism is resistant to the antibiotic.

**antibiotic sensitivity or susceptibility** Ability of the antibiotic to inhibit growth of a microorganism.

**antibody** Protein substance, found in the plasma or other body fluids, that is formed as the result of antigenic stimulation and is specific for the antigen against which it is formed. In blood banking, antibodies are present in commercially prepared serum, called antiserum.

**antibody titer** Amount of antibody present or required to produce a reaction with a particular amount of another substance; concentration of antibody.

**anticoagulant** Prevents coagulation of blood.

**antidiuretic hormone (ADH)** A hormone that regulates urine volume by increasing the amount of water reabsorbed by the kidney.

**antigen** Foreign (different from "self") substance that, when introduced into the body of a person lacking the antigen, results in an immune response and formation of a corresponding antibody. In blood banking, antigens are generally, but not always, found on the red cell membrane.

**antigen-antibody ratio** Number of antibody molecules in relation to the number of antigen sites per cell.

**antihuman globulin (AHG) test (AGT) or reaction** Method of detecting the presence of all human isoantibodies by using a specially prepared antiserum to human immunoglobulin and/or complement. May be a direct (DAT) or indirect (IAT) test. Also known as the Coombs' reaction or test.

**antinuclear antibodies (ANA)** Circulating immunoglobulins that react with the whole nucleus or nuclear components; frequently assayed by using indirect fluorescent antibody (IFA) techniques.

**antiserum** Serum containing antibodies. In blood banking, a special highly purified preparation of antibodies used as a reagent to show the presence of antigen on red blood cells.

**anuria** The complete absence of urine formation.

**aperture iris diaphragm** The part of the microscope located at the bottom of the Abbé condenser, under the lens but within the condenser body; controls the amount of light passing through the material under observation; can be opened or closed to adjust contrast by means of a lever.

**aplastic** Condition when the bone marrow is suppressed or unable to function normally in cell production.

**Apt test** Test for maternal hemoglobin ingestion in newborn infants.

**arithmetic logic unit** A component of the central processing unit (CPU) of a computer.

**arthrocentesis** Collection of synovial fluid from a joint by needle aspiration.

**ASCII** See American Standard Code for Information Exchange.

**ascorbic acid (vitamin C)** A strong reducing substance that may interfere with several of the reagent strip tests used in urinalysis, especially tests for blood and glucose.

**atherosclerosis**  Condition of "hardening of the arteries," in which plaques of cholesterol, lipids, and cellular debris collect in the inner layers of the walls of large- and medium-sized arteries.

**autoantibodies**  Antibodies directed against self-antigens.

**autoclave**  Apparatus for effecting sterilization by using steam under pressure; when it is used with an automatic regulating pressure gauge, the degree of heat to which the contents are subjected is automatically regulated also.

**automated cell counters**  Instruments designed to repeatedly and automatically count the numbers of formed cellular elements present in a blood specimen, usually the erythrocytes, leukocytes, and platelets.

**automated differential counters**  Instruments designed to repeatedly and automatically determine the types and percentages of leukocytes present in a blood specimen.

**automated hematocrit**  The hematocrit result obtained when a multiparameter instrument is used for hematology determinations. The result is computed from measured red cell volume.

**automatic pipettes**  Devices used to repeatedly and accurately measure volumes of standard solutions, reagents, specimens, or other liquid substances.

**automatic pipetting devices**  See automatic pipettes.

**azotemia**  Significantly increased concentrations of urea and creatinine in the blood.

**B**

**B lymphocyte**  Blood cell that matures in the bone marrow; undergoes transformation to plasma cell that produces antibodies or immunoglobulins.

**bacilli**  Rod-shaped bacteria.

**bacteremia**  Presence of bacteria in blood; bacteria can be cultured from the blood.

**bacteriology**  The study of bacteria.

**bacteriuria**  Presence of bacteria in the urine.

**balance the centrifuge**  To make certain that weight is distributed evenly on opposite sides of the centrifuge to prevent breakage of contents being centrifuged.

**bar-code readers**  Optical reading devices that convert a series of black lines into a sequence of numbers or letters for entry into a computer (e.g., names of patients, identification numbers, tests requested).

**bar coding**  A sample recognition system whereby the bar codes—a series of black lines or bars on a label, for example—can be electronically read. Bar codes contain information such as name, hospital number, date, and other patient demographic data; see bar-code readers.

**barrier precautions**  Personal protective devices (e.g., gloves, gowns) placed between blood or other body fluid specimen and the person handling it, to prevent transmission of infectious agents borne by specimens. See also personal protective equipment.

**basic first aid**  Immediate care given after an injury, before treatment is started by trained medical personnel.

**basophilia**  An increase in the number of basophils.

**basophilic**  Base loving. The acidic cell components, such as nuclei and cytoplasmic RNA, that stain blue-violet by methylene azure in polychrome stains.

**basophilic stippling**  The presence of dark blue granules evenly distributed throughout the red cell in Wright-stained blood films.

**batch or run**  A collection of any number of specimens to be analyzed at any one time, plus control specimens, standard solutions, and so forth.

**batch analyzers**  Analyzer that can test a batch of samples simultaneously for one particular analyte at a time; are designed to analyze a number of different analytes, but only one at a time.

**bedside testing**  Capillary blood samples can be used to perform rapid testing procedures (many are utilizing commercial products) at the bedside; a common test is the glucose blood test, done for management of diabetes mellitus patients; see also point-of-care testing (POCT).

**Beer's law, Beer-Lambert law**  In a solution, color intensity at a constant depth is directly proportional to concentration.

**Benedict's qualitative test** A copper reduction test for reducing sugars (substances) in urine; the basis of the Clinitest Tablet Test.

**beta hemolysis** Clear or complete hemolysis.

**bilirubin** Vivid yellow pigment; major byproduct of normal red blood cell destruction.

**bilirubin glucuronide, direct bilirubin, conjugated bilirubin** Water-soluble form of bilirubin; formed by conjugation with glucuronic acid in the liver.

**biochemical properties and reactions** Properties are characteristics (e.g., molecular weight, melting point) present in various types of chemicals; reactions involve the conversion of one chemical species, the reactant, to another chemical species, the product.

**biohazard symbol** Symbol or term denoting any infectious material or agent that presents a possible health risk.

**biohazard containers** All infectious materials are handled as potential biohazards. These special containers should be used for all blood, other body fluids, and tissues, and disposable materials contaminated with them; they should be tagged "Biohazard" or bear the standard biohazard symbol.

**biohazard waste** See infectious waste.

**biometrics** The science of statistics applied to biological observations.

**biosafety cabinet** Protective workplace device used to control the presence of infectious agents in the air.

**birefringence** Ability of an object or crystal to rotate or polarize light.

**blank solution** Solution containing all the components, including solvents and solutes, except the compound to be measured.

**bleeding time (BT)** The time required for cessation of bleeding after a standardized capillary puncture to a capillary bed; dependent on capillary integrity, numbers of platelets, and platelet function.

**blood banking** The procedures involved in collecting, storing, processing, and distributing blood.

**blood spot collection** Collection of capillary blood onto a filter paper; example, spot collections for neonatal screening programs.

**blood transfusion** Technique of replacing whole blood and/or its components.

**blood-borne pathogens** Infectious agents or pathogens carried by blood and blood products.

**Board of Registry of the American Society of Clinical Pathologists (ASCP)** Offers an examination and certification for medical laboratory personnel.

**body cavity fluids** Fluids normally found in small amounts in various cavities or body spaces (e.g., cerebrospinal, pleural, abdominal, pericardial, peritoneal, and synovial fluid). In certain conditions, such fluid is aspirated and assayed.

**body tube** The part of the microscope through which the light passes to the ocular.

**brightfield microscope** Illumination system used in the common clinical microscope.

**broth media** Culture media that are in a broth or liquid form in a tube.

**buffy coat** One of the three layers of normal anticoagulated blood. A thin grayish-white layer on top of the packed red blood cells, consisting of leukocytes and platelets, which normally makes up 1% of the total blood volume.

**buret** Long cylindrical graduated tube with a stopcock delivery closing on one end, used to control the delivery of the flow of liquid from the device; used to deliver measured quantities of fluid or solutions.

**C**

**calibrated cuvettes** Tubes or cuvettes that have been optically matched so that the same solution in each will give the same reading on the photometer.

**calibration** Means by which glassware or other laboratory apparatus is checked to determine the exact units it will measure or deliver by relating them to a known concentration of an analyte.

**calibration mark** Mark on volumetric glassware that indicates the point from which the volume is measured.

**calculi** Kidney or renal stones.

**CAP quality assurance program** Provided by CAP to assist a laboratory in organizing and managing its quality assurance program under CAP.

**capillary blood (peripheral blood) collection** Blood drawn from the capillary bed by means of puncturing the skin; example, a finger or heel puncture.

**capillary pipette** Small glass or plastic tube used to collect small amounts of capillary blood, usually directly from a capillary puncture.

**capillary tube density gradient** Method of cell enumeration whereby cells, upon centrifugation, settle in different layers because of their different densities; they are further expanded, stained, and magnified to derive the results of the counts.

**carcinogens** Substance that can cause the development of cancerous growths in living tissues.

**casts** Structures that result from solidification of Tamm-Horsfall mucoprotein in the lumen of the kidney tubules; they form a mold, or cast, of the tubule and trap other material that may be present when they are formed. Several types exist. They represent a biopsy of the kidney and are clinically significant.

**catabolism** The phase of metabolism in which fats are broken down for energy.

**cathode ray tube (CRT), terminal, video display unit** Television-like screen device used to monitor input, output, and general status of a computer system.

**cell-mediated (cellular) response** Involves actions of T lymphocytes and their subsets, together with plasma cells and macrophages.

**Celsius scale** Scale used to measure temperature in the metric system; outdated term for this scale is centigrade.

**Centers for Disease Control and Prevention (CDC)** Carries out mandated public health laws and reporting requirements.

**central memory** A component of the central processing unit (CPU) of a computer; provides storage and rapid access for information (data).

**central processing unit (CPU)** The part of the computer that controls and performs the execution of programs or instructions.

**centralized laboratory** A central location in a health care facility where all laboratory testing is done.

**centrifugation** Separation of a solid material from a liquid by application of increased gravitational force by rapid rotating or spinning.

**cerebrospinal fluid (CSF)** Extravascular fluid that surrounds the brain and spinal cord. Formed by the choroid plexus in the ventricles of the brain and found within the subarachnoid space, the central canal of the spinal cord, and the four ventricles of the brain.

**cervical mucus test** See Fern test.

**chain of custody** When results of laboratory testing are to be used in a court of law, a specific chain of documentation is required, whereby all steps of the testing are recorded, from specimen collection to the issuing of the results report.

**chemical hygiene plan** Outlines the specific work practices and procedures necessary to protect workers from any health hazards associated with use of hazardous chemicals.

**chloride shift** When carbon dioxide leaves the plasma and chloride diffuses or shifts out of the red cells to replace it; can take place when plasma and red cells are not separated in a timely manner.

**chromasia** Term used to describe the staining reaction of red cells in the Wright-stained blood film.

**chromatography** Method of analysis in which the solutes, dissolved in a common solvent, are separated from one another by differential distribution of the solutes between two phases (a mobile phase and a stationary phase).

**chromosome** Threadlike structure within the nucleus of each cell, made up of genes. Chromosomes exist in pairs in all cells except sex cells. Each species has a specific number of paired chromosomes.

**chylomicrons** Small droplets of lipoproteins that give blood specimens a characteristic milky appearance, when present.

**CLIA '88** See Clinical Laboratory Improvement Amendments of 1988 (CLIA '88).

**clinical immunology** Study of antigen-antibody reactions in vitro.

**clinical laboratory assistant (CLA)** See clinical laboratory technician (CLT).

**Clinical Laboratory Improvement Amendments of 1988 (CLIA '88)** Standards set for all laboratories to ensure quality patient care; provisions include requirements for quality control and assurance, for the use of proficiency tests, and for certain levels of personnel to perform and supervise work done in the clinical laboratory.

**clinical laboratory scientist (CLS)** Formerly known as a medical technologist (MT); usually has earned a bachelor of science degree in medical technology or clinical laboratory science.

**clinical laboratory technician (CLT)** Category of laboratory personnel; this group usually has some formal laboratory training, as from a technical school or other vocational training program; CLTs usually have some limitations as to the complexity of laboratory testing they are trained to do.

**clinical pathology** Medical discipline by which clinical laboratory science and technology are applied to the care of patients.

**clone** Cell originating from a single ancestral parent cell.

**clot** Formation of a fibrin network; a thrombus.

**clot retraction** Clot becomes smaller.

**clue cells** Vaginal squamous epithelial cells that are covered or encrusted with *Gardnerella vaginalis.*

**coagglutination** To enhance visibility of agglutination, antibodies are bound to a particle.

**coagulation** Mechanism whereby after injury to a blood vessel, plasma coagulation factors, tissue factors, and calcium work together on the surface of platelets to form a fibrin clot.

**coagulation cascade** Process of coagulation, in which a series of biochemical reactions occur, converting inactive substances to active forms that in turn activate other substances; carefully controlled process responding to injury while maintaining normal blood circulation.

**coagulation factors** Proteins engaged in formation of a fibrin clot from fibrinogen.

**coagulation system** See coagulation cascade.

**cocci** Bacteria that are round.

**coefficient of variation (CV)** Used to compare the standard deviations of two samples; in percent, the CV is equal to the standard deviation divided by the mean.

**cofactors** Proteins that accelerate the reactions of the enzymes involved in the coagulation process.

**College of American Pathologists (CAP)** Professional organization of pathologists; one responsibility is to certify clinical laboratories.

**colony forming unit, culture (CFU-C)** Multipotential hematopoietic (myeloid) stem cell.

**colony forming unit, lymphoid (CFU-L)** Committed lymphoid stem cell.

**colony forming unit, spleen (CFU-S)** Uncommitted pluripotential stem cell; also colony forming unit, lymphoid-myeloid (CFU-LM).

**colony forming units (CFU)** In microbiology, colony count; in hematology, a pluripotential, undifferentiated stem cell that is stimulated to proliferate and differentiate into colonies of a specific cell type.

**colony stimulating factor (CSF)** Factor required for hematopoietic stem cells to multiply and differentiate.

**colorimetry** Technique used to determine the concentration of a substance by the variation in intensity of its color.

**commensal state** Situation in which parasite and host exist together with no harm coming to the host.

**Commission on Office Laboratory Accreditation (COLA)** Provides accreditation for physician office laboratories; has been deemed HCFA-approved.

**common pathway** Final stages of the coagulation cascade, beginning with the convergence of the extrinsic and intrinsic pathways (factor X) and ending with formation of the fibrin clot.